The Practice of Chinese Medicine

To my son Sebastian who patiently kept me company throughout
the writing of this book.

For Churchill Livingstone

Publisher: Mary Law
Project editor: Dinah Thom
Production controller: Neil Dickson
Sales promotion executive: Hilary Brown

中藥鍼灸治療學

The Practice of Chinese Medicine

The Treatment of Diseases with Acupuncture and Chinese Herbs

Giovanni Maciocia CAc(Nanjing)

Acupuncturist and Medical Herbalist. Lecturer at the Norsk Akupunktur Skole, Oslo, Norway. Lecturer at the Acupuncture Foundation of Ireland, Dublin, Republic of Ireland. Guest Lecturer at Pacific College of Oriental Medicine, San Diego, USA. Guest Lecturer at Scuola Italo-Cinese di Agopuntura (Associazione Medici Agopuntori Bolognesi), Bologna, Italy. Honorary lecturer at the Nanjing College of Traditional Chinese Medicine, Nanjing, People's Republic of China.

Foreword by

Professor Zhou Zhong Ying

Former President, Nanjing College of Traditional Chinese Medicine, Nanjing

CHURCHILL LIVINGSTONE
EDINBURGH LONDON MADRID MELBOURNE NEW YORK AND TOKYO 1994

CHURCHILL LIVINGSTONE
Medical Division of Longman Group UK Limited

Distributed in the United States of America by
Churchill Livingstone Inc., 650 Avenue of the Americas,
New York, N. Y. 10011, and by associated companies,
branches and representatives throughout the world.

First published 1994
  Reprinted 1994 (twice)

ISBN 0-443-043051

British Library Cataloguing in Publication Data
A catalogue record for this book is available from the
British Library.

Library of Congress Cataloging in Publication Data
A catalogue record for this book is available from the
Library of Congress.

The
publisher's
policy is to use
**paper manufactured
from sustainable forests**

Produced by Longman Singapore Publishers (Pte) Ltd.
Printed in Singapore

Contents

Cross reference of diseases and patterns

Cross reference of patterns and diseases

Hypochondrial pain, 419
Constipation, 475
Parkinson's disease, 657
Pre-menstrual tension, 765

LIVER-YIN DEFICIENCY

Asthma, 105
Mental-emotional problems, 197
Insomnia, 281
Tiredness, 315
Hypochondrial pain, 419
Parkinson's disease, 657

LIVER-YIN DEFICIENCY WITH EMPTY-HEAT

Mental-emotional problems, 197

STASIS OF LIVER-BLOOD

Headaches, 1
Mental-emotional problems, 197
Hypochondrial pain, 419
Abdominal pain, 431
Dysmenorrhoea, 735

Heart

HEART-QI DEFICIENCY

Tiredness, 315

HEART-YANG DEFICIENCY

Tiredness, 315
Chest Painful Obstruction Syndrome, 359
Oedema, 537

HEART-BLOOD DEFICIENCY

Headaches, 1
Mental-emotional problems, 197
Tinnitus, 305
Tiredness, 315

HEART-BLOOD STASIS

Mental-emotional problems, 197
Chest Painful Obstruction Syndrome, 359

HEART-YIN DEFICIENCY

Mental-emotional problems, 197
Insomnia, 281
Tiredness, 315

HEART-FIRE

Mental-emotional problems, 197
Insomnia, 281
Painful-Urination Syndrome, 493

PHLEGM-HEAT HARASSING THE MIND (HEART)

Mental-emotional problems, 197
Insomnia, 281

Lungs

WIND-COLD INVADING THE LUNGS

Headaches, 1
Breathlessness, 67
Asthma, 105
Allergic rhinitis, 143
Cough, 171
Common cold and influenza, 777

WIND-HEAT INVADING THE LUNGS

Headaches, 1
Asthma, 105
Allergic rhinitis, 143
Sinusitis, 163
Cough, 171
Common cold and influenza, 777

WIND-DAMPNESS

Headaches, 1
Common cold and influenza, 777

Foreword

Traditional Chinese internal medicine is the basis of all specialities of Chinese medicine. It systematically reflects Chinese medicine's method of determining treatment on the basis of differentiation of patterns. Doctors of all departments of Chinese medicine must have a good command of it.

"The Practice of Chinese Medicine: The Treatment of Diseases with Acupuncture and Chinese Herbs" written by Giovanni Maciocia discusses in detail the basic theories of the internal medicine and treatment of 34 common diseases with acupuncture and Chinese herbs. This book describes common methods of differentiation of patterns and treatment of diseases by systematically discussing their aetiology, pathology, treatment principles, acupuncture points and Chinese herbal treatment; in addition, it combines traditional theories with the author's own clinical experience. Giovanni Maciocia has established his own ideas concerning allergic rhinitis and asthma, atopic eczema and post-viral fatigue syndrome, which are new not only in China but also in the West.

Over the past few decades, there has been a great surge of interest world-wide in Chinese herbal medicine and acupuncture. Many people in different parts of the world have begun to study Chinese medicine. The publication of this book will certainly help the integration of Western medicine with Chinese medicine which, being free of side-effects, will bring additional benefits to people in the West.

Giovanni Maciocia has studied Chinese medicine in my college three times, so he is an alumnus of ours. During his stay in China, he studied conscientiously and respected his teachers and clinical instructors. He has flexibly applied what he has learnt in China to the conditions in the West, and successfully treated a large number of patients. Students and practitioners both in and outside China speak highly of his contributions to the popularization of Chinese medicine in the West.

This book is not only a textbook for students of Chinese medicine, but also a reference book for practitioners in the West. I believe this book will be very influential in spreading Chinese medicine throughout the world.

Z.Z.Y.

Preface

This book is intended to be the companion volume to the "Foundations of Chinese Medicine", setting out the application of the theory of Chinese medicine to the treatment of specific diseases with both acupuncture and Chinese herbs.

The discussion is centred around the old Chinese disease–symptoms, e.g. "headache", "dizziness", "abdominal pain", etc. Although these are normally referred to as "diseases" in Chinese medicine, they are symptoms rather than diseases in a Western medical sense. In a few cases, however, I do discuss actual diseases as defined in Western medicine; these are asthma, allergic rhinitis, sinusitis, nephritis, myalgic encephalomyelitis, Parkinson's disease, multiple sclerosis, the common cold and influenza.

This textbook sets out the treatment for 34 common diseases. With four exceptions — asthma, allergic rhinitis, myalgic encephalomyelitis (ME) and multiple sclerosis — all appear in textbooks of Chinese medicine.

The theory of allergic asthma and allergic rhinitis presented in this book is entirely new; of course, it is far from perfect and will need constant revision according to clinical experience and research. The theory of ME, similarly new, is based on my own clinical experience, although the concepts of "residual pathogenic factor" and "Latent Heat" on which it is based are very old.

New, too, is the theory of multiple sclerosis (MS), but this is mostly based on the pathology and symptomatology of Atrophy Syndrome.

The chapter on "Tiredness" is based on the old symptom of "*xu-lao*" which means "exhaustion", but I have departed from the traditional approach in so far as I have included the Excess causes of tiredness, something which is not done in the Chinese discussion of *xu-lao*.

A table of cross references after the table of contents lists the patterns found in each disease. For those who work mostly from patterns rather than diseases, another table lists the diseases in which a particular pattern appears.

Although Chinese medicine treats each individual as a whole rather than treating the "diseases" from which that patient is suffering, and explores the patterns of disharmony, life-style, environment, family situation, emotional life, diet, sexual habits, work routine and exercise, it is still important to discuss the treatment of individual diseases since treatment techniques vary enormously; for example, the treatment of Wind-stroke calls for specific techniques and approaches which are quite different from those used for, say, insomnia. The use of these techniques is not in contradiction with whatever other approach or philosophy a particular practitioner may follow and I therefore hope that this textbook can be of use to practitioners of many different orientations.

Another important reason for discussing individual diseases is their particular and specific pathology and aetiology: it is only by under-standing the distinctive pathology and aetiology that we can advise the patient on life-style, work, emotional life, sexual habits, diet and exercise. Educating the patient in these areas is as important as the treatment imparted, as it gives the patient responsibility for his or her own health and so can prevent recurrence of the problem.

The acupuncture points indicated for each pattern are *not* formulae but only the possible points from which the practitioner can choose when determining an acupuncture treatment. There are a few exceptions and these are indicated as "general prescription" or "ancient prescription". The principles of combination of acupuncture points are discussed in Appendix I and the reader is strongly advised to read this as it discusses how to formulate a harmonious point combination by balancing Yin-Yang, Front-Back, Top-Bottom, and Left Right. Just as a beautiful painting must have vibrant colours, expert technique and balanced composition, a good acupuncture treatment must be based on a deft needle technique, a skilful choice of points according to their action, and a balanced and harmonious combination of such points. This last aspect is discussed in Appendix I.

The herbal treatment of each disease is based on several modern Chinese textbooks and integrated with the treatment found in ancient classics (see bibliography). The main modern textbook followed was that used in all colleges of Chinese Medicine in China, i.e. "Chinese Internal Medicine" (*Zhong Yi Nei Ke Xue* 中医内科学) by Zhang Bo Yu (1986).

I should make some comments on the dosages of the herbal prescriptions. The dosages shown are mostly those from modern and old Chinese books. In my practice I use much lower dosages and these are reflected in the case histories, the average for each herb being about 4 g. I find that these reduced dosages work very well. As for the mode of administration of the herbs, I use, almost exclusively, decoctions as I find these give the best therapeutic results. In my practice in England the patients' compliance is very high indeed (about 95%) and even most children manage to take decoctions (albeit disguised in a variety of ways). In children under 3 years of age the decoction can be substantially diluted and given throughout the day. In children over 3, honey can be added to the decoction: strictly speaking, the addition of honey alters the taste of the decoction and brings in honey's own properties, but in practice I think it is better for a child to take the herbs with honey than not to take them at all. Other ways of coaxing children to take decoctions include offering them a biscuit (cookie) or a favourite drink immediately after they have swallowed the mixture. However, I find that one of the best ways of getting children over 3 years to take a decoction is by involving them in the dispensing of the herbs: the child is fascinated by the different shapes, textures and smells of the herbs and loves helping to dispense the herbs and putting them in the bags. Involving a young patient in this way ensures that when the child drinks the decoction it is not an alien preparation but something the child relates to the actual herbs he or she helped to dispense. This method is of course time-consuming for the practitioner but it is also great fun.

Whenever possible, I have indicated patent remedies which can be used for each pattern. This section of the book is mostly for the benefit of acupuncturists who do not use Chinese herbs, as an experienced Chinese herbalist would choose a patent remedy according to his or her own knowledge and experience. I have evaluated the therapeutic effect of patent remedies according to their ingredients and sometimes quite independently of the actions and indications given by the manufacturer. For this reason, a patent remedy may occasionally be suggested for a condition quite different from the ones for which it is normally given. To help the acupuncturist select the fitting remedy I have given the tongue (and sometimes pulse) presentation appropriate to each remedy: this is an important guideline to the choice of the correct remedy and the reader's attention is drawn to it. The reader should also note that some patent remedies may contain substances which are illegal in certain countries: this could be either because they are toxic (such as Zhu Sha *Cinnabaris*) or because they are of animal origin from protected species. The mention of such patent remedies in this book does not signify an endorsement of their use, and the reader is strongly advised to enquire about the laws governing the use of certain herbs in his or her country. Each practitioner should therefore satisfy himself or herself as to the suitability of a particular patent remedy.

Dosages of the patent remedies have not been given because they may come in different form and size of pills: the practitioner should therefore check dosages and contraindications in textbooks of patent remedies such as Fratkin's "Chinese Herbal Patent Formulas" or Zhu's "Chinese Prepared Medicines", which are both mentioned in the bibliography.

All the case histories are drawn from my own practice and the reader is invited to study them as they show how prescriptions are adapted to the individual's particular disharmony, and also how acupuncture points are chosen and combined.

For reasons of length, this book omits the discussion of skin diseases and paediatric diseases, while the discussion of gynaecology is limited to dysmenorrhoea, menorrhagia and pre-menstrual tension: it is hoped that gynaecology will form the subject of a future book.

Finally, each chapter includes the Western differentiation of the symptom discussed, e.g. the possible causes of headaches in Western medicine. Of course this is not intended to be a replacement of a good book on Western clinical medicine (some are mentioned in the bibliography): it is simply meant to provide the practitioner in a clinical setting with a quick check-list of the possible Western causes of that particular symptom. This is important because we should know when to refer a patient to a Western medical doctor or specialist for a further diagnosis. For example, a patient may come to us complaining of urinary difficulty and we should know when to suspect a prostate carcinoma. The second reason for familiarizing ourselves with the Western differentiation of symptoms is prognosis. Although Chinese medicine is excellent at providing not only a diagnosis but also a reasonable prognosis by carefully examining symptoms, signs, tongue and pulse, in many cases the prognosis depends also on the Western diagnosis. For example, it makes a big difference to prognosis whether tingling in a limb is caused by a "simple" Liver-Blood deficiency or by the beginning of multiple sclerosis.

I sincerely hope that this book will be of practical use to practitioners in various countries in order to develop Chinese medicine and help it to take its rightful place in modern medicine.

Amersham, 1994   G. M.

Acknowledgements

I acknowledge with sincere thanks the many people who, in one way or another, helped me to write this book.

The most important period in my professional training was spent at the Nanjing College of Traditional Chinese Medicine and I am deeply indebted to its directors, teachers and other members of staff for the care and patience in sharing their profound knowledge with me. I am also grateful to the teaching staff of the Jiangsu Province Hospital for Traditional Chinese Medicine where my clinical training took place.

Dr J. H. F. Shen was and continues to be an inspiration. I owe him a debt of gratitude for communicating his diagnostic skills to me.

I would like to acknowledge that I also owe much to Dr Chen Jing Hua. Her ideas on asthma sparked off my new theory about this disease, although any shortcomings in this theory are of course entirely my responsibility.

Dr Ted Kaptchuk provided my first introduction to Chinese herbs and for that I am very grateful.

I wish to thank Mr You Ben Lin of the Nanjing College of Traditional Chinese Medicine who drew the characters for the title page with great skill and elegance. I am grateful to Mr Huang Zi Qiang who drew the Chinese characters that appear at the head of each chapter.

I am indebted to Francesca Diebschlag for editing and proof-reading my manuscript with great care and for providing useful suggestions.

I am grateful to Alan Papier and Peter Deadman for reading some of the chapters and making useful suggestions.

I would like to thank the staff of Churchill Livingstone for their expertise, efficiency and courtesy: in particular, I am grateful to Mary Law, Inta Ozols and Dinah Thom for their help and support with this project.

Finally, this book would not have come into being without my wife's continuous support, suggestions and inspiration.

G. M.

Note on the translation of Chinese medical terms

The terminology used in this book generally follows that used in the "Foundations of Chinese Medicine". As in this book, I have opted for translating all Chinese medical terms with the exception of *Yin*, *Yang* and *Qi*. I have also continued using capitals for the terms which are specific to Chinese medicine. For example, "Blood" indicates one of the vital substances of Chinese medicine, whereas "blood" denotes the liquid flowing in the blood vessels; e.g."In Blood deficiency the menstrual blood may be pale".

I have changed a few of the terms appearing in the "Foundations of Chinese Medicine". I now translate *men* as "a feeling of oppression" (previously translated as "a feeling of stuffiness"), and *pi* as "a feeling of stuffiness". These terms and their diagnostic significance are explained in detail in chapter 14. I translate *Lin* disease as "Painful-Urination Syndrome" rather than "Difficult Urination Syndrome".

The translation of *Shen* deserves a special mention. I still translate that as "Mind" when it refers to the mental and psychological faculties pertaining to the Heart, but as "Spirit" when it indicates the complex of the mental–spiritual aspects of all the five Yin organs (i.e. Ethereal Soul, Corporeal Soul, Intellect, Will-Power and the Mind itself). This is explained in detail in chapter 9.

A glossary with Chinese characters, pinyin names and English translation appears on p. 905.

Plates

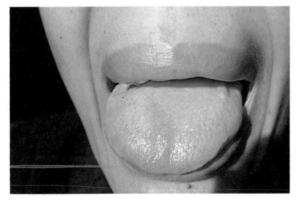

Plate 3.1 Breathlessness case history: woman, 48, p. 81

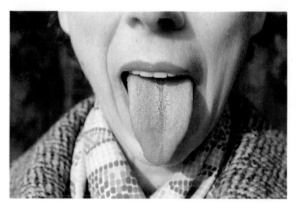

Plate 3.2 Breathlessness case history: woman, 42, p. 82

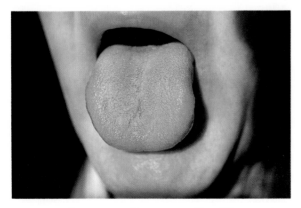

Plate 4.1 Wheezing case history: man, 58, p. 97

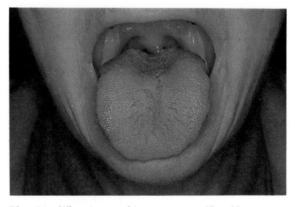

Plate 4.2 Wheezing case history: woman, 45, p. 99

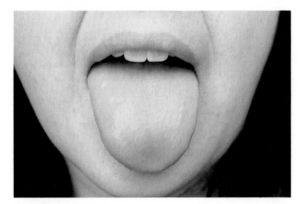

Plate 5.1   Asthma case history: woman, 35, p. 134

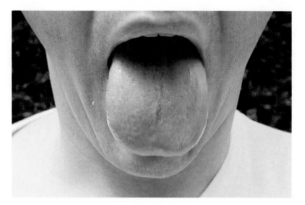

Plate 5.2   Asthma case history: man, 33, p. 138

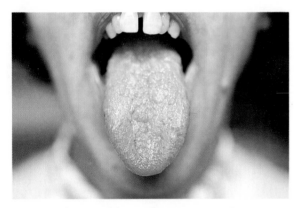

Plate 8.1   Cough case history: woman, 80, p. 185

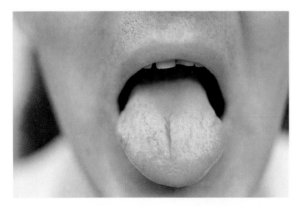

Plate 9.1   Mental-emotional problem: tongue shape in severe mental illness, p. 221

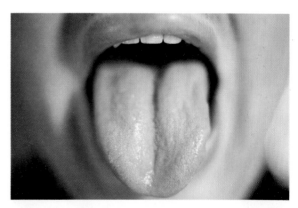

Plate 9.2   Mental-emotional problem case history, man, 51, p. 227

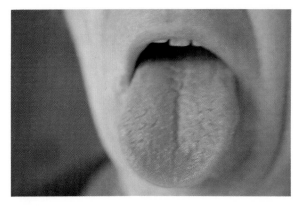

Plate 9.3 Mental-emotional problem case history, man, 39, p. 243

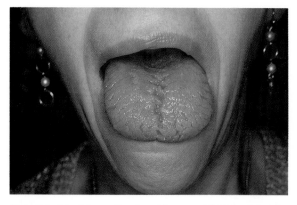

Plate 9.4 Mental-emotional problem case history, woman, 52, p. 253

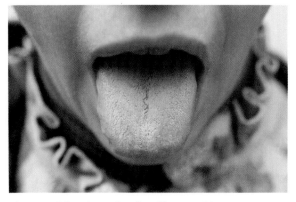

Plate 9.5 Mental-emotional problem case history, woman, 40, p. 261

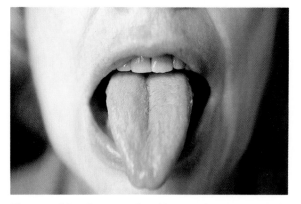

Plate 9.6 Mental-emotional problem case history, woman, 54, p. 263

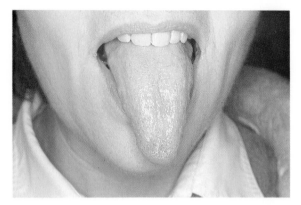

Plate 9.7   Mental-emotional problem case history, woman, 46, p. 270

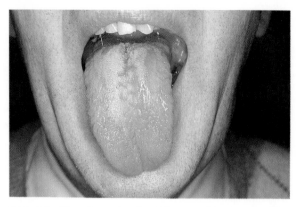

Plate 9.8   Mental-emotional problem case history, man, 35, p. 272

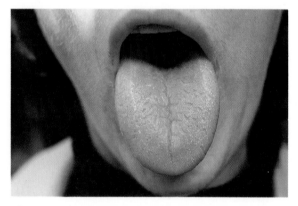

Plate 9.9   Mental-emotional problem case history, woman, 39, p. 274

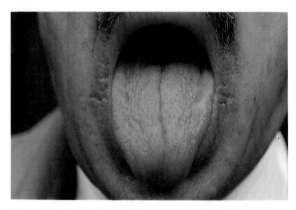

Plate 10.1   Insomnia case history, man, 61, p. 297

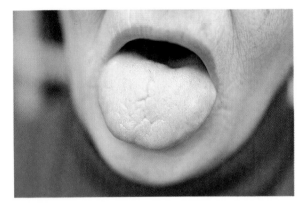

Plate 12.1   Tiredness case history, woman, 61, p. 329

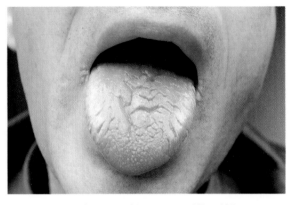

Plate 12.2   Tiredness case history, man, 37, p. 336

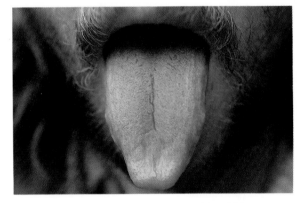

Plate 12.3   Tiredness case history, man, 28, p. 344

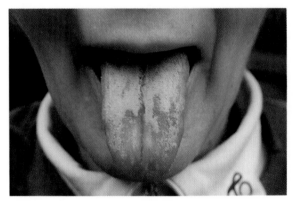

Plate 12.4   Tiredness case history, woman, 42, p. 355

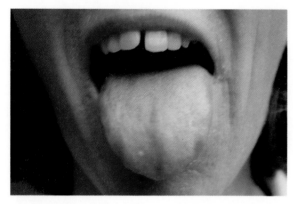

Plate 13.1   Chest Painful Obstruction Syndrome case history, woman, 59, p. 369

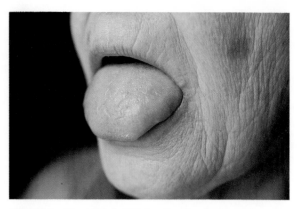

Plate 13.2   Chest Painful Obstruction Syndrome case history, woman, 70, p. 374

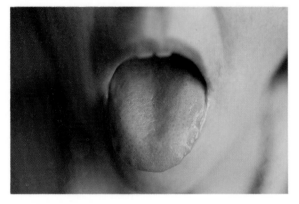

Plate 14.1   Epigastric pain case history, woman, 45, p. 394

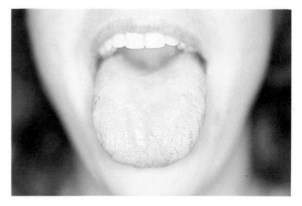

Plate 14.2   Epigastric pain case history, woman, 47, p. 412

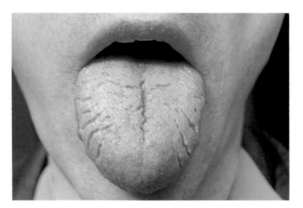

Plate 14.3   Epigastric pain case history, man, 37, p. 414

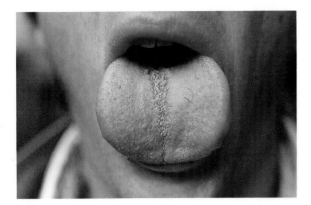

Plate 16.1   Abdominal pain case history, man, 40, p. 443

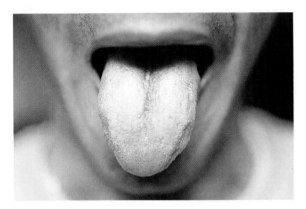

Plate 18.1   Diarrhoea case history, man, 37, p. 466

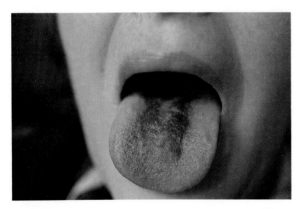

Plate 19.1   Constipation case history, woman, 62, p. 482

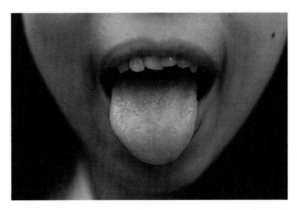

Plate 19.2   Constipation case history, woman, 39, p. 486

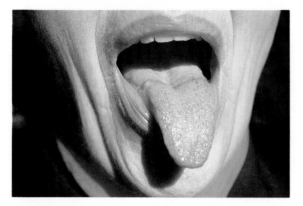

Plate 20.1 Painful-Urination Syndrome case history, woman, 30, p. 503

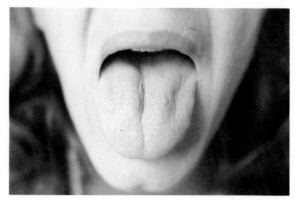

Plate 20.2 Painful-Urination Syndrome case history, woman, 47, p. 511

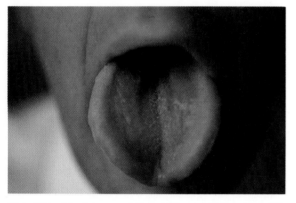

Plate 25.1 Myalgic encephalomyelitis case history, man, 33, p. 639

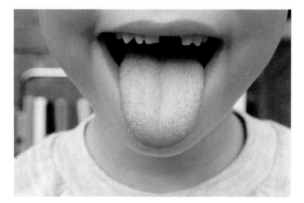

Plate 34.1 Common cold and influenza case history, boy, 6, p. 790

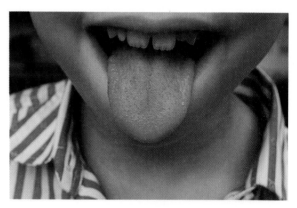

Plate 34.2 Common cold and influenza case history, boy, 7, p. 797

Headaches 1

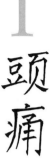

Headache is one of the most common symptoms encountered in clinical practice. There are few people who have never experienced a headache at some time or other of their life. The discussion of the treatment of headaches will include that of migraine and will be based on the following headings:

- Aetiology
- Channels
- Diagnosis
- Identification of patterns
- Treatment.

Aetiology

Any of the causes of disease normally considered in Chinese Medicine can play a part in the aetiology of headaches.

1. CONSTITUTION

The constitutional body condition inherited from our parents depends on three factors:

1. The parents' health in general
2. The parents' health at the time of conception
3. The conditions of the mother's pregnancy.

Any of these factors can affect the body condition and become a cause of headaches later in life. Persistent and recurrent headaches that start in childhood (usually between about 7 and 10) strongly indicate the presence of a constitutional factor of disease. If the parents' Qi and Essence are weak, the resulting Pre-Heaven Essence of the child will also be weak. Similarly if the parents conceive when too old. This can result in headaches deriving from a Kidney or Liver deficiency starting during childhood. A hereditary Kidney or Liver weakness manifests with enuresis or frequent urination, lack of vitality, dull headaches and frequently, myopia.

Even though the parents' general health may be good, if it is poor at the time of the child's conception (perhaps through overwork, excessive sexual activity, excessive consumption of alcohol, or use of certain medications or drugs such as cannabis or cocaine), this will result in the child having a weak constitution and in the possibility of its suffering from headaches. In this case, the weakness will affect not the Kidneys or Liver, but any of the other organs, i.e. Spleen, Lungs or Heart, depending on the particular condition which is negatively affecting the parents' health. For example, if the parents' health is poor at the time of conception from overwork it may be a cause of hereditary Spleen weakness in the child. The excessive consumption of alcohol or the use of drugs or certain medicines may cause a hereditary weakness of the child's Heart or Lungs. A hereditary Spleen weakness in a child may manifest with poor muscle tone, physical weakness, digestive problems, and, in severe cases, Child Nutritional Impairment (*Gan*). In this case the headaches will be on the forehead and be related to food intake.

A hereditary Lung weakness in a child may manifest with a tendency to catching colds and respiratory infections, whooping cough, asthma, eczema, pale complexion, a thin chest and a pulse in both Front positions which when felt is more medial and running upwards towards the thumb (Fig. 1.1).

A hereditary Heart weakness in a child may manifest with dream-disturbed sleep, nervousness and a relatively deep midline crack on the tongue. Young children (under 3) may wake up crying at night. In such cases, the headaches are usually on the forehead or in the whole head.

The condition of the mother during the pregnancy can affect the foetus. For example, an accident to the mother can cause headaches for the child. A shock during pregnancy can also cause a child to suffer headaches deriving from Heart deficiency. This will also manifest with a bluish tinge on the child's forehead and chin.

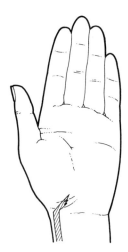

Fig. 1.1   Pulse picture in hereditary Lung weakness

2. EMOTIONS

Emotional causes of disease are of course extremely frequent causes of headaches.

ANGER

Many different emotions fall under the broad term of "anger" in Chinese Medicine. These are frustration, resentment and pent-up grudges. All these cause the rising of Liver-Yang or Liver-Fire. Among the emotional causes of headaches this is by far the most common one. It will give rise to headaches from Liver-Yang rising or Liver-Fire blazing. These headaches are typically situated on the Gall-Bladder channel on the temple or side of the head.

WORRY

Worrying excessively knots Qi, in particular Lung and Heart Qi. This is often an indirect cause of headaches as the deficiency of Lung-Qi (Metal in the 5-Element model) may allow Liver-Yang to rise (Wood in the 5-Element model) and cause headaches.

Worry may also be a direct cause of headaches, which are usually situated on the forehead or the top of the head, and are dull in character.

FEAR

A chronic state of anxiety and fear depletes the Kidneys and causes headaches either directly from Kidney deficiency (in this case affecting the whole head) or indirectly when the Kidney deficiency leads to the rising of Liver-Yang.

SHOCK

Shock "suspends" Qi and it affects Heart, Lung and Spleen Qi. It will usually cause headaches affecting the whole head.

EXCESSIVE MENTAL WORK

Although this is obviously not an "emotion" it is usually discussed with the emotional causes of disease. Excessive mental activity is a frequent cause of chronic headaches in children. Although this may seem strange at first, it does occur frequently when a bright child attends an academically-demanding school with high parent expectations. This sets a pattern early in life of long hours of mental work and concentration combined with the worry of doing well, that leads to severe headaches or migraine. The long hours of reading by themselves (and nowadays work at a computer monitor) strain the eyes and lead to headaches.

3. OVERWORK

Working too long hours without adequate rest weakens Spleen-Qi and, in the long run, Kidney-Yin. This is the most common cause of Yin deficiency in Western industrial societies. The deficiency of Kidney-Yin will give rise to headaches in the whole head, or it will lead to Liver-Yang rising and causing migraine-type headaches on one side of the head on the Gall-Bladder channel.

4. EXCESSIVE SEXUAL ACTIVITY

This is a common cause of headaches, particularly in men. Under normal circumstances the temporary loss of Kidney-Essence resulting from sexual activity is quickly restored and so sexual activity will not lead to disease. When sexual activity is too frequent however, there is no time for the Kidney-Essence to be restored and this results in deficiency of Kidney energy (either Yin or Yang depending on the constitution of the person). An old Daoist saying declares: "*Sleeping alone is better than taking 100 tonics*"!

Men are affected by excessive sexual activity more than women. Too many childbirths in too short a time weaken the uterus and the Kidneys in women. This is an important cause of depletion of Kidney-Essence in women, somewhat equivalent to excessive sexual activity in men (see below).

By depleting the Kidneys, excessive sexual activity is a frequent cause of headaches either on the occiput or the whole head. Indeed, if someone experiences a headache and dizziness following sexual intercourse, it is a certain sign that that particular level of sexual activity is excessive and it should be moderated.

It is of course impossible to define what is "excessive" sexual activity as this is entirely relative and depends on the person's constitution and strength of Essence.[1]

5. DIET

Diet has a direct and profound influence on the aetiology of headaches. Dietary irregularities may cause headaches by affecting different organs. First of all, not eating enough in itself will obviously cause headaches from general deficiency of Qi and Blood, usually occurring on the top of the head. This situation occurs when people follow too strict a diet adhering to rigid "rules" and consequently lacking essential nourishment. On the other extreme, over-eating obstructs Stomach-Qi and weakens the Spleen leading to headaches on the forehead which are usually sharp in character.

Excessive consumption of hot-energy foods such as curries, spices, pepper (black, white or red), red meat and alcohol causes Liver-Fire and/or Stomach-Heat. Liver-Fire will result in lateral headaches and Stomach-Heat in frontal headaches, both of which are sharp in character.

The excessive consumption of Damp-producing foods affects the Spleen and leads to Dampness which may cause dull headaches on the forehead and a typical feeling of heaviness in the head. Damp-producing foods include all greasy foods, fried foods, milk, cheese, butter, cream, ice-cream, bananas, peanuts, sweets and white sugar.

Too much salt in the diet will cause a Kidney deficiency and may result in dull headaches in the whole head or on the occiput. A diet based on tinned or processed foods is often heavy in salt because this is added to many such foods: bacon, sausages, cereals, tinned soups, smoked fish and many others.

An excessive consumption of sour foods affects the Liver and is also a frequent cause of headaches. Sour foods include yoghurt, grapefruit and its juice, cooking apples, pickles, vinegar, spinach, rhubarb, gooseberries, redcurrants, etc.

The way in which food is eaten also influences the energy of the internal organs. Eating too quickly or while discussing work, leads to retention of food in the Stomach and to sharp headaches on the forehead. Eating irregularly or too late at night induces a deficiency of Stomach-Yin and may cause dull headaches on the forehead (see also chapter 14, "Epigastric Pain").

It should be remembered that the principles of Chinese diet were developed over 2000 years ago. They do not take into account modern discoveries about food and, most of all, do not consider the role of chemicals in food. Food has never been subjected to so much chemical manipulation as in the past 30 years or so. As far as headaches are concerned, they can be very much affected by chemicals in food. For example, it is well known that monosodium glutamate (found in Chinese restaurant food) can cause headaches. The possibility of a sensitivity to certain chemicals should therefore always be kept in mind when investigating the aetiology of headaches.

Finally, certain of the foods we consume are not found in a Chinese diet at all and for this reason are not even mentioned in books on diet. Cocoa (and chocolate) and coffee are cases in point. Both of these can aggravate headaches or precipitate a migraine attack. In particular, an excessive consumption of coffee is a frequent cause of chronic headaches in our society and, in my experience, any chronic-headache sufferer always benefits greatly from not drinking coffee at all.[2]

6. ACCIDENTS

Severe accidents and falls which affect the head can cause stasis of Blood in a particular area of the head. This is a frequent cause of chronic headache. Whenever the headaches a patient suffers always occur in the same part of the head and usually in a small area, then the possibility of an old trauma to the head should be considered. The patient may not be aware of or remember an old fall or accident and not relate it to the headaches. A single, large purple spot near the tip of the tongue may indicate an old trauma in the head region.

In particular, a trauma to the head may not cause headaches immediately after it, but these can start years later when a new cause of disease intervenes. For example, a child may fall on the head and be mildly concussed. Many years later, he or she may experience emotional problems related to anger or frustration which cause Liver-Yang to rise. In such a case, the headache from Liver-Yang rising will settle in the area of the head where the old trauma occurred and will always affect such an area.

7. CHILDBIRTH

Too many childbirths too close together seriously weaken Liver, Kidneys, and the Directing Vessel in a woman. A deficiency of Liver and Kidneys can give rise to Empty-type headaches from Kidney-Essence not reaching the head; the deficiency of Liver and Kidneys may also induce Liver-Yang to rise and therefore cause headaches of this type.

It is important to remember that miscarriages also count as "childbirth" as far as causes of disease are concerned. A miscarriage is as depleting as childbirth: in fact, some Chinese doctors even say that miscarriages are more depleting than childbirth. This is because, first of all, there may be more blood loss in a miscarriage than in childbirth; secondly, after a miscarriage there is an abrupt alteration of the hormone levels; thirdly, a miscarriage (especially a late one) is emotionally very distressing and the mother often has deep feelings of loss, and even failure.

8. EXTERNAL PATHOGENIC FACTORS

The main external pathogenic factors which cause headaches are Wind and Dampness.

Wind affects the top part of the body and is a very frequent cause of acute headaches which may arise independently without other symptoms, or may occur together with the symptoms of invasion of Wind-Cold. External Wind also affects the neck muscles causing a pronounced stiffness. Wind is normally a cause of acute headaches, but repeated invasions of Wind may give rise to chronic headaches and stiffness of the neck and shoulders (called "Head-Wind").

External Dampness can also affect the head even though this particular pathogenic factor normally invades the lower part of the body. However, acute invasions of Dampness easily affect the Middle Burner: from here, Dampness may rise to the head and prevent the clear Yang from reaching the head and clearing the head's orifices.

Channels

The "Correct Seal of Medical Circles" says:

The head is like Heaven [being at the top]: the clear Qi of the three Yang channels [Greater Yang, Lesser Yang and Bright Yang] and the six Yang organs as well as the Blood and Essence of the three Yin channels [Greater Yin, Lesser Yin and Terminal Yin] and the five Yin organs, all reach it. It is affected by the six external pathogenic climates as well as by internal pathogenic factors.[3]

The head is the highest part of the body not only anatomically but also energetically accord-

ing to the flow of Qi in the 12 channels. It is, in fact, the area of maximum potential of energy in the circulation of Qi in the channels. Qi circulates in the channels because there is a difference of potential between the chest and the head. If we consider the first four channels, for example, we see that Qi starts at the chest area in the Lung channel: this is the area of minimum potential of energy. In order to understand this we can visualize a certain amount of water at the bottom of a hill, where its potential of producing energy is minimal. If we slowly carry this water up the hill, gradually its potential of producing energy will increase, as we know. When the water reaches the top of the hill, its potential of producing (hydroelectric) energy will be maximum. The bottom of the hill corresponds to the chest, half-way up the hill corresponds to the hands (or feet) and the top of the hill corresponds to the head. Thus, from the Lung channel in the chest, Qi starts to move upwards towards the head. At the fingertips, Qi changes polarity, i.e. it flows from the Yin Lung channel to the Yang Large Intestine channel, but it is still flowing towards the head and its potential is increasing. When it reaches the head the potential is at its maximum and it then starts decreasing as it flows towards the feet. At the feet, Qi changes polarity, i.e. it flows from the Yang Stomach channel to the Yin Spleen channel, but its potential is still decreasing as it flows towards the chest area. When it

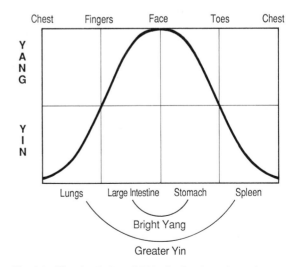

Fig. 1.2 The circulation of Qi in the first four channels

reaches the chest the potential is minimum (the water has reached the bottom of the hill again). The Qi from the Spleen channel then connects internally with the Heart channel and a new 4-channel cycle starts in exactly the same way. The cycle of Qi in the first four channels can be seen in Figure 1.2. Figure 1.3 shows the circulation of Qi in the 12 channels.

The implication of all this is that the head is the area of maximum potential of Qi and therefore intrinsically prone to rising of energy (or pathogenic factors) to the top, for example, the rising of Liver-Yang, Liver-Fire, Liver-Wind, or Heart-Fire. Conversely, clear Yang Qi failing to rise to the top may lead to the obstruction of the head by Phlegm or Dampness.

The head is also the area of concentration of Yang energy as all the Yang channels directly meet and join up in the head. In fact, as far as the superficial pathways are concerned, only Yang channels reach the head. For this reason the head is variously called *"the confluence of Yang"* or *"the Palace of Yang"* or *"the Palace of clear Yang"*[4].

However, Yin Qi obviously also reaches the head but only internally. Of the Yin channels only the Heart and Liver reach the head internally (deep pathway). All the other Yin channels reach the head indirectly via their divergent channels as each Yin divergent channel merges with its related Yang divergent channel at the neck area (Fig. 1.4). Thus both the clear Yang from the Yang organs and the pure essences from the Yin organs reach the head.

As far as headaches are concerned, the two Yang channels which are most frequently involved are the Gall-Bladder and Bladder. Of the Yin channels, the two most frequently involved are Liver and Kidneys.

Diagnosis

Headaches can be diagnosed from two perspectives: from the point of view of channels or internal organs. Both of these are equally relevant in clinical practice particularly from the acupuncturist's perspective. I will discuss the main diagnostic pointers from three viewpoints:

1. Diagnosis according to channels
2. Diagnosis according to type of pain
3. Diagnosis according to amelioration and aggravation.

The diagnosis according to the internal organs will be discussed under the next heading, "Identification of patterns".

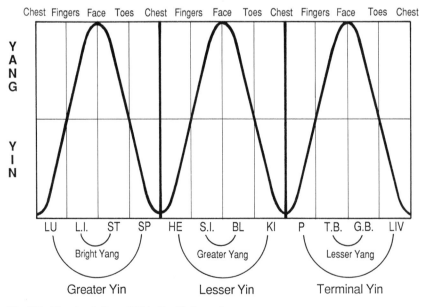

Fig. 1.3   The circulation of Qi in the 12 channels

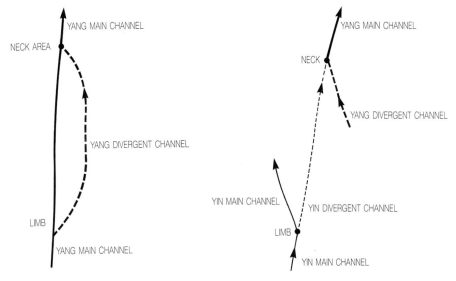

Fig. 1.4   Connection between Yin and Yang divergent channels

DIAGNOSIS ACCORDING TO CHANNELS

The "Medical Talks from the Deserted Cottage" says:

The Greater Yang type of headache affects the occiput, the Bright Yang type affects the forehead, the Lesser Yang type affects the sides of the head . . . the Terminal Yin type affects the top of the head . . . the Greater and Lesser Yin do not ascend to the head, but Phlegm can prevent Qi from descending and the pure Yang from ascending freely to the head.[5]

This classification provides a useful guideline in clinical practice for a quick identification of the channel involved in a given type of headache (Fig. 1.5).

However, this is only a broad guideline which first of all needs to be further refined, and secondly needs to be integrated with the identification of internal-organ patterns. For example, while a headache on the top of the head often involves the Terminal-Yin channel, i.e. the Liver channel, it can be due to either Liver-Yang rising or Liver-Blood deficiency. Furthermore, a headache on the top of the head can also be due to deficient Qi and/or Blood unable to reach the

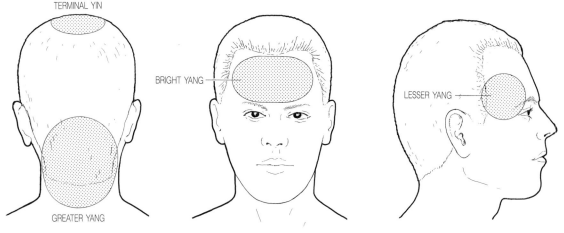

Fig. 1.5   Headache areas

head, and not necessarily reflect a Liver channel involvement at all.

A further analysis of the channel affecting various head areas in headaches is as follows.

TOP OF THE HEAD

The Liver channel reaches the top of the head internally and is the most frequent cause of headache there (Fig. 1.6).

A headache on top of the head is most often due to deficient Liver-Blood being unable to reach the area. This headache will improve if the patient lies down and it will be dull in character. In a few cases a headache in this area may be due to Liver-Yang rising, in which case it will be sharp in character.

There are also other causes of headache in this area not related to the Liver channel, such as deficient Qi and Blood unable to reach the top and Heart-Blood deficiency.

A headache on the top of the head only, should not be confused with one that affects the top but starts all the way from the base of the occiput. This type of headache is due to the Bladder channel.

SIDES OF THE HEAD

This area corresponds to the Gall-Bladder channel and a headache here is most frequently due to Liver-Yang, Liver-Fire or Liver-Wind rising (Fig. 1.7). This headache is sharp and throbbing in character.

ONE SIDE ONLY

This area also corresponds to the Gall-Bladder channel and a headache here is also due to either Liver-Yang or Liver-Fire rising. It is said in Chinese Medicine that a headache on the left side is more likely to result from a Deficiency and one on the right side to result from an Excess, but this is by no means a completely reliable rule.

TEMPLES

This area also corresponds to the Gall-Bladder channel and a headache most frequently affects one side only. This headache is usually due to Liver-Yang, Liver-Fire or Liver-Wind rising and is throbbing in character (Fig. 1.8).

BEHIND THE EYES

This is a very frequent location for migraine. The headache is due to Liver-Blood deficiency if the pain is dull, or to Liver-Yang rising if the pain is sharp and severe.

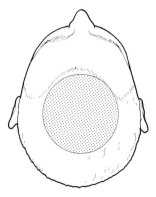

Fig. 1.6 Liver-channel headache area

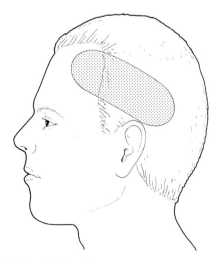

Fig. 1.7 Sides of the head area

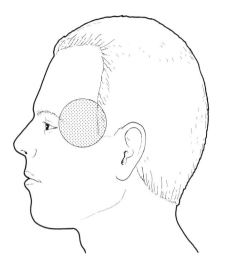

Fig. 1.8 Temple area

FOREHEAD

Headaches in this area are usually related to the Stomach. They can indicate either Stomach deficiency if the pain is dull or Stomach-Heat if it is sharp.

A very frequent cause of frontal headaches is either Dampness or Phlegm being retained in the head and preventing the clear Yang from ascending to the head to brighten the sense orifices. For this reason this type of headache is associated with a heavy sensation of the head, a muzzy feeling of the head, and a lack of concentration. If Phlegm is causing the headache the person will also experience dizziness and blurred vision.

In a few cases, frontal headaches can be due to a residual pathogenic factor, such as external Wind, which has not been expelled after an invasion of exterior Wind-Cold or Wind-Heat.

BACK OF THE HEAD (OCCIPUT)

Chronic headaches in this area are usually due to a Kidney deficiency manifesting on the Bladder channel.

Acute headaches here are due to invasion of external Wind (usually Wind-Cold) and form a typical feature of the Greater Yang pattern within the 6-Stage pattern identification (see Ap-

pendix 2). This type of headache is accompanied by great stiffness of the back of the neck.

In a few cases, occipital headache can be associated with a Bladder pattern, such as Damp-Heat in the Bladder, in which case the pain will be sharp.

WHOLE HEAD

Chronic headaches in this area are due to Kidney-Essence deficiency. The Kidney-Essence nourishes the brain and when it is deficient it lacks nourishment. This can give rise to dull headaches in the whole head accompanied by a feeling of emptiness of the head.

Acute headaches affecting the whole head are due to invasion of external Wind (which can be either Wind-Cold or Wind-Heat). These are severe and sharp in character, sometimes accompanied by a pulling sensation.

Thus there is generally a correlation between the pattern related to a specific type of headache and the channel involved. For example, the pattern of Liver-Yang rising will give rise to headaches on the Gall-Bladder channel, while the pattern of Kidney deficiency will cause headaches on the Bladder channel. However, there can be exceptions. This happens in situations when more than one pattern is involved. For example, a person may suffer from a chronic Kidney deficiency leading to the rising of Liver-Yang. If the Kidney deficiency is very long-standing and the Bladder channel on the head is affected, it is possible for Liver-Yang type of headaches (i.e. very sharp and throbbing in character) to manifest on the Bladder channel on the occiput.

It should also be remembered that headaches frequently occur in different parts of the head at different times. This is not unusual and is simply due to the coexistence of two different patterns causing headaches. For example, Liver-Blood deficiency can give rise to Liver-Yang rising. In this case a person may suffer from dull headaches on top of the head reflecting the Liver-Blood deficiency, occasionally changing into sharp and throbbing headaches on one temple reflecting the Liver-Yang rising.

If the area of the headache changes all the time and the headache is experienced in different parts of the head at different times, it either indicates the presence of Liver-Wind, in which case the pain will be accompanied by a pulling sensation, or the presence of Phlegm, in which case the pain will be accompanied by a heavy sensation of the head.

DIAGNOSIS ACCORDING TO TYPE OF PAIN

Generally, a dull ache indicates an Empty condition, while a sharp pain indicates a Full condition from the 8-Principle perspective. A sudden onset tends to indicate an exterior invasion, whilst a gradual onset tends to indicate an interior one. Empty conditions causing dull headaches include deficiency of Qi and/or Blood, Liver-Blood deficiency and Kidney deficiency. Full conditions include Liver-Yang rising, Liver-Fire blazing, Liver-Wind, Phlegm, stasis of Blood and Stomach Heat.

DULL

A dull headache is due to one of the deficiencies outlined above.

FEELING OF HEAVINESS

This is characteristic of Dampness or Phlegm obstructing the head and preventing the clear Yang Qi from ascending to the head and the turbid Yin Qi from descending. The head typically feels heavy, muzzy and as if it were wrapped in a cloth. The person would also find it difficult to concentrate and think, especially in the morning.

Both Dampness and Phlegm may cause the above sensations but Phlegm is more obstructive and it clouds the "orifices" and sense organs, causing dizziness and blurred vision. These last two symptoms distinguish Phlegm from Dampness in the head.

DISTENDING PAIN

This is a typical Chinese expression which will be seldom used by Western patients (or at least in Anglo-Saxon languages). The most frequently recurrent expressions regarding this type of pain are "throbbing", "bursting" and "pulsating", all of which correspond to "distending". This sensation is typical of a Liver-related headache which could be from Liver-Yang or Liver-Fire.

However, a distending pain can also be due to exterior Wind-Heat, in which case it will affect the whole head, whereas in the case of Liver-Yang or Liver-Fire it will most probably affect one or both sides of the head.

STIFF

A pronounced stiffness of the occiput usually indicates an invasion of exterior Wind-Cold. A chronic headache with stiffness of the top of the shoulders and neck usually indicates Liver-Yang rising.

PULLING

A pulling type of sensation indicates internal Liver-Wind.

STABBING, BORING

This sensation is very intense and fixed in one place and it indicates Blood stasis. It occurs only in chronic headaches. A description also used in this context is "splitting headache".

FEELING OF EMPTINESS

A sensation of emptiness of the brain indicates deficiency of Kidney (Yin or Yang).

We can summarize the different types of headaches according to patterns:

Wind-Cold: severe occipital with pronounced stiffness
Wind-Heat: severe, distending, in the whole head
Wind-Damp: feeling of heaviness as if head were wrapped

Liver-Yang, Liver-Fire: distending
Liver-Wind: pulling
Stasis of Blood: stabbing, splitting, boring
Phlegm: heavy sensation as if head were wrapped, dizziness
Dampness: heavy sensation as if head were wrapped
Qi-Blood deficiency: dull
Kidney deficiency: feeling of emptiness.

DIAGNOSIS ACCORDING TO AMELIORATION AND AGGRAVATION

The factors which make a headache better or worse may give an indication of the condition causing the headache.

TIME OF DAY

Chronic headaches which are worse in day-time indicate either deficiency of Qi/Yang or Dampness.

Chronic headaches which are worse in the evening or at night indicate deficiency of Blood or Yin (which may be causing Yang rising).

ACTIVITY/REST

Headaches that get worse with activity are due to deficiency of Qi or Blood, whilst headaches that improve with light exercise may be due to Liver-Yang rising or Phlegm.

Headaches that improve with rest and lying down are due to deficiency of Qi or Blood, whilst headaches that worsen with lying down are due to Dampness or Phlegm.

WEATHER

Headaches which get worse with heat may be due to Liver-Yang or Liver-Fire rising, whilst headaches that get worse with cold may be due to deficiency of Yang. If they worsen with damp weather, it is a clear indication that they are due to Dampness or Phlegm.

A headache that improves temporarily with the application of cold (for example, cold water) may be due to Liver-Yang or Liver-Fire.

EMOTIONS

Headaches which worsen with anger are due to Liver-Yang or Liver-Fire. Headaches which get worse when the person suddenly relaxes (the typical weekend headache) are due to Liver-Yang rising. Headaches which worsen with a sudden excitement may be due to Liver-Yang rising.

SEXUAL ACTIVITY

Chronic headaches that are aggravated after sexual activity (culminating in ejaculation for men or orgasm for women) clearly indicate a deficiency of the Kidneys.

In rare cases, headaches may be ameliorated by sexual activity, which indicates Liver-Fire.

FOOD

Barring the vast subject of intolerance of certain foods, headaches which get worse after eating indicate Dampness, Phlegm, retention of food or Stomach-Heat.

Headaches which get better with eating indicate deficiency of Qi or Blood. Headaches which are aggravated by the consumption of sour foods (such as oranges, grapefruit, vinegar, etc.) are due to Liver-Yang rising.

POSTURE

If a headache improves when the patient is lying down it is due to a Deficiency; if it worsens when lying down (and improves when sitting) it is due to an Excess. For example, severe headaches from Liver-Yang rising usually get better sitting up and the patient dislikes lying down.

MENSTRUATION

Many types of headaches are closely affected by

the menstrual function. Headaches which precede the onset of the period are usually due to Liver-Yang rising. If they worsen during the period, they may be due to Liver-Fire or stasis of Blood. If they occur towards the end of the period, they indicate Blood Deficiency.

PRESSURE

If the person dislikes pressure on the part of the head where the headache occurs, it indicates an Excess condition. Conversely, if the headache improves with pressure, it indicates a Deficiency condition.

Differentiation and treatment

When identifying patterns for the treatment of headaches the first differentiation to make is between exterior and interior headaches. From an 8-Principle perspective, exterior headaches are of Excess-type by definition. Within the interior headaches, it is important to differentiate between Deficiency or Excess type. Zhang Jie Bin in his "Classic of Categories" says that all headaches are simply due to either too much or too little Qi in the head: the former is an Excess-type, the latter a Deficiency-type. He says: *"When the head is painful, it indicates a deficiency below and an excess above ... When Qi cannot ascend, the head aches ... when Qi does not ascend, the brain is empty".*[6]

The patterns discussed will be:

EXTERIOR

Wind-Cold
Wind-Heat
Wind-Dampness

INTERIOR

EXCESS-TYPE

Liver-Yang
Liver-Fire

Liver-Wind
Liver-Qi Stagnation
Stagnation of Cold in the Liver channel
Dampness
Turbid Phlegm
Turbid Phlegm-Wind
Retention of Food
Stasis of Blood
Stomach-Heat

DEFICIENCY-TYPE

Qi Deficiency
Blood Deficiency
Kidney Deficiency

GENERAL PRINCIPLES

TREATING THE ROOT OR THE MANIFESTATION

The question of treating the Root or the Manifestation is particularly important in the case of headaches. There are three possible courses of action.

1. TREATING BOTH THE ROOT AND THE MANIFESTATION

This is the most common approach. In most cases it is possible and necessary to deal with both the Root and the Manifestation simultaneously. For example, if a headache is due to Liver-Yang rising deriving from Kidney-Yin deficiency, the most obvious course of action is to tonify the Kidneys and subdue Liver-Yang simultaneously.

However, even if both Root and Manifestation are treated at the same time, it is often necessary to place the emphasis on one rather than the other. If the headaches are very severe with very frequent attacks, it may be necessary to concentrate one's attention on treating the Manifestation rather than the Root. In the example given above, if the headaches caused by Liver-Yang rising are very severe and frequent, it would be important to direct one's attention to treating the Manifestation first, i.e. subduing Liver-Yang.

On the other hand, if the Manifestation is not causing very severe headaches, then it might be sufficient to give primary importance to treatment of the Root. For example, if a person suffers from mild headaches from Qi deficiency, one would concentrate one's attention on treating the Root, i.e. tonify Qi.

2. TREATING THE MANIFESTATION FIRST, THE ROOT SECOND

This approach is necessary when the headaches caused by the Manifestation are extremely severe and frequent so as to impede any form of normal life. For example, if the headaches from Liver-Yang are of such intensity and frequency, one would concentrate one's attention first on treating the Manifestation only, i.e. subdue Liver-Yang. Once the severity and the frequency of the headaches have been reduced, then one can start treating the Root too.

3. TREATING THE ROOT ONLY

This is possible when the headaches are mild and infrequent. These headaches are usually deficient in nature; for example, mild headaches from Qi or Blood deficiency. In these cases it might be enough to concentrate simply on tonifying Qi or Blood, so that the headaches will gradually disappear.

POINT SELECTION

In the treatment of headaches it is essential to combine local with distal points. The more chronic or intense the headache the more local points are required. Local points are also especially required when a chronic headache appears always in the same spot. This indicates a local stasis of Blood which always calls for the use of local points to disperse it.

Generally speaking, distal points are chosen according to the pattern characterizing the headache and according to the channel involved. The two may not necessarily coincide. For example, a Liver-Yang headache nearly always manifests on the Gall-Bladder channel. We might therefore choose as distal points LIV-3 Taichong according to the pattern and G.B.-43 Xiaxi according to the channel.

Local points are mostly chosen according to the channel involved. For example, for headaches on the Gall-Bladder channel, one might choose G.B.-6 Xuanli as local point. Some local points may be chosen according to the location of the headache irrespective of the pattern. For example:

- Frontal headache: Du-23 Shangxing and G.B.-14 Yangbai
- Headache on vertex: Du-20 Baihui and Du-21 Qianding
- Occipital headache: BL-10 Tianzhu and Du-19 Houding
- Temporal headache: G.B.-8 Shuaigu and Taiyang.

However, local points may also be chosen according to the pattern. In the example above, if the headache on the Gall-Bladder channel is caused by Liver-Yang rising, in addition to points on the Gall-Bladder channel, we might also use Du-20 Baihui as the internal pathway if the Liver channel reaches up to that point.

The same principles apply to herbal therapy. The "local" herbs, i.e. those that specifically affect the head, are chosen according to the channel involved (but to a certain extent also according to the pattern) and the "distal" herbs, i.e. those that treat the condition causing the headaches, are chosen according to the pattern. For example, in frontal headaches from Liver-Qi stagnation and Spleen deficiency, Bai Zhi *Radix Angelicae dahuricae* can be selected as a "local" herb to affect the forehead, while the Xiao Yao San *Free and Easy Wanderer Powder* could be selected as the main prescription to deal with the pattern causing the headaches, i.e. stagnation of Liver-Qi.

EXTERIOR HEADACHES

Headaches from exterior origin are due to invasion of exterior Wind. Wind affects the top part of the body and a headache is one of its main manifestations. Headaches from exterior Wind are of the Excess-type by definition as they are characterized by the presence of Wind. Exterior Wind combines with other pathogenic factors to give rise to Wind-Cold, Wind-Heat, or Wind-Dampness.

1. WIND-COLD

Wind-Cold invades the Greater Yang channels first and manifests with a headache and stiffness on the occiput, where these channels flow. Cold contracts and tightens the sinews and slows down the circulation of Defensive Qi, hence the typical feeling of stiffness at the back of the neck.

This headache is obviously of acute onset and can be very severe but it will last only a short time, i.e. for the duration of time that the Wind-Cold is on the Exterior. Once the pathogenic factor penetrates the Interior, this type of headache goes. There are exceptions, however, as in a few cases when the external Wind-Cold is not expelled it can settle in the muscles and give rise to chronic headaches.

In acute cases, apart from the headache, there would also be generalized aches of the whole body as the exterior Wind-Cold obstructs the free circulation of Defensive Qi in the muscles.

Other symptoms and signs include: aversion to cold, shivers, possibly a fever, stiff and achy shoulders, absence of thirst, some breathlessness, cough, sneezing, a runny nose with a white discharge or a blocked nose, pale urine and a Floating-Tight pulse.

TREATMENT PRINCIPLE

Release the Exterior, expel Wind, scatter Cold, remove obstruction from the channels.

ACUPUNCTURE

General prescription: LU-7 Lieque, G.B.-20 Fengchi, Du-16 Fengfu, BL-10 Tianzhu. All with reducing method.

Explanation

The above points have been selected for their action in expelling Wind-Cold with particular reference to the headache deriving from Wind-Cold. Several other points might have been chosen to release the Exterior without a specific action on headaches such as, for example, BL-12 Fengmen and BL-13 Feishu (see also chapter 34 "Common Cold and Influenza").

- **LU-7** is the main point to release the Exterior and expel Wind-Cold. In addition, it especially affects the head and relieves headaches. For this reason, it can be used for headaches from Wind-Cold, Wind-Heat and also Turbid Phlegm.
- **G.B.-20** expels Wind in the head.
- **Du-16** expels Wind in the head and treats the Greater Yang-channel area.
- **BL-10** is used as a local point pertaining to the Greater Yang-channel area which is usually affected in invasion of Wind-Cold.

Other points

- **Du-20** Baihui can be used if the headache is not specifically on the occiput but affects the whole head.
- **S.I.-3** Houxi eliminates Wind and affects the Greater Yang area.
- **S.I.-3** and **BL-62** Shenmai in combination open the Governing Vessel, eliminate Wind and affect the Greater Yang area.
- **BL-67** Zhiyin and **BL-66** Tonggu can be selected to affect the Greater Yang area if the headache is on the occiput. These two points are the Well and Spring points respectively and as such are good in Full patterns to eliminate pathogenic factors. Also, being at the tip of the foot, they will affect the head, according to the principle that points at one end will affect the opposite end.
- **BL-60** Kunlun is used if the headache affects also the lower part of the neck and the top of the shoulders.
- **Du-8** Jinsuo eliminates both interior and exterior Wind and relaxes the muscles and tendons of the top of the shoulders as its name implies ("Tendon spasm").

HERBAL TREATMENT

Prescription

CHUAN XIONG CHA TIAO SAN
Ligusticum-Green Tea Regulating Powder
Chuan Xiong *Rhizoma Ligustici wallichii* 6 g
Qiang Huo *Radix et Rhizoma Notopterygii* 6 g
Bai Zhi *Radix Angelicae dahuricae* 6 g
Jing Jie *Herba seu Flos Schizonepetae tenuifoliae* 6 g
Xi Xin *Herba Asari cum radice* 3 g
Fang Feng *Radix Ledebouriellae sesloidis* 6 g
Bo He *Herba Menthae* 3 g
Gan Cao *Radix Glycyrrhizae uralensis* 3 g
Qing Cha (Green Tea) *Folia Cameliae*

Explanation

This prescription is aimed at treating specifically the headache deriving from Wind-Cold, and not so much at releasing the Exterior although it will do that too.

- **Chuan Xiong, Qiang Huo** and **Bai Zhi** are aimed at treating the Greater Yang area and expelling Wind.
- **Jing Jie, Xi Xin** and **Fang Feng** expel Wind-Cold.
- **Bo He** expels Wind-Heat and is added here first of all to expel Wind, and secondly because it affects the head and relieves headaches.
- **Gan Cao** harmonizes and balances the other herbs.
- **Green Tea** is an integral part of the prescription to clear upwards towards the eyes and head, thus relieving the headache. It is also added because it is cool and thus will balance out the majority of the other herbs which are quite warm.

Variations

If there are pronounced symptoms and signs of invasion of the Defensive-Qi portion by Wind-Cold (such as sneezing, cough and breathlessness), then the Ma Huang Tang *Ephedra Decoction* can be used with suitable additions to affect the headache.

Herbs

Several herbs can be considered. We can classify the herbs according to the area affected, i.e. Greater Yang, Lesser Yang or Bright Yang. These are:

- Greater Yang: Du Huo *Radix Angelicae pubescentis*, Qiang Huo *Radix et Rhizoma Notopterygii*, Chuan Xiong *Rhizoma Ligustici wallichii* and Gao Ben *Rhizoma et Radix Ligustici sinensis*.
- Lesser Yang: Chai Hu *Radix Bupleuri*, Huang Qin *Radix Scutellariae baicalensis* and Qing Hao *Herba Artemisiae apiaceae*.
- Bright Yang: Sheng Ma *Rhizoma Cimicifugae*, Ge Gen *Radix Puerariae* and Bai Zhi *Radix Angelicae dahuricae*.

(a) Patent remedy

CHUAN XIONG CHA TIAO WAN
Ligusticum-Green Tea Regulating Pill
Chuan Xiong *Rhizoma Ligustici wallichii*
Qiang Huo *Radix et Rhizoma Notopterygii*
Bai Zhi *Radix Angelicae dahuricae*
Jing Jie *Herba seu Flos Schizonepetae tenuifoliae*
Xi Xin *Herba Asari cum radice*
Fang Feng *Radix Ledebouriellae sesloidis*
Bo He *Herba Menthae*
Gan Cao *Radix Glycyrrhizae uralensis*
Qing Cha (Green Tea) *Folia Cameliae*

Explanation

This pill has the same ingredients and functions as the above prescription. It is suitable to treat acute headaches from invasion of external Wind-Cold. For best results, the pills should be swallowed with a hot fresh-ginger decoction.

(b) Patent remedy

TONG XUAN LI FEI WAN
Penetrating Dispersing and Regulating the Lungs Pill
Ma Huang *Herba Ephedrae*
Zhi Ke *Fructus Citri aurantii*
Jie Geng *Radix Platycodi grandiflori*
Fu Ling *Sclerotium Poriae cocos*
Qian Hu *Radix Peucedani*
Huang Qin *Radix Scutellariae baicalensis*
Chen Pi *Pericarpium Citri reticulatae*

Gan Cao *Radix Glycyrrhizae uralensis*
Ban Xia *Rhizoma Pinelliae ternatae*
Xing Ren *Semen Pruni armeniacae*
Zi Su Ye *Folium Perillae frutescentis*

Explanation

This remedy can be used to treat a headache from an invasion of external Wind-Cold although its main use is to restore the dispersing and descending of Lung-Qi and resolve Phlegm. If it used for a headache best results are obtained with the large-soft pills which should be chewed.

2. WIND-HEAT

Wind-Heat obstructs the clear orifices in the head and leads to a headache which is felt inside the head and is distending in character. It can be very severe and cause the head to feel as if it was being "cracked".

This headache, like that from Wind-Cold, also has an acute onset and can last only while the pathogenic factor is in the Exterior.

Other symptoms and signs include: aversion to cold, shivers, fever, slight thirst, runny nose with a yellow discharge, a sore throat, possibly swollen tonsils, red eyes, slightly dark urine, slightly red sides or tip of the tongue and Floating-Rapid pulse. The aversion to cold and shivers would be less pronounced than in Wind-Cold and the fever would be more pronounced.

TREATMENT PRINCIPLE

Release the Exterior, clear Heat, expel Wind and remove obstruction from the channels.

ACUPUNCTURE

General prescription: L.I.-4 Hegu, G.B.-20 Fengchi, Du-16 Fengfu, Du-14 Dazhui, T.B.-5 Waiguan. All with reducing method.

Explanation

- **L.I.-4** releases the Exterior, expels Wind-Heat

and is a special point to affect the head and face.
- **G.B.-20** and **Du-16** expel Wind from the head.
- **Du-14** expels Wind, clears Heat and relieves headache.
- **T.B.-5** expels Wind-Heat and relieves headache.

Other points

- **Du-20** Baihui expels Wind and relieves headache. It is particularly used if the headache affects the whole head.
- **L.I.-11** Quchi expels Wind-Heat and is used if the symptoms and signs of Heat are pronounced.
- **T.B.-16** Tianyou expels Wind-Heat and, in particular, it relieves headache.

HERBAL TREATMENT

(a) Prescription

SANG JU YIN
Morus-Chrysanthemum Decoction
Sang Ye *Folium Mori albae* 6 g
Ju Hua *Flos Chrysanthemi morifolii* 3 g
Bo He *Herba Menthae* 3 g
Xing Ren *Semen Pruni armeniacae* 6 g
Jie Geng *Radix Platycodi grandiflori* 6 g
Lian Qiao *Fructus Forsythiae suspensae* 6 g
Lu Gen *Rhizoma Phragmitis communis* 6 g
Gan Cao *Radix Glycyrrhizae uralensis* 3 g

Explanation

This is the main prescription to expel Wind-Heat in mild cases. If headache is the predominant symptom, the prescription would have to be adapted by adding some herbs specific for headaches out of those listed below.

- **Sang Ye** and **Ju Hua** expel Wind-Heat. They are both light herbs and will float to the Upper Burner. Ju Hua, in particular, will relieve any headache.
- **Bo He**, **Jie Geng** and **Xing Ren** help the two main herbs to expel Wind-Heat and stimulate the descending of Lung-Qi. In particular, Jie Geng and Bo He will relieve the headache.

- **Lian Qiao** and **Lu Gen** expel Wind-Heat and promote fluids to relieve thirst.
- **Gan Cao** harmonizes.

(b) Prescription

JU HUA CHA TIAO SAN
Chrysanthemum-Green Tea Regulating Powder
Chuan Xiong Cha Tiao San prescription plus:
Ju Hua *Flos Chrysanthemi morifolii* 6 g
Jiang Can *Bombix batryticatus* 6 g

Explanation

This prescription combines the Chuan Xiong Cha Tiao San *Ligusticum-Green Tea Regulating Powder* as a whole which expels Wind-Cold, with two herbs that expel Wind-Heat and are specific for headaches.

- **Ju Hua** expels Wind-Heat and specifically relieves headaches.
- **Jiang Can** expels Wind-Heat and is also specific for headaches deriving from Wind-Heat invasion.

Herbs

- **Man Jing Zi** *Fructus Viticis* expels Wind-Heat and is specific for headaches.
- **Ge Gen** *Radix Puerariae* expels Wind-Heat and releases the muscles and sinews, making it specific to relieve the ache and stiffness of the neck and shoulders from invasion of exterior Wind.
- **Bo He** *Herba Menthae* and **Ju Hua** *Flos Chrysanthemi morifolii* expel Wind-Heat. They are light and aromatic and affect the head specifically. They also relieve headaches from Liver-Yang rising. Ju Hua, in addition, specifically affects the eyes and would therefore be indicated when the headache is situated around the eyes, or if the eyes are red.

(i) Patent remedy

SANG JU GAN MAO PIAN
Morus-Chrysanthemum Common Cold Tablet
Sang Ye *Folium Mori albae* 6 g
Ju Hua *Flos Chrysanthemi morifolii* 3 g
Bo He *Herba Menthae* 3 g
Xing Ren *Semen Pruni armeniacae* 6 g
Jie Geng *Radix Platycodi grandiflori* 6 g
Lian Qiao *Fructus Forsythiae suspensae* 6 g
Lu Gen *Rhizoma Phragmitis communis* 6 g
Gan Cao *Radix Glycyrrhizae uralensis* 3 g

Explanation

This tablet has the same ingredients and functions as the prescription Sang Ju Yin *Morus-Chrysanthemum Decoction*. The presence of Sang Ye, Ju Hua and Bo He, all herbs which affect the head, makes it suitable for headaches from Wind-Heat.

This formula is quite mild, so it is suitable only for light cases.

(ii) Patent remedy

YIN QIAO JIE DU PIAN
Lonicera-Forsythia Expelling Poison Tablet
Jin Yin Hua *Flos Lonicerae japonicae*
Lian Qiao *Fructus Forsythiae suspensae*
Jie Geng *Radix Platycodi grandiflori*
Niu Bang Zi *Fructus Arctii lappae*
Bo He *Herba Menthae*
Jing Jie *Herba seu Flos Schizonepetae tenuifoliae*
Zhu Ye *Herba Lophatheri gracilis*
Dan Dou Chi *Semen Sojae praeparatum*
Gan Cao *Radix Glycyrrhizae uralensis*

Explanation

This well-known tablet can be used for headaches from Wind-Heat due to the presence of Bo He and Jing Jie. This formula is stronger than Sang Ju Yin and is therefore suitable for more severe cases of Wind-Heat.

(iii) Patent remedy

LING YANG SHANG FENG LING
Cornu Antelopis Influenza Formula
Ling Yang Jiao *Cornu Antelopis*
Tian Hua Fen *Radix Trichosanthis*
Lian Qiao *Fructus Forsythiae suspensae*
Zhu Yu *Herba Lophatheri gracilis*
Jing Jie *Herba seu Flos Schizonepetae tenuifoliae*

Ge Gen *Radix Puerariae*
Gan Cao *Radix Glycyrrhizae uralensis*
Jin Yin Hua *Flos Lonicerae japonicae*
Niu Bang Zi *Fructus Arctii lappae*
Bo He *Herba Menthae*

Explanation

This remedy is similar in composition to the previous one, Yin Qiao Jie Du Pian *Lonicera-Forsythia Expelling Poison Tablet*, but it is particularly suitable for headaches from Wind-Heat due to the presence of Ling Yang Jiao which expels Wind and Ge Gen which relaxes the sinews. It is therefore excellent for severe headache and stiffness of the neck from an invasion of Wind-Heat.

3. WIND-DAMPNESS

This is a type of Wind-Cold but combined with Dampness. Dampness obstructs the clear orifices of the head and gives rise to a headache with a typical feeling of heaviness. The head feels muzzy, as if it was wrapped in a cloth. This sensation would be aggravated by damp weather. Dampness prevents the clear Yang from reaching the head and brightening the orifices and the turbid Yin from descending. This causes the typical muzzy feeling, heavy head, poor concentration and heavy eyes.

Other symptoms and signs include: aversion to cold, shivers, possibly a fever, a sensation of oppression in the chest and epigastrium, a feeling of heaviness of the whole body, a runny nose with a white discharge, a sticky tongue coating and a Floating-Slippery pulse.

TREATMENT PRINCIPLE

Release the Exterior, expel Wind, resolve Dampness and remove obstruction from the channels.

ACUPUNCTURE

General prescription: LU-7 Lieque, L.I.-6 Pianli, SP-6 Sanyinjiao, ST-8 Touwei, Du-23 Shangxing. Reducing method on all points.

Explanation

– **LU-7** releases the Exterior and stimulates the Lungs' dispersing and descending of fluids. It will therefore simultaneously expel Wind and resolve exterior Dampness. It is also a specific point for headaches.
– **L.I.-6** releases the Exterior and also stimulates the Lungs' descending of fluids from the Upper Burner. It is the Connecting point of the Large Intestine Connecting channel which flows up to the jaw and ear thus relieving any headache in this region.
– **SP-6** resolves Dampness.
– **ST-8** is the main local point on the head to resolve Dampness affecting the head and is specific for dull headaches with a feeling of the head being wrapped.
– **Du-23** relieves headaches on the forehead and eyes.

HERBAL TREATMENT

Prescription

QIANG HUO SHENG SHI TANG
Notopterygium Dispelling Dampness Decoction
Qiang Huo *Radix et Rhizoma Notopterygii* 6 g
Du Huo *Radix Angelicae pubescentis* 6 g
Fang Feng *Radix Ledebouriellae sesloidis* 6 g
Gao Ben *Rhizoma Ligustici sinensis* 6 g
Chuan Xiong *Rhizoma Ligustici wallichii* 3 g
Man Jing Zi *Fructus Viticis* 6 g
Zhi Gan Cao *Radix Glycyrrhizae uralensis praeparata* 3 g

Explanation

– **Qiang Huo** is the main herb as it releases the Exterior, expels Wind-Cold and Dampness and specifically affects the channels of the upper back and neck.
– **Du Huo** assists Qiang Huo in expelling Wind-Damp.
– **Fang Feng** and **Gao Ben** both expel Wind-Cold. Fang Feng also expels Dampness and relieves headache while Gao Ben specifically affects the channels of the back thus helping Qiang Huo to relieve the headache.

- **Chuan Xiong** expels Wind and helps to relieve the headache.
- **Man Jing Zi** expels Wind-Heat and is specific for exterior headaches.
- **Gan Cao** harmonizes.

Herbs

- **Bai Zhi** *Radix Angelicae dahuricae* expels Wind from the head and face and is specific for headaches of this type.
- **Huo Xiang** *Herba Agastachis* is a fragrant herb that resolves exterior Dampness. It is aromatic and light and therefore affects the head.
- **Cang Zhu** *Rhizoma Atractylodis lanceae* is also a fragrant herb that resolves Dampness and is particularly indicated for headaches.

Patent remedy

HUO XIANG ZHENG QI WAN
Agastache Upright Qi Pill
Huo Xiang *Herba Agastachis*
Zi Su Ye *Folium Perillae frutescentis*
Bai Zhi *Radix Angelicae dahuricae*
Ban Xia *Rhizoma Pinelliae ternatae*
Chen Pi *Pericarpium Citri reticulatae*
Bai Zhu *Rhizoma Atractylodis macrocephalae*
Fu Ling *Sclerotium Poriae cocos*
Hou Po *Cortex Magnoliae officinalis*
Da Fu Pi *Pericarpium Arecae*
Jie Geng *Radix Platycodi grandiflori*
Sheng Jiang *Rhizoma Zingiberis officinalis recens*
Da Zao *Fructus Ziziphi jujubae*
Zhi Gan Cao *Radix Glycyrrhizae uralensis praeparata*

Explanation

This pill is suitable to treat headaches from invasion of external Dampness (both Cold-Dampness and Damp-Heat). This type of headache occurs on the forehead and is accompanied by a heavy sensation of the head.

This remedy can also be used for a Dampness-type headache from other causes, such as food poisoning, for example.

The tongue presentation appropriate to this remedy is a sticky-white coating.

INTERIOR HEADACHES

Interior headaches can be due to a very great variety of causes. The most important distinction to make is that between Deficiency or Excess headaches. Once this differentiation has been made, one must identify which organ and channel are involved, bearing in mind that these two do not always coincide in the pathogenesis of headaches. For example, most headaches due to Liver-Yang rising manifest on the Gall-Bladder channel but some may not. This point will be clarified shortly as we discuss the treatment methods.

The four organs which are most directly involved in the pathogenesis of headaches are the Spleen, Stomach, Liver and Kidneys. The aetiology and pathology of interior headaches are represented in Figure 1.9.

EXCESS HEADACHES

All these headaches are characterized by the presence of an Excess in the head leading to obstruction in the circulation of Qi and local stasis of Blood in the head, giving rise to headaches. This Excess can take the form of Liver-Yang or Liver-Fire, Phlegm, Dampness and Blood stasis. Being due to an Excess, the pain in the head is severe compared to that of Deficiency headaches.

1. LIVER-YANG RISING

This is probably the most common of all interior headaches. It arises when the Yang of the Liver "rebels" upwards creating an excess of Yang in the head. It is in the nature of Liver-Qi and Liver-Yang to flow freely upwards but in pathological circumstances this movement can be excessive and give rise to headaches. As we have seen, the Liver main channel is one of only two (together with the Heart channel) to flow to the head internally, all other Yin channels reaching the head via their respective divergent channels.

The most frequent cause of this type of headache is emotional. Emotions of anger (whether it

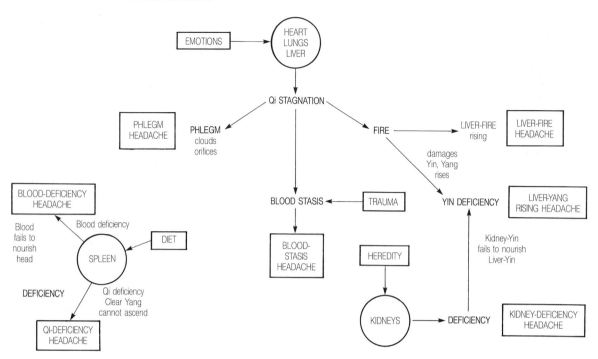

Fig. 1.9 Aetiology and pathology of interior headaches

is manifested or repressed), frustration or resentment over a long period of time can cause the excessive rising of Liver-Yang.

Liver-Yang rising is usually due to one of four situations:

(a) Liver-Blood Deficiency
(b) Liver-Yin Deficiency
(c) Liver- and Kidney-Yin Deficiency
(d) Liver/Kidney-Yin and Kidney-Yang Deficiency.

Liver-Blood deficiency is a common cause of the rising of Liver-Yang. Blood is part of Yin and is stored in the Liver. The Blood of the Liver roots and anchors the Yang of the Liver. Hence if Liver-Blood is deficient, Liver-Yang may "escape" upwards to disturb the head.

Liver-Yin deficiency is practically the same as Liver-Blood deficiency, dry eyes being one of the main signs to distinguish it from Liver-Blood deficiency.

The Liver and Kidneys share a common root and a deficiency of one often affects the other. Liver-Blood deficiency may in the long run fail to nourish the Kidney-Essence which may become deficient. Conversely, a deficient Kidney-Essence may fail to produce Blood and lead to Liver-Blood deficiency. Both Blood and Essence pertain to Yin, and Liver- and Kidney-Yin deficiency thus lead to the excessive rising of Liver-Yang.

In a few cases, Liver-Yang rising may also derive from Kidney-Yang deficiency. This is only an apparent paradox. The Kidneys are the source of all the Yin and Yang energies in the human body. There is a close interaction between the Yin and the Yang of the Kidneys and the two cannot be separated. Thus, it is not uncommon for deficiency of both Kidney-Yin and Kidney-Yang to appear simultaneously. Of course the deficiency of Yin and Yang within the Kidneys is never in a 50/50 proportion, but one is always predominant. The tongue-body colour always shows the predominant deficiency: if it is Pale it indicates a predominance of Kidney-Yang deficiency and if it is Red it indicates a predominance of Kidney-Yin deficiency.

When Kidney-Yang is deficient over a long period of time it can induce a lesser deficiency of Kidney-Yin which, in turn, may lead to Liver-

Yang rising. This explains how a person may have several symptoms and signs of Kidney-Yang deficiency (such as frequent-pale urination, chilliness, a Pale-Swollen tongue and a Deep and Slow pulse), only one symptom of Kidney-Yin deficiency (such as night sweating) and some symptoms of Liver-Yang rising (such as headaches, irritability and dizziness).

The headache from Liver-Yang rising is intense, severe, throbbing or distending in character. Some patients also describe it as "pulsating", "pounding" or "bursting". It usually affects either or both sides of the head along the Gall-Bladder channel, or the temple or eyebrow. Frequently, it is felt behind one or both eyes (Fig. 1.10). It may also occur on a small area around the point G.B.-14 Yangbai.

The headache from Liver-Yang rising is frequently accompanied by nausea or vomiting. These are due to Liver-Qi invading the Stomach and preventing Stomach-Qi from descending. In a few cases, it is also accompanied by diarrhoea due to Liver-Qi invading the Spleen and impairing its transformation and transportation activity.

The Liver-Yang headache is usually better sitting up and often a person will prefer to lie in bed propped up by several pillows.

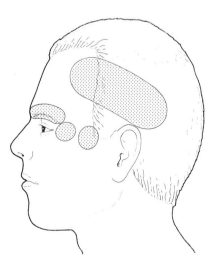

(Areas of LIV-Yang headache)

Fig. 1.10 Areas of Liver-Yang headache

Other common symptoms with headaches from Liver-Yang are visual disturbances. The person may see flashing lights or auras or the vision may be blurred.

This type of headache is often the cause of the "weekend headaches". These occur in people who work excessively long hours and under considerable tension during the week which somehow "masks" the condition of Liver-Yang. Once they suddenly stop work at weekends, the inactivity makes Liver-Yang flare upwards to cause the headache.

Other manifestations of Liver-Yang rising include dizziness, tinnitus, deafness, a dry throat, insomnia, irritability, a Red tongue-body and a Wiry pulse. The pulse may be Wiry only on the left side or even only on the left Middle position. It is important to realize that the tongue and pulse can be different, depending on whether the headache stems from Liver-Blood or Kidney/Liver-Yin deficiency. If it stems from Liver-Blood deficiency the tongue body may be Pale and Thin, whereas if it stems from Kidney/Liver-Yin deficiency the tongue body will be Red and Peeled. Finally, in the few cases when Liver-Yang rising derives from Kidney-Yang deficiency, the tongue body will be Pale and Swollen and the pulse Deep and Slow.

Treatment principle

Pacify the Liver, subdue rebellious Yang, nourish Liver-Blood or Liver-Yin and/or Kidney-Yin as appropriate.

Acupuncture

General prescription: LIV-3 Taichong, LIV-8 Ququan, SP-6 Sanyinjiao, T.B.-5 Waiguan, G.B.-20 Fengchi, Taiyang extra point. In case of Liver and Kidney Yin deficiency add KI-3 Taixi.

Reducing method on LIV-3, T.B.-5 and G.B.-20, reinforcing method on LIV-8, SP-6 and KI-3. Even method on Taiyang. If the condition is very chronic, even method can be applied to the points that are normally reduced.

Explanation

– **LIV-3** is the main distal point to pacify the

Liver and subdue Yang rising. It is also the main distal point for this type of headache. It should be needled at an appropriate depth (at least 0.5 cun) and usually reduced. In acute cases it should be rather vigorously reduced or at least manipulated repeatedly at intervals during the treatment, for example 4–5 times during 20 minutes. For very severe acute headaches when the pulse is extremely Wiry the needles should be left in a fairly long time, i.e. longer than 20 minutes, up to 1 hour. Many of the patients with this type of headache dislike lying down during an acute attack and should therefore be treated propped-up in a comfortable position.

The more chronic the condition, the less one needs to reduce this point and in very chronic cases it is enough to apply manipulation with even method.

LIV-3 will affect a Liver-Yang headache no matter where the headache is situated.

- **LIV-8** is reinforced to nourish Liver-Blood and/or Liver-Yin. Liver-Yang rising always derives from a deficiency of Liver-Blood (or Liver-Yin) and/or Kidney-Yin. It is therefore necessary to use points to nourish Liver-Blood and/or tonify Kidney-Yin.
- **SP-6** is tonified to nourish Liver-Blood. Being the meeting point of Liver, Spleen and Kidney channels, it will also help to pacify the Liver. It also calms the Mind and helps to promote sleep. This is important in chronic headaches because if the person does not sleep well, it will be much more difficult to cure the headaches.
- **T.B.-5** is reduced to subdue Liver-Yang and affect the side of the head. The use of this point is based on the relationship existing between the Triple Burner and Gall-Bladder channels, both pertaining to the Lesser Yang channel system. The relationship between Yang hand and foot channels is very close indeed because they meet superficially on the head region and merge into one another. For this reason, in practice they are almost interchangeable. In this case, T.B.-5 is chosen to affect the Lesser Yang area (which includes the Gall-Bladder channel area) on the head where the Liver-Yang headache usually occurs.

But why do we choose the Triple Burner instead of the Gall-Bladder channel, and why T.B.-5 in preference to other points on that channel? If a choice exists between Yang hand or foot channels (as it normally does) to affect their common-influence area, the hand channel points have a more moderate effect than those of the foot channels. Thus T.B.-5 has a milder effect than, say, G.B.-43. The choice between Yang hand or foot channel points can therefore be guided by the severity of the symptoms: in severe cases Yang foot-channel points will be used. Of course, both hand- and foot-channel points can be used simultaneously for an even stronger effect.

T.B.-5 is used in preference to other points on this channel because it is the Connecting point and, as such, is especially suited to treat channel problems. This point is therefore used not so much to subdue Liver-Yang at internal-organ level, but to pacify rebellious Yang within the Lesser Yang channels area. Specifically, T.B.-5 will affect headaches in the temple area.

- **G.B.-20** is used as an adjacent point to subdue Liver-Yang. It subdues Liver-Yang and Liver-Wind and is specific for headaches from these two causes. It will also relax the muscles of the upper neck and brighten the eyes, both of which actions will help chronic headaches.

This point is needled at least 0.5 cun deep with the needles pointed towards the opposite eye. This direction can, however, be changed and the needle directed towards the eye on the same side in order to treat a unilateral headache on that side. This point, contrary to points situated further up the neck and skull, can be manipulated with reducing method. It can be needled with the patient lying down and reached without the patient having to sit up.

- **Taiyang** is an extra point on the temple. It is specific to subdue Liver-Yang when it causes temporal headaches. It is used only if the headache is situated on the temple, otherwise different local points are selected. It is manipulated with even method.

Other points

Many other points can be used according to the location of the headache.

Distal points:

- **P-6** Neiguan is used as a distal point for various reasons. First of all, the Pericardium channel is connected to the Liver channel within the Terminal Yin. P-6 will therefore indirectly help to subdue Liver-Yang and calm the Mind and Ethereal Soul at the same time. P-6 is also the Connecting point of the Pericardium channel and it therefore connects with the Triple Burner channel. For this reason it affects the Triple Burner channel on the head and can contribute to subduing Liver-Yang rising affecting the Lesser Yang channels. For this effect P-6 can be combined with Yangchi T.B.-4. This combination is very effective for headaches on the Lesser Yang channel area (i.e. temples, sides of the head and lateral side of the neck) especially in women. Finally, a condition of Liver-Yang rising is frequently associated with stress and a highly-strung disposition. P-6 will help to harmonize the Liver and calm the Mind and Ethereal Soul, especially in women.

- **LU-7** Lieque is a special point for headaches. It is not specific for Liver-Yang headaches but it can be used here for two reasons. First of all, it will affect any type of headache and secondly, it can tonify the Lungs when the deficiency of Lung-Qi is contributing to the rebellious rising of Liver-Yang. In 5-Element terms this corresponds to "Metal failing to control Wood". This situation is quite common and is reflected in the pulse, the right Front position being very weak and the left Middle position very Wiry. Often, there may be no other symptoms or signs of Lung deficiency apart from the pulse.

- **G.B.-43** Xiaxi is the Spring point of the Gall-Bladder channel. As such, it is used in Full patterns to eliminate pathogenic factors. In this case, it can be used to subdue Liver-Yang and remove obstructions from the Gall-Bladder channel in the head. Being on the foot, it can treat the opposite end, i.e. the head. Specifically, it will affect the temple and eye area.

Local points:

- **G.B.-4** Hanyan, **G.B.-5** Xuanlu and **G.B.-6** Xuanli are all very important local points for headaches on the Gall-Bladder channel on the side of the head deriving from Liver-Yang rising. They are needled horizontally (i.e. just under the skin with the needle at an angle of about 15 degrees) usually pointing backwards. These local points should always be used at some time during the course of treatment especially if the headache is very chronic and always appearing in that particular area.

- **G.B.-8** Shuaigu is an effective local point for headaches around the ear-area and the upper part of the lateral side of the neck. It is needled horizontally backwards.

- **G.B.-9** Tianchong is a very important local point for headaches on the sides of the head. In addition, it also has a general effect in calming the Mind and Ethereal Soul and subduing Liver-Yang. This point would be chosen when the person is very tense and is troubled by long-standing emotional problems.

- **G.B.-13** Benshen is used when the headache is on one side of the forehead, usually around G.B.-14. Besides subduing Liver-Yang, G.B.-13 has a powerful effect in calming the Mind and Ethereal Soul and helping sleep. The difference between G.B.-9 and G.B.-13 is that the former is used for emotional problems deriving from feelings of resentment and frustration, while the latter is better for calming the Mind when the person is extremely tense and cannot sleep.

- **G.B.-14** Yangbai is simply used when the headache is situated around this point. Some headaches from Liver-Yang rising are situated on the forehead on one side around this point and they feel like a nail being driven in.

- **G.B.-21** Jianjing is used as an adjuvant point when the top of the shoulders are very tense and stiff as so often happens in those who suffer from chronic headaches. The repeated use of this point is very good for relaxing the neck muscles.

- **BL-2** Zanzhu is used when the headache occurs around the eyes, or on the forehead extending down to the eyes.
- **Yuyao**, an extra point in the middle of the eyebrow, can be used when the headache occurs around or behind the eyes, especially when Liver-Yang rising stems from Liver-Blood deficiency.
- **G.B.-1** Tongziliao is used when the headache occurs around the temples and outer corners of the eyes.

Ancient formula

Du-20 Baihui, Du-21 Qianting, Du-24 Shenting, Du-23 Shangxing, T.B.-23 Sizhukong, G.B.-20 Fengchi, L.I.-4 Hegu, BL-2 Zanzhu, ST-8 Touwei ("Great Compendium of Acupuncture").[7]

Herbal treatment

(a) Prescription

TIAN MA GOU TENG YIN
Gastrodia-Uncaria Decoction
Tian Ma *Rhizoma Gastrodiae elatae* 9 g
Gou Teng *Ramulus Uncariae* 9 g
Shi Jue Ming *Concha Haliotidis* 6 g
Sang Ji Sheng *Ramulus Loranthi* 9 g
Du Zhong *Radix Eucommiae ulmoidis* 9 g
Chuan Niu Xi *Radix Cyathulae* 9 g
Zhi Zi *Fructus Gardeniae jasminoidis* 6 g
Huang Qin *Radix Scutellariae baicalensis* 9 g
Yi Mu Cao *Herba Leonori heterophylli* 9 g
Ye Jiao Teng *Caulis Polygoni multiflori* 9 g
Fu Shen *Sclerotium Poriae cocos pararadicis* 6 g

Explanation

This prescription is very widely used for headaches from Liver-Yang rising.

- **Tian Ma**, **Gou Teng** and **Shi Jue Ming** subdue Liver-Yang and Liver-Wind. All three of these herbs are specific for headaches from Liver-Yang rising.
- **Sang Ji Sheng** nourishes Liver-Blood. This is necessary as Liver-Yang rising frequently derives from Liver-Blood deficiency.
- **Du Zhong** tonifies the Kidneys. This is

necessary as Liver-Yang rising often derives from Kidney deficiency.
- **Chuan Niu Xi** nourishes Liver and Kidneys and is included for the reasons mentioned above with the previous two herbs.
- **Zhi Zi** and **Huang Qin** are included to clear any condition of Liver-Fire that there might be. In particular, Huang Qin clears upwards and will help to alleviate any signs of Liver-Fire in the Upper Burner such as red and sore eyes and headache.
- **Yi Mu Cao** moves and harmonizes Liver-Blood and, by so doing, it pacifies rebellious Liver-Qi.
- **Ye Jiao Teng** and **Fu Shen** are included to calm the Mind and Ethereal Soul and promote sleep. This is necessary to deal with the irritability that often accompanies Liver-Yang rising. It is also a general principle that it is good to promote sleep in persons suffering from chronic headaches as lack of sleep will constantly hinder progress in the treatment.

(b) Prescription

ZHEN GAN XI FENG TANG
Pacifying the Liver and Subduing Wind Decoction
Huai Niu Xi *Radix Achyrantis* 15 g
Dai Zhe Shi *Haematitum* 15 g
Long Gu *Os Draconis* 12 g
Mu Li *Concha Ostreae* 12 g
Gui Ban *Plastrum Testudinis* 12 g
Xuan Shen *Radix Scrophulariae ningpoensis* 12 g
Tian Men Dong *Tuber Asparagi cochinchinensis* 12 g
Bai Shao *Radix Paeoniae albae* 12 g
Yin Chen Hao *Herba Artemisiae capillaris* 6 g
Chuan Lian Zi *Fructus Meliae toosendan* 6 g
Mai Ya *Fructus Hordei vulgaris germinatus* 6 g
Gan Cao *Radix Glycyrrhizae uralensis* 6 g

Explanation

- **Niu Xi** nourishes the Liver and Kidneys and therefore reinforces the "root" in order to subdue Yang.
- **Dai Zhe Shi**, **Long Gu**, **Mu Li** and **Gui Ban** are all sinking substances that subdue Liver-

Yang. In addition, Gui Ban also strongly tonifies the Yin.

- **Xuan Shen**, **Tian Men Dong** and **Bai Shao** are added to nourish Yin. In addition, Bai Shao also pacifies the Liver and stops pain.
- **Yin Chen Hao** and **Chuan Lian Zi** are included to direct the prescription to the Liver channel.
- **Mai Ya** is added to help the stomach as the prescription includes mineral substances that are difficult to digest such as Dai Zhe Shi.
- **Gan Cao** harmonizes.

The main difference between this prescription and the previous one is that the latter nourishes the Yin more and is therefore suitable when there is a pronounced deficiency of Liver- and Kidney-Yin. Note that Dai Zhe Shi is not suitable for long-term use and is contra-indicated in pregnancy. It could be eliminated from this prescription or replaced with Zhen Zhu Mu *Concha margaritiferae* which is also a sinking substance that subdues Liver-Yang.

(c) Prescription

LING JIAO GOU TENG TANG
Cornu Antelopis-Uncaria Decoction
Ling Yang Jiao *Cornu Antelopis* 4.5 g
Gou Teng *Ramulus Uncariae* 9 g
Sang Ye *Folium Mori albae* 6 g
Ju Hua *Flos Chrysanthemi morifolii* 9 g
Bai Shao *Radix Paeoniae albae* 9 g
Sheng Di Huang *Radix Rehmanniae glutinosae* 15 g
Fu Shen *Sclerotium Poriae cocos pararadicis* 9 g
Chuan Bei Mu *Bulbus Fritillariae cirrhosae* 12 g
Zhu Ru *Caulis Bambusae in Taeniis* 15 g
Gan Cao *Radix Glycyrrhizae uralensis* 2.5 g

Explanation

- **Ling Yang Jiao** and **Gou Teng** subdue Liver-Yang and Liver-Wind. These are the emperor herbs in the prescription.
- **Sang Ye** and **Ju Hua** are the minister herbs to assist the first two to subdue Liver-Yang.
- **Sheng Di** and **Bai Shao** are the assistant herbs to nourish Yin, as Liver-Yang derives from deficiency of Liver-Yin or Liver-Blood.

- **Bei Mu** and **Zhu Ru** are also assistant herbs and are included here to resolve any Phlegm-Heat that might arise from Liver-Fire burning the fluids.
- **Fu Shen** calms the Mind.
- **Gan Cao** harmonizes.

If Liver-Yang rising stems from Liver-Blood deficiency, the Si Wu Tang (*Four Substances Decoction*) could be added to any of the above prescriptions. If it stems from Liver-Yin deficiency, Yi Guan Jian *One Linking Decoction* could be added. If it stems from Kidney-Yin deficiency, Liu Wei Di Huang Wan *Six-Ingredient Rehmannia Pill* or Zuo Gui Wan *Restoring the Left [Kidney] Pill* could be added.

Herbs

- **Tian Ma** *Rhizoma Gastrodiae elatae* is *the* herb for Liver-Yang headache. It subdues Liver-Yang and Liver-Wind and specifically treats headaches.
- **Gou Teng** *Ramulus Uncariae* also subdues Liver-Yang and Liver-Wind and treats headaches. In addition and in contrast to Tian Ma, it is cool and clears Liver-Heat.
- **Bai Ji Li** *Fructus Tribuli terrestris* subdues Liver-Yang and Liver-Wind and is specific for headaches especially if situated around the eyes. It is warm, bitter and pungent and therefore to be used with caution in Yin deficiency.
- **Ju Hua** *Flos Chrysanthemi morifolii* subdues Liver-Yang and is one of the most frequently used herbs for this type of headache, especially if located around the eyes. It is frequently added to other prescriptions for headaches from other causes simply to direct the prescription to the head.
- **Shi Jue Ming** *Concha Haliotidis* subdues Liver-Yang and Liver-Wind and is specific for headaches. It is also cold and it therefore clears Liver-Fire.
- **Ling Yang Jiao** *Cornu Antelopis* subdues Liver-Wind and Liver-Yang and can be used for chronic headaches.
- **Bai Shao** *Radix Paeoniae albae* harmonizes the Liver and is a very important herb for pain

from many different Liver disharmonies. It promotes the smooth flow of Liver-Qi but it also subdues Liver-Yang and hence it can be used for headaches. It generally soothes and harmonizes (as it also nourishes Blood and Yin) and therefore stops pain, especially in combination with Gan Cao.

- **Gan Cao** *Radix Glycyrrhizae uralensis*, besides its other functions, can be used for chronic headaches from Liver-Yang because it is sweet in nature. The sweet flavour harmonizes and pacifies the Liver and therefore contributes to stopping pain, especially in combination with Bai Shao. The "Simple Questions" in chapter 22 says: "*For pain of Liver origin, [herbs with] sweet taste should be used to pacify the Liver*".[8]

- **Long Gu** *Os Draconis* sinks Liver-Yang, calms the Mind and settles the Ethereal Soul.

- **Mu Li** *Concha Ostreae* sinks Liver-Yang, calms the Mind, settles the Ethereal Soul and is suitable to treat Liver-Yang headaches. This substance and the previous one also nourish the Yin.

- **Suan Zao Ren** *Semen Ziziphi spinosae* is an important addition to prescription for headaches from Liver-Yang. It subdues Liver-Yang and is excellent for calming the Mind, settling the Ethereal Soul and allaying the irritability typical of Liver-Yang rising. It is particularly indicated for headaches from Liver-Yang as it enters the Liver and Gall-Bladder channel. Furthermore, if a person suffering from chronic headaches does not sleep well, this will definitely hinder the treatment. This herb is therefore important as it promotes sleep.

(i) Patent remedy

JIANG YA WAN
Lowering [Blood] Pressure Pill
Yi Mu Cao *Herba Leonori heterophylli*
Huai Niu Xi *Radix Achyranthis bidentatae*
Sheng Di Huang *Radix Rehmanniae glutinosae*
E Jiao *Gelatinum Corii Asini*
Dang Gui *Radix Angelicae sinensis*
Gou Teng *Ramulus Uncariae*
Chen Xiang *Lignum Aquilariae*

Chuan Xiong *Radix Ligustici wallichii*
Xia Ku Cao *Spica Prunellae vulgaris*
Mu Dan Pi *Cortex Moutan radicis*
Tian Ma *Rhizoma Gastrodiae elatae*
Da Huang *Rhizoma Rhei*
Hu Po *Succinum*
Huang Lian *Rhizoma Coptidis*
Ling Yang Jiao *Cornu Antelopis*

Explanation

This remedy is suitable for headaches from Liver-Yang rising against a background of Liver-Yin deficiency.

The tongue presentation appropriate to this remedy is a Red body with rootless coating.

Due to the presence of Da Huang, this remedy should not be used for too long (i.e. not more than a few weeks at a stretch).

(ii) Patent remedy

TIAN MA SHOU WU PIAN
Gastrodia-Polygonum Pill
Tian Ma *Rhizoma Gastrodiae elatae*
Shou Wu *Radix Polygoni multiflori*
Yin Yang Huo *Herba Epimedii*
Ren Shen *Radix Ginseng*

Explanation

This remedy is for headaches from Liver-Yang rising on a background of Qi and Blood deficiency.

The tongue presentation appropriate to this remedy is a Pale and Thin body.

(iii) Patent remedy

TIAN MA QU FENG BU PIAN
Gastrodia Expelling Wind and Tonifying Tablet
Tian Ma *Rhizoma Gastrodiae elatae*
Dang Gui *Radix Angelicae sinensis*
Sheng Di Huang *Radix Rehmanniae glutinosae*
Rou Gui *Cortex Cinnamomi cassiae*
Huai Niu Xi *Radix Achyranthis bidentatae*
Du Zhong *Cortex Eucommiae ulmoidis*
Qiang Huo *Radix et Rhizoma Notopterygii*
Bai Fu Zi *Rhizoma Thyphonii gigantei*

Explanation

This tablet is suitable for headaches from Liver-Yang rising on a background of deficiency of both Kidney-Yin and Kidney-Yang. This situation, more frequent in women, is not at all uncommon. When there is a deficiency of both Kidney-Yin and Kidney-Yang, it is the deficient Kidney-Yin that induces Liver-Yang to rise.

The tongue presentation appropriate to this remedy is a Pale, Swollen and wet tongue body.

Case history

A 32-year-old woman had been suffering from migraine for the past 8 years. The headaches occurred on the top of the head and behind the eyes. They started with a dull pain and increased in intensity to a severe character, accompanied by nausea, vomiting and diarrhoea. They were better lying down. By the time she sought treatment they occurred almost every day. Her tongue was Pale and Thin and her pulse was Weak on the right side and slightly Wiry on the left.

Diagnosis
Liver-Yang rising stemming from Liver-Blood deficiency. The Liver-Blood deficiency is apparent from the Pale and Thin tongue and Weak pulse. The dullness of some of the headaches and the fact that they improve lying down indicates that they are due to a deficiency, in this case of Liver-Blood. The location of the headaches on top of the head, also indicates Liver-Blood deficiency. Liver-Yang rising accounts for the more severe headaches and the vomiting and diarrhoea, due to Liver-Qi invading Stomach and Spleen, preventing Stomach-Qi from descending (vomiting) and Spleen-Qi from ascending (diarrhoea).

Treatment principle
Nourish Liver-Blood and subdue Liver-Yang. In this case, although the severe headaches are due to Liver-Yang rising, the pattern is still primarily one of deficiency, as evidenced by the tongue. For this reason, the treatment was aimed primarily at nourishing Liver-Blood.

Acupuncture
The main points used were:
P-6 Neiguan, T.B.-4 Yangchi, ST-36 Zusanli, LIV-8 Ququan, SP-6 Sanyinjiao and LIV-3 Taichong.

The first two points were used with even method, LIV-3 was reduced and all the other were reinforced. Warming needle was applied to ST-36.

Explanation
- **P-6** was used to regulate Liver-Blood, calm the Mind and settle the Ethereal Soul.
- **T.B.-4** was used in conjunction with Neiguan P-6 as a combination of Connecting and Source point. This combination strengthens the effect of P-6, while it also regulates the Lesser Yang channels. In addition, Yangchi T.B.-4 has a general tonifying effect.
- **ST-36** and **SP-6** were used to nourish Blood.
- **LIV-8** was used to nourish Liver-Blood.
- **LIV-3** was used to subdue Liver-Yang.

Herbal treatment
The prescription used was a variation of Si Wu Tang *Four Substances Decoction* to nourish Liver-Blood. This prescription was chosen in preference to one of those to subdue Liver-Yang, because the condition was deemed to be primarily one of deficiency (of Liver-Blood). Herbs were added to subdue Liver-Yang. The prescription used was:

Dang Gui *Radix Angelicae sinensis* 9 g
Bai Shao *Radix Paeoniae albae* 6 g
Chuan Xiong *Radix Ligustici wallichii* 6 g
Shu Di Huang *Radix Rehmanniae glutinosae praeparata* 6 g
Shi Jue Ming *Concha Haliotidis* 9 g
Gou Teng *Ramulus Uncariae* 6 g
Man Jing Zi *Fructus Viticis* 4 g
Ju Hua *Flos Chrysanthemi morifolii* 3 g

Explanation
- The first four herbs are the *Four Substances Decoction* to nourish Liver-Blood.
- Shi Jue Ming, Ju Hua and Gou Teng were added to subdue Liver-Yang.
- Man Jing Zi was added to treat the headaches.

This patient had a remarkable improvement after only one treatment and her headache more or less went after three acupuncture treatments and three courses of 10 decoctions each.

2. LIVER-FIRE

Liver-Fire differs from Liver-Yang in so far as it is characterized by the presence of an actual pathogenic factor, i.e. Fire. Liver-Yang is characterized by an imbalance between Yin and Yang, without any actual pathogenic factor. Many of the symptoms and signs of Liver-Yang rising are seen in Liver-Fire too. These are dizziness, tinnitus, deafness, irritability, headache, a dry throat, insomnia and a Wiry pulse. In addition to these, Liver-Fire is characterized by thirst, a bitter taste, scanty-dark urine, constipation with dry stools, red eyes and a Red tongue with yellow coating. Liver-Fire is a purely Excess pattern, while Liver-Yang rising is a combined Excess-Deficiency pattern.

The headache from Liver-Fire is similar in nature to that from Liver-Yang, being throbbing, distending, pulsating or bursting. It is, however, even more intense, tends to be more fixed in one place, and is more frequently accompanied by nausea or vomiting.

Principle of treatment

Pacify the Liver, clear Fire.

Acupuncture

General prescription: LIV-2 Xingjian, SP-6 Sanyinjiao, T.B.-5 Waiguan, G.B.-38 Yangfu, G.B.-20 Fengchi, Taiyang extra point. Distal points with reducing method, local points with even method.

Explanation

- **LIV-2** is the main distal point to clear Liver-Fire. Being the Spring point, it clears Heat.
- **SP-6** is used to nourish Yin, to prevent injury of Yin from Liver-Fire.
- **T.B.-5** is used as a distal point affecting the Lesser Yang channels. See the explanation given for this point under Liver-Yang rising.
- **G.B.-38** clears Liver and Gall-Bladder Fire and treats unilateral headaches especially if situated around an eye. It is especially good for very chronic migraine.
- **G.B.-20** expels Wind from the head and subdues Liver-Fire. See explanation given under Liver-Yang rising.
- **Taiyang:** see explanation given under Liver-Yang rising.

Other points

- **G.B.-43** Xiaxi: being the Spring point, it clears Gall-Bladder Heat and is suitable if the headache is located around or behind one eye.
- **G.B.-44** Qiaoyin clears Gall-Bladder Heat and is suitable if the headache is located on the side of the head.

- **L.I.-11** Quchi is used if there are pronounced signs of Heat, such as thirst, a bitter taste, a feeling of heat, a Deep-Red tongue body with yellow coating and a Rapid pulse.

All the local points mentioned under Liver-Yang rising are equally applicable in the treatment of Liver-Fire headaches.

Herbal treatment

Prescription

LONG DAN XIE GAN TANG
Gentiana Draining the Liver Decoction
Long Dan Cao *Radix Gentianae scabrae* 6 g
Huang Qin *Radix Scutellariae baicalensis* 9 g
Shan Zhi Zi *Fructus Gardeniae jasminoidis* 9 g
Ze Xie *Rhizoma Alismatis orientalis* 9 g
Mu Tong *Caulis Akebiae* 9 g
Che Qian Zi *Semen Plantaginis* 9 g
Sheng Di Huang *Radix Rehmanniae glutinosae* 12 g
Dang Gui *Radix Angelicae sinensis* 9 g
Chai Hu *Radix Bupleuri* 9 g
Gan Cao *Radix Glycyrrhizae uralensis* 3 g

Explanation

- **Long Dan Cao** is the emperor herb in this prescription as it clears Liver-Fire. It is particularly effective at clearing Liver-Fire in the head and ears and is therefore suitable for headaches. It also clears Damp-Heat in the Lower Burner and this is another use of this prescription.
- **Huang Qin** and **Shan Zhi Zi** clear Liver-Heat and are the minister herbs to help Long Dan Cao. They also clear Damp-Heat.
- **Ze Xie**, **Mu Tong** and **Che Qian Zi** are assistant herbs. They are cool and have a diuretic action to expel Damp-Heat. Besides clearing Damp-Heat in the Lower Burner, they are included to drain Fire via urination.
- **Sheng Di** and **Dang Gui** are included to nourish Yin, so as to prevent injury of Yin from Fire.
- **Chai Hu** is used as a messenger herb to direct the prescription to the Liver channel.
- **Gan Cao** harmonizes.

Herbs

- **Long Dan Cao** *Radix Gentianae scabrae* is the main herb to clear Liver-Fire. It is especially suited to the treatment of headaches as it acts on the area around the ears and eyes.
- **Xia Ku Cao** *Spica Prunellae vulgaris* clears Liver-Fire and affects the head.
- **Jue Ming Zi** *Semen Cassiae torae* clears Liver-Fire and affects the eyes. It is therefore suitable for Liver-Fire headaches around one eye.

(a) Patent remedy

LONG DAN XIE GAN WAN
Gentiana Draining the Liver Pill
This pill has the same ingredients and functions as the above prescription.

The tongue presentation appropriate to this remedy is a Red tongue with redder sides and a yellow coating.

(b) Patent remedy

HUANG LIAN YANG GAN WAN
Coptis-Goat's Liver Pill
Huang Lian *Rhizoma Coptidis*
Mi Meng Hua *Flos Buddleiae officinalis*
Jue Ming Zi *Semen Cassiae torae*
Shi Jue Ming *Concha Haliotidis*
Chong Wei Zi *Semen Leonori heterophylli*
Ye Ming Sha *Excrementum Vespertilionis*
Long Dan Cao *Radix Gentianae scabrae*
Huang Bo *Cortex Phellodendri*
Huang Qin *Radix Scutellariae baicalensis*
Hu Huang Lian *Radix Picrorhizae*
Chai Hu *Radix Bupleuri*
Qing Pi *Pericarpium Citri reticulatae viridae*
Mu Zei *Herba Equiseti hieinalis*
Yang Gan *Iecur Caprae seu Ovis*

Explanation

This pill is suitable for headaches from Liver-Fire with constipation. It is especially indicated for headaches occurring behind the eyes.

The tongue presentation appropriate to this remedy is the same as that for the previous remedy except that the coating would be much drier.

Case history

A 33-year-old woman had been suffering from chronic migraine for several years. The headaches were frequent and intense and occurred over the right eye. They were throbbing in character and aggravated by lying down. They were accompanied by nausea, a feeling of heat, thirst and a bitter taste. The headaches improved during pregnancy and worsened after childbirth.

The periods were regular and normal, but she experienced pre-menstrual tension manifesting with irritability, mood-swings and weeping.

She had also been suffering from alopecia at 7, 14 and 21 years of age when the hair suddenly fell out in clumps and then regrew each time. In the past, she had suffered from severe depression.

Her pulse was Wiry and her tongue was slightly Red, dry, rather peeled in the centre, with cracks in the central area.

Diagnosis

The present condition is one of Liver-Fire rising causing the migraine. This is evidenced by the Red and dry tongue, Wiry pulse and the feeling of heat, thirst and bitter taste. Had the tongue not been dry and Red and had there been no thirst and bitter taste, the diagnosis would have been Liver-Yang rising. In this case, the Liver-Fire was beginning to injure the Yin of the Stomach as evidenced by the centre of the tongue being slightly peeled and cracked.

She must have been suffering from Liver-Qi stagnation as well preceding the development of Liver-Fire as shown by the previous period of depression and pre-menstrual tension.

The alopecia was due to Liver-Wind (which develops from Liver-Fire). When the hair falls out suddenly and in clumps, it indicates Liver-Wind. It is interesting that the alopecia occurred regularly at 7-year intervals (7, 14 and 21), coinciding exactly with a girl's development cycles described in the first chapter of the "Simple Questions". The fact that the migraine improved during pregnancy and worsened after childbirth indicates a Kidney deficiency, but this is the only sign of it in this case.

Treatment principle

Clear Liver-Fire, subdue Liver-Wind, nourish Stomach and Kidney-Yin, calm the Mind and settle the Ethereal Soul.

Treatment

This patient was treated with acupuncture only and the main points used were:
T.B.-5 Waiguan, P-6 Neiguan, ST-36 Zusanli, SP-6 Sanyinjiao, KI-3 Taixi, LIV-2 Xingjian.
Other points used at other times included:
Ren-12 Zhongwan, LU-7 Lieque and KI-6 Zhaohai in combination, G.B.-43 Xiaxi, KI-9 Zhubin, G.B.-20 Fengchi, Yuyao and G.B.-1 Tongziliao.

Explanation

- **T.B.-5** was used on the right side as a distal point to affect the Lesser-Yang channels where the headaches manifested.
- **P-6** was used on the left side (to balance T.B.-5) to regulate the Liver (by virtue of the connection between Pericardium and Liver within the Terminal Yin) and to calm the Mind and settle the Ethereal Soul. The combination of these two points for chronic headaches on the Lesser Yang channels from either Liver-Yang or Liver-Fire rising, is very effective to affect the area of the headache, regulate the Liver and calm the Mind. In addition, T.B.-5 will regulate the Gall-Bladder and P-6 will regulate the Liver. Since the Triple Burner pertains to the Lesser Yang which is the "hinge" of the Yang channels, and the Pericardium pertains to the Terminal Yin which is the "hinge" of the Yin channels, these two points will also regulate Yin and Yang, Defensive and Nutritive Qi, the Exterior and Interior, and Yin- and Yang-Linking Vessels.
- **ST-36** and **SP-6** were used to tonify Stomach-Yin. SP-6, in addition, will also regulate the Liver and calm the Mind.
- **KI-3** was used to nourish the Kidneys and Liver-Yin. Although in this case it is Liver-Fire that is injuring Yin (and not the other way round) it is still important to nourish the Kidneys since Liver and Kidneys have a "common source", and tonifying the Kidney points will help to regulate the Liver.
- **LIV-2** was used with reducing method to clear Liver-Fire.
- **Ren-12** was used to nourish Stomach-Yin.
- **LU-7** and **KI-6** in combination open the Directing Vessel. This was done to nourish the Kidneys and regulate the Uterus.
- **G.B.-43** was used with reducing method to clear the Gall-Bladder channel, where the headaches occurred.
- **KI-9** was used to nourish the Kidneys and calm the Mind. This point has a powerful calming action.
- **G.B.-20** was used as an adjacent point to subdue Liver-Fire and Liver-Wind.
- **Yuyao** is the extra point in the middle of the eyebrow and was used as a local point.
- **G.B.-1** was also used as a local point to clear the Gall-Bladder channel.

3. LIVER-WIND

The headache from Liver-Wind is pulling in character and affects the whole head rather than the sides. It is accompanied by severe giddiness.

Other possible manifestations include a slight shaking of the head, numbness, or tremor of a limb. The pulse and tongue will vary according to whether the Liver-Wind derives from Liver-Fire or from Liver-Blood deficiency.

Treatment principle

Pacify the Liver, extinguish Wind.

Acupuncture

General prescription: LIV-3 Taichong, SP-6 Sanyinjiao, G.B.-20 Fengchi, Du-16 Fengfu, Du-20 Baihui. Reducing method, except on SP-6 which should be tonified.

Explanation

- **LIV-3** subdues Liver-Wind.
- **SP-6** is tonified to nourish Yin and Blood which is always necessary in order to subdue internal Wind.
- **G.B.-20** subdues Wind (both internal and external).
- **Du-16** and **Du-20** subdue internal Wind and relieve headache.

Other points

- **S.I.-3** Houxi and **BL-62** Shenmai in combination open the Governing Vessel and subdue internal Wind agitating within it and causing headaches. In men these two points can be used on their own, whilst in women they are best combined with the points to open the Directing Vessel, i.e. LU-7 Lieque and KI-6 Zhaohai.

Any of the local points mentioned for the Liver-Yang type of headache can be used for the Liver-Wind type too.

Herbal treatment

(a) Prescription

TIAN MA GOU TENG YIN
Gastrodia-Uncaria Decoction

(b) Prescription

ZHEN GAN XI FENG TANG
Calming the Liver and Subduing Wind Decoction

Both these prescriptions have been discussed under Liver-Yang rising.

Herbs

- **Bai Ji Li** *Fructus Tribuli terrestris* extinguishes internal Wind and treats headaches, especially around the eyes.
- **Di Long** *Lumbricus* subdues internal Wind and is used for chronic headaches of this type, especially in old people.
- **Quan Xie** *Buthus martensi* is used for severe and chronic headaches from internal Wind.

Patent remedies

All the patent remedies mentioned for headaches from Liver-Yang rising are also suitable for those from Liver-Wind.

4. LIVER-QI STAGNATION

This type of headache usually occurs on the forehead or temples. It is frequently associated with a Stomach disharmony such as retention of food in the Stomach. The type of ache resembles that from Stomach deficiency but it is more intense. It is not, however, throbbing like that from Liver-Yang rising. Another characteristic of it is that it moves from one side to the other.

The headache from Liver-Qi stagnation is typically caused by anxiety and stress. Other manifestations include hypochondrial pain or distension, nervous tension, poor digestion, belching, flatulence, abdominal distension, small-bitty stools, sighing and a Wiry pulse.

Treatment principle

Pacify the Liver, eliminate stagnation, calm the Mind and settle the Ethereal Soul.

Acupuncture

General prescription: LIV-3 Taichong, G.B.-34 Yanglingquan, L.I.-4 Hegu, ST-36 Zusanli, Du-24 Shenting, Taiyang. LIV-3, G.B.-34 and L.I.-4 with reducing method. ST-36 with reinforcing method and the local points with even method.

Explanation

- **LIV-3** pacifies the Liver and eliminates stagnation. It is chosen out of all other Liver-channel points because it is the best to affect the head.
- **G.B.-34** relieves stagnation of Liver-Qi. In combination with Du-24, it eliminates stagnation of Liver-Qi in the head.
- **L.I.-4** is chosen because it will combine with LIV-3 to eliminate stagnation of Liver-Qi in the head. It also calms the Mind which is important since stagnation of Liver-Qi is normally caused by emotional problems.
- **ST-36** is used because the headache is caused by the influence of Liver-Qi stagnation on the Stomach channel in the head.
- **Du-24** and **Taiyang** in combination with G.B.-34 relieve stagnation of Liver-Qi in the head. Du-24, in addition, also calms the Mind.

Other points

- **LIV-14** Qimen can be added to help to eliminate stagnation of Liver-Qi.
- **Yintang** is an extra point that can be used as a local point for headaches on the forehead. It also calms the Mind and promotes sleep.

Herbal treatment

Prescription

XIAO YAO SAN
Free and Easy Wanderer Powder
Bo He *Herba Menthae* 3 g
Chai Hu *Radix Bupleuri* 9 g
Dang Gui *Radix Angelicae sinensis* 9 g
Bai Shao *Radix Paeoniae albae* 12 g
Bai Zhu *Rhizoma Atractylodis macrocephalae* 9 g
Fu Ling *Sclerotium Poriae cocos* 15 g
Gan Cao *Radix Glycyrrhizae uralensis* 6 g
Sheng Jiang *Rhizoma Zingiberis officinalis recens* 3 slices

Explanation

- **Bo He** and **Chai Hu** eliminate stagnation of Liver-Qi. Although Chai Hu is, strictly speaking, contraindicated in headaches, the overall effect of the formula is such that it can be used for headaches from Liver-Qi stagnation, especially with the addition of other herbs which make Qi descend, such as Chen Xiang *Lignum Aquilariae*.

- **Dang Gui** and **Bai Shao** nourish Liver-Blood, which will contribute to the pacifying of Liver-Qi. In addition, Bai Shao also pacifies and harmonizes the Liver.
- **Bai Zhu** and **Fu Ling** tonify Spleen-Qi and eliminate Dampness.
- **Gan Cao** and **Sheng Jiang** harmonize.

Herbs

- **Mu Xiang** *Radix Saussureae* moves Qi in the Stomach, Spleen, Intestines and Gall-Bladder. Because it enters the Gall-Bladder it can relieve headaches from Liver-Qi stagnation.
- **Ju Hua** *Flos Chrysanthemi morifolii* subdues Liver-Yang and can be added as a symptomatic herb to relieve the headache.
- **Sang Ye** *Folium Mori albae* has the same function as Ju Hua.
- **Zhi Shi** *Fructus Citri aurantii immaturus* moves Qi and makes Qi descend. For this reason it is a suitable addition to treat headaches from Liver-Qi stagnation.
- **Yan Hu Suo** *Rhizoma Corydalis yanhusuo* moves Qi and Blood of Stomach and Liver and is particularly good for stopping pain.
- **Chen Xiang** *Lignum Aquilariae* moves Qi and has a strong effect in subduing rebellious Qi. For this reason, it is suitable to treat headaches.

Patent remedy

SHU GAN WAN
Pacifying the Liver Pill
Chuan Lian Zi *Fructus Meliae toosendan*
Jiang Huang *Rhizoma Curcumae longae*
Chen Xiang *Lignum Aquilariae*
Yan Hu Suo *Rhizoma Corydalis yanhusuo*
Mu Xiang *Radix Saussureae*
Bai Dou Kou *Fructus Amomi cardamomi*
Bai Shao *Radix Paeoniae albae*
Fu Ling *Sclerotium Poriae cocos*
Zhi Ke *Fructus Citri aurantii*

Chen Pi *Pericarpium Citri reticulatae*
Sha Ren *Fructus seu Semen Amomi*
Hou Po *Cortex Magnoliae officinalis*

Explanation

This remedy can be used for headaches from Liver-Qi stagnation. It contains Chen Xiang which also makes Qi descend.

Note that there is another version of this pill by the same name, which omits Chuan Lian Zi and Fu Ling and adds Xiang Fu *Rhizoma Cyperi rotundi*, Gan Cao *Radix Glycyrrhizae uralensis*, Mu Dan Pi *Cortex Moutan radicis*, Chai Hu *Radix Bupleuri*, Fu Shou *Fructus Citri sarcodactylis*, Qing Pi *Pericarpium Citri reticulatae viridae*, Xiang Yuan *Fructus Citri medicae* and Tan Xiang *Lignum Santali albi*. This can be used for headaches too, but it is slightly less suitable than the former version as it contains Chai Hu which is contra-indicated for headaches.

5. STAGNATION OF COLD IN THE LIVER CHANNEL

This is quite a rare type of headache. It is caused by Cold in the Liver channel rebelling upwards to reach the head. It is called "Terminal-Yin headache". The ache is intense and is experienced at the top of the head. It is associated with a feeling of cold, vomiting, cold limbs and a Wiry pulse.

Treatment principle

Pacify and warm the Liver, expel Cold, subdue rebellious Qi.

Acupuncture

General prescription: LIV-3 Taichong, Du-20 Baihui. Reducing method on LIV-3 followed by application of moxa on the needle. Even method on Du-20.

Explanation

- **LIV-3** pacifies the Liver and subdues

rebellious Liver-Qi and is an important distal point for headaches from Liver disharmonies.

– **Du-20** is used (with needle) as a local point to disperse the stagnation of Liver-Qi in the vertex.

Herbal treatment

(a) Prescription

WU ZHU YU TANG
Evodia Decoction
Wu Zhu Yu *Fructus Evodiae rutaecarpae* 3 g
Ren Shen (or **Dang Shen**) *Radix Ginseng* 6 g
Sheng Jiang *Rhizoma Zingiberis officinalis recens* 18 g
Da Zao *Fructus Ziziphi jujubae* 4 pieces

Explanation

– **Wu Zhu Yu** warms the Liver and subdues rebellious ascending Qi. It is the main herb in this prescription.
– **Ren Shen** (or **Dang Shen**) tonifies the Stomach.
– **Sheng Jiang** helps to expel Cold and stop vomiting.
– **Da Zao** harmonizes and also helps Ren Shen to tonify the Stomach.

(b) Prescription

CHEN XIANG JIANG QI SAN
Aquilaria Subduing Qi Powder
Chen Xiang *Lignum Aquilariae* 3 g
Sha Ren *Fructus seu Semen Amomi* 4 g
Xiang Fu *Rhizoma Cyperi rotundi* 6 g
Zhi Gan Cao *Radix Glycyrrhizae uralensis praeparata* 3 g
Sheng Jiang *Rhizoma Zingiberis officinalis recens* 3 slices

Explanation

– **Chen Xiang** is the main herb and is used here to subdue rebellious Qi.
– **Sha Ren** and **Xiang Fu** move Qi and help Chen Xiang to subdue it.
– **Zhi Gan Cao** regulates and warms.
– **Sheng Jiang** warms.

Herbs

– **Chuan Xiong** *Radix Ligustici wallichii* enters the Liver and treats headaches.
– **Dang Gui** *Radix Angelicae sinensis* enters the Liver channel.
– **Rou Gui** *Cortex Cinnamomi cassiae* is very warm and expels Cold.
– **Gui Zhi** *Ramulus Cinnamomi cassiae* is warming and enters the channels and blood vessels.

Case history

A 38-year-old man had been suffering from migraine headaches for the past five years. The headaches occurred over the whole head and were dull but intense in character. They were better lying down, worse from stress and worse from exposure to light. They were accompanied by nausea and vomiting without bringing up much food and a feeling of cold.

He also experienced some hypochondrial pain extending to the back, elicited by intake of fatty foods. He was also prone to belching and constipation.

His tongue was of a normal colour and was Swollen with a dirty coating. His pulse was Wiry and Slow.

Diagnosis
The headaches were clearly due to stagnation of Cold in the Liver channel as evidenced by the feeling of cold, the location of the headache, the dry vomiting and the Wiry-Slow pulse. The hypochondrial pain, belching and constipation were due to stagnation of Liver-Qi. In addition, there was also Spleen-Qi deficiency with accumulation of Phlegm, as indicated by the Swollen tongue and dirty coating.

Principle of treatment
In this case it is necessary to move Liver-Qi and eliminate Cold.

Acupuncture
The main points used were:
LU-7 Lieque, ST-40 Fenglong, G.B.-34 Yanglingquan and LIV-3 Taichong. The first two points were used with even method, and the latter two with reducing method. Moxa was used on LIV-3. In order to reduce the number of needles and create a balanced and dynamic combination of points, LU-7 was used on the right side, ST-40 on the left side, G.B.-34 on the right side and LIV-3 on the left. The sides could have been inverted too, but the above was worked out so that G.B.-34 would be on the right side to treat the hypochondrial pain which was on the right side.

Explanation
– **LU-7** was used to facilitate the flow of clear Qi up to the head.

- **ST-40** was used to tonify the Spleen and eliminate Phlegm.
- **G.B.-34** was used to move Liver-Qi and eliminate stagnation.
- **LIV-3** was used to move Liver-Qi and moxa was used on it to expel Cold from the Liver channel.

Herbal treatment
The prescription used was a variation of Wu Zhu Yu Tang *Evodia Decoction:*

Wu Zhu Yu *Fructus Evodiae rutaecarpae* 3 g
Dang Shen *Radix Codonopsis pilosulae* 6 g
Sheng Jiang *Rhizoma Zingiberis officinalis recens* 3 slices
Gan Cao *Radix Glycyrrhizae uralensis* 3 g
Gui Zhi *Ramulus Cinnamomi cassiae* 3 g
Chen Pi *Pericarpium Citri reticulatae* 3 g
Yin Chen Hao *Herba Artemisia capillaris* 3 g
Da Zao *Fructus Ziziphi jujubae* 3 dates

Explanation
Wu Zhu Yu, Dang Shen, Sheng Jiang, and Da Zao are all part of the Wu Zhu Yu Tang.

- **Gui Zhi** was added to help to expel Cold. It also enters the blood vessels and channels and would therefore help the headaches.
- **Chen Pi** was added to help to eliminate Phlegm.
- **Yin Chen Hao** was added as a messenger herb to direct the prescription to the Liver channel.
- **Gan Cao** was added to harmonize the prescription.

This man's headache stopped completely after 3 months.

6. DAMPNESS

Internal Dampness is a very frequent cause of headaches, particularly in damp countries such as the British Isles. Although Dampness has a natural tendency to settle in the Lower Burner as it is heavy in nature, it can affect the head too. This happens in chronic cases when Dampness obstructs the Middle Burner, prevents Stomach-Qi from descending and interferes with the normal movement of Qi in the Middle. Because of this long-term stagnation of Dampness in the Middle, the obstruction gradually spreads upwards as well and it fills the head.

Once in the head, Dampness prevents the clear Yang from ascending to brighten the sense orifices and the turbid Yin from descending away from the head. The result is that the sense orifices are clouded by Dampness. This causes a headache which is dull and feels as if the head were wrapped in a cloth or full of cotton wool.

There is also a sensation of heaviness of the head and a difficulty in thinking. These symptoms are worse in the mornings. The headache may affect the whole head or it could be on the forehead only. In a few cases the Dampness may be affecting the Gall-Bladder channel, in which case the headaches would occur on the temples or sides of the head.

Other symptoms include persistent catarrh, sometimes sinusitis, nausea, lack of appetite, a feeling of fullness of the chest and epigastrium, a thick-sticky tongue coating and a Slippery pulse. If the Dampness is very chronic and the Spleen very deficient, the pulse may be Weak-Floating, i.e. it feels Weak, it is slightly Floating especially on the right Middle position and is soft.

Internal Dampness arises from a deficiency of Spleen-Qi failing to transform and transport fluids which accumulate into Dampness. It can also derive from retention of external Dampness over a long period of time.

Treatment principle

Resolve Dampness, stimulate ascending of clear Yang, tonify Stomach and Spleen.

Acupuncture

General prescription: SP-3 Taibai, L.I.-4 Hegu, LU-7 Lieque, Ren-12 Zhongwan, BL-20 Pishu, ST-8 Touwei. Reducing method on SP-3 and L.I.-4, even method on ST-8, reinforcing method on LU-7, BL-20 and Ren-12.

Explanation

- **SP-3** is a general point to eliminate Dampness in any part of the body. Being towards the extremity of the channel, it specifically affects the head.
- **L.I.-4** can eliminate pathogenic factors from the face and forehead area.
- **LU-7** is specific for headaches and is used to stimulate the ascending of clear Yang to the head.
- **Ren-12** and **BL-20** are used to tonify the Spleen to eliminate Dampness.
- **ST-8** is the main local point to eliminate

Dampness from the head and is specific for this type of headache.

Other points

- **Du-20** Baihui is used if the headache is accompanied by a marked cloudiness of the head. It stimulates the ascending of clear Yang to the head.
- **Du-24** Shenting can be used as a local point to eliminate Dampness from the forehead.
- **Du-23** Shangxing can be used if the headache is located around the eyes.
- **Yintang** can be used as a local point if the headache is located on the forehead.
- **SP-6** Sanyinjiao and **SP-9** Yinlingquan can be used as distal points to eliminate Dampness.
- **BL-21** Weishu can be added to strengthen the Stomach and Spleen to eliminate Dampness. It is especially good if the person suffers from chronic tiredness.

Herbal treatment

(a) Prescription

QIANG HUO SHENG SHI TANG
Notopterygium Dispelling Dampness Decoction
Qiang Huo *Radix et Rhizoma Notopterygii* 6 g
Du Huo *Radix Angelicae pubescentis* 6 g
Fang Feng *Radix Ledebouriellae sesloidis* 6 g
Gao Ben *Rhizoma Ligustici sinensis* 6 g
Chuan Xiong *Rhizoma Ligustici wallichii* 3 g
Man Jing Zi *Fructus Viticis* 6 g
Zhi Gan Cao *Radix Glycyrrhizae uralensis praeparata* 3 g

Explanation

- **Qiang Huo** and **Du Huo** are the main herbs. They both eliminate Dampness, the former from the upper part of the body and the latter from the lower part. They potentiate each other. In this case, Qiang Huo is the more important herb to reach the upper part of the Greater Yang channels and treat the headache. Its dose could therefore be increased in respect of that of Du Huo.
- **Fang Feng** and **Gao Ben** are the minister herbs and both eliminate Wind and Dampness from the Greater Yang channels.

In particular Gao Ben is specific for the upper part of the body and head.
- **Chuan Xiong** and **Man Jing Zi** eliminate Wind from the head and stop headaches.
- **Gan Cao** harmonizes.

(b) Prescription

YIN CHEN WU LING SAN
Artemisia capillaris Five Ling Powder
Yin Chen Hao *Herba Artemisiae capillaris* 10 g
Wu Ling San *Five Ling Powder* 5 g

Explanation

This is a variation of the Wu Ling San *Five Ling Powder* and the above are the dosages for a powder. If the crude herbs are used, the dosage of Yin Chen Hao would be considerably higher than the other herbs.

- **Yin Chen Hao** is the main herb in the prescription to enter the Gall-Bladder and resolve Dampness from it. In the case of headaches, this herb would direct the prescription to the Gall-Bladder channel.
- **Wu Ling San**: the whole prescription is to eliminate Dampness and resolve oedema.

This prescription is suitable for headaches from Dampness affecting the Gall-Bladder rather than the Stomach and Spleen. It is thus used for more intense headaches on the temples or sides of the head rather than the forehead which the previous formula addresses.

It should be noted that there is nothing in these two prescriptions to strengthen the Spleen. For chronic headaches from Dampness, these prescriptions should be integrated with another to tonify the Spleen (for example, the Si Jun Zi Tang *Four Gentlemen Decoction*). In severe cases, the prescriptions could be used on their own first to eliminate Dampness, and then adapted with the addition of some herbs to tonify the Spleen (such as Bai Zhu *Rhizoma Atractylodis macrocephalae*).

Patent remedy

HUO XIANG ZHENG QI WAN
Agastache Upright Qi Pill

Explanation

The ingredients and functions of this pill have already been explained above under "Dampness" in the section on exterior headaches.

It can be used also to treat headaches from interior Dampness. This remedy treats only the Dampness and does not tonify the Spleen.

Case history

A 52-year-old woman had been suffering from headaches for the past three years. The headaches occurred mostly on the forehead and face, but also on the top of the head. They started after a fast and were worse in daytime. They were accompanied by a feeling of muzziness of the head. There was *no* dizziness.

She had also been suffering from chronic catarrh and rhinitis for the past 25 years. She had a chronic ache in the lower back and her urination was too frequent. She felt tired. The bowels were constipated, not having a movement every day. When she did have a movement, it was sometimes loose. She felt generally cold. The Pulse was Deep and Weak on the whole, and slightly Slippery on the right side. Her tongue was Pale and Swollen with a sticky-yellow coating.

The diagnosis was Spleen- and Kidney-Yang deficiency leading to Dampness obstructing the head. The headaches had all the typical features of Dampness: they were dull in character, with a feeling of muzziness of the head and occurred mostly on the forehead. The absence of dizziness indicates Dampness as opposed to Phlegm. The presence of Dampness is confirmed by the chronic catarrh and rhinitis, the slippery quality of the pulse and the sticky tongue coating. The Kidney-Yang deficiency is indicated by the lower back ache, frequent urination, cold feeling and the Deep pulse, while the Spleen-Yang deficiency is indicated by the tiredness, the cold feeling, the Weak pulse and the Pale tongue. The constipation is due to deficient Kidney-Yang unable to move the stools: this is confirmed by the fact that the stools were not dry and that they were indeed sometimes loose.

It is interesting that the headaches should start after a fast. She had obviously suffered from Dampness for a long time as evidenced by the chronic catarrh and rhinitis. Being on a fast weakened the Spleen which became even more unable to transform and transport and therefore led to more Dampness. A person with Spleen deficiency should only fast under very controlled conditions and lead up to the fast by very gradually reducing the quantity of food eaten. Similarly, one should break the fast very gradually. Only if done under these conditions, can a fast be beneficial. The treatment was based on both acupuncture and herbal therapy.

Treatment principle
Tonify Spleen- and Kidney-Yang and resolve Dampness.

Acupuncture
The main points used were: LU-7 Lieque, L.I.-4 Hegu, Ren-12 Zhongwan, ST-36 Zusanli, SP-3 Taibai and KI-7 Fuliu. LU-7, L.I.-4 and SP-3 were needled with even method while the others were needled with reinforcing method. Moxa was used on ST-36 and KI-7.

Other points used included: Ren-9 Shuifen, SP-6 Sanyinjiao, BL-20 Pishu, BL-23 Shenshu, ST-8 Touwei.

Explanation
- **LU-7** and **L.I.-4** were used to open the channels of the head and face and remove obstructions. They would also stimulate the rising of clear Yang to the head.
- **Ren-12**, **ST-36,** and **BL-20** were used to tonify the Spleen.
- **BL-23** and **KI-7** were used to tonify the Kidneys.
- **SP-3**, **SP-6** and **Ren-9** were used to resolve Dampness.
- **ST-8** was used as a local point. It is the best local point to resolve Dampness in the head.

Herbal treatment
The prescription was based on a variation of **Qiang Huo Sheng Shi Tang** with the addition of:

Huo Xiang *Herba Agastachis* 3 g
Pei Lan *Herba Eupatorii fortunei* 3 g
Chen Pi *Pericarpium Citri reticulatae* 3 g
Bai Zhu *Rhizoma Atractylodis macrocephalae* 6 g
Du Zhong *Cortex Eucommiae ulmoidis* 6 g
Cang Zhu *Rhizoma Atractylodis lanceae* 3 g

Explanation
- **Huo Xiang** and **Pei Lan** were added as fragrant herbs to resolve Dampness. Being fragrant and light they would also affect the head and face and relieve the headaches.
- **Cang Zhu** is another fragrant herb to resolve Dampness and it is frequently used for headaches.
- **Chen Pi** was added to help to resolve Dampness and move Qi. Moving Qi is nearly always necessary to help to resolve Dampness.
- **Bai Zhu** was added to tonify the Spleen.
- **Du Zhong** was used to tonify Kidney-Yang. Being slightly pungent, it would also help to relieve the backache.

This patient's headaches were cured after 6 months' treatment.

7. TURBID PHLEGM

Phlegm is similar to Dampness in nature and it also derives from deficiency of Spleen-Qi. The headache from Phlegm is similar to that from Dampness, i.e. it is dull and is accompanied by a feeling of heaviness and muzziness. However, Phlegm is more obstructive than Dampness and it clouds the sense orifices more. This results in blurred vision and dizziness which are not present with Dampness.

Other manifestations include catarrh on the chest, a feeling of fullness and oppression of the chest, a sticky tongue coating and a Slippery pulse.

Treatment principle

Resolve Phlegm, harmonize the Middle.

Acupuncture

General prescription: ST-40 Fenglong, L.I.-4 Hegu, LU-7 Lieque, ST-8 Touwei, Du-20 Baihui. Reducing method on ST-40 and L.I.-4, reinforcing method on LU-7, even method on ST-8 and Du-20.

Explanation

– **ST-40** is the main point to resolve Phlegm.
– **L.I.-4** is used as a distal point to eliminate pathogenic factors from the face and head.
– **LU-7** is used as a distal point to stimulate the ascending of clear Yang to the head.
– **ST-8** is a local point for headaches from Phlegm (or Dampness).
– **Du-20** is used to stimulate the ascending of clear Yang to the head.

Other points

– **ST-36** Zusanli can be added as a distal point to tonify the Spleen and resolve Phlegm. It is important to use it if the person feels very tired.
– **SP-6** Sanyinjiao eliminates Dampness and helps to resolve Phlegm.
– **SP-3** Taibai eliminates Dampness and helps to resolve Phlegm. Being at the extremity of the channel, it affects the head.
– **L.I.-11** Quchi can be used if the Phlegm is associated with Heat.
– **Du-23** Shangxing can be used as a local point especially if the eyes are affected.

– **Yintang** can be used as a local point if the headache is on the forehead.

Herbal treatment

Prescription

BAN XIA BAI ZHU TIAN MA TANG
Pinellia-Atractylodes-Gastrodia Decoction
Ban Xia *Rhizoma Pinelliae ternatae* 9 g
Tian Ma *Rhizoma Gastrodiae elatae* 6 g
Bai Zhu *Rhizoma Atractylodis macrocephalae* 15 g
Fu Ling *Sclerotium Poriae cocos* 6 g
Chen Pi *Pericarpium Citri reticulatae* 6 g
Gan Cao *Rhizoma Glycyrrhizae uralensis* 4 g
Sheng Jiang *Rhizoma Zingiberis officinalis recens* 1 slice
Da Zao *Fructus Ziziphi jujubae* 2 pieces

Explanation

– **Fa Ban Xia** resolves Phlegm, makes Qi descend and stops vomiting.
– **Tian Ma** subdues internal Wind and stops headaches. These two herbs are the emperor herbs, one to resolve Phlegm, the other to subdue Wind. Thus, they treat Wind-Phlegm causing headache and dizziness. Li Dong Yuan in the "Discussion on Stomach and Spleen" says: *"Headaches due to Phlegm cannot be treated without Ban Xia and headaches with dizziness due to Wind cannot be treated without Tian Ma".*[9] Even though this prescription is actually for Wind-Phlegm, it is the prescription of choice because it includes Tian Ma which is an important herb for headaches.
– **Bai Zhu** strengthens the Spleen and dries Dampness. This helps Ban Xia to resolve Phlegm. It is the minister herb.
– **Fu Ling** and **Chen Pi** resolve Dampness and therefore also help Ban Xia to resolve Phlegm. They are assistant herbs.
– **Gan Cao** harmonizes.
– **Da Zao** and **Sheng Jiang** harmonize the Middle and mildly strengthen the Spleen to resolve Phlegm.

Herbs

– **Dan Nan Xing** *Rhizoma Arisaematis praeparata*

is a warm herb to resolve Phlegm and subdue internal Wind and is therefore suitable to treat headaches of this type. It is particularly suitable if the headaches move from one side to the other.

- **Bai Fu Zi** *Rhizoma Typhonii gigantei* is another warm herb to resolve Phlegm and could be added particularly if Phlegm is associated with Cold and is difficult to eliminate.
- **Jiang Can** *Bombyx batryticatus* subdues Wind and treats headaches. It is particularly useful in cases of very chronic headaches from Wind-Phlegm in old people.
- **Quan Xie** *Buthus martensi* is indicated for headaches from Wind-Phlegm and is particularly useful for chronic headaches of this type in old people.

Patent remedy

ER CHEN WAN
Two Old Pill
Fa Ban Xia *Rhizoma Pinelliae ternatae*
Chen Pi *Pericarpium Citri reticulatae*
Fu Ling *Sclerotium Poriae cocos*
Zhi Gan Cao *Radix Glycyrrhizae uralensis praeparata*
Sheng Jiang *Rhizoma Zingiberis officinalis recens*
Wu Mei *Fructus Pruni Mume*

Explanation

This pill is not specific for headaches from Phlegm, but it is a remedy for Phlegm in general. It can therefore be used as an adjunctive to one's acupuncture treatment.

The tongue presentation appropriate to this remedy is a Swollen tongue body with a sticky-white coating.

Case history

A man of 48 had been suffering from headaches for 10 years. The headaches occurred around the forehead and were dull in character. They were accompanied by a feeling of cloudiness, heaviness and dizziness. He also suffered from extreme tiredness and a lack of sexual drive. He felt cold easily. His pulse was Deep and Slippery and his tongue was Pale with swollen sides and a very thick-sticky yellow coating.

Diagnosis

The headaches were clearly caused by Turbid-Phlegm obstructing the head orifices and preventing the clear Yang from rising. This caused the typical feeling of cloudiness, heaviness and dizziness. Dizziness in particular, distinguishes it from Dampness. The Phlegm arose from a background of Spleen-Yang deficiency (Pale tongue with swollen sides, Deep pulse, feeling cold, tiredness and lack of sexual drive). Lack of sexual drive is not always due to Kidney deficiency: in this case, in fact, it was due to Spleen deficiency.

Treatment principle

In this case, due to the chronicity of the condition, attention was directed at treating both the Root and the Manifestation simultaneously. This involved both tonifying the body's Qi and eliminating the pathogenic factors (in this case Phlegm). This patient was treated with acupuncture only.

Acupuncture

The main points used were Ren-12 Zhongwan, ST-8 Touwei, LU-7 Lieque, L.I.-4 Hegu, ST-36 Zusanli, BL-20 Pishu, ST-40 Fenglong and SP-3 Taibai.

ST-40 and ST-8 were needled with even method while all the other points were needled with reinforcing method.

Explanation

- **Ren-12**, **ST-36**, **BL-20** and **SP-3** were reinforced to tonify the Spleen. Moxa was used on ST-36 to tonify Spleen-Yang.
- **LU-7** and **L.I.-4** were used to stimulate the rising of clear Yang to the head and open the head orifices.
- **ST-8** is the main local point for headaches from Phlegm or Dampness.
- **ST-40** was used with even method to resolve Phlegm.

8. TURBID PHLEGM-WIND

This pattern is similar to the previous one and it simply corresponds to a combined condition of Phlegm and internal Wind. It is only seen in old people and it may indicate the likelihood of Wind-stroke.

Treatment principle

Resolve Phlegm, subdue Wind, pacify the Liver.

Acupuncture

General prescription: ST-40 Fenglong, L.I.-4 Hegu,

LIV-3 Taichong, S.I.-3 Houxi, BL-62 Shenmai, ST-8 Touwei, Du-20 Baihui, G.B.-20 Fengchi. Reducing method on ST-40, L.I.-4, LIV-3 and G.B.-20, even method on S.I.-3, BL-62, ST-8 and Du-20.

Explanation

- **ST-40**, **L.I.-4**, **ST-8**, and **Du-20**: the use of these points has already been explained under the Phlegm-type headache.
- **LIV-3** subdues Wind and is an important point to relieve this type of headache. In combination with Hegu L.I.-4, it subdues Wind from the face and head.
- **S.I.-3** and **BL-62** in combination open the Governing vessel and subdue Wind. In particular, by opening the Governing vessel they will also relieve the headache.
- **G.B.-20** subdues Wind and relieves headaches.

Other points

- **G.B.-39** Xuanzhong subdues internal Wind and will relieve headaches of this type along the Gall-Bladder channel.
- **Du-16** Fengfu subdues internal Wind and removes obstructions from the Governing vessel.

All the other points mentioned under the Turbid-Phlegm type are applicable to the Wind-Phlegm type too.

Herbal treatment

The same prescription as for the Turbid-Phlegm type is applicable, i.e. Ban Xia Bai Zhu Tian Ma Tang (*Pinellia-Atractylodes-Gastrodia Decoction*). Substances that subdue internal Wind such as Quan Xie *Buthus Martensis* and Jiang Can *Bombyx batryticatus* should definitely be added. Alternatively, this prescription can be integrated with one to subdue Liver-Wind such as Tian Ma Gou Teng Yin G*astrodia-Uncaria Decoction* or Zhen Gan Xi Feng Tang *Pacifying the Liver and Subduing Wind Decoction*.

Herbs

- **Di Long** *Lumbricus* subdues Wind and

removes obstructions from the channels. It is particularly useful for chronic Wind-Phlegm in old people.

All the other herbs mentioned for the Turbid-Phlegm type are also indicated.

Patent remedy

NIU HUANG JIANG YA WAN
Calculus Bovis Lowering [Blood] Pressure Pill
Ling Yang Jiao *Cornu Antelopis*
Niu Huang *Calculus Bovis*
Zhen Zhu *Margarita*
Bing Pian *Borneol*
Yu Jin *Tuber Curcumae*
Huang Qi *Radix Astragali membranacei*

Explanation

Although this remedy does not resolve Phlegm, it does open the orifices and subdues internal Wind. Opening the orifices is a method of treatment which is often used in conjunction with resolving Phlegm to brighten the upper orifices and relieve headache and dizziness. Subduing internal Wind will also help to allay headaches.

The tongue presentation appropriate to this remedy is a Swollen tongue body with a dirty-sticky coating.

9. RETENTION OF FOOD

This type of headache is experienced on the forehead and can be intense. It is obviously related to food intake and it will be aggravated by eating. It is frequently encountered as an acute headache after a dietary indiscretion.

Other manifestations include a feeling of fullness of the epigastrium, sour regurgitation, belching, foul breath, a thick-sticky tongue coating and a Slippery pulse.

Treatment principle

Resolve retention of food, stimulate the descending of Stomach-Qi, promote digestion, harmonize the Middle.

Acupuncture

General prescription: Ren-10 Xiawan, ST-21 Liangmen, P-6 Neiguan, ST-34 Liangqiu, ST-45 Lidui, L.I.-4 Hegu, ST-8 Touwei. Even method on Ren-10, ST-21 and ST-8, reducing method on the others.

Explanation

- **Ren-10** stimulates the descending of Stomach-Qi and the movement of food downwards from the Stomach.
- **ST-21** resolves stagnant food and stops epigastric pain.
- **P-6** stimulates the descending of Stomach-Qi.
- **ST-34** relieves retention of food and stops pain.
- **ST-45** relieves retention of food. It is also chosen here as, being at the extremity of the channel, it will affect the head.
- **L.I.-4** is chosen to clear obstruction from the face and head.
- **ST-8** is chosen as a local point for Stomach-channel problems manifesting on the head.

Other points

- **ST-44** Neiting can be chosen as a distal point to eliminate obstructions from the Stomach, especially if the retention of food is associated with Heat. Being near the extremity of the channel it will also affect the head.
- **SP-4** Gongsun relieves retention of food.
- **Ren-13** Shangwan is used if there are marked symptoms of ascending Stomach-Qi such as belching, sour regurgitation, nausea or vomiting.
- **ST-36** Zusanli is used if the retention of food is associated with a deficient condition of the Stomach.
- **ST-40** Fenglong is used if the retention of food is severe and long-standing and the tongue has a very thick and sticky coating.

Herbal treatment

(a) Prescription

BAO HE WAN
Preserving and Harmonizing Pill

Shan Zha *Fructus Crataegi* 9 g
Shen Qu *Massa Fermentata medicinalis* 6 g
Lai Fu Zi *Semen Raphani sativi* 6 g
Ban Xia *Rhizoma Pinelliae ternatae* 6 g
Chen Pi *Pericarpum Citri reticulatae* 3 g
Fu Ling *Sclerotium Poriae cocos* 6 g
Lian Qiao *Fructus Forsythiae suspensae* 6 g

Explanation

- **Shan Zha** promotes digestion and resolves retention of food (particularly of meat and fatty foods).
- **Shen Qu** strengthens the Spleen and promotes digestion (particularly of alcohol and fermented foods).
- **Lai Fu Zi** makes Qi descend and promotes digestion (particularly of cereals).
- **Fa Ban Xia** and **Chen Pi** move Qi, resolve stagnation, harmonize the Stomach and stop vomiting.
- **Fu Ling** resolves Dampness and strengthens the Spleen.
- **Lian Qiao** clears Heat as retention of food in the Stomach can easily give rise to Heat.

(b) Prescription

XIANG SHA ZHI ZHU WAN
Saussurea-Amomum-Citrus-Atractylodes Pill
Mu Xiang *Radix Saussureae* 4.5 g
Sha Ren *Fructus seu Semen Amomi* 4.5 g
Zhi Shi *Fructus Citri aurantii immaturus* 4.5 g
Chen Pi *Pericarpium Citri reticulatae* 3 g
Ban Xia *Rhizoma Pinelliae ternatae* 6 g
Bai Zhu *Rhizoma Atractylodis macrocephalae* 6 g
Bo He *Herba Menthae* 3 g

Explanation

- **Mu Xiang**, **Sha Ren** and **Zhi Shi** move Qi and thus help to resolve stagnation of food. Zhi Shi has a descending movement and therefore helps to move food downwards.
- **Chen Pi** resolves Dampness and moves Qi.
- **Ban Xia** resolves Phlegm and helps Chen Pi to resolve Dampness. It also harmonizes the Stomach, subdues rebellious Stomach-Qi and stops nausea and vomiting.

- **Bai Zhu** tonifies Stomach-Qi and resolves Dampness.
- **Bo He** is aromatic and helps to resolve stagnation of food.

This prescription is used in preference to the previous one if there are pronounced symptoms of rebellious Stomach-Qi such as belching, nausea, or vomiting.

Herbs

- **Da Huang** *Radix Rhei* is used if retention of food is accompanied by constipation.
- **Huo Xiang** *Herba Agastachis* can be used to transform Dampness in the Middle. Being light and aromatic, it will help headaches from retention of food.
- **Cang Zhu** *Rhizoma Atractylodis lanceae* is an aromatic herb to transform Dampness and it relieves headaches.
- **Zi Su Ye** *Folia Perillae frutescentis* harmonizes the Middle. It is a floating herb and will relieve headaches from retention of food.
- **Fang Feng** *Radix Ledebouriellae sesloidis* expels Wind and Dampness, it is a floating herb and is used for headaches.
- **Bo He** *Herba Menthae* clears the head, is light and aromatic and would therefore help to relieve this type of headache, especially if retention of food is accompanied by Heat.

Patent remedy

BAO HE WAN
Preserving and Harmonizing Pill
Shan Zha *Fructus Crataegi*
Shen Qu *Massa Fermentata medicinalis*
Lai Fu Zi *Semen Raphani sativi*
Ban Xia *Rhizoma Pinelliae ternatae*
Chen Pi *Pericarpum Citri reticulatae*
Fu Ling *Sclerotium Poriae cocos*
Lian Qiao *Fructus Forsythiae suspensae*

Explanation

This pill has the same ingredients and functions as the homonymous prescription.

The tongue presentation appropriate to this remedy is a thick-sticky coating which may be white or yellow.

10. STASIS OF BLOOD

This type of pattern is seen only in very chronic headaches. Stasis of Blood derives from long-standing stagnation of Liver-Qi. In the case of headaches, it also often derives from local stasis of Blood in the head caused by trauma. This may be due to an old fall or accident, often one which the person has forgotten about. If a headache always occurs on the same spot without fail, stasis of Blood from trauma should be suspected.

The headache from stasis of Blood is very severe and intense. It is stabbing or boring in character and patients will often describe it as a "nail being driven into the head". It is fixed in its location.

It is more common in old people or in women with stasis of Blood associated with deficiency and dryness of Blood. Other manifestations include: dark complexion, hypochondrial or abdominal pain and, in women, painful periods with dark-clotted blood. The pulse will be Firm, Wiry, or Choppy and the tongue will be Purple. In case of a past accident to the head, the pulse may be very Weak on the Front position of both left and right side and the tongue may have a purple spot on the tip whilst the rest of the tongue body is normal in colour. This is due to the fact that the tongue body reflects, apart from the internal organs, areas of the body. Thus the tip of the tongue corresponds to the head and an isolated purple spot there may indicate a past trauma to the head, while a normal colour of the rest of the tongue indicates there is not a generalized stasis of Blood.

Treatment principle

Move Blood, open the orifices.

Acupuncture

General prescription: L.I.-11 Quchi, L.I.-4 Hegu, SP-6 Sanyinjiao, LIV-3 Taichong, Ah Shi points. Reducing or even method on all points.

Explanation

- **L.I.-11** besides cooling Blood, also moves Blood and benefits sinews.
- **L.I.-4** in combination with LIV-3, expels pathogenic factors from the head and moves Blood.
- **SP-6** moves Blood.
- **LIV-3** moves Blood and alleviates headaches.
- **Ah Shi** points on the head are an important and essential part of the treatment. The choice of local points is made simply according to the location of the headaches and a clear differentiation of the channel involved.

Other points

- **T.B.-5** Waiguan moves Qi and is especially indicated for headaches on the side of the head.
- **SP-10** Xuehai is used if there is general stasis of Blood.
- **BL-18** Ganshu is indicated if there are marked symptoms of Liver-Blood stasis.
- **BL-2** Zanzhu is for stasis of Blood in the eye.
- **Taiyang** is for stasis of Blood in the temples.
- **T.B.-18** Qimai is for stasis of Blood in the occiput.
- **Sishencong**, extra point, for stasis of Blood on the vertex.

It should be emphasized that stasis of Blood does not arise independently but it may stem from various conditions, such as Qi stagnation, Blood deficiency, Blood-Heat, internal Cold and Qi deficiency. The treatment should obviously be aimed at treating the condition underlying the stasis of Blood.

Herbal treatment

(a) Prescription

TONG QIAO HUA XUE TANG
Opening the Orifices and Moving Blood Decoction
Chi Shao *Radix Paeoniae rubrae* 3 g
Chuan Xiong *Rhizoma Ligustici wallichii* 3 g
Tao Ren *Semen Persicae* 9 g
Hong Hua *Flos Carthami tinctorii* 9 g
She Xiang *Secretio Moschus moschiferi* .15 g
Cong Bai *Herba Allii* 3 g

Hong Zao *Fructus Ziziphi jujubae* 7 red dates
Sheng Jiang *Rhizoma Zingiberis officinalis recens* 3 slices
Rice wine

Explanation

- **Chi Shao**, **Chuan Xiong**, **Tao Ren** and **Hong Hua** move Blood. In particular, Chuan Xiong moves Blood, expels Wind and is a major herb for headaches.
- **She Xiang** opens the orifices. Since this substance is extremely expensive it could be replaced by the much cheaper Shi Chang Pu *Rhizoma Acori graminei*. The dose of the latter herb would of course be higher, e.g. 6–9 g.
- **Cong Bai**, **Sheng Jiang** and **rice wine** penetrate the Yang and help to open the orifices. They also reach upwards and will help to relieve headaches.
- **Hong Zao** nourishes Blood and harmonizes.

This prescription is specific for headaches from stasis of Blood and is applicable for chronic headaches, especially, but not exclusively, in old people with a dark complexion. It is also suitable for women with Blood that is deficient, dry and stagnant and for children suffering from Child Nutritional Impairment (*Gan* disease).

(b) Prescription

TAO HONG SI WU TANG
Persica-Carthamus Four Substances Decoction
Shu Di Huang *Radix Rehmanniae glutinosae praeparata* 12 g
Dang Gui *Radix Angelicae sinensis* 10 g
Bai Shao *Radix Paeoniae albae* 12 g
Chuan Xiong *Radix Ligustici wallichii* 8 g
Tao Ren *Semen Persicae* 6 g
Hong Hua *Flos Carthami tinctorii* 6 g

Explanation

- **Si Wu Tang** nourishes and moves Blood.
- **Tao Ren** and **Hong Hua** move Blood. These two herbs are frequently used in combination to move Blood as one is a seed and therefore sinking, the other a light flower and therefore

floating and ascending. The combination and opposition of sinking and ascending movements sets the Blood in motion.

Herbs

- **Chuan Xiong** *Radix Ligustici wallichii* moves Blood and, more specifically, the Qi portion of Blood, and is an important herb for headaches.
- **Hong Hua** *Flos Carthami tinctorii* moves Blood and, being a flower and very light, it has a floating movement and affects the top part of the body.
- **San Qi** *Radix Pseudoginseng* moves Blood (besides stopping bleeding) and is frequently used for chronic headaches, especially in combination with Tian Ma *Rhizoma Gastrodiae elatae*.
- **Yan Hu Suo** *Rhizoma Corydalis yanhusuo* moves Qi and Blood and is a major herb to stop pain.

(i) Patent remedy

YAN HU SUO ZHI TONG PIAN
Corydalis Stopping Pain Tablet
Yan Hu Suo *Rhizoma Corydalis yanhusuo*

Explanation

This remedy, consisting only of one herb, can be used for chronic headaches from stasis of Blood. Yan Hu Suo moves Blood and has excellent analgesic properties.

The tongue presentation appropriate to this remedy is a slightly Purple body.

(ii) Patent remedy

WU JIN WAN
Black Gold Pill
Yi Mu Cao *Herba Leonori heterophylli*
San Leng *Rhizoma Sparganii*
E Zhu *Rhizoma Curcumae zedoariae*
Xiang Fu *Rhizoma Cyperi rotundi*
Yan Hu Suo *Rhizoma Corydalis yanhusuo*
Wu Zhu Yu *Fructus Evodiae rutaecarpae*

Xiao Hui Xiang *Fructus Foeniculi vulgaris*
Mu Xiang *Radix Saussureae*
Bai Shao *Radix Paeoniae albae*
Chuan Xiong *Radix Ligustici wallichii*
Dang Gui *Radix Angelicae sinensis*
Shu Di Huang *Radix Rehmanniae glutinosae praeparata*
Bu Gu Zhi *Fructus Psoraleae corylifoliae*
Pu Huang *Pollen Typhae*
Ai Ye Tan *Folium Artemisiae carbonisatum*

Explanation

This pill is suitable for headaches from Blood stasis against a background of Blood deficiency and internal Cold. It is particularly indicated for women as it contains the Yi Mu Si Wu Tang *Leonorus Four Substances Decoction*.

Please note that this pill contains herbs (such as San Leng and E Zhu) which strongly move Blood: indeed, they pertain to the category of herbs which "break" Blood. In order to use this pill, therefore, one must be absolutely certain of the diagnosis, i.e. a very severe and chronic stasis of Blood manifesting with a very Purple (Bluish-Purple) tongue and a dark-purple complexion.

(iii) Patent remedy

JIN GU DIE SHANG WAN
Muscle and Bone Traumatic Injury Pill
San Qi *Radix Notoginseng*
Xue Jie *Sanguis Draconis*
Dang Gui *Radix Angelicae sinensis*
Ru Xiang *Gummi Olibanum*
Mo Yao *Myrrha*
Hong Hua *Flos Carthami tinctorii*

Explanation

Although this pill is primarily for traumatic injury of sinews and bones (such as sport injuries), it can be used to treat headaches from stasis of Blood as its chief ingredient, San Qi, is particularly good for headaches.

The tongue presentation appropriate to this remedy is a Purple body.

(iv) Patent remedy

YUNNAN TE CHAN TIAN QI PIAN
Yunnan Specially-Prepared Notoginseng Tablet
San Qi *Radix Notoginseng*

Explanation

This tablet can be used for headaches from Blood stasis as its only ingredient, San Qi, moves Blood and treats headaches.

This remedy is available also as a powder called Sheng Tian Qi Fen *Fresh Notoginseng Powder*.

The tongue presentation appropriate to this remedy is a slightly Purple body.

(v) Patent remedy

TONG JING WAN
Penetrating Menses Pill
E Zhu *Rhizoma Curcumae zedoariae*
San Leng *Rhizoma Sparganii*
Chi Shao *Radix Paeoniae rubrae*
Hong Hua *Flos Carthami tinctorii*
Chuan Xiong *Radix Ligustici wallichii*
Dang Gui *Radix Angelicae sinensis*
Dan Shen *Radix Salviae miltiorrhizae*

Explanation

Although this pill is primarily to move Blood and regulate menstruation, it can be used for headaches from stasis of Blood as two of its ingredients, Chuan Xiong and Hong Hua, relieve headaches.

Please note that this remedy has the same *pinyin* spelling, but different meaning and ingredients, as the other remedy Tong Jing Wan which means "dysmenorrhoea pill".

The tongue presentation appropriate to this remedy is a Reddish-Purple body.

Table 1.1 compares and contrasts the above five remedies for headaches from stasis of Blood.

Case history

A 31-year-old woman had been suffering from chronic headaches since her childhood. The headaches occurred on either side of the head (along the Gall-Bladder channel) and settling behind either eyeball. The pain was severe and stabbing in nature and was accompanied by vomiting and diarrhoea. Her periods were scanty. Her tongue was Pale and slightly Bluish-Purple, with dark-swollen veins underneath it. Her pulse was Deep and Minute.

Diagnosis
This pattern presents a combination of Liver-Yang rising and stasis of Blood in the head. The headaches occurring along the Gall-Bladder channel are a manifestation of Liver-Yang rising. The vomiting and diarrhoea are due to Liver-Qi stagnation invading Stomach and Spleen preventing the former from descending (hence vomiting) and the latter from ascending (hence diarrhoea).

In this case, Liver-Yang rising derives from deficiency of Blood as evidenced by the scanty periods, Pale tongue and Minute pulse.

In addition, the long-standing headaches led to stasis of Blood in the head, hence the stabbing nature of the pain and the Bluish-Purple tongue with dark-distended veins underneath.

Principle of treatment
In this case it is possible to treat both the Root

Table. 1.1 Comparison of remedies for Blood-stasis headaches.

Remedy	Pattern	Symptoms	Tongue
YAN HU SUO ZHI TONG PIAN	Blood stasis	General Blood-stasis symptoms	Purple
WU JIN WAN	Blood stasis, Blood deficiency, Internal Cold	Irregular-painful periods with clots, chilliness, tiredness, dry skin, headaches before periods	Bluish-Purple
JIN GU DIE SHANG WAN	Blood stasis in channels and limbs	Pain in limbs	Purple, Stiff
YUNNAN TE CHAN TIAN QI PIAN	Blood stasis	General Blood-stasis symptoms	Purple
TONG JING WAN	Blood stasis in uterus	Irregular-painful periods with clots, headaches before periods	Reddish-Purple

(deficiency of Liver-Blood) and the Manifestation (stasis of Blood in the head and rising of Liver-Yang). It is therefore necessary to nourish Liver-Blood, move Blood and subdue Liver-Yang.

Acupuncture
The main points used were T.B.-5 Waiguan, P-6 Neiguan, Ren-4 Guanyuan, LIV-8 Ququan, LIV-3 Taichong, SP-6 Sanyinjiao, G.B.-1 Tongziliao and SP-10 Xuehai.

Ren-4, LIV-8 and SP-6 were needled with reinforcing method to nourish Liver-Blood. The other points were needled with even method to move Blood and subdue Liver-Yang.

Explanation
- **Ren-4**, **LIV-8** and **SP-6** were reinforced to nourish Liver-Blood.
- **T.B.-5** was chosen as a distal point to affect the Gall-Bladder channel on the head and subdue Liver-Yang.
- **P-6** was chosen to move Blood in the head.
- **G.B.-1** was chosen as a local point to move Blood in the head.
- **LIV-3** subdues Liver-Yang.
- **SP-10** moves Blood.

Herbal treatment
The prescription chosen was a variation of Tao Hong Si Wu Tang *Prunus-Carthamus Four Substances Decoction* mentioned above.

The only variations made to this prescription were increasing the dosage of Chuan Xiong *Radix Ligustici wallichii* and adding Tian Ma *Rhizoma Gastrodiae elatae* to subdue Liver-Yang.

This patient was completely cured of her headaches in one year. Acupuncture was administered once a month and she took the herbal decoction for 6 months, though with occasional breaks during that time.

11. STOMACH-HEAT

This type of headache occurs on the forehead and it can be acute or chronic. If it appears in the course of a febrile disease it corresponds to the Bright-Yang stage within the 6-Stage patterns of diseases caused by exterior Cold. The Bright-Yang stage is characterized by Heat in the Stomach which may cause intense headache on the forehead. Other symptoms include profuse sweating, intense thirst, fever and an Overflowing-Rapid pulse.

In chronic cases, this type of headache is due to a long-standing condition of Stomach-Heat. This is usually caused by the excessive consumption of hot-energy foods such as meat, spices, fried foods and alcohol. This type of headache is intense and is felt across the forehead. It may be elicited by the consumption of too hot foods or simply by over-eating. Other manifestations include thirst with desire to drink cold water, dry stools, possibly epigastric pain, a thick-yellow tongue coating and a Slippery and Overflowing pulse on the right Middle position.

Treatment principle

Clear Heat, clear the Stomach, subdue rebellious Qi.

Acupuncture

General prescription: ST-44 Neiting, L.I.-4 Hegu, Yintang extra point. Reducing method on ST-44 and L.I.-4 and even method on Yintang.

Explanation

- **ST-44** is the main point to clear Stomach-Heat. Also, being towards the lower extremity of the channel, it will affect the other end, i.e. the head.
- **L.I.-4** clears Heat and affects the head and forehead.
- **Yintang** is used as a local point for headaches on the forehead.

Other points

- **ST-34** Liangqiu is the Accumulation point of the Stomach channel and, as such, it stops pain.
- **Du-23** Shangxing can be used as a local point to affect the forehead and eyes.
- **ST-8** Touwei can be used as a local point for headaches on the forehead.

Herbal treatment

Prescription

QING WEI SAN
Clearing the Stomach Powder
Huang Lian *Rhizoma Coptidis* 5 g
Sheng Di Huang *Radix Rehmanniae glutinosae* 12 g

Mu Dan Pi *Cortex Moutan radicis* 9 g
Dang Gui *Radix Angelicae sinensis* 6 g
Sheng Ma *Rhizoma Cimicifugae* 6 g

Explanation

- **Huang Lian** clears Stomach-Heat.
- **Sheng Di** cools Blood and nourishes Yin.
- **Mu Dan Pi** cools Blood and clears Heat.
- **Dang Gui** nourishes and harmonizes Blood.
- **Sheng Ma** clears Stomach-Heat.

Herbs

- **Shi Gao** *Gypsum* clears Stomach-Heat at the Qi level.
- **Zhi Mu** *Radix Anemarrhenae asphodeloidis* clears Stomach-Heat and nourishes Yin.
- **Zhu Ye** *Herba Lophatheri gracilis* clears Stomach-Heat especially when manifesting in the face region.
- **Lu Gen** *Rhizoma Phragmitis communis* clears Stomach-Heat and promotes fluids. It is especially indicated if thirst is pronounced. It is light and floating and will therefore affect the head.

(a) Patent remedy

HUANG LIAN SHANG QING WAN (PIAN)
Coptis Upward-Clearing Pill (Tablet)
Huang Lian *Rhizoma Coptidis*
Chuan Xiong *Radix Ligustici wallichii*
Jing Jie *Herba seu Flos Schizonepetae tenuifoliae*
Fang Feng *Radix Ledebouriellae sesloidis*
Huang Qin *Radix Scutellariae baicalensis*
Jie Geng *Radix Platycodi grandiflori*
Shi Gao *Gypsum fibrosum*
Ju Hua *Flos Chrysanthemi morifolii*
Bai Zhi *Radix Angelicae dahuricae*
Gan Cao *Radix Glycyrrhizae uralensis*
Da Huang *Rhizoma Rhei*
Man Jing Zi *Fructus Viticis*
Lian Qiao *Fructus Forsythiae suspensae*
Xuan Fu Hua *Flos Inulae*
Huang Bo *Cortex Phellodendri*
Bo He *Herba Menthae*
Zhi Zi *Fructus Gardeniae jasminoidis*

Explanation

This pill is for Stomach-Fire rather than Stomach-Heat. It drains Stomach-Fire by moving downwards (with Da Huang) and it is used for symptoms of Fire-Poison in the head deriving from Stomach-Fire. These are: mouth ulcers, parotitis, fever, headache, swollen-red-painful gums, tonsillitis, conjunctivitis, etc.

This remedy can be used for Stomach-Fire headaches due to the presence of several herbs which relieve headaches: these are Chuan Xiong, Jing Jie, Fang Feng, Ju Hua, Bai Zhi, Man Jing Zi and Bo He.

Before using this pill it is essential that one understands its nature and effect clearly. First of all, it moves downwards and it should only be used if the tongue is Red and has a thick-yellow and dry coating. Secondly, it should be stopped if diarrhoea occurs. Thirdly, it is only for acute headaches and is not at all suitable for long-term use. Fourthly, it is for Stomach-Fire rather than Stomach-Heat and therefore there should be such symptoms as constipation or dry stools, a dry tongue coating, dark urine, a red face, thirst and a Deep-Full pulse.

(b) Patent remedy

SHUANG LIAO HOU FENG SAN
Double-Ingredient Throat-Wind Powder
Niu Huang *Calculus Bovis*
Bing Pian *Borneol*
Gan Cao *Radix Glycyrrhizae uralensis*
Qing Dai *Indigo naturalis*
Zhen Zhu *Margarita*
Huang Lian *Rhizoma Coptidis*
Shan Dou Gen *Radix Sophorae subprostratae*

Explanation

Although this remedy is primarily for throat infections occurring on a background of Stomach-Heat, it can be used also for Stomach-Heat headaches and especially sinus headaches.

The tongue presentation appropriate to this remedy is a sticky-yellow coating.

DEFICIENCY HEADACHES

Deficiency headaches are due to not enough

Qi or Blood reaching the head. In the case of Qi deficiency, Qi fails to reach the head to brighten the orifices and in the case of Blood deficiency, Blood fails to nourish the brain.

All Deficiency headaches are characterized by a dull ache and by coming in bouts. The headaches are relieved by rest and aggravated by excessive work.

The three main types of Deficiency headaches are:

– Qi deficiency
– Blood deficiency
– Kidney deficiency.

1. QI DEFICIENCY

This headache is due to deficient Qi failing to ascend to the head to brighten the orifices. It can be due to deficiency of Qi of the Stomach, Spleen, Lungs or Heart. It may manifest in the whole head or frequently on the forehead only, especially when it is due to Stomach-Qi deficiency.

This headache comes in bouts, it is dull in nature and is alleviated by rest and aggravated by excessive work. It is also better lying down and is worse in the mornings.

Other manifestations include poor appetite, tiredness, loose stools, slight breathlessness and an Empty pulse. In case of Heart-Qi deficiency there would also be some slight palpitations and breathlessness on exertion. The "Simple Questions" in chapter 18 says that in headaches from deficiency of Qi of the Heart or Lungs, the Front position pulse (of both right and left) can feel Short, i.e. not quite reaching the top of the pulse position.[10]

Treatment principle

Tonify and raise Qi.

Acupuncture

General prescription: ST-36 Zusanli, Ren-6 Qihai, SP-6 Sanyinjiao, Du-20 Baihui. All with reinforcing method. Du-20 with direct moxibustion.

Explanation

– **ST-36** and **SP-6** in combination strongly tonify Qi.
– **Ren-6** tonifies and raises Qi.
– **Du-20** raises Yang.

Other points

– **L.I.-4** Hegu when reinforced in combination with ST-36, can tonify and raise Qi. For this reason it would be particularly indicated if the headache is on the forehead since this is the area affected by this point.
– **BL-7** Tongtian can be used as a local point to raise Qi, especially if there is some deficiency of the Kidneys.
– **BL-20** Pishu can be used to tonify and raise Qi since this is a function of Spleen-Qi.

Herbal treatment

Prescription

BU ZHONG YI QI TANG
Tonifying the Centre and Benefiting Qi Decoction
Huang Qi *Radix Astragali membranacei* 12 g
Ren Shen *Radix Ginseng* 9 g
Bai Zhu *Rhizoma Atractylodis macrocephalae* 9 g
Dang Gui *Radix Angelicae sinensis* 6 g
Chen Pi *Pericarpium Citri reticulatae* 6 g
Sheng Ma *Rhizoma Cimicifugae* 3 g
Chai Hu *Radix Bupleuri* 3 g

Explanation

– **Huang Qi, Dang Shen, Bai Zhu** and **Zhi Gan Cao** tonify and raise Qi.
– **Chen Pi** regulates Qi and prevents the stagnation that may derive from excessive tonification.
– **Dang Gui** tonifies Blood to help to tonify Qi.
– **Sheng Ma** and **Chai Hu** raise Qi.

Other herbs

– **Ren Shen** *Radix Ginseng* is stronger than Dang Shen *Radix Codonopsis pilosulae* in tonifying and raising Qi. The original prescription actually includes Ren Shen rather than Dang Shen, but the latter is frequently substituted for the former because of cost.

Patent remedy

BU ZHONG YI QI WAN
Tonifying the Centre and Benefiting Qi Pill

This pill has the same ingredients and func-tions as the homonymous prescription.

The tongue presentation appropriate to this remedy is a slightly Pale body.

2. BLOOD DEFICIENCY

This headache is due to deficient Blood failing to reach the head and nourish the brain. It is slightly more severe in nature than the Qi-defi-ciency headache. It typically affects the top of the head and is related to Blood deficiency of the Liver or Heart. It is often worse in the afternoon or evening and is accompanied by poor memory and lack of concentration. In women, it often oc-curs at the end of the period, as the temporary blood loss aggravates the Blood deficiency. This headache is also better lying down.

Principle of treatment

Nourish Blood, tonify and raise Qi.

Acupuncture

General prescription: ST-36 Zusanli, SP-6 Sanyinjiao, BL-20 Pishu, LIV-8 Ququan, Ren-4 Guanyuan, Du-20 Baihui, BL-15 Xinshu. Tonifying method on all points.

Explanation

- **ST-36**, **SP-6** and **BL-20** nourish Blood and tonify Qi.
- **LIV-8** nourishes Liver-Blood.
- **Ren-4** nourishes Blood.
- **Du-20** raises Qi.
- **HE-5** nourishes Heart-Blood. It is necessary to tonify Heart-Blood as deficient Heart-Blood not reaching the head is often a feature of this type of headache.

Other points

- **BL-20** Pishu and **BL-18** Ganshu in combination nourish Liver-Blood.
- **Yuyao** is indicated as a local point if the headaches occur behind the eyes.

Herbal treatment

(a) Prescription

BA ZHEN TANG
Eight Precious Decoction
Dang Gui *Radix Angelicae sinensis* 10 g
Chuan Xiong *Radix Ligustici wallichii* 5 g
Bai Shao *Radix Paeoniae albae* 8 g
Shu Di Huang *Radix Rehmanniae glutinosae prae-eparata* 15 g
Ren Shen *Radix Ginseng* 3 g
Bai Zhu *Rhizoma Atractylodis macrocephalae* 10 g
Fu Ling *Sclerotium Poriae cocos* 8 g
Zhi Gan Cao *Radix Glycyrrhizae uralensis prae-parata* 5 g

Explanation

- The first four herbs make the Si Wu Tang *Four Substances Decoction* which nourishes Blood, and the last four make the Si Jun Zi Tang *Four Gentlemen Decoction* which tonifies Qi.

(b) Prescription

SHI QUAN DA BU TANG
Ten Complete Great Tonification Decoction
Ba Zhen Tang *Eight Precious Decoction* plus:
Huang Qi *Radix Astragali membranacei* 8 g
Rou Gui *Cortex Cinnamomi cassiae* 4 g

Explanation

- **Ba Zhen Tang** tonifies Qi and nourishes Blood.
- **Huang Qi** tonifies and raises Qi.
- **Rou Gui** warms the Yang and tonifies the Original Qi.

This prescription is better indicated for head-aches as it contains Huang Qi *Radix Astra-gali membranacei* which tonifies and raises Qi.

However, since it contains Rou Gui *Cortex Cinnamomi cassiae* which is very hot, it is only indicated if there are manifestations of internal Cold.

Herbs

- **Sang Ji Sheng** *Ramulus Loranthi* nourishes Liver-Blood.
- **Shou Wu** *Radix Polygoni multiflori* nourishes Blood and is particularly indicated in chronic cases of Blood deficiency with manifestations of dryness (e.g. dry skin, dry hair and dry eyes).
- **Gou Qi Zi** *Fructus Lycii chinensis* nourishes Blood and benefits the eyes. It is therefore particularly indicated if the headaches occur behind the eyes.
- **Long Yang Rou** *Arillus Euphoriae longanae* nourishes Blood and promotes sleep. It is therefore indicated if the Blood deficiency causes insomnia.
- **Chuan Xiong** *Radix Ligustici wallichii*. This is of course already included in the above two prescriptions, but its dosage could be increased since it is an important and specific herb for headaches.

(i) Patent remedy

BA ZHEN WAN
Eight Precious Pill

This well-known pill has the same ingredients and functions as the homonymous prescription.

The tongue presentation appropriate to this remedy is a Pale and Thin body.

(ii) Patent remedy

SHI QUAN DA BU WAN
Ten Complete Great Tonification Pill
Ba Zhen Wan *Eight Precious Pill*
Huang Qi *Radix Astragali membranacei*
Rou Gui *Cortex Cinnamomi cassiae*

This remedy has the same ingredients and functions as the prescription with the same name.

The tongue presentation appropriate to this remedy is a Pale, Thin, and slightly wet body.

3. KIDNEY DEFICIENCY

This headache is due to deficient Kidney-Essence failing to reach the head and nourish the brain. It may manifest with deficiency of Kidney-Yin or Kidney-Yang as the Essence has a Yin and a Yang aspect. The headache is experienced inside the brain and not in any specific place and is accompanied by dizziness and a feeling of emptiness of the brain. When the Kidney deficiency affects the Bladder channel, the headache may also occur on the occiput.

The headache from Kidney-Yang deficiency is somewhat milder and more similar to that from Qi deficiency, whilst that from Kidney-Yin deficiency is more severe and feels deeper in the head. In both cases the headache may occur after sexual activity.

Other manifestations depend on whether there is a deficiency of Kidney-Yin or Kidney-Yang. In case of Kidney-Yin deficiency there will be a feeling of heat in the evening, scanty urination, dizziness, tinnitus, soreness of the lower back, slight constipation, a Red tongue without coating and a Floating-Empty pulse.

In case of Kidney-Yang deficiency there will be a feeling of cold, soreness of the lower back and knees, abundant-pale urination, a Pale tongue and a Deep and Weak pulse.

Treatment principle

Tonify the Kidneys, nourish Marrow.

Acupuncture

General prescription: KI-3 Taixi, ST-36 Zusanli, SP-6 Sanyinjiao, Du-20 Baihui, G.B.-19 Naokong.
For Kidney-Yin deficiency: Ren-4 Guanyuan.
For Kidney-Yang deficiency: BL-23 Shenshu.

All points should be reinforced. Moxa can be used on KI-3, unless there are pronounced symptoms of Empty-Heat. In case of Kidney-Yang deficiency moxa *must* be used on BL-23. Direct moxa can also be used on Du-20.

Explanation

- **KI-3** tonifies both Kidney-Yin and Kidney-Yang and the Original Qi.

- **ST-36** and **SP-6** tonify Qi and Blood which will help to tonify Yin. SP-6 also tonifies Yin.
- **Du-20** attracts Qi up towards the head and nourishes Marrow.
- **G.B.-19** attracts Kidney-Essence up to the brain, fills Marrow, and is a specific local point for headache from Kidney deficiency. Its name means "empty brain".
- **Ren-4** nourishes Kidney-Yin.
- **BL-23** tonifies Kidney-Yang.

Other points

- **BL-60** Kunlun can be used as a distal point to affect the Bladder channel, especially if the headaches are along this channel on the occiput.
- **BL-10** Tianzhu can be used as an adjacent point if the headaches occur on the Bladder channel on the occiput.
- **BL-7** Tongtian can be used as a local point.
- **Du-17** Naohu can be used as an adjacent point to nourish Marrow.

Ancient formula

Du-23 Shangxing, G.B.-20 Fengchi, G.B.-19 Naokong, BL-10 Tianzhu, HE-3 Shaohai ("Great Compendium of Acupuncture").[11]

Herbal treatment

The difference in treatment between Kidney-Yin and Kidney-Yang deficiency is more marked in herbal medicine than it is in acupuncture.

Kidney-Yang Deficiency

(a) Prescription

YOU GUI WAN
Restoring the Right [Kidney] Pill
Fu Zi *Radix Aconiti carmichaeli praeparata* 3 g
Rou Gui *Cortex Cinnamomi cassiae* 3 g
Du Zhong *Cortex Eucommiae ulmoidis* 6 g
Shan Zhu Yu *Fructus Corni officinalis* 4.5 g
Tu Si Zi *Semen Cuscutae* 6 g
Lu Jiao Jiao *Colla Cornu Cervi* 6 g
Shu Di Huang *Radix Rehmanniae glutinosae praeparata* 12 g

Shan Yao *Radix Dioscoreae oppositae* 6 g
Gou Qi Zi *Fructus Lycii chinensis* 6 g
Dang Gui *Radix Angelicae sinensis* 4.5 g

Explanation
- **Shu Di Huang, Shan Yao** and **Shan Zhu Yu** nourish Kidneys, Stomach and Liver respectively and are a contracted form of the Liu Wei Di Huang Wan *Six-Ingredient Rehmannia Pill*, to nourish Kidney-Yin.
- **Tu Si Zi, Lu Jiao Jiao** and **Du Zhong** tonify Kidney-Yang. Lu Jiao Jiao also nourishes Blood.
- **Gou Qi Zi** and **Dang Gui** nourish Blood.
- **Rou Gui** and **Fu Zi** tonify Kidney-Yang and the Fire of the Gate of Vitality and expel internal Cold.

This formula is particularly indicated for women.

(b) Prescription

JIN GUI SHEN QI WAN
Golden Chest Kidney-Qi Pill
Fu Zi *Radix Aconiti carmichaeli praeparata* 3 g
Gui Zhi *Ramulus Cinnamomi cassiae* 3 g
Shu Di Huang *Radix Rehmanniae glutinosae praeparata* 24 g
Shan Zhu Yu *Fructus Corni officinalis* 12 g
Shan Yao *Radix Dioscoreae oppositae* 12 g
Ze Xie *Rhizoma Alismatis orientalis* 9 g
Mu Dan Pi *Cortex Moutan radicis* 9 g
Fu Ling *Sclerotium Poriae cocos* 9 g

Explanation   This prescription consists of the Liu Wei Di Huang Wan *Six-Ingredient Rehmannia Pill* which nourishes Kidney-Yin, with the addition of:

- **Fu Zi** and **Rou Gui** which strongly tonify and warm Kidney-Yang and tonify the Fire of the Gate of Vitality.

Kidney-Yin Deficiency

(a) Prescription

ZUO GUI WAN
Restoring the Left [Kidney] Pill
Shu Di Huang *Radix Rehmanniae glutinosae praeparata* 15 g
Shan Yao *Radix Dioscoreae oppositae* 9 g

Shan Zhu Yu *Fructus Corni officinalis* 9 g
Gou Qi Zi *Fructus Lycii chinensis* 9 g
Chuan Niu Xi *Radix Cyathulae* 6 g
Tu Si Zi *Semen Cuscutae* 9 g
Lu Jiao *Cornu Cervi* 9 g
Gui Ban Jiao *Colla Plastri Testudinis* 9 g

Explanation
- **Shi Di Huang**, **Shan Yao**, **Shan Zhu Yu** and **Gui Ban Jiao** nourish Kidney-Yin.
- **Gou Qi Zi** nourishes Blood and Yin.
- **Niu Xi** moves Blood and nourishes Liver and Kidneys.
- **Tu Si Zi** and **Lu Jiao** tonify Kidney-Yang.

This formula is particularly indicated for women.

(b) Prescription

LIU WEI DI HUANG WAN
Six-Ingredient Rehmannia Pill
Shu Di Huang *Radix Rehmanniae glutinosae praeparata* 24 g
Shan Zhu Yu *Fructus Corni officinalis* 12 g
Shan Yao *Radix Dioscoreae oppositae* 12 g
Ze Xie *Rhizoma Alismatis orientalis* 9 g
Mu Dan Pi *Cortex Moutan radicis* 9 g
Fu Ling *Sclerotium Poriae cocos* 9 g

Explanation
- **Shu Di Huang** nourishes the Kidneys.
- **Shan Zhu Yu** nourishes the Liver.
- **Shan Yao** nourishes Stomach and Kidneys.
- **Ze Xie** clears Empty-Heat from the Kidneys.
- **Mu Dan Pi** clears Liver-Heat.
- **Fu Ling** drains Dampness from the Stomach.

Herbs
- **Hei Zhi Ma** *Semen Sesami indici* nourishes Liver and Kidney Yin and it extinguishes Wind. It is specific for headaches from Liver and Kidney Yin deficiency.
- **Du Huo** *Radix Angelicae pubescentis* expels Wind-Damp and enters the Bladder channel of the back. It is indicated for headaches from deficiency of Kidney-Yang.
- **Qiang Huo** *Radix Notopterygi* expels Wind-Damp and enters the Bladder channel of the shoulders and neck. It is indicated for headaches from deficiency of Kidney-Yang.

- **Du Zhong** *Radix Eucommiae ulmoidis* tonifies the Kidneys and expels Wind-Damp from the Bladder channel. Indicated for headaches from deficiency of Kidney-Yang.
- **Yu Zhu** *Rhizoma Polygonati odorati* nourishes Stomach-Yin. In addition, it extinguishes Wind and softens and relaxes the sinews. It would therefore help headaches from deficiency of Kidney-Yin.
- **Sang Ji Sheng** *Ramus Loranthi* nourishes Liver and Kidneys and expels Wind-Damp. It is indicated for headaches from Kidney and Liver Yin deficiency.

(c) Prescription

QI JU DI HUANG WAN
Lycium-Chrysanthemum-Rehmannia Pill
Gou Qi Zi *Fructus Lycii chinensis* 9 g
Ju Hua *Flos Chrysanthemi morifolii* 6 g
Shu Di Huang *Radix Rehmanniae glutinosae praeparata* 24 g
Shan Zhu Yu *Fructus Corni officinalis* 12 g
Shan Yao *Radix Dioscoreae oppositae* 12 g
Ze Xie *Rhizoma Alismatis orientalis* 9 g
Mu Dan Pi *Cortex Moutan radicis* 9 g
Fu Ling *Sclerotium Poriae cocos* 9 g

Explanation
- **Gou Qi Zi** nourishes Liver-Blood and Liver-Yin and brightens the eyes.
- **Ju Hua** brightens the eyes, subdues Liver-Yang and relieves headaches.
- The other six herbs constitute the Liu Wei Di Huang Wan.

This prescription nourishes Liver- and Kidney-Yin, subdues Liver-Yang, brightens the eyes and is particularly indicated for headaches as it contains Ju Hua.

(i) Patent remedy

JIN GUI SHEN QI WAN
Golden Chest Kidney-Qi Pill

This pill has the same ingredients and functions as the homonymous prescription.

The tongue presentation appropriate to this remedy is a Pale and wet body.

(ii) Patent remedy

QI JU DI HUANG WAN

Lycium-Chrysanthemum-Rehmannia Pill
Gou Qi Zi *Fructus Lycii chinensis*
Ju Hua *Flos Chrysanthemi morifolii*
Shu Di Huang *Radix Rehmanniae glutinosae prae-parata*
Shan Zhu Yu *Fructus Corni officinalis*
Shan Yao *Radix Dioscoreae oppositae*
Ze Xie *Rhizoma Alismatis orientalis*
Mu Dan Pi *Cortex Moutan radicis*
Fu Ling *Sclerotium Poriae cocos*

Explanation   This pill has the same ingredients and functions as the homonymous prescription. It is very effective for Liver-Yang headaches occurring on a background of Liver- and/or Kidney-Yin deficiency.

The tongue presentation appropriate to this remedy is a Red body without coating or with a rootless coating.

Case history

A woman of 45 complained of persistent headaches on the back of the neck and head extending over the top of the head to the eyes. She also suffered from lower back-ache. She had been experiencing these symptoms for two years since she had a kidney infection. She had been diagnosed as having pyelonephritis and was put on antibiotics. She also had a tendency to constipation and the urine was scanty and dark at times. She sweated at night on most nights. Her tongue was slightly Red with a yellow coating which was thick on the root and rather rootless in the centre. Her pulse was Fine and very slightly Wiry in both Rear positions.

Diagnosis
The headaches were of a Deficiency nature and were caused by Kidney-Yin deficiency. They clearly occurred along the Bladder channel. Her main condition was one of Kidney-Yin deficiency (lower back-ache, night-sweating, dark-scanty urine, constipation, Fine pulse and Red tongue) with Damp-Heat in the Bladder (thick-yellow coating on the root of the tongue, slightly Wiry pulse on both Rear positions). In addition, there was also some Stomach-Yin deficiency (slightly rootless tongue coating).

Principle of treatment
First resolve Damp-Heat from the Bladder, then nourish Kidney-Yin.

Acupuncture
The main points used initially were LU-7 Lieque and KI-6 Zhaohai (Directing Vessel), SP-6 Sanyinjiao and SP-9 Yinlingquan. Later on (after a few weeks), other points were added such as Ren-12 Zhongwan, ST-36 Zusanli, BL-10 Tianzhu, BL-60 Kunlun and KI-3 Taixi.

Explanation
– **LU-7** Lieque and **KI-6** Zhaohai open the Directing Vessel and nourish Kidney-Yin.
– **SP-6** Sanyinjiao and **SP-9** Yinlingquan resolve Damp-Heat in the Lower Burner.
– **Ren-12** Zhongwan and **ST-36** Zusanli were used to nourish Stomach-Yin.
– **BL-10** Tianzhu was used as a local point to relieve the headaches along the Bladder channel.
– **BL-60** Kunlun was used as a distal point to open the Bladder channel and relieve the headaches.
– **KI-3** Taixi was used to nourish Kidney-Yin.

Herbal treatment
Two prescriptions were used. Applying the principle of treating the Manifestation before the Root in this case, a variation of Ba Zheng San *Eight Upright Powder* was used first for a few weeks to resolve Damp-Heat in the Bladder. This was followed by a variation of the Zhi Bo Ba Wei Wan *Anemarrhena-Phellodendron Eight-Ingredient Pill* to nourish Kidney-Yin and resolve Damp-Heat simultaneously.

The variation of the *Eight Upright Powder* used was:

– **Che Qian Zi** *Semen Plantaginis* 6 g
– **Shan Zhi Zi** *Fructus Gardeniae jasminoidis* 4 g
– **Mu Tong** *Caulis Akebiae* 3 g
– **Da Huang** *Radix Rhei* 3 g
– **Bian Xu** *Herba Polygoni avicularis* 4 g
– **Fu Ling** *Sclerotium Poriae cocos* 6 g
– **Zhu Ling** *Sclerotim Polypori umbellati* 6 g
– **Gui Zhi** *Ramulus Cinnamomi cassiae* 2 g
– **Yi Yi Ren** *Semen Coicis lachryma jobi* 6 g
– **Bai Zhu** *Radix Atractylodis macrocephalae* 4 g

The variation of the *Anemarrhena-Phellodendron Eight-Ingredient Pill* was:

– **Zhi Mu** *Rhizoma Anemarrhenae asphodeloidis* 3 g
– **Huang Bo** *Cortex Phellodendri* 6 g
– **Shu Di Huang** *Radix Rehmanniae glutinosae praeparata* 9 g
– **Ze Xie** *Rhizoma Alismatis orientalis* 3 g
– **Shan Yao** *Radix Dioscoreae oppositae* 6 g
– **Fu Ling** *Sclerotium Poriae cocos* 6 g
– **Shan Zhu Yu** *Fructus Corni officinalis* 4 g
– **Mu Dan Pi** *Cortex Moutan radicis* 3 g
– **Bai Zhu** *Radix Atractylodis macrocephalae* 6 g
– **Dang Shen** *Radix Codonopsis pilosulae* 6 g
– **Sang Ji Sheng** *Ramulus Loranthi* 6 g

Explanation
The first prescription was used to resolve Damp-Heat from the Lower Burner. Qu Mai *Herba Dianthi*, Hua

Shi *Talcum*, Deng Xin Cao *Medulla Junci* and Gan Cao *Radix Glycyrrhizae uralensis* were omitted as there was no burning on urination. Fu Ling *Sclerotium Poriae cocos*, Zhu Ling *Sclerotium Polypori umbellati* and Yi Yi Ren *Semen Coicis lachryma jobi* were added to help to eliminate Dampness. Bai Zhu *Rhizoma Atractylodis macrocephalae* was added to tonify the Spleen and help to drain Dampness.

The second prescription was used to nourish Kidney-Yin and simultaneously eliminate Damp-Heat from the Lower Burner.

To this was added Bai Zhu *Rhizoma Atractylodis macrocephalae* and Dang Shen *Radix Codonopsis pilosulae* to tonify the Spleen, and Sang Ji Sheng *Ramulus Loranthi* to nourish Liver and Kidney and expel Wind-Dampness. This last herb would help to stop the back pains.

This patient achieved a complete improvement of her condition after 6 months of treatment.

Prognosis and prevention

Both acupuncture and Chinese herbs are extremely effective for headaches and migraine. Results, however, are not necessarily always achieved quickly. Obviously the longer a person has been suffering from headaches, the longer it will take to treat them. Very often we see patients who have been suffering from headaches for 20 years or more: in these cases the treatment will necessarily take many months or even over a year.

The three most difficult types of headaches to treat are those from Phlegm, Wind-Phlegm and stasis of Blood.

As for prevention, this follows logically from what was said about aetiology. A person who is prone to headaches or someone who has been successfully treated for headaches should refrain from excessive sexual activity and overwork. They should have enough rest and sleep and they should avoid eating sour foods (as defined above in this chapter) and drinking coffee. If they suffer from a deficiency they should have enough rest, and especially lie down for a short time after lunch.

If a person has been successfully treated for headaches from Liver-Yang, Liver-Fire, Liver-Qi stagnation or Liver-Wind, they should pay attention to their emotional state and avoid getting angry.

Western differential diagnosis

SYNOPSIS OF CAUSES

1. INTRACRANIAL

(a) INFLAMMATORY

Meningitis

(b) NON-INFLAMMATORY

  (i) Vascular

    Migraine, cerebral haemorrhage

  (ii) Neoplastic

    Cerebral tumour

  (iii) Hypertensive

    Essential hypertension, secondary hypertension (glomerulo-nephritis)

2. CRANIAL

Sinusitis, otitis media

3. EXTRA-CRANIAL

Glaucoma, cervical spondylosis, trigeminal neuralgia

SYMPTOMATOLOGY

1. INTRACRANIAL

(a) INFLAMMATORY

Meningitis

This is an inflammation of the meninges occurring during a febrile disease. It strikes infants, children or young adults. Two thirds of cases occur before the age of 5.

Meningitis often starts during a viral infection such as influenza or a bacterial infection such as a respiratory or ear infection.

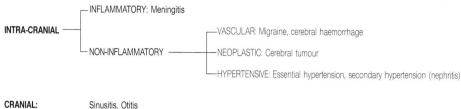

INTRA-CRANIAL ─┬─ INFLAMMATORY: Meningitis

└─ NON-INFLAMMATORY ─┬─ VASCULAR: Migraine, cerebral haemorrhage

─ NEOPLASTIC: Cerebral tumour

─ HYPERTENSIVE: Essential hypertension, secondary hypertension (nephritis)

CRANIAL: Sinusitis, Otitis

EXTRA-CRANIAL: Glaucoma, cervical spondylosis, trigeminal neuralgia

Fig. 1.11   Synopsis of causes of headache

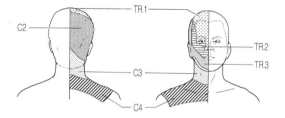

Fig. 1.12   Nerves to head

The main manifestations are a severe headache, fever, vomiting, neck rigidity and, in severe cases, mental confusion.

The Brudzinski sign is positive: with the patient supine and the chest held firmly to the bed, try to flex the neck. In meningitis, this procedure causes involuntary flexion of the hips (Fig. 1.13).

The diagnosis of headache from meningitis is obvious from its acute onset, the age of the patient, the fever and the neck rigidity. The headache is generalized, radiating to the neck (Fig. 1.14).

(b) NON-INFLAMMATORY

(i) Vascular

Migraine

This is the most frequent cause of recurrent headaches. It consists in an initial constriction of the head arteries (giving rise to prodromal symptoms) followed by vasodilatation and distension of the vessels (which causes a throbbing pain). The main manifestations are a unilateral, severe and throbbing pain, photophobia, nausea and possibly vomiting.

The attacks are precipitated by stress, cheese, chocolate, red wine and the contraceptive pill.

The headache is located around the eye, radiating to the side of the head; it is unilateral or bilateral (Fig. 1.15).

Cerebral (sub-arachnoid) haemorrhage

This is more frequent in males over 40. The main manifestations are an intense head pain,

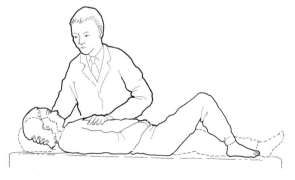

Fig. 1.13   Brudzinski sign

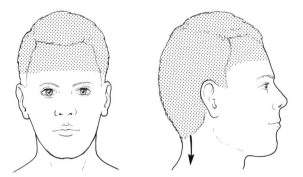

Fig. 1.14   Location of headache in meningitis

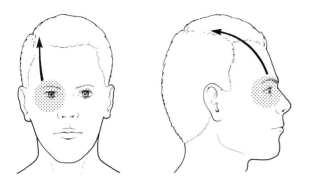

Fig. 1.15 Location of headache in migraine

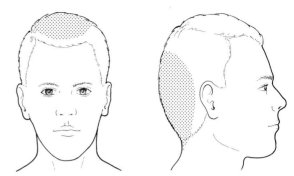

Fig. 1.17 Location of headache in hypertension

neck rigidity and vomiting followed by loss of consciousness.

(ii) Neoplastic

Cerebral tumour

This is an uncommon cause of headache but if a person develops headaches which become *progressively* worse in terms of frequency, duration and intensity and are accompanied by vertigo, vomiting and intellectual impairment, a cerebral tumour should be suspected. The headache eventually becomes continuous (Fig. 1.16).

The "grasp reflex" may be observed: if an object is put on the palm of the hand between thumb and index finger, the patient will automatically grasp it. This reflex action is only present on the side opposite to the location of the tumour.

(iii) Hypertensive

Essential hypertension

This indicates a persistent high blood pressure without an apparent cause. It occurs in persons between 40 and 70.

The main manifestations are a vertical (on top of the head) or occipital headache, occipital stiffness, giddiness, tinnitus, irritability and, in a few cases, epistaxis. The main sign is, of course, a raised diastolic and/or systolic blood pressure. However, it is not at all uncommon to see patients with raised blood pressure without any of the above symptoms. The headache from hypertension can occur either on the top of the head or on the occiput and is accompanied by a pronounced stiffness of the neck muscles (Fig. 1.17).

Secondary hypertension

This a raised blood pressure secondary to other factors, the most frequent of them being chronic glomerulo-nephritis (see ch. 22, "Oedema").

The main manifestations, apart from a raised blood pressure and a headache, are an ache in the loins, tiredness, oedema and albuminuria.

2. CRANIAL

SINUSITIS

This is a common complaint in industrialized countries. It is characterized by inflammation of the sinuses.

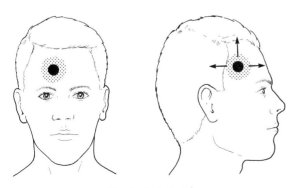

Fig. 1.16 Location of headache in brain tumour

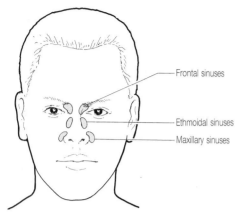

Fig. 1.18   Location of headache in sinusitis

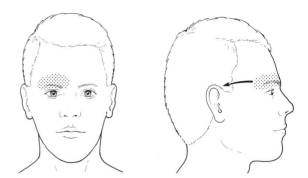

Fig. 1.20   Location of headache in glaucoma

The headache from sinusitis is easily distinguished from that from other causes as it is clearly located on the face in correspondence with the frontal, ethmoidal or maxillary sinuses (Fig. 1.18).

Other manifestations include a runny nose, a post-nasal discharge and a characteristic feeling of muzziness of the face.

OTITIS

This may be a cause of headache in a small child. Very often the child may not be able to distinguish the source of pain and may complain of a "headache" when he or she has an earache.

The diagnosis is fairly obvious as this type of headache will occur in a small child during a febrile disease and there may be a discharge from the ear (Fig. 1.19).

3. EXTRA-CRANIAL

GLAUCOMA

This consists in a raised intra-ocular fluid pressure. It is rare before middle-age. It may cause a headache around or behind the eyes which is easily mistaken for migraine. It is usually worse in the evening and is accompanied by the appearance of "halos" around lights and blurred vision (Fig. 1.20).

CERVICAL SPONDYLOSIS

This term includes arthritis of the cervical spine or cervical disc degeneration. This causes an occipital headache with ache extending to the top of the shoulders and neck (Fig. 1.21). There is marked tenderness on pressure on the neck and shoulder muscles.

X-rays of the cervical spine usually show a

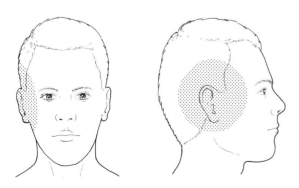

Fig. 1.19   Location of headache in otitis

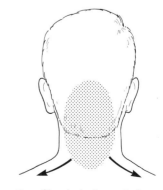

Fig. 1.21   Location of headache in cervical spondylosis

narrowing of the intervertebral spaces and osteophyte formation.

TRIGEMINAL NEURALGIA

This is an inflammation of one or more of the three trigeminal nerves (which are part of the cranial nerves). It is usually seen in the elderly. The pain is unilateral and it is usually very intense lasting for a short time. The pain can occur on the forehead and eye, cheek or temple and jaw according to the nerve involved (Fig. 1.22).

Finally, a word should be said about Western medication for headaches. Of all the various drugs used for migraine, ergotamine tartrate (Cafergot) is, in my opinion, the most detrimental one. It not only produces side-effects such as nausea and tingling of the limbs, but, in my opinion, its long-term use only makes the headaches more frequent. This occurs for two reasons: first of all, ergotamine tartrate (with a chemical structure somewhat similar to LSD) is a powerful vaso-constrictor (this stops the acute headache), but vaso-constriction is inevitably followed by vaso-dilatation which is going to

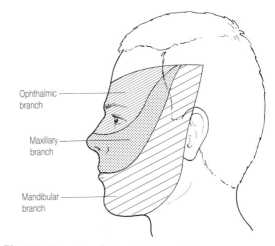

Fig. 1.22 Location of trigeminal neuralgia

cause the next headache. Secondly, most preparations of ergotamine tartrate also include caffeine which is also a vaso-constrictor, but, as for ergotamine, vaso-constriction is only followed by a worse vaso-dilatation. The role of caffeine in headaches has already been discussed in this chapter (see also note 2). For these reasons, I always advise patients who take this medication, to come off it if at all possible. There is no danger in stopping this drug abruptly.

Table 1.2 Synopsis of causes of headaches.

Disease	Pathology	Symptoms	Signs
Meningitis	Inflammation of meninges	Severe headache, vomiting	Rigidity of neck, fever
Migraine	First contraction, then dilation of the arteries	Unilateral headache, photophobia, vomiting	Red eyes
Sub-arachnoid haemorrhage	Bleeding between arachnoid and pia mater from aneurysm	Sudden, violent headache, vomiting, confusion	Loss of consciousness, rigidity of neck, dilated pupils, rapid pulse, hemiplegia
Cerebral tumour	Tumour of brain	Headache, vertigo, poor memory, vomiting	Slow pulse, "grasp reflex"
Essential hypertension	Raised blood pressure	Headache on top or on occiput, giddiness, tinnitus	Occipital stiffness, retinal arteriosclerosis
Nephritis-hypertension	Inflammation of kidney parenchyma	Headache	Oedema, scanty urination, albuminuria, pale face, raised blood pressure
Sinusitis	Inflammation of sinuses	Facial pain	Runny nose
Otitis media	Ear infection	Pain around ear and mastoid	Discharge from ear
Glaucoma	Raised intra-ocular pressure	Blurred vision, headache around eyes, halos around lights	
Cervical spondylosis	Arthritis of cervical spine or degeneration of cervical discs	Headache and ache of neck muscles, stiffness	Tenderness of neck muscles on pressure, "creaking" neck
Trigeminal neuralgia	Inflammation of trigeminal nerves	Intense facial pain in short bursts	

END NOTES

1. For a more detailed discussion of this subject see Maciocia G 1989 The Foundations of Chinese Medicine, Churchill Livingstone, Edinburgh, p. 137.
2. 1970 Journal of the American Medical Association 213:628. An article in this journal states that caffeine is one of the more frequent causes of chronic headaches.
3. Wu Zhan Ren-Yu Zhi Gao 1987 Correct Seal of Medical Circles (*Yi Lin Zheng Yin* 医林正印), Jiangsu Science Publishing House, Nanjing. Written by Ma Zhao Sheng and first published in 1605.
4. 1979 The Yellow Emperor's Classic of Internal Medicine — Simple Questions (*Huang Ti Nei Jing Su Wen* 黄帝内经素问), People's Health Publishing House, Beijing Ch. 17, p. 98. First published *c.* 100 BC.
5. Lu Yi Hua 1897 Medical Talk from the Deserted Cottage (*Leng Hu Yi Hua* 冷庐医话), cited in 1981 Differentiation of Diseases and Patterns in Internal Medicine, Heilongjiang People's Publishing House, p. 331.
6. Zhang Jie Bin 1982 Classic of Categories (*Lei Jing* 类经), People's Health Publishing House, Beijing, p. 325. First published 1624.
7. Cited in Yang Jia San 1989 Acupuncture (*Zhen Jiu Xue* 针灸学), People's Health Publishing House, Beijing, p. 614.
8. Simple Questions, p. 141.
9. Li Dong Yuan 1976 Discussion on Stomach and Spleen (*Pi Wei Lun* 脾胃论), People's Publishing House, p. 362. First published 1249.
10. Simple Questions, Ch. 18, p. 111.
11. Cited in Acupuncture, p. 614.

Dizziness 2

眩
晕

Dizziness in Chinese medicine is called *Xuan Yun*. *Xuan* means "blurred vision", while *Yun* means "dizziness". This symptom may range from a very slight dizziness, sometimes only on changing posture, to very severe vertigo with loss of balance when everything around the patient seems to be spinning. The term "dizziness" also includes the very common sensation of "muzziness" or "fuzziness" and a heavy feeling as if the head was full of cotton wool with inability to think properly and concentrate.

The first reference to dizziness occurs in the "Yellow Emperor's Classic of Internal Medicine" which links it to various patterns. The "Simple Questions" in chapter 74 relates it to Liver-Wind: *"Wind causes dizziness and it pertains to the Liver."*[1] The "Spiritual Axis" in chapter 28 attributes dizziness to Qi not reaching the head: *"When the Qi of the Upper Burner is deficient, the brain is not full . . . [this causes] dizziness and blurred vision."*[2] In chapter 33 it relates it to deficiency of the Sea of Marrow: *"When the Sea of Marrow is deficient . . . there is dizziness."*[3]

Zhu Dan Xi in "Essential Methods of Dan Xi" (1347) relates dizziness to Phlegm and goes as far as saying *"There is no dizziness without Phlegm."*[4] He therefore advocates resolving Phlegm as the main method of treating dizziness. Zhang Jing Yue, on the other hand, in his book "The Complete Book of Jing Yue" (1634) relates dizziness to Deficiency and says: *"Deficiency above causes dizziness"* and *"There is no dizziness without Deficiency."*[5] He therefore recommends tonifying as the main method of treating dizziness.

The differentiation and treatment of dizziness together with those of Headaches can be used to treat hypertension.

Aetiology and pathology

1. EMOTIONAL STRAIN

Anger, frustration, resentment, bottled-up hatred and any other emotion which affects the Liver may cause Liver-Yang to rise. This is a common cause of dizziness of the Full type.

On the other hand, prolonged stagnation of Qi from emotional strain often gives rise to Fire, in this case Liver-Fire which may also cause dizziness. Moreover, Liver-Fire may generate Wind which causes even more intense dizziness, to the point of loss of balance.

2. OVERWORK OR EXCESSIVE SEXUAL ACTIVITY

Overwork and/or excessive sexual activity over many years without adequate rest weakens the Kidneys. These fail to generate enough Marrow to nourish the brain and dizziness results. This is dizziness of the Empty type.

3. DIET

Excessive consumption of greasy foods or dairy products or simply irregular eating may weaken the Spleen and lead to Dampness and Phlegm. When this is associated with a deficiency of Qi in the Upper Burner, the clear Qi cannot rise to the head and turbid Phlegm stagnates there giving rise to dizziness, blurred vision and a sensation of muzziness and heaviness of the head.

As for pathology, the most important distinction to be made in dizziness is that between Deficiency and Excess. The sensation of dizziness quite simply arises either because not enough Qi reaches the head (Deficiency type) or because there is a pathogenic factor in the head which prevents the clear Yang from reaching the head (Excess type).

The main deficiencies which give rise to dizziness are those of Qi and Blood or Kidney-Essence. The main pathogenic factors causing dizziness are Liver-Yang, Liver-Fire, Liver-Wind and Phlegm.

Dizziness deriving from a deficiency is slight and is associated with blurred vision. It may occur only on change of posture. When caused by a Full condition, dizziness is more severe, in serious cases causing loss of balance. When Phlegm is the cause of dizziness it is associated with blurred vision and a sensation of heaviness and muzziness of the head together with an inability to concentrate.

Differentiation and treatment

There are four main patterns causing dizziness:

EXCESS PATTERNS

Liver-Yang, Liver-Fire or Liver-Wind rising
Turbid Phlegm in the head

DEFICIENCY PATTERNS

Qi and Blood Deficiency
Kidney-Essence Deficiency

EXCESS CONDITIONS

1. LIVER-YANG, LIVER-FIRE OR LIVER-WIND RISING

CLINICAL MANIFESTATIONS

Liver-Yang

Quite severe dizziness, tinnitus, red face, irritability, propensity to outbursts of anger, headache.
Tongue: slightly Red sides.
Pulse: Wiry.

Liver-Fire

Red face, thirst, bitter taste, dry stools, scanty dark urine, Red tongue with dry-yellow coating and a Rapid-Wiry-Full pulse.

Liver-Wind

More severe dizziness, vertigo and loss of balance, tremors.

TREATMENT PRINCIPLE

Subdue Liver-Yang, nourish Liver-Yin or Liver-Blood and Kidney-Yin if necessary.
Liver-Fire: drain Liver-Fire.
Liver-Wind: subdue Liver-Wind.

ACUPUNCTURE

LIV-3 Taichong, G.B.-20 Fengchi, T.B.-5 Waiguan, Du-16 Fengfu, S.I.-3 Houxi, LIV-2 Xingjian, P-6 Neiguan, LIV-8 Ququan, SP-6 Sanyinjiao, KI-3 Taixi. Reducing method on all points, except LIV-8 and KI-3 which should be reinforced.

Explanation

– **LIV-3** and **G.B.-20** subdue Liver-Yang. G.B.-20 is specific for dizziness.
– **T.B.-5** helps to subdue Liver-Yang.
– **Du-16** and **S.I.-3** subdue Liver-Wind.
– **LIV-2** clears Liver-Fire.
– **P-6** indirectly helps to subdue Liver-Yang, calms the Mind and settles the Ethereal Soul.
– **LIV-8** and **SP-6** nourish Liver-Blood.
– **KI-3** nourishes Kidney-Yin.

HERBAL TREATMENT

Prescription

TIAN MA GOU TENG YIN
Gastrodia-Uncaria Decoction
Tian Ma *Rhizoma Gastrodiae elatae* 9 g
Gou Teng *Ramulus Uncariae* 9 g
Shi Jue Ming *Concha Haliotidis* 6 g
Sang Ji Sheng *Ramulus Loranthi* 9 g
Du Zhong *Radix Eucommiae ulmoidis* 9 g
Chuan Niu Xi *Radix Cyathulae* 9 g
Zhi Zi *Fructus Gardeniae jasminoidis* 6 g
Huang Qin *Radix Scutellariae baicalensis* 9 g
Yi Mu Cao *Herba Leonori heterophylli* 9 g
Ye Jiao Teng *Caulis Polygoni multiflori* 9 g
Fu Shen *Sclerotium Poriae cocos pararadicis* 6 g

Explanation

This formula, which has already been explained in the chapter on Headaches (ch. 1), subdues Liver-Yang and nourishes Liver and Kidneys. It is widely used for dizziness from Liver-Yang or Liver-Wind rising.

Variations

– If there are symptoms and signs of Liver-Fire

(indicated above) either add Long Dan Cao *Radix Gentianae scabrae* or use Long Dan Xie Gan Tang *Gentiana Draining the Liver Decoction* instead, adding Tian Ma *Rhizoma Gastrodiae elatae*, Gou Teng *Ramulus Uncariae* and Shi Jue Ming *Concha Haliotidis*.
– If there is Liver-Wind add Di Long *Pheretima aspergillum*, Zhen Zhu Mu *Concha margaritiferae* and Mu Li *Concha Ostreae*.

Case history

A 70-year-old man had been suffering from vertigo for several years. He was very unsteady on his feet and often used a shopping trolley to steady himself while walking. His blood pressure was raised and he occasionally had blurred vision. His nails were very dry and withered, his complexion was dark and his skin dry. His tongue was Reddish-Purple with a thin yellow coating in the centre but no coating elsewhere. The tongue was also Stiff and dry. His pulse was very Full and Wiry.

Diagnosis
His condition was clearly due to Liver-Yang rising with an underlying deficiency of Liver-Yin. The vertigo was due to Liver-Yang rising which was also reflected in the pulse quality, while Liver-Yin deficiency was evidenced by the blurred vision, the dry skin, the dry and withered nails and the Stiff tongue.

Principle of treatment
The principle of treatment adopted was therefore to nourish Liver-Yin and subdue Liver-Yang.

Acupuncture
The main points used were G.B.-20 Fengchi, T.B.-5 Waiguan, L.I.-4 Hegu and LIV-3 Taichong with even method and LIV-8 Ququan, SP-6 Sanyinjiao and KI-3 with reinforcing method.

Explanation
– **G.B.-20** subdues Liver-Yang and relieves dizziness.
– **T.B.-5** subdues Liver-Yang.
– **L.I.-4**, together with LIV-3, subdues Liver-Yang from the head.
– **LIV-3** subdues Liver-Yang and Liver-Wind.
– **LIV-8**, **SP-6** and **KI-3** nourish Liver-Yin.

Herbal treatment
No herbs were prescribed but only the patent remedy Jiang Ya Wan *Lowering [Blood] Pressure Pill* which subdues Liver-Yang and Liver-Wind and nourishes Liver- and Kidney-Yin.

After six treatments his blood pressure became normal and his dizziness was much relieved. Due to his age and the chronic nature of the condition he continues to receive treatment once a month.

2. TURBID PHLEGM IN THE HEAD

CLINICAL MANIFESTATIONS

Dizziness, a feeling of heaviness and muzziness of the head as if it were full of cotton wool, difficulty in thinking and concentrating especially in the morning, a feeling of oppression of the chest, nausea, poor appetite, a sticky taste.
Tongue: Swollen with a sticky coating.
Pulse: Slippery.

This condition is due to Phlegm obstructing the head so that the clear Yang cannot rise to it and turbid Qi cannot descend. The above manifestations are purely those due to Phlegm. Obviously, the more chronic the condition, the more there will be manifestations of Spleen deficiency.

TREATMENT PRINCIPLE

Dry Dampness, resolve Phlegm, strengthen the Spleen and harmonize the Stomach.

ACUPUNCTURE

Ren-12 Zhongwan, ST-36 Zusanli, SP-3 Taibai, BL-20 Pishu, BL-21 Weishu, Ren-9 Shuifen, SP-9 Yinlingquan, ST-40 Fenglong, ST-41 Jiexi, L.I.-4 Hegu, ST-8 Touwei, Du-20 Baihui. Reinforcing method on Ren-12, ST-36, SP-3, BL-20 and BL-21. Reducing or even method on the others.

Explanation

- **Ren-12, ST-36, SP-3, BL-20** and **BL-21** tonify Stomach and Spleen to resolve Phlegm.
- **Ren-9, SP-9, ST-40** and **ST-41** resolve Dampness and Phlegm.
- **L.I.-4** is used to affect the Stomach channels in the face and regulate the ascending of clear Yang and descending of turbid Qi.
- **ST-8** is a local point specific to resolve Phlegm from the head.

- **Du-20** facilitates the rising of clear Yang to the head.

HERBAL TREATMENT

Prescription

BAN XIA BAI ZHU TIAN MA TANG
Pinellia-Atractylodes-Gastrodia Decoction
Ban Xia *Rhizoma Pinelliae ternatae* 9 g
Tian Ma *Rhizoma Gastrodiae elatae* 6 g
Bai Zhu *Rhizoma Atractylodis macrocephalae* 15 g
Fu Ling *Sclerotium Poriae cocos* 6 g
Chen Pi *Pericarpium Citri reticulatae* 6 g
Gan Cao *Rhizoma Glycyrrhizae uralensis* 4 g
Sheng Jiang *Rhizoma Zingiberis officinalis recens* 1 slice
Da Zao *Fructus Ziziphi jujubae* 2 pieces

Explanation

This formula, which has already been explained in the chapter on Headaches (ch. 1), is specific to resolve Phlegm from the head.

Variations

- To enhance this formula's resolving Phlegm effect add Shi Chang Pu *Rhizoma Acori graminei* to open the orifices and help the descending of turbid Qi.
- If there is a pronounced feeling of nausea add Zhu Ru *Caulis Bambusae in Taeniis*.
- If there is a feeling of fullness in the epigastrium add Bai Dou Kou *Fructus Cardamomi rotundi* and Sha Ren *Fructus seu Semen Amomi*.
- If there is Phlegm and Heat (mental restlessness, headache, bitter taste and a Rapid-Wiry pulse) add Zhu Ru *Caulis Bambusae in Taeniis*, Gua Lou *Semen Trichosanthis* and Huang Qin *Radix Scutellariae baicalensis*, and remove Bai Zhu.
  Alternatively, use Wen Dan Tang *Warming the Gall-Bladder Decoction* especially if the tongue has a Stomach-crack in the centre with a rough-yellow coating inside it and the tongue-body is Red. If this formula is used add Huang Qin *Radix Scutellariae baicalensis*, Huang Lian *Rhizoma Coptidis* and Shi Chang Pu *Rhizoma Acori graminei* to it.

DEFICIENCY CONDITIONS

1. QI AND BLOOD DEFICIENCY

CLINICAL MANIFESTATIONS

Slight dizziness, sometimes only on change of posture, tiredness, dull-pale face, poor memory, insomnia, palpitations, depression, poor appetite.
Tongue: Pale and Thin.
Pulse: Choppy or Fine.
   This is essentially a deficiency of Spleen- and Heart-Blood.

TREATMENT PRINCIPLE

Tonify Qi and nourish Blood, strengthen Stomach and Spleen.

ACUPUNCTURE

ST-36 Zusanli, SP-6 Sanyinjiao, Ren-12 Zhongwan, BL-20 Pishu, BL-21 Weishu, Du-20 Baihui, Ren-6 Qihai, BL-15 Xinshu. Reinforcing method. Moxa should be used.

Explanation

- **ST-36**, **SP-6**, **Ren-12**, **BL-20** and **BL-21** strengthen the Stomach and Spleen and nourish Blood.
- **Du-20** facilitates the rising of clear Qi to the head and relieves dizziness.
- **Ren-6** tonifies Qi in general.
- **BL-15** nourishes Heart-Blood.

HERBAL TREATMENT

Prescription

GUI PI TANG
Tonifying the Spleen Decoction
Ren Shen *Radix Ginseng* 6 g or **Dang Shen** *Radix Codonopsis pilosulae* 12 g
Huang Qi *Radix Astragali membranacei* 15 g
Bai Zhu *Rhizoma Atractylodis macrocephalae* 12 g
Dang Gui *Radix Angelicae sinensis* 6 g
Fu Shen *Sclerotium Poriae cocos pararadicis* 9 g

Suan Zao Ren *Semen Ziziphi spinosae* 9 g
Long Yan Rou *Arillus Euphoriae longanae* 12 g
Yuan Zhi *Radix Polygalae tenuifoliae* 9 g
Mu Xiang *Radix Saussureae* 6 g
Zhi Gan Cao *Radix Glycyrrhizae uralensis praeparata* 4 g
Sheng Jiang *Rhizoma Zingiberis officinalis recens* 3 slices
Hong Zao *Fructus Ziziphi jujubae* 5 dates

Explanation

This formula tonifies Qi and Blood, strengthens Spleen and Heart, and nourishes the brain.

- **Ren Shen**, **Huang Qi** and **Bai Zhu** tonify Qi.
- **Dang Gui** nourishes Blood.
- **Fu Shen** combines with the Qi tonics to prevent Dampness. It also calms the Mind.
- **Suan Zao Ren**, **Long Yan Rou** and **Yuan Zhi** nourish the Heart and calm the Mind.
- **Mu Xiang** moves Qi and is used to counterbalance the cloying nature of the Qi and Blood tonics.
- **Zhi Gan Cao** helps the Qi tonics to tonify Qi and harmonizes.
- **Sheng Jiang** and **Hong Zao** harmonize the formula, harmonize Defensive and Nutritive Qi and help to tonify Spleen-Qi.

Variations

- If a deficiency of Stomach and Spleen in making Blood is more pronounced than a deficiency of Liver-Blood, reduce the dosage of Dang Gui, increase that of Mu Xiang and add Fu Ling *Sclerotium Poriae cocos*, Yi Yi Ren *Semen Coicis lachryma jobi* and Sha Ren *Fructus seu Semen Amomi*.
- If there are symptoms of Cold and epigastric pain add Gui Zhi *Ramulus Cinnamomi cassiae* and Bai Shao *Radix Paeoniae albae*.
- If Blood deficiency is pronounced add Shu Di Huang *Radix Rehmanniae glutinosae praeparata*.
- If Qi deficiency is more pronounced remove Dang Gui and Long Yang Rou and increase the dosage of Huang Qi. Alternatively, use Bu Zhong Yi Qi Tang *Tonifying the Centre and Benefiting Qi Decoction* instead.

2. KIDNEY DEFICIENCY

CLINICAL MANIFESTATIONS

Persistent dizziness with a feeling of emptiness in the brain, tinnitus, depression, exhaustion, waking up during the night, poor memory, sore back and knees.

Tongue: Pale if Yang deficiency, Red and Peeled if Yin deficiency.

Pulse: Deep and Weak if Yang deficiency, Floating-Empty if Yin deficiency.

This is essentially a deficiency of Kidney-Essence; the Essence is failing to nourish Marrow and the brain. This results in a deficiency of the Sea of Marrow, one of the main symptoms of which is dizziness. As the Essence has both a Yin and a Yang aspect, its deficiency may manifest with symptoms of either Kidney-Yang or Kidney-Yin deficiency.

TREATMENT PRINCIPLE

Tonify Kidney-Yang or Kidney-Yin, strengthen the Essence and nourish the Sea of Marrow.

ACUPUNCTURE

Ren-4 Guanyuan, KI-3 Taixi, BL-23 Shenshu, BL-52 Zhishi, S.I.-3 Houxi and BL-62 Shenmai, Du-16 Fengfu, Du-17 Naohu, Du-20 Baihui, G.B.-39 Xuanzhong. Reinforcing method. Use moxa in Kidney-Yang deficiency.

Explanation

- **Ren-4**, **KI-3**, **BL-23** and **BL-52** strengthen Kidney-Yang or Yin (depending on whether moxa is used or not) and nourish the Essence.
- **S.I.-3** and **BL-62**, better for Kidney-Yang deficiency, strengthen the Governing Vessel and nourish Marrow and the brain.
- **Du-16** and **Du-20** are points of the Sea of Marrow according to chapter 33 of the "Spiritual Axis".[6] They stimulate the rising of Qi to the brain and nourish Marrow.
- **Du-17**, called "Brain Window", nourishes Marrow and relieves giddiness.

- **G.B.-39** is the Gathering point of Marrow and therefore nourishes Marrow and relieves dizziness from Kidney deficiency.

HERBAL TREATMENT

(a) Prescription

ZUO GUI WAN
Restoring the Left [Kidney] Pill
Shu Di Huang *Radix Rehmanniae glutinosae praeparata* 15 g
Shan Yao *Radix Dioscoreae oppositae* 9 g
Shan Zhu Yu *Fructus Corni officinalis* 9 g
Gou Qi Zi *Fructus Lycii chinensis* 9 g
Chuan Niu Xi *Radix Cyathulae* 6 g
Tu Si Zi *Semen Cuscutae* 9 g
Lu Jiao *Cornu Cervi* 9 g
Gui Ban Jiao *Colla Plastri Testudinis* 9 g

Explanation

This formula, which has already been explained in the chapter on Headaches (ch. 1), tonifies Kidney-Yin and nourishes the Essence and Marrow. In particular, Lu Jiao and Lu Jiao Jiao (see below) nourish Marrow and the brain. It is particularly suited to women.

Variations

- If there are symptoms of Empty-Heat add Zhi Mu *Rhizoma Anemarrhenae asphodeloidis* and Huang Bo *Cortex Phellodendri*.

(b) Prescription

YOU GUI WAN
Restoring the Right [Kidney] Pill
Fu Zi *Radix Aconiti carmichaeli praeparata* 3 g
Rou Gui *Cortex Cinnamomi cassiae* 3 g
Du Zhong *Cortex Eucommiae ulmoidis* 6 g
Shan Zhu Yu *Fructus Corni officinalis* 4.5 g
Tu Si Zi *Semen Cuscutae* 6 g
Lu Jiao Jiao *Colla Cornu Cervi* 6 g
Shu Di Huang *Radix Rehmanniae glutinosae praeparata* 12 g
Shan Yao *Radix Dioscoreae oppositae* 6 g
Gou Qi Zi *Fructus Lycii chinensis* 6 g
Dang Gui *Radix Angelicae sinensis* 4.5 g

Explanation

This formula, which has already been explained in the chapter on Headaches (ch. 1), tonifies Kidney-Yang. In particular, Lu Jiao Jiao nourishes Marrow.

Case history

A 31-year-old man had been suffering from severe dizziness, slight deafness and tinnitus for one year. His condition had been diagnosed as Meniere's disease. He sometimes sweated at night and felt generally exhausted. He had had a bout of dizziness ten years previously. He also suffered from headaches of a throbbing character on the temples with flickery eyes.

His tongue was slightly Red and the coating was too thin. His pulse was Empty on the deep level and Wiry on both Rear positions.

Diagnosis

This is a clear case of Kidney-Yin deficiency (night-sweating, exhaustion, tongue without enough coating, pulse Empty on the deep level) and Liver-Yang rising (throbbing headache, flickery eyes, Wiry pulse). Thus this is a combined condition of Deficiency (of Kidney-Yin) and Excess (Liver-Yang rising). The dizziness and tinnitus can be accounted for by both Kidney-Yin deficiency and Liver-Yang rising.

Treatment principle

Nourish Kidney-Yin and subdue Liver-Yang.

Herbal treatment

This patient, who had been referred to me by his acupuncturist, sought herbal treatment. The formula used was a variation of Liu Wei Di Huang Wan *Six-Ingredient Rehmannia Pill*:

Shu Di Huang *Radix Rehmanniae glutinosae praeparata* 9 g
Shan Yao *Radix Dioscoreae oppositae* 6 g
Shan Zhu Yu *Fructus Corni officinalis* 4.5 g
Ze Xie *Rhizoma Alismatis orientalis* 4 g
Mu Dan Pi *Cortex Moutan radicis* 4 g
Fu Ling *Sclerotium Poriae cocos* 4.5 g
Shi Jue Ming *Concha Haliotidis* 12 g
Gou Teng *Ramulus Uncariae* 6 g
Tian Ma *Rhizoma Gastrodiae elatae* 6 g
Zhi Gan Cao *Radix Glycyrrhizae uralensis praeparata* 3 g

Explanation

- The first six herbs constitute the Liu Wei Di Huang Wan which nourishes Kidney-Yin.
- **Shi Jue Ming**, **Gou Teng** and **Tian Ma** subdue Liver-Yang.
- **Gan Cao** harmonizes.

Western differentiation

The causes of vertigo in Western medicine may be classified according to the sites which may be:

- Ear
- Eighth cranial nerve
- Brainstem.

EAR

Causes in the ear include wax, otitis media, acute labyrinthitis, Ménière's disease and postural vertigo.

The two most common causes of severe vertigo are acute labyrinthitis and Ménière's disease.

1. ACUTE LABYRINTHITIS

This occurs during an acute febrile disease such as influenza. The patient develops a sense of whirling with a sudden onset. Nausea and vomiting may occur. The patient has to lie flat and the slightest movement brings on the vertigo. The symptoms gradually subside and disappear in 3 to 6 weeks. There is no accompanying tinnitus or hearing loss.

2. MENIERE'S DISEASE

This is characterized by recurring bouts of sudden vertigo, tinnitus and deafness. In the intervals between bouts the patient has complete freedom from vertigo, but the tinnitus and deafness continue.

EIGHTH CRANIAL NERVE

This can be affected by acute meningitis, trauma and tumours. Damage to the eighth nerve produces vertigo, nystagmus (involuntary rapid movement of the eyeball) and hearing loss.

BRAINSTEM

This can be affected by infections (encephalitis,

meningitis), trauma, thrombosis of the posteroinferior cerebellar artery and multiple sclerosis.

Damage to the brainstem causes vertigo and nystagmus but no hearing loss.

Transient vertigo may be caused by a vascular spasm.

END NOTES

1. 1979 The Yellow Emperor's Classic of Internal Medicine — Simple Questions (*Huang Ti Nei Jing Su Wen* 黄帝内经素问), People's Health Publishing House, Beijing, p. 538. First published *c.* 100 BC.
2. 1981 Spiritual Axis (*Ling Shu Jing* 灵枢经), People's Health Publishing House, Beijing, p. 68. First published *c.* 100 BC.
3. Ibid., p. 72.
4. Zhu Dan Xi 1347 Essential Methods of Dan Xi (*Dan Xi Xin Fa* 丹溪心法), cited in Internal Medicine, p. 204.
5. Zhang Jing Yue 1959 The Complete Book of Jing Yue (*Jing Yue Quan Shu* 景岳全书), Shanghai Science Publishing House, Shanghai, p. 320. First published in 1624.
6. Spiritual Axis, p. 73.

Breathlessness ("Chuan") 3 喘 证

Breathlessness was called *"Chuan"* in Chinese Medicine. *Chuan* means "to pant". The symptoms and signs of breathlessness have been described in the "Yellow Emperor's Classic of Internal Medicine". In fact, the "Simple Questions" says in chapter 22: *"When the Lungs are diseased there is panting, cough, breathlessness, pain in the shoulders and back and sweating . . .".*[1] In chapter 62 it says: *"When Qi is in excess [in the chest, tr.] there is panting, cough and breathlessness; when Qi is deficient there is difficulty in breathing with shallow breath".*[2] The "Spiritual Axis" in chapter 20 says: *"When the pathogenic factor is in the Lungs the skin is painful, there are feelings of heat and cold, panting, sweating, cough and pain in the shoulders".*[3]

The "Prescriptions of the Golden Chest" (AD 220) in chapter 7 indicates "panting" as breathlessness at rest with inability to lie down. It also includes a "sound in the throat like a moorhen".[4]

Thus, the term "panting" in Chinese Medicine includes difficulty in breathing, breathing with an open mouth, lifting of the shoulders when breathing and inability to lie down. This could be an acute or chronic state.

Aetiology

1. EXTERNAL PATHOGENIC FACTORS

Invasion of Wind-Cold or Wind-Heat are an important causative factor of breathlessness in many ways. First of all, they can both cause acute breathlessness. Wind-Cold (or Wind-Heat) obstruct the Lungs and prevent its dispersing and descending of Qi: this results in an accumulation of Qi in the chest and breathlessness.

Secondly, an invasion of Wind-Cold or Wind-Heat can trigger off an acute attack in patients suffering from chronic breathlessness.

Thirdly, external Wind in itself is a frequent initial cause for the beginning of what eventually becomes chronic breathlessness. This is especially true in children. If a child suffers from an invasion of Wind-Cold or Wind-Heat (or repeated invasions) and this is not expelled properly (either through lack of treatment, or through improper treatment such as treatment with antibiotics), the external pathogenic factor lodges itself in the Interior and it continuously obstructs the descending of Lung-Qi causing chronic breathlessness.

A frequent consequence of an invasion of Wind is interior Lung-Heat or Phlegm-Heat. Wind-Heat has a strong tendency to create interior Heat from its early stages by its drying action. Wind-Cold too, can turn into Heat once in the Interior. If there is a pre-existing condition of Lung-Heat, Wind-Cold can "lock" the Heat in the Lungs giving rise to breathlessness. As Lung-Qi fails to descend, fluids cannot be transformed and they accumulate into Phlegm. Phlegm of course, becomes a powerful cause of breathlessness in itself as it further obstructs the descending of Lung-Qi in the chest.

Phlegm-Heat in the Interior also obstructs the ascending of Spleen-Qi and the descending of Stomach-Qi so that fluids cannot be transformed properly. This further contributes to forming Phlegm or Dampness. For these reasons, Dampness or Phlegm are a very common result of any acute disease which becomes protracted.

The possibility of the development of breathlessness from repeated invasions of external Wind (which occurs especially but not exclusively in children) is a further reason to treat all such invasions seriously and actively expel the pathogenic factor while it is still on the Exterior.

2. DIET

The excessive consumption of fats, dairy foods, sweets, sugar and raw-cold foods impairs the transformation and transportation of food essences and fluids by the Spleen. As fluids are not transformed, this eventually leads to the formation of Phlegm which settles in the Lungs. In the Lungs, Phlegm obstructs the descending of Qi and causes breathlessness.

This an extremely common aetiological factor of breathlessness in Western societies, especially due to the excessive consumption of dairy foods such as milk, cheese, butter and cream.

In babies, breathlessness can be caused by weaning too early and feeding heavy foods which the very young digestive system cannot digest. This easily leads to the accumulation of Phlegm.

3. EMOTIONAL PROBLEMS

Worry, pensiveness or brooding over a long period of time weaken the Lung and Spleen. Lung-Qi becomes obstructed and this leads to breathlessness. Spleen-Qi is weakened, fluids are not transformed properly and this leads to Phlegm which is a contributing factor in chronic breathlessness.

Anger, frustration, irritation, resentment over a long period of time cause Liver-Yang or Liver-Fire to rise. This can rise to invade the Lungs and obstruct the descending of Lung-Qi. In 5-Element terms this is called "Wood insulting Metal". This is a fairly common cause of breathlessness particularly in tense young people or children who are in a stressful family situation.

4. FATIGUE, CHRONIC ILLNESS

Overwork over a long period of time weakens Kidney-Yin. A deficiency of Kidney-Yin leads to the impairment of various Kidney functions, in this case that of receiving Qi. Thus the deficient Kidneys cannot receive and grasp Qi, Qi rebels upwards and obstructs the descending of Lung-Qi. This leads to a situation of Excess above and Deficiency below and therefore chronic breathlessness.

Physical overexertion over a long period of time, or standing for too long, weakens Kidney-Yang which cannot receive and hold Qi down. This leads to chronic breathlessness in exactly the same way as outlined above. Thus a Kidney deficiency (whether of Yin or Yang) is nearly always present in chronic breathlessness. For this reason Ye Tian Shi (1667-1746) said of breathlessness: *"If the Lungs are the cause, it is of the Excess type; if the Kidneys are the cause, it is of the Deficiency type"*.[5]

A chronic deficiency of Lung-Qi or Lung-Yin such as one following an external invasion of Wind, prevents Lung-Qi from descending and therefore leads to chronic cough and breathlessness.

Pathology

As outlined above, the causes of breathlessness centre around the Lungs and Kidneys primarily. The Lungs, which govern Qi, are always involved as in breathlessness Lung-Qi fails to descend. Lung-Qi fails to descend when it is obstructed by exterior Wind or by Phlegm, or when it is deficient.

The Kidneys are the root of Qi and receive and hold Qi down. Lung and Kidney work in coordination for proper breathing as Lung-Qi descends to the Kidneys and the Kidneys hold it down. The Lungs control exhalation and the Kidney inhalation. Thus in chronic breathlessness a difficulty in inhalation indicates Kidney deficiency, whilst a difficulty in exhalation points to a Lung deficiency. Although the pattern of Kidneys not receiving Qi, which is typical of chronic breathlessness, is a Yang-deficiency pattern, both Kidney-Yin and Kidney-Yang deficiency can lead to chronic breathlessness.

Other organs are involved in breathlessness too. A deficiency of the Spleen leads to the formation of Phlegm which obstructs the descending of Lung-Qi. Phlegm is often present, especially in bronchitic breathlessness.

Liver-Yang or Liver-Fire rising can impair the descending of Lung-Qi and lead to chronic breathlessness.

In very chronic cases in old people, the Heart may also be involved in two ways. First of all, the Heart vessels fill the lungs and Lung-Qi moves Blood. If Lung-Qi is deficient, Blood is not moved and it stagnates in the lungs. This leads to right-heart failure due to retention of fluids in the lungs. Secondly, Kidney-Yang is the basis for Heart-Yang. When Kidney-Yang is deficient, the Fire of Ming Men fails to warm the Heart, fluids are not transformed and accumulate in the Lungs and Heart. This is manifested with a profuse expectoration of white, watery, dilute and frothy sputum. There will also be a pronounced feeling of oppression of the chest and palpitations. It is called "Kidney-Yang deficient with Water overflowing to Lungs and Heart". In even more chronic cases, the deficient Heart-Yang fails to move Blood in the chest and the stagnant fluids in the chest further obstruct Blood. This leads to stasis of Blood in the chest with symptoms of chest pain, cyanotic lips, dark nails and a Purple and Swollen tongue.

Thus we can summarize the aetiology and pathology of chronic breathlessness with a diagram (Fig. 3.1).

Differentiation and treatment

For the treatment of breathlessness it is most important to differentiate Excess from Deficiency. In Excess-type of breathlessness, breathing is shallow and long, the person exhales quickly with a loud noise, there are loud wheezing sounds, there may be a cough and the pulse is Slippery or Tight and Full. In Deficiency-type of breathlessness, breathing is short and rapid, the person inhales quickly with a low noise and the pulse is Weak.

The "Complete Book of Jing Yue" (1624) says:

In Excess-breathlessness breathing is long, there is a

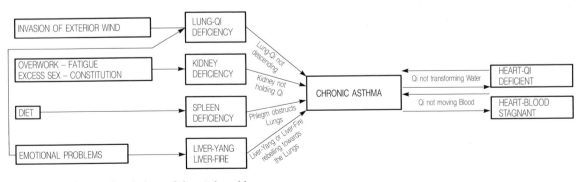

Fig. 3.1 Aetiology and pathology of chronic breathlessness

feeling of oppression of the chest, the breathing sounds are loud, the person cannot hold the breath in and breathes out quickly. In Deficiency-breathlessness breathing is short, the person is flustered, Qi is weak, breathing sounds are weak, breathing is interrupted and is worse on exertion . . . .[6]

For the treatment of Excess conditions one concentrates on treating the Manifestation and on expelling pathogenic factors. For the treatment of Deficiency cases one concentrates on treating the Root and tonifying the body's Qi. For example, in breathlessness from Phlegm-Heat (the Manifestation), even though it is a Spleen deficiency (the Root) that leads to Phlegm, the first priority is to resolve Phlegm and clear Heat rather than tonifying the Spleen. On the other hand, in chronic breathlessness from deficiency of Lungs and Kidneys (the Root), the primary task is to tonify Lungs and Kidneys and only secondarily relieve breathlessness and possibly resolve Phlegm (the Manifestation).

The patterns analyzed will be:

EXCESS

Wind-Cold invading the Lungs
Wind-Cold on the Exterior, Phlegm-Fluids in the Interior
Cold on the Exterior, Heat in the Interior
Phlegm-Heat in the Lungs
Turbid Phlegm in the Lungs
Lung-Qi Obstructed
Liver-Fire invading the Lungs

DEFICIENCY

Lung-Qi Deficiency
Lung-Yin Deficiency
Lung and Kidney Deficiency
Lung- and Kidney-Yin Deficiency
Lung- and Kidney-Yang Deficiency
Lung-, Heart- and Kidney-Yang Deficiency

EXCESS

1. WIND-COLD INVADING THE LUNGS

CLINICAL MANIFESTATIONS

Aversion to cold, shivering, fever, cough, breath-

lessness, a feeling of oppression of the chest, thin-white mucus, headache, no sweating.
Pulse: Floating-Tight.

External Wind-Cold invades the Lung's Defensive-Qi energetic layer and it impairs the dispersing and descending of Lung-Qi: this causes the breathlessness and cough.

This situation corresponds either to an acute attack of breathlessness or an acute exacerbation of chronic breathlessness. At this acute stage, the treatment must always be aimed at releasing the Exterior and expelling Wind-Cold even in chronic breathlessness.

TREATMENT PRINCIPLE

Release the Exterior, restore the dispersing and descending of Lung-Qi, expel Wind-Cold.

ACUPUNCTURE

LU-7 Lieque, LU-6 Kongzui, BL-12 Fengmen, BL-13 Feishu, Dingchuan extra-point. All with reducing method, cupping on BL-12 and BL-13. Direct moxa with cones is applicable to BL-12 *after* needling and cupping.

Explanation

- **LU-7** releases the Exterior, expels Wind-Cold and restores the descending of Lung-Qi.
- **LU-6**, Accumulation point, is used for acute Lung patterns and it stops breathlessness.
- **BL-12** and **BL-13** with cupping release the Exterior and restore the dispersing and descending of Lung-Qi. Moxa can be applied after needling and cupping if Cold is predominant.
- **Dingchuan** (0.5 *cun* lateral to Du-14 Dazhui) stops acute breathlessness.

HERBAL TREATMENT

Prescription

MA HUANG TANG
Ephedra Decoction

Ma Huang *Herba Ephedrae* 6 g
Gui Zhi *Ramulus Cinnamomi cassiae* 4 g
Xing Ren *Semen Pruni armeniacae* 9 g
Zhi Gan Cao *Radix Glycyrrhizae uralensis praeparata* 3 g

Explanation

This is *the* decoction to release the Exterior and expel Wind-Cold. It has a strong scattering effect and it makes Lung-Qi disperse and descend. It is particularly indicated for acute breathlessness.

This prescription has a definite warm energy and, in order to use it, one should be absolutely certain that the pathogenic factor is Wind-Cold rather than Wind-Heat.

Variations

– In case of Cold-Phlegm in the Lungs add Ban Xia *Rhizoma Pinelliae ternatae*, Chen Pi *Pericarpium Citri reticulatae*, Su Zi *Fructus Perillae frutescentis*, Zi Wan *Radix Asteris tatarici* and Bai Qian *Radix et Rhizoma Cynanchii Stautoni*.
– In case of sweating (which indicates the predominance of Wind within Wind-Cold) use: Gui Zhi Jia Hou Po Xing Zi Tang *Ramulus Cinnamomi Decoction plus Magnolia and Prunus*:
Gui Zhi *Ramulus Cinnamomi cassiae* 9 g
Bai Shao *Radix Paeoniae albae* 9 g
Zhi Gan Cao *Radix Glycyrrhizae uralensis praeparata* 6 g
Sheng Jiang *Rhizoma Zingiberis recens* 9 g
Da Zao *Fructus Ziziphi jujubae* 3 dates
Hou Po *Cortex Magnoliae officinalis* 4 g
Xing Ren *Semen Pruni armeniacae* 6 g

This prescription releases the Exterior by harmonizing Defensive and Nutritive Qi, it relieves fullness of the chest and stops breathlessness.

2. WIND-COLD ON THE EXTERIOR, PHLEGM-FLUIDS IN THE INTERIOR

CLINICAL MANIFESTATIONS

Aversion to cold, fever, shivering, headache, no sweating, breathlessness, cough with profuse white-watery sputum, difficulty in lying down, swelling of the limbs.
Tongue: sticky-white coating.
Pulse: Floating.

This corresponds to an invasion of exterior Wind-Cold in a person with a pre-existing condition of Phelgm-Fluids in the Interior. It is a common situation in an acute exacerbation of chronic breathlessness.

Besides the typical symptoms and signs of exterior invasion (aversion to cold, shivering, fever, headache, no sweating and Floating pulse), there are symptoms of retention of Phlegm-Fluids in the Interior, i.e. breathlessness, cough with expectoration of profuse white-watery sputum and sticky tongue coating. The swelling of the limbs is due to Phlegm-Fluids retained subcutaneously. The person finds it difficult to lie down because of the Phlegm-Fluids stagnating in the chest.

TREATMENT PRINCIPLE

Release the Exterior, expel Wind-Cold, restore the descending of Lung-Qi, resolve Phlegm.

ACUPUNCTURE

LU-7 Lieque, LU-6 Kongzui, LU-5 Chize, BL-12 Fengmen, BL-13 Feishu, Dingchuan extra-point, P-6 Neiguan, ST-40 Fenglong, Ren-22 Tiantu. All with reducing or even method.

Explanation

– **LU-7** releases the Exterior and expels Wind-Cold.
– **LU-6**, Accumulation point, relieves breathlessness.
– **LU-5** resolves Phlegm from the Lungs.
– **BL-12** and **BL-13** with cupping (with or without needling) release the Exterior.
– **Dingchuan** stops acute breathlessness.
– **P-6** opens the chest, relieves a feeling of oppression of the chest and helps breathing.

- **ST-40** resolves Phlegm and opens the chest.
- **Ren-22** stimulates the descending of Lung-Qi and resolves Phlegm.

HERBAL TREATMENT

Prescription

XIAO QING LONG TANG
Small Green Dragon Decoction
Ma Huang *Herba Ephedrae* 9 g
Gui Zhi *Ramulus Cinnamomi cassiae* 6 g
Xi Xin *Herba Asari cum radice* 3 g
Gan Jiang *Rhizoma Zingiberis officinalis* 3 g
Fa Ban Xia *Rhizoma Pinelliae ternatae* 9 g
Bai Shao *Radix Paeoniae albae* 9 g
Wu Wei Zi *Fructus Schisandrae chinensis* 3 g
Zhi Gan Cao *Radix Glycyrrhizae uralensis praeparata* 6 g

Explanation

This decoction simultaneously releases the Exterior and resolves Phlegm-Fluids in the Interior.

- **Ma Huang** and **Gui Zhi** release the Exterior and expel Wind-Cold.
- **Xi Xin** and **Gan Jiang** are very warm and drying and resolve Phlegm-Fluids and Cold-Phlegm.
- **Ban Xia** resolves Phlegm.
- **Bai Shao** and **Wu Wei Zi** are absorbing and are added to moderate and balance the scattering and drying action of the other herbs.
- **Gan Cao** harmonizes.

3. COLD ON THE EXTERIOR, HEAT IN THE INTERIOR

CLINICAL MANIFESTATIONS

Breathlessness, distension or pain in the chest, coarse breathing, runny nose, cough, vomiting of sticky phlegm, feeling of heat, cold limbs, irritability, aches, thirst.
Tongue: Red, coating white or yellow.
Pulse: Slippery-Rapid.

This corresponds to the second stage of an invasion of Wind-Cold, when Wind-Cold is still on the Exterior, but interior Heat has already formed. Alternatively, it could occur in an invasion of Wind-Cold in a person with a pre-existing condition of interior Heat. It can therefore either be an acute attack of breathlessness, or an acute exacerbation of chronic breathlessness precipitated by an invasion of Wind-Cold on a background of interior Lung-Heat.

There are some symptoms of Cold on the Exterior such as cold limbs, aches and runny nose, and some of interior Heat (of the Lungs) such as irritability, feeling of heat, coarse breathing, thirst, Rapid pulse and Red tongue.

TREATMENT PRINCIPLE

Clear Heat, restore the descending of Lung-Qi.

ACUPUNCTURE

LU-7 Lieque, LU-6 Kongzui, LU-10 Yuji, L.I.-11 Quchi, LU-1 Zhongfu. Reducing or even method.

Explanation

- **LU-7** restores the descending of Lung-Qi.
- **LU-6** relieves acute breathlessness.
- **LU-10** clears Lung-Heat.
- **LU-1**, Front Collecting point, clears Lung-Heat, relieves fullness of the chest and stops breathlessness.
- **L.I.-11** clears Heat.

HERBAL TREATMENT

Prescription

MA XING SHI GAN TANG
Ephedra-Prunus-Gypsum-Glycyrrhiza Decoction
Ma Huang *Herba Ephedrae* 5 g
Xing Ren *Semen Pruni armeniacae* 9 g
Shi Gao *Gypsum fibrosum* 18 g
Zhi Gan Cao *Radix Glycyrrhizae uralensis praeparata* 6 g

Explanation

- **Ma Huang** and **Xing Ren** restore the descending of Lung-Qi, stop breathlessness and expel Wind-Cold.
- **Shi Gao** clears interior Lung-Heat.
- **Gan Cao** harmonizes.

Variations

- In case of profuse phlegm add Huang Qin *Radix Scutellariae baicalensis*, Sang Bai Pi *Cortex Mori radicis* and Gua Lou *Semen Trichosanthis*.

Patent remedy

ZHI SOU DING CHUAN WAN
Stopping Cough and Calming Breathlessness Pill
Ma Huang *Herba Ephedrae*
Xing Ren *Semen Pruni armeniacae*
Shi Gao *Gypsum fibrosum*
Zhi Gan Cao *Radix Glycyrrhizae uralensis praeparata*

Explanation

This remedy has the same ingredients and functions as the homonymous prescription above.

The tongue presentation appropriate to this remedy is a Red body with a yellow coating.

4. PHLEGM-HEAT IN THE LUNGS

CLINICAL MANIFESTATIONS

Cough, breathlessness, pain in the chest, profuse sticky-yellow or blood-tinged sputum, irritability, uncomfortable feeling in the chest, feeling of heat, sweating, thirst, red face, dry throat, dark urine, constipation.
Tongue: Red with sticky-yellow coating.
Pulse: Slippery-Rapid.

This corresponds to the stage following an invasion of Wind-Cold or Wind-Heat, when the pathogenic factor turns into Heat and it settles in the Lungs. All the symptoms point to Lung-Heat.

TREATMENT PRINCIPLE

Clear Heat, resolve Phlegm, clear the Lungs.

ACUPUNCTURE

LU-5 Chize, LU-1 Zhongfu, L.I.-11 Quchi, ST-40 Fenglong, DU-14 Dazhui. Reducing method, no moxa.

Explanation

- **LU-5** clears Lung-Heat.
- **LU-1** clears Lung-Heat and relieves fullness and pain in the chest.
- **L.I.-11** clears Heat.
- **ST-40** resolves Phlegm.
- **Du-14** clears Heat.

HERBAL TREATMENT

Prescription

SANG BAI PI TANG
Cortex Mori Decoction
Sang Bai Pi *Cortex Mori albae radicis* 9 g
Huang Qin *Radix Scutellariae baicalensis* 6 g
Huang Lian *Rhizoma Coptidis* 3 g
Zhi Zi *Fructus Gardeniae jasminoidis* 4 g
Chuan Bei Mu *Bulbus Fritillariae cirrhosae* 4 g
Xing Ren *Semen Pruni armeniacae* 6 g
Su Zi *Fructus Perillae frutescentis* 6 g
Fa Ban Xia *Rhizoma Pinelliae ternatae* 6 g

Explanation

- **Sang Bai Pi**, **Huang Qin**, **Huang Lian** and **Zhi Zi** clear Heat, clear the Lungs and restore the descending of Lung-Qi.
- **Bei Mu**, **Xing Ren**, **Su Zi** and **Ban Xia**, resolve Phlegm, restore the descending of Lung-Qi and stop breathlessness.

Variations

- In case of high fever add Shi Gao *Gypsum fibrosum* and Zhi Mu *Rhizoma Anemarrhenae asphodeloidis*.
- In case of profuse phlegm add Hai Ge Ke *Concha Cyclinae sinensis*.
- In case of intense thirst add Tian Hua Fen *Radix Trichosanthis*.
- In case of severe breathlessness with inability

to lie down and sticky phlegm add Da Huang *Radix Rhei* and Mang Xiao *Mirabilitum*.
– If phlegm tastes of bile add Yu Xing Cao *Herba Houttuyniae cordatae*, Dong Gua Zi *Semen Benincasae hispidae*, Yi Yi Ren *Semen Coicis lachryma-jobi* and Lu Gen *Rhizoma Phragmitis communis*.

Patent remedy

QING QI HUA TAN WAN
Clearing Qi and Resolving Phlegm Pill
Dan Nan Xing *Rhizoma Arisaematis praeparata*
Gua Lou *Semen Trichosanthis*
Huang Qin *Radix Scutellariae baicalensis*
Zhi Shi *Fructus Citri aurantii immaturus*
Chen Pi *Pericarpium Citri reticulatae*
Fu Ling *Sclerotium Poriae cocos*
Xing Ren *Semen Pruni armeniacae*
Ban Xia *Rhizoma Pinelliae ternatae*

Explanation

This remedy resolves Phlegm, clears Lung-Heat and restores the descending of Lung-Qi.

The tongue presentation appropriate to this remedy is a Red body with a sticky-yellow coating.

5. TURBID PHLEGM IN THE LUNGS

CLINICAL MANIFESTATIONS

Breathlessness, difficulty in breathing out, a feeling of oppression and fullness of the chest, cough with profuse sticky-white sputum, vomiting or nausea, sticky taste, no thirst.
Tongue: thick-sticky-white coating.
Pulse: Slippery-Full.

This condition is characterized by retention of Damp-Phlegm in the Lungs. Damp-Phlegm severely obstructs the descending of Lung-Qi resulting in cough and breathlessness. Phlegm also impairs the circulation of Qi in the chest, thus causing a feeling of oppression and fullness of the chest and nausea or vomiting (as it also prevents the descending of Stomach-Qi).

TREATMENT PRINCIPLE

Resolve Phlegm, restore the descending of Lung-Qi.

ACUPUNCTURE

LU-5 Chize, LU-7 Lieque, LU-1 Zhongfu, P-6 Neiguan, ST-40 Fenglong, BL-13 Feishu, BL-20 Pishu. Reducing or even method.

Explanation

– **LU-5** and **LU-7** expel Damp-Phlegm from the Lungs and restore the descending of Lung-Qi.
– **LU-1** relieves the feeling of oppression of the chest.
– **P-6** relieves fullness of the chest, stops nausea or vomiting and opens the chest, facilitating the expulsion of phlegm.

HERBAL TREATMENT

Prescription

ER CHEN TANG and SAN ZI YANG QIN TANG
Two Old Decoction and *Three-Seed Nourishing the Parents Decoction*
Fa Ban Xia *Rhizoma Pinelliae ternatae* 15 g
Chen Pi *Pericarpium Citri reticulatae* 15 g
Fu Ling *Sclerotium Poriae cocos* 9 g
Zhi Gan Cao *Radix Glycyrrhizae uralensis praeparata* 5 g
Sheng Jiang *Rhizoma Zingiberis recens* 3 g
Wu Mei *Fructus Mume* one prune
Su Zi *Fructus Perillae frutescentis* 9 g
Bai Jie Zi *Semen Sinapis albae* 6 g
Lai Fu Zi *Semen Raphani sativi* 9 g

Explanation

– The first six herbs compose the Er Chen Tang *Two Old Decoction* which resolves Damp-Phlegm. The last three herbs make up the San Zi Yang Qin Tang *Three-Seed Nourishing the Parents Decoction*. This decoction was especially formulated for chronic Damp-

Phlegm in the chest in old people (hence its name). Within this prescription, **Su Zi** makes Lung-Qi descend and stops cough and breathlessness, **Bai Jie Zi** is warm and resolves Cold-Phlegm in the Lungs and **Lai Fu Zi** is a digestive herb which will help to resolve Phlegm.

Variations

– In case of severe breathlessness, other herbs which make Lung-Qi descend such as Xing Ren *Semen Pruni armeniacae* should be added.
– In case of profuse phlegm add Cang Zhu *Rhizoma Atractylodis lanceae* and Hou Po *Cortex Magnoliae officinalis*.

Patent remedy

ER CHEN WAN
Two Old Decoction
Ban Xia *Rhizoma Pinelliae ternatae*
Chen Pi *Pericarpium Citri reticulatae*
Fu Ling *Sclerotium Poriae cocos*
Zhi Gan Cao *Radix Glycyrrhizae uralensis praeparata*
Sheng Jiang *Rhizoma Zingiberis officinalis recens*
Wu Mei *Fructus Pruni mume*

Explanation

This remedy resolves Damp-Phlegm. The tongue presentation appropriate to this remedy is a sticky-dirty coating.

6. LUNG-QI OBSTRUCTED

CLINICAL MANIFESTATIONS

Sudden attacks of breathlessness precipitated by emotional problems, no wheezing sounds, feeling of suffocation or constriction in the throat, a feeling of oppression or pain in the chest, palpitations, restless sleep.
Tongue: Red sides.
Pulse: Wiry.

This condition is due to stagnant Liver-Qi rebelling upwards towards the chest. Rebellious Liver-Qi impairs the descending of Lung-Qi and causes breathlessness. This is typically caused by emotional problems and the attacks are brought on by some stressful situation. The feeling of constriction or suffocation in the throat is due to stagnation of Liver-Qi and obstruction of the throat by Qi-Phlegm, i.e. a very rarefied type of Phlegm to the point of being nearly like Qi.

TREATMENT PRINCIPLE

Soothe the Liver, move Qi, restore the descending of Lung-Qi, stop breathlessness.

ACUPUNCTURE

LIV-3 Taichong, LIV-14 Qimen, SP-4 Gongsun and P-6 Neiguan, LU-1 Zhongfu, Ren-17 Shanzhong, LU-7 Lieque, HE-7 Shenmen, ST-40 Fenglong.

Explanation

– **LIV-3** and **LIV-14** soothe the Liver and relieve stagnation. LIV-14, in particular, will relieve stagnation of Qi in the chest.
– **SP-4** and **P-6** in combination, open the Penetrating Vessel, free the chest and subdue rebellious Qi in the chest.
– **LU-1**, **Ren-17** and **LU-7** restore the descending of Lung-Qi, free the chest and relieve fullness.
– **ST-40** is used to resolve Qi-Phlegm.
– **HE-7** calms the Mind.

HERBAL TREATMENT

Prescription

WU MO YIN ZI
Five Powders Decoction
Chen Xiang *Lignum Aquilariae* 6 g
Mu Xiang *Radix Saussureae* 3 g
Bing Lang *Semen Arecae catechu* 6 g
Wu Yao *Radix Linderae strychnifoliae* 6 g
Zhi Shi *Fructus Aurantii immaturus* 6 g
White Wine

Bai He *Bulbus Lilii* 6 g
He Huan Pi *Cortex Albizziae julibrissin* 6 g
Suan Zao Ren *Semen Ziziphi spinosae* 6 g
Yuan Zhi *Radix Polygalae tenuifoliae* 6 g

Explanation

– **Chen Xiang, Mu Xiang, Bing Lang, Wu Yao, Zhi Shi** and **white wine** relieve stagnation, restore the descending of Qi and stop breathlessness.
– **Bai He, He Huan Pi, Suan Zao Ren** and **Yuan Zhi** calm the Mind and soothe the Liver.

7. LIVER-FIRE INVADING THE LUNGS

CLINICAL MANIFESTATIONS

Breathlessness attacks precipitated by emotional stress, a feeling of oppression of the chest, chest pain, dream-disturbed sleep, short temper, thirst, bitter taste, dark urine, constipation, head-ache, red eyes and face.
Tongue: Red, redder and swollen on the sides, yellow coating.
Pulse: Wiry and Rapid.

This condition includes aspects of the previ-ous one, i.e. rebellious Liver-Qi invading the chest and obstructing the descending of Lung-Qi. In this case, however, it is Liver-Fire that carries Liver-Qi upwards towards the chest. Since Fire dries up the body fluids, there is thirst, dark urine and constipation. Fire also af-fects the Mind causing dream-disturbed sleep.

This type of breathlessness is fairly frequent in children.

TREATMENT PRINCIPLE

Soothe the Liver, drain Fire, restore the de-scending of Lung-Qi.

ACUPUNCTURE

LIV-2 Xingjian, LIV-14 Qimen, LU-7 Lieque,

Ren-17 Shanzhong, LU-1 Zhongfu, BL-18 Ganshu, BL-13 Feishu. Reducing or even method.

Explanation

– **LIV-2** clears Liver-Fire.
– **LIV-14** soothes the Liver and relieves stagnation of Qi in the chest and ribs.
– **LU-7, BL-13** and **Ren-17** restore the descending of Lung-Qi.
– **LU-1** relieves fullness and pain in the chest.
– **BL-18** clears Liver-Fire.

HERBAL TREATMENT

Prescription

LONG DAN XIE GAN TANG Variation
Gentiana Draining the Liver Decoction
Long Dan Cao *Radix Gentianae scabrae* 9 g
Huang Qin *Radix Scutellariae baicalensis* 4 g
Shan Zhi Zi *Fructus Gardeniae jasminoidis* 4 g
Ze Xie *Rhizoma Alismatis orientalis* 6 g
Mu Tong *Caulis Akebiae* 3 g
Sheng Di Huang *Radix Rehmanniae glutinosae* 6 g
Chai Hu *Radix Bupleuri* 6 g
Suan Zao Ren *Semen Ziziphi spinosae* 6 g
Sang Bai Pi *Cortex Mori albae radicis* 6 g
Di Gu Pi *Cortex Lycii radicis* 6 g
Su Zi *Fructus Perillae frutescentis* 6 g
Zhi Gan Cao *Radix Glycyrrhizae uralensis prae-parata* 3 g

Explanation

This is a variation of Long Dan Xie Gan Tang *Gentiana Draining the Liver Decoction* which clears Liver-Fire.

– **Sang Bai Pi, Di Gu Pi** and **Su Zi** restore the descending of Lung-Qi and clear Heat in the chest.

Patent remedy

QING FEI YI HUO PIAN
Clearing the Lungs and Eliminating Fire Tablet
Huang Qin *Radix Scutellariae baicalensis*
Shan Zhi Zi *Fructus Gardeniae jasminoidis*
Da Huang *Rhizoma Rhei*

Qian Hu *Radix Peucedani*
Ku Shen *Radix Sophorae flavescentis*
Tian Hua Fen *Radix Trichosanthis*
Jie Geng *Radix Platycodi grandiflori*
Zhi Mu *Radix Anemarrhenae asphodeloidis*

Explanation

This remedy clears Lung-Heat and drains Liver-Fire by purging. It must be used only for Fire as opposed to Heat: the symptoms are intense thirst, severe irritability, constipation with dry stools and a dark urine. There may also be blood-tinged sputum.

The tongue presentation appropriate to this remedy is a Red body with a very dry, dark-yellow or brown coating.

Case history

A 33-year-old woman had been suffering from breathlessness for the previous two years. She found it difficult to breathe out and her attacks were elicited by emotional stress. She also felt easily thirsty and experienced a bitter taste in her mouth occasionally. She had frequent headaches on the temples of a throbbing nature and she felt generally wound-up and frustrated. She also felt easily hot and occasionally had palpitations. Her pulse was Wiry and her tongue was Red with redder sides and tip, with a shallow midline Heart-crack. The sides also had red points.

Diagnosis
This was a very clear case of breathlessness due to Liver-Fire rebelling upwards towards the chest and obstructing the Lungs. It was also clearly due to emotional tensions mostly to do with her relationship with her father. Although Liver-Fire was the main problem, there was also some Heart-Fire as shown by the shallow Heart-crack, red tip of the tongue and palpitations.

Treatment
She was treated with herbs only with the following variation of Long Dan Xie Gan Tang *Gentiana Draining the Liver Decoction*.

Long Dan Cao *Radix Gentianae scabrae* 6 g
Huang Qin *Radix Scutellariae baicalensis* 4 g
Shan Zhi Zi *Fructus Gardeniae jasminoidis* 4 g
Ze Xie *Rhizoma Alismatis orientalis* 6 g
Mu Tong *Caulis Akebiae* 3 g
Sheng Di Huang *Radix Rehmanniae glutinosae* 6 g
Chai Hu *Radix Bupleuri* 6 g
Suan Zao Ren *Semen Ziziphi spinosae* 6 g

He Huan Pi *Cortex Albizziae julibrissin* 6 g
Hou Po *Cortex Magnoliae officinalis* 3 g
Su Zi *Fructus Perillae frutescentis* 6 g
Zhi Gan Cao *Radix Glycyrrhizae uralensis praeparata* 3 g

This is almost like the original decoction with the addition of Suan Zao Ren *Semen Ziziphi spinosae* and He Huan Pi *Cortex Albizziae julibrissin* to calm the Mind, and Hou Po *Cortex Magnoliae officinalis* to relieve fullness of the chest and also to calm the Mind.

The treatment stopped her breathlessness and helped her to calm down and achieve a more balanced emotional life.

DEFICIENCY

Breathlessness of the Deficiency-type is characterized by Lung and Kidney deficiency since the Lungs govern Qi and the Kidneys are the root of Qi. The Lungs control exhalation and the Kidneys inhalation.

In addition to these two organs, the Spleen is often deficient leading to the formation of Phlegm which obstructs the Lungs. In very chronic cases, Heart-Qi becomes weak since Lung-Qi fails to move Blood. This also leads to stasis of Blood in the chest manifested with cyanotic lips, chest pain and purple tongue.

All the Deficiency types of breathlessness correspond to chronic cases.

1. LUNG-QI DEFICIENCY

CLINICAL MANIFESTATIONS

Shortness of breath, weak lung sounds, slight rattling sound in the throat, sweating, chilliness, pale face, weak voice, expectoration of scanty phlegm.
Tongue: Pale.
Pulse: Weak, especially on the right Front position.

TREATMENT PRINCIPLE

Tonify the Lungs, strengthen Qi, restore the descending of Lung-Qi.

Acupuncture

LU-7 Lieque, LU-9 Taiyuan, BL-13 Feishu, Du-12

Shenzhu, Ren-12 Zhongwan, Ren-6 Qihai, ST-36 Zusanli. Reinforcing method.

Explanation

- **LU-9** and **LU-7** tonify the Lungs and restore the descending of Lung-Qi.
- **BL-13** and **Du-12** tonify Lung-Qi. Direct moxa can be used.
- **Ren-12** and **Ren-6** tonify Qi in general and they are also concentration points along the Lung channel which starts over Ren-12 and flows down to Ren-6 before coursing back upwards.
- **ST-36** tonifies Stomach and Spleen and this helps the Lungs according to the principle of "strengthening Earth to tonify Metal".

HERBAL TREATMENT

Prescription

BU FEI TANG
Tonifying the Lungs Decoction
Ren Shen *Radix Ginseng* 9 g
Huang Qi *Radix Astragali membranacei* 12 g
Shu Di Huang *Radix Rehmanniae glutinosae prae-parata* 12 g
Wu Wei Zi *Fructus Schisandrae chinensis* 6 g
Zi Wan *Radix Asteris tatarici* 9 g
Sang Bai Pi *Cortex Mori albae radicis* 6 g

Explanation

- **Ren Shen** and **Huang Qi** are the chief ingredients to tonify Lung-Qi and firm the Defensive Qi.
- **Shu Di Huang** nourishes Blood and tonifies the Kidneys to grasp Qi.
- **Wu Wei Zi** tonifies the Lungs and also helps the Kidneys to grasp Qi.
- **Zi Wan** and **Sang Bai Pi** restore the descending of Lung-Qi and stop cough and breathlessness.

Patent remedy

PING CHUAN WAN
Calming Breathlessness Pill

Dang Shen *Radix Codonopsis pilosulae*
Dong Chong Xia Cao *Sclerotium Cordicipitis chinensis*
Ge Jie *Gecko*
Xing Ren *Semen Pruni armeniacae*
Chen Pi *Pericarpium Citri reticulatae*
Gan Cao *Radix Glycyrrhizae uralensis*
Sang Bai Pi *Cortex Radicis Mori albae*
Bai Qian *Radix et Rhizoma Cynanchii stautoni*
Meng Shi *Lapis Chloritis*
Wu Zhi Mao Tao *Radix Fici simplicissimae*
Man Hu Tui Zi *Semen Elaeagni glabrae thunbergii*

Explanation

This remedy mostly tonifies Lung- and Spleen-Qi and restores the descending of Lung-Qi. However, it has quite a broad action as it also tonifies the Kidney's grasping of Qi and mildly nourishes Lung-Yin.

The tongue presentation appropriate to this remedy is a Pale tongue.

2. LUNG-YIN DEFICIENCY

CLINICAL MANIFESTATIONS

Shortness of breath, chronic breathlessness, sweating at night, 5-palm heat, dry throat, dry cough with scanty sputum, malar flush.
Tongue: Red and dry without coating, or Red with coating and transversal cracks in the Lung area.
Pulse: Floating-Empty or Fine, Rapid and Weak in the right Front position.

Lung-Yin deficiency can occur in combination with Lung-Qi deficiency. Yin-deficiency is more common in old people. Only in very advanced cases the tongue would be completely without coating. In other cases it could have a rootless coating or lack a coating only in the front part.

TREATMENT PRINCIPLE

Nourish Lung-Yin and restore the descending of Lung-Qi.

ACUPUNCTURE

LU-9 Taiyuan, LU-7 Lieque and KI-6 Zhaohai in combination, BL-43 Gaohuangshu, Ren-4 Guanyuan, BL-13 Feishu, Du-12 Shenzhu. Reinforcing method.

Explanation

- **LU-9** tonifies Lung-Yin.
- **LU-7** and **KI-6** open the Directing Vessel, nourish Yin, restore the descending of Lung-Qi and benefit the throat. The combination of these two points is excellent in cases of chronic breathlessness from Lung-Yin deficiency or both Lung- and Kidney-Yin deficiency.
- **BL-43** nourishes Lung-Yin and is particularly effective in very chronic diseases.
- **BL-13** and **Du-12** tonify Lung-Qi.
- **Ren-4** nourishes Yin in general and strengthens the Kidney's grasping of Qi.

HERBAL TREATMENT

Prescription

SHENG MAI SAN
Generating the Pulse Powder
Ren Shen *Radix Ginseng* 9 g
Mai Men Dong *Tuber Ophiopogonis japonici* 9 g
Wu Wei Zi *Fructus Schisandrae chinensis* 3 g

Explanation

- **Ren Shen** tonifies Lung-Qi.
- **Mai Men Dong** nourishes Lung-Yin.
- **Wu Wei Zi** nourishes Lung-Yin and absorbs leakage (such as night sweating).

This is the best prescription to tonify Lung-Yin. However, in cases of chronic breathlessness, herbs that restore the descending of Lung-Qi such as Xing Ren *Semen Pruni armeniacae* or Su Zi *Fructus Perillae frutescentis* should be added. Alternatively, this prescription could simply be combined with the previous one. They would combine particularly well also because they have two herbs in common (Ren Shen *Radix* Ginseng and Wu Wei Zi *Fructus Schisandrae chinensis*).

Patent remedy

LI FEI WAN
Benefiting the Lungs Pill
Dong Chong Xia Cao *Sclerotium Cordicipitis chinensis*
Ge Jie *Gecko*
Bai He *Bulbus Lilii*
Wu Wei Zi *Fructus Schisandrae chinensis*
Bai Ji *Rhizoma Bletillae striatae*
Bai Bu *Radix Stemonae*
Mu Li *Concha Ostreae*
Pi Pa Ye *Folium Eriobotryae japonicae*
Gan Cao *Radix Glycyrrhizae uralensis*

Explanation

This remedy nourishes Lung-Yin and benefits fluids. The tongue presentation appropriate to this remedy is a body which is Red in the front without coating.

3. LUNG AND KIDNEY DEFICIENCY

CLINICAL MANIFESTATIONS

Chronic breathlessness, attacks brought on by exertion, difficulty in inhalation, loss of weight, depression, oedema of ankles, cold limbs, sore back, dizziness, weak knees.
Tongue: Pale, Swollen.
Pulse: Deep, Weak, Slow.

This corresponds to Yang deficiency of both Lungs and Kidneys, with the Kidneys unable to grasp Qi. This results in the situation described in Chinese medicine as "Fullness above and Emptiness below", i.e. deficiency of the Kidneys with relative Fullness in the Lungs.

This pattern is due to Kidney-Yang deficiency hence the oedema of ankles, cold limbs, weak knees, dizziness, depression, Pale and Swollen tongue and Deep and Weak pulse. As Kidneys control inhalation, typically the patient would find it more difficult to breathe in.

TREATMENT PRINCIPLE

Tonify and warm the Kidneys, stimulate the descending of Lung-Qi.

Acupuncture

BL-23 Shenshu, BL-13 Feishu, Du-4 Mingmen, KI-7 Fuliu, KI-25 Shencang, KI-3 Taixi, LU-7 Lieque. Reinforcing method, moxa.

Explanation

– **BL-23** and **KI-7** tonify KI-Yang.
– **Du-4** tonifies the Fire of the Gate of Vitality. Used with moxa it strongly tonifies Yang.
– **KI-3**, source point, tonifies the Kidneys.
– **KI-25** is an important local point to relieve fullness of the chest and breathlessness caused by Kidney deficiency.
– **LU-7** stimulates the descending of Lung-Qi.

Herbal treatment

(a) Prescription

JIN GUI SHEN QI WAN
Golden Chest Kidney-Qi Pill
Fu Zi *Radix Aconiti carmichaeli praeparata* 3 g
Gui Zhi *Ramulus Cinnamomi cassiae* 3 g
Shu Di Huang *Radix Rehmanniae glutinosae praeparata* 24 g
Shan Zhu Yu *Fructus Corni officinalis* 12 g
Shan Yao *Radix Dioscoreae oppositae* 12 g
Ze Xie *Rhizoma Alismatis orientalis* 9 g
Mu Dan Pi *Cortex Moutan radicis* 9 g
Fu Ling *Sclerotium Poriae cocos* 9 g

Explanation

This is the classical formula to tonify and warm Kidney-Yang, derived from Zhang's "Discussion of Cold-induced Diseases" of the Han dynasty. Later versions of this formula replace Gui Zhi *Ramulus Cinnamomi cassiae* with Rou Gui *Cortex Cinnamomi cassiae*.

Variations

When used for chronic Kidney-breathlessness,

some herbs which promote the descending of Lung-Qi should be added, such as Su Zi *Fructus Perillae frutescentis* or Xing Ren *Semen Pruni armeniacae*.

(b) Prescription

SHEN GE SAN
Panax-Gecko Powder
Ren Shen *Radix Ginseng* 12 g
Ge Jie *Gecko* 12 g

Explanation

– **Ren Shen** tonifies the Original Qi.
– **Ge Jie** tonifies Kidney-Yang and it specifically promotes the Kidney function of grasping Qi.

This formula can be used when the symptoms of Yang deficiency are not very pronounced.

(c) Prescription

SU ZI JIANG QI TANG
Perilla Seed Lowering Qi Decoction
Su Zi *Fructus Perillae frutescentis* 9 g
Fa Ban Xia *Rhizoma Pinelliae ternatae* 9 g
Hou Po *Cortex Magnoliae officinalis* 6 g
Qian Hu *Radix Peucedani* 6 g
Rou Gui *Cortex Cinnamomi cassiae* 3 g
Dang Gui *Radix Angelicae sinensis* 6 g
Sheng Jiang *Rhizoma Zingiberis recens* 2 slices
Su Ye *Folium Perillae frutescentis* 5 leaves
Zhi Gan Cao *Radix Glycyrrhizae uralensis praeparata* 6 g
Da Zao *Fructus Ziziphi jujubae* one date

Explanation

– **Su Zi** is the emperor herb used to promote the descending of Lung-Qi and stop breathlessness.
– **Ban Xia**, **Qian Hu** and **Hou Po** resolve Phlegm, calm breathlessness and relieve fullness of the chest. They are the minister herbs and, together with the emperor herb, treat "Fullness above".
– **Rou Gui** warms the Kidneys, expels Cold, stimulates the Kidney grasping of Qi and therefore calms breathlessness.

– **Dang Gui** nourishes the Blood and tonifies the Liver. Together with Rou Gui, which tonifies the Kidneys, it tonifies the "Emptiness below". It also stops cough and subdues rebellious Qi.
– **Sheng Jiang** and **Su Ye** are the assistant herbs and they scatter Cold and help to calm breathlessness by subduing rebellious Qi.
– **Zhi Gan Cao** and **Da Zao**, messenger herbs, harmonize the Middle.

This prescription differs from the previous two in that it deals with both the "Emptiness below" and the "Fullness above". It is therefore better indicated when there is pronounced fullness of the chest with expectoration of white phlegm and cough. It deals with both the Manifestation (accumulation of Qi in the Lungs) and the Root (deficiency of the Kidneys).

Variations

– If Qi rebels upwards and there is a feeling of movement under the umbilicus, add Chen Xiang *Lignum Aquilariae*.

Patent remedy

SU ZI JIANG QI WAN
Perilla-seed Descending Qi Pill
Su Zi *Fructus Perillae frutescentis*
Ban Xia *Rhizoma Pinelliae ternatae*
Hou Po *Cortex Magnoliae officinalis*
Qian Hu *Radix Peucedani*
Chen Pi *Pericarpium Citri reticulatae*
Chen Xiang *Lignum Aquilariae*
Dang Gui *Radix Angelicae sinensis*
Sheng Jiang *Rhizoma Zingiberis officinalis recens*
Da Zao *Fructus Ziziphi jujubae*
Gan Cao *Radix Glycyrrhizae uralensis*

Explanation

This remedy is similar in composition to the homonymous formula. It restores the descending of Lung-Qi and tonifies Kidney-Yang.

The tongue presentation appropriate to this remedy is a Pale and Swollen body.

Case history

A 48-year-old woman had been suffering from breathlessness for the previous 10 years. She found it difficult to breathe in and was worse at night. The breathlessness seemed to have started after being caught in a dust storm in the Middle East, after which she contracted broncho-pneumonia. She had had pneumonia previously as a child. She also experienced fluid retention in the abdomen and ankles for the previous ten years. She was often constipated and felt cold, especially in the legs.

Her pulse was Fine and Deep and particularly Weak in both Rear positions. Her tongue was Pale and Swollen and had a sticky-white coating (Plate 3.1).

Diagnosis
This is a clear condition of breathlessness from Lung- and Kidney-Yang deficiency. She obviously had had a weakness in the Lungs since childhood deriving from the pneumonia, later aggravated by the bronchio-pneumonia 10 years before. Due to her age, the Kidney energy started to decline and, combining with the Lung deficiency, triggered off the onset of her breathlessness. The Kidney-Yang deficiency is confirmed by the fluid retention, the constipation, the cold feeling of the legs and the very Weak pulse on both Rear positions.

Treatment
This lady was treated with both acupuncture and herbs. The acupuncture treatment was very simple, basically aimed at tonifying the Lungs and Kidneys with **ST-36** Zusanli, **SP-6** Sanyinjiao, **BL-13** Feishu, **Du-12** Shenzhu and **BL-23** Shenshu. In addition to these points, the Directing vessel opening points were used every time, i.e. **LU-7** Lieque on the right and **KI-6** Zhaohai on the left to tonify Lungs and Kidneys.

The herbal prescription used was a variation of Su Zi Jiang Qi Tang *Perilla Seed Lowering Qi Decoction*:

Su Zi *Semen Perillae frutescentis* 6 g
Fa Ban Xia *Rhizoma Pinelliae ternatae* 6 g
Qian Hu *Radix Peucedani* 4 g
Hou Po *Cortex Magnoliae officinalis* 4 g
Rou Gui *Cortex Cinnamomi cassiae* 1.5 g
Dang Gui *Radix Angelicae sinensis* 6 g
Rou Cong Rong *Herba Cistanchis* 6 g
Zhi Gan Cao *Radix Glycyrrhizae uralensis praeparata* 3 g

The combination of acupuncture and Chinese herbs produced an immediate improvement which then continued steadily until most of her symptoms were relieved after a few months.

Case history

A 42-year-old lady suffered from breathlessness since

the age of 7. It had got worse since moving to an old and dusty house 13 years previously. She found it difficult to breathe in, was worse at night and worse from exposure to cold or dust. She also suffered from lower back-ache and dizziness. She had two children and her breathlessness had been better during both pregnancies. She felt cold easily and her ankles often swelled up.

When she was 6 months old she contracted whooping cough which lasted for a long time.

Her pulse was Deep and Weak, especially on both Rear positions (Kidneys). Her tongue was Red, Stiff and had a shallow Stomach crack with a yellow coating (Plate 3.2).

Diagnosis
The breathlessness was due to a deficiency of the Yang of both Lungs and Kidneys. Originally, it may have been due to a Lung deficiency only, following the weakening of the Lungs from whooping cough. Later on, the onset of Kidney deficiency contributed to the breathlessness. Difficulty in breathing in, feeling cold, back-ache, swollen ankles, dizziness and Weak pulse on Rear positions, all indicated Kidney (Yang) deficiency. The fact that she got better during the pregnancies also pointed to a Kidney deficiency. However, the tongue pointed to another co-existing condition of Heat and Phlegm. The deficient Lung and Kidneys failing to transform fluids led to the formation of Phlegm which further aggravated the breathlessness. After a long time, Phlegm easily leads to the formation of Heat. Thus, this case shows a clear combination of Deficiency (of Lungs and Kidneys) and Excess (Phlegm-Heat in the Lungs) and of Cold (from Kidney-Yang deficiency) and Heat (in the Lungs). The Root is the deficiency of Lung- and Kidney-Yang while the Phlegm-Heat in the Lungs is the Manifestation.

Treatment
Since this is an internal condition we can treat both the Root and the Manifestation simultaneously, i.e. tonifying Lung- and Kidney-Yang, restoring the descending of Lung-Qi and resolving Phlegm and clearing Heat. As the pathogenic factor is internal, we can simultaneously tonify the body's Qi (i.e. Lung- and Kidney-Yang) and expel the pathogenic factor (i.e. Phlegm-Heat).

She was treated with acupuncture only using the following points at various times during 12 months of treatment:

- **Ren-12** Zhongwan, **Ren-9** Shuifen and **ST-40** Fenglong were used to resolve Phlegm. In addition, ST-40, in combination with P-6 Neiguan, opens the chest and helps breathing.
- **P-6** Neiguan was used to open the chest and alleviate breathlessness.
- **Directing vessel** (i.e. LU-7 Lieque on the right and KI-6 Zhaohai on the left) was used several times to

restore the descending of Lung-Qi and stimulate the Kidney's grasping of Qi. This extraordinary vessel is very important for the treatment of chronic breathlessness from Lung and Kidney deficiency.
- **BL-13** Feishu, **BL-20** Pishu and **BL-23** Shenshu were used to tonify and warm Lungs, Spleen and Kidneys with needles and moxa.
- **LU-5** Chize was used to clear Heat and resolve Phlegm from the Lungs.
- **KI-7** Fuliu and **SP-6** Sanyinjiao were used to tonify Spleen and Kidney-Yang and resolve oedema. Needles and moxa were used.

This patient's attacks of breathlessness drastically decreased in intensity and frequency over a 12-month period of treatment.

Case history

A 39-year-old woman suffered from breathlessness since the age of 4. She found it difficult to breathe in, sweated easily in daytime and felt usually cold. She felt easily tired and also suffered from what was diagnosed as allergic rhinitis. Her nose was almost always running (white mucus) and she frequently sneezed when exposed to dust and dogs or cats. She also had myomas in the uterus which occasionally caused bleeding in between periods. The blood was not dark and there were no clots.

Her pulse was generally Weak and her tongue was Pale, with swollen edges (of the Spleen-type), a dirty coating all over and two deep transversal cracks in the Lung area.

Diagnosis
This breathlessness is also due to Lung- and Kidney-Yang deficiency. It started in childhood with a Lung deficiency most probably due to repeated invasions of Wind not treated properly (see two transversal Lung cracks). It later affected the Kidneys as well becoming unable to grasp Qi. The Spleen is also deficient as evidenced by the tiredness, the swelling on the edges of the tongue and the Weak pulse. Symptoms of Lung deficiency are the breathlessness and the daytime sweating. The difficulty in breathing in is due to Kidney deficiency. Besides this, there is also Phlegm deriving from the deficiency of Spleen, Lungs and Kidneys. The Phlegm can be observed in the swelling of the tongue, the dirty tongue coating and the myomas in the uterus. These could also be due to stasis of Blood but this is not the case here as the blood is not dark with clots.

Treatment
In this case, as in the previous one, the condition is internal and we can treat both the Root (deficiency of Yang of the Spleen, Lungs and Kidneys) and the Manifestation (Phlegm). On the one hand, one can tonify the body's Qi and on the other one can resolve Phlegm.

This woman was treated with acupuncture only with the following selection of points over a period of 8 months:

- **Directing vessel** (i.e. LU-7 Lieque on the right and KI-6 Zhaohai on the left). This combination of points opens the Directing Vessel, restores the descending of Lung-Qi and stimulates the grasping of Qi by the Kidneys.
- **Ren-12** Zhongwan, **Ren-9** Shuifen and **ST-40** Fenglong to resolve Phlegm.
- **ST-36** Zusanli and **BL-20** Pishu with needles and moxa to warm and tonify the Spleen.
- **BL-13** Feishu and **Du-12** Shenzhu to tonify and warm the Lungs.
- **BL-23** Shenshu and **KI-7** Fuliu to tonify and warm the Kidneys.
- **L.I.-20** Yingxiang to expel Wind and stop sneezing.

4. LUNG- AND KIDNEY-YIN DEFICIENCY

CLINICAL MANIFESTATIONS

Chronic breathlessness, difficulty in breathing in, dry throat, dry cough, night sweating, 5-palm heat, malar flush.
Tongue: Red without coating, cracks in Lung area, dry.
Pulse: Floating-Empty.

Generally speaking, the Kidney's grasping Qi is a Yang function. However, when Kidney-Yin is deficient, it also fails to grasp Qi leading to breathlessness.

TREATMENT PRINCIPLE

Nourish Yin, strengthen Lung and Kidneys, calm breathlessness.

ACUPUNCTURE

LU-9 Taiyuan, Ren-17 Shanzhong, ST-36 Zusanli, SP-6 Sanyinjiao, Ren-12 Zhongwan, Ren-4 Guanyuan, KI-3 Taixi, LU-7 Lieque and KI-6 Zhaohai in combination, KI-25 Shencang.

Explanation

- **LU-9** and **Ren-17** tonify the Lungs and promote the descending of Lung-Qi.

- **ST-36** and **Ren-12** strengthen Earth to reinforce Metal.
- **SP-6** and **Ren-4** nourish Yin.
- **KI-3** nourishes the Kidneys.
- **LU-7** and **KI-6** nourish Kidney-Yin, restore the descending of Lung-Qi, and benefit the throat. They open the Directing Vessel and are ideal for this type of breathlessness.
- **KI-25** is a local point to stimulate the Kidney grasping of Qi in chronic breathlessness from Kidney deficiency.

HERBAL TREATMENT

(a) Prescription

BA XIAN CHANG SHOU WAN
Eight Immortals Longevity Pill
Shu Di Huang *Radix Rehmanniae glutinosae prae-parata* 24 g
Shan Zhu Yu *Fructus Corni officinalis* 12 g
Shan Yao *Radix Dioscoreae oppositae* 12 g
Ze Xie *Rhizoma Alismatis orientalis* 9 g
Mu Dan Pi *Cortex Moutan radicis* 9 g
Fu Ling *Sclerotium Poriae cocos* 9 g
Mai Men Dong *Tuber Ophiopogonis japonici* 9 g
Wu Wei Zi *Fructus Schisandrae chinensis* 6 g

Explanation

This is the main formula for deficiency of both Lung and Kidney Yin. It is a variation of Liu Wei Di Huang Wan *Six-Ingredient Rehmannia Pill* (which nourishes Liver and Kidney Yin) with the addition of Mai Men Dong *Tuber Ophiopogonis japonici* and Wu Wei Zi *Fructus Schisandrae chinensis* to nourish Lung-Yin and absorb leakages (such as night sweating).

Variations

To treat chronic breathlessness, one or two herbs to stimulate the descending of Lung-Qi should be added, as indicated for the previous prescriptions.

- In case of symptoms of rising Yang (such as dizziness and headaches) add Long Gu *Os Draconis* and Mu Li *Concha Ostreae*.

(b) Prescription

EMPIRICAL PRESCRIPTION BY DR DONG JIAN HUA[7]

Dong Chong Xia Cao *Sclerotium Cordicipitis chinensis* 5 g

Sheng Di Huang *Radix Rehmanniae glutinosae* 12 g

Shu Di Huang *Radix Rehmanniae glutinosae praeparata* 12 g

Shan Zhu Yu *Fructus Corni officinalis* 6 g

Zi Shi Ying *Fluoritum* 15 g

Chen Xiang *Lignum Aquilariae* 0.9 g

Chuan Xiong *Radix Ligustici wallichii* 6 g

Wu Wei Zi *Fructus Schisandrae chinensis* 6 g

Xing Ren *Semen Pruni armeniacae* 6 g

Sha Ren *Fructus seu Semen Amomi* 3 g

Explanation

- **Dong Chong Xia Cao** tonifies both Kidney-Yin and Kidney-Yang as well as Lung-Yin.
- **Sheng Di Huang**, **Shu Di Huang** and **Shan Zhu Yu** tonify the Kidneys and Liver.
- **Zi Shi Ying** and **Chen Xiang** strongly promote the descending of Lung-Qi and stop breathlessness.
- **Chuan Xiong** enters the Blood portion in order to open up the Qi passages for Qi to descend.
- **Wu Wei Zi** tonifies the Lungs.
- **Xing Ren** helps to stimulate the descending of Lung-Qi.
- **Sha Ren** resolves Dampness and is here to counterbalance the "stickiness" of the Liver and Kidney tonics in the prescription.

Patent remedy

BA XIAN CHANG SHOU WAN
Eight-Immortal Longevity Pill
Mai Men Dong *Tuber Ophiopogonis japonici*
Wu Wei Zi *Fructus Schisandrae chinensis*
Shu Di Huang *Radix Rehmanniae glutinosae praeparata*
Shan Yao *Radix Dioscoreae oppositae*
Shan Zhu Yu *Fructus Corni officinalis*
Ze Xie *Rhizoma Alismatis orientalis*
Fu Ling *Sclerotium Poriae cocos*
Mu Dan Pi *Cortex Moutan radicis*

Explanation

This remedy has the same ingredients and functions as the homonymous prescription above.

The tongue presentation appropriate to this remedy is a Red tongue without coating.

Case history

A 43-year-old man complained of hay fever and breathlessness for the past 18 years. He found it difficult to breathe in and often sweated at night. His lower back was sore and he suffered from slight tinnitus in one ear. His throat was dry. His pulse was slightly Floating-Empty in general and Weak in the right Front position. His tongue was slightly Red, with rootless coating and dry.

Diagnosis
This man's breathlessness was due to Lung- and Kidney-Yin deficiency. The Lung-Yin deficiency is evident from the dry throat and the rootless coating on the tongue. The Kidney-Yin deficiency caused the back-ache, tinnitus, difficulty in breathing in, night sweating and Floating-Empty pulse.

Treatment
A variation of Ba Xian Chang Shou Wan *Eight Immortals Longevity Pill* was used:

Shu Di Huang *Radix Rehmanniae glutinosae praeparata* 12 g
Shan Zhu Yu *Fructus Corni officinalis* 4 g
Shan Yao *Radix Dioscoreae oppositae* 6 g
Ze Xie *Rhizoma Alismatis orientalis* 4 g
Mu Dan Pi *Cortex Moutan radicis* 4 g
Fu Ling *Sclerotium Poriae cocos* 6 g
Mai Men Dong *Tuber Ophiopogonis japonici* 6 g
Wu Wei Zi *Fructus Schisandrae chinensis* 4 g
Xing Ren *Semen Pruni armeniacae* 4 g
Su Zi *Semen Perillae frutescentis* 6 g
Zhi Gan Cao *Radix Glycyrrhizae uralensis praeparata* 3 g

5. LUNG AND KIDNEY YANG DEFICIENCY, FLUIDS OVERFLOWING TO HEART AND LUNGS

CLINICAL MANIFESTATIONS

Chronic breathlessness, cough with expectoration of white-watery sputum, a feeling of oppression of the chest, palpitations, oedema, scanty urination, chilliness.
Tongue: Pale, Swollen, wet.
Pulse: Deep-Weak-Slow.

This condition is due to deficiency of Yang of Lung and Kidneys leading to the accumulation of Phlegm-Fluids in the Lungs and Heart. The expectoration of white-watery sputum is typical of Phlegm-Fluids.

TREATMENT PRINCIPLE

Tonify and warm Lung and Kidneys, resolve Phlegm-Fluids, stimulate the descending of Lung-Qi.

ACUPUNCTURE

LU-7 Lieque, L.I.-6 Pianli, Ren-17 Shanzhong, Ren-12 Zhongwan, Ren-9 Shuifen, KI-7 Fuliu, Ren-6 Qihai, SP-6 Sanyinjiao, ST-40 Fenglong, P-6 Neiguan, BL-20 Pishu, BL-23 Shenshu, BL-22 Sanjiaoshu, BL-13 Feishu, BL-15 Xinshu. All with reinforcing method except for LU-7, L.I.-6 and Ren-9 which should be needled with even method. Moxa.

Explanation

- **LU-7**, **L.I.-6** and **Ren-17** stimulate the descending of Lung-Qi and open the Lung Water passages to resolve oedema.
- **Ren-12**, **Ren-9** and **Ren-6** tonify Qi and resolve oedema.
- **KI-7** and **SP-6** tonify the Kidneys and resolve oedema.
- **ST-40** resolves Phlegm.
- **P-6** opens the chest thus relieving the feeling of oppression of the chest and tonifies Heart-Yang.
- **BL-20**, **BL-23** and **BL-22** tonify Spleen and Kidney Yang and stimulate the transformation of fluids in the Lower Burner to resolve oedema.
- **BL-13** and **BL-15** tonify Lung and Heart Yang.

HERBAL TREATMENT

Prescription

ZHEN WU TANG Variation
True Warrior Decoction

Fu Zi *Radix Aconiti carmichaeli praeparata* 10 g
Bai Zhu *Rhizoma Atractylodis macrocephalae* 12 g
Fu Ling *Sclerotium Poriae cocos* 15 g
Bai Shao *Radix Paeoniae albae* 6 g
Sheng Jiang *Rhizoma Zingiberis officinalis recens* 3 slices
Gui Zhi *Ramulus Cinnamomi cassiae* 6 g
Huang Qi *Radix Astragali membranacei* 12 g
Fang Ji *Radix Stephaniae tetrandae* 9 g
Xing Ren *Semen Pruni armeniacae* 6 g

Explanation

- The Zhen Wu Tang *True Warrior Decoction* tonifies and warms Spleen- and Kidney-Yang and resolves Phlegm-Fluids.
- **Gui Zhi** warms Yang to move fluids and resolve oedema.
- **Huang Qi** tonifies Lung-Qi and stimulates the Lungs to disperse and descend fluids. It also opens the Lung's Water passages and resolves oedema.
- **Fang Ji** resolves oedema.
- **Xing Ren** stimulates the descending of Lung-Qi and relieves breathlessness.

Variations

- In case of Heart-Yang deficiency as well, with Phlegm-Fluids in the Heart leading to stasis of Blood (purple face, cyanotic lips, dark nails, Purple tongue) add Dan Shen *Radix Salviae miltiorrhizae*, Hong Hua *Flos Carthami tinctorii*, Tao Ren *Semen Persicae* and Chuan Xiong *Rhizoma Ligustici wallichii*.

Patent remedy

JIN GUI SHEN QI WAN
Golden Chest Kidney-Qi Pill
Gui Zhi *Ramulus Cinnamomi cassiae* (or Rou Gui *Cortex Cinnamomi cassiae*)
Fu Zi *Radix Aconiti carmichaeli praeparata*
Shu Di Huang *Radix Rehmanniae glutinosae praeparata*
Shan Yao *Radix Dioscoreae oppositae*
Shan Zhu Yu *Fructus Corni officinalis*
Ze Xie *Rhizoma Alismatis orientalis*

Fu Ling *Sclerotium Poriae cocos*
Mu Dan Pi *Cortex Moutan radicis*

Explanation

This remedy treats only the Root, i.e. tonifies Kidney-Yang, and not the Manifestation (Water overflowing to Heart and Lungs).

The tongue presentation appropriate to this remedy is a Pale and wet body.

6. LUNG-, HEART- AND KIDNEY-YANG DEFICIENCY, FLUIDS OVERFLOWING TO HEART

CLINICAL MANIFESTATIONS

Chronic breathlessness, a feeling of oppression and pain of the chest, nausea, cyanotic lips, purple face and nails, expectoration of white-watery sputum, difficulty in lying down, oedema, chilliness, backache, weak knees, scanty but pale urine.
Tongue: Bluish-Purple and Swollen.
Pulse: Deep-Slow-Knotted.

This condition only occurs in old people suffering from chronic breathlessness. It is characterized by deficiency of Yang of Lungs, Kidneys and Heart leading to the formation of Phlegm-Fluids (manifesting with white-watery expectoration). These overflow to Lungs and Heart. In the Lungs they further impair the descending of Lung-Qi and aggravate the breathlessness. In the Heart they obstruct the circulation of Blood in the chest leading to pain in the chest and cyanotic colour of face, nails, lips and tongue. The deficiency of Kidney-Yang causes back-ache, weak knees and scanty urination.

TREATMENT PRINCIPLE

Tonify and warm Lungs, Heart and Kidneys, resolve Phlegm, restore the descending of Lung-Qi, move Blood and eliminate stasis.

ACUPUNCTURE

LU-7 Lieque, L.I.-6 Pianli, Ren-17 Shanzhong, Ren-12 Zhongwan, Ren-9 Shuifen, KI-7 Fuliu, Ren-6 Qihai, SP-6 Sanyinjiao, ST-40 Fenglong, P-6 Neiguan, BL-20 Pishu, BL-23 Shenshu, BL-22 Sanjiaoshu, BL-13 Feishu, BL-15 Xinshu, BL-17 Geshu, SP-10 Xuehai.

Reinforcing method except on LU-7, L.I.-6, Ren-9, SP-6 and ST-40 which should be needled with even method. Moxa.

Explanation

- **LU-7**, **L.I.-6** and **Ren-17** stimulate the descending of Lung-Qi and open the Lung's Water passages to resolve oedema.
- **Ren-12**, **Ren-9** and **Ren-6** tonify Qi and resolve oedema.
- **KI-7** and **SP-6** tonify the Kidneys and resolve oedema.
- **ST-40** resolves Phlegm.
- **P-6** opens the chest thus relieving the feeling of oppression and tonifies Heart-Yang.
- **BL-20**, **BL-23** and **BL-22** tonify Spleen and Kidney-Yang and stimulate the transformation of fluids in the Lower Burner to resolve oedema.
- **BL-13** and **BL-15** tonify Lung and Heart Yang.
- **BL-17** and **SP-10** move Blood and eliminate stasis.

HERBAL TREATMENT

Prescription

LING GUI ZHU GAN TANG, LING GAN WU WEI JIANG XIN TANG and ZHEN WU TANG (Variation)
Poria-Ramulus Cinnamomi-Atractylodes-Glycyrrhiza Decoction, Poria-Glycyrrhiza-Schisandra-Zingiber-Asarum Decoction and *True Warrior Decoction*
Fu Ling *Sclerotium Poriae cocos* 15 g
Gui Zhi *Ramulus Cinnamomi cassiae* 9 g
Bai Zhu *Rhizoma Atractylodis macrocephalae* 9 g
Zhi Gan Cao *Radix Glycyrrhizae uralensis praeparata* 6 g
Wu Wei Zi *Fructus Schisandrae chinensis* 6 g
Gan Jiang *Rhizoma Zingiberis officinalis* 3 g
Xi Xin *Herba Asari cum radice* 1.5 g
Fu Zi *Radix Aconiti carmichaeli praeparata* 6 g
Bai Shao *Radix Paeoniae albae* 6 g

Dan Shen *Radix Salviae miltiorrhizae* 6 g
Chuan Xiong *Radix Ligustici wallichii* 6 g
Sang Bai Pi *Cortex Mori albae radicis* 6 g
Su Zi *Fructus Perillae frutescentis* 6 g

Explanation

Although this is a variation of three prescriptions, there is quite an overlap of ingredients among the three prescriptions so that the total ingredients are not too many.

- The first prescription Ling Gui Zhu Gan Tang (*Poria-Ramulus Cinnamomi-Atractylodes-Glycyrrhiza Decoction*) tonifies Spleen-Yang and resolves Phlegm-Fluids in the chest. It alleviates nausea, a feeling of oppression of the chest and breathlessness.
- The second prescription Ling Gan Wu Wei Jiang Xin Tang (*Poria-Glycyrrhiza-Schisandra-Zingiber-Asarum Decoction*) warms the Lungs, resolves Phlegm-Fluids and relieves breathlessness and a feeling of oppression of the chest.
- The third prescription, used for the previous pattern, tonifies Spleen- and Kidney-Yang and resolves oedema.
- To these three prescriptions was added **Chuan Xiong** and **Dan Shen** to move Blood in the chest and eliminate stasis, and **Sang Bai Pi** and **Su Zi** to restore the descending of Lung-Qi.

Patent remedy

JIN GUI SHEN QI WAN
Golden Chest Kidney-Qi Pill

Explanation

As mentioned above, this remedy treats only the Root and, actually, only part of the Root, i.e. Kidney-Yang deficiency. It does not treat the Manifestation.

Case history

A 75-year-old woman suffered from breathlessness for 40 years. The breathlessness started after double pneumonia and collapse of a lung. She was treated with Prednisolone for many years. She found it difficult to breathe in or out, had a sensation of oppression of the chest and slight nausea. Her lips were slightly cyanotic and she expectorated white-watery sputum. She felt easily cold and her back and knees ached. Occasionally she felt palpitations.

Her tongue was very Pale but also Bluish on the sides (chest area) and very Swollen. Her pulse was Deep, Weak and Slow. It was particularly Weak on both Rear positions.

Diagnosis
This condition is due to extreme deficiency of Yang of the Lungs, Heart, Spleen and Kidneys, leading to Phlegm-Fluids in the Lungs and Heart.

Treatment
Due to her age and the prolonged use of Prednisolone her condition could only be improved but not cured. She was treated with herbal medicine using a variation of Ling Gui Zhu Gan Tang, Ling Gan Wu Wei Jiang Xin Tang and Zhen Wu Tang (*Poria-Ramulus Cinnamomi-Atractylodes-Glycyrrhiza Decoction, Poria-Glycyrrhiza-Schisandra-Zingiber-Asarum Decoction* and *True Warrior Decoction*).

Fu Ling *Sclerotium Poriae cocos* 10 g
Gui Zhi *Ramulus Cinnamomi cassiae* 3 g
Bai Zhu *Rhizoma Atractylodis macrocephalae* 9 g
Zhi Gan Cao *Radix Glycyrrhizae uralensis praeparata* 3 g
Wu Wei Zi *Fructus Schisandrae chinensis* 4 g
Gan Jiang *Rhizoma Zingiberis officinalis* 1.5 g
Fu Zi *Radix Aconiti carmichaeli praeparata* 3 g
Bai Shao *Radix Paeoniae albae* 6 g
Dan Shen *Radix Salviae miltiorrhizae* 4 g
Chuan Xiong *Radix Ligustici wallichii* 4 g
Sang Bai Pi *Cortex Mori albae radicis* 6 g
Su Zi *Fructus Perillae frutescentis* 6 g
Xing Ren *Semen Pruni armeniacae* 4 g

Prognosis and prevention

Both acupuncture and herbal medicine are effective in treating breathlessness. The kind of results obtained depend on the duration of the disease and the condition of the patient. Generally speaking, acute patterns respond very quickly while chronic conditions obviously respond slowly.

For example, the first three patterns described, i.e. Wind-Cold invading the Lungs, Wind-Cold on the Exterior, Phlegm-Fluids in the Interior and Cold on the Exterior, Heat in the Interior are acute conditions and should therefore respond to treatment in a few sessions with a combination of acupuncture and herbs. The other Excess patterns of Phlegm-Heat in the Lungs, Turbid Phlegm in the Lungs, Lung-Qi Obstructed and Liver-Fire invading the Lungs will take longer to treat, between a few weeks and a few months depending on the severity of the condition. The most difficult to treat out of these four patterns is that of Turbid Phlegm in the Lungs.

Of the Deficiency patterns, the most difficult to treat is that of Lung-, Heart- and Kidney-Yang Deficiency. This is a very chronic condition which only occurs in old people and is characterized by the presence of Phlegm-Fluids affecting both Heart and Lungs. Phlegm-Fluids is a type of Phlegm which is always very difficult to treat.

As for the relative importance of acupuncture and herbs, in general herbs are necessary whenever there is Phlegm as they are better than acupuncture at resolving Phlegm. Acupuncture on its own gives particularly good results in the two Liver-related patterns, i.e. Lung-Qi Obstructed and Liver-Fire insulting the Lungs.

As for prevention, after a successful treatment it is important to take certain preventive measures so that the breathlessness will not recur.

DIET

A person who has been successfully treated for breathlessness should abstain from eating dairy foods (milk, cheese, butter, cream, yoghurt, ice-cream) because these tend to form Phlegm which easily settles in the Lungs and obstructs breathing. For the same reason, greasy and fried foods should be kept to a minimum.

It is also best to advise the patient not to eat too much fresh fruit and raw vegetables. Although in moderation these foods are beneficial, in excess they also tend to form Phlegm and injure Yang. This advice is particularly important for those patients whose breathlessness was caused by deficiency of Yang.

LIFE HABITS

Persons who suffered from breathlessness

should take great care in protecting themselves adequately from wind and cold. All too often the dictates of fashion are not conducive to sensible dressing. Patients who have been suffering from breathlessness should especially take care to protect the upper back and chest.

PREVENTIVE TREATMENT

Both moxa and herbs can be used to prevent a recurrence of breathlessness.

Indirect moxibustion with garlic can be applied in the summertime at 10-day intervals on the following three groups of points:

FIRST GROUP

– Extra-point Bai Lao (on the occiput one *cun* below the hairline and one *cun* from the midline).
– BL-13 Feishu
– BL-43 Gaohuangshu

SECOND GROUP

– Du-14 Dazhui
– BL-12 Fengmen
– BL-20 Pishu

THIRD GROUP

– BL-11 Dashu
– BL-13 Feishu
– BL-23 Shenshu

A herbal plaster can also be applied on the same three groups of points at the same interval in summertime. The herbs used for the plaster are:

– Bai Jie Zi *Semen Sinapis albae*
– Xi Xin *Herba Asari cum radice*
– Gan Sui *Radix Euphorbiae Kansui*
– She Xiang *Secretio Moschus moschiferi*
– Yan Hu Suo *Rhizoma Corydalis yanhusuo.*

Grind these herbs (She Xiang can be omitted as it is very expensive) into a powder in a coffee-grinder, add ginger juice and honey, shape into tiny pieces (about the size of an "O"), place on a plaster and stick this on the acupuncture points. Keep the plasters on *not more* than 2 hours as the herbs are blistering.

Patients who are prone to Lung-Qi deficiency could take a course of Yu Ping Feng San *Jade Wind Screen Powder* towards the end of August of each year.

Patients who are prone to Kidney deficiency can take the Jin Gui Shen Qi Wan *Golden Chest Kidney-Qi Pill* (as a pill) during the winter months. In case of Kidney-Yin deficiency, they should take Liu Wei Di Huang Wan *Six-Ingredient Rehmannia Pill* instead.

Western differential diagnosis

Dyspnoea (breathlessness) can have many different causes in Western medicine. However, apart from general causes such as anemia, they all relate either to the lungs or heart.

In fact, breathlessness can arise either from a disease of the lungs themselves (such as asthma, bronchitis or emphysema), or from a heart disease affecting the lungs (such as left ventricular heart failure).

The most common causes of chronic breathlessness can be summarized with a diagram (Fig. 3.2).

1. CAUSES IN LUNGS

(a) ASTHMA

This consists in the constriction of the bronchi on exhalation. It may arise during childhood in atopic individuals, i.e. those who easily form antibodies to commonly-encountered allergens such as house dust, pollen or house-dust mites. Such patients often suffer from other allergic diseases such as allergic rhinitis or atopic eczema. This is called early-onset or extrinsic asthma and will be discussed in a separate chapter (ch. 5). In other cases, it starts in later life in non-atopic individuals and is called late-onset or intrisic asthma. This type of asthma is not due to an allergic reaction.

In both types the main manifestations are breathlessness on exertion and wheezing and coughing which may be worse at night.

(b) CHRONIC BRONCHITIS

This is due to narrowing of the bronchioles by mucus and oedema of mucous membranes within the lungs. It is this narrowing that causes the breathlessness.

This condition occurs in middle-aged or elderly people and the main distinguishing sign to differentiate it from asthma is a chronic productive cough with abundant expectoration. It also differs from asthma in so far as the breathlessness is often worse in the morning (rather than at night as in asthma). Another feature of this condition is the propensity to frequent chest infections.

With time, chronic bronchitis may lead to emphysema, i.e. overdistension of the alveoli.

(c) EMPHYSEMA

This condition is due to a permanent and irreversible overdistension of the alveoli. It frequently develops from chronic bronchitis as explained above. After years of overdistension, an increasing proportion of the alveolar wall disintegrates with progressive obliteration of the vascular bed of the lungs. This is the most common cause of right ventricular heart failure, which, in itself, also causes breathlessness.

The main clinical features are breathlessness first on exertion and, with time, also at rest. In severe cases the breathlessness is constant, the chest movements are limited, the breath sounds inaudible and there may be cyanosis.

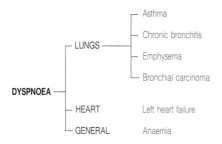

Fig. 3.2 Causes of chronic breathlessness

Emphysema can be clearly differentiated from asthma as the breathlessness is constant, whereas in asthma, it comes in bouts. It can be differentiated from chronic bronchitis as there is no cough nor abundant sputum.

The differentiation between asthma, chronic bronchitis and emphysema is important for prognosis as the first two react well to acupuncture and herbal treatment, whilst emphysema less so (Table 3.1).

(d) CARCINOMA OF BRONCHI

This is statistically the most common of all carcinomas and it accounts for 40% of all male deaths from malignant disease.

The main clinical manifestations are a cough, with scanty sputum which may be blood-tinged, chest pain and breathlessness, although this may appear only in quite late stages.

2. CAUSES IN HEART

LEFT HEART FAILURE

When the left ventricle of the heart loses strength of contraction blood accumulates behind the left ventricle in the pulmonary veins and lungs. The resulting pulmonary congestion reduces the supply of oxygen to the alveoli and causes breathlessness.

Left ventricular failure may be caused by:

– Cardiac infarction
– Aortic disease
– Mitral incompetence
– Essential hypertension.

The patient is severely breathless on exertion and has to sit up in bed to breathe, gasping for breath. He or she may wake up suddenly and feel hot. The breathlessness gets progressively worse until it is constant. There may also be a cough at night with watery-frothy sputum, palpitations, giddiness, nausea, vomiting, diarrhoea and abdominal pain. The phenomenon of "pulsus alternans" may be heard on the sphygmomanometer: at the upper limit only half the heart beats come through but when the pressure is lowered by 10 mm or more all the beats become audible. For example, at 180 mm the pulse rate may appear to be 50, whilst at 160 mm it is 100.

3. GENERAL CAUSES

ANAEMIA

Breathlessness on exertion is a feature of anaemia.

The causes of breathlessness are summarized in Table 3.2.

Table 3.1   Comparison of asthma, chronic bronchitis and emphysema

	Asthma	Chronic bronchitis	Emphysema
Frequency	Bouts of dyspnoea	Bouts of dyspnoea with chest infections	Constant dyspnoea
Time	Worse of night	Worse in the morning	All the time
Allergies	Yes	No	No
Sputum	No	Yes	Yes

Table 3.2   Synopsis of causes of breathlessness

Disease	Pathology	Symptoms	Signs
Asthma	Bronchospasm	Bouts of dyspnoea	Wheezing sound
Chronic bronchitis	Narrowing of bronchi by mucus	Dyspnoea, stuffiness of chest	Cough with abundant sputum
Emphysema	Distension of alveoli	Constant dyspnoea	Thin chest
Carcinoma of bronchi	Tumour obstructing bronchi	Chest pain, cough, dyspnoea, tiredness, poor appetite	Blood-tinged sputum, weight loss
Left heart failure	Blood accumulating in lungs and pulmonary vein	Dyspnoea on exertion, gasping for breath, palpitations, giddiness, nausea, vomiting	Watery-frothy sputum, intervals of apnoea lasting 20–30 seconds, "pulsus alternans"
Anemia	Reduced red blood cells	Dyspnoea, tiredness	Pallor

END NOTES

1. 1979 The Yellow Emperor's Classic of Internal Medicine — Simple Questions (*Huang Ti Nei Jing Su Wen* 黄帝内经素问), People's Health Publishing House, Beijing, p. 147. First published *c.* 100 BC.

2. Ibid., p. 336.

3. 1981 Spiritual Axis (*Ling Shu Jing* 灵枢经), People's Health Publishing House, Beijing, p. 55. First published *c.* 100 BC.

4. He Ren 1979 A Popular Guide to the Essential Prescriptions of the Golden Chest (*Jin Gui Yao Lue Tong Su Jiang Hua* 金匮要略通俗讲话), Shanghai Science Publishing House, Shanghai, p. 46. The "Essential Prescriptions of the Golden Chest" itself by Zhang Zhong Jing was published *c.* AD 200.

5. Cited in Zhang Bo Yu 1986 Internal Medicine (*Zhong Yi Nei Ke Xue* 中医内科学), Shanghai Science Publishing House, p. 66.

6. Zhang Jing Yue (or Zhang Jie Bin) 1959 Complete Book of Jing Yue (*Jing Yue Quan Shu* 景岳全书), Shanghai Science Publishing House, p. 345. First published 1624.

7. Tian Hai He 1990 Dr Dong Jian Hua's Experience in Treating Asthma. In Journal of Traditional Chinese Medicine (*Zhong Yi Za Zhi* 中医杂志), All-China Association of Traditional Chinese Medicine, vol. 31, no. 6, p. 18.

Wheezing ("Xíao") 4 哮证

"*Xiao*" indicates a wheezing sound which may resemble that of whistling, snoring or sawing. It is usually accompanied by breathlessness with an inability to breathe when lying down.

The "Prescriptions of the Golden Chest" by Dr Zhang Zhong Jing was the first book to refer to wheezing: "*For cough with a moor-hen sound in the throat, use Belamcanda-Ephedra Decoction.*"[1] The "moor-hen sound in the throat" is wheezing. In later times wheezing was also variously described as "hidden Yin", "sip cough", "howling wheezing" and "snoring wheezing".

In subsequent dynasties the symptoms of wheezing (*Xiao*) and breathlessness (*Chuan*) were not differentiated. Dr Zhu Dan Xi (1281–1358) was the first to use the term "*Xiao-Chuan*" and considered it due to Phlegm. He therefore indicated that the main principle of treatment was to tonify the body's Qi and, in acute cases, expel pathogenic factors.

The book "Orthodox Medical Record" (1515) by Dr Yu Tuan distinguishes between Wheezing (*Xiao*) and Breathlessness (*Chuan*) for the first time:

Wheezing is named after its sound, Breathlessness after the breath. If breathing is rapid and there is a sound in the throat like a moor-hen, it is Wheezing [Xiao]; if breathing is rapid continuously and there is breathlessness, it is called Breathlessness [Chuan].[2]

The "Case Reports for Clinical Practice" (1766) by Dr Ye Gui differentiates the two conditions by saying:

If the pathogenic factor is expelled, breathlessness [Chuan] stops and will never return . . . In wheezing [Xiao], the pathogenic factor is hidden in the Interior and in the Lungs, it is sometimes active and sometimes quiescent, and there are frequent episodes over many years.[3]

Doctors of subsequent dynasties reverted to considering Wheezing and Breathlessness as one condition.

In modern China they are also considered together and modern books usually say that they may correspond to the two separate conditions of "bronchial asthma" or "asthmatic bronchitis" (chronic bronchitis leading to breathlessness).

There are different types of asthma and they may be summarized in three groups:

1. Allergic (or atopic) asthma which starts in early childhood and is often associated with eczema: this will be discussed in a separate chapter (ch. 5).

2. Asthma which starts early during childhood after repeated invasions of external Wind leading to chest infections.

3. Asthma which starts later in life as a consequence of repeated invasions of exterior Wind, irregular diet, emotional strain, overwork and excessive sexual activity.

The symptom of "Wheezing" discussed in this chapter corresponds to nos 2. and 3. above.

Aetiology

1. EXTERNAL PATHOGENIC FACTORS

External Wind-Cold or Wind-Heat may invade the body, penetrate deeper and settle in the Lungs. Here they obstruct Lung-Qi, which then cannot transform fluids; and the fluids accumulate into Phlegm.

2. DIET

The excessive consumption of cold, sour, or sweet-greasy foods injures the Spleen so that it cannot transform and transport food essences properly. When this happens, Phlegm forms, it accumulates in the Lungs, obstructs Lung-Qi and causes wheezing. Old books distinguished "food-wheezing", "sugar-wheezing" or "sour-wheezing" according to the particular type of food responsible.

3. WEAK BODY CONDITION

A weakened body condition after a long illness (which in children may happen after measles or whooping cough) may deplete Lung-Qi and Spleen-Qi. When this happens, fluids are not tranformed properly and Phlegm forms.

If the Yin of the body is depleted, Empty-Heat arises; this evaporates and condenses fluids into Phlegm.

Pathology

The main pathological factor in Wheezing is "hidden Phlegm" stored in the Lungs. The upwards movement of Phlegm propelled by rebellious Qi narrows the airways and causes wheezing. The "Supplement to Diagnosis and Treatment" (1687) by Li Yong Cui says:

Chronic wheezing and breathlessness are due to: 1) obstruction of Qi in the Interior; 2) an attack of an exterior pathogenic factor; 3) sticky Phlegm in the diaphragm. These three factors combine to obstruct the Qi passages and when breath is forced out there is a wheezing sound.[4]

Factors which may trigger the upwards movement of rebellious Qi and Phlegm are weather changes, diet, emotional stress and overwork.

Phlegm may be cold or hot. *Cold Phlegm* may derive from frequent exposure to cold which injures the Lungs or from excessive consumption of cold foods which injure Spleen-Yang. Cold Phlegm is more likely to be stirred by external pathogenic factors. It both derives from and causes Yang deficiency.

Hot Phlegm may derive from excessive consumption of sour, sweet, or greasy foods. Yin deficiency may contribute to forming Phlegm-Heat.

In chronic cases Cold Phlegm injures Spleen-Yang while Hot Phlegm injures Lung-Yin. The disease becomes therefore characterized by a combination of Fullness (Phlegm) and Emptiness (of the Lungs, Spleen or Kidneys). Deficient Lungs, Spleen and Kidney may in turn all lead to Phlegm. In particular, if Kidney-Yang is deficient there will be Cold Phlegm; if Kidney-Yin is deficient there will be Phlegm-Heat.

In severe and prolonged cases, when the deficient Lungs fail to control the blood vessels and harmonize the channels, Heart-Blood cannot circulate properly, the Fire of the Gate of Vitality cannot rise to the Heart and this causes a deficiency of Heart-Yang.

Differentiation and treatment

In order to apply the correct principle of treatment a clear distinction must be made between the acute and chronic phases. In general one follows the principle of treating the Manifestation during the acute phase, and the Root during the chronic phase. This means that in the acute phase one must expel pathogenic factors, resolve Phlegm and restore the descending of Lung-Qi. During the chronic phase attention should be turned to tonifying the body's Qi, particularly of the Lungs, Spleen or Kidneys.

In some chronic cases, it may be necessary to treat both Manifestation and Root simultaneously.

The patterns discussed are:

ACUTE PHASE

Cold Phlegm
Hot Phlegm

CHRONIC PHASE

Lung Deficiency
Spleen Deficiency
Kidney Deficiency

ACUTE PHASE

This includes not only treatment during the actual acute attack but also treatment during a period of time when attacks are frequent. The main differentiation to be made is that between Cold or Hot Phlegm and the main principle of treatment is to resolve Phlegm and restore the descending of Lung-Qi.

1. COLD PHLEGM

CLINICAL MANIFESTATIONS

Rapid breathing, wheezing, a feeling of fullness and oppression of the chest, cough, scanty phlegm, a bluish-white complexion, no thirst, or a desire for warm drinks, feeling cold, worse in cold weather.
Tongue: Swollen with a sticky-white coating.
Pulse: Tight and Slippery.

TREATMENT PRINCIPLE

Warm the Lungs, scatter Cold, resolve Phlegm, relieve breathlessness.

ACUPUNCTURE

LU-7 Lieque, BL-13 Feishu, LU-1 Zhongfu, LU-6 Kongzui, Ren-22 Tiantu, Ren-17 Shanzhong, ST-40 Fenglong, P-6 Neiguan. All with reducing or even method. Moxa is applicable.

Explanation

- **LU-7, BL-13** and **LU-1** restore the descending of Lung-Qi and stop wheezing.
- **LU-6**, Accumulation point, stops wheezing and breathlessness in acute cases.
- **Ren-22** restores the descending of Lung-Qi and resolves Phlegm.
- **Ren-17** moves Qi in the chest and affects the Lung channel. With direct moxa, it can dispel Cold from the Lungs.
- **ST-40** and **P-6** open the chest, relieve breathlessness and resolve Phlegm.

HERBAL TREATMENT

Prescription

SHE GAN MA HUANG TANG
Belamcanda-Ephedra Decoction
She Gan *Rhizoma Belamcandae chinensis* 6 g
Ma Huang *Herba Ephedrae* 9 g
Gan Jiang *Rhizoma Zingiberis officinalis* 3 g
Xi Xin *Herba Asari cum radice* 3 g
Ban Xia *Rhizoma Pinelliae ternatae* 9 g
Zi Wan *Radix Asteris tatarici* 6 g
Kuan Dong Hua *Flos Tussilaginis farfarae* 6 g
Gan Cao *Radix Glycyrrhizae uralensis* 3 g
Wu Wei Zi *Fructus Schisandrae chinensis* 3 g
Da Zao *Fructus Ziziphi jujubae* 3 dates

Explanation

- **She Gan** and **Ma Huang** restore the descending of Lung-Qi, stop wheezing, resolve Phlegm, calm breathlessness and benefit the throat.
- **Gan Jiang**, **Xi Xin** and **Ban Xia** warm the Lungs and resolve Cold Phlegm.
- **Zi Wan**, **Kuan Dong Hua** and **Gan Cao** resolve Phlegm and stop cough.
- **Wu Wei Zi** absorbs Lung-Qi and moderates the scattering effect of the other herbs (especially Ma Huang and Xi Xin).
- **Da Zao** harmonizes.

Variations

- If there are symptoms of exterior Cold and internal Phlegm-Fluids, use Xiao Qing Long Tang *Small Green Dragon Decoction* instead.
- In a chronic case with Yang deficiency and frequent attacks with wheezing that sounds like low snoring, breathing not rapid, watery sputum, a dull-pale complexion, cold sweating, a Deep pulse and a Pale tongue, one must treat both the Manifestation and the Root simultaneously. One must resolve Phlegm and restore the descending of Lung-Qi on one hand, and tonify Kidney-Yang on the other hand. This therapeutic aim may be achieved by using Su Zi Jiang Qi Tang *Perilla Seed Lowering Qi Decoction*. Add to this formula: Dang Shen *Radix Codonopsis pilosulae*, Hu Tao Rou *Semen Juglandis regiae* and Qi Dai *Umbilical cord* to tonify Spleen and Kidneys, and Chen Xiang *Lignum Aquilariae* to restore the descending of Lung-Qi.
- In cases of very severe symptoms of Yang deficiency (such as severe chilliness and a very Pale and wet tongue) add Fu Zi *Radix Aconiti carmichaeli praeparata*.

2. HOT PHLEGM

CLINICAL MANIFESTATIONS

Wheezing with a loud noise, breathlessness, distended chest, cough, yellow-sticky sputum, irritability, sweating, a red face, a bitter taste, thirst, a feeling of heat.
Tongue: Red with a yellow-sticky coating.
Pulse: Slippery-Rapid.

TREATMENT PRINCIPLE

Clear Heat, restore the descending of Lung-Qi, resolve Phlegm, stop wheezing.

ACUPUNCTURE

LU-5 Chize, LU-10 Yuji, LU-6 Kongzui, BL-13 Feishu, LU-1 Zhongfu, L.I.-11 Quchi, P-5 Jianshi, ST-40 Fenglong, Ren-22 Tiantu.

Explanation

- **LU-5** resolves Phlegm-Heat from the Lungs.
- **LU-10** clears Lung-Heat.
- **LU-6**, Accumulation point, stops wheezing and breathlessness in acute cases.
- **LU-1** and **BL-13**, Front-Collecting and Back-Transporting point respectively, clear Lung-Heat and restore the descending of Lung-Qi, especially in acute cases.
- **L.I.-11** clears Heat.
- **P-5** and **ST-40** resolve Phlegm and open the chest.
- **Ren-22** resolves Phlegm, restores the descending of Lung-Qi and benefits the throat.

HERBAL TREATMENT

Prescription

DING CHUAN TANG
Stopping Breathlessness Decoction
Ma Huang *Herba Ephedrae* 9 g
Huang Qin *Radix Scutellariae baicalensis* 6 g
Sang Bai Pi *Cortex Mori albae radicis* 9 g
Xing Ren *Semen Pruni armeniacae* 9 g
Ban Xia *Rhizoma Pinelliae ternatae* 9 g
Kuan Dong Hua *Flos Tussilaginis farfarae* 9 g
Su Zi *Fructus Perillae frutescentis* 6 g
Bai Guo *Semen Ginkgo bilobae* 9 g
Gan Cao *Radix Glycyrrhizae uralensis* 3 g

Explanation

- **Ma Huang** and **Bai Guo** are coordinated: one is scattering, the other sour and absorbing. The two together restore the dispersing and descending of Lung-Qi and stop wheezing.
- **Huang Qin** and **Sang Bai Pi** clear Lung-Heat and also restore the descending of Lung-Qi.
- **Xing Ren** and **Su Zi** restore the descending of Lung-Qi and stop wheezing.
- **Ban Xia** resolves Phlegm and subdues rebellious Qi.
- **Kuan Dong Hua** stops cough and wheezing.
- **Gan Cao** harmonizes.

Variations

- If there are simultaneous symptoms of exterior Cold add Gui Zhi *Ramulus Cinnamomi cassiae* and Sheng Jiang *Rhizoma Zingiberis officinalis recens*.
- If there are symptoms of Fire (as opposed to Heat) such as constipation, dark urine, dry stools, dry mouth and a dry-yellow tongue coating, add Da Huang *Rhizoma Rhei* and Mang Xiao *Mirabilitum*.
- If there is vomiting of sticky-yellow phlegm add Zhi Mu *Radix Anemarrhenae asphodeloidis*, Hai Ge Ke *Concha Cyclinae sinensis* and She Gan *Rhizoma Belamcandae chinensis*.
- If Heat has injured the Yin add Mai Men Dong Tang *Ophiopogon Decoction*.
- If Phlegm is the main problem without any clear-cut hot or cold symptom, use San Zi Yang Qin Tang *Three-Seed Nourishing the Parents Decoction*.

(a) Patent remedy

ZHI SOU DING CHUAN WAN
Stopping Cough and Calming Breathlessness Pill
Ma Huang *Herba Ephedrae*
Xing Ren *Semen Pruni armeniacae*
Shi Gao *Gypsum fibrosum*
Zhi Gan Cao *Radix Glycyrrhizae uralensis praeparata*

Explanation

This remedy corresponds to the prescription for combined Greater Yang and Bright Yang patterns of the Six Stages from the "Discussion of Cold-induced Diseases". However, its main impact is to clear Lung-Heat and restore the descending of Lung-Qi.

The tongue presentation appropriate to this remedy is a Red body in the front part.

Case history

A 58-year-old man had been suffering from asthma for 6 years. At the time of consultation, the asthma was very severe with frequent attacks every day. He was using a Ventolin inhaler, Becoforte (corticosteroid) spray and cortico-steroids orally. His chest felt extremely tight and he could not lie down. He was prone to chest infections, developing expectoration of yellow sputum. He also experienced epigastric fullness and distension. His tongue was slightly Red, with swollen edges (of the Spleen-type) and a sticky coating (Plate 4.1). His pulse was Rapid, Full and Slippery.

Diagnosis
This is non-allergic late-onset asthma from Hot Phlegm against a background of Spleen deficiency.

Treatment principle
Since the attacks are severe and frequent, this is treated as an acute case and attention must be turned to treating the Manifestation, i.e. resolve Phlegm, clear Heat and restore the descending of Lung-Qi.

Treatment
This patient was treated with acupuncture only. He had to be treated every other day initially, followed by a gradual spacing-out of treatments. The main points used were:

- **SP-4** Gongsun and **P-6** Neiguan, open the Penetrating Vessel, relax the chest and subdue rebellious Stomach-Qi. The Lung and Stomach channels are closely connected and rebellious Stomach-Qi will adversely affect Lung-Qi.
- **LU-5** Chize, **LU-7** Lieque and **LU-6** Kongzui restore the descending of Lung-Qi. LU-6, Accumulation point, is specific for acute cases. LU-5 also clears Phlegm from the Lungs.
- **LU-1** Zhongfu and **BL-13** Feishu, Front-Collecting and Back-Transporting points respectively, clear Lung-Heat and restore the descending of Lung-Qi.
- **ST-40** Fenglong and **SP-6** Sanyinjiao resolve Phlegm. ST-40 also opens the chest and eases breathing.
- **Dingchuan**, extra point 0.5 *cun* lateral to Du-14 Dazhui, is an empirical point for acute asthma.

With treatment on alternate days, he started to improve gradually. The treatment was slowed down by his use of oral cortico-steroids. However, these were gradually reduced and discontinued after 3 months. As he started to improve, after 3 months the treatment included some tonification of the Spleen (with Ren-12 Zhongwan, BL-20 Pishu and ST-36 Zusanli) and the use of the patent remedy Ping Chuan Wan *Calming Breathlessness Pill* which tonifies Spleen and Kidneys and restores the descending of Lung-Qi.

CHRONIC PHASE

During the chronic phase the main priority is to tonify Lungs, Spleen, or Kidneys.

1. LUNG DEFICIENCY

CLINICAL MANIFESTATIONS

Sweating, chilliness, propensity to catching colds, sneezing, a runny nose, shortness of breath, slight wheezing with a low sound, a slight cough.
Tongue: Pale.
Pulse: Weak.

TREATMENT PRINCIPLE

Tonify the Lungs and consolidate the Exterior.

ACUPUNCTURE

LU-9 Taiyuan, ST-36 Zusanli, Ren-6 Qihai, BL-13 Feishu, Du-12 Shenzhu, LU-7 Lieque. All with reinforcing method.

Explanation

- **LU-9**, **BL-13** and **Du-12** tonify Lung-Qi and consolidate the Exterior.
- **ST-36** and **Ren-6** tonify Qi in general.
- **LU-7** restores the descending of Lung-Qi and stops wheezing and cough.

HERBAL TREATMENT

Prescription

YU PING FENG SAN
Jade Wind Screen Powder

Huang Qi *Radix Astragali membranacei* 30 g
Bai Zhu *Rhizoma Atractylodis macrocephalae* 60 g
Fang Feng *Radix Ledebouriellae sesloidis* 30 g

Explanation

- **Huang Qi** and **Bai Zhu** tonify Lung-Qi and consolidate the Exterior.
- **Fang Feng**, in combination with the previous two, consolidates the Exterior and prevents invasion of exterior Wind.

Note that the above dosages are for making a batch of powder and not a decoction.

Variations

- If there are Cold symptoms add Gui Zhi *Ramulus Cinnamomi cassiae*, Bai Shao *Radix Paeoniae albae*, Sheng Jiang *Rhizoma Zingiberis officinalis recens* and Da Zao *Fructus Ziziphi jujubae*.
- If there is both Qi and Yin deficiency add Sheng Mai San *Generating the Pulse Decoction*.

2. SPLEEN DEFICIENCY

CLINICAL MANIFESTATIONS

Slight wheezing that has a low sound, poor appetite, slight abdominal distension, intolerance to certain foods, tiredness, shortness of breath, dislike of speaking, desire to lie down, weariness.
Tongue: Pale.
Pulse: Weak.

TREATMENT PRINCIPLE

Tonify the Spleen and resolve Phlegm.

ACUPUNCTURE

ST-36 Zusanli, SP-3 Taibai, BL-20 Pishu, BL-21 Weishu, Ren-12 Zhongwan, ST-40 Fenglong, LU-7 Lieque, LU-9 Taiyuan, BL-13 Feishu, Ren-6 Qihai. All with reinforcing method. Moxa is applicable.

Explanation

- **ST-36**, **SP-3**, **BL-20**, **BL-21** and **Ren-12** tonify Stomach and Spleen.
- **ST-40** resolves Phlegm.
- **LU-7** restores the descending of Lung-Qi.
- **LU-9** and **BL-13** tonify Lung-Qi.
- **Ren-6** tonifies Qi in general.

HERBAL TREATMENT

Prescription

LIU JUN ZI TANG
Six Gentlemen Decoction
Ren Shen *Radix Ginseng* 10 g
Bai Zhu *Rhizoma Atractylodis macrocephalae* 9 g
Fu Ling *Sclerotium Poriae cocos* 9 g
Zhi Gan Cao *Radix Glycyrrhizae uralensis prae-parata* 6 g
Chen Pi *Pericarpium Citri reticulatae* 9 g
Ban Xia *Rhizoma Pinelliae ternatae* 12 g

Explanation

- **Ren Shen**, **Bai Zhu**, **Fu Ling** and **Gan Cao** tonify Qi.
- **Chen Pi** and **Ban Xia** resolve Dampness.

Variations

- If there are pronounced symptoms of Cold add Gui Zhi *Ramulus Cinnamomi cassiae* and Gan Jiang *Rhizoma Zingiberis officinalis*.

Patent remedy

QI GUAN YAN KE SOU TAN CHUAN WAN
Bronchial Cough, Phlegm and Dyspnoea Pill
Qian Hu *Radix Peucedani*
Xing Ren *Semen Pruni armeniacae*
Yuan Zhi *Radix Polygalae tenuifoliae*
Sang Ye *Folium Mori albae*
Chuan Bei Mu *Bulbus Fritillariae cirrhosae*
Chen Pi *Pericarpium Citri reticulatae*
Pi Pa Ye *Folium Eriobotryae japonicae*
Kuan Dong Hua *Flos Tussilaginis farfarae*
Dang Shen *Radix Codonopsis pilosulae*
Ma Dou Ling *Fructus Aristolochiae*
Wu Wei Zi *Fructus Schisandrae chinensis*

Sheng Jiang *Rhizoma Zingiberis officinalis recens*
Da Zao *Fructus Ziziphi jujubae*

Explanation

This pill tonifies Spleen-Qi, resolves Phlegm and stimulates the descending of Lung-Qi. It is suitable for chronic wheezing with a background of Spleen deficiency and Phlegm. It is appropriate for both Cold or Hot Phlegm.

Case history

A 45-year-old woman had been suffering from asthma for 8 years since she stopped smoking. She found it difficult to breathe in and had a constant nasal discharge. She constantly felt catarrh in her throat and chest and sometimes coughed up some sticky-yellow phlegm. She often experienced a feeling of oppression of the chest and slight nausea. She was slightly deaf in one ear and her urine was rather pale. She often complained of bad digestion, slight thirst and acid regurgitation. She frequently had hiccups for long periods of time.

She was overweight, particularly around her stomach and abdomen. Her tongue body was of a normal colour although slightly Purple on the sides (chest area), was very Swollen, and with a Stomach crack in the middle with a rough, dirty-yellow coating in it (Plate 4.2). Her pulse was definitely Slippery on the whole and slightly Weak on the right side.

Diagnosis
This is a clear case of retention of Phlegm-Heat with a background of Spleen deficiency. The symptoms of Phlegm-Heat are: expectoration of sticky-yellow phlegm, nasal discharge, feeling of oppression of the chest, nausea, overweight body, Swollen tongue and Slippery pulse. Although this is Phlegm-Heat because the mucus is yellow, the Heat is only slight and the predominant aspect is the Phlegm rather than Heat.

There is also a slight, secondary Kidney-Yang deficiency as shown by the slight deafness and pale urine.

A third pathological condition is the retention of Phlegm-Heat in the Stomach as shown by the acid regurgitation, bad digestion and Stomach crack with rough, yellow coating inside it. The presence of Phlegm-Heat induced Stomach-Qi to rebel upwards causing frequent hiccups. The rebelling upwards of Stomach-Qi contributed to the asthma.

The fact that her asthma started after *stopping* smoking is puzzling but interesting. One possible explanation could be that the conditions to cause asthma were already present but tobacco, which has a hot and *drying* energy, constantly dried up Phlegm, thus delaying the onset of the disease. A sudden cessation of smoking means that the drying action of tobacco is abruptly withdrawn and Phlegm therefore overflows profusely.

Treatment principle
Since this is a chronic condition the treatment principle is to treat Root and Manifestation simultaneously, i.e. tonify the body's Qi and expel pathogenic factors. Treating the Root involves primarily tonifying Spleen-Qi and secondarily tonifying Kidney-Yang. Treating the Manifestation involves resolving Phlegm from the Lungs, restoring the descending of Lung-Qi, resolving Phlegm-Heat from the Stomach and subduing rebellious Stomach-Qi.

Treatment
This patient was treated with both acupuncture and herbs. The acupuncture treatment was focused on tonifying the Spleen, restoring the descending of Lung-Qi and subduing Stomach-Qi.
The main points used at various times were:

- **SP-4** Gongsun on the right and **P-6** Neiguan on the left, to open the Penetrating Vessel and subdue rebellious Stomach-Qi. The Lung and Stomach channels are closely connected and Qi rebelling upwards in one channel easily affects the other. It was therefore important in this case to subdue Stomach-Qi as well as stimulate the descending of Lung-Qi. The Penetrating Vessel is excellent to subdue rebellious Stomach-Qi, especially in overweight people.
- **ST-40** Fenglong to resolve Phlegm and open the chest.
- **Ren-12** Zhongwan, **BL-20** Pishu and **Ren-9** Shuifen to tonify the Spleen and resolve Phlegm.
- **LU-7** Lieque, **Ren-22** Tiantu and **LU-5** Chize to restore the descending of Lung-Qi.
- **BL-23** Shenshu and **KI-7** Fuliu to tonify Kidney-Yang.

Since acupuncture was aimed at treating the Root by tonifying the Spleen and Kidneys, the herbs were used mainly to treat the Manifestation, i.e. to resolve Phlegm, as they are better than acupuncture at doing this. The main formula used was a variation of Wen Dan Tang *Warming the Gall-Bladder Decoction* which resolves Phlegm-Heat from both Lungs and Stomach:

Zhu Ru *Caulis Bambusae in Taeniis* 6 g
Zhi Shi *Fructus Citri aurantii immaturus* 6 g
Ban Xia *Rhizoma Pinelliae ternatae* 6 g
Fu Ling *Sclerotium Poriae cocos* 6 g
Chen Pi *Pericarpium Citri reticulatae* 4 g
Sheng Jiang *Rhizoma Zingiberis officinalis recens* 3 slices
Da Zao *Fructus Ziziphi jujubae* 3 dates
Xing Ren *Semen Pruni armeniacae* 4 g
Su Zi *Fructus Perillae frutescentis* 6 g
Hou Po *Cortex Magnoliae officinalis* 4 g

Explanation
- The first seven herbs constitute the Wen Dan Tang which resolves Phlegm-Heat.
- **Xing Ren** and **Su Zi** restore the descending of Lung-Qi.
- **Hou Po** moves Qi and relieves fullness and oppression of the chest.

As the treatment progressed and she improved, a few herbs to strengthen the Spleen were added, such as Bai Zhu *Rhizoma Atractylodis macrocephalae* and the dosage of Fu Ling *Sclerotium Poriae cocos* was increased.
This patient achieved great improvement in 9 months of treatment.

3. KIDNEY DEFICIENCY

CLINICAL MANIFESTATIONS

Shortness of breath, slight wheezing that has a low sound, greater difficulty in breathing in, absent-mindedness, poor memory, tinnitus, weakness and soreness of the lower back, breathlessness on exertion.
Kidney-Yang deficiency: chilliness, Pale tongue, Deep-Weak pulse.
Kidney-Yin deficiency: feeling of heat, Red tongue without coating, Floating-Empty pulse.

TREATMENT PRINCIPLE

Tonify the Kidneys, strengthen the Kidney's grasping of Qi.

ACUPUNCTURE

KI-3 Taixi, SP-6 Sanyinjiao, Ren-4 Guanyuan, BL-23 Shenshu, BL-13 Feishu, Du-12 Shenzhu, KI-25 Shencang. All with reinforcing method. Use moxa for Kidney-Yang deficiency.

Explanation

- **KI-3**, **SP-6**, **Ren-4** and **BL-23** tonify the Kidneys.
- **BL-13** and **Du-12** strengthen the Lungs.
- **KI-25** is an important local point to relieve wheezing due to a Kidney deficiency.

HERBAL TREATMENT

(a) Prescription

Kidney-Yang deficiency

JIN GUI SHEN QI WAN
Golden Chest Kidney-Qi Pill
Fu Zi *Radix Aconiti carmichaeli praeparata* 3 g
Gui Zhi *Ramulus Cinnamomi cassiae* 3 g
Shu Di Huang *Radix Rehmanniae glutinosae praeparata* 24 g
Shan Zhu Yu *Fructus Corni officinalis* 12 g
Shan Yao *Radix Dioscoreae oppositae* 12 g
Ze Xie *Rhizoma Alismatis orientalis* 9 g
Mu Dan Pi *Cortex Moutan radicis* 9 g
Fu Ling *Sclerotium Poriae cocos* 9 g

Variations

– For severe Yang deficiency add Bu Gu Zhi
  Fructus Psoraleae corylifoliae and Lu Jiao *Cornu cervi*.
– To strengthen the Kidney's grasping of Qi
  add Hu Tao Rou *Semen Juglandis regiae*.

Kidney-Yin deficiency

MAI WEI DI HUANG WAN (BA XIAN CHANG SHOU WAN)
Ophiopogon-Schisandra-Rehmannia Pill (Eight Immortals Longevity Pill)
Shu Di Huang *Radix Rehmanniae glutinosae praeparata* 24 g
Shan Zhu Yu *Fructus Corni officinalis* 12 g
Shan Yao *Radix Dioscoreae oppositae* 12 g
Ze Xie *Rhizoma Alismatis orientalis* 9 g
Mu Dan Pi *Cortex Moutan radicis* 9 g
Fu Ling *Sclerotium Poriae cocos* 9 g
Mai Men Dong *Tuber Ophiopogonis japonici* 6 g
Wu Wei Zi *Fructus Schisandrae chinensis* 6 g

Variation

– To strengthen the Kidney's grasping of Qi
  add Hu Tao Rou *Semen Juglandis regiae* and Zi
  He Che *Placenta hominis*.

(i) Patent remedy

BA XIAN CHANG SHOU WAN
Eight Immortals Longevity Pill

Explanation

This pill has the same ingredients and indications as the above formula.

The tongue presentation appropriate to this remedy is a Red body without coating in the front part.

(ii) Patent remedy

LI FEI WAN (or LI FEI TANG YI PIAN)
Benefiting the Lungs Pill (Benefiting the Lungs Sugar-coated Tablet)
Dong Chong Xia Cao *Sclerotium Cordicipitis chinensis*
Ge Jie *Gecko*
Bai He *Bulbus Lilii*
Wu Wei Zi *Fructus Schisandrae chinensis*
Bai Ji *Rhizoma Bletillae striatae*
Bai Bu *Radix Stemonae*
Mu Li *Concha Ostreae*
Pi Pa Ye *Folium Eriobotryae japonicae*
Gan Cao *Radix Glycyrrhizae uralensis*

Explanation

This pill nourishes Lung and Kidney-Yin and stimulates the descending of Lung-Qi.

It is suitable for the chronic stage of wheezing, when the wheezing attacks are slight and infrequent on a background of Kidney-Yin deficiency.

The tongue presentation appropriate to this remedy is a Red body without coating or with rootless coating.

(iii) Patent remedy

PING CHUAN WAN
Calming Breathlessness Pill
Dang Shen *Radix Codonopsis pilosulae*
Dong Chong Xia Cao *Sclerotium Cordicipitis chinensis*
Ge Jie *Gecko*
Xing Ren *Semen Pruni armeniacae*
Chen Pi *Pericarpium Citri reticulatae*
Gan Cao *Radix Glycyrrhizae uralensis*
Sang Bai Pi *Cortex Radicis Mori albae*
Bai Qian *Radix et Rhizoma Cynanchii stautoni*
Meng Shi *Lapis Chloritis*

Wu Zhi Mao Tao *Radix Fici simplicissimae*
Man Hu Tui Zi *Semen Elaeagni glabrae Thunb.*

Explanation

This pill tonifies Kidney-Yang and Spleen-Qi and stimulates the descending of Lung-Qi. It is suitable for chronic wheezing from a deficiency of Kidney-Yang.

The tongue presentation appropriate to this remedy is a Pale body.

Case history

A 42-year-old woman had been suffering from asthma for 10 years. It started after the birth of her second child. She experienced a feeling of oppression of the chest and sometimes coughed up some yellow phlegm.

She also suffered from lower back-ache and often felt dizzy. Occasionally she experienced tinnitus and her urine was pale and frequent. She felt very tired.

Her tongue was slightly Pale but with a yellow coating and her pulse was Deep and Weak, especially on both Kidney positions.

Diagnosis
This is a clear case of asthma from deficiency of Kidney-Yang, with the Kidneys not grasping Qi. There is also some Phlegm-Heat (yellow sputum and yellow tongue coating), but not significant.

Treatment principle
The treatment principle must therefore be aimed primarily at strengthening Kidney-Yang and secondarily at tonifying the Spleen and resolving Phlegm.

Treatment
This patient was treated only with acupuncture. The main points used were:

- **BL-23** Shenshu, **Ren-4** Guanyuan and **KI-3** Taixi, with moxa, to tonify Kidney-Yang.
- **LU-7** Lieque on the right and **KI-6** Zhaohai on the left, to open the Directing Vessel, tonify the Kidneys and restore the descending of Lung-Qi.
- **LU-5** Chize and **Ren-22** Tiantu to restore the descending of Lung-Qi.
- **BL-20** Pishu and **Ren-12** Zhongwan to tonify the Spleen.
- **ST-40** Fenglong and **SP-6** Sanyinjiao to resolve Phlegm.
- **P-6** Neiguan to open the chest and relieve breathlessness.

This patient was treated every two weeks (as she lived quite far away) for 18 months, after which time there was an improvement of about 80% in her condition and she experienced only occasional breathlessness.

Prognosis and prevention

Apart from obvious reference to tongue and pulse, the prognosis in the symptom of Wheezing must be based on a Western differentiation. The main conditions that give rise to wheezing are acute and chronic bronchitis and asthma (see below) and the prognosis varies considerably in each of these diseases.

Acute bronchitis is the easiest to treat and it normally manifests with symptoms of Hot Phlegm described above. It corresponds to the Qi level (affecting the Lungs) within the Four-Level Identification of Patterns. The treatment of this condition is discussed in further detail in the chapter on "Common Cold and Influenza" (ch. 34).

Generally speaking, this condition responds extremely well to acupuncture and Chinese herbs which should bring about an improvement within days, and it is not usually necessary to resort to antibiotics. These damage Stomach-Yin and often lead to a residual Heat in the Lungs which predisposes the patient to further invasions of Wind. When such a vicious circle of exterior invasions of Wind, chest infections, antibiotics, residual Heat in the Lungs and further invasions of Wind takes hold, wheezing may become chronic.

Chronic bronchitis also responds extremely well to acupuncture and Chinese herbs but it will obviously take much longer to treat. The length of treatment will depend on the age of the patient and the duration and severity of the disease, but it will certainly take months rather than weeks. Chronic bronchitis should be treated by attending to the Root and Manifestation simultaneously, i.e. tonify the body's Qi and expel pathogenic factors. Tonifying the body's Qi will involve tonifying the Lungs, Spleen, or Kidneys, or a combination of these and expelling pathogenic factors will involve resolving Phlegm and either scattering Cold or clearing Heat, depending on whether there is Hot Phlegm or Cold

Phlegm. The differentiation and treatment of this condition are discussed in further detail in the chapters on "Cough" (ch. 8) and "Common Cold and Influenza" (ch. 34).

The prognosis of *asthma* depends on the age of the patient and the type of asthma. Early-onset, allergic asthma which is associated with eczema is the most difficult to treat because it stems from an inborn deficiency of the Lung and Kidney's Defensive-Qi systems (see ch. 5). From a Western point of view, it is due to an inborn excessive level of IgE antibodies. The treatment of this condition will certainly take several months and, depending on the severity, even years.

Non-allergic, early-onset asthma is easier to treat, especially in children. In most cases, treatment should not take more than a few weeks. This condition is due to repeated invasions of Wind leading to retention of Phlegm in the Lungs which obstructs the dispersing and descending of Lung-Qi. The foremost principle of treatment in children is to resolve Phlegm, restore the descending of Lung-Qi and relieve stagnation of food. Retention of food is very common in children and the stagnation in the Middle Burner predisposes the child to retention of Phlegm in the Upper Burner. It is thus beneficial to relieve stagnation of food with digestive herbs such as Mai Ya *Fructus Hordei vulgaris germinatus*, Gu Ya *Fructus Oryzae sativae germinatus*, Lai Fu Zi *Semen Raphani sativi*, Shan Zha *Fructus Crataegi*, Shen Qu *Massa Fermentata Medicinalis* and Ji Nei Jin *Endothelium Corneum gigeraiae galli*.

Late-onset asthma in adults stands somewhat in between the previous two types in terms of prognosis: it is easier to treat than allergic asthma, but more difficult than non-allergic early-onset asthma in children. Late-onset asthma in adults is usually characterized by a deficiency of Lungs, Spleen, or Kidneys or a combination of these, and retention of Phlegm. The treatment principle is therefore based on treating the Root (i.e. tonifying the body's Qi) and the Manifestation simultaneously (i.e. resolving Phlegm and restoring the descending of Lung-Qi). The treatment will take several months at least. In some cases asthma is caused by Liver-Qi stagnation or Liver-Fire (from emotional strain) obstructing the descending of Lung-Qi. This type of asthma is usually easier to treat and is discussed in chapter 5.

As for prevention, this also differs according to the condition causing wheezing.

Acute bronchitis cannot really be prevented as it is due to an invasion of exterior Wind.

The main way of preventing *chronic bronchitis* is to avoid the set of circumstances leading to the vicious circle outlined above. This means that any acute invasion of Wind should never be underestimated and should be treated promptly, preferably avoiding antibiotics. The patient should also avoid dairy products and greasy foods which facilitate the formation of Phlegm. He or she should also regulate their eating habits so that meals are taken at regular times.

As for *asthma*, preventive measures for allergic asthma will be described in the chapter on "Asthma" (ch. 5) and these apply to other types of asthma as well.

Western differentiation

A wheezing sound is a sign of bronchiolar narrowing by spasm, oedema of the epithelium, retained mucus, or all three acting together. Wheezes are therefore like musical sounds produced by the rapid passage of air through a narrowed bronchus.

Wheezes appear in obstructive lung diseases. They usually occur on exhalation but may also appear on inhalation. The state of bronchiolar narrowing on expiration can be diagnosed by measuring the maximum volume of air which can be blown out in a second. This is called Forced Expiratory Volume (FEV) and is a way of assessing the respiratory disability in diseases such as asthma, emphysema or chronic bronchitis. If a peak-flow meter is not available, a simpler test can be carried out by asking the patient to blow out a lighted match without pursing the lips. A patient who is unable to do so and wheezes audibly in the attempt, is suffering from obstructive airway disease. Another way of eliciting a wheeze is to press on the sternum while the patient breathes out.

A wheeze is called *polyphonic* when it is composed of different sounds with different pitches all starting and stopping at the same time, and *monophonic* when it is composed of single sounds, each with its own pitch. A persistent, single, monophonic wheeze may indicate obstruction of a bronchus by tumour.

The main conditions which may cause wheezing are acute and chronic bronchitis and asthma.

ACUTE BRONCHITIS

This is an inflammation of the trachea and bronchi caused by various pyogenic organisms such as *Strept. pneumoniae*, *H. influenzae* or *Staph. pyogenes*.

The main clinical manifestations include a cough which is productive of mucoid, viscid sputum in the beginning, then becoming more copious and purulent, breathlessness, wheezing, a feeling of tightness of the chest, fever and leucocytosis.

CHRONIC BRONCHITIS

This condition is characterized by repeated attacks of cough during winter, gradually increasing in frequency until the cough becomes almost constant. Other manifestations include wheezing, tightness of the chest, tenacious, mucoid, purulent sputum and breathlessness.

ASTHMA

The pathology and clinical manifestations of this disease will be described in detail in the chapter on allergic asthma (ch. 5).

END NOTES

1. Duan Guang Zhou et al 1986 A manual of the Essential Prescriptions of the Golden Chest (*Jin Gui Yao Lue Shou Ce* 金匱要略手册), Science Publishing House, p. 21. The "Essential Prescriptions of the Golden Chest" itself by Zhang Zhong Jing was first published *c.* AD 220.

2. Cited in Zhang Bo Yu 1986 Internal Medicine, p. 59.
3. Ibid., p. 59.
4. Ibid., p. 59.

Asthma 5

哮
喘

In this chapter I will concentrate on the treatment of allergic or "atopic" asthma, also called early-onset or extrinsic asthma. The incidence of atopic asthma (and of eczema which is associated with it) has steadily increased in industrialized countries in the past decades. In spite of the introduction of several new drugs for the treatment of asthma, severe asthma is still by far the most common chronic debilitating disease in childhood and its mortality rate has not declined. Indeed, some researchers are investigating the possibility that the long-term use of some anti-asthma drugs such as bronchodilators may be detrimental and may even have increased the mortality rate from this disease, which, in the USA, has increased by 45% in the past 10 years.

The theoretical framework of Chinese medicine and its approach to treatment focus on symptoms rather than diseases. For example, textbooks of Chinese internal medicine discuss the treatment of "epigastric pain", "chest pain", "constipation", etc. Western internal medicine, on the contrary, discusses only the treatment of recognized "diseases" such as "stomach ulcer", "coronary heart disease", "diverticulitis", etc.

We generally treat specific Western diseases by referring to a corresponding Chinese symptom. For example, in order to treat a person with a stomach ulcer, we can clearly use the differentiation and treatment of "epigastric pain" in Chinese medicine. In some cases, the correspondence is less obvious. For example, in order to differentiate and treat hypertension, we generally need to refer to the differentiation and treatment of "Headache" and "Dizziness" in Chinese medicine.

Asthma is a well-defined disease with very specific and characteristic aetiology and pathology. In order to diagnose and treat it properly with Chinese medicine, we must identify the symptom to which it most closely corresponds in the Chinese framework. All textbooks of Chinese medicine, whether Chinese or Western, say that asthma corresponds to the symptom of "*Xiao-Chuan*" as defined in Chinese medicine. The reason for this is probably also semantic as the Chinese word for "asthma" *is xiao-chuan* and, in terminology, there is no way of distinguishing between allergic asthma and chronic breathlessness from other causes. I propose that:

1. *Xiao* (Wheezing) and *Chuan* (Breathlessness) are two separate symptoms
2. Allergic asthma does *not* correspond to either of them (although it is somewhat

closer to *Xiao* than *Chuan*) and the differentiation and treatment of *Xiao* or *Chuan* cannot be applied to asthma.

In order to ascertain the correspondence and differences between *Xiao-Chuan* and asthma we have to discuss the three following aspects:

1. The pathology and aetiology of allergic asthma in Western medicine
2. The connections and differences between *Xiao-Chuan* and allergic asthma
3. A new theory of allergic asthma in Chinese medicine.

Pathology and aetiology of allergic asthma in Western medicine

PATHOLOGY

The pathology of asthma is characterized by a partial obstruction of airflow in the airways. This is caused by a temporary narrowing of the bronchi by muscle spasm followed by mucosal swelling. The bronchial narrowing interferes with ventilation and raises the resistance to airflow in the bronchi. This is more marked on exhalation and it causes air to be trapped in the lungs. The narrowed bronchi can no longer be effectively cleared of mucus by coughing.

In allergic asthma, the bronchospasm is caused by an allergic reaction due to immune hypersensitivity. This is also called anaphylactic or Type-I reaction. Only IgE (reaginic) antibodies produce Type-I reactions. As these antibodies adhere strongly to tissues (and particularly to mast cells in the tissues), they are often called tissue-sensitizing antibodies. Anaphylactic crises in asthma are caused by an antigen-antibody reaction on the surface of the mast cells in the bronchi. This activates a series of enzymes which leads to the release of certain chemical substances from the mast cells, such as histamine, serotonin, bradykinin and prostaglandins. The IgE-dependent release of mast-cell products not only provokes acute bronchospasm but also

contributes to the development of the late-phase asthmatic reaction (Fig. 5.1).

IgG antibodies account for 73% of Ig antibodies in serum and they can prevent IgE-mediated allergic reactions. They are the only antibodies that are transported across the placenta to reach the foetal circulation. This factor is quite significant in explaining the aetiology of allergic asthma from a Chinese medical perspective, as will be discussed later.

Bronchospasm from an allergic reaction, however, is only one aspect of the pathology of asthma, chronic inflammation of the bronchial mucosa being another. The mucosa is inflamed and oedematous, and there are infiltrating in-

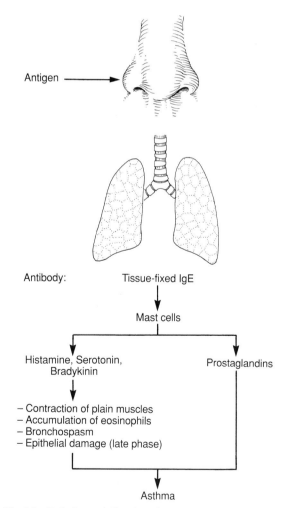

Fig. 5.1   Pathology of allergic asthma

flammatory cells. There is an excess of eosino-phils which lead to destruction of epithelial cells with consequent exposure of irritant receptors on the basement membrane. This, in turn, leads to an increase in bronchial responsiveness from allergic stimulation.[1]

AETIOLOGY

There are two types of asthma: the early-onset type which is also called extrinsic or atopic asthma, and the late-onset type which is also called intrinsic asthma. As the names imply, the early-onset one usually starts during childhood while the late-onset one starts later on in life. Our discussion will concentrate mostly on the allergic, early-onset type.

Early-onset asthma has the following charac-teristics:

1. it starts during early childhood
2. it appears to run in families
3. it is often associated with eczema from birth
4. individuals who suffer from this type of asthma have whealing skin reactions to common allergens
5. they also have antibodies in their serum which could be transferred to the skin of non-sensitized people to cause the same whealing skin reactions.

Individuals who suffer from allergic asthma with the above characteristics are called "atopic" and they have levels of IgE immunoglobulins up to six times higher than those found in patients suffering from non-atopic asthma. Atopic in-dividuals have a hereditary predisposition to anaphylactic (or Type-I) reactions.

Many different allergens are implicated but the main ones are faecal particles of house-dust mites, pollen, fungal spores, feathers, animal dander and cats' saliva. Once the mast cells have been primed by exposure to these allergens and high levels of IgE immunoglobulins adhere to them, they also become hypersensitive to other non-specific allergens such as smoke, tobacco smoke, petrol fumes, dust, atmospheric pollut-ants, perfumes, etc. Occasionally an allergic re-action in the bronchi can be elicited by ingested

allergens from food such as shellfish, fish, eggs, milk, yeast or wheat which reach the bronchi via the bloodstream.

It should be noted here that asthma that starts during early childhood is not necessarily atopic asthma. In other words, an early onset is not the only criterion for defining asthma as "allergic" or "atopic". The familial incidence, its connec-tion with eczema and the typical whealing skin reactions on inhalation of allergens are other important features necessary to diagnose atopic asthma.

There are cases of asthma starting in early childhood without an allergic basis. This hap-pens especially when a small child suffers from an upper respiratory infection (invasion of Wind-Cold or Wind-Heat) which is either not treated properly or treated with antibiotics. If Wind is not expelled properly, it lodges itself in the Lungs and impairs the dispersing and de-scending of Lung-Qi resulting in breathlessness and Phlegm. On the other hand, the presence of Wind and Phlegm in the Lungs predisposes the child to further invasions of external Wind which make the situation worse. Thus, a vicious cycle sets in when the child is progressively weakened and prone to invasions of external Wind and the breathlessness gets gradually worse. This chapter, however, will concentrate primarily on discussing the typical allergic asthma, as non-allergic asthma can be diagnosed and treated mostly according to the guidelines given for "Wheezing" (ch. 4).

Late-onset asthma, also called intrinsic asthma, normally starts later in life and is due to bron-chial hyper-reactivity. In this case there is no familial history of asthma and no eczema. Late-onset asthma occurs in non-atopic individuals and, although in some cases it may be triggered by certain allergens, it does not present all the typical traits of atopic asthma. In other cases it would appear that external allergens play no part in the aetiology of this disease.

The diagnosis of asthma is done on the basis of lung function tests (FEV = forced expiratory volume), peak-flow charts (PEFR = Peak Expira-tory Flow Rate), exercise tests, histamine pro-vocation tests and skin tests (inhalation of an allergen which produces large wheals on the skin also triggers off asthma). Sputum and blood tests are done to exclude bronchitis as large numbers of eosinophils in the sputum point to bronchitis. X-rays have no diagnostic value in asthma as they show no particular feature in this disease.

CLINICAL FEATURES

Asthma is characterized by wheezing attacks with shortness of breath which are usually worse at night. Sometimes there is a dry cough which is also worse at night. The onset is sudden and is preceded by tightness of the chest. The dyspnoea and wheezing occur mainly on exhalation with fixing of the shoulder-girdle. The patient likes to sit up.

DIFFERENTIAL DIAGNOSIS

Patients with asthma can have similar symptoms to those suffering from airflow limitation from chronic bronchitis and emphysema. Table 5.1 illustrates the features of asthma, chronic bronchitis and emphysema.

CHRONIC BRONCHITIS

This disease is characterized by hypertrophy of mucus-secreting glands in the bronchial tree. In advanced cases the bronchi themselves are inflamed and there is pus with infection.

The clinical features include breathlessness and a cough on most days. There is also wheezing and the cough is productive of abundant sputum. This may become purulent from time to time indicating a bacterial infection which often supervenes in chronic bronchitis.

EMPHYSEMA

This disease is characterized by distension and damage of bronchioles and/or alveoli.

There is breathlessness on exertion and wheezing which is almost constant.

BRONCHIECTASIS

This disease is characterized by dilatation of the bronchi with production of large amounts of sputum. There are recurrent episodes of fever or pneumonia.

It may develop from pneumonia or whooping cough.

Connections and differences between asthma and Xiao-Chuan

EARLY-ONSET ASTHMA

Let us start by analysing the gaps in the Chinese view of *Xiao-Chuan* in relation to asthma. We will look at the three areas of aetiology, pathology and differentiation/treatment.

Table 5.1 Differentiation of asthma, chronic bronchitis and emphysema

	Asthma	Chronic bronchitis	Emphysema
Pathology	Bronchospasm	Narrowing of bronchi by mucus	Distension of alveoli and/or bronchioles
Signs	Wheezing	Productive cough with profuse sputum	Thin chest
Symptoms	Bouts of dyspnoea	Dyspnoea, stuffiness of the chest	Constant dyspnoea
Frequency	Bouts of dyspnoea	Bouts of dyspnoea with chest infections	Constant dyspnoea
Time	Worse at night	Worse in the morning	All the time
Allergies	Yes	No	No
Sputum	No	Yes, abundant	Yes
Eczema	Yes	No	No

AETIOLOGY

It will be remembered that the main aetiological factors mentioned in the theory of Wheezing and Breathlessness are:

- external pathogenic factors
- diet
- emotional problems
- fatigue, chronic illness and excessive sexual activity.

Let us now examine each of these aetiological factors in relation to asthma and also any gaps in the traditional aetiology of *Xiao-Chuan*.

1. A fundamental gap in the traditional theory of *Xiao-Chuan* is that it has no concept of allergy as an aetiological factor in asthma, though early-onset asthma is so clearly related to an allergic immune hypersensitivity. A few modern Chinese books briefly refer to the allergic nature of asthma but they still apply the theory of *Xiao-Chuan* for its treatment.

2. Most books say that asthma attacks are elicited by invasion of external pathogenic factors such as Wind-Cold or Wind-Heat. While this is true in some cases, it is certainly not true in all.

3. The theory of *Xiao-Chuan* mentions the excessive consumption of sour, greasy, or cold foods as an aetiological factor. While this is certainly true in late-onset asthma, it cannot be true when asthma starts in early childhood. Very few children, if any, are likely to eat such foods in excess.

4. Dairy foods, which certainly are a possible aetiological factor in asthma, are not mentioned in the aetiology of *Xiao-Chuan* simply because they are not eaten in China. Intolerance to milk is an important aetiological factor in asthma.

5. Overwork and excessive sexual activity as mentioned in the theory of *Xiao-Chuan* are clearly not an aetiological factor in children with asthma, although they may play a part in the case of adults with late-onset asthma.

6. Emotional stress such as worry, brooding and pensiveness mentioned in the theory of *Xiao-Chuan* is certainly not an aetiological factor in very young children with early-onset asthma. Of course children may be subject to emotional stress from early age but not in the same sense as adults.

One of the aetiological factors of *Xiao-Chuan* which does apply to early-onset asthma is a weak body-condition. In young children this may be caused by a severe attack of measles, whooping cough, or pneumonia.

PATHOLOGY

1. Phlegm is central to the pathology of both *Xiao* and *Chuan*. In both conditions, wheezing and breathlessness are caused by Phlegm obstructing the airways. The wheezing sound is due to rebellious Qi ascending along the airways obstructed by Phlegm.

Phlegm is not, however, the main pathogenic factor in asthma. In this disease, wheezing and breathlessness are due to narrowing of the airways from bronchospasm following an allergic reaction. The narrowed bronchi cannot be properly cleared of mucus by coughing. Seen from this point of view, Phlegm is therefore the result rather than the cause of the condition.

The old Chinese doctors had to attribute narrowing of the airways to Phlegm as they could not know the mechanism of broncho-constriction from parasympathetic stimulation. Interestingly, old Western medicine also attributed asthma to obstruction of the airways by mucus. John Miller wrote in 1769: *"The superfluous serum, which ought to be thrown out by expiration, is accumulated: . . . the organs of respiration are weakened"*.[2] Robert Bree (1807) saw asthma as *". . . an extraordinary effort to get rid of some peccant and irritating matter existing in the air tubes"*.[3] Other doctors, however, understood as early as 1868 that wheezing and breathlessness in asthma were due to bronchospasm rather than obstruction from phlegm and that this was the result rather than the cause of asthma. Dr Henry Hyde Salter in fact said: *"The fact is, Dr Bree mistook the effect [i.e. phlegm] for the cause"*.[4] As far back as 1786 some doctors perceived the allergic nature of asthma even though they could not explain it fully. Dr William Withering (who pioneered the use of foxglove extracts for congestive cardiac failure) wrote in 1786 that asthma might be cured by living in large rooms from which curtains and feather beds had been removed.[5]

Two other elements which are not consistent with Phlegm being the main factor in asthma are the tongue and the pulse. If Phlegm were the main pathological factor in asthma, then the tongue should be Swollen with a sticky coating and the pulse Slippery. This is very often not the case. In early-onset asthma, the tongue is not usually Swollen (it is often Thin) and the pulse not Slippery (it is often Tight).

Another factor that rules out Phlegm as a pathogenic factor in asthma is the fact that, in between attacks, an asthmatic person is often quite normal. Indeed, there are some athletes who are asthmatic. If Phlegm obstructs the Lungs, however, wheezing and breathlessness are constant and they persist until Phlegm is completely eliminated. Thus doctor Ye Gui in "Case Reports for Clinical Practice" (1766) correctly says: *"If the pathogenic factor is expelled, breathlessness [Chuan] stops and will never return . . . In wheezing [Xiao], the pathogenic factor is hidden in the Interior and in the Lungs, it is sometimes active and sometimes quiescent, and there are frequent episodes over many years"*.[6] This confirms that Phlegm is the main causative factor in Breathlessness (*Chuan*): once Phlegm is eliminated, the breathlessness goes completely. In Wheezing (*Xiao*), which is closer to asthma, the pathogenic factor is hidden in the Lungs and it becomes active in bouts causing asthma attacks.

What is the pathogenic factor in asthma then? Basically, it is Wind: not exterior Wind as such invading the Lungs, nor interior Wind, but a kind of chronic (exterior) Wind lodged in the bronchi and periodically leading to bronchospasm. The attacks are elicited by exposure to allergens or cold weather or by emotional stress. The nature of this Wind as a pathogenic factor in asthma will be expanded on shortly.

It is also interesting that X-rays have no diagnostic value in asthma. This seems to confirm that Wind, and not Phlegm, is the main pathogenic factor in asthma. Wind is a non-substantial pathogenic factor and, as such, it naturally would not show on an X-ray whereas Phlegm, a substantial pathogenic factor, would.

Of course, in a person with early-onset asthma, after many years the pathology becomes more complicated and other factors, including Phlegm, may play a role. This happens under the influence of several aetiological factors such as overwork, emotional stress, excessive sexual activity and irregular diet, all factors which are not present in childhood.

2. The pathology of *Xiao-Chuan* does not contemplate infantile eczema which so often accompanies or precedes early-onset asthma. And yet the connection between eczema and early-onset asthma is very close and clinically extremely frequent. Chinese medical theory can easily explain this connection via the Lungs which are involved in breathing and control the skin. Strangely, this connection between Lungs and skin does not seem to be used in the diagnosis and treatment of infantile eczema.

The connection between asthma and eczema is also easily observed in the whealing reaction occuring on the skin of atopic individuals from inhalation of allergens.

DIFFERENTIATION AND TREATMENT

In order to discuss the differences and connections between asthma and *Xiao-Chuan*, it is better to deal with *Xiao* and *Chuan* separately.

XIAO

It will be remembered that the main patterns in *Xiao* are:

During attacks	*In between attacks*
– Cold Phlegm	Lung Deficiency
– Hot Phlegm	Spleen Deficiency
	Kidney Deficiency

1. The differentiation of treatment during or in between attacks is important and is used in the treatment of asthma.

2. The distinction between Cold Phlegm and Hot Phlegm is useful in the treatment of asthma to differentiate between two basic types with Cold or Heat even though there is no Phlegm.

CHUAN

It will be remembered that the main patterns in *Chuan* are:

Full
- Invasion of Wind-Cold
- Wind-Cold on Exterior, Phlegm-Fluids in Interior
- Cold on Exterior, Heat in Interior
- Phlegm-Heat in Lungs
- Turbid Phlegm in Lungs
- Lung-Qi obstructed

Empty
Lung Deficiency
Kidney Deficiency

1. External Wind-Cold can trigger off an acute attack of asthma. From a Western point of view too, it is well known that viral infections can trigger off allergic asthma in sensitized individuals.[7] Furthermore, activation of mast cells causing bronchoconstriction may be elicited not only by allergens but also by exercise, cold air and hyperventilation.[8]

An invasion of external Wind which is not expelled properly or is suppressed with antibiotics may also cause the beginning of asthma in non-atopic children.

2. Exterior Wind-Cold with interior Phlegm-Fluids usually occurs only in adults as Phlegm-Fluid is a chronic condition which only develops over many years.

3. The pattern of Cold on the Exterior and Heat in the Interior corresponds not to asthma but to an acute chest infection.

4. Phlegm-Heat in the Lungs corresponds not to asthma but to acute bronchitis, pneumonia, or febrile episodes of bronchiectasis.

5. Turbid Phlegm corresponds not to asthma but to a severe chest infection with sepsis.

6. Lung-Qi obstructed corresponds to an acute attack of asthma in adults from emotional stress affecting the Liver. It does not correspond to early-onset asthma.

7. *Chuan* from Lung deficiency corresponds to chronic asthma.

8. *Chuan* from Kidney deficiency corresponds to asthma or emphysema in old people, not the early-onset asthma.

LATE-ONSET ASTHMA

Late-onset asthma is not allergic and occurs without eczema. As its name implies, it starts later in life, usually during the 30s or 40s.

For the treatment of this disease, the theory of *Xiao-Chuan* can be applied. Late-onset asthma is characterized more often by Spleen deficiency manifesting with a Swollen tongue.

A new theory of asthma

Since, as we have seen, the theory of *Xiao-Chuan* is not adequate to diagnose and treat allergic asthma (and eczema), we must attempt to develop a new theory of asthma in Chinese medicine. It should be stressed here that the following is by no means a definitive new theory of asthma and that it will need much refining and revising according to clinical experience.

This discussion will concentrate on the diagnosis and treatment of early-onset asthma, also called extrinsic or atopic asthma. One of the reasons why the theory of *Xiao-Chuan* does not quite apply to asthma is simply that atopic asthma probably did not exist in ancient China. Even in modern times, it is relatively rare in China and the Far East and its incidence is far higher in Western countries. The development of allergic asthma must obviously be related to Western life-style as, in Chinese people who live in the West and adopt a Western life-style, the incidence of allergic asthma is the same as for Westerners.[9]

AETIOLOGY AND PATHOLOGY

Two main factors play a role in the pathogenesis of asthma: the first is a deficiency of both Lung and Kidney's Defensive-Qi systems and the other is Wind. The former accounts for the Root of the disease, the latter for its Manifestation.

LUNG AND KIDNEY'S DEFENSIVE-QI SYSTEMS DEFICIENCY

The Lungs spread Defensive-Qi to skin and muscles and the Kidneys are the root of the Defensive-Qi. Defensive-Qi is Yang in nature and it warms skin and muscles. Kidney-Yang is the source of all Yang energies of the body: it is in this sense that it is the root of Defensive-Qi. The Kidneys are paired with the Bladder and Kidney-Yang provides Qi to the Bladder for its transformation of fluids. In the process of this transformation a clear part of the fluids flows upwards, along the Bladder channel in the back to the skin and muscles where they mingle with Defensive-Qi. This is another indirect way in which Kidney-Yang is the root of Defensive-Qi.

Besides this, both the Bladder channel and the Governing vessel, which spread Defensive-Qi all over the back in the Greater Yang area, are connected to the Kidneys. It will be remembered that the Governing vessel starts from the Kidneys themselves. Furthermore, the "Spiritual Axis" in chapter 71 says: *The Defensive Qi flows in the Yang in daytime and in the Yin at night-time, starting from the muscles portion of the Kidney channel, flowing to the 5 Yin and 6 Yang organs*.[10] Interestingly, the "Correction of Errors in Medicine" (1831) by Wang Qing Ren has diagrams showing "Defensive-Qi-gathering vessels" emerging from the Kidneys.[11] Thus, resistance to pathogenic factors (which include allergens) is dependent not only on the Lungs but to a great extent also on the Kidneys.

However, the type of deficiency involved in allergic asthma is a deficiency of only one aspect of the Kidney functions, i.e. in connection with Defensive-Qi. It could be called deficiency of the Kidney's Defensive-Qi system, similar to the Lung's Defensive-Qi system. This Kidney deficiency involves only this aspect of its functions and therefore not many other symptoms and signs are present. For example, a child or teenager with allergic asthma would not have dizziness, deafness, tinnitus, back-ache, week knees or night-sweating.

The traditional theories of Wheezing (*Xiao*) and Breathlessness (*Chuan*) both contemplate a Kidney deficiency as a factor in asthma, but only for its late stages in chronic cases. In allergic asthma, on the contrary, there is a deficiency of the Kidney Defensive-Qi system from the beginning. In children also, prolonged wheezing and cough may induce a Kidney deficiency which is therefore the consequence of a Lung pathology; in atopic asthma, however, a Kidney deficiency is the *cause* of the condition, and the cause for chronic Wind to be lodged in the chest.

It is interesting to note that atopic asthma often improves during pregnancy.[12] This confirms the involvement of the Kidneys in atopic asthma as a Kidney deficiency sometimes improves during pregnancy.

Thus the immune hyper-reactivity which is at the basis of asthma is due to a deficiency of both Lung and Kidney's Defensive-Qi systems. The Kidneys influence the immune system not only through the connection between Kidney-Yang and Defensive-Qi, but also because the Kidney-Essence, through the Governing, Penetrating and Directing vessels, is partly responsible for protection from external pathogenic factors. Western physiology confirms this role of the Kidneys in the immune defences since all cells involved in the immune response are derived from a common stem cell in the marrow (which is a product of the Kidney-Essence). This is illustrated in Figure 5.2.

How does a deficiency of the Kidney's Defensive-Qi system arise? It may derive from:

(a) hereditary constitutional weakness
(b) problems to the mother during pregnancy such as a shock, smoking, drinking alcohol, or using drugs
(c) problems at childbirth such as foetal distress and induction
(d) immunizations.

It has been shown recently that maternal smoking during pregnancy may result in increased levels of IgE antibodies in the cord blood of the newborn baby.[13] Some drugs taken during pregnancy have also been shown to predispose infants to atopic disease. For example, a double-blind placebo control study showed that children exposed *in utero* to beta-adrenergic receptor-blocking drugs taken for toxicosis of pregnancy, had elevated IgE levels in the cord

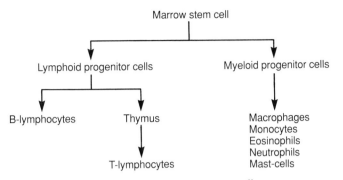

Fig. 5.2   Marrow stem cells and immune-system cells

blood and developed clinical allergy during the first four years of life significantly more often than the children of placebo-treated control mothers.[14]

Apart from a constitutional Kidney-Defensive-Qi system weakness which may be hereditary or developed *in utero* as in points (a) and (b) above, the period of time during the actual birth has a bearing on the development of the Lung and Kidney's Defensive-Qi systems. Studies have shown that stress during the neonatal period may increase the risk of development of allergy later in life.[15]

In particular, premature severing of the umbilical cord may interrupt the vital flow of hormones and immune cells from the placenta to the offspring and the excretion of waste products from the baby to the placenta. As mentioned earlier, IgG immunoglobulins which prevent IgE-mediated allergic reactions, are the only immunoglobulins that are transported across the placenta to reach the foetal circulation. It is therefore possible that a premature severance of the umbilical cord may lead to a deficiency of IgG immunoglobulins in the baby and therefore a predisposition to IgE-mediated allergic reactions later in life. In fact, levels of IgE antibodies are already higher at birth in infants who later develop atopic disease.[16] As IgE antibodies do not cross the placental barrier they must be of foetal origin. Their elevated levels therefore suggest a spontaneous antibody formation which is not efficiently suppressed by the IgG immunoglobulins.

There is an interesting connection here with the traditional Chinese use of placenta and um-

bilical cord for the treatment of asthma in children. In modern China, some doctors inject placenta extract in the points LU-6 Kongzui, ST-40 Fenglong and BL-23 Shenshu to treat allergic asthma. This seems to confirm that an interruption in the two-way flow of hormones, immune cells and wastes between the placenta and the baby during childbirth is one of the causes of a deficiency of the Kidney's Defensive-Qi system. Dr Kiiko Matsumoto also attributes allergies and asthma to the premature severing of the umbilical cord.[17] Finally, the very last development of lungs and kidneys takes place in the birth canal and in babies delivered by Caesarian section there is a higher incidence of allergic asthma.

Immunizations may sometimes trigger off atopic asthma and/or eczema in susceptible individuals. Animal studies have demonstrated that pertussis bacteria induce IgE antibody formation. It is therefore possible that pertussis immunization may induce excessive levels of IgE antibodies: this effect would be enhanced if immunization is given during the pollen season.[18]

It has also been reported that general anaesthesia in infants may be associated with later development of respiratory tract allergy.[19]

Breastfed infants may also be sensitized by minute amounts of foreign proteins (such as from cow's milk, eggs and fish) present in the maternal milk. Studies have shown that atopic dermatitis was significantly lower in the babies of mothers avoiding the above foods during the first six months of breastfeeding.[20]

The deficiency of the Lung and Kidney's Defensive-Qi systems may also play a role in the pathogenesis of eczema in babies and very young children. The relationship between the Lungs and skin is well known in Chinese medicine and yet, as mentioned above, it is seldom used to explain the linkage between asthma and atopic eczema in children. The Kidneys also influence the skin. The Lungs influence the skin in as much as they spread Defensive-Qi and fluids to the skin and control the pores. The Kidneys control the condition and lustre of the skin. The same deficiency of the Kidney's Defensive-Qi system that leads to IgE-mediated allergic asthma, causes eczema lesions on the skin. From a Chinese perspective, the Kidneys fail to nourish the skin, leading to either Wind-Heat or Damp-Heat.

Furthermore, there is a close relationship between the Kidney-Essence and the Lung's Corporeal Soul. The Corporeal Soul is closely linked to the Essence and is described in chapter 8 of the "Spiritual Axis" as the *"exiting and entering of the Essence"*.[21] The Corporeal Soul derives from the mother and arises soon after the Pre-natal Essence of a newly-conceived being is formed. It could be described as the manifestation of the Essence in the sphere of sensations and feelings. The Corporeal Soul provides movement to the Essence, i.e. it brings the Essence into play in all physiological processes of the body. The Corporeal Soul is the closest to the Essence and, as such, is responsible for the first physiological processes after birth. Zhang Jie Bin says: *"In the beginning of life ears, eyes and Heart perceive, hands and feet move and breathing starts: all this is due to the sharpness of the Corporeal Soul".*[22] He also says: *"The Corporeal Soul can move and do things and [when it is active] pain and itching can be felt."* This shows that the Corporeal Soul is responsible for sensations and itching and is therefore closely related to the skin through which such sensations are experienced. This explains the somatic expression on the skin of emotional tensions which affect the Corporeal Soul via the Mind and the connection between Corporeal Soul, Lungs and skin.

The relationship between Corporeal Soul and Essence may therefore explain the eruption of atopic eczema and asthma in babies. From the Chinese point of view, eczema in babies is due to the surfacing of toxic Heat from the uterus: it is therefore closely linked with the Pre-natal Essence of the baby. Since the Essence is related to the Corporeal Soul which manifests on the skin (itching and pain), the toxic Heat from the uterus erupts on the baby's skin in the form of eczema. Asthma can be explained in the same way as the deficient Essence of the baby fails to root its Corporeal Soul and therefore its Lungs.

WIND AS MAIN PATHOGENIC FACTOR IN ASTHMA

Having discussed the role of the Lung and Kidney's Defensive-Qi systems as the Root in asthma, we can now turn our attention to Wind as the main Manifestation of this disease.

Wind is the main pathogenic factor in asthma: not in the sense of an invasion of external Wind, but as a kind of chronic external Wind locked in the bronchi. The Lungs are the most exterior of the Yin organs as they control the skin. The bronchial mucosa could be seen as an extension of the skin. Thus, just as Wind invades the skin, it may invade the bronchi, lodge itself there and cause bronchospasm. Even from a Western point of view, animal studies suggest that the pathological features of skin and pulmonary actions are very similar.[23]

This can happen only against a background of deficiency of the Lung and Kidney's Defensive-Qi systems which allows Wind to lodge in the bronchi for a long time. Thus, asthma is characterized by Wind, a non-substantial pathogenic factor. This may explain how X-rays have no diagnostic value in asthma as they may show phlegm but not "Wind", and also how in asthmatic children or young people the tongue is nearly always not Swollen and the pulse not Slippery as one would expect were Phlegm the main pathogenic factor; instead, the tongue is often Thin and the pulse Tight.

The Chinese idea of Wind may be compared to the Western concept of allergens. The inhalation of dust, faecal matter from house-dust mites, pollen and animal dander could be compared to invasion of "Wind" as conceived in Chinese medicine. In fact, the Chinese character for Wind includes the radical for "insect" or "worm", i.e. comparable to allergens and germs carried by the wind.

Thus, the main problem in asthma is a deficiency of the Lung and Kidney's Defensive-Qi systems which allows Wind to penetrate and lodge itself in the bronchi causing bouts of bronchospasm. When Dr Ye Gui (1766) said, as mentioned above, that *"in breathlessness [Chuan] if the pathogenic factor [Phlegm] is expelled it will never return . . . in wheezing [Xiao] the pathogenic factor is hidden in the Interior and in the Lungs . . . and there are frequent episodes over the years"*, he correctly highlighted the difference between wheezing (*Xiao*) and breathlessness (*Chuan*). Breathlessness is due to Phlegm and once this is resolved, the condition is cured permanently. Allergic asthma is due to Wind in the bronchi causing periodic bouts of wheezing. The reason this is difficult to expel is not that it is particularly deep in the Interior, but that it is linked to a deficiency of the Lung and Kidney's Defensive-Qi systems. Until this deficiency is addressed, the Wind cannot be expelled.

Another phenomenon which points to Wind rather than Phlegm as the main pathogenic factor in asthma is the remarkable effectiveness of acupuncture in stopping an acute asthma attack. This is because Wind is a non-substantial pathogenic factor and, as such, more responsive to acupuncture treatment. When Phlegm is the main pathogenic factor as in chronic bronchitis, acupuncture has only a limited efficacy in relieving breathlessness in the short term as it obviously takes a long time to resolve Phlegm.

As for late-onset asthma, although this is usually not allergic, its pathology is similar, with the Root being the deficiency of Lung and Kidney's Defensive-Qi systems and the Manifestation being Wind lodged in the bronchi. The aetiology is different since the Kidney deficiency is induced by overwork, excessive sexual activity and a natural decline of Kidney-Qi in middle age, rather than being congenital. Thus the Kidney's Defensive-Qi system is affected not from birth, but by life-style. Many patients with late-onset asthma, especially men, often find the condition worse after sexual activity.

In late-onset asthma, a Spleen deficiency, caused by irregular diet, is often present and therefore there is some Phlegm as well. This manifests with a Swollen tongue.

Late-onset asthma is also characterized by a more frequent involvement of the Liver, caused by emotional stress, in the pathogenesis of the condition.

DIFFERENTIATION AND TREATMENT

The differentiation made in Wheezing (ch. 4) between treatment during attacks and treatment in between attacks is applicable to asthma. The differentiation made in Breathlessness (ch. 3) between Deficiency and Excess conditions is not applicable to asthma since this is always characterized by both a Deficiency (of the Lung and Kidney's Defensive-Qi systems) and an Excess (Wind).

The main patterns seen in asthma are as follows:

During attacks	*In between attacks*
Wind-Cold	Lung and Kidney's Defensive-Qi systems Deficiency
Wind-Heat	

In the treatment of asthma, especially acute cases, it is important also to calm the Mind. This is a useful principle of treatment, as acute asthma is due to bronchospasm from overstimulation of the parasympathetic nervous system. The herbs and acupuncture points which "calm the Mind" also have a regulating effect on the nervous system. For example, the point Du-24 Shenting, which calms the Mind, is widely used to calm asthma.

DURING ATTACKS

The treatments discussed below apply not only to the actual acute attack, but also to a period of time when attacks are frequent.

The two patterns of Wind-Cold and Wind-Heat may correspond to an asthma attack elicited by an actual invasion of Wind with all its relevant symptoms, or to a picture of symptoms and signs due to a pre-existing Wind in the bronchi which is mimicking an invasion of Wind.

If there were an actual invasion of Wind, there would be aversion to cold, shivering and possibly fever (especially in Wind-Heat). The pulse would be Floating. The patterns described below, however, presume an acute attack of asthma manifesting with certain symptoms of Wind, but without an actual invasion of external Wind.

Even if there is not an actual invasion of external Wind, the treatment principle is to "release the Exterior" as herbs that release the Exterior also expel Wind from the Lungs in allergic asthma.

The patterns occurring during attacks discussed will be:

Wind-Cold (without sweating)
Wind-Cold (with sweating)
Wind-Heat

WIND-COLD (without sweating)

Clinical manifestations

Sudden wheezing and breathlessness with difficulty in breathing out, no sweating, tightness of the chest, pale face, feeling cold, sneezing, cough, no thirst, attack elicited by cold weather, stiffness of shoulders and neck.
Pulse: Tight.

Treatment principle

Release the Exterior, expel Wind-Cold, calm asthma, calm the Mind.

Acupuncture

Dingchuan, BL-12 Fengmen, BL-13 Feishu, Ren-22 Tiantu, LU-7 Lieque, LU-6 Kongzui, HE-7 Shenmen, Ren-15 Jiuwei, G.B.-20 Fengchi, G.B.-21 Jianjing. Reducing method. Cupping is applicable to BL-12 and BL-13.

Explanation

– **Dingchuan** stops acute asthma.
– **BL-12** expels Wind.
– **BL-13**, **Ren-22** and **LU-7** restore the descending of Lung-Qi.

– **LU-6**, Accumulation point, stops acute asthma.
– **HE-7** and **Ren-15** calm the Mind. He-7 also makes Qi descend and Ren-15 relieves fullness in the chest.
– **G.B.-20** and **G.B. -21** relax the neck and shoulders, which is important to drop the shoulder-girdle and help breathing.
– **G.B.-21** also makes Qi descend.

Herbal treatment

1. Prescription

MA HUANG TANG
Ephedra Decoction
Ma Huang *Herba Ephedrae* 6 g
Gui Zhi *Ramulus Cinnamomi cassiae* 4 g
Xing Ren *Semen Pruni armeniacae* 6 g
Zhi Gan Cao *Radix Glycyrrhizae uralensis praeparata* 3 g

Explanation

This is the standard formula for Wind-Cold and the Greater Yang stage of the 6 Stages from the "Discussion of Cold-induced Diseases".

– **Ma Huang** releases the Exterior, scatters Cold, restores the dispersing and descending of Lung-Qi and stops asthma.
– **Gui Zhi** helps Ma Huang to release the Exterior and scatter Cold.
– **Xing Ren** helps Ma Huang to restore the descending of Lung-Qi.
– **Zhi Gan Cao** harmonizes and moderates the scattering effect of Ma Huang.

2. Prescription

HUA GAI SAN
Glorious Lid Decoction
Ma Huang *Herba Ephedrae* 6 g
Xing Ren *Semen Pruni armeniacae* 9 g
Su Zi *Fructus Perillae frutescentis* 9 g
Sang Bai Pi *Cortex Mori albae radicis* 6 g
Chen Pi *Pericarpium Citri reticulatae* 6 g
Fu Ling *Sclerotium Poriae cocos* 9 g
Gan Cao *Radix Glycyrrhizae uralensis* 3 g

Explanation

- **Ma Huang** releases the Exterior, scatters Cold, restores the dispersing and descending of Lung-Qi and stops asthma.
- **Xing Ren**, **Su Zi** and **Sang Bai Pi** restore the descending of Lung-Qi by relieving fullness in the Middle.
- **Chen Pi** and **Fu Ling** resolve Dampness and harmonize the Centre.
- **Gan Cao** harmonizes.

This formula is better for asthma as it has a stronger Qi-descending effect.

Variations

- For acute asthma increase the dosage of Su Zi *Fructus Perillae frutescentis* and add Xuan Fu Hua *Flos Inulae* to restore the descending of Lung-Qi.
- If there is an actual invasion of exterior Wind-Cold add Fang Feng *Radix Ledebouriellae sesloidis* and Jing Jie *Herba seu Flos Schizonepetae tenuifoliae*.

WIND-COLD (with sweating)

Clinical manifestations

Slight sweating, asthma attack with breathlessness and wheezing, less noisy than previous case, not so much chilliness, a feeling of tightness of the chest, pale face.
Pulse: Tight-Slow.

Treatment principle

Release the Exterior, harmonize Nutritive and Defensive Qi, calm asthma, calm the Mind.

Acupuncture

Dingchuan, BL-12 Fengmen, BL-13 Feishu, Ren-22 Tiantu, LU-6 Konzui, ST-36 Zusanli, SP-6 Sanyinjiao, HE-7 Shenmen, Ren-15 Jiuwei. Reducing method except for ST-36 and SP-6 which should be needled with even method to harmonize Nutritive and Defensive Qi. Cupping is applicable on BL-12.

Explanation

- **Dingchuan** stops acute asthma.
- **BL-12** and **BL-13** expel Wind and restore the dispersing and descending of Lung-Qi.
- **Ren-22** restores the descending of Lung-Qi and stops asthma.
- **LU-6**, Accumulation point, stops acute asthma.
- **ST-36** and **SP-6** harmonize Nutritive and Defensive Qi.
- **HE-7** and **Ren-15** calm the Mind. HE-7 also restores the descending of Qi as Heart-Qi, similarly to Lung-Qi, also has a descending movement. The descending of Heart-Qi will also help breathing. Ren-15 also relieves fullness in the chest.

Herbal treatment

Prescription

GUI ZHI JIA HOU PO XING ZI TANG
Ramulus Cinnamomi Decoction plus Magnolia and Prunus
Gui Zhi *Ramulus Cinnamomi cassiae* 9 g
Bai Shao *Radix Paeoniae albae* 9 g
Zhi Gan Cao *Radix Glycyrrhizae uralensis praeparata* 6 g
Sheng Jiang *Rhizoma Zingiberis officinalis recens* 9 g
Da Zao *Fructus Ziziphi jujubae* 3 dates
Hou Po *Cortex Magnoliae officinalis* 6 g
Xing Ren *Semen Pruni armeniacae* 6 g

Explanation

The first five herbs constitute the Gui Zhi Tang *Ramulus Cinnamomi Decoction* which is the standard decoction for expelling Wind-Cold by harmonizing Nutritive and Defensive Qi. It is used instead of Ma Huang Tang *Ephedra Decoction* when the patient is sweating slightly, which indicates a deficiency of Nutritive-Qi.

- **Hou Po** and **Xing Ren** are added to restore the descending of Lung-Qi.

Variations

- If there is an acute invasion of external Wind-Cold add Fang Feng *Radix Ledebouriellae sesloidis* and Jing Jie *Herba seu Flos Schizonepetae tenuifoliae.*

- To strengthen the descending action of Lung-Qi add Su Zi *Fructus Perillae frutescentis* and Xuan Fu Hua *Flos Inulae.*
- If there are some symptoms of interior Heat just beginning add Shi Gao *Gypsum fibrosum.*

Patent remedy

QI GUAN YAN KE SOU TAN CHUAN WAN
Bronchial Cough, Phlegm and Dyspnoea Pill
Qian Hu *Radix Peucedani*
Xing Ren *Semen Pruni armeniacae*
Yuan Zhi *Radix Polygalae tenuifoliae*
Sang Ye *Folium Mori albae*
Chuan Bei Mu *Bulbus Fritillariae cirrhosae*
Chen Pi *Pericarpium Citri reticulatae*
Pi Pa Ye *Folium Eriobotryae japonicae*
Kuan Dong Hua *Flos Tussilaginis farfarae*
Dang Shen *Radix Codonopsis pilosulae*
Ma Dou Ling *Fructus Aristolochiae*
Wu Wei Zi *Fructus Schisandrae chinensis*
Sheng Jiang *Rhizoma Zingiberis officinalis recens*
Da Zao *Fructus Ziziphi jujubae*

Explanation

This pill harmonizes Nutritive and Defensive Qi, restores the descending of Lung-Qi, resolves Phlegm, stops cough and relieves asthma.

WIND-HEAT

Clinical manifestations

Fever and aversion to cold (if true exterior invasion, otherwise feeling of heat), headache, tightness of the chest, loud wheezing, barking cough, asthma, mental restlessness, slight thirst.
Tongue: Red sides towards the front.
Pulse: Rapid.

Treatment principle

Release the Exterior, restore the descending of Lung-Qi, expel Wind-Heat, calm asthma, calm the Mind.

Acupuncture

LU-5 Chize, LU-7 Lieque, LU-1 Zhongfu, BL-13 Feishu, LU-6 Kongzui, LU-11 Shaoshang, Dingchuan, HE-7 Shenmen, Ren-15 Jiuwei. Reducing method, no moxa.

Explanation

- **LU-5** clears Lung-Heat.
- **LU-7**, **LU-1** and **BL-13** restore the descending of Lung-Qi.
- **LU-6**, Accumulation point, stops acute asthma.
- **LU-11** expels Wind-Heat and eases the throat.
- **Dingchuan** stops acute asthma.
- **HE-7** and **Ren-15** calm the Mind.

Herbal treatment

1. Prescription

SANG JU YIN
Morus-Chrysanthemum Decoction
Sang Ye *Folium Mori albae* 7.5 g
Ju Hua *Flos Chrysanthemi morifolii* 3 g
Bo He *Herba Menthae* 2.5 g
Jie Geng *Radix Platycodi grandiflori* 6 g
Xing Ren *Semen Pruni armeniacae* 6 g
Lian Qiao *Fructus Forsythiae suspensae* 5 g
Ou Gen *Rhizoma Nelumbinis nuciferae* 6 g
Gan Cao *Radix Glycyrrhizae uralensis* 2.5 g

Explanation

- **Sang Ye** and **Ju Hua** restore the descending of Lung-Qi, expel Wind-Heat and clear the Upper Burner.
- **Bo He** helps to clear the Upper Burner and expels Wind-Heat.
- **Jie Geng** and **Xing Ren** are coordinated: one circulates, the other makes Lung-Qi descend. In combination, they regulate Lung-Qi and stop cough and asthma.
- **Lian Qiao** clears Heat above the diaphragm.
- **Ou Gen** clears Heat and promotes fluids.
- **Gan Cao** harmonizes and resolves toxins.

2. Prescription

DING CHUAN TANG
Stopping Breathlessness Decoction

Ma Huang *Herba Ephedrae* 9 g
Bai Guo *Semen Ginkgo bilobae* 9 g
Huang Qin *Radix Scutellariae baicalensis* 6 g
Sang Bai Pi *Cortex Mori albae radicis* 9 g
Xing Ren *Semen Pruni armeniacae* 9 g
Ban Xia *Rhizoma Pinelliae ternatae* 9 g
Kuan Dong Hua *Flos Tussilaginis farfarae* 9 g
Su Zi *Fructus Perillae frutescentis* 6 g
Gan Cao *Radix Glycyrrhizae uralensis* 3 g

Explanation

This formula is stronger than the previous one and it is used if Heat is more prevalent. It also has a stronger effect in calming asthma.

- **Ma Huang** and **Bai Guo** are combined to restore the descending of Lung-Qi and stop asthma. They are coordinated since the former scatters and the latter absorbs.
- **Huang Qin** and **Sang Bai Pi** clear Lung-Heat and restore the descending of Lung-Qi.
- **Xing Ren**, **Ban Xia**, **Kuan Dong Hua** and **Su Zi** restore the descending of Lung-Qi, subdue rebellious Qi and calm cough and asthma.
- **Gan Cao** harmonizes.

Variations

- A small dose of Ma Huang may be added even if it is hot in order to calm asthma.
- If there is pronounced irritability increase the dosage of Huang Qin *Radix Scutellariae baicalensis* and add Dan Dou Chi *Semen Sojae praeparatum*.
- If symptoms of interior Heat are beginning add Shi Gao *Gypsum fibrosum*.

(a) Patent remedy

ZHI SOU DING CHUAN WAN
Stopping Cough and Calming Breathlessness Pill
Ma Huang *Herba Ephedrae*
Xing Ren *Semen Pruni armeniacae*
Shi Gao *Gypsum fibrosum*
Gan Cao *Radix Glycyrrhizae uralensis*

Explanation

This pill corresponds to the formula Ma Xing Shi

Gan Tang *Ephedra-Prunus-Gypsum-Glycyrrhiza Decoction* from the "Discussion on Cold-induced Diseases" for the combined patterns of Greater Yang and Bright Yang of the Six Levels. However, it may also be used for invasions of Wind-Heat when Heat is pronounced. In this case, Ma Huang and Xing Ren will relieve asthma.

(b) Patent remedy

XIAO CHUAN CHONG JI
Asthma Granules
Da Qing Ye *Folium Isatidis seu Baphicacanthi*
Ping Di Mu (also called Zi Jin Niu) *Folium Ardisiae japonicae*
Qian Hu *Radix Peucedani*
Sang Bai Pi *Cortex Mori albae radicis*
Ban Xia *Rhizoma Pinelliae ternatae*
Xuan Fu Hua *Flos Inulae*
Zhi Gan Cao *Radix Glycyrrhizae uralensis praeparata*
Ma Huang *Herba Ephedrae*
Bai Guo *Semen Ginkgo bilobae*

Explanation

These granules (dissolved in hot water) are suitable for an acute asthma attack following an invasion of Wind-Heat, especially if of viral origin as Da Qing Ye has anti-viral properties. Ma Huang helps to relieve asthma and the remedy is suitable for Wind-Heat even though Ma Huang is warm because its dosage within the formula is much smaller than the other ingredients.

This remedy is better than the previous one for relieving asthma specifically and for acute viral infections.

Note

Acupuncture is important in acute attacks of asthma as it usually is very effective. As for herbal medicine, some doctors use a small dose of Ma Huang *Herba Ephedrae* for its adrenergic properties even if there are some Heat signs.

Ma Huang yields many different alkaloids among which are ephedrine and psi-ephedrine. Ephedrine is alfa-adrenergic and psi-ephedrine is beta-adrenergic. An alfa-adrenergic effect produces vasoconstriction and a rise in the blood pressure, whilst a beta-adrenergic effect induces dilation of the bronchi, and increases the respiration rate and cardiac output and rate.

The balance of alkaloids in the natural plant is such that none of the undesirable effects of the isolated alkaloids has been observed from administration of Ephedra itself.

For this reason, many doctors use a small dose of Ma Huang in any acute asthma attack. Ma Huang may be combined with many different herbs for different situations. Some of the herbs with which it is combined are listed below:

- Cold: Gui Zhi *Ramulus Cinnamomi cassiae*
- Heat: Shi Gao *Gypsum fibrosum*
- Lung-Heat: Sang Bai Pi *Cortex Mori albae radicis*
- Rebellious Qi: Xing Ren *Semen Pruni armeniacae*
- Phlegm: She Gan *Rhizoma Belamcandae chinensis*
- Stagnation of Qi in the chest: Hou Po *Cortex Magnoliae officinalis*
- Qi deficiency: Dang Shen *Radix Codonopsis pilosulae*
- Kidney deficiency: Shu Di Huang *Radix Rehmanniae glutinosae praeparata*
- Lung-Yin deficiency: Bei Sha Shen *Radix Glehniae littoralis* or Wu Wei Zi *Fructus Schisandrae chinensis*
- Kidney-Yang deficiency: Fu Zi *Radix Aconiti carmichaeli praeparata*.

IN BETWEEN ATTACKS

This refers to periods of time when asthma attacks are very infrequent, or when the asthma is controlled by the occasional use of inhalers. At this stage, some asthma attacks are typically elicited by exposure to cats, dogs, pollen or dust causing wheezing, breathlessness and tightness of the chest.

If the patient is using inhalers there is no conflict with Chinese herbs or acupuncture and these can be used concurrently. Indeed, the frequency with which the patient needs to use the inhalers can be a very useful benchmark to gauge the efficacy of the treatment.

The priority of treatment in between attacks is to treat the Root, i.e. tonify the Lung and Kidney's Defensive-Qi systems. At the same time, the Manifestation (i.e. Wind in the bronchi obstructing the descending of Lung-Qi) should not be overlooked, so that each formula should always include some herbs to expel Wind and make Lung-Qi descend.

Within the scope of Lung and Kidney deficiency there may be many variations, with different degrees of deficiency between Lung and Kidneys and, within the Kidneys, between deficiency of Yang or Yin.

Some Chinese doctors treat chronic asthma in between attacks simply by tonifying Lung, Spleen, or Kidneys or a combination of these with the addition of small doses of Ma Huang *Herba Ephedrae* and Xing Ren *Semen Pruni armeniacae*.[24] This runs contrary to traditional theory according to which Ma Huang should be used strictly for Full conditions since it has a scattering effect. However, in small doses (3 grams) and combined with tonics, it can be used in chronic Deficiency-asthma for its strong adrenergic properties. Furthermore, in order to decrease its scattering effect, one could use honey-toasted Ma Huang.

Some doctors also use Dan Shen *Radix Salviae miltiorrhizae* in chronic cases of asthma to move Blood in the chest. Interestingly, modern research shows that Dan Shen reduces levels of IgE immunoglobulins which are responsible for the antigen-antibody reaction which triggers off an asthma attack.[25]

The following formulae are all aimed at tonifying the Lung and Kidney's Defensive-Qi systems with several variations to account for varying involvement of Lungs or Kidneys and deficiency of Yin or Yang. All the formulae without exception should be modified with the following two aims in mind:

1. Tonify the Kidney's Defensive-Qi system with such herbs as Tu Si Zi *Semen Cuscutae*, Du Zhong *Cortex Eucommiae ulmoidis*, Bu Gu Zhi *Fructus Psoraleae corylifoliae*, Hu Tao Rou *Semen Juglandis regiae* or Shu Di Huang *Radix Rehmanniae glutinosae praeparata*. A small dose of a

Kidney-Yang-tonic herb may be added even in Yin deficiency in order to bolster the Kidney's Defensive-Qi system.

2. Stimulate the descending of Lung-Qi and expel Wind with such herbs as Xing Ren *Semen Pruni armeniacae*, Su Zi *Fructus Perillae frutescentis*, Xuan Fu Hua *Flos Inulae* and Fang Feng *Radix Ledebouriellae sesloidis*.

3. Use herbs which have an anti-allergy effect such as Wu Wei Zi *Fructus Schisandrae chinensis* and Wu Mei *Fructus Pruni mume*.

The above modifications apply to all the following formulae and will therefore not be repeated in each case.

For each formula, the pattern and clinical manifestations will be given. These are in addition to the pattern and clinical manifestations of deficiency of Lung and Kidney's Defensive-Qi systems present in all cases and which are essentially asthma, wheezing, tightness of the chest and, in some cases, eczema.

ACUPUNCTURE

The aims of treatment with acupuncture are:

(a) Tonify the Lung and Kidney's Defensive-Qi systems
(b) Restore the descending of Lung-Qi
(c) Calm the Mind
(d) In late-onset asthma, tonify the Spleen.

The points to use for the above aims are:

(a) BL-23 Shenshu, Ren-4 Guanyuan, BL-52 Zhishi, Ren-8 Shenque with moxa cones on salt, KI-16 Huangshu, LU-9 Taiyuan and BL-13 Feishu to tonify Lung and Kidney's Defensive-Qi systems
(b) LU-7 Lieque, LU-5 Chize, Ren-17 Shanzhong and BL-13 Feishu to restore the descending of Lung-Qi
(c) Du-24 Shenting, HE-7 Shenmen, DU-19 Houding and Ren-15 Jiuwei to calm the Mind
(d) ST-36 Zusanli, ST-40 Fenglong, Ren-12 Zhongwan, BL-20 Pishu and BL-21 Weishu to tonify the Spleen.

The patterns discussed under the various formulae in this section are:

Lung-Qi Deficiency
Lung-Qi and Lung-Yin Deficiency
Lung-Qi and Kidney-Yang Deficiency
Lung-Yin Deficiency
Lung- and Kidney-Yin Deficiency

HERBAL TREATMENT

1. Prescription

YU PING FENG SAN
Jade Wind Screen Decoction
Huang Qi *Radix Astragali membranacei* 9 g
Fang Feng *Radix Ledebouriellae sesloidis* 9 g
Bai Zhu *Rhizoma Atractylodis macrocephalae* 12 g

Pattern

Lung-Qi deficiency.

Clinical manifestations

Sweating, pale face, weak voice, prone to catching colds, sneezing, runny nose, shortness of breath, attacks of asthma elicited by pollen or dust, allergic rhinitis.
Pulse: Empty.

Explanation

– **Huang Qi** tonifies Lung-Qi and consolidates the Exterior.
– **Fang Feng** expels Wind and, in combination with Huang Qi, consolidates the Exterior to prevent invasion of Wind.
– **Bai Zhu** helps Huang Qi to tonify Lung-Qi.

2. Prescription

SHENG MAI SAN
Generating the Pulse Powder
Ren Shen *Radix Ginseng* 10 g
Mai Men Dong *Tuber Ophiopogonis japonici* 15 g
Wu Wei Zi *Fructus Schisandrae chinensis* 6 g

Pattern

Lung-Qi and Lung-Yin deficiency.

Clinical manifestations

Attacks of asthma at night, tightness of the chest, wheezing, dry cough, dry throat, weak voice, night-sweating, tiredness, prone to catching colds, pale face, palpitations.
Tongue: dry, slightly Red in the Lung area.
Pulse: Floating-Empty.

Explanation

- **Ren Shen** tonifies Lung-Qi.
- **Mai Men Dong** and **Wu Wei Zi** nourish Lung-Yin and promote fluids.

3. Prescription

REN SHEN GE JIE SAN
Ginseng-Gecko Powder
Ge Jie *Gecko* 9 g
Zhi Gan Cao *Radix Glycyrrhizae uralensis praeparata* 9 g
Ren Shen *Radix Ginseng* 6 g
Fu Ling *Sclerotium Poriae cocos* 6 g
Chuan Bei Mu *Bulbus Fritillariae cirrhosae* 6 g
Sang Bai Pi *Cortex Mori albae radicis* 6 g
Xing Ren *Semen Pruni armeniacae* 9 g
Zhi Mu *Radix Anemarrhenae asphodeloidis* 6 g

Pattern

Lung-Qi and Kidney-Yang deficiency.

Clinical manifestations

Asthma attacks worse at night, tightness of the chest, chilliness, oedema of the face, tiredness, back-ache, depression, husky voice.
Tongue: Pale.
Pulse: Weak-Deep-Slow.

Explanation

- **Ge Jie** tonifies the Lung and Kidney's Defensive-Qi system, strengthens the Kidney function of grasping Qi and stops asthma.
- **Zhi Gan Cao** tonifies Qi.
- **Ren Shen** and **Fu Ling** tonify Lung-Qi.
- **Chuan Bei Mu**, **Sang Bai Pi** and **Xing Ren** stimulate the descending of Lung-Qi.

- **Zhi Mu** prevents any Heat deriving from excessive tonification of Yang and it also strengthens the Kidney function of grasping Qi.

Variations

- If the person is very thin one can add Placenta pills.

4. Prescription

REN SHEN HU TAO TANG
Ginseng-Juglans Decoction
Ren Shen *Radix Ginseng* 4.5 g
Hu Tao Ren *Semen Juglandis regiae* 5 pieces
Sheng Jiang *Rhizoma Zingiberis officinalis recens* 5 slices

Pattern

Lung-Qi and Kidney-Yang deficiency.

Clinical manifestations

Daytime sweating, infrequent attacks of asthma, chilliness, back-ache, frequent-pale urination, pale face, tiredness.
Tongue: Pale.
Pulse: Deep-Weak.

Explanation

- **Ren Shen** tonifies Lung-Qi.
- **Hu Tao Rou** tonifies Kidney-Yang and strengthens the Kidney's function of grasping Qi.
- **Sheng Jiang** warms the channels.

5. Prescription

DING CHUAN SAN
Stopping Breathlessness Powder
Hong Shen *Radix Ginseng* 6 g
Ge Jie *Gecko* 6 g
Bei Sha Shen *Radix Glehniae littoralis* 6 g
Wu Wei Zi *Fructus Schisandrae chinensis* 4 g
Mai Men Dong *Tuber Ophiopogonis japonici* 6 g
Chen Pi *Pericarpium Citri reticulatae* 3 g
Zi He Che *Placenta hominis* 9 g

Pattern

Lung-Qi and Kidney-Yang deficiency with pronounced Cold.

Clinical manifestations

Infrequent attacks of asthma elicited by exposure to cold, wheezing, chilliness, frequent-pale urination, tiredness, depression.
Tongue: Pale, wet.
Pulse: Deep-Weak-Slow.

Explanation

- **Hong Shen** (Red Ginseng) tonifies Yang, the Lungs and the Original Qi.
- **Ge Jie** tonifies Kidney-Yang and strengthens the Kidney's function of grasping Qi.
- **Bei Sha Shen**, **Wu Wei Zi** and **Mai Men Dong** nourish Yin and absorb fluids to moderate the heating influence of the first two substances.
- **Chen Pi** combines with Hong Sheng to prevent Dampness.
- **Zi He Che** tonifies the Essence and strengthens the Kidney's function of grasping Qi.

6. Prescription

SHA SHEN MAI DONG TANG
Glehnia-Ophiopogon Decoction
Bei Sha Shen *Radix Glehniae littoralis* 9 g
Mai Men Dong *Tuber Ophiopogonis japonici* 9 g
Tian Hua Fen *Radix Trichosanthis* 9 g
Sang Ye *Folium Mori albae* 9 g
Bian Dou *Semen Dolichoris lablab* 9 g
Yu Zhu *Rhizoma Polygonati odorati* 12 g
Gan Cao *Radix Glycyrrhizae uralensis* 3 g

Pattern

Lung-Yin and Stomach-Yin deficiency with dryness and some Empty-Heat.

Clinical manifestations

Mild attacks of asthma at night, dry cough, dry throat, breathlessness on exertion, slight night-sweating.

Tongue: Red, without coating in the front part.
Pulse: Floating-Empty on the right Front position.

Explanation

- **Bei Sha Shen** and **Mai Men Dong** nourish Lung-Yin.
- **Tian Hua Fen** promotes fluids and clears dryness.
- **Sang Ye** promotes the descending of Lung-Qi and benefits the throat.
- **Bian Dou** tonifies the Spleen and is used according to the principle of strengthening the Earth to tonify Metal.
- **Yu Zhu** clears Empty-Heat and benefits fluids.
- **Gan Cao** harmonizes.

This formula is also suitable to treat either late-onset asthma with Lung-Yin deficiency or asthma attacks from injury of Lung-Yin in children after a febrile Warm disease.

6(a) Prescription

MAI MEN DONG TANG
Ophiopogon Decoction
Mai Men Dong *Tuber Ophiopogonis japonici* 15 g
Dang Shen *Radix Codonopsis pilosulae* 12 g
Ban Xia *Rhizoma Pinelliae ternatae* 6 g
Gan Cao *Radix Glycyrrhizae uralensis* 3 g
Geng Mi *Semen Oryzae* 15 g
Da Zao *Fructus Ziziphi jujubae* 4 dates

Pattern

Lung-Yin deficiency, no dryness and no Empty-Heat.

Clinical manifestations

Same as above but with fewer symptoms of Dryness.

Explanation

- **Mai Men Dong** nourishes Lung-Yin.
- **Dang Shen** tonifies the Spleen according to

the principle of strengthening the Earth to tonify Metal.
- **Ban Xia** counteracts any Phlegm or Dampness deriving from tonification of Yin.
- **Gan Cao**, **Geng Mi** and **Da Zao** tonify Qi and harmonize.

Variations

- If the asthma attacks are relatively frequent add Xuan Fu Hua *Flos Inulae* and Sang Bai Pi *Cortex Mori albae radicis* to restore the descending of Lung-Qi.

Patent remedy

LI FEI WAN
Benefiting the Lungs Pill
Dong Chong Xia Cao *Sclerotium Cordicipitis chinensis*
Ge Jie *Gecko*
Bai He *Bulbus Lilii*
Wu Wei Zi *Fructus Schisandrae chinensis*
Bai Ji *Rhizoma Bletillae striatae*
Bai Bu *Radix Stemonae*
Mu Li *Concha Ostreae*
Pi Pa Ye *Folium Eriobotryae japonicae*
Gan Cao *Radix Glycyrrhizae uralensis*

Explanation

This pill, sometimes also called Li Fei Tang or just Li Fei, nourishes Lung-Yin and strengthens the Lung and Kidney's Defensive-Qi systems. It is absorbing and is therefore good for night-sweating from Lung-Yin deficiency. It also contains stopping-bleeding herbs (Bai Ji) and can therefore be used if there is expectoration of scanty, blood-specked sputum.

The tongue presentation appropriate to this remedy is a Red body in the front.

7. Prescription

BAI HE GU JIN TANG
Lilium Consolidating Metal Decoction
Bai He *Bulbus Lilii* 15 g
Mai Men Dong *Tuber Ophiopogonis japonici* 9 g
Xuan Shen *Radix Scrophulariae ningpoensis* 9 g

Sheng Di Huang *Radix Rehmanniae glutinosae* 9 g
Shu Di Huang *Radix Rehmanniae glutinosae praeparata* 9 g
Dang Gui *Radix Angelicae sinensis* 6 g
Bai Shao *Radix Paeoniae albae* 9 g
Jie Geng *Radix Platycodi grandiflori* 6 g
Chuan Bei Mu *Bulbus Fritillariae cirrhosae* 6 g
Gan Cao *Radix Glycyrrhizae uralensis* 3 g

Pattern

Lung and Kidney-Yin deficiency.

Clinical manifestations

Chronic asthma with infrequent attacks which usually occur at night, wheezing, breathlessness on exertion, dry throat, night sweating, backache, tinnitus, dry cough, 5-palm heat.
Tongue: Red and without coating in the front part.
Pulse: Floating-Empty.

Explanation

- **Bai He** and **Mai Men Dong** nourish Lung-Yin.
- **Xuan Sheng Shen Di** and **Shu Di** nourish Kidney-Yin and clear any Empty-Heat.
- **Dang Gui** and **Bai Shao** nourish Blood to help nourish Yin. Dang Gui also stops cough.
- **Jie Geng** restores the descending of Lung-Qi, benefits the throat and stops cough.
- **Bei Mu** clears Lung-Heat, restores the descending of Lung-Qi and calms cough and asthma.
- **Gan Cao** harmonizes.

(a) Patent remedy

BAI HE GU JIN WAN
Lilium Consolidating Metal Pill
Same ingredients and functions as the above decoction.

(b) Patent remedy

PING CHUAN WAN
Calming Breathlessness Pill
Dang Shen *Radix Codonopsis pilosulae*

Ge Jie *Gecko*
Dong Chong Xia Cao *Sclerotium Cordicipitis chinensis*
Xing Ren *Semen Pruni armeniacae*
Chen Pi *Pericarpium Citri reticulatae*
Gan Cao *Radix Glycyrrhizae uralensis*
Sang Bai Pi *Cortex Mori albae radicis*
Bai Qian *Radix et Rhizoma Cynanchii stautoni*
Meng Shi *Lapis Chloriti*
Wu Zhi Mao Tao *Radix Fici simplicissimae*
Man Hu Tui Zi *Semen Elaeagni glabrae thunbergii*

Explanation

This pill tonifies Qi, strengthens the Lung and Kidney's Defensive-Qi systems, nourishes Lung-Yin and restores the descending of Lung-Qi. It is quite similar in effect to the previous one: they differ in that Bai He Gu Jin Wan is more moistening and slightly less tonifying than Ping Chuan Wan. This latter pill is also more specific for asthma as it contains Ge Jie and it also tonifies Spleen-Qi as it contains Dang Shen.

The tongue presentation appropriate to this remedy is a Pale body.

8. Prescription

SU ZI JIANG QI TANG
Perilla Seed Lowering Qi Decoction
Su Zi *Fructus Perillae frutescentis* 9 g
Ban Xia *Rhizoma Pinelliae ternatae* 9 g
Hou Po *Cortex Magnoliae officinalis* 6 g
Qian Hu *Radix Peucedani* 6 g
Rou Gui *Cortex Cinnamomi cassiae* 3 g
Dang Gui *Radix Angelicae sinensis* 6 g
Sheng Jiang *Rhizoma Zingiberis officinalis recens* 2 slices
Su Ye *Folium Perillae frutescentis* 5 leaves
Da Zao *Fructus Ziziphi jujubae* 3 dates
Gan Cao *Radix Glycyrrhizae uralensis* 3 g

Pattern

Lung-Qi and Kidney-Yang deficiency with internal Cold.

Clinical manifestations

Chronic asthma with infrequent attacks occurring mostly in daytime, chilliness, wheezing, back-ache, frequent-pale urination, oedema of ankles.
Tongue: Pale, wet.
Pulse: Deep-Weak-Slow.

Explanation

- **Su Zi** restores the descending of Lung-Qi and calms asthma.
- **Ban Xia**, **Hou Po** and **Qian Hu** restore the descending of Lung-Qi, resolve Phlegm and relieve fullness in the chest.
- **Rou Gui** warms the Kidney and tonifies the Fire of the Gate of Vitality to strengthen the Kidney's grasping of Qi.
- **Dang Gui** tonifies Liver-Blood to strengthen the Original Qi.
- **Sheng Jiang** and **Su Ye** help to make Lung-Qi descend and harmonize the Stomach.
- **Da Zao** and **Gan Cao** harmonize.

THE LIVER AND ASTHMA

The Liver is also involved in the pathogenesis of asthma especially in the late-onset type. In early onset asthma, emotional stress affecting the Liver can often be a triggering factor for an attack.

The Liver can play a role in the pathology of asthma in three possible ways:

1. Stagnant Liver-Qi may rebel upwards in the chest and obstruct the descending of Lung-Qi. From a 5-Element perspective this is called "Wood insulting Metal".

2. Liver-Fire may also rebel upwards in the chest and similarly obstruct the descending of Lung-Qi. This is also called "Wood insulting Metal". In addition, Liver-Fire may dry up the Lung fluids.

3. Deficient Liver-Yin may fail to nourish the Kidneys and this may lead to the Kidneys not grasping it. Furthermore, a deficiency of Kidney-Yin may lead to dryness in the Lungs.

Stagnant Liver-Qi derives from emotional problems such as repressed anger, frustration and resentment over a long period of time. After some years, stagnant Liver-Qi may easily turn to Liver-Fire. Liver-Yin deficiency may also derive from emotional problems such as sadness. In addition, in women, it may be induced by childbirth and overwork.

The three main Liver patterns affecting asthma are therefore:

Liver-Qi stagnant insulting the Lungs
Liver-Fire insulting the Lungs
Liver-Yin deficiency.

1. LIVER-QI STAGNANT INSULTING THE LUNGS

CLINICAL MANIFESTATIONS

Asthma attacks elicited by emotional stress, a feeling of oppression and distension of the chest and hypochondrium.
Tongue: the tongue body may not change in colour except in long-standing cases when the sides might be Red.
Pulse: Wiry.

TREATMENT PRINCIPLE

Soothe the Liver, regulate Qi, restore the descending of Lung-Qi, calm the mind.

ACUPUNCTURE

SP-4 Gongsun, P-6 Neiguan, LIV-14 Qimen, Ren-17 Shanzhong, BL-18 Ganshu with reducing or even method. These points are in addition to those mentioned above for the various types of deficiency of Lung and Kidney's Defensive-Qi systems.

Explanation

– **SP-4** and **P-6** in combination open the Penetrating Vessel, relieve fullness in the chest and subdue rebellious Qi in the chest. In addition, P-6 calms the Mind and indirectly moves Liver-Qi as the Pericardium and Liver

channel are connected within the Terminal Yin channels.
– **LIV-14** and **BL-18**, Front-Collecting and Back-Transporting point of the Liver respectively, move Liver-Qi.
– **Ren-17** moves Qi in the chest and restores the descending of Lung-Qi.

HERBAL TREATMENT

Prescription

CHEN XIANG JIANG QI SAN
Aquilaria Subduing Qi Powder
Chen Xiang *Lignum Aquilariae* 3 g
Sha Ren *Fructus seu Semen Amomi* 4 g
Xiang Fu *Rhizoma Cyperi rotundi* 6 g
Zhi Gan Cao *Radix Glycyrrhizae uralensis praeparata* 3 g
Sheng Jiang *Rhizoma Zingiberis officinalis recens* 3 slices

Explanation

– **Chen Xiang** restores the descending of Lung-Qi.
– **Sha Ren** and **Xiang Fu** move Liver-Qi.
– **Zhi Gan Cao** and **Sheng Jiang** harmonize.

Herbs

In cases when Liver-Qi stagnation plays a role in asthma, any of the formulae mentioned above for deficiency of the Lung and Kidney's Defensive-Qi systems, can be modified with the addition of herbs such as Qing Pi *Pericarpium Citri reticulatae viridae*, Mu Xiang *Radix Saussureae*, Yu Jin *Tuber Curcumae*, Zhi Ke *Fructus Citri aurantii* and He Huan Pi *Cortex Albizziae julibrissin*.

2. LIVER-FIRE INSULTING THE LUNGS

CLINICAL MANIFESTATIONS

Loud wheezing, attacks of asthma elicited by emotional strain, irritability, propensity to outbursts of anger, hypochondrial and chest fullness and distension, bitter taste, thirst.

Tongue: Red with redder sides and yellow coating.
Pulse: Wiry-Rapid.

TREATMENT PRINCIPLE

Clear the Liver, clear Fire, subdue rebellious Qi, restore the descending of Lung-Qi and calm the Mind.

ACUPUNCTURE

LIV-2 Xingjian, LIV-14 Qimen, BL-18 Ganshu, P-6 Neiguan, LU-7 Lieque. Reducing or even method. These points are to be used in addition to those mentioned previously for the various patterns of asthma.

Explanation

- **LIV-2** is the main point to clear Liver-Fire.
- **LIV-14** and **BL-18** clear Liver-Fire and move Liver-Qi.
- **P-6** regulates the Liver, opens the chest, eases breathing and calms the Mind.
- **LU-7** restores the descending of Lung-Qi.

HERBAL TREATMENT

(a) Prescription

LONG DAN XIE GAN TANG
Gentiana Draining the Liver Decoction
Long Dan Cao *Radix Gentianae scabrae* 6 g
Huang Qin *Radix Scutellariae baicalensis* 9 g
Shan Zhi Zi *Fructus Gardeniae jasminoidis* 9 g
Ze Xie *Rhizoma Alismatis orientalis* 9 g
Mu Tong *Caulis Akebiae* 9 g
Che Qian Zi *Semen Plantaginis* 9 g
Sheng Di Huang *Radix Rehmanniae glutinosae* 12 g
Dang Gui *Radix Angelicae sinensis* 9 g
Chai Hu *Radix Bupleuri* 9 g
Gan Cao *Radix Glycyrrhizae uralensis* 3 g

Explanation

This is the most important formula to clear Liver-Fire and it has already been explained in the chapter on Headaches (ch. 1).

Variations

When this formula is used for Liver-Fire insulting the Lungs in asthma, one needs to add some herbs to restore the descending of Lung-Qi such as Xuan Fu Hua *Flos Inulae*, Xing Ren *Semen Pruni armeniacae* and Su Zi *Fructus Perillae frutescentis*.

(b) Prescription

Empirical formula[26]
Ma Huang *Herba Ephedrae* 3 g
Zi Wan *Radix Asteris tatarici* 9 g
Pi Pa Ye *Folium Eriobotryae japonicae* 9 g
Zhe Bei Mu *Bulbus Fritillariae thunbergii* 9 g
Xing Ren *Semen Pruni armeniacae* 6 g
Qian Hu *Radix Peucedani* 9 g
Sang Bai Pi *Cortex Mori albae radicis* 6 g
Ban Xia *Rhizoma Pinelliae ternatae* 6 g
Chen Pi *Pericarpium Citri reticulatae* 4.5 g
Yu Jin *Tuber Curcumae* 6 g
Shan Zhi Zi *Fructus Gardeniae jasminoidis* 6 g
Lian Qiao *Fructus Forsythiae suspensae* 6 g

Explanation

- **Ma Huang** restores the dispersing and descending of Lung-Qi and calms asthma. It is used here in a small dose to calm asthma even though it is a warm herb.
- **Zi Wan**, **Pi Pa Ye**, **Bei Mu**, **Xing Ren**, **Qian Hu** and **Sang Bai Pi** restore the descending of Lung-Qi, resolve Phlegm and calm asthma.
- **Ban Xia** resolves Phlegm and subdues rebellious Qi.
- **Chen Pi** and **Yu Jin** move Qi and regulate the Liver.
- **Zhi Zi** and **Lian Qiao** clear Liver-Heat.

Herbs

If one were to use one of the formulae for deficiency of the Lung and Kidney's Defensive-Qi systems mentioned above, then herbs to clear Liver-Fire should be added, e.g. Long Dan Cao *Radix Gentianae scabrae*.

3. LIVER-YIN DEFICIENCY

CLINICAL MANIFESTATIONS

Infrequent asthma attacks at night, dry throat, dry cough, blurred vision, dry eyes, hypochondriac and chest distension. Floating-Empty pulse and Red tongue without coating.

TREATMENT PRINCIPLE

Nourish Liver-Yin, move Liver-Qi, restore the descending of Lung-Qi and calm the Mind.

ACUPUNCTURE

LIV-8 Ququan, SP-6 Sanyinjiao, KI-3 Taixi, Ren-4 Guanyuan, P-6 Neiguan and SP-4 Gongsun. Reinforcing method. These points are used in addition to the ones previously mentioned for deficiency of the Lung and Kidney's Defensive-Qi systems.

Explanation

- **LIV-8** and **Ren-4** nourish Liver-Yin.
- **SP-6** and **KI-3** nourish Kidney-Yin, which helps to nourish Liver-Yin.
- **P-6** and **SP-4** open the Yin Linking vessels, nourish Liver-Blood, open the chest and calm the Mind.

HERBAL TREATMENT

Prescription

YI GUAN JIAN
One Linking Decoction
Bei Sha Shen *Radix Glehniae littoralis* 10 g
Mai Men Dong *Tuber Ophiopogonis japonici* 10 g
Dang Gui *Radix Angelicae sinensis* 10 g
Sheng Di Huang *Radix Rehmanniae glutinosae* 30 g
Gou Qi Zi *Fructus Lycii chinensis* 12 g
Chuan Lian Zi *Fructus Meliae toosendan* 5 g

Explanation

- **Bei Sha Shen** and **Mai Men Dong** nourish Lung-Yin.

- **Dang Gui**, **Sheng Di** and **Gou Qi Zi** nourish Liver-Yin.
- **Chuan Lian Zi** moves Liver-Qi. It is one of the few cold moving Qi-herbs.

Variations

When used for chronic asthma, herbs to restore the descending of Lung-Qi should be added such as Xuan Fu Hua *Flos Inulae*, Xing Ren *Semen Pruni armeniacae* and Su Zi *Fructus Perillae frutescentis*.

Herbs

If one were to use one of the formulae for deficiency of the Lung and Kidney's Defensive-Qi systems, then some herbs to nourish Liver-Yin should be added, such as Sheng Di Huang *Radix Rehmanniae glutinosae*, Gou Qi Zi *Fructus Lycii chinensis*, Nu Zhen Zi *Fructus Ligustri lucidi* and Sang Ji Sheng *Ramulus Loranthi*.

ECZEMA

Eczema from a very early age or even from birth often accompanies or precedes the development of allergic asthma. The two symptoms of eczema and asthma have the same allergic root as is easily demonstrated by the whealing skin reactions occurring on inhalation of allergens in individuals suffering from extrinsic asthma.

From the point of view of Chinese pathology eczema is also due to an inborn deficiency of the Lung and Kidney's Defensive-Qi systems. The relationship between the Lungs and skin is well known and yet, when discussing the pathology of skin diseases, Chinese books always seem to stress more the role of Blood (and Liver) in connection with the skin. In the case of atopic eczema and asthma, the connection between the Lungs and the skin could not be clearer. These two symptoms are very clearly related and often one will appear as the other improves. For example, often eczema appears first at a very early age or even from birth, to be followed later by asthma when the child is about 4 or 5 years old. This pattern is more likely to occur if the eczema is suppressed with the application of cortisone creams. The reverse may also occur when asthma appears first and then apparently improves only to be followed by eczema.

The relationship between skin diseases and the Lungs can also be observed in the action of many of the herbs which are used to expel Wind in skin diseases. The same herbs which expel Wind from the skin in eczema or rashes also stimulate the dispersing and descending of Lung-Qi in exterior conditions. The following are some examples with their action on the skin in brackets:

- Fang Feng *Radix Ledebouriellae sesloidis* (clears Wind-Damp)
- Jing Jie *Herba seu Flos Schizonepetae tenuifoliae* (clears Wind)
- Chan Tui *Periostracum Cicadae* (clears Wind-Heat)
- Ge Gen *Radix Puerariae* (expresses rashes)
- Ma Huang *Herba Ephedrae* (clears Wind-Cold)
- Bai Zhi *Radix Angelicae dahuricae* (expresses pus from skin)
- Cang Er Zi *Fructus Xanthii* (clears Wind)
- Bo He *Herba Menthae* (expresses rashes)
- Niu Bang Zi *Fructus Arctii lappae* (expresses rashes, reduces erythema)
- Fu Ping *Herba Lemnae seu Spirodelae* (expresses rashes)
- Sheng Ma *Rhizoma Cimicifugae* (expresses rashes).

There are also other herbs which act on the Lungs and affect the skin:

- Bei Sha Shen *Radix Glehniae littoralis*, which tonifies Lung-Yin, is used a lot for chronic skin diseases especially if there is dryness
- Wu Wei Zi *Fructus Schisandrae chinensis*, which tonifies Lung-Yin and promotes the Lung's fluids, is also used frequently for chronic skin diseases with dryness
- Sang Bai Pi *Cortex Mori albae radicis*, which restores the descending of Lung-Qi and resolves Phlegm-Heat from the Lungs, is used in chronic skin diseases with Damp-Heat.

Thus, there is a very close relationship between the Lungs, and in particular the Lung's Defensive-Qi system, and the skin.

The Kidneys also play a role in the pathogenesis of eczema. First of all, whilst the Lungs control the skin in the sense of being linked to its pores, the Kidneys nourish and moisten the skin. Secondly, as mentioned before, the Kidney-Essence is closely bound with the Corporeal Soul of the Lungs which manifests on the skin and which is responsible for sensations of itching and pain on the skin. An inborn defect of the Kidney-Essence, such as occurs in atopic asthma and eczema, can therefore affect the Corporeal Soul and the skin. Thirdly, the Extraordinary Vessels, especially the Penetrating and Directing Vessels, nourish the skin through a network of secondary vessels all over the body. Since these two vessels arise from the Kidneys and spread the Kidney-Essence to the skin, they provide a further link between the Kidneys and the skin. Li Shi Zhen in his work "A Study of the Eight Extraordinary Vessels" (1578) says: "...when the Qi of the channels overflows, it flows into the Extraordinary Vessels...warming the organs internally and irrigating the space between the skin and muscles externally".[27] The Penetrating Vessel also moistens the skin. The "Spiritual Axis" in chapter 65 says: "... if the Blood [of the Penetrating Vessel] is abundant the skin is moist ...".[28] Skin pigmentation also depends on the Extraordinary Vessels. That is why darker pigmentation is concentrated along the pathway of the Extraordinary Vessels (Directing and Penetrating Vessels) such as genitals, the midline between pubis and umbilicus and nipples. In fact, the pigmentation on the midline between pubis and umbilicus (Directing Vessel) often becomes darker during pregnancy.[29]

Another example of the relationship between Kidneys and skin is the development of nephritis from a blood infection deriving from a skin disease.

There are two basic types of eczema in babies, one characterized by Wind-Heat (called "dry foetus") and the other characterized by Damp-Heat (called "damp foetus"). They are both due to a deficiency of Lung and Kidney's Defensive Qi systems but with varying degrees of involvement of the Lungs or Kidneys. The Wind-Heat type is more due to the Lungs, whilst the Damp-Heat type is more related to the Kidneys.

As for the treatment, the aim depends on whether the asthma or the eczema is the predominant problem. If asthma is the predominant problem, one would simply use one of the formulae indicated above and add some herbs to treat the eczema according to type:

Wind-Heat	Damp-Heat
Jing Jie	Fang Feng
Chan Tui	Bai Xian Pi
Bo He	Ge Gen
Bai Xian Pi	Bai Zhi
	Niu Bang Zi
	Sheng Ma

All these herbs are suitable for babies or young children. Eczema from Wind-Heat is characterized by skin lesions which are very dry, red and itchy, with the itchiness being spread all over the body and moving from place to place. Eczema from Damp-Heat is characterized by skin lesions which are moist, oozing fluid, red and itchy, with the itchiness being more confined to specific parts of the body, often the forearm and lower leg.

If eczema is the main problem, then one must use one of the following formulae and modify them with the addition of herbs to restore the descending of Lung-Qi such as Su Zi *Fructus Perillae frutescentis*, Xing Ren *Semen Pruni armeniacae*, Sang Bai Pi *Cortex Mori albae radicis*, Pi Pa Ye *Folium Eriobotryae japonicae*, or Xuan Fu Hua *Flos Inulae*. In particular, Pi Pa Ye and Sang Bai Pi are suitable to restore the descending of Lung-Qi and they also clear Damp-Heat from the skin.

ACUTE ECZEMA

WIND-HEAT

Acupuncture

T.B.-6 Zhigou, G.B.-31 Fengshi, BL-12 Fengmen, L.I.-11 Quchi, L.I.-4 Hegu, Du-14 Dazhui, SP-10 Xuehai, SP-6 Sanyinjiao, LIV-2 Xingjian, HE-8 Shaofu, HE-7 Shenmen, P-4 Ximen, Zhiyangxue extra point, LU-7 Lieque and KI-6 Zhaohai, LU-9 Taiyuan, KI-3 Taixi, Sifeng. Reducing method on all points except SP-6, LU-7, KI-6, LU-9 and KI-3 which should be reinforced. No moxa.

Explanation

- **T.B.-6** and **G.B.-31** are the main points to expel Wind-Heat from the skin.
- **BL-12** helps to expel Wind.
- **L.I.-11** and **L.I.-4** expel Wind-Heat and cool Blood.
- **Du-14** is used if Heat is pronounced.
- **SP-10** and **SP-6** cool and nourish Blood. This is necessary according to the principle of "harmonizing Blood in order to expel Wind".
- **LIV-2** is used if there are signs of Liver-Heat. It also helps to expel Wind.
- **HE-8**, **HE-7** and **P-4** stop itching and one of these points is used if this symptom is pronounced.
- **Zhiyangxue**, extra point, stops itching. It is situated two *cun* directly above L.I.-11 on the Large Intestine channel.
- **LU-7** and **KI-6** in combination, open the Directing Vessel, tonify the Lung and Kidney's Defensive-Qi systems, nourish the Essence and benefit the skin. These points are used in women. In men, use:
- **LU-9** and **KI-3** tonify the Lung and Kidney's Defensive-Qi systems and benefit the skin.
- **Sifeng**, extra point, can be pricked in infants for acute Wind-Heat. It is located in the cracks of the fingers.

Herbal treatment

Prescription

XIAO FENG SAN
Clearing Wind Powder
Jing Jie *Herba seu Flos Schizonepetae tenuifoliae* 3 g
Fang Feng *Radix Ledebouriellae sesloidis* 3 g
Chan Tui *Periostracum Cicadae* 3 g
Niu Bang Zi *Fructus Arctii lappae* 3 g
Ku Shen *Radix Sophorae flavescentis* 3 g
Mu Tong *Caulis Akebiae* 1.5 g
Cang Zhu *Rhizoma Atractylodis lanceae* 3 g
Sheng Di Huang *Radix Rehmanniae glutinosae* 5 g
Shi Gao *Gypsum fibrosum* 10 g
Zhi Mu *Radix Anemarrhenae asphodeloidis* 3 g
Dang Gui *Radix Angelicae sinensis* 3 g
Hei Zhi Ma *Semen Sesami indici* 3 g
Gan Cao *Radix Glycyrrhizae uralensis* 3 g

Explanation

– **Jing Jie**, **Fang Feng**, **Chan Tui** and **Niu Bang Zi** clear Wind-Heat from the skin and release the Exterior.
– **Ku Shen**, **Mu Tong** and **Cang Zhu** resolve Damp-Heat.
– **Sheng Di**, **Shi Gao** and **Zhi Mu** clear Heat and cool Blood.
– **Dang Gui** enters the Blood and directs all the herbs to the Blood portion in order to cool Blood in the skin.
– **Hei Zhi Ma** nourishes Blood and moistens the skin.
– **Gan Cao** harmonizes.

Variations

– In very chronic conditions, there may be a pronounced deficiency and dryness of the Blood. In these cases, the herbs which resolve Dampness (Ku Shen, Mu Tong, and Cang Zhu) can be eliminated or reduced in dosage, and the herbs which nourish Blood (Sheng Di and Dang Gui) should be increased in dosage. Furthermore, Shou Wu *Radix Polygoni multiflori* should be added.

DAMP-HEAT

Acupuncture

L.I.-11 Quchi, SP-9 Yinlingquan, SP-6 Sanyinjiao, Du-14 Dazhui, SP-10 Xuehai, Ren-12 Zhongwan, BL-20 Pishu, LU-7 Lieque and KI-6 Zhaohai, LU-9 Taiyuan, KI-3 Taixi, Sifeng. Reducing method except on Ren-12, BL-20, LU-7, KI-6, LU-9 and KI-3 which should be reinforced. No moxa.

Explanation

– **L.I.-11**, **SP-9** and **SP-6** resolve Damp-Heat.
– **Du-14** and **SP-10** clear Heat and cool Blood.
– **Ren-12** and **BL-20** tonify the Spleen to resolve Dampness.
– **LU-7** and **KI-6** in combination, open the Directing Vessel, tonify the Lung and Kidney's Defensive-Qi systems, nourish the Essence and benefit the skin. These points are used in women. In men, use:

– **LU-9** and **KI-3** tonify the Lung and Kidney's Defensive-Qi systems and benefit the skin.
– **Sifeng,** in infants, expels Damp-Heat.

Herbal treatment

1. Prescription

BI XIE SHEN SHI TANG
Dioscorea Draining Dampness Decoction
Bi Xie *Rhizoma Dioscoreae hypoglaucae* 9 g
Yi Yi Ren *Semen Coicis lachryma jobi* 15 g
Huang Bo *Cortex Phellodendri* 6 g
Fu Ling *Sclerotium Poriae cocos* 9 g
Ze Xie *Rhizoma Alismatis orientalis* 6 g
Hua Shi *Talcum* 9 g
Mu Tong *Caulis Akebiae* 3 g
Mu Dan Pi *Cortex Moutan radicis* 6 g

Explanation

– **Mu Dan Pi** cools Blood.
– All the other herbs drain Damp-Heat.

2. Prescription

CHU SHI WEI LING TANG
Eliminating Dampness Stomach "Ling" Decoction
Cang Zhu *Rhizoma Atractylodis lanceae* 6 g
Hou Po *Cortex Magnoliae officinalis* 4 g
Mu Tong *Caulis Akebiae* 2 g
Zhu Ling *Sclerotium Polypori umbellati* 6 g
Ze Xie *Rhizoma Alismatis orientalis* 6 g
Hua Shi *Talcum* 6 g
Yi Yi Ren *Semen Coicis lachryma jobi* 12 g
Shan Zhi Zi *Fructus Gardeniae jasminoidis* 4 g

Explanation

– **Cang Zhu** and **Hou Po** fragrantly resolve Dampness.
– **Mu Tong**, **Zhu Ling**, **Ze Xie**, **Hua Shi** and **Yi Ren** drain Dampness and clear Heat.
– **Shan Zhi Zi** clears Damp-Heat.

3. Prescription

QING RE SHEN SHI TANG
Clearing Heat and Draining Dampness Decoction
Huang Qin *Radix Scutellariae baicalensis* 3 g

Huang Bo *Cortex Phellodendri* 3 g
Ku Shen *Radix Sophorae flavescentis* 3 g
Bai Xian Pi *Cortex Dictami dasycarpi radicis* 3 g
Ban Lan Gen *Radix Isatidis seu Baphicacanthi* 5 g
Sheng Di Huang *Radix Rehmanniae glutinosae* 5 g
Fu Ling *Sclerotium Poriae cocos* 3 g
Hua Shi *Talcum* 5 g
Zhu Ye *Herba Lophatheri gracilis* 3 g

Explanation

- **Huang Qin**, **Huang Bo** and **Ku Shen** drain Damp-Heat.
- **Bai Xian Pi** and **Ban Lan Gen** clear Damp-Heat and resolve Fire-Poison.
- **Sheng Di** cools Blood.
- **Fu Ling** and **Hua Shi** drain Dampness.
- **Zhu Ye** clears Heat.

These three formulae for acute eczema may be differentiated in Table 5.2.

CHRONIC ECZEMA

WIND-HEAT (WITH BLOOD DEFICIENCY)

Acupuncture

T.B.-6 Zhigou, G.B.-31 Fengshi, BL-12 Fengmen, L.I.-11 Quchi, L.I.-4 Hegu, Du-14 Dazhui, SP-10 Xuehai, SP-6 Sanyinjiao, LIV-2 Xingjian, HE-8 Shaofu, Zhiyangxue extra point, LU-7 Lieque and KI-6 Zhaohai, LU-9 Taiyuan, KI-3 Taixi, ST-36 Zusanli, BL-17 Geshu, LIV-8 Ququan, Ren-4 Guanyuan. Even method on all points except SP-6, LU-7, KI-6, LU-9, KI-3, ST-36, BL-17, LIV-8 and Ren-4 which should be reinforced. No moxa.

Table 5.2   Differentiation of acute eczema formulae

	Bi Xie Shen Shi Tang	Chu Shi Wei Ling Tang	Qing Re Shen Shi Tang
Action	Drain Damp-Heat via urine	Drain Damp-Heat via urine and relieve epigastric fullness	Drain Damp-Heat and resolve Fire-Poison
Skin	Moist-red skin lesions	Moist-red skin lesions, eczema more on legs	Pustular-red skin lesions

Explanation

- **T.B.-6** and **G.B.-31** are the main points to expel Wind-Heat from the skin.
- **BL-12** helps to expel Wind.
- **L.I.-11** and **L.I.-4** expel Wind-Heat and cool Blood.
- **Du-14** is used if Heat is pronounced.
- **SP-10** and **SP-6** cool and nourish Blood. This is necessary according to the principle of "harmonizing Blood in order to expel Wind".
- **LIV-2** is used if there are signs of Liver-Heat. It also helps to expel Wind.
- **HE-8** stops itching and is used if itching is pronounced.
- **Zhiyangxue**, extra point, stops itching. It is situated two *cun* directly above L.I.-11 on the Large Intestine channel.
- **LU-7** and **KI-6** in combination, open the Directing Vessel, tonify the Lung and Kidney's Defensive-Qi systems, nourish the Essence and benefit the skin. These points are used in women.
- **LU-9** and **KI-3** tonify the Lung and Kidney's Defensive-Qi systems and benefit the skin.
- **ST-36** and **BL-17** nourish Blood.
- **LIV-8** and **Ren-4** are reinforced if there are symptoms of Liver-Blood deficiency.

Herbal treatment

1. Prescription

YANG XUE DING FENG TANG
Nourishing Blood and Clearing Wind Decoction
Sheng Di Huang *Radix Rehmanniae glutinosae* 12 g
Dang Gui *Radix Angelicae sinensis* 9 g
Shou Wu *Radix Polygoni multiflori* 9 g
Tian Men Dong *Tuber Asparagi cochinchinensis* 6 g
Mai Men Dong *Tuber Ophiopogonis japonici* 6 g
Chi Shao *Radix Paeoniae rubrae* 6 g
Chuan Xiong *Radix Ligustici wallichii* 4 g
Mu Dan Pi *Cortex Moutan radicis* 4 g
Jiang Can *Bombyx batryticatus* 3 g
Shan Zhi Zi *Fructus Gardeniae jasminoidis* 4 g

Explanation

- **Sheng Di**, **Dang Gui** and **Shou Wu** nourish Blood.

– **Tian Men Dong** and **Mai Men Dong** nourish Yin to help to nourish Blood.
– **Chi Shao**, **Chuan Xiong** and **Mu Dan Pi** move and cool Blood.
– **Jiang Can** clears Wind.
– **Zhi Zi** clears Heat.

This formula is for chronic eczema from Wind-Heat in the Blood affecting the skin against a background of Blood deficiency. The skin lesions are not very red and the skin is very dry and itchy.

2. Prescription

XIAO FENG CHONG JI
Clearing Wind Decoction
Jing Jie *Herba seu Flos Schizonepetae tenuifoliae* 6 g
Chan Tui *Periostracum Cicadae* 6 g
Niu Bang Zi *Fructus Arctii lappae* 4 g
Dang Gui *Radix Angelicae sinensis* 9 g
Hei Zhi Ma *Semen Sesami indici* 6 g
Sheng Di Huang *Radix Rehmanniae glutinosae* 9 g
Ku Shen *Radix Sophorae flavescentis* 9 g
Cang Zhu *Rhizoma Atractylodis lanceae* 4 g
Mu Tong *Caulis Akebiae* 2 g
Zhi Mu *Radix Anemarrhenae asphodeloidis* 4 g
Shi Gao *Gypsum fibrosum* 12 g
Gan Cao *Radix Glycyrrhizae uralensis* 3 g

Explanation

– **Jing Jie**, **Chan Tui** and **Niu Bang Zi** clear Wind-Heat from the skin.
– **Dang Gui**, **Sheng Di** and **Hei Zhi** nourish Blood.
– **Ku Shen**, **Cang Zhu** and **Mu Tong** drain Dampness.
– **Zhi Mu** and **Shi Gao** clear Heat and cool Blood.
– **Gan Cao** harmonizes.

This formula is for a more complex condition than the previous one. It is for chronic eczema from both Wind-Heat and some Damp-Heat against a background of Blood deficiency with some Blood-Heat. The skin lesions are quite red, not too itchy, dry but frequently turning moist.

DAMP-HEAT

Acupuncture

L.I.-11 Quchi, SP-9 Yinlingquan, SP-6 Sanyinjiao, Du-14 Dazhui, SP-10 Xuehai, Zhiyangxue, Ren-12 Zhongwan, BL-20 Pishu, LU-7 Lieque and KI-6 Zhaohai, LU-9 Taiyuan, KI-3 Taixi. Reducing method except on Ren-12, BL-20, LU-7, KI-6, LU-9 and KI-3 which should be reinforced. No moxa.

Explanation

– **L.I.-11**, **SP-9** and **SP-6** resolve Damp-Heat.
– **Du-14** and **SP-10** clear Heat and cool Blood.
– **Zhiyangxue**, extra point located two *cun* above L.I.-11, stops itching.
– **Ren-12** and **BL-20** tonify the Spleen to resolve Dampness.
– **LU-7** and **KI-6** in combination, open the Directing Vessel, tonify the Lung and Kidney's Defensive-Qi systems, nourish the Essence and benefit the skin. These points are used in women.
– **LU-9** and **KI-3** tonify the Lung and Kidney's Defensive-Qi systems and benefit the skin.

Herbal treatment

Prescription

SAN FENG CHU SHI TANG
Scattering Wind and Eliminating Dampness Decoction
Huang Bo *Cortex Phellodendri* 6 g
Cang Zhu *Rhizoma Atractylodis lanceae* 6 g
Fang Feng *Radix Ledebouriellae sesloidis* 6 g
Xi Xian Cao *Herba Siegesbeckiae orientalis* 4 g
Cang Er Zi *Fructus Xanthii* 4 g
Fu Ping *Herba Lemnae seu Spirodelae* 4 g
Bai Xian Pi *Cortex Dictami dasycarpi radicis* 6 g
She Chuang Zi *Semen Cnidii monnieri* 4 g

Explanation

– **Huang Bo** and **Cang Zhu** drain Dampness.
– **Fang Feng**, **Xi Xian Cao**, **Cang Er Zi**, **Fu Ping** and **Bai Xian Pi** clear Wind from the skin and resolve Dampness.

– **She Chuang Zi** drains Dampness and clears Heat. It is specific for chronic skin diseases.

This formula is for chronic eczema from Damp-Heat with dark lesions usually in a limited area oozing fluid and with a thick-rough skin.

EXTERNAL TREATMENT

The application of herbs externally is very beneficial for chronic eczema. The herbs may be boiled in the usual way except with a much larger quantity of water and then strained. The resulting liquid may then be poured in a shallow bath and let the patient bathe in this water.

A common formula for external use is:

DA HUANG *Rhizoma Rhei*
HUANG QIN *Radix Scutellariae baicalensis*
HUANG BO *Cortex Phellodendri*
KU SHEN *Radix Sophorae flavescentis*
JU HUA *Flos Chrysanthemi morifolii*
ZI HUA DI DING *Herba Violae cum radice*

Case history

A 35-year-old woman had been suffering from eczema since she was 3 months old. Over the years, she used all sorts of steroid creams. She had had three children and, during each of her gestations, her eczema was always worse in the first 3 months of pregnancy, better in the last 6 months and worse after childbirth. It was mostly on the limbs and face (around her mouth). It consisted of papules (red spots) which were very itchy. They then turned into pustules and oozed a liquid.

She had also been suffering from asthma since the age of 3 after pneumonia. Her wheezing attacks were triggered by dust, house-dust mites, animals' fur, dairy products and shellfish. She also suffered from hay fever (seasonal allergic rhinitis).

She occasionally had mild tinnitus. Her pulse was unremarkable, only slightly Weak on the right Front and the left Rear positions. Her tongue was also unremarkable with slightly Swollen sides (Plate 5.1). This is a good example of how the tongue is often unremarkable in patients with atopic asthma, seemingly confirming that Wind and not Phlegm is the main pathological feature of asthma.

Diagnosis
Asthma, seasonal allergic rhinitis and eczema from Lung and Kidney's Defensive-Qi systems deficiency

from birth. Kidney-Essence affecting the Lung-Corporeal Soul which, in turn, affected the skin. The Kidney deficiency is also clearly shown by the aggravation during the first 3 months of pregnancy, amelioration in the last 6 months and again aggravation after childbirth. The relatively normal pulse and tongue show that the Kidney deficiency only involves the Kidney Defensive-Qi system and not other aspects of the Kidney functions. The eczema is of the chronic Damp-Heat type. The eliciting of asthma attacks from certain foods points to Large Intestine Heat.

Principle of treatment
Her main problem at the time of consultation was the eczema rather than the asthma, the attacks of which were quite infrequent. The principle of treatment adopted was therefore to clear Wind in the skin, resolve Damp-Heat, cool Blood, tonify the Lung and Kidney's Defensive-Qi systems and stimulate the descending of Lung-Qi.

Herbal treatment
The prescriptions chosen were those for chronic Damp-Heat with some variations to tonify the Kidney's Defensive-Qi system. The formula was a variation of San Feng Chu Shi Tang *Scattering Wind and Eliminating Dampness Decoctions* and Chu Shi Wei Ling Tang *Eliminating Dampness Stomach "Ling" Decoction* with the addition of herbs to tonify the Lung and Kidney's Defensive-Qi systems and to stimulate the descending of Lung-Qi:

Huang Bo *Cortex Phellodendri* 4 g
Cang Zhu *Rhizoma Atractylodis lanceae* 4 g
Fang Feng *Radix Ledebouriellae sesloidis* 4 g
Bai Xian Pi *Cortex Dictami dasycarpi radicis* 6 g
She Chuang Zi *Semen Cnidii monnieri* 4 g
Zhu Ling *Sclerotium Polypori umbellati* 4 g
Fu Ling *Sclerotium Poriae cocos* 6 g
Yi Yi Ren *Semen Coicis lachryma jobi* 9 g
Chen Pi *Pericarpium Citri reticulatae* 3 g
Ze Xie *Rhizoma Alismatis orientalis* 4 g
Shou Wu *Radix Polygoni multiflori* 9 g
Sheng Di Huang *Radix Rehmanniae glutinosae* 9 g
Tu Si Zi *Semen Cuscutae* 6 g
Bu Gu Zhi *Fructus Psoraleae corylifoliae* 4 g
Mai Men Dong *Tuber Ophiopogonis japonici* 6 g
Bai He *Bulbus Lilii* 6 g
Sang Bai Pi *Cortex Mori albae radicis* 4 g
Gan Cao *Radix Glycyrrhizae uralensis* 3 g

Explanation
– **Huang Bo** and **Cang Zhu** resolve Damp-Heat.
– **Fang Feng** resolves Dampness and expels Wind.
– **Bai Xian Pi** and **She Chuang Zi** expel Wind and resolve Dampness and Fire-Poison. They are both very important herbs for skin diseases.
– **Zhu Ling**, **Fu Ling**, **Yi Yi Ren**, **Chen Pi** and **Ze Xie** drain Dampness via urination.

- **Shou Wu** and **Sheng Di** nourish and cool Blood.
- **Tu Si Zi** and **Bu Gu Zhi** tonify the Kidney's Defensive-Qi system.
- **Mai Dong** and **Bai He** tonify the Lung's Defensive-Qi system and will also help to regenerate new skin.
- **Sang Bai Pi** restores the descending of Lung-Qi and also helps the skin.
- **Gan Cao** harmonizes.

Acupuncture
LU-7 Lieque and KI-6 Zhaohai, KI-16 Huangshu, KI-3 Taixi, BL-23 Shenshu, L.I.-11 Quchi, SP-10 Xuehai, SP-9 Yinglingquan, BL-13 Feishu, DU-12 Shenzhu.

Explanation
- **LU-7** and **KI-6** tonify Lung and Kidneys, benefit the Essence and the Corporeal Soul, nourish the skin and stimulate the descending of Lung-Qi.
- **KI-16**, **KI-3** and **BL-23** tonify the Kidney's Defensive-Qi system. In particular, KI-16 also benefits the Essence and therefore acts at a deep level to correct the inborn deficiency of the Kidney's Defensive-Qi system. In a way, it is the acupuncture equivalent of the herbal use of placenta and umbilical cord for asthma.
- **L.I.-11** and **SP-10** cool Blood and clear Heat from the skin.
- **SP-9** resolves Damp-Heat.
- **BL-13** and **Du-12** tonify the Lung's Defensive-Qi system.

This woman's eczema cleared up almost completely after 9 months' treatment mostly with herbal medicine and infrequent acupuncture treatment.

Case history

A 19-year-old woman had been suffering from eczema and asthma since the age of 2. At the time of consultation both the eczema and asthma were still very bad. She had to use Ventolin and Becotide every day for her asthma and had used steroid creams in the past for her eczema. Her asthma attacks were elicited by exposure to cats and house-dust mites. She also sweated at night and her bowels opened only every other day. Apart from this, she had no other symptoms. She was very thin and shy. Her skin was very dry, red and itchy. The pulse and tongue were unremarkable as they often are in atopic asthma.

Diagnosis
This is a very typical case of atopic asthma and eczema from deficiency of the Lung and Kidney's Defensive-Qi systems in a highly allergic individual. There is some Lung-Yin deficiency as shown by the night-sweating and constipation.

Treatment principle
Tonify the Lung and Kidney's Defensive-Qi systems,

nourish Lung-Yin, nourish Blood, moisten the skin, clear Wind from the skin and expel Wind from the chest. She had only herbal treatment and the formula used initially was:

Mai Men Dong *Tuber Ophiopogonis japonici* 6 g
Bai He *Bulbus Lilii* 6 g
Su Zi *Fructus Perillae frutescentis* 4 g
Xing Ren *Semen Pruni armeniacae* 4 g
Fang Feng *Radix Ledebouriellae sesloidis* 4 g
Tu Si Zi *Semen Cuscutae* 6 g
Du Zhong *Cortex Eucommiae ulmoidis* 4 g
Nu Zhen Zi *Fructus Ligustri lucidi* 4 g
Shou Wu *Radix Polygoni multiflori* 9 g
Dang Gui *Radix Angelicae sinensis* 6 g
Bai Xian Pi *Cortex Dictami dasycarpi radicis* 6 g
Chan Tui *Periostracum Cicadae* 4 g
Nan Sha Shen *Radix Adenophorae* 4 g
Huo Ma Ren *Semen Cannabis sativae* 4 g
Hei Zhi Ma *Semen Sesami indici* 6 g
Hong Hua *Flos Carthami tinctorii* 3 g
Gan Cao *Radix Glycyrrhizae uralensis* 3 g

Explanation
- **Mai Dong** and **Bai He** nourish Lung-Yin and tonify the Lung's Defensive-Qi system.
- **Su Zi** and **Xing Ren** restore the descending of Lung-Yin.
- **Fang Feng** expels Wind from the chest.
- **Tu Si Zi** and **Du Zhong** tonify the Kidney's Defensive-Qi system.
- **Nu Zhen Zi**, **Shou Wu** and **Dang Gui** nourish Blood and the skin.
- **Bai Xian Pi** and **Chan Tui** clear Wind-Heat from the skin.
- **Nan Sha Shen**, **Huo Ma Ren** and **Hei Zhi Ma** moisten the skin and promote the bowel movements.
- **Hong Hua** moves Blood and, being a light petal, it has a floating movement and therefore carries the other herbs towards the surface, i.e. the skin.
- **Gan Cao** harmonizes and detoxifies.

This patient is still being treated and the eczema and asthma are gradually improving.

Case history

A 23-year old woman had been suffering from asthma since she was 4 years old. She used Ventolin and Becotide. Her asthma attacks were elicited by exposure to dogs, cats and house-dust mites. She also suffered mildly from eczema only when exposed to inhaled or ingested allergens. She usually felt tired, her lower back ached and her bowels opened only every two or three days. Her sleep was not good, waking up frequently during the night. Her periods lasted 7 to 8 days and she suffered from pre-menstrual tension. Her pulse was slightly Weak in the left Rear position and slightly Wiry in the left Middle position. Her tongue was Red on the sides and tip.

Diagnosis
This is again a clear case of Lung and Kidney's Defensive-Qi systems being deficient from birth. There are, however, other factors and notably some Liver-Yang rising (red sides of the tongue and pre-menstrual tension) and some Kidney-Yin deficiency (constipation, back-ache and insomnia).

Treatment principle
The principle of treatment was to tonify the Lung and Kidney's Defensive-Qi systems, nourish Kidney-Yin, restore the descending of Lung-Qi, expel Wind and subdue Liver-Yang.

Herbal treatment
The formula used was a variation of Bai He Gu Jin Tang *Lilium Consolidating Metal Decoction*:

Bai He *Bulbus Lilii* 15 g
Mai Men Dong *Tuber Ophiopogonis japonici* 9 g
Shu Di Huang *Radix Rehmanniae glutinosae praeparata* 9 g
Dang Gui *Radix Angelicae sinensis* 6 g
Bai Shao *Radix Paeoniae albae* 9 g
Jie Geng *Radix Platycodi grandiflori* 6 g
Chuan Bei Mu *Bulbus Fritillariae cirrhosae* 6 g
Fang Feng *Radix Ledebouriellae sesloidis* 4 g
Tu Si Zi *Semen Cuscutae* 6 g
Bu Gu Zhi *Fructus Psoraleae corylifoliae* 4 g
Xing Ren *Semen Pruni armeniacae* 3 g
Su Zi *Fructus Perillae frutescentis* 4 g
Suan Zao Ren *Semen Ziziphi spinosae* 4 g
Gan Cao *Radix Glycyrrhizae uralensis* 3 g

Explanation
- **Bai He** and **Mai Men Dong** nourish Lung-Yin and tonify the Lung's Defensive-Qi system.
- **Shu Di** tonifies the Kidney's function of grasping Qi.
- **Dang Gui**, **Bai Shao** and **Suan Zao Ren** harmonize the Liver, subdue Liver-Yang and calm the Mind.
- **Jie Geng**, **Chuan Bei Mu**, **Xing Ren** and **Su Zi** restore the descending of Lung-Qi and calm asthma.
- **Fang Feng** expels Wind.
- **Tu Si Zi** and **Bu Gu Zhi** tonify the Kidney's Defensive-Qi system.
- **Gan Cao** harmonizes.

Case history

A 30-year-old woman had been suffering from eczema and asthma since birth. She used Ventolin and Becloforte inhalers every day and also took Phyllocontin tablets. As a baby, she was given steroids for the asthma, but these made the eczema worse. She used cortisone creams for her eczema from the age of 7. The eczema seemed to clear during her school years but returned with a vengeance at around 20. When she came for treatment, it was extremely bad. It covered practically the whole body, and was worse on her face, chest and limbs. The skin was very red, very dry, thick, coarse and itchy. Although the skin was dry, the eczema lesions would also weep occasionally. She also suffered from seasonal allergic rhinitis (hay fever) and her mouth often felt dry. There were no other obvious symptoms and signs and her urine and stools were normal. Her tongue was slightly Pale, Thin and dry. Her pulse was Weak, Choppy and both Rear positions (Kidneys) were particularly Weak.

Diagnosis
This is also a clear case of inborn deficiency of Lung and Kidney's Defensive-Qi systems. The pulse confirms the Kidney weakness. Due to the long duration of the illness, there is also some Blood deficiency (as the Kidneys also contribute to making Blood) which, leading to the development of Wind-Heat in the skin, aggravates the eczema. The Blood deficiency is clearly shown by the tongue being Pale, Thin and dry. The eczema is primarily of the Wind-Heat type although there is some Damp-Heat as well because it is sometimes weepy.

Treatment principle
Since the eczema was by far the most distressing problem at the time, attention was turned to treating it first. The aim of treatment was to tonify the Lung and Kidney's Defensive-Qi systems, expel Wind from the chest, nourish Blood, clear Wind-Heat from the skin and restore the descending of Lung-Qi. The formula used was a variation of Yang Xue Ding Feng Tang *Nourishing Blood and Clearing Wind Decoction*:

Sheng Di Huang *Radix Rehmanniae glutinosae* 12 g
Dang Gui *Radix Angelicae sinensis* 9 g
Shou Wu *Radix Polygoni multiflori* 9 g
Tian Men Dong *Tuber Asparagi cochinchinensis* 9 g
Mai Men Dong *Tuber Ophiopogonis japonici* 6 g
Chi Shao *Radix Paeoniae rubrae* 6 g
Mu Dan Pi *Cortex Moutan radicis* 4 g
Shan Zhi Zi *Fructus Gardeniae jasminoidis* 4 g
Chan Tui *Periostracum Cicadae* 6 g
Jing Jie *Herba seu Flos Schizonepetae tenuifoliae* 4 g
Fang Feng *Radix Ledebouriellae sesloidis* 4 g
Tu Si Zi *Semen Cuscutae* 6 g
Bu Gu Zhi *Fructus Psoraleae corylifoliae* 4 g
Xing Ren *Semen Pruni armeniacae* 4 g
Su Zi *Fructus Perillae frutescentis* 4 g
Gan Cao *Radix Glycyrrhizae uralensis* 4 g

Explanation
- **Sheng Di Huang**, **Dang Gui** and **Shou Wu** nourish Blood. Sheng Di also cools Blood.
- **Tian Dong** and **Mai Dong** nourish Yin to help to nourish Blood and they moisten, Mai Dong also

tonifies the Lungs. They also tonify the Lung's Defensive-Qi system.
– **Chi Shao, Dan Pi** and **Zhi Zi** clear Heat and cool Blood to help to clear Heat from the skin.
– **Jing Jie** and **Chan Tui** clear Wind-Heat from the skin.
– **Fang Feng** expels Wind from the chest.
– **Tu Si Zi** and **Bu Gu Zhi** tonify the Kidney's Defensive-Qi system.
– **Su Zi** and **Xing Ren** restore the descending of Lung-Qi.
– **Gan Cao** harmonizes and detoxifies.

This patient is slowly improving and the treatment is still in progress.

Case history

A 28-year-old woman had been suffering from asthma since she was 7 years old. The attacks were worse at night and were elicited by exposure to cold, dogs, cats or horses. She had to resort to using a Ventolin inhaler every day. She also suffered from seasonal allergic rhinitis (hay fever). She generally felt cold and her hands and feet were cold. Her tongue was slightly Pale and her pulse was Slow and Weak especially on the right Rear position.

Diagnosis
This is yet another case of deficiency of the Lung and Kidney's Defensive-Qi system on a background of Kidney-Yang deficiency as is very clear from the general cold feeling, the Pale tongue and the Weak pulse on the right Rear position.

Treatment principle
The principle of treatment was to tonify the Lung and Kidney's Defensive-Qi systems, strengthen Kidney-Yang, expel Wind and restore the descending of Lung-Qi. The formula used was a variation of Su Zi Jiang Qi Tang *Perilla-Seed Lowering Qi Decoction*:

Su Zi *Fructus Perillae frutescentis* 9 g
Su Ye *Folium Perillae frutescentis* 5 leaves
Ban Xia *Rhizoma Pinelliae ternatae* 9 g
Hou Po *Cortex Magnoliae officinalis* 6 g
Fang Feng *Radix Ledebouriellae sesloidis* 4 g
Rou Gui *Cortex Cinnamomi cassiae* 3 g
Dang Gui *Radix Angelicae sinensis* 6 g
Tu Si Zi *Semen Cuscutae* 6 g
Xu Duan *Radix Dipsaci* 4 g
Sheng Jiang *Rhizoma Zingiberis officinalis recens* 2 slices
Zhi Gan Cao *Radix Glycyrrhizae uralensis praeparata* 6 g
Da Zao *Fructus Ziziphi jujubae* 1 date

Explanation
– **Su Zi** and **Su Ye** restore the descending of Lung-Qi.
– **Ban Xia** and **Hou Po** subdue rebellious Qi and relieve fullness in the chest.
– **Fang Feng** expels Wind from the chest.

– **Rou Gui** and **Dang Gui** tonify Kidney-Yang and the Liver to strengthen the Lower Burner.
– **Tu Si Zi** and **Xu Duan** tonify the Kidney's Defensive-Qi system and strengthen Kidney-Yang.
– **Sheng Jiang, Gan Cao** and **Da Zao** harmonize.

Case history

A 40-year-old woman had been suffering from asthma since her early 20s. The attacks started following a deep emotional trauma. She used Ventolin and Becotide inhalers four times a day. At the time of consultation, she was also on corticorsteroids orally (Prednisolone). She was not seemingly allergic to any substance nor did she suffer from allergic rhinitis.

In addition to asthma she also had a lot of catarrh with a profuse, sticky-yellow nasal discharge.

She said that when under stress she became very tense and weak; her hands became cold and she felt unable to cope. She also complained of pre-menstrual tension and hypochondrial and abdominal distension.

Her tongue was Red, redder on the sides and tip with a yellow coating. Her pulse was Wiry on the left side.

Diagnosis
This asthma is not allergic but of the late-onset type and it is very clearly related to a Liver disharmony. Stagnation of Liver-Qi, over a long period of time, has turned into Liver-Fire and this has obstructed the descending of Lung-Qi in the chest giving rise to asthma. The presence of Liver-Fire is obvious from the Red tongue body with redder sides.

The thick-yellow nasal discharge is a case of rhinorrhoea (*Bi Yuan*) from Liver and Gall-Bladder Fire rising to the nose.

Treatment principle
Move Liver-Qi, clear Liver-Fire, restore the descending of Lung-Qi, calm the Mind and settle the Ethereal Soul.

Herbal treatment
This patient was treated only with herbs. The formula chosen was a variation of Si Ni San *Four Rebellious Powder* which moves Liver-Qi and Xie Bai San *Draining Whiteness Powder* which clears Lung-Heat and restores the descending of Lung-Qi. Si Ni San was chosen because it was Liver-Qi stagnation which led to Liver-Fire. The method to be adopted therefore is not to *drain* Liver-Fire with bitter and cold herbs, but to *clear* Liver-Fire with pungent herbs which open Qi and bitter herbs which drain. A further reason for choosing Si Ni San was because the patient had cold hands when under emotional strain, one of the symptoms of this formula.

The formula used was:

Chai Hu *Radix Bupleuri* 6 g

Bai Shao *Radix Paeoniae albae* 9 g
Gan Cao *Radix Glycyrrhizae uralensis* 4.5 g
Zhi Shi *Fructus Citri aurantii immaturus* 6 g
Hou Po *Cortex Magnoliae officinalis* 4.5 g
Shan Zhi Zi *Fructus Gardeniae jasminoidis* 4 g
Sang Bai Pi *Cortex Mori albae radicis* 6 g
Di Gu Pi *Cortex Lycii chinensis radicis* 4 g
Su Zi *Fructus Perillae frutescentis* 6 g
Xing Ren *Semen Pruni armeniacae* 6 g
Suan Zao Ren *Semen Ziziphi spinosae* 4 g
Yuan Zhi *Radix Polygalae tenuifoliae* 4 g

Explanation
- **Chai Hu**, **Bai Shao**, **Gan Cao** and **Zhi Shi**
  constitute the Si Ni San which moves Liver-Qi and
  calms the Mind.
- **Hou Po**, a pungent herb, was added to help to
  move Qi and open the chest. It will therefore help
  breathing and has also a good calming effect on the
  Mind.
- **Zhi Zi**, a bitter herb to clear, was added to clear
  Liver-Fire.
- **Sang Bai Pi** and **Di Gu Pi** constitute the Xie Bai San
  which clears Lung-Heat and restores the
  descending of Lung-Qi.
- **Su Zi** and **Xing Ren** restore the descending of
  Lung-Qi and relieve asthma.
- **Suan Zao Ren** and **Yuan Zhi** calm the Mind and
  settle the Ethereal Soul.

This patient was treated with this basic formula, with
some variations along the way, and she reacted very
well, reaching almost a complete cure after 9 months.

Case history

A 33-year-old man had been suffering from asthma
since he was 1. He got better during his teenage years
but then worse again from 20 onwards. His asthma
attacks were brought on by exposure to dust, house-
dust mites and cats. He had to resort to using a
Ventolin inhaler every day. Apart from his asthma, he
had hardly any other symptoms. He had to urinate at
night.

His tongue-body colour was nearly normal and
only very slightly Pale, its body was Swollen, and
there was a Stomach crack (Plate 5.2). His pulse was
slightly Weak on the right side.

Diagnosis
This is another case of deficiency of the Lung and
Kidney's Defensive-Qi systems, especially of the
Lung's. In addition, there was a deficiency of the
Stomach and Spleen as evidenced by the Weak pulse
on the right, the Stomach crack on the tongue and the
Swollen tongue body.

Treatment principle
Tonify the Lung and Kidney's Defensive-Qi systems
and strengthen the Spleen.

Herbal treatment
This patient was treated only with herbs and the
formula used was a variation of Ren Shen Ge Jie San
Ginseng-Gecko Powder:

Ge Jie *Gecko* 4 g (as a powder)
Zhi Gan Cao *Radix Glycyrrhizae uralensis praeparata* 4 g
Ren Shen *Radix Ginseng* 6 g
Fu Ling *Sclerotium Poriae cocos* 6 g
Chuan Bei Mu *Bulbus Fritillariae cirrhosae* 6 g
Sang Bai Pi *Cortex Mori albae radicis* 6 g
Xing Ren *Semen Pruni armeniacae* 9 g
Huang Qi *Radix Astragali membranacei* 6 g
Mai Men Dong *Tuber Ophiopogonis japonici* 3 g

Explanation
This formula tonifies the Lung and Kidney's
Defensive-Qi systems, strengthens the Spleen and
restores the descending of Lung-Qi.

- The first seven herbs constitute the original
  prescription.
- **Zhi Mu** was eliminated from the original formula
  as there are no signs of Heat.
- **Huang Qi** and **Mai Men Dong** were added to
  tonify the Lung's Defensive-Qi system further.

This patient is still being treated and he is gradually
reducing the use of his inhaler.

Prognosis and prevention

The treatment of allergic asthma will necessarily
take a long time as the disease is always based,
as we have seen, on an inborn deficiency of
Lung and Kidney's Defensive-Qi systems. In
most cases, the treatment may need many
months if not years to produce lasting results.
Both acupuncture and Chinese herbs are equally
effective in combination or independently. If
children can be treated fairly early after the development of the disease, the course of treatment
will be much shorter. If the patient is on bronchodilator inhalers (such as Ventolin) it is not
necessary to make a conscious effort to stop
them as the need to use them will automatically
decrease as the treatment progresses. As for oral
steroids, it is much better if the patient can reduce them very gradually as soon as possible as
they have many side-effects, the main one being
that of inducing a deficiency of the Kidneys in
the long run. As allergic asthma is based on a
deficiency of the Kidney's Defensive-Qi system,
oral steroids, although affording relief in the

short run, can only make it worse in the long run.

If asthma is accompanied by eczema and the patient is using steroid creams, these should be stopped. This means, and the patient should be warned, that the eczema may temporarily become worse. This aggravation can and should be counteracted, however, by the use of herbs externally as described above. This is important to do to gain the patient's confidence in the treatment.

After successfully treating a patient with asthma it is important to take preventive measures to avoid its recurrence.

Adults should be advised to have enough rest and avoid excessive sexual activity. Children (or rather their parents) should be advised to avoid eating excessive amounts of dairy foods, sweets and greasy-fried foods. They should also take great care to avoid exposure to cold and wind without proper clothing.

Both adults and children should be treated immediately at the first signs of invasion of external Wind since this may easily precipitate an attack of asthma in susceptible individuals.

If there is eczema, they should never eat shellfish such as shrimps, prawns, crab and lobster. They should also avoid eating spinach and mushrooms, dairy products, fried-greasy foods, spicy foods and alcohol.

Certain herbal formulae may also be given, especially during the early autumn. By "autumn" is meant here autumn according to the Chinese calendar following which equinoxes and solstices mark not the beginning but roughly the middle of each season. Thus early "autumn" would be towards the end of August.

The following are some of the formulae used:

1. Prescription

Dang Shen *Radix Codonopsis pilosulae* 60 g
Ge Jie *Gecko* 2 geckos
Ma Huang *Herba Ephedrae* 30 g
Xing Ren *Semen Pruni armeniacae* 100 g
Gan Cao *Radix Glycyrrhizae uralensis* 50 g
Sheng Jiang *Rhizoma Zingiberis officinalis recens* 60 g
Hong Zao *Fructus Ziziphi jujubae* 120 g

These are the proportions to make roughly 500 g of powder. Grind the above ingredients very finely in a coffee-grinder and give one teaspoonful a day to be swallowed with hot water after a meal.

2. Placenta pills may be used, especially for thin children, combined with the following formulae (in pill form):

– Yu Ping Feng San *Jade Wind Screen Powder* for deficiency of the Lung's Defensive-Qi system
– Liu Jun Zi Wan *Six Gentlemen Pill* for Spleen deficiency
– Jin Gui Shen Qi Wan *Golden Chest Kidney-Qi Pill* for deficiency of the Kidney's Defensive-Qi system on a background of Yang deficiency
– Mai Wei Di Huang Wan *Ophiopogon-Schisandra-Rehmannia Pill* for deficiency of the Kidney's Defensive-Qi system against a background of Yin deficiency.

3. Prescription

Ren Shen *Radix Ginseng*
Ge Jie *Gecko*

In equal doses as a powder. One teaspoonful once a day with hot water after breakfast.

4. Prescription (for external use)

Bai Jie Zi *Semen Sinapsis albae* 12 g
Yan Hu Suo *Rhizoma Corydalis yanhusuo* 12 g
Xi Xin *Herba Asari cum radice* 21 g
Gan Sui *Radix Euphorbiae kansui* 12 g
She Xiang *Secretio Moschus moschiferi* 0.15 g

Grind the above herbs into a fine powder, mix with fresh ginger juice, shape into small cones and apply with plaster on the following points: BL-13 Feishu, BL-43 Gaohuangshu and DU-14 Dazhui. Remove after 2 hours. Apply two or three times in August for the reason explained above.

5. Acupuncture

Reinforce the following points with moxa (unless there is Yin deficiency):

- BL-13 Feishu, DU-12 Shenzhu and BL-43 Gaohuangshu to strengthen the Lung's Defensive-Qi system. Use these points in late August
- BL-23 Shenshu, Ren-4 Guanyuan and KI-16 Huangshu to strengthen the Kidney's Defensive-Qi system. Use these points in late October.

Western drug therapy

Since most patients with asthma we treat are bound to be on some kind of medication, it is important to understand their mode of action and how they affect our treatment.

The three main approaches to drug treatment of asthma in Western medicine are:

1. anti-allergic drugs
2. bronchodilators
3. corticosteroids.

Each of these drugs acts on a certain stage of the pathological process that leads to asthma.

1. ANTI-ALLERGIC DRUGS (INTAL)

These act by stabilizing the mast cells in the bronchi and reducing their sensitivity to allergen stimulation. They are used only as a prophylactic in the prevention and not the treatment of asthma. They seem to be more effective in children than in adults.

They do not affect the treatment with acupuncture or herbs and do not produce any appreciable change in the pulse or tongue.

2. BRONCHODILATORS (VENTOLIN)

These act by stimulating the adrenergic receptors in the sympathethic nerves to the bronchi and thus causing bronchodilation. The most widely-used ones are the beta2-adrenoceptor stimulants as they are more selective and produce fewer side-effects than adrenaline or teophylline (which stimulate both alfa- and beta-adrenoceptors). Even these, however, have side-effects and, in particular, they may stimulate the heart producing tachycardia.

From the point of view of Chinese diagnosis, selective bronchodilators such as salbutamol (Ventolin) do not affect the tongue although they may make the Heart pulse slightly Overflowing. Other brochodilators such as isoprenaline (Iso-Autohaler) and orciprenaline (Alupent) have more side-effects on the heart and besides making the Heart pulse Overflowing, they may also make the tip of the tongue red.

The use of bronchodilator inhalers may be integrated with acupuncture and herbal treatment. Indeed, they may provide a useful benchmark of the efficacy of our treatment as the patient gradually reduces the frequency of use of inhalers.

3. CORTICOSTEROIDS (BECOTIDE)

These act by reducing bronchial mucosal inflammation and hypersecretion of mucus. They are given either orally, such as prednisolone, or by inhalation, such as beclomethasone (Becotide and Becloforte respectively). When given orally they produce many more side-effects.

From a Chinese perspective, they produce Heat and weaken the Kidneys. They definitely affect the tongue making it Red and Swollen. They also affect the pulse as the Kidney position becomes Weak and the pulse is generally more

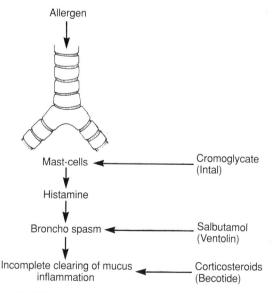

Fig. 5.3 Mode and site of action of anti-allergy agents, bronchodilators and corticosteroids

rapid than normal. Although they can be combined with acupuncture and herbal treatment, corticosteroids slow down the effects of our treatment somewhat. In the course of our treatment, it is necessary to tonify the Kidneys even more by using points such as BL-23 Shenshu and herbs such as Shu Di Huang *Radix Rehmanniae glutinosae praeparata* and Sheng Di Huang *Radix Rehmanniae glutinosae*.

The mode and site of action of the above three drugs may be summarized in a diagram (Fig. 5.3).

END NOTES

1. A. B. Kay 1989 Allergy and Asthma, Blackwell Scientific Publications, p. 153.
2. Niels Mygind 1990 Rhinitis and Asthma, Munksgaard, p. 10.
3. Ibid., p. 10.
4. Ibid., p. 10.
5. Ibid., p. 14. Dr Withering also advocated "coffee made very strong" as the prime reliever of asthma. This is in accordance with the modern use of sympathomimetic agents to promote bronchodilation. Caffeine is a xanthine with sympathomimetic effects.
6. Cited in Zhang Bo Yu 1986 Internal Medicine (*Zhong Yi Nei Ke Xue* 中医内科学), Shanghai Science Publishing House, Shanghai, p. 59.
7. Allergy and Asthma, p. 104.
8. Ibid., p. 159.
9. Parveen J. Kumar and Michael L. Clark 1987 Clinical Medicine, Baillière Tindall, London, p. 586.
10. 1981 Spiritual Axis (*Ling Shu Jing* 灵枢经), People's Health Publishing House, Beijing. First published *c.* 100 BC, p. 126.
11. B. J. Andrews in Journal of Chinese Medicine, no. 35, January 1991, p. 31.
12. Rhinitis and Asthma, p. 252.
13. Ibid., p. 113.
14. Allergy and Asthma, p. 107.
15. Ibid., p. 114.
16. Rhinitis and Asthma, p. 102.
17. Kiiko Matsumoto 1990 Presentation at Pacific Symposium of Oriental Medicine.
18. Rhinitis and Asthma, p. 112.
19. Allergy and Asthma, p. 107.
20. Ibid., p. 108.
21. Spiritual Axis, p. 23.
22. Zhang Jie Bin 1982 Classic of Categories (*Lei Jing* 类经), People's Health Publishing House, Beijing. First published 1624, p. 63.
23. Allergy and Asthma, p. 162.
24. Shi Zi Guang 1988 Essential Clinical Experience of Famous Modern Doctors — Asthma (*Dang Dai Ming Yi Ling Zhen Jing Hua* 当代名医临证精华), Ancient Chinese Medical Texts Publishing House, p. 96.
25. Journal of Chinese Medicine (*Zhong Yi Za Zhi* 中医杂志), vol. 32, no. 12, p. 4.
26. Essential Clinical Experience of Famous Contemporary Doctors, p. 180.
27. Wang Luo Zhen 1985 A Compilation of the "Study of the Eight Extraordinary Vessels" (*Qi Jing Ba Mai Kao Jiao Zhu* 奇经八脉考校注), Shanghai Science Publishing House, p. 1. The "Study of the Eight Extraordinary Vessels" itself by Li Shi Zhen was first published in 1578.
28. Spiritual Axis, p. 120.
29. E. De Giacomo 1991 Rivista Italiana di Medicina Tradizionale Cinese (Italian Journal of Chinese Medicine) no. 3, p. 10.

Allergic rhinitis 6

过
敏
性
鼻
炎

The approach to the diagnosis and treatment of allergic rhinitis presents similar problems to that of asthma. Since "allergic rhinitis" is a disease defined according to Western medicine, we need to establish which symptom it might correspond to in the Chinese medical literature. Most books, both Chinese and English-language ones, correlate allergic rhinitis to the Chinese symptom of "*Bi Yuan*" which literally means "nose-pool". We need first to ascertain whether there is such a correspondence and whether the theory of "*Bi Yuan*" may be used to differentiate and diagnose allergic rhinitis. As for asthma, we shall therefore discuss the following items:

– Allergic rhinitis in Western medicine
– The theory of *Bi Yuan* in Chinese medicine
– Differences between allergic rhinitis and *Bi Yuan*
– A new theory of allergic rhinitis in Chinese medicine.

Allergic rhinitis in Western medicine

The main clinical manifestations of allergic rhinitis are nasal congestion, a watery nasal discharge and sneezing. In a few cases it affects the eyes and the conjunctiva may become red and itchy. In 20% of cases there is also asthma in conjunction with the rhinitis.

AETIOLOGY

Allergic rhinitis is due to an antigen-antibody reaction in the nasal mucosa. If the antigens responsible are only pollen particles then it is called seasonal allergic rhinitis (hay fever). If the antigens are dust, house-dust mites' faecal matter, fungal spores and animal dander, it is called perennial allergic rhinitis. As for furry animals such as dogs and cats, the most allergenic substances are protein from their skin, urine and saliva. In perennial rhinitis the nose becomes more reactive to non-specific stimuli such as cigarette smoke, petrol fumes, perfumes and, in the case of acupuncturists, moxa smoke.

PATHOLOGY

Allergic rhinitis develops as a result of the inter-action between the inhaled allergen and adjacent molecules of IgE antibodies. These adhere to the surface of the mast cells which line the nasal epithelium with the first exposure to the offending allergen. After the first exposure, the mast cells are "primed", i.e. high levels of IgE antibodies adhere to their surface. With subsequent exposure to allergens, the IgE antibodies provoke an "explosion" in the mast cells with the massive release of histamine. Histamine itself causes an increase in permeability of the epithelium allowing allergens to reach IgE-primed mast cells. Sneezing results from overstimulation of the afferent nerve endings and starts within minutes of the allergens entering the nose. This is followed by a greatly increased nasal secretion and eventually nasal blockage about 15-20 minutes after contact with the allergen.

This pathological process is similar to that of asthma, the main difference being that histamine plays a more important role in the development of allergic rhinitis than of asthma. In fact, anti-histamines are effective for allergic rhinitis but are of little value for asthma.

A higher number of mast cells is present in the nasal mucosa of individuals with rhinitis and they probably increase as allergen stimulation continues. This accounts for the increasing re-sponsiveness of the nose to lower amounts of allergens.

The grossly swollen mucosa in allergic rhinitis may obstruct drainage from the sinuses causing sinusitis in half the patients. Thus, infection of the paranasal sinuses is a frequent complication and consequence of allergic rhinitis. This is an important point to remember when discussing the differences between allergic rhinitis and *Bi Yuan*. Some individuals may also lose the sense of taste and smell.

The antigen-antibody reaction is illustrated in Figure 6.1 in which the allergen in question is pollen granules.

The Western treatment of allergic rhinitis

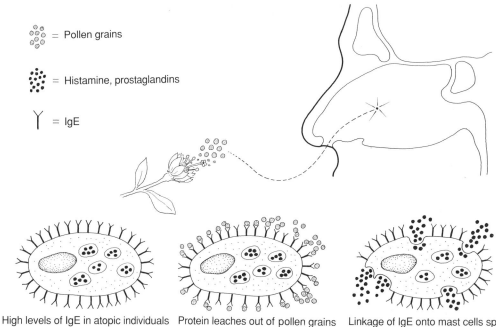

High levels of IgE in atopic individuals attached to mast cells in respiratory tract

Protein leaches out of pollen grains and binds IgE antibodies onto mast cells

Linkage of IgE onto mast cells sparks off "explosion" in them. Histamine and prostaglandins (amongst others) leak from the cells. These cause sneezing, congestion and itching.

Fig. 6.1 Antigen-antibody reaction in allergic rhinitis

relies mostly on the use of antihistamine agents. These work by preventing histamine from reaching its site of action, i.e. the H_1 receptors and hence they are called H_1-receptor blockers. Side-effects include sedation, dizziness, fatigue, insomnia, nervousness, gastro-intestinal disturbances. Failure to respond to antihistamines is due to the fact that active substances other than histamine are released in allergic states.

Steroids by nasal inhalation are also used for allergic rhinitis: these do not seem to have the same general, systemic effect of oral steroids.

The Chinese theory of "Bi Yuan"

The main clinical manifestations usually mentioned in connection with *Bi Yuan* are a purulent nasal discharge with a foul smell, a stuffed nose, a runny nose, headache and sneezing.

AETIOLOGY AND PATHOLOGY

"*Bi Yuan*" is due to repeated invasions of Wind-Cold in the Lung channel which are not treated properly. After some time, Cold turns into Heat, the Lung cannot disperse and descend Qi and local stagnation of Qi and Blood develops in the nose. All these factors lead to nasal discharge. The Gall-Bladder channel carries Heat upwards to the brain, and as the Governing Vessel also flows into the brain and the nose, this therefore causes a purulent yellow nasal discharge. In Chinese medicine this condition was in fact also called "brain flooding" or "brain discharge".

Thus two channels and organs are involved: Lungs and Gall-Bladder. After several years, the Spleen will usually also become involved and a Spleen deficiency leading to Dampness further aggravates the condition.

The Manifestation of this condition consists of symptoms of Wind-Cold or Wind-Heat. The Root of the condition is a deficiency of the Lung in dispersing and descending Qi and, in some cases, Gall-Bladder Heat.

The treatment is variously aimed at expelling Wind-Cold, clearing Gall-Bladder Heat or clearing Spleen-Heat according to the pattern involved.

The main patterns encountered in *Bi Yuan* are:

– Lung invaded by Wind-Cold
– Lung invaded by Wind-Heat
– Liver and Gall-Bladder Heat
– Lung-Heat
– Spleen-Heat.

1. LUNG INVADED BY WIND-COLD

Stuffed nose, runny nose with clear mucus, slight headache, sneezing.

2. LUNG INVADED BY WIND-HEAT

Sneezing, stuffed nose, runny nose with thick-yellow discharge, itchy nose and throat, redness and swelling around the nose, itchy eyes.

3. LIVER AND GALL-BLADDER HEAT

Dry nose, runny nose with yellow-sticky-purulent and foul-smelling discharge, diminished sense of smell, bitter taste, dry throat, headache.

4. LUNG-HEAT

Stuffed nose, runny nose with yellow foul-smelling discharge which may contain blood, dry mouth, feeling of heat.

5. SPLEEN-HEAT

Stuffed nose, runny nose with yellow foul-smelling discharge, diminished sense of smell, feeling of heaviness of the head, headache, bitter and sticky taste.

Differences between allergic rhinitis and Bi Yuan

The use of the theory of *Bi Yuan* to treat allergic rhinitis presents several problems.

1. The theory of *Bi Yuan* presents no clear explanation of the allergic nature of rhinitis and no explanation of its aetiology.

2. Some of the patterns described in *Bi Yuan* are not allergic rhinitis but sinusitis. In fact, all of them, except for Lung invaded by Wind-Cold, include runny nose with a yellow, sticky, purulent and foul-smelling discharge. This is very clearly a symptom of sinusitis, not rhinitis, as it is the infection of the sinuses, not rhinitis, that produces the yellow and purulent discharge.

A new theory of allergic rhinitis

Allergic rhinitis is due to an over-reactivity of the immune system to certain allergens. Like asthma, this is due, from the Chinese point of view, to a deficiency of the Lung and Kidney's Defensive-Qi systems, combined with retention of chronic Wind in the nose.

AETIOLOGY

The deficiency of Lung and Kidney's Defensive-Qi systems is either hereditary or due to problems during the pregnancy or childbirth. The aetiological factors are exactly the same as for asthma (see chapter 5).

Repeated invasions of Wind which are not treated properly, combined with a pre-existing deficiency of Lung and Kidney's Defensive-Qi systems, lead to the retention of what could be described as chronic Wind in the nose, similar to what happens in asthma when Wind is retained in the chest.

PATHOLOGY

Allergic rhinitis is therefore characterized by two factors: a deficiency of Lung and Kidney's Defensive-Qi systems and retention of Wind in the nose. As mentioned for asthma, a deficiency of the Kidney's Defensive-Qi system involves only this particular aspect of its function and not others. One would not expect therefore to see

symptoms such as tinnitus, dizziness, night-sweating, weak back and legs, etc. Even more than asthma, allergic rhinitis is due to a Kidney deficiency. This is so because, in allergic rhinitis, the Kidneys are involved not only in the Root of the disease, but also in the Manifestation via the Governing Vessel. The Governing Vessel emerges from between the Kidneys and flows up the spine to the top of the head and then down to the nose and lips. It is therefore the channel connection between the Kidneys and the nose. For this reason the Kidneys are responsible not only for breathing, due to their function of grasping Qi, but also sneezing.

Thus the hyper-reactivity of the immune response of allergic rhinitis is due to a deficiency of the Kidney's Defensive-Qi system and Governing Vessel. With regard to the role of the Governing Vessel in allergic rhinitis, it is interesting that many of the herbs which Li Shi Zhen connected with this vessel are expelling-Wind herbs which act on the nose. These herbs are Fang Feng *Radix Ledebouriellae sesloidis*, Cang Er Zi *Fructus Xanthii*, Jing Jie *Herba seu Flos Schizonepetae tenuifoliae*, Qiang Huo *Radix et Rhizoma Notopterygii*, Xi Xin *Herba Asari cum radice* and Gao Ben *Rhizoma et Radix Ligustici sinensis*.[2]

The symptoms and signs of allergic rhinitis are those of Wind-Cold as the nasal discharge is always white and watery. This indicates a deficiency of Defensive Qi which is spread by the Lungs but has its root in the Kidneys.[3] Thus, although some books do refer to a Kidney deficiency as the Root of allergic rhinitis, the Kidneys are responsible not only for the Root of this disease (because of the deficiency of the Kidney's Defensive-Qi system), but also for the Manifestation through their direct connection with the Defensive-Qi and sneezing.

Allergic rhinitis often starts in early childhood but it may also start later in life, with a progressive decline of Kidney-Qi or perhaps with a decline of Kidney-Qi connected to the beginning of sexual activity. In fact, in men over 40 suffering from allergic rhinitis there is often a direct connection between sexual activity and an attack of rhinitis. Thus, although rhinitis is obviously a much less severe disease than asthma, when compared with it, it indicates a more severe deficiency of the Kidneys.

As for the difference between seasonal and perennial allergic rhinitis (hay fever), the latter simply occurs when there is a more severe Kidney deficiency.

Obviously, in patients aged 50 or over the pathology will be complicated by other factors, the most common of which is a Spleen deficiency which produces more mucus and therefore a runny nose.

As for the Manifestation, the main pathogenic factor is Wind invading the Lung channel in the nose. However, this is due not only to repeated invasions of Wind, as in the theory of *Bi Yuan*, but primarily to the inherent deficiency of the Kidney's Defensive-Qi system and Governing Vessel in the nose which "mimics" symptoms of invasion of Wind-Cold. Sneezing itself is also directly due to the Kidneys and not necessarily to Wind.

TREATMENT

As for treatment, it is important to distinguish seasonal from perennial rhinitis. In seasonal rhinitis we should apply different principles of treatment according to the season. In perennial rhinitis, the principle of treatment is irrespective of the season.

The discussion of the treatment will therefore be structured in the following way:

SEASONAL ALLERGIC RHINITIS

Treatment of the Manifestation

1. Wind-Cold
2. Wind-Heat

Treatment of the Root

Deficiency of Lung and Kidney's Defensive-Qi systems and the Governing Vessel

PERENNIAL ALLERGIC RHINITIS

Deficiency of Lung and Kidney's Defensive-Qi systems and the Governing Vessel.

SEASONAL ALLERGIC RHINITIS

In seasonal rhinitis one must adapt the treatment according to the season. During the pollen season, attention is directed at treating the Manifestation, i.e. expelling Wind-Cold or Wind-Heat. Outside the summer season, attention is directed at treating the Root, i.e. tonifying the Lung and Kidney's Defensive-Qi systems and strengthening the Governing Vessel.

TREATMENT OF THE MANIFESTATION

1. Wind-Cold

Clinical manifestations

Sneezing, profuse runny nose with white-watery discharge, pale complexion, stuffed nose, slight headache, no thirst.

Treatment principle

Expel Wind-Cold and restore the dispersing and descending of Lung-Qi.

Acupuncture

BL-12 Fengmen, BL-13 Feishu, LU-7 Lieque, L.I.-20 Yingxiang, Bitong, Du-23 Shangxing, G.B.-20 Fengchi, Yintang. Reducing or even method. Cupping is applicable on BL-12 and BL-13.

Explanation

- **BL-12**, **BL-13** and **LU-7** restore the dispersing and descending of Lung-Qi and expel Wind. BL-12 is particularly effective with cupping.
- **L.I.-20**, **Bitong** and **Yintang** are local points to expel Wind from the nose and to stop itching and sneezing.
- **Du-23** and **G.B.-20** are adjacent points to expel Wind from the head. Du-23, in particular, expels Wind from the nose and stops nasal discharge.

Herbal treatment

(a) Prescription

XIAO QING LONG TANG
Small Green Dragon Decoction

Ma Huang *Herba Ephedrae* 9 g
Gui Zhi *Ramulus Cinnamomi cassiae* 6 g
Xi Xin *Herba Asari cum radice* 3 g
Gan Jiang *Rhizoma Zingiberis officinalis* 3 g
Ban Xia *Rhizoma Pinelliae ternatae* 9 g
Bai Shao *Radix Paeoniae albae* 9 g
Wu Wei Zi *Fructus Schisandrae chinensis* 3 g
Zhi Gan Cao *Radix Glycyrrhizae uralensis prae-parata* 6 g

Explanation
- **Ma Huang** and **Gui Zhi** release the Exterior, expel Wind-Cold and stop sneezing.
- **Xi Xin**, **Gan Jiang** and **Ban Xia** resolve Phlegm, in particular when it manifests with white-watery discharges.
- **Bai Shao** and **Wu Wei Zi**, which are sour and absorbing, counterbalance the pungent and scattering flavour of Ma Huang and Gui Zhi and prevent injury of Yin.
- **Gan Cao** harmonizes.

Variations
- In case of very itchy and runny nose add Xin Yi Hua *Flos Magnoliae liliflorae*, Cang Er Zi *Fructus Xanthii* and Bai Zhi *Radix Angelicae dahuricae*.

(b) Prescription

CANG ER ZI SAN
Xanthium Powder
Cang Er Zi *Fructus Xanthii* 7.5 g
Xin Yi Hua *Flos Magnoliae liliflorae* 15 g
Bai Zhi *Radix Angelicae dahuricae* 30 g
Bo He *Herba Menthae* 1.5 g

Explanation
- **Cang Er Zi** and **Xin Yi Hua** are specific to expel Wind from the nose and they stop itchiness of the nose and sneezing.
- **Bai Zhi** also acts on the nose to expel Wind and Dampness.
- **Bo He** is light and fragrant and flows upwards to expel Wind.

This formula is applicable if sneezing rather than runny nose is the main problem. As it is composed of only four herbs, it may also be added as a unit to other formulae when sneezing is a predominant problem.

(c) Prescription

MA HUANG TANG
Ephedra Decoction
Ma Huang *Herba Ephedrae* 6 g
Gui Zhi *Ramulus Cinnamomi cassiae* 4 g
Xing Ren *Semen Pruni armeniacae* 9 g
Zhi Gan Cao *Radix Glycyrrhizae uralensis prae-parata* 3 g

Explanation   This formula is used if there are pronounced symptoms of Wind-Cold such as chilliness, absence of sweating and a Floating-Tight pulse.

(d) Prescription

GUI ZHI TANG
Ramulus Cinnamomi Decoction
Gui Zhi *Ramulus Cinnamomi cassiae* 9 g
Bai Shao *Radix Paeoniae albae* 9 g
Sheng Jiang *Rhizoma Zingiberis officinalis recens* 9 g
Da Zao *Fructus Ziziphi jujubae* 3 dates
Zhi Gan Cao *Radix Glycyrrhizae uralensis prae-parata* 6 g

Explanation
- **Gui Zhi** is pungent and releases the Exterior.
- **Bai Shao** is sour and absorbing and nourishes Nutritive Qi. The combination of Gui Zhi and Bai Shao expels Wind by harmonizing Defensive and Nutritive Qi. The slight sweating is a symptom of deficiency of Nutritive Qi.
- **Sheng Jiang** and **Da Zao** perform the same function as Gui Zhi and Bai Shao respectively and they therefore help the first two to harmonize Nutritive and Defensive Qi.
- **Gan Cao** harmonizes.

This formula is used if there are symptoms of Wind-Cold with slight sweating.

(e) Prescription

TONG XUAN LI FEI TANG
Dispersing, Descending and Regulating Lung-Qi Decoction
Zi Su Ye *Folium Perillae frutescentis* 6 g
Ma Huang *Herba Ephedrae* 6 g

Xing Ren *Semen Pruni armeniacae* 6 g
Zhi Ke *Fructus Citri aurantii* 6 g
Jie Geng *Radix Platycodi grandiflori* 4 g
Qian Hu *Radix Peucedani* 4 g
Chen Pi *Pericarpium Citri reticulatae* 3 g
Fu Ling *Sclerotium Poriae cocos* 6 g
Ban Xia *Rhizoma Pinelliae ternatae* 6 g
Huang Qin *Radix Scutellariae baicalensis* 3 g
Gan Cao *Radix Glycyrrhizae uralensis* 3 g

Explanation
- **Su Ye** and **Ma Huang** expel Wind-Cold, release the Exterior and stimulate the dispersing of Lung-Qi.
- **Xing Ren**, **Zhi Ke** and **Jie Geng** restore the descending of Lung-Qi.
- **Qian Hu**, **Chen Pi**, **Fu Ling** and **Ban Xia** resolve Phlegm.
- **Huang Qin** clears the Lungs.
- **Gan Cao** harmonizes.

This formula is used if there is a profuse discharge from the nose, sneezing, a cough and possibly a headache.

(f) Prescription

JIA WEI XIANG SU SAN
New Cyperus-Perilla Powder
Zi Su Ye *Folium Perillae frutescentis* 5 g
Jing Jie *Herba seu Flos Schizonepetae tenuifoliae* 3 g
Fang Feng *Radix Ledebouriellae sesloidis* 3 g
Qin Jiao *Radix Gentianae macrophyllae* 3 g
Man Jing Zi *Fructus Viticis* 3 g
Xiang Fu *Rhizoma Cyperi rotundi* 4 g
Chuan Xiong *Radix Ligustici wallichii* 1.5 g
Chen Pi *Pericarpium Citri reticulatae* 4 g
Gan Cao *Radix Glycyrrhizae uralensis* 2.5 g

Explanation
- **Su Ye** and **Jing Jie** expel Wind and release the Exterior.
- **Fang Feng** and **Qin Jiao** relax the muscles and tendons.
- **Man Jing Zi** expels Wind and stops headaches.
- **Xiang Fu** and **Chen Pi** move Qi.
- **Chuan Xiong** moves Blood and expels Wind.
- **Gan Cao** harmonizes.

This prescription is used if there is stiffness of the shoulders, a headache and sneezing. It is suitable for a more chronic condition which has led to stagnation of Qi and Blood in the head and shoulders.

(i) Patent remedy

TONG XUAN LI FEI WAN
Penetrating, Dispersing and Regulating the Lungs Pill
Ma Huang *Herba Ephedrae*
Zhi Ke *Fructus Citri aurantii*
Jie Geng *Radix Platycodi grandiflori*
Fu Ling *Sclerotium Poriae cocos*
Qian Hu *Radix Peucedani*
Huang Qin *Radix Scutellariae baicalensis*
Chen Pi *Pericarpium Citri reticulatae*
Gan Cao *Radix Glycyrrhizae uralensis*
Ban Xia *Rhizoma Pinelliae ternatae*
Xing Ren *Semen Pruni armeniacae*
Zi Su Ye *Folium Perillae frutescentis*

Explanation This pill has the same ingredients and functions as the prescription of the same name mentioned above. It is very effective to treat the symptoms of hay fever especially when there is a runny nose with a profuse white-watery discharge.

The tongue presentation appropriate to this remedy is a white coating.

(ii) Patent remedy

WU SHI CHA
Midday Tea
Huo Xiang *Herba Agastachis*
Bai Zhi *Radix Angelicae dahuricae*
Zi Su Ye *Folium Perillae frutescentis*
Fang Feng *Radix Ledebouriellae sesloidis*
Qiang Huo *Radix et Rhizoma Notopterygii*
Chai Hu *Radix Bupleuri*
Zhi Shi *Fructus Citri aurantii immaturus*
Chen Pi *Pericarpium Citri reticulatae*
Shan Zha *Fructus Crataegi*
Mai Ya *Fructus Hordei vulgaris germinatus*
Shen Qu *Massa Fermentata Medicinalis*
Hou Po *Cortex Magnoliae officinalis*
Cang Zhu *Rhizoma Atractylodis lanceae*
Qian Hu *Radix Peucedani*
Jie Geng *Radix Platycodi grandiflori*

Gan Cao *Radix Glycyrrhizae uralensis*
Hong Cha *Black tea*

Explanation   This tea also treats the symptoms of hay fever such as sneezing and a profuse white-watery nasal discharge, especially if they are associated with epigastric fullness.

The tongue presentation appropriate to this remedy is a thick-sticky coating.

(iii) Patent remedy

CHUAN XIONG CHA TIAO WAN
Ligusticum-Green Tea Regulating Pill
Chuan Xiong *Radix Ligustici wallichii*
Qiang Huo *Radix et Rhizoma Notopterygii*
Bai Zhi *Radix Angelicae dahuricae*
Jing Jie *Herba seu Flos Schizonepetae tenuifoliae*
Xi Xin *Herba Asari cum radice*
Fang Feng *Radix Ledebouriellae sesloidis*
Bo He *Herba Menthae*
Gan Cao *Radix Glycyrrhizae uralensis*
Qing Cha (Green Tea) *Folia Cameliae*

Explanation   This pill treats mostly the headache deriving from Wind-Cold. However, it also treats the manifestations of hay fever such as sneezing and a profuse runny nose with a white-watery discharge.

2. Wind-Heat

Clinical manifestations

Sneezing, runny nose with white and watery discharge, itchy throat, itchy-red eyes, slight thirst.

Treatment principle

Expel Wind, clear Heat, restore the dispersing and descending of Lung-Qi.

Acupuncture

BL-12 Fengmen, BL-13 Feishu, L.I.-4 Hegu, L.I.-11 Quchi, L.I.-20 Yingxiang, Bitong, Yintang. Reducing or even method. Cupping is applicable on BL-12 and BL-13.

Explanation

– **BL-12** and **BL-13** restore the dispersing and descending of Lung-Qi.
– **L.I.-4** and **L.I.-11** expel Wind and clear Heat.
– **L.I.-20**, **Bitong** and **Yintang** are local points to expel Wind from the nose.

Herbal treatment

(a) Prescription

SANG JU YIN
Morus-Chrysanthemum Decoction
Sang Ye *Folium Mori albae* 6 g
Ju Hua *Flos Chrysanthemi morifolii* 3 g
Bo He *Herba Menthae* 3 g
Xing Ren *Semen Pruni armeniacae* 6 g
Jie Geng *Radix Platycodi grandiflori* 6 g
Lian Qiao *Fructus Forsythiae suspensae* 6 g
Lu Gen *Rhizoma Phragmitis communis* 6 g
Gan Cao *Radix Glycyrrhizae uralensis* 3 g

Explanation

– **Sang Ye** and **Ju Hua** expel Wind-Heat and restore the descending of Lung-Qi.
– **Bo He** expels Wind-Heat.
– **Xing Ren** and **Jie Geng** restore the descending of Lung-Qi.
– **Lian Qiao** and **Lu Gen** clear Heat.
– **Gan Cao** harmonizes.

This is a general formula for Wind-Heat, especially affecting the throat and causing itchy throat and a cough.

Variations

– If there is pronounced sneezing add Cang Er Zi *Fructus Xanthii*, Xin Yi Hua *Flos Magnoliae liliflorae* and Bai Zhi *Radix Angelicae dahuricae*.

(b) Prescription

CHAI GE JIE JI TANG
Bupleurum-Pueraria Relaxing the Tendons Decoction
Ge Gen *Radix Puerariae* 9 g
Chai Hu *Radix Bupleuri* 6 g
Qiang Huo *Radix et Rhizoma Notopterygii* 3 g
Bai Zhi *Radix Angelicae dahuricae* 3 g
Huang Qin *Radix Scutellariae baicalensis* 6 g

Shi Gao *Gypsum fibrosum* 5 g
Jie Geng *Radix Platycodi grandiflori* 3 g
Bai Shao *Radix Paeoniae albae* 6 g
Gan Cao *Radix Glycyrrhizae uralensis* 3 g

Explanation
- **Ge Gen** and **Chai Hu** expel Wind-Heat and relax the tendons.
- **Qiang Huo** and **Bai Zhi** expel Wind and release the Exterior. Bai Zhi, in particular, reaches the nose to expel Wind and resolve mucus.
- **Huang Qin** and **Shi Gao** clear Heat.
- **Jie Geng** restores the descending of Lung-Qi.
- **Bai Shao** and **Gan Cao** harmonize the Nutritive Qi.

This formula is used for sneezing with symptoms of Wind-Heat and some interior Heat.

(i) Patent remedy

SANG JU GAN MAO PIAN
Morus-Chrysanthemum Common Cold Tablet
Sang Ye *Folium Mori albae*
Ju Hua *Flos Chrysanthemi morifolii*
Bo He *Herba Menthae*
Xing Ren *Semen Pruni armeniacae*
Jie Geng *Radix Platycodi grandiflori*
Lian Qiao *Fructus Forsythiae suspensae*
Lu Gen *Rhizoma Phragmitis communis*
Gan Cao *Radix Glycyrrhizae uralensis*

Explanation This tablet has the same ingredients and functions as Sang Ju Yin *Morus-Chrysanthemum Decoction* mentioned above. It is particularly good to treat hay-fever manifestations such as itchy throat and eyes.

(ii) Patent remedy

YIN QIAO JIE DU WAN (PIAN)
Lonicera-Forsythia Expelling Poison Pill (or Tablet)
Jin Yin Hua *Flos Lonicerae japonicae*
Lian Qiao *Fructus Forsythiae suspensae*
Jie Geng *Radix Platycodi grandiflori*
Niu Bang Zi *Fructus Arctii lappae*
Bo He *Herba Menthae*
Jing Jie *Herba seu Flos Schizonepetae tenuifoliae*
Zhu Ye *Herba Lophatheri gracilis*

Dan Dou Chi *Semen Sojae praeparatum*
Gan Cao *Radix Glycyrrhizae uralensis*

Explanation This very well-known pill is suitable for a wide range of hay-fever symptoms associated with Wind-Heat: itchy throat and eyes, watery eyes and sneezing. Note that even when it is associated with Wind-Heat, hay fever usually manifests with a nasal discharge which is white and watery.

The tongue presentation appropriate to this remedy is slightly Red sides and/or front part.

(iii) Patent remedy

GAN MAO DAN
Common Cold Pill
Jin Yin Hua *Flos Lonicerae japonicae*
Lian Qiao *Fructus Forsythiae suspensae*
Shan Zhi Zi *Fructus Gardeniae jasminoidis*
Lu Gen *Rhizoma Phragmitis communis*
Chi Shao *Radix Paeoniae rubrae*
Bai Mao Gen *Rhizoma Imperatae cylindricae*
Dan Dou Chi *Semen Sojae praeparatum*
Bo He *Herba Menthae*
Sang Ye *Folium Mori albae*
Jing Jie *Herba seu Flos Schizonepetae tenuifoliae*
Zi Wan *Radix Asteris tatarici*
Jie Geng *Radix Platycodi grandiflori*
Chen Pi *Pericarpium Citri reticulatae*

Explanation This pill is similar to the Yin Qiao Jie Du Wan *Lonicera-Forsythia Expelling Poison Pill* except that it is more wide-ranging in action (affecting the throat as well) and is more cooling: it is therefore suitable when symptoms and signs of Heat are pronounced, such as Red sides of the tongue and thirst.

TREATMENT OF THE ROOT

In seasonal rhinitis, attention should be directed at treating the Root of the disease at any time outside the pollen season. The best time to do it is actually towards the end of the summer and beginning of Autumn, i.e. August, September and October.

In treating the Root, the aim is to tonify the Lung and Kidney's Defensive-Qi systems and strengthen the Governing Vessel. As the rhinitis is seasonal, there is no need to treat the Manifestation.

Herbs which strengthen the Governing Vessel include Lu Rong *Cornu Cervi parvum*, Lu Jiao *Cornu Cervi*, Lu Jiao Jiao *Colla Cornu Cervi* and Gui Ban *Plastrum Testudinis*. Lu Rong, Lu Jiao and Lu Jiao Jiao are particularly important to treat allergic rhinitis as they tonify Kidney-Yang without creating too much Heat, strengthen the Governing Vessel, and bolster the Lung and Kidney's Defensive-Qi systems. By entering the Governing Vessel and tonifying the Kidneys, they treat both the Root and the Manifestation of the disease. Lu Jiao Jiao is particularly applicable to women as it additionally nourishes Blood. Lu Rong, in particular, strengthens the Governing Vessel, tonifies Yang without drying, nourishes the Essence and Marrow and strengthens tendons and bones. In other words, it strengthens both the Yin and Yang aspects of the Governing Vessel and of the Essence. Lu Rong and Lu Jiao could be taken in pill form with the patent remedy Quan Lu Wan *Whole-Deer Pill* (see below).

Gui Ban nourishes the Directing Vessel and is particularly used in women, in combination with Lu Jiao or Lu Jiao Jiao, to strengthen both Governing and Directing Vessels. With acupuncture in women, this is achieved by using the opening and secondary points of both the Governing and Directing Vessels. Thus, in a woman, one would needle S.I.-3 Houxi on the right, BL-62 Shenmai on the left, LU-7 Lieque on the left and KI-6 Zhaohai on the right in this order.

Li Shi Zhen indicates the following herbs for the Governing Vessel:

Rou Gui *Cortex Cinnamomi cassiae*
Gui Zhi *Ramulus Cinnamomi cassiae*
Fu Zi *Radix Aconiti carmichaeli praeparata*
Du Huo *Radix Angelicae pubescentis*
Qiang Huo *Radix et Rhizoma Notopterygii*
Fang Feng *Radix Ledebouriellae sesloidis*
Jing Jie *Herba seu Flos Schizonepetae tenuifoliae*
Xi Xin *Herba Asari cum radice*
Gao Ben *Rhizoma et Radix Ligustici sinensis*
Cang Er Zi *Fructus Xanthii*[4]

The first three herbs tonify the Original Qi, from which the Governing Vessel originates,

and strengthen the Fire of the Gate of Vitality. Du Huo strengthens the back and expels Wind-Damp from the lower back. All the other herbs affect the Governing Vessel in its upper part along the nose. In fact all these herbs expel Wind from the nose and restore the dispersing of Lung-Qi.

Deficiency of Lung and Kidney's Defensive-Qi systems and the Governing Vessel

Clinical manifestations

Pale complexion, weak back, propensity to catching colds, Pale tongue, Weak-Deep pulse.

Treatment principle

Tonify the Lung and Kidney's Defensive-Qi systems and strengthen the Governing Vessel.

Acupuncture

Du-4 Mingmen, Ren-4 Guanyuan with moxa, BL-23 Shenshu, KI-3 Taixi, BL-13 Feishu, Du-12 Shenzhu, Du-24 Shenting, Du-23 Shangxing, G.B.-20 Fengchi, Du-14 Dazhui with moxa, S.I.-3 Houxi and BL-62 Shenmai (in women combined with LU-7 Lieque and KI-6 Zhaohai). Reinforcing method, except on the head points which should be needled with even method.

Explanation

- **Du-4** and **Ren-4**, in combination, with moxa strengthen the Governing Vessel. Ren-4 is used because the internal pathway of the Governing Vessel actually runs along the front midline of the body under the Directing Vessel. The use of Du-4 and Ren-4, therefore, tonifies both the Yang and the Yin aspects of the Governing Vessel.
- **BL-23**, **KI-3**, **BL-13** and **Du-12** tonify the Lung and Kidney's Defensive-Qi systems.
- **Du-24** and **Du-23** expel Wind from the nose, strengthen the Governing Vessel locally and stop nasal discharge.
- **G.B.-20** is an adjacent point to expel Wind. In order to affect the nose, it should be needled with the tip of the needle pointing towards the nostril of the same side.

- **Du-14** with moxa strengthens the Governing Vessel in its upper part.
- **S.I.-3** and **BL-62** open the Governing Vessel. The points are crossed over with S.I.-3 on the left side for men and right for women and BL-62 on the right side for men and left for women. In women, it is preferable to combine the Governing Vessel with the Directing Vessel: one would therefore needle S.I.-3 on the right, BL-62 on the left, LU-7 on the left and KI-6 on the right.

Herbal treatment

Prescription

YI DU YANG YUAN TANG
Benefiting the Governing Vessel and Nourishing the Original Qi Decoction
Gui Ban *Plastrum Testudinis* 15 g
Shu Di Huang *Radix Rehmanniae glutinosae praeparata* 9 g
Rou Cong Rong *Herba Cistanchis* 9 g
Bu Gu Zhi *Fructus Psoraleae corylifoliae* 6 g
Lu Jiao Jiao *Colla Cornu Cervi* 3 g
Wu Wei Zi *Fructus Schisandrae chinensis* 3 g
Zhi Mu *Radix Anemarrhenae asphodeloidis* 3 g
Huang Bo *Cortex Phellodendri* 3 g

Explanation
- **Gui Ban** and **Shu Di** nourish the Directing and Governing Vessels and strengthen the Kidneys. They also nourish the Kidney-Essence which is the substantial foundation of Kidney-Yang.
- **Rou Cong Rong**, **Bu Gu Zhi** and **Lu Jiao Jiao** tonify Kidney-Yang and strengthen the Lung and Kidney's Defensive-Qi systems. Lu Jiao Jiao also strengthens the Governing Vessel.
- **Wu Wei Zi** nourishes the Essence and strengthens the Lungs.
- **Zhi Mu** and **Huang Bo** are included to prevent any excessive Heat which might derive from tonification of Yang by the other herbs.

Variations
- If there are pronounced symptoms of Cold and deficiency of Kidney-Yang add Rou Gui *Cortex Cinnamomi cassiae.*
- If there is a propensity to catching colds add

Huang Qi *Radix Astragali membranacei*, Bai Zhu *Rhizoma Atractylodis macrocephalae* and Fang Feng *Radix Ledebouriellae sesloidis.*
- If there is a nasal discharge and a sticky tongue coating add Bai Zhu *Rhizoma Atractylodis macrocephalae*, Ban Xia *Rhizoma Pinelliae ternatae* and Fu Ling *Sclerotium Poriae cocos.*

The above formula is particularly suited to allergic rhinitis as it tonifies the Lung and Kidney's Defensive-Qi systems, strengthens the Governing Vessel and nourishes the Essence. However, any Kidney-Yang-tonifying formula may be used modified with the addition of the following ingredients:

(a) Herbs which strengthen the Governing Vessel, such as Lu Rong *Cornu Cervi parvum*, Lu Jiao *Cornu Cervi* or Lu Jiao Jiao *Colla Cornu Cervi* in women.

(b) Herbs which nourish the Essence and Marrow such as Gui Ban *Plastrum Testudinis*, Tu Si Zi *Semen Cuscutae*, Gou Qi Zi *Fructus Lycii chinensis*, Placenta *Placenta hominis* or Wu Wei Zi *Fructus Schisandrae chinensis.*

(c) Herbs to tonify the Lung's Defensive-Qi system such as Huang Qi *Radix Astragali membranacei*, Mai Men Dong *Tuber Ophiopogonis japonici* and Bei Sha Shen *Radix Glehniae littoralis.*

(d) If necessary, add one or two herbs, in small doses, to prevent over-heating from the hot herbs which tonify Kidney-Yang. For example, Zhi Mu *Radix Anemarrhenae asphodeloidis* and Huang Bo *Cortex Phellodendri.*

In women, it is necessary to strengthen the Directing as well as the Governing Vessel with such herbs as Sheng Di Huang *Radix Rehmanniae glutinosae*, Gui Ban *Plastrum Testudinis*, Bie Jia *Carapax Trionycis* or E Jiao *Gelatinum Corii Asini.*

Although allergic rhinitis in itself indicates a deficiency of Lung and Kidney's Defensive-Qi systems, especially in people over 40, this may be combined with a Kidney-Yin deficiency. In such cases, it is better to start from a prescription to nourish Kidney-Yin such as Liu Wei Di Huang Wan *Six-Ingredient Rehmannia Pill* and modify it with the addition of herbs to tonify

Lung and Kidney's Defensive-Qi systems and strengthen the Governing Vessel as indicated above.

Finally, if there are symptoms and signs of Spleen deficiency, simply add Bai Zhu *Rhizoma Atractylodis macrocephalae*, Huang Qi *Radix Astragali membranacei* and Fu Ling *Sclerotium Poriae cocos*.

Many other formulae can be used according to the patient's body condition and these are illustrated below when discussing the treatment of perennial rhinitis.

Patent remedy

QUAN LU WAN
Whole-Deer Pill
Lu Rou *Caro Cervi*
Lu Rong *Cornu Cervi parvum*
Lu Wei *Penis et testis Cervi*
Lu Shen *Renes Cervi*
Lu Jiao Jiao *Colla Cornu Cervi*
Ren Shen *Radix Ginseng*
Bai Zhu *Rhizoma Atractylodis macrocephalae*
Fu Ling *Sclerotium Poriae cocos*
Gan Cao *Radix Glycyrrhizae uralensis*
Dang Gui *Radix Angelicae sinensis*
Chuan Xiong *Radix Ligustici wallichii*
Shu Di Huang *Radix Rehmanniae glutinosae praeparata*
Huang Qi *Radix Astragali membranacei*
Gou Qi Zi *Fructus Lycii chinensis*
Du Zhong *Cortex Eucommiae ulmoidis*
Niu Xi *Radix Achyranthis bidentatae seu Cyathulae*
Xu Duan *Radix Dipsaci*
Rou Cong Rong *Herba Cistanchis*
Suo Yang *Herba Cynomorii songarici*
Ba Ji Tian *Radix Morindae officinalis*
Tian Men Dong *Tuber Asparagi cochinchinensis*
Mai Men Dong *Tuber Ophiopogonis japonici*
Wu Wei Zi *Fructus Schisandrae chinensis*
Chen Xiang *Lignum Aquilariae*
Chen Pi *Pericarpium Citri reticulatae*

Explanation This is an excellent pill to strengthen Kidney-Yang and tonify the Lung and Kidney's Defensive-Qi systems. It can be used to treat the Root-cause of seasonal allergic rhinitis. It should be remembered, however, that it is hot in energy and should be used with caution if there is some Heat in the body (for example, Damp-Heat in the Bladder) or if there is, in addition to a Kidney-Yang deficiency, also a slight Kidney-Yin deficiency. In the latter case, this remedy can be combined with a lesser dose of one to nourish Kidney-Yin. For example, the main remedy Quan Lu Wan could be taken in the morning and midday (8 pills each time), and the Liu Wei Di Huang Wan *Six-Ingredient Rehmannia Pill* could be taken in the evening in a lesser dose (6 pills only).

PERENNIAL ALLERGIC RHINITIS

To treat perennial rhinitis one must treat both the Root and the Manifestation simultaneously because the symptoms are evident the whole year round.

TREATMENT PRINCIPLE

Tonify the Lung and Kidney's Defensive-Qi systems, strengthen the Governing Vessel, consolidate the Exterior and expel Wind.

ACUPUNCTURE

- BL-13 Feishu, Du-12 Shenzhu, Ren-12 Zhongwan, ST-36 Zusanli, LU-7 Lieque, LU-9 Taiyuan, with reinforcing method, to tonify the Lung's Defensive-Qi system.
- L.I.-4 Hegu, L.I.-20 Yingxiang, Bitong, Du-23 Shangxing, with even method, to expel Wind from the nose.
- All other Kidney and Governing Vessel as indicated above for treatment of the Root of seasonal rhinitis.

HERBAL TREATMENT

There are many suitable formulae and they should all be modified with the addition of the following types of herbs:

(a) Herbs to tonify the Lung and Kidney's Defensive-Qi such as Du Zhong *Cortex Eucommiae* ulmoidis, Xu Duan *Radix Dipsaci* or Bu Gu Zhi *Fructus Psoraleae corylifoliae*.

(b) Herbs which strengthen the Governing Vessel, such as Lu Rong *Cornu Cervi parvum*, Lu Jiao *Cornu Cervi* or Lu Jiao Jiao *Colla Cornu Cervi* in women.

(c) Herbs to tonify the Lung's Defensive-Qi system such as Huang Qi *Radix Astragali membranacei*, Mai Men Dong *Tuber Ophiopogonis japonici* and Bei Sha Shen *Radix Glehniae littoralis*.

(d) Herbs which expel Wind from the nose and stop nasal discharge such as Fang Feng *Radix Ledebouriellae sesloidis*, Jing Jie *Herba seu Flos Schizonepetae tenuifoliae*, Cang Er Zi *Fructus Xanthii*, Xin Yi Hua *Flos Magnoliae liliflorae* and Xi Xin *Herba Asari cum radice*.

(e) Herbs which nourish the Essence and Marrow such as Gui Ban *Plastrum Testudinis*, Tu Si Zi *Semen Cuscutae*, Gou Qi Zi *Fructus Lycii chinensis*, Placenta *Placenta hominis* or Wu Wei Zi *Fructus Schisandrae chinensis*.

(f) If necessary, add one or two herbs, in small doses, to prevent overheating from the hot herbs which tonify Kidney-Yang. For example, Zhi Mu *Radix Anemarrhenae asphodeloidis* and Huang Bo *Cortex Phellodendri*.

The comments made above on the treatment of the Root of seasonal allergic rhinitis, apply also to the treatment of perennial rhinitis:

(a) In women, it is necessary to strengthen the Directing as well as the Governing Vessel with such herbs as Sheng Di Huang *Radix Rehmanniae glutinosae*, Gui Ban *Plastrum Testudinis*, Bie Jia *Carapax Trionycis* or E Jiao *Gelatinum Corii Asini*.

(b) If there is a background of Kidney-Yin deficiency or a deficiency of both Kidney-Yang and Yin, it is better to start from a prescription to nourish Kidney-Yin such as Liu Wei Di Huang Wan *Six-Ingredient Rehmannia Pill* and modify it with the addition of herbs to tonify Lung and Kidney's Defensive-Qi systems and strengthen the Governing Vessel as indicated above.

(c) If there are symptoms and signs of Spleen deficiency, simply add Bai Zhu *Rhizoma Atrac-*

tylodis macrocephalae, Huang Qi *Radix Astragali membranacei* and Fu Ling *Sclerotium Poriae cocos*.

1. Prescription

YU PING FENG SAN
Jade Wind Screen Powder
Huang Qi *Radix Astragali membranacei* 30 g
Bai Zhu *Rhizoma Atractylodis macrocephalae* 60 g
Fang Feng *Radix Ledebouriellae sesloidis* 30 g

Explanation

This is a very simple and effective formula to tonify Lung-Qi and consolidate the Exterior (with Fang Feng).

2. Prescription

SHEN SU YIN
Ginseng-Perilla Decoction
Ren Shen *Radix Ginseng* 9 g
Zi Su Ye *Folium Perillae frutescentis* 3 g
Ge Gen *Radix Puerariae* 9 g
Qian Hu *Radix Peucedani* 3 g
Ban Xia *Rhizoma Pinelliae ternatae* 6 g
Fu Ling *Sclerotium Poriae cocos* 9 g
Chen Pi *Pericarpium Citri reticulatae* 3 g
Zhi Ke *Fructus Citri aurantii* 6 g
Jie Geng *Radix Platycodi grandiflori* 6 g
Zhi Gan Cao *Radix Glycyrrhizae uralensis praeparata* 3 g
Sheng Jiang *Rhizoma Zingiberis officinalis recens* 3 g
Da Zao *Fructus Ziziphi jujubae* 4 dates

Explanation

– **Dang Shen** tonifies Lung and Spleen-Qi.
– **Su Ye** restores the dispersing and descending of Lung-Qi.
– **Ge Gen** expels Wind.
– **Qian Hu**, **Ban Xia**, **Fu Ling** and **Chen Pi** resolve Phlegm.
– **Jie Geng** and **Zhi Ke** restore the descending of Lung-Qi.
– **Sheng Jiang** expels Wind.
– **Da Zao** helps Dang Shen to tonify Qi.
– **Gan Cao** harmonizes.

This formula is suitable if there is some Spleen deficiency as well and Phlegm with a profuse nasal discharge.

3. Prescription

REN SHEN BAI DU SAN
Ginseng Expelling Poison Powder
Ren Shen *Radix Ginseng* 9 g
Fu Ling *Sclerotium Poriae cocos* 9 g
Zhi Gan Cao *Radix Glycyrrhizae uralensis praeparata* 3 g
Qiang Huo *Radix et Rhizoma Notopterygii* 3 g
Du Huo *Radix Angelicae pubescentis* 6 g
Chuan Xiong *Radix Ligustici wallichii* 6 g
Sheng Jiang *Rhizoma Zingiberis officinalis recens* 3 slices
Chai Hu *Radix Bupleuri* 6 g
Bo He *Herba Menthae* 3 g
Qian Hu *Radix Peucedani* 9 g
Zhi Ke *Fructus Citri aurantii* 6 g
Jie Geng *Radix Platycodi grandiflori* 4 g

Explanation

- **Dang Shen**, **Fu Ling** and **Gan Cao** tonify Qi and strengthen Lungs and Spleen.
- **Qiang Huo**, **Du Huo**, **Chuan Xiong** and **Sheng Jiang** expel Wind and Dampness and expel Wind from the Governing Vessel. Qiang Huo and Chuan Xiong direct the herbs upwards to the head. Qiang Huo and Du Huo enter the Governing Vessel.
- **Chai Hu** and **Bo He** expel Wind and also direct the herbs upwards to the head.
- **Qian Hu**, **Zhi Ke** and **Jie Geng** restore the descending of Lung-Qi and resolve Phlegm.

This prescription is suitable if there is some Spleen deficiency with Phlegm and pronounced stiffness of the muscles of the top of the shoulders and neck.

4. Prescription

JIA JIAN YU ZHU TANG
Variation of Polygonatum Decoction
Yu Zhu *Rhizoma Polygonati odorati* 12 g
Dan Dou Chi *Semen Sojae praeparatum* 9 g
Cong Bai *Herba Allii fistulosi* 15 g

Bo He *Herba Menthae* 6 g
Jie Geng *Radix Platycodi grandiflori* 6 g
Bai Wei *Radix Cynanchi* 6 g
Gan Cao *Radix Glycyrrhizae uralensis* 3 g
Da Zao *Fructus Ziziphi jujubae* 3 g

Explanation

- **Yu Zhu** and **Bai Wei** nourish Stomach-Yin and clear Stomach Empty-Heat.
- **Dan Dou Chi** and **Cong Bai** release the Exterior and stop sneezing.
- **Bo He** and **Jie Geng** release the Exterior and restore the dispersing and descending of Lung-Qi.
- **Gan Cao** and **Da Zao** tonify Qi and harmonize.

This formula is used if there is a background of Stomach-Yin deficiency.

5. Prescription

WU JI SAN
Five Accumulations Powder
Ma Huang *Herba Ephedrae* 4 g
Bai Zhi *Radix Angelicae dahuricae* 3 g
Cong Bai *Herba Allii fistulosi* 4 g
Sheng Jiang *Rhizoma Zingiberis officinalis recens* 3 slices
Cang Zhu *Rhizoma Atractylodis lanceae* 12 g
Hou Po *Cortex Magnoliae officinalis* 3 g
Chen Pi *Pericarpium Citri reticulatae* 4 g
Gan Cao *Radix Glycyrrhizae uralensis* 3 g
Ban Xia *Rhizoma Pinelliae ternatae* 3 g
Fu Ling *Sclerotium Poriae cocos* 3 g
Jie Geng *Radix Platycodi grandiflori* 6 g
Zhi Ke *Fructus Citri aurantii* 4 g
Gan Jiang *Rhizoma Zingiberis officinalis* 2 g
Rou Gui *Cortex Cinnamomi cassiae* 2 g
Dang Gui *Radix Angelicae sinensis* 3 g
Bai Shao *Radix Paeoniae albae* 3 g
Chuan Xiong *Radix Ligustici wallichii* 3 g

Explanation

- **Ma Huang**, **Bai Zhi**, **Cong Bai** and **Sheng Jiang** release the Exterior, expel Wind, restore the dispersing of Lung-Qi and stop nasal discharge and itching.

- **Cang Zhu**, **Hou Po**, **Chen Pi**, and **Gan Cao** tonify the Stomach and dry Dampness. These herbs form the formula Ping Wei San *Balancing the Stomach Powder*.
- **Ban Xia**, and **Fu Ling** dry Dampness and resolve Phlegm. Together with Chen Pi and Gan Cao above they form the prescription Er Chen Tang *Two Old Decoction*.
- **Jie Geng** and **Zhi Ke** restore the descending of Lung-Qi.
- **Gan Jiang** and **Rou Gui** warm the Middle and dry up watery phlegm and nasal discharge.
- **Dang Gui**, **Bai Shao** and **Chuan Xiong**, a contracted version of the Si Wu Tang *Four-Substance Decoction*, harmonize Blood.

This formula is suitable for very chronic allergic rhinitis with Spleen and Stomach Yang deficiency and some stasis of Blood. It is particularly suitable for women.

6. Prescription

GUI ZHI REN SHEN TANG
Ramulus Cinnamomi-Ginseng Decoction
Gui Zhi *Ramulus Cinnamomi cassiae* 12 g
Gan Jiang *Rhizoma Zingiberis officinalis* 9 g
Zhi Gan Cao *Radix Glycyrrhizae uralensis praeparata* 12 g
Ren Shen *Radix Ginseng* 15 g
Bai Zhu *Rhizoma Atractylodis macrocephalae* 9 g

Explanation

- **Gui Zhi** and **Gan Jiang** resolve Cold Phlegm and stop nasal discharge. Gui Zhi also expels Wind.
- **Zhi Gan Cao**, **Dang Shen** and **Bai Zhu** tonify Lung- and Spleen-Qi.

This prescription is for deficiency of Lung- and Spleen-Yang with Phlegm and profuse runny nose with very watery and white discharge.

7. Prescription

MA HUANG FU ZI XI XIN TANG
Ephedra-Aconitum-Asarum Decoction

Ma Huang *Herba Ephedrae* 6 g
Fu Zi *Radix Aconiti carmichaeli praeparata* 9 g
Xi Xin *Herba Asari cum radice* 6 g

Explanation

- **Ma Huang** and **Xi Xin** release the Exterior, expel Wind-Cold, restore the dispersing and descending of Lung-Qi and resolve Cold Phlegm.
- **Fu Zi** tonifies Kidney-Yang and scatters internal Cold.

This formula is suitable if there is severe Kidney-Yang deficiency and internal Cold with profuse white-watery discharge from the nose. It may be used as a unit added to other prescriptions for Yang deficiency. In this case, much smaller doses should be used; for example, reduced by two thirds.

8. Prescription

ZAI ZAO SAN
Renewal Powder
Dang Shen *Radix Codonopsis pilosulae* 12 g
Huang Qi *Radix Astragali membranacei* 15 g
Fu Zi *Radix Aconiti carmichaeli praeparata* 6 g
Qiang Huo *Radix et Rhizoma Notopterygii* 6 g
Fang Feng *Radix Ledebouriellae sesloidis* 6 g
Chuan Xiong *Radix Ligustici wallichii* 6 g
Xi Xin *Herba Asari cum radice* 3 g
Gui Zhi *Ramulus Cinnamomi cassiae* 6 g
Bai Shao *Radix Paeoniae albae* 6 g
Gan Cao *Radix Glycyrrhizae uralensis* 3 g
Sheng Jiang *Rhizoma Zingiberis officinalis recens* 6 g
Da Zao *Fructus Ziziphi jujubae* 3 dates

Explanation

- **Dang Shen**, **Huang Qi** and **Fu Zi** tonify Yang, consolidate the Exterior and stop sweating.
- **Qiang Huo**, **Fang Feng**, **Chuan Xiong** and **Xi Xin** expel Wind and stop nasal discharge and itching.
- **Gui Zhi** and **Bai Shao** harmonize Nutritive and Defensive Qi and stop sweating.

– **Sheng Jiang** and **Da Zao** help the previous two herbs to harmonize Nutritive and Defensive Qi.
– **Gan Cao** harmonizes.

This formula is for deficiency of Yang of the Spleen, Lungs and Kidneys with a profuse nasal discharge and sweating.

9. Prescription

YI DU YANG YUAN TANG
Benefiting the Governing Vessel and Nourishing the Original Qi Decoction
Gui Ban *Plastrum Testudinis* 15 g
Shu Di Huang *Radix Rehmanniae glutinosae praeparata* 9 g
Rou Cong Rong *Herba Cistanchis* 9 g
Bu Gu Zhi *Fructus Psoraleae corylifoliae* 6 g
Lu Jiao Jiao *Colla Cornu Cervi* 3 g
Wu Wei Zi *Fructus Schisandrae chinensis* 3 g
Zhi Mu *Radix Anemarrhenae asphodeloidis* 3 g
Huang Bo *Cortex Phellodendri* 3 g

Explanation

This formula strengthens the Governing Vessel and tonifies the Kidney's Defensive-Qi system. It has already been discussed above in connection with treatment of the Root of seasonal rhinitis.

Variations

These variations apply to all the above formulae.

– If there is profuse sneezing and nasal discharge add Fang Feng *Radix Ledebouriellae sesloidis*, Cang Er Zi *Fructus Xanthii* and Xi Xin *Herba Asari cum radice*. This last herb is used in a small dose such as 1.5 g.
– If there is profuse nasal discharge add Bai Zhi *Radix Angelicae dahuricae*, Xi Xin *Herba Asari cum radice* and Gan Jiang *Rhizoma Zingiberis officinalis*.
– If there are symptoms of Wind-Heat use Ju Hua *Flos Chrysanthemi morifolii* and Chan Tui *Periostracum Cicadae*.
– If there are headaches add Ju Hua *Flos Chrysanthemi morifolii*, Ge Gen *Radix Puerariae* and Man Jing Zi *Fructus Viticis*.

– If there is sweating use Gui Zhi Tang *Ramulus Cinnamomi Decoction*.
– If there is Spleen deficiency and Phlegm add Bai Zhu *Rhizoma Atractylodis macrocephalae*, Fu Ling *Sclerotium Poriae cocos* and Ban Xia *Rhizoma Pinelliae ternatae*.

(a) Patent remedy

GE JIE DA BU WAN
Gecko Big Tonifying Pill
Ge Jie *Gecko*
Dang Shen *Radix Codonopsis pilosulae*
Huang Qi *Radix Astragali membranacei*
Gou Qi Zi *Fructus Lycii chinensis*
Dang Gui *Radix Angelicae sinensis*
Fu Ling *Sclerotium Poriae cocos*
Shu Di Huang *Radix Rehmanniae glutinosae praeparata*
Nu Zhen Zi *Fructus Ligustri lucidi*
Gan Cao *Radix Glycyrrhizae uralensis*
Shan Yao *Radix Dioscoreae oppositae*
Mu Gua *Fructus Chaenomelis lagenariae*
Ba Ji Tian *Radix Morindae officinalis*
Bai Zhi *Radix Angelicae dahuricae*
Xu Duan *Radix Dipsaci*
Du Zhong *Cortex Eucommiae ulmoidis*
Huang Jing *Rhizoma Polygonati*
Gu Sui Bu *Rhizoma Gusuibu*

Explanation

This pill tonifies Qi and Blood, tonifies Kidney-Yang and strengthens the Lungs. It can be used to tonify the Lung and Kidney's Defensive-Qi systems in perennial rhinitis.

The tongue presentation appropriate to this remedy is a Pale and wet body.

(b) Patent remedy

HE CHE DA ZAO WAN
Placenta Great Fortifying Pill
Gui Ban *Plastrum Testudinis*
Shu Di Huang *Radix Rehmanniae glutinosae praeparata*
Dang Shen *Radix Codonopsis pilosulae*
Huang Bo *Cortex Phellodendri*
Du Zhong *Cortex Eucommiae ulmoidis*

Zi He Che *Placenta hominis*
Niu Xi *Radix Achyranthis bidentatae seu Cyathulae*
Tian Men Dong *Tuber Asparagi cochinchinensis*
Mai Men Dong *Tuber Ophiopogonis japonici*
Fu Ling *Sclerotium Poriae cocos*
Sha Ren *Fructus seu Semen Amomi*

Explanation

This pill nourishes Blood and Yin, tonifies the Kidney-Essence and strengthens the Lung's Defensive-Qi system.

It can be used for perennial allergic rhinitis from deficiency of the Lung and Kidney's Defensive-Qi systems against a background of Blood and Yin deficiency. The presence of animal substances such as Gui Ban and Zi He Che is particularly beneficial to tonify the Kidney's Defensive-Qi system.

The tongue presentation appropriate to this remedy is a Red body without coating.

(c) Patent remedy

REN SHEN LU RONG WAN
Ginseng-Deer Antler Pill
Ren Shen *Radix Ginseng*
Du Zhong *Cortex Eucommiae ulmoidis*
Ba Ji Tian *Radix Morindae officinalis*
Huang Qi *Radix Astragali membranacei*
Lu Rong *Cornu Cervi parvum*
Dang Gui *Radix Angelicae sinensis*
Niu Xi *Radix Achyranthis bidentatae seu Cyathulae*
Long Yan Rou *Arillus Euphoriae longanae*

Explanation

This pill tonifies Lung-Qi and Kidney-Yang and strengthens the Lung and Kidney's Defensive-Qi systems.

The tongue presentation appropriate to this remedy is a Pale body.

(d) Patent remedy

GE JIE BU SHEN WAN
Gecko Tonifying the Kidneys Pill
Ge Jie *Gecko*
Lu Rong *Cornu Cervi parvum*

Ren Shen *Radix Ginseng*
Huang Qi *Radix Astragali membranacei*
Du Zhong *Cortex Eucommiae ulmoidis*
Gou Shen *Testis et Penis Canis*
Dong Chong Xia Cao *Sclerotium Cordicipitis chinensis*
Gou Qi Zi *Fructus Lycii chinensis*
Fu Ling *Sclerotium Poriae cocos*
Bai Zhu *Rhizoma Atractylodis macrocephalae*

Explanation

This pill tonifies Lung-Qi and Kidney-Yang and strengthens the Lung and Kidney's Defensive-Qi systems. It also mildly nourishes Lung-Yin.

The tongue presentation appropriate to this remedy is a Pale body.

Case history

A 33-year-old woman had been suffering from allergic rhinitis since the age of 18. She sneezed and her nose ran (white-watery discharge) when exposed to dust, cats, and dogs. She also sneezed and "came out in blotches" on drinking tea, coffee, wine, spirits, or eating certain foods such as cheese, butter, chocolate, fats and spices.

She suffered from frequent urination and her need to urinate sometimes became urgent. She described it as "cystitis" but there was no burning and the urine was pale. This symptom had started only a few months previously. She had also been suffering from back-ache for the previous 6 years.

Her pulse was Weak and Deep and both Rear positions were Weak. Her tongue was Pale and slightly bluish with teeth-marks and a yellow coating on the root.

Diagnosis
Perennial rhinitis from deficiency of Lung and Kidney's Defensive-Qi systems, particularly Kidneys and specifically Kidney-Yang (hence the back-ache, frequent-urgent urination and Pale-Bluish tongue). The fact that she also sneezed on eating certain foods indicates that there was some Heat in the Large Intestine (hence the yellow tongue coating on the root).

She obviously had a Lung and Kidney's Defensive-Qi systems deficiency from birth: the back-ache and frequent urination appeared later with the physiological decline of Kidney-Qi.

Treatment
Since this is perennial rhinitis one must treat both Root and Manifestation simultaneously with a

formula that tonifies Kidney-Yang. However, this patient was treated primarily with acupuncture with:

- **LU-7** Lieque and **KI-6** Zhaohai to open the Directing Vessel and tonify Lungs and Kidneys;
- **ST-36** Zusanli and **SP-6** Sanyinjiao to tonify Qi in general;
- **BL-23** Shenshu, **KI-7** Fuliu, **Ren-4** Guanyuan and **KI-16** Huangshu to tonify Kidney-Yang and the Kidney-Essence;
- **BL-13** Feishu and **Du-12** Shenzhu to tonify the Lung's Defensive-Qi system;
- **SP-9** Yinlingquan and **BL-25** Dachangshu to clear Large Intestine Heat;
- **Du-23** Shangxing and **L.I.-20** Yingxiang to expel Wind from the nose.

Additionally, she was given the patent remedy Quan Lu Wan *Whole-Deer Pill*. The combination of acupuncture and this patent remedy produced a complete cure of her condition.

Case history

A 25-year-old woman had been suffering from hay fever (seasonal allergic rhinitis) "for as long as she could remember". During the summer season she sneezed and had itchy eyes and throat.

She also suffered from eczema at the sides of her nose and on her chin. The eruptions were papule-like (red spots) at first and they then turned dry and flaky some weeks later. The spots were red and itchy and worse with exposure to the sun.

Her pulse was only slightly Weak and the left Rear position was weaker. Her tongue had a normal colour with a slightly sticky coating.

Diagnosis
Seasonal rhinitis from deficiency of Lung and Kidney's Defensive-Qi systems. Eczema from same cause.

Treatment
The aim of the treatment is to tonify Lung and Kidney's Defensive-Qi systems and clear Wind-Heat from the Lung's Defensive-Qi system (skin). The formula chosen was a variation of Yi Du Yang Yuan Tang *Benefiting the Governing Vessel and Nourishing the Original Qi Decoction*:

Gui Ban *Plastrum Testudinis* 15 g
Shu Di Huang *Radix Rehmanniae glutinosae praeparata* 9 g
Bu Gu Zhi *Fructus Psoraleae corylifoliae* 6 g
Lu Jiao Jiao *Colla Cornu Cervi* 4 g
Wu Wei Zi *Fructus Schisandrae chinensis* 3 g
Zhi Mu *Radix Anemarrhenae asphodeloidis* 3 g
Fang Feng *Radix Ledebouriellae sesloidis* 4 g
Chan Tui *Periostracum Cicadae* 4 g
Bai Xian Pi *Cortex Dictami dasycarpi radicis* 6 g

Explanation
- **Gui Ban** and **Shu Di Huang** nourish the Kidney-Essence and strengthen the Directing Vessel.
- **Bu Gu Zhi** and **Lu Jiao Jiao** tonify the Kidney's Defensive-Qi system and strengthen the Governing Vessel.
- **Wu Wei Zi** tonifies the Lung's Defensive-Qi system.
- **Zhi Mu** clears Heat.
- **Fang Feng**, **Chan Tui** and **Bai Xian Pi** clear Wind-Heat from the skin.

This formula and subsequent variations produced a considerable improvement over six months.

Case history

A 44-year-old man had suffered from seasonal rhinitis since the age of 22. The main manifestations were sneezing, sensitive eyes and a runny nose with a white-watery discharge except in the morning when it was thick-yellow.

His pulse was only slightly Weak and the left Rear position was weaker. His tongue was Pale and Swollen.

Diagnosis
Seasonal rhinitis from Lung and Kidney's Defensive-Qi systems deficiency. The Pale and Swollen tongue also indicates a deficiency of Spleen-Yang which often occurs in such cases after 40. The sticky-yellow mucus in the mornings indicates that the sinuses have been affected due to swelling of the nasal mucosa preventing proper drainage.

Treatment
The main aim (outside the season) is to tonify Lung and Kidney's Defensive-Qi systems and Spleen-Yang. The formula used was a variation of Yi Du Yang Yuan Tang *Benefiting the Governing Vessel and Nourishing the Original Qi Decoction*:

Gui Ban *Plastrum Testudinis* 15 g
Shu Di Huang *Radix Rehmanniae glutinosae praeparata* 9 g
Bu Gu Zhi *Fructus Psoraleae corylifoliae* 6 g
Lu Jiao *Cornu Cervi* 9 g
Wu Wei Zi *Fructus Schisandrae chinensis* 3 g
Zhi Mu *Radix Anemarrhenae asphodeloidis* 3 g
Huang Qi *Radix Astragali membranacei* 9 g
Fang Feng *Radix Ledebouriellae sesloidis* 4g
Bai Zhu *Rhizoma Atractylodis macrocephalae* 6 g
Fu Ling *Sclerotium Poriae cocos* 6 g

Explanation
- **Shu Di** and **Gui Ban** nourish the Kidney-Essence.
- **Bu Gu Zhi** and **Lu Jiao** tonify the Kidney's Defensive-Qi system and strengthen the Governing Vessel.

– **Wu Wei Zi** and **Huang Qi** tonify the Lung's Defensive-Qi system.
– **Zhi Mu** clears Heat.
– **Fang Feng** expels Wind from the nose.

– **Bai Zhu** and **Fu Ling** tonify the Spleen and drain Dampness.

This formula produced an improvement after a short time. The patient is still under treatment.

END NOTES

1. Although most Western books and articles correlate allergic rhinitis with *Bi Yuan* 鼻渊 , there is in Chinese medicine another disease-symptom called *Bi Qiu* 鼻鼽 which corresponds more closely to allergic rhinitis. *Qiu* actually indicates "a thin, clear nasal discharge". In fact, the main symptoms and signs of *Bi Qiu* are sneezing, an itchy nose, and a white-watery nasal discharge; its pathology is Lung-Qi, Spleen-Qi or Kidney-Yang deficiency.

2. Wang Luo Zhen 1985 A Compilation of the "Study of the Eight Extraordinary Vessels" (*Qi Jing Ba Mai Kao Jiao Zhu* 奇经八脉考校注), Shanghai Science Publishing House, Shanghai, p. 89. The "Study of the Eight

Extraordinary Vessels" itself was written by Li Shi Zhen and first published in 1578.

3. Another interesting connection between the Kidneys and rhinitis could be observed in the use by some Chinese doctors of injection of cortisone in the point BL-12 Fengmen with far fewer side-effects than in a systemic administration of cortisone. If we view cortisone as a kind of "Kidney tonic", it would make sense to inject it in the point BL-12 which expels Wind and spreads Defensive-Qi in the Exterior.

4. A Compilation of the "Study of the Eight Extraordinary Vessels", p. 89.

Sinusitis 7

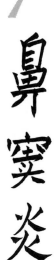

The sinuses are mucosa-lined cavities in the skull communicating with the nasal cavities. There are four pairs of sinuses, i.e. the ethmoidal, frontal, maxillary and sphenoidal sinuses. The frontal and maxillary sinuses, especially the latter ones, are more prone to infection and inflammation. Figures 7.1 and 7.2 show the location of frontal and maxillary sinuses in relation to nasal cavities while Figure 7.3 shows the areas overlying such sinuses for clinical examination.

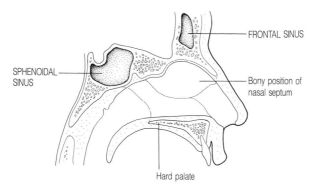
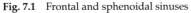

Fig. 7.1 Frontal and sphenoidal sinuses

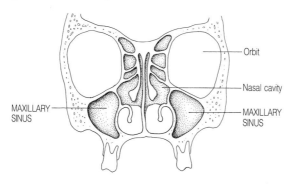

Fig. 7.2 Maxillary sinuses (Cross section, anterior view)

163

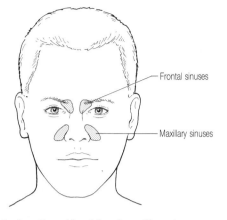

Fig. 7.3   Location of frontal and maxillary sinuses

The condition of sinusitis broadly corresponds to the old Chinese medical category of *Bi Yuan* which literally means "nose pool". As we have seen in the chapter on allergic rhinitis, the differentiation and treatment of *Bi Yuan* are often used to diagnose and treat allergic rhinitis, which is a mistake since *Bi Yuan* corresponds more closely to sinusitis.

Bi Yuan is sometimes also called *Nao Lou* which means "brain discharge" since the profuse and purulent discharge from the nose was considered to come from the brain. Interestingly, Hippocrates and his disciples also thought that the evil humour (of sinusitis) arose in the brain and from there descended into the nasal cavities.[1] It was not until 1672 that Richard Lower demonstrated in his book "De Catarrhis" that it was anatomically impossible for respiratory catarrh to originate in the brain:

. . . since the opinion has generally persisted amongst learned doctors everywhere that catarrh . . . comes from the cerebrum I shall . . . attempt to prove the contrary. People claim that the fluid collected in the ventricles of the brain oozes down into the nostrils solely by the cribriform plate, and into the palate by the pituitary gland; but I shall prove that the structure of these parts is such that neither is possible.[2]

It is interesting to note that, when seen from the viewpoint of Chinese medicine, the assumption that nasal discharges originate from the brain is obviously anatomically wrong but physiologically possible since the Gall-Bladder channel flows through the brain.

The main symptoms of sinusitis are a purulent, yellow nasal discharge from the front and the back of the nose (into the throat), a stuffed nose, a frontal headache, facial pain and a feeling of muzziness and heaviness of the head. There may be local tenderness over the maxillary or frontal sinuses.

Aetiology and pathology

1. REPEATED INVASIONS OF WIND-HEAT OR WIND-COLD

Repeated invasions of external Wind, whether Wind-Heat or Wind-Cold but more frequently Wind-Heat, impair the dispersing and descending of Lung-Qi in the nasal passages so that fluids stagnate in the nose and sinuses. The long-term stagnation of fluids leads to Phlegm and Heat which manifest with a yellow, purulent nasal discharge.

Repeated invasions of external Wind are the main cause of sinusitis especially when the person does not take care or have extra rest during such invasions.

From a Western medical perspective, infections from the common cold or influenza viruses frequently cause secondary infections in the sinuses, especially the maxillary sinuses. For anatomical reasons, sinus infection is liable to become chronic. In fact, the openings through which the maxillary sinuses communicate with the nasal cavities are narrow, and inflammatory oedema of the mucosa lining them often prevents adequate drainage of the infected sinuses. As a result, resolution of sinus infection is often slow and incomplete so that, when the next viral infection from common cold or influenza occurs, the already infected and inflamed sinuses will be affected again. Thus, repeated infections by the common cold or influenza viruses will lead to chronic sinusitis.

2. DIET

Excessive consumption of greasy-hot foods leading to Phlegm and Heat may predispose one to sinusitis. This type of food may lead to the formation of Damp-Heat in the Stomach and Spleen which may be carried upwards to the sinuses via the Stomach channel.

However, this can only be a predisposing factor in the development of sinusitis, the repeated invasions of Wind being the necessary condition.

Differentiation and treatment

The patterns discussed will be:

1. Wind-Heat
2. Lung-Heat
3. Liver and Gall-Bladder Fire
4. Stomach and Spleen Damp-Heat.

It should be remembered that all the above patterns are of the Excess type and the formulae used are aimed at expelling pathogenic factors. However, in chronic cases, there is always an underlying deficiency, especially of the Spleen, which needs to be addressed. In such cases, all the formulae indicated below need to be modified with the addition of Spleen-Qi tonic herbs such as Bai Zhu *Rhizoma Atractylodis macrocephalae*, Dang Shen *Radix Codonopsis pilosulae*, or Huang Qi *Radix Astragali membranacei*.

With acupuncture, the points indicated below will have to be integrated by the addition of points to tonify the Spleen such as ST-36 Zusanli and BL-20 Pishu.

1. WIND-HEAT

CLINICAL MANIFESTATIONS

Stuffed nose, yellow-sticky or purulent nasal discharge, headache, diminished sense of smell, aversion to cold and fever.
Tongue: Red sides and/or front.
Pulse: Floating-Rapid.

This corresponds to an acute attack of sinusitis following an invasion of Wind-Heat.

TREATMENT PRINCIPLE

Release the Exterior, expel Wind-Heat and restore the dispersing and descending of Lung-Qi.

ACUPUNCTURE

L.I.–11 Quchi, L.I.–4 Hegu, L.I.–20 Yingxiang, Bitong, Du-23 Shangxing, BL-12 Fengmen. Reducing method.

EXPLANATION

- **L.I.-11** expels Wind-Heat and clears Heat.
- **L.I.-4** expels Wind-Heat and clears the nose.
- **L.I.-20** and **Bitong** (extra point) expel Wind and clear the nose and sinuses.
- **Du-23** opens the nose and expels Wind. It should be needled horizontally forwards.
- **BL-12**, with cupping, expels Wind.

HERBAL TREATMENT

(a) PRESCRIPTION

Empirical prescription
He Ye *Folium Nelumbinis nuciferae* 6 g
Niu Bang Zi *Fructus Arctii lappae* 6 g
Bo He *Herba Menthae* 6 g
Shi Chang Pu *Rhizoma Acori graminei* 6 g
Shi Gao *Gypsum fibrosum* 12 g
Lian Qiao *Fructus Forsythiae suspensae* 6 g
Xuan Shen *Radix Scrophulariae ningpoensis* 4.5 g
Jie Geng *Radix Platycodi grandiflori* 4.5 g
Xin Yi Hua *Flos Magnoliae liliflorae* 4.5 g

Explanation

- **He Ye**, **Niu Bang Zi** and **Bo He** expel Wind-Heat.
- **Shi Chang Pu** opens the nasal orifice and separates turbid from clear.
- **Shi Gao**, **Lian Qiao** and **Xuan Shen** clear Heat. Xuan Shen is included also to prevent injury of Yin from Heat.
- **Jie Geng** restores the descending of Lung-Qi.
- **Xin Yi Hua** expels Wind and opens the nose.

(b) PRESCRIPTION

Empirical prescription
Xin Yi Hua *Flos Magnoliae liliflorae* 9 g

Bai Zhi *Radix Angelicae dahuricae* 9 g
Chai Hu *Radix Bupleuri* 6 g
Jing Jie *Herba seu Flos Schizonepetae tenuifoliae* 4.5 g
Bo He *Herba Menthae* 6 g
Jie Geng *Radix Platycodi grandiflori* 6 g
Ma Huang *Herba Ephedrae* 6 g
Huang Qin *Radix Scutellariae baicalensis* 6 g
Shan Zhi Zi *Fructus Gardeniae jasminoidis* 6 g
Long Dan Cao *Radix Gentianae scabrae* 6 g
Yu Xing Cao *Herba Houttuyniae cordatae* 9 g
Jin Yin Hua *Flos Lonicerae japonicae* 9 g
Gua Lou *Semen Trichosanthis* 6 g
Chuan Xiong *Radix Ligustici wallichii* 4.5 g

Explanation

This formula has a stronger effect than the previous one in clearing Damp-Heat and Fire-Poison and is therefore used when there is a profuse sticky-yellow or purulent nasal discharge.

– **Xin Yi Hua** and **Bai Zhi** direct the prescription to the nose and sinuses. They also expel Wind.
– **Chai Hu**, **Jing Jie**, **Bo He**, **Jie Geng** and **Ma Huang** expel Wind and restore the dispersing and descending of Lung-Qi. Chai Hu and Jie Geng also direct the other herbs upwards.
– **Huang Qin**, **Zhi Zi** and **Long Dan Cao** resolve Damp-Heat.
– **Yu Xing Cao** and **Jin Yin Hua** resolve Fire-Poison.
– **Gua Lou** resolves Phlegm-Heat.
– **Chuan Xiong** expels Wind.

2. LUNG-HEAT

CLINICAL MANIFESTATIONS

Sticky-yellow or purulent nasal discharge, tenderness over maxillary sinuses, flushed face, feeling of heat, thirst, headache.
Tongue: Red with sticky-yellow coating.
Pulse: Slippery and Full, though possibly only on the right Front position.
This is a condition of chronic sinusitis when repeated invasions of Wind-Heat have impaired the dispersing and descending function of the Lungs so that fluids stagnate in the sinuses and give rise to Phlegm-Heat.

PRINCIPLE OF TREATMENT

Restore the dispersing and descending of Lung-Qi, clear Lung-Heat.

ACUPUNCTURE

L.I.–11 Quchi, L.I.–4 Hegu, LU-10 Yuji, LU-7 Lieque, L.I.-20 Yingxiang, Bitong, Du-14 Dazhui. Reducing method.

EXPLANATION

– **L.I.-11** clears Heat.
– **L.I.-4** opens the nose.
– **LU-10** clears Lung-Heat and opens the nose.
– **LU-7** restores the dispersing and descending of Lung-Qi.
– **L.I.-20** and **Bitong** open the nose and expel Wind.
– **Du-14** is added if the symptoms of Heat are pronounced.

HERBAL TREATMENT

PRESCRIPTION

XIN YI QING FEI YIN
Magnolia Clearing the Lungs Decoction
Xin Yi Hua *Flos Magnoliae liliflorae* 9 g
Huang Qin *Radix Scutellariae baicalensis* 9 g
Shan Zhi Zi *Fructus Gardeniae jasminoidis* 6 g
Shi Gao *Gypsum fibrosum* 12 g
Zhi Mu *Radix Anemarrhenae asphodeloidis* 6 g
Jin Yin Hua *Flos Lonicerae japonicae* 6 g
Yu Xing Cao *Herba Houttuyniae cordatae* 6 g
Mai Men Dong *Tuber Ophiopogonis japonici* 6 g

Explanation

– **Xin Yi Hua** directs the formula to the nose and sinuses.
– **Huang Qin**, **Zhi Zi**, **Shi Gao** and **Zhi Mu** clear Lung-Heat.

– **Jin Yin Hua** and **Yu Xing Cao** resolve Fire-Poison. Their dosage is increased if there is a profuse purulent discharge from the nose.
– **Mai Dong** prevents injury of Lung-Yin from Heat.

3. LIVER AND GALL-BLADDER FIRE

CLINICAL MANIFESTATIONS

Yellow-purulent nasal discharge, bloodshot eyes, red face, headache on temples and cheeks, dizziness, a bitter taste, dry stools, irritability.
Tongue: Red with redder sides, sticky-yellow coating.
Pulse: Wiry, Slippery and Rapid.

This condition is due to Liver and Gall-Bladder Fire rising to the nose and the brain. Fire condenses the fluids in the nose and leads to Phlegm-Heat. The Gall-Bladder channel flows through the brain and Gall-Bladder Fire causes what is considered to be a discharge of purulent fluid from the brain.

TREATMENT PRINCIPLE

Clear Liver and Gall-Bladder Fire, restore the descending of Lung-Qi.

ACUPUNCTURE

LIV-2 Xingjian, G.B.-43 Xiaxi, LU-7 Lieque, L.I.-4 Hegu, Bitong, G.B.-15 Toulinqi. Reducing method.

EXPLANATION

– **LIV-2** clears Liver-Fire.
– **G.B.-43** clears Gall-Bladder Fire.
– **LU-7** restores the descending of Lung-Qi.
– **L.I.-4** and **Bitong** open the nose and the sinuses.
– **G.B.-15** is a local point to clear the Gall-Bladder channel. It affects the eyes and the sinuses.

HERBAL TREATMENT

(a) PRESCRIPTION

QING GAN TOU DING TANG

Clearing the Liver and Penetrating the Crown (of the head) Decoction
Ling Yang Jiao *Cornu Antelopis* 4.5 g
Shi Jue Ming *Concha Haliotidis* 12 g
Chan Tui *Periostracum Cicadae* 4.5 g
Sang Ye *Folium Mori albae* 6 g
Bo He *Herba Menthae* 3 g
Xia Ku Cao *Spica Prunellae vulgaris* 6 g
Mu Dan Pi *Cortex Moutan radicis* 4.5 g
Xuan Shen *Radix Scrophulariae ningpoensis* 3 g
Jie Geng *Radix Platycodi grandiflori* 3 g
Chen Pi *Pericarpium Citri reticulatae* 3 g

Explanation

– **Ling Yang Jiao, Shi Jue Ming, Chan Tui, Sang Ye** and **Bo He** subdue Liver-Yang and expel Wind.
– **Xia Ku Cao** clears Liver-Fire.
– **Mu Dan Pi** and **Xuan Shen** clear Heat and cool Blood. Xuan Shen also prevents injury of Yin from Heat.
– **Jie Geng** restores the descending of Lung-Qi and directs the other herbs upwards.
– **Chen Pi** helps to digest the ingredients of the prescriptions.

(b) PRESCRIPTION

LONG DAN BI YUAN FANG

Gentiana "Nose Pool" Formula
Long Dan Cao *Radix Gentianae scabrae* 6 g
Huang Qin *Radix Scutellariae baicalensis* 6 g
Xia Ku Cao *Spica Prunellae vulgaris* 6 g
Yu Xing Cao *Herba Houttuyniae cordatae* 9 g
Ju Hua *Flos Chrysanthemi morifolii* 6 g
Bai Zhi *Radix Angelicae dahuricae* 6 g
Cang Er Zi *Fructus Xanthii* 6 g
Huo Xiang *Herba Agastachis* 4.5 g
Yi Yi Ren *Semen Coicis lachryma jobi* 15 g
Che Qian Zi *Semen Plantaginis* 6 g
Jie Geng *Radix Platycodi grandiflori* 6 g

Explanation

– **Long Dan Cao, Huang Qin** and **Xia Ku Cao** drain Liver-Fire.
– **Yu Xing Cao** resolves Fire-Poison and opens the sinuses.
– **Ju Hua, Bai Zhi, Cang Er Zi** and **Huo Xiang**

expel Wind. Cang Er Zi and Bai Zhi open the nose and the sinuses.
- **Yi Yi Ren** and **Che Qian Zi** drain Heat via urination.
- **Jie Geng** restores the descending of Lung-Qi and directs the other herbs upwards.

4. STOMACH AND SPLEEN DAMP-HEAT

CLINICAL MANIFESTATIONS

Sticky-yellow nasal discharge, red cheeks, thirst, dry lips, impaired sense of smell, a feeling of heaviness and muzziness of the head, a frontal headache, a sticky taste, a feeling of oppression of the chest and epigastrium.
Tongue: sticky-yellow coating in the centre.
Pulse: Slippery.

TREATMENT PRINCIPLE

Clear Heat, resolve Dampness, harmonize the Stomach, tonify the Spleen.

ACUPUNCTURE

Ren-12 Zhongwan, BL-20 Pishu, Ren-9 Shuifen, SP-9 Yinlingquan, BL-22 Sanjiaoshu, L.I.-11 Quchi, L.I.-4 Hegu, Ren-13 Shangwan, Bitong. Even method, except on the first two points which should be reinforced.

EXPLANATION

- **Ren-12** and **BL-20** tonify the Spleen to resolve Dampness.
- **Ren-9**, **SP-9** and **BL-22** resolve Dampness.
- **L.I.-11** resolves Damp-Heat.
- **L.I.-4** opens the nose and harmonizes the Stomach.
- **Ren-13** harmonizes the Stomach and regulates the Upper Burner.
- **Bitong** opens the nose and the sinuses.

HERBAL TREATMENT

PRESCRIPTION

CANG ER BI DOU YAN FANG
Xanthium Sinusitis Formula

Cang Er Zi *Fructus Xanthii* 9 g
Huang Qin *Radix Scutellariae baicalensis* 9 g
Pu Gong Ying *Herba Taraxaci mongolici cum radice* 6 g
Ge Gen *Radix Puerariae* 9 g
Jie Geng *Radix Platycodi grandiflori* 6 g
Bai Zhi *Radix Angelicae dahuricae* 3 g
Che Qian Zi *Semen Plantaginis* 9 g
Gan Cao *Radix Glycyrrhizae uralensis* 3 g

Explanation

- **Cang Er Zi** directs the formula to the nose and sinuses.
- **Huang Qin** and **Pu Gong Ying** clear Damp-Heat and harmonize the Stomach.
- **Ge Gen** clears Stomach-Heat.
- **Jie Geng** restores the descending of Lung-Qi.
- **Bai Zhi** opens the nose and sinuses.
- **Che Qian Zi** drains Dampness via urination.
- **Gan Cao** harmonizes.

Variations

- If there is Stomach-Fire with constipation or dry stools add Da Huang *Rhizoma Rhei.*

(i) PATENT REMEDY

HUO DAN WAN
Agastache-Bile Pill
Huo Xiang *Herba Agastachis*
Zhu Dan *Pig's bile*
This remedy is suitable for most types of sinusitis in conjunction with acupuncture treatment.

(ii) PATENT REMEDY

BI YAN PIAN
Rhinitis Tablet
Cang Er Zi *Fructus Xanthii*
Xin Yi Hua *Flos Magnoliae liliflorae*
Gan Cao *Radix Glycyrrhizae uralensis*
Huang Bo *Cortex Phellodendri*

Jie Geng *Radix Platycodi grandiflori*
Wu Wei Zi *Fructus Schisandrae chinensis*
Lian Qiao *Fructus Forsythiae suspensae*
Bai Zhi *Radix Angelicae dahuricae*
Zhi Mu *Radix Anemarrhenae asphodeloidis*
Ju Hua *Flos Chrysanthemi morifolii*
Fang Feng *Radix Ledebouriellae sesloidis*
Jing Jie *Herba seu Flos Schizonepetae tenuifoliae*

Although this remedy is called "Rhinitis Tablet", it is better indicated for sinusitis than for rhinitis. It should be used only if there are signs of Heat with a sticky-yellow nasal discharge. If the nasal discharge is white and watery, then the condition is not sinusitis but rhinitis and this remedy will not help much.

Prognosis

Sinusitis is a stubborn, chronic disease which requires long-term treatment. The more obvious the signs of Fire-Poison, the longer it will take to treat. It is important to attend to any underlying deficiency as well as clearing Heat, resolving Damp-Heat or Fire-Poison. The most likely deficiencies are those of Lung-Qi and Stomach and Spleen Qi. If both acupuncture and herbal medicine are used, it is possible to use acupuncture to tonify any underlying deficiency and herbal medicine to clear pathogenic factors (Heat, Damp-Heat or Fire-Poison).

END NOTES

1. N. Mygind et al 1990 Rhinitis and Asthma: Similarities and Differences, Munksgaard, Lund, Sweden, p. 10.

2. Ibid., p. 10.

Cough 8

咳
嗽

Cough is mentioned in the "Yellow Emperor's Classic" where a whole chapter is dedicated to it. The two characters of its Chinese name, *Ke Sou*, originally referred to two different types of cough. The "Collection of Life-Saving Pathologies from the Simple Questions" (1186) says:

"Ke" denotes cough with a sound but without phlegm: this indicates injury of the Lungs. "Sou" denotes cough with phlegm but without sound: this indicates that the Spleen is obstructed by Phlegm. "Ke-Sou" therefore denotes a cough with both sound and phlegm due to injury of the Lungs and Phlegm from the Spleen.[1]

Chapter 23 of the "Simple Questions" relates different sounds to different organs and it says: *"Diseases of Qi manifest . . . in the Lungs with cough . . . ."[2]*

Chapter 38 of the "Simple Questions", entirely dedicated to cough, says that cough does not depend only on the Lungs but may be caused by each of the five Yin organs:

Lung-cough [is accompanied by] breathlessness and spitting of blood; Heart-cough by pain in the heart region and a feeling of an obstruction in the throat; Liver-cough by hypochondrial fullness and pain . . . Kidney-cough by backache . . . Spleen-cough by right hypochondrial pain . . .[3]

It then goes on to say that when cough is prolonged it may transmit from the Yin organs to their related Yang organs:

When the cough of the five Yin organs persists for a long time it will be transmitted to the six Yang organs. If a Spleen-cough persists for a long time it will transmit to the Stomach . . . [causing] vomiting on coughing . . . If a Liver-cough persists for a long time it will transmit to the Gall-Bladder . . . [causing] coughing of bile. If a Lung-cough persists for a long time, it will transmit to the Large Intestine . . . [causing] bowel incontinence on coughing. If a Heart-cough persists for a long time it will transmit to the Small Intestine . . . [causing] flatulence on coughing. If a Kidney-cough persists for a long time it will transmit to the Bladder . . . [causing] incontinence of urine on coughing. Any chronic cough will affect the Triple Burner . . . [causing] cough with abdominal fullness and no desire to eat or drink.[4]

The same chapter clearly attributes cough to a combination of invasion of an external pathogenic factor and improper diet:

The skin is in relation with the Lungs; when an external pathogenic factor [Wind-Cold] invades the skin, it progresses to the Lungs. When cold food and drinks enter the Stomach, they go upwards to the Lungs via the Lung channel [which starts in the Middle Burner] and give rise to Cold in the Lungs. The combination of exterior and interior Cold causes cough in the Lungs.[5]

The chapter on cough ends by giving indications for treatment: *"For cough of the Yin organs needle the [Back] Transporting points; for cough of the Yang organs needle the Sea points; for cough with oedema needle the River points."*[6] The "Complete Book of Jing Yue" (1624) distinguishes cough caused by invasion of an external pathogenic factor from that due to an internal disharmony.[7]

Aetiology and pathology

1. EXTERNAL PATHOGENIC FACTORS

External Wind is the main cause of exterior coughs. Wind penetrates the skin and the Defensive-Qi portion which is controlled by the Lungs. It therefore impairs the descending of Lung-Qi and causes cough. This is an exterior type of cough which, with proper treatment, disappears rather quickly without leaving any consequence.

Wind combines with other pathogenic factors and the most likely to cause a cough are Wind-Cold, Wind-Heat and Wind-Dryness.

Wind-Cold invades the skin and Defensive-Qi portion impairing the descending of Lung-Qi and thus causing cough.

Wind-Heat enters via the nose and mouth and affects the throat. It causes a cough by invading the Lung channel in the throat and preventing the descending of Lung-Qi. The cough caused by Wind-Heat is of a drier type than that caused by Wind-Cold.

Wind-Dryness, rare in the British Isles but rather prevalent in the American South-West, also invades the Lung channel in the throat and causes a very dry and ticklish cough. Besides impairing the descending of Lung-Qi, Wind-Dry-ness also dries up the Lung's fluids and the resulting cough is more persistent than that caused by Wind-Cold or Wind-Heat.

2. EMOTIONAL STRESS

Worry is a frequent emotional cause of cough. It affects the Lungs directly and it knots Qi preventing the descending of Lung-Qi. This type of cough would be dry and irritating.

Prolonged anger, frustration, or resentment lead to stagnation of Liver-Qi and, over a long period of time, to Liver-Fire. This may invade the Lungs and prevent the descending of Lung-Qi, causing cough.

3. DIET

Excessive consumption of sweets, greasy foods and dairy foods may lead to the formation of Phlegm which settles in the Lungs and prevents Lung-Qi from descending. This causes a cough with profuse expectoration.

Excessive consumption of hot foods, alcohol and fried-greasy foods leads to the formation of Heat and Phlegm. Phlegm settles in the Lungs and impairs the descending of Lung-Qi, while Heat dries up the Lung fluids. Both these processes cause cough.

4. CHRONIC ILLNESS

A chronic illness affecting the Lungs weakens Lung-Qi and/or Lung-Yin. The deficient Lung-Qi fails to descend and causes a chronic cough of the Empty type.

Thus the pathology of cough is always characterized by Lung-Qi failing to descend. This may happen either because the Lungs are obstructed by an exterior or interior pathogenic factor (Full-type) or because Lung-Qi is deficient and fails to descend properly (Empty-type). Pathogenic factors in the Lungs which impair the descending of Qi include external Wind, Heat, Phlegm, stagnation of Qi and Liver-Fire. In such cases when Qi fails to descend because of a pathogenic factor, it is said to be "rebelling upwards". All the old classics convey this idea of cough being caused by rebellious Qi. The "Simple Questions" in chapter 10 says: *"Cough consists in Qi rebelling upwards."*[8] The "Prescriptions of the Golden Chest" by Zhang Zhong Ying says: *"Cough is due to Qi rebelling upwards."*[9] External coughs are therefore by definition of the Full type.

Interior coughs may be of the Deficiency or Excess type and the main pathology in the Excess type is Phlegm or Fire. Phlegm combines with Heat or Cold and Fire may be of the Excess or Deficiency type.

Thus coughs may be classified in various ways. Using Fullness and Emptiness, we may classify them as follows:

FULL-TYPE	EMPTY-TYPE
EXTERIOR	Lung-Qi Deficiency
	Lung-Yin Deficiency
Wind-Cold	
Wind-Heat	
Wind-Dryness	
INTERIOR	
Damp-Phlegm	
Phlegm-Heat	
Fire	
Phlegm-Fluids	

Using Exterior and Interior, we may classify coughs as follows:

EXTERIOR	INTERIOR
Wind-Cold	*FULL*
Wind-Heat	
Wind-Dryness	Damp-Phlegm
	Phlegm-Heat
	Fire
	Phlegm-Fluids
	EMPTY
	Lung-Qi Deficiency
	Lung-Yin Deficiency

However, I prefer to classify coughs as acute or chronic, since this factor is clinically more significant. In fact, when presented with a patient with cough the first thing to ascertain is whether the cough is acute or chronic. Once this has been ascertained, one needs to establish whether the cough is external or internal. Acute coughs may be external or internal but are always of the Full type, while chronic coughs may be of the Full or Empty type.

The train of thought and guideline for interrogation of the patient may be represented with a diagram (Fig. 8.1).

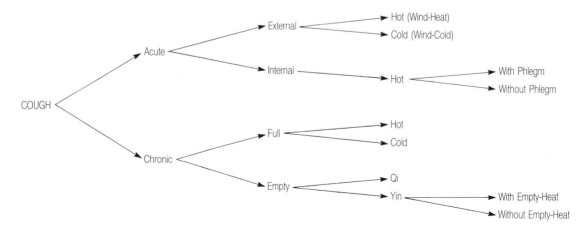

Fig. 8.1 Classification of cough and guideline for interrogation

Diagnosis

Cough can be diagnosed according to its sound, the time of occurrence and the character of any sputum.

SOUND

As a general rule, a weak-sounding cough indicates Deficiency while a loud cough indicates Excess.

A barking cough denotes Heat while a loose, rattling cough indicates the presence of Phlegm.

TIME OF DAY

A cough which occurs only in the late afternoon or evening indicates Yin deficiency.

A cough which is worse in the morning is usually due to Phlegm.

SPUTUM

A cough without sputum indicates either Deficiency or Heat.

If there is abundant sputum, it is due to Phlegm. A yellow sputum denotes Heat, while white sputum denotes Cold. White sputum may be sticky or dilute: if it is sticky it indicates the prevalence of Dampness and Phlegm over Cold, while if it is dilute, it indicates the prevalence of Cold over Dampness or Phlegm.

Blood-tinged sputum indicates either Full- or Empty-Heat. Greenish sputum indicates Heat, whilst white, very watery and frothy sputum indicates Phlegm-Fluids.

Differentiation and treatment

As mentioned above, we shall classify coughs into acute or chronic. Acute cases are usually characterized by Fullness, while chronic cases may be of the Full or Empty type. Fullness and Emptiness, however, often combine. Zhang Jing Yue says in the "Complete Book of Jing Yue" (1634):

Coughs of external origin are very frequent [and are characterized by] some Deficiency within the Fullness, hence one must tonify somewhat as well as expelling [pathogenic factors]. In coughs of internal origin there is some Fullness within Emptiness, hence one must clear and moisten simultaneously.[10]

ACUTE

By acute is meant a cough of a few days' or, at most, a few weeks' duration. The most important fact to establish when seeing a patient suffering from acute cough is whether the cough is external or internal. All acute coughs are originally due to invasion of external Wind but the external pathogenic factor may become internal in only a few days while the cough is still at the acute stage.

The differentiation of patterns according to the 4 Levels provides the clinical framework for the symptomatology of invasions of external Wind turning into interior Heat. For example, within the 4 Levels patterns, invasion of Wind-Heat may cause a cough (together with shivering, fever, aversion to cold, body aches and a Floating-Rapid pulse). If Wind-Heat penetrates into the Interior it gives rise to the pattern of Lung-Heat with a barking cough (together with high fever, thirst, sweating, and a Big pulse). Within the 6 Stages patterns, although a change from Wind-Cold to interior Lung-Heat is not contemplated, it *does* happen in practice. Thus, acute Lung-Heat with cough in the course of a febrile disease may derive either from Wind-Heat or Wind-Cold, although the former is more likely.

Thus, when presented with a patient with acute cough, the crucial distinction must be made between exterior or interior cough. Apart from many other symptoms, this differentiation may be made very simply on the basis of the patient's feelings of cold or heat. If the patient shivers and feels aversion to cold, and this feeling is not alleviated by wrapping up, it indicates an exterior pattern, i.e. the pathogenic factor is still on the Exterior.

If the patient feels aversion to heat and is generally hot, very thirsty and restless, it indicates an interior pattern of Heat, i.e. the pathogenic factor is in the Interior and it has turned into Heat. The presence of cough, breathlessness, some chest pain and possibly flaring of the alae nasi indicate the location of Heat in the Lungs.

After establishing the character of exterior or interior cough, we must differentiate the pattern further in each case. If it is exterior, we must ascertain whether it is Wind-Cold or Wind-Heat. If it is interior, it is due to Lung-Heat and we must ascertain whether there is just Lung-Heat or Lung Phlegm-Heat (see Fig. 8.2).

The acute patterns to be discussed are:

EXTERIOR

Invasion of Wind-Cold
Invasion of Wind-Heat
Invasion of Wind-Dryness

INTERIOR

Lung-Heat
Lung Phlegm-Heat

EXTERIOR

1. INVASION OF WIND-COLD

Clinical manifestations

Cough, slight breathlessness, sneezing, runny nose with white discharge, aversion to cold, shivers, no temperature or one that is only slightly raised, no sweating, body aches, stiff neck, headache and pale urine.

Tongue: there may be no evident change.
Pulse: Floating-Tight.

This is the typical pattern of invasion of Wind-Cold with prevalence of Cold. It corresponds to the Greater-Yang pattern with prevalence of Cold within the 6 Stages.

Treatment principle

Release the Exterior, restore the dispersing and descending of Lung-Qi, expel Wind, scatter Cold by promoting sweating and stop cough.

Acupuncture

LU-7 Lieque, BL-12 Fengmen, BL-13 Feishu, L.I.-4 Hegu, KI-7 Fuliu, LU-6 Kongzui. Reducing method, cupping is applicable on BL-12 and BL-13.

Explanation

– **LU-7** releases the Exterior, restores the descending of Lung-Qi and stops cough.
– **BL-12** expels exterior Wind and releases the Exterior. It is very effective with cupping.
– **BL-13** releases the Exterior, restores the descending of Lung-Qi and stops cough. Cupping is also applicable on this point.
– **L.I.-4** (reduced) and **KI-7** (reinforced), in combination, promote sweating to release the Exterior.
– **LU-6**, Accumulation point, stops acute cough.

Herbal treatment

(a) Prescription

MA HUANG TANG
Ephedra Decoction

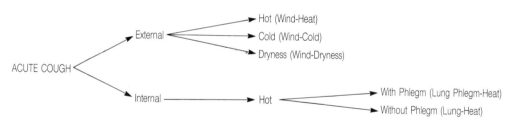

Fig. 8.2 Patterns in acute cough

Ma Huang *Herba Ephedrae* 6 g
Gui Zhi *Ramulus Cinnamomi cassiae* 4 g
Xing Ren *Semen Pruni armeniacae* 9 g
Zhi Gan Cao *Radix Glycyrrhizae uralensis prae-parata* 3 g

Explanation

– **Ma Huang**, the emperor herb in the formula, expels Wind, scatters Cold, promotes sweating, releases the Exterior, restores the dispersing and descending of Lung-Qi and stops cough and breathlessness.
– **Gui Zhi**, the minister herb, helps Ma Huang to scatter Cold and expel Wind.
– **Xing Ren**, assistant herb, specifically restores the descending of Lung-Qi and stops cough.
– **Gan Cao**, messenger herb, harmonizes and tempers the scattering effect of Ma Huang.

Variations

– To enhance the antitussive effect add Kuan Dong Hua *Flos Tussilaginis farfarae*, especially treated with honey, and increase the dosage of Xing Ren.

(b) Prescription

SAN AO TANG and ZHI SOU SAN
Three Break Decoction and *Stopping Cough Powder*
Ma Huang *Herba Ephedrae* 6 g
Xing Ren *Semen Pruni armeniacae* 9 g
Zhi Gan Cao *Radix Glycyrrhizae uralensis prae-parata* 3 g
Jing Jie *Herba seu Flos Schizonepetae tenuifoliae* 6 g
Jie Geng *Radix Platycodi grandiflori* 4.5 g
Bai Qian *Radix et Rhizoma Cynanchii stautoni* 6 g
Chen Pi *Pericarpium Citri reticulatae* 3 g
Bai Bu *Radix Stemonae* 6 g
Zi Wan *Radix Asteris tatarici* 6 g

Explanation

– The first three herbs comprise the first formula which is simply a variation of Ma Huang Tang *Ephedra Decoction* without Gui Zhi. This formula releases the Exterior, expels Wind, scatters Cold, restores the descending of Lung-Qi and stops cough.

– **Jing Jie** and **Jie Geng** release the Exterior and restore the descending of Lung-Qi. Jie Geng stops cough.
– **Bai Qian** and **Chen Pi** resolve Phlegm.
– **Bai Bu** and **Zi Wan** stop cough.

Variations

– If there is a lot of sputum, stuffiness of the chest and a sticky tongue coating (signs of Phlegm) add Ban Xia *Rhizoma Pinelliae ternatae*, Hou Po *Cortex Magnoliae officinalis* and Fu Ling *Sclerotium Poriae cocos*.
– If there are Heat signs such as thirst and red sides of the tongue add Shi Gao *Gypsum fibrosum*, San Bai Pi *Cortex Mori albae radicis* and Huang Qin *Radix Scutellariae baicalensis*.

(i) Patent remedy

MA XING ZHI KE PIAN
Ephedra-Prunus Cough Tablet
Ma Huang *Herba Ephedrae*
Xing Ren *Semen Pruni armeniacae*
Shi Gao *Gypsum fibrosum*
Gan Cao *Radix Glycyrrhizae uralensis*
Jie Geng *Radix Platycodi grandiflori*
Chen Pi *Pericarpium Citri reticulatae*
Hua Shi *Talcum*
Feng Mi *Honey*

Explanation

This tablet expels Wind-Cold and restores the descending of Lung-Qi. It can be used for acute cough from Wind-Cold; however, as it also contains cold substances such as Shi Gao and Hua Shi, it can be used also for cough from Wind-Heat.

(ii) Patent remedy

TONG XUAN LI FEI WAN
Penetrating Dispersing and Regulating the Lungs Pill
Ma Huang *Herba Ephedrae*
Zhi Ke *Fructus Citri aurantii*
Jie Geng *Radix Platycodi grandiflori*
Fu Ling *Sclerotium Poriae cocos*
Qian Hu *Radix Peucedani*

Huang Qin *Radix Scutellariae baicalensis*
Chen Pi *Pericarpium Citri reticulatae*
Gan Cao *Radix Glycyrrhizae uralensis*
Ban Xia *Rhizoma Pinelliae ternatae*
Xing Ren *Semen Pruni armeniacae*
Zi Su Ye *Folium Perillae frutescentis*

Explanation

This pill also expels Wind-Cold and restores the descending of Lung-Qi. While the former remedy only restores the descending of Lung-Qi, this one also releases the Exterior. It is indicated for an acute cough from Wind-Cold, especially with production of white sputum.

2. INVASION OF WIND-HEAT

Clinical manifestations

Dry cough with a tickling sensation in the throat, aversion to cold, shivers, fever, sore throat, slight sweating, body aches, headache, runny nose with yellow discharge, sneezing, slight thirst and slightly dark urine.
Tongue: slightly Red sides and/or front part.
Pulse: Floating-Rapid.

Treatment principle

Release the Exterior, expel Wind, clear Heat, restore the descending of Lung-Qi and stop cough.

Acupuncture

LU-7 Lieque, L.I.-4 Hegu, BL-12 Fengmen, BL-13 Feishu, L.I.-11 Quchi, LU-11 Shaoshang, Du-14 Dazhui, LU-6 Kongzui. All with reducing method; cupping is applicable to BL-12 and BL-13.

Explanation

- **LU-7** and **BL-13** release the Exterior, expel Wind, restore the descending of Lung-Qi and stop cough.
- **L.I.-4** expels Wind-Heat.
- **BL-12** releases the Exterior.
- **L.I.-11** expels Wind-Heat.
- **LU-11** expels Wind-Heat and is used if there is a sore throat and swollen tonsils.

- **Du-14** is used if symptoms of Heat are pronounced.
- **LU-6**, Accumulation point, stops acute cough.

Herbal treatment

Prescription

SANG JU YIN
Morus-Chrysanthemum Decoction
Sang Ye *Folium Mori albae* 6 g
Ju Hua *Flos Chrysanthemi morifolii* 3 g
Bo He *Herba Menthae* 3 g
Xing Ren *Semen Pruni armeniacae* 6 g
Jie Geng *Radix Platycodi grandiflori* 6 g
Lian Qiao *Fructus Forsythiae suspensae* 6 g
Lu Gen *Rhizoma Phragmitis communis* 6 g
Gan Cao *Radix Glycyrrhizae uralensis* 3 g

Explanation

- **Sang Ye**, **Ju Hua** and **Bo He** release the Exterior and expel Wind-Heat. Sang Ye, in particular, restores the descending of Lung-Qi and stops cough.
- **Xing Ren** and **Jie Geng** restore the descending of Lung-Qi and stop cough.
- **Lian Qiao** and **Lu Gen** clear Heat and stop thirst.
- **Gan Cao** harmonizes and resolves Fire-Poison (in case of very inflamed throat and inflamed-swollen tonsils).

Variations

- In case of pronounced Heat signs add Huang Qin *Radix Scutellariae baicalensis* and Zhi Mu *Radix Anemarrhenae asphodeloidis*.
- In case of very sore throat and hoarse voice add She Gan *Rhizoma Belamcandae chinensis* and Chi Shao *Radix Paeoniae rubrae*.
- If Heat has begun to injure the Lung fluids causing dry mouth and throat add Nan Sha Shen *Radix Adenophorae* and Tian Hua Fen *Radix Trichosanthis*.

Patent remedy

SANG JU GAN MAO PIAN
Morus-Chrysanthemum Common Cold Tablet

Sang Ye *Folium Mori albae*
Ju Hua *Flos Chrysanthemi morifolii*
Bo He *Herba Menthae*
Xing Ren *Semen Pruni armeniacae*
Jie Geng *Radix Platycodi grandiflori*
Lian Qiao *Fructus Forsythiae suspensae*
Lu Gen *Rhizoma Phragmitis communis*
Gan Cao *Radix Glycyrrhizae uralensis*

Explanation

This tablet releases the Exterior, expels Wind-Heat and restores the descending of Lung-Qi. It can be used for acute cough from Wind-Heat.

3. INVASION OF WIND-DRYNESS

Clinical manifestations

Dry and ticklish cough, dry-itchy-sore throat, sore sensation in the upper chest (trachea), dry lips, dry mouth, stuffed nose, headache, slight aversion to cold and slight shivers.
Tongue: slightly Red sides and/or front part.
Pulse: Floating.

Treatment principle

Release the Exterior, restore the descending of Lung-Qi, promote fluids and stop cough.

Acupuncture

LU-7 Lieque, LU-9 Taiyuan, Ren-12 Zhongwan, KI-6 Zhaohai, SP-6 Sanyinjiao. All with reinforcing method except for LU-7 which should be needled with reducing method.

Explanation

- **LU-7** releases the Exterior and restores the descending of Lung-Qi to stop cough.
- **LU-9** nourishes the Lung's fluids.
- **Ren-12**, the point marking the beginning of the Lung-channel's internal pathway, promotes fluids.
- **KI-6** promotes fluids and benefits and moistens the throat.
- **SP-6** promotes fluids.

Herbal treatment

Prescription

SANG XING TANG
Morus-Prunus Decoction
Sang Ye *Folium Mori albae* 9 g
Xing Ren *Semen Pruni armeniacae* 9 g
Dan Dou Chi *Semen Sojae praeparatum* 9 g
Zhi Zi *Fructus Gardeniae jasminoidis* 6 g
Zhe Bei Mu *Bulbus Fritillariae thunbergii* 6 g
Nan Sha Shen *Radix Adenophorae* 6 g
Li Pi *Pericarpium Fructi Pyri* 6 g

Explanation

- **Sang Ye** and **Xing Ren** restore the descending of Lung-Qi and stop cough.
- **Dan Dou Chi** and **Zhi Zi** clear Heat and stop irritability deriving from Heat.
- **Zhe Bei Mu** resolves Phlegm and stops cough.
- **Nan Sha Shen** and **Li Pi** (pear skin) promote fluids.

Variations

- If the fluids have been severely injured add Mai Men Dong *Tuber Ophiopogonis japonici* and Yu Zhu *Rhizoma Polygonati odorati*.
- If symptoms of Heat are pronounced add Shi Gao *Gypsum fibrosum* and Zhi Mu *Radix Anemarrhenae asphodeloidis*.
- If there is coughing of scanty, blood-flecked sputum add Bai Mao Gen *Rhizoma Imperatae cylindricae*.
- If Dryness is accompanied by symptoms of Wind-Cold (normally it is accompanied by Wind-Heat) use:

XING SU SAN
Prunus-Perilla Leaf Powder
Xing Ren *Semen Pruni armeniacae* 9 g
Zi Su Ye *Folium Perillae frutescentis* 6 g
Jie Geng *Radix Platycodi grandiflori* 4.5 g
Chen Pi *Pericarpium Citri reticulatae* 3 g
Ban Xia *Rhizoma Pinelliae ternatae* 6 g
Fu Ling *Sclerotium Poriae cocos* 6 g
Zhi Ke *Fructus Citri aurantii* 6 g
Qian Hu *Radix Peucedani* 6 g

Sheng Jiang *Rhizoma Zingiberis officinalis recens* 3 slices
Gan Cao *Radix Glycyrrhizae uralensis* 3 g
Da Zao *Fructus Ziziphi jujubae* 3 dates

Case history

A 41-year-old man had contracted an upper respiratory infection while holidaying in the Rocky Mountains in summertime. At the time, this manifested with symptoms of Wind-Heat and Dryness, i.e. aversion to cold, a slight temperature, a dry cough, a dry and itchy sensation of the throat and a headache. He came for treatment on his return from his holiday when he still had a dry persistent, and ticklish cough which was keeping him awake at night.

Diagnosis
This was originally an attack of Wind-Heat-Dryness which had then dried up the Lung's fluids and left him with some Dryness.

Treatment
The principle of treatment adopted was to moisten the Lungs, promote fluids and restore the descending of Lung-Qi. Although this was not an Exterior pattern any longer, I used a variation of Sang Xing Tang *Morus-Prunus Decoction* as this prescription does not contain many herbs which release the Exterior. The variation used was:

Sang Ye *Folium Mori albae* 6 g
Xing Ren *Semen Pruni armeniacae* 6 g
Dan Dou Chi *Semen Sojae praeparatum* 4 g
Zhi Zi *Fructus Gardeniae jasminoidis* 3 g
Zhe Bei Mu *Bulbus Fritillariae thunbergii* 6 g
Nan Sha Shen *Radix Adenophorae* 6 g
Li Pi *Pericarpium Fructi Pyri* 6 g
Tian Hua Fen *Radix Trichosanthis* 6 g
Yu Zhu *Rhizoma Polygonati odorati* 6 g
Kuan Dong Hua (honey-treated) *Flos Tussilaginis farfarae* 9g

Explanation
– **Sang Ye** and **Xing Ren** are the two main herbs to restore the descending of Lung-Qi.
– **Dan Dou Chi** and **Zhi Zi** clear any residual Heat. Their dosage was reduced as there was no sign of much Heat left; they were left in, however, to prevent any residual Heat forming.
– **Zhe Bei Mu** helps to restore the descending of Lung-Qi and stop cough.
– **Sha Shen**, **Li Pi**, **Tian Hua Fen** and **Yu Zhu** promote fluids and moisten the Lungs and throat.
– **Kuan Dong Hua** restores the descending of Lung-Qi and stops cough. Its antitussive effect is enhanced by toasting with honey.

Only three doses of this decoction were enough to stop the cough completely.

INTERIOR

1. LUNG-HEAT

Clinical manifestations

Barking cough, chest pain, breathlessness, fever, thirst, sweating, flaring of alae nasi, restlessness and a feeling of heat.
Tongue: Red with yellow coating.
Pulse: Rapid and Overflowing.

This corresponds to the pattern "Heat in the diaphragm" within the Qi Level of the 4-Level identification of patterns.

Treatment principle

Clear Lung-Heat, restore the descending of Lung-Qi and stop cough.

Acupuncture

LU-5 Chize, LU-1 Zhongfu, Du-14 Dazhui, LU-6 Kongzui and L.I.-11 Quchi. Reducing method.

Explanation
– **LU-5** clears Lung-Heat and restores the descending of Lung-Qi.
– **LU-1** clears Lung-Heat and treats acute patterns of the Lungs.
– **Du-14** clears Heat.
– **LU-6**, Accumulation point, treats acute patterns of the Lungs and stops cough.
– **L.I.-11** clears Heat.

Herbal treatment

Prescription

MA XING SHI GAN TANG
Ephedra-Prunus-Gypsum-Glycyrrhiza Decoction
Ma Huang *Herba Ephedrae* 5 g
Xing Ren *Semen Pruni armeniacae* 9 g
Shi Gao *Gypsum fibrosum* 18 g
Zhi Gan Cao *Radix Glycyrrhizae uralensis prae-parata* 6 g

Explanation
– **Ma Huang** restores the descending of Lung-

Qi and stops cough and breathlessness. Even though it is a hot herb, it is used here in combination with Shi Gao *Gypsum fibrosum* which is very cold.
- **Xing Ren** restores the descending of Lung-Qi and stops cough.
- **Shi Gao** clears Heat at the Qi Level. It clears Lung and Stomach Heat.
- **Zhi Gan Cao** harmonizes and tempers the scattering effect of Ma Huang *Herba Ephedrae*.

Variations

- To enhance the antitussive effect of the formula add Sang Bai Pi *Cortex Mori albae radicis*, Pi Pa Ye *Folium Eriobotryae japonicae* and Kuan Dong Hua *Flos Tussilaginis farfarae*.
- To enhance the Lung-clearing effect add Huang Qin *Radix Scutellariae baicalensis*.

(i) Patent remedy

ZHI SOU DING CHUAN WAN
Stopping Cough and Calming Breathlessness Pill
Ma Huang *Herba Ephedrae*
Xing Ren *Semen Pruni armeniacae*
Shi Gao *Gypsum fibrosum*
Zhi Gan Cao *Radix Glycyrrhizae uralensis praeparata*

Explanation

This pill has the same ingredients and functions as the prescription Ma Xing Shi Gan Tang *Ephedra-Prunus-Gypsum-Glycyrrhiza Decoction* above.

(ii) Patent remedy

MA XING ZHI KE PIAN
Ephedra-Prunus Cough Tablet
Ma Huang *Herba Ephedrae*
Xing Ren *Semen Pruni armeniacae*
Shi Gao *Gypsum fibrosum*
Gan Cao *Radix Glycyrrhizae uralensis*
Jie Geng *Radix Platycodi grandiflori*
Chen Pi *Pericarpium Citri reticulatae*
Hua Shi *Talcum*
Feng Mi *Honey*

Explanation

This tablet, already mentioned above under Wind-Cold, may be used also for Lung-Heat as it combines Ma Huang to restore the descending of Lung-Qi, with Shi Gao to clear Lung-Heat.

2. LUNG PHLEGM-HEAT

Clinical manifestations

Barking cough with expectoration of profuse-sticky-yellow sputum, fever, restlessness, thirst, feeling of heat and a sensation of oppression in the chest.
Tongue: Red with a sticky-yellow coating.
Pulse: Rapid and Slippery.

This corresponds to Lung-Heat at the Qi Level within the 4-Level identification of patterns, but with the presence of Phlegm in addition to Heat. Wind-Heat easily leads to Phlegm as it quickly dries up the body fluids which condense into Phlegm.

Treatment principle

Clear Lung-Heat, resolve Phlegm, restore the descending of Lung-Qi and stop cough.

Acupuncture

LU-5 Chize, LU-1 Zhongfu, Ren-12 Zhongwan, Ren-9 Shuifen, ST-40 Fenglong, SP-6 Sanyinjiao, LU-6 Kongzui, Du-14 Dazhui, L.I.-11 Quchi, T.B.-6 Sanyangluo and SP-15 Daheng. All with reducing method except Ren-12 which should be reinforced.

Explanation

- **LU-5** expels Phlegm and clears Heat from the Lungs.
- **LU-1** and **LU-6**, Front-Collecting point and Accumulation point respectively, are used for acute cases: they clear Lung-Heat and stop cough.
- **Ren-12**, **Ren-9**, **ST-40** and **SP-6** resolve Phlegm.

- **Du-14** and **L.I.-11** clear Heat.
- **T.B.-6** and **SP-15** clear Heat and move downwards.

Herbal treatment

(a) Prescription

QING QI HUA TAN TANG
Clearing Qi and Resolving Phlegm Decoction
Dan Nan Xing *Rhizoma Arisaematis praeparata* 12 g
Gua Lou *Semen Trichosanthis* 9 g
Huang Qin *Radix Scutellariae baicalensis* 9 g
Zhi Shi *Fructus Citri aurantii immaturus* 9 g
Chen Pi *Pericarpium Citri reticulatae* 9 g
Fu Ling *Sclerotium Poriae cocos* 9 g
Xing Ren *Semen Pruni armeniacae* 9 g
Ban Xia *Rhizoma Pinelliae ternatae* 12 g

Explanation

- **Nan Xing**, **Gua Lou** and **Ban Xia** resolve Phlegm.
- **Huang Qin** clears Lung-Heat.
- **Zhi Shi** moves Qi in the chest and helps to resolve Phlegm.
- **Chen Pi** and **Fu Ling** resolve Dampness which helps to resolve Phlegm. Together with Ban Xia, they form the Er Chen Tang *Two Old Decoction*.
- **Xing Ren** restores the descending of Lung-Qi and stops cough.

(b) Prescription

XIAO XIAN XIONG TANG
Small Sinking [Qi of the] Chest Decoction
Huang Lian *Rhizoma Coptidis* 6 g
Ban Xia *Rhizoma Pinelliae ternatae* 12 g
Gua Lou *Semen Trichosanthis* 30 g

Explanation

- **Huang Lian** is bitter, clears Heat and makes Qi descend.
- **Ban Xia** is pungent and resolves Phlegm. These two herbs are combined according to the principle of using bitter herbs to make Qi descend and pungent ones to open. The

combination of these two flavours clears Heat at the Qi Level.
- **Gua Lou** resolves Phlegm-Heat.

The main difference between these two formulae is that the former is better at resolving Phlegm (and therefore used for profuse expectoration), while the latter is better to make Qi descend in the chest (and therefore used for a feeling of oppression in the chest).

(c) Prescription

GUN TAN WAN
Chasing away Phlegm Pill
Da Huang *Rhizoma Rhei* 15 g
Mang Xiao *Mirabilitum* 3 g
Huang Qin *Radix Scutellariae baicalensis* 15 g
Chen Xiang *Lignum Aquilariae* 3 g

Explanation

- **Da Huang** and **Mang Xiao** drain Fire by moving downwards.
- **Huang Qin** drains Lung-Fire.
- **Chen Xiang** has a strong sinking movement and makes Lung-Qi descend.

This is a strong formula for Lung-Fire as opposed to Lung-Heat. Although Heat and Fire are the same in nature, there are differences between them, the main one being that Heat is more superficial and less intense than Fire. This distinction is not very significant or important in acupuncture but it is crucial when herbal medicine is used. For Heat, one uses pungent-cold herbs (such as Shi Gao *Gypsum fibrosum*) to *clear it* by pushing it outwards. Fire is more intense and is knotted deep inside in the Interior of the body: one therefore *drains it* with bitter-cold herbs (such as Huang Qin *Radix Scutellariae baicalensis* or Long Dan Cao *Radix Gentianae scabrae*) and, if the stools are dry, with moving-downward herbs such as Da Huang *Rhizoma Rhei*. Some of the clinical manifestations of Heat and Fire overlap such as a feeling of heat, thirst, sweating, a red face, a Red tongue and a Rapid pulse. Fire, however, is more drying, affects the Mind more and may cause bleeding. Thus, in addition to the above manifestations, Fire also causes mental restlessness, dark urine, dry stools, very dry tongue coating, a bitter taste, dry mouth and a deeper pulse.

In this case, there is Lung-Fire as opposed to Lung-Heat and the manifestations would be: a barking cough with profuse yellow-purulent or blood-flecked expectoration, fever, constipation or dry stools, dark urine, a red face, dry mouth, mental restlessness, a Red tongue with a thick-dry-yellow or dark brown or even black coating and a Deep-Full and Rapid pulse. In such a case, clearing Heat is not enough; we need to drain Fire by moving downwards, which is what this formula does.

Variations

– To enhance the antitussive effect add Kuan Dong Hua *Flos Tussilaginis farfarae*, Sang Bai Pi *Cortex Mori albae radicis* and Xing Ren *Semen Pruni armeniacae*.

(i) Patent remedy

QING QI HUA TAN WAN
Clearing Qi and Resolving Phlegm Pill
Dan Nan Xing *Rhizoma Arisaematis praeparata*
Gua Lou *Semen Trichosanthis*
Huang Qin *Radix Scutellariae baicalensis*
Zhi Shi *Fructus Citri aurantii immaturus*
Chen Pi *Pericarpium Citri reticulatae*
Fu Ling *Sclerotium Poriae cocos*
Xing Ren *Semen Pruni armeniacae*
Ban Xia *Rhizoma Pinelliae ternatae*

Explanation

This pill has the same ingredients and functions as the homonymous prescription. It clears Lung-Heat and resolves Phlegm. It is ideal for acute Phlegm-Heat in the Lungs following an invasion of Wind-Heat.

The tongue presentation appropriate to this remedy is a Red tongue with a sticky-yellow coating; the tongue-body may be Red only in the front part.

(ii) Patent remedy

QING FEI YI HUO PIAN
Clearing the Lungs and Eliminating Fire Tablet

Huang Qin *Radix Scutellariae baicalensis*
Shan Zhi Zi *Fructus Gardeniae jasminoidis*
Da Huang *Rhizoma Rhei*
Qian Hu *Radix Peucedani*
Ku Shen *Radix Sophorae flavescentis*
Tian Hua Fen *Radix Trichosanthis*
Jie Geng *Radix Platycodi grandiflori*
Zhi Mu *Radix Anemarrhenae asphodeloidis*

Explanation

This tablet drains Lung-Fire (as opposed to clearing Lung-Heat) and is suitable to treat an acute cough following an invasion of Wind-Heat when there are symptoms of Fire such as a very dry tongue-coating, dry stools or constipation and a Deep-Full and Rapid pulse.

For a further explanation of the difference between Lung-Heat and Lung-Fire, see the discussion under the prescription Gun Tan Wan *Chasing away Phlegm Pill* above.

Case history

A 2-year-old girl had contracted an upper respiratory infection which had been treated with antibiotics. Her mother took her to me for treatment about one week into the antibiotic treatment as she was not getting better. Although the initial temperature had gone, she now had a barking cough productive of yellow sputum; she also wheezed slightly, was restless and slept badly. Her tongue had a sticky-yellow coating and was Red in the front part.

Diagnosis
This is a typical example of progression of an external pathogenic factor into the Interior due to treatment with antibiotics (see also ch. 34). The pathogenic factor is now interior Phlegm-Heat obstructing the Lungs.

Treatment
The treatment aim was to resolve Phlegm, clear Lung-Heat, restore the descending of Lung-Qi and stop cough and wheezing. She was treated only with herbal decoctions and the one used was a variation of Qing Qi Hua Tan Tang *Clearing Qi and Resolving Phlegm Decoction*:

Dan Nan Xing *Rhizoma Arisaematis praeparata* 3 g
Gua Lou *Semen Trichosanthis* 6 g
Huang Qin *Radix Scutellariae baicalensis* 4 g
Zhi Shi *Fructus Citri aurantii immaturus* 3 g
Chen Pi *Pericarpium Citri reticulatae* 3 g

Fu Ling *Sclerotium Poriae cocos* 6 g
Xing Ren *Semen Pruni armeniacae* 4 g
Ban Xia *Rhizoma Pinelliae ternatae* 6 g
Su Zi *Fructus Perillae frutescentis* 4 g
Sang Bai Pi *Cortex Mori albae radicis* 4 g
Kuan Dong Hua (honey-treated) *Flos Tussilaginis farfarae* 6 g

Explanation
- The first eight herbs constitute the Qing Qi Hua Tan Tang which resolves Phlegm and clears Lung-Heat.
- **Su Zi** and **Sang Bai Pi** were added to restore the descending of Lung-Qi.
- **Kuan Dong Hua**, especially good when honey-treated, restores the descending of Lung-Qi and stops cough.

The decoction was given to the little girl well diluted with water and mixed with some honey in small amounts throughout the day. She improved completely after one week. Her treatment was followed up with a decoction to tonify the Spleen and resolve Phlegm (the Liu Jun Zi Tang *Six Gentlemen Decoction*) in order to prevent any recurrence.

CHRONIC

Chronic cough may be of the Full or Empty type. The main patterns are:

EXCESS	DEFICIENCY
Damp-Phlegm	Lung-Qi Deficiency
Phlegm-Heat	Lung-Yin Deficiency
Phlegm-Fluids	Lung-Dryness
Liver-Fire	

The pathology of chronic coughs is characterized by involvement of other organs besides the Lungs. The organs involved for each pattern are as follows:

- Damp-Phlegm: Spleen-Qi or Spleen-Yang Deficiency
- Phlegm-Heat: Spleen-Qi Deficiency
- Phlegm-Fluids: Spleen- and Kidney-Yang Deficiency
- Liver-Fire insulting the Lungs: Liver-Fire
- Lung-Qi Deficiency: Spleen-Qi Deficiency
- Lung-Yin Deficiency: Kidney-Yin Deficiency
- Lung-Dryness: Stomach-Yin Deficiency.

EXCESS TYPE

1. DAMP-PHLEGM IN THE LUNGS

Clinical manifestations

Repeated attacks of cough, profuse expectoration of white-sticky sputum, breathlessness, worse in the mornings and after eating, a sensation of oppression in the chest, a feeling of fullness of the epigastrium, nausea, poor appetite, tiredness, a feeling of heaviness and loose stools.
Tongue: Pale or normal with a sticky-thick-white coating.
Pulse: Slippery.

Treatment principle

Dry Dampness, resolve Phlegm, tonify the Spleen, restore the descending of Lung-Qi and stop cough.

Acupuncture

LU-5 Chize, Ren-12 Zhongwan, Ren-9 Shuifen, ST-40 Fenglong, SP-6 Sanyinjiao, BL-20 Pishu, ST-36 Zusanli, BL-13 Feishu. Reinforcing method on ST-36, Ren-12 and BL-20, reducing method on the others. Moxa is applicable.

Explanation

- **LU-5** resolves Phlegm from the Lungs and restores the descending of Lung-Qi.
- **Ren-12**, **Ren-9**, **ST-40** and **SP-6** resolve Dampness and Phlegm.
- **BL-20** and **ST-36** tonify the Spleen to resolve Phlegm.
- **BL-13**, Back-Transporting point, is used for chronic patterns and restores the descending of Lung-Qi.

Herbal treatment

Prescription

ER CHEN TANG and SAN ZI YANG QIN TANG
Two Old Decoction and *Three-Seed Nourishing the Parents Decoction*
Ban Xia *Rhizoma Pinelliae ternatae* 15 g

Chen Pi *Pericarpium Citri reticulatae* 15 g
Fu Ling *Sclerotium Poriae cocos* 9 g
Zhi Gan Cao *Radix Glycyrrhizae uralensis prae-parata* 5 g
Sheng Jiang *Rhizoma Zingiberis officinalis recens* 3 g
Wu Mei *Fructus Pruni mume* 1 prune
Su Zi *Fructus Perillae frutescentis* 9 g
Bai Jie Zi *Semen Sinapis albae* 6 g
Lai Fu Zi *Semen Raphani sativi* 9 g

Explanation

– The Er Chen Tang is used to resolve Damp-Phlegm. Damp-Phlegm is characterized by profuse-sticky sputum and a feeling of oppression and heaviness of the chest.
– The formula San Zi Yang Qin Tang is used to resolve Cold Phlegm accompanied by retention of food. Cold Phlegm is characterized by watery-white sputum and a pronounced feeling of cold. Su Zi within this formula also restores the descending of Lung-Qi and stops cough.

This pattern nearly always occurs on a background of Spleen-Qi or Spleen-Yang deficiency. In such cases, it is necessary to add some Spleen tonics such as Bai Zhu *Rhizoma Atractylodis macrocephalae* and, if there is Spleen-Yang deficiency, Gan Jiang *Rhizoma Zingiberis officinalis*.

Variations

– To enhance the antitussive effect add Kuan Dong Hua *Flos Tussilaginis farfarae* and Xing Ren *Semen Pruni armeniacae*.
– In cases of pronounced Dampness add Cang Zhu *Rhizoma Atractylodis lanceae* and Hou Po *Cortex Magnoliae officinalis*.
– If there are symptoms of Cold Phlegm (see above) add Gan Jiang *Rhizoma Zingiberis officinalis* and Xi Xin *Herba Asari cum radice*.
– If there is a pronounced deficiency of the Spleen add Bai Zhu *Rhizoma Atractylodis macrocephalae* and Dang Shen *Radix Codonopsis pilosulae*.
– After the Phlegm has been successfully resolved, use the Liu Jun Zi Tang *Six Gentlemen Decoction* to consolidate the results by strengthening the Spleen.
– If the attacks of cough are elicited by frequent colds, add Huang Qi *Radix Astragali membranacei* and Fang Feng *Radix Ledebouriellae sesloidis*.

Patent remedy

ER CHEN WAN
Two Old Pill
Ban Xia *Rhizoma Pinelliae ternatae*
Chen Pi *Pericarpium Citri reticulatae*
Fu Ling *Sclerotium Poriae cocos*
Zhi Gan Cao *Radix Glycyrrhizae uralensis prae-parata*
Sheng Jiang *Rhizoma Zingiberis officinalis recens*
Wu Mei *Fructus Pruni mume*

Explanation

This well-known pill resolves Damp-Phlegm, i.e. Phlegm characterized by expectoration of profuse sticky-white sputum.

Please note that this pill only deals with the Manifestation (chronic Phlegm), and not with the Root, which is Spleen deficiency. In order to treat also the Root, this pill combines well with the Liu Jun Zi Wan *Six Gentlemen Pill* which tonifies Spleen-Qi and resolves Dampness.

The tongue presentation appropriate to this remedy is a white-sticky coating.

2. PHLEGM-HEAT IN THE LUNGS

Clinical manifestations

Repeated attacks of a barking cough with profuse expectoration of yellow or blood-flecked purulent sputum, breathlessness, rattling sound in the throat, a sensation of oppression in the chest, red face, tiredness, poor appetite, feeling of heat, dry mouth and thirst.
Tongue: Red with a sticky-yellow coating.
Pulse: Slippery and Rapid or Weak-Floating, slightly Slippery and Rapid.

This condition is similar to Phlegm-Heat cough at the acute stage. It differs from it in so far as it is a chronic condition occurring on a background of Spleen deficiency.

Treatment principle

Clear Heat, resolve Phlegm, tonify the Spleen, restore the descending of Lung-Qi and stop cough.

Acupuncture

LU-5 Chize, Ren-12 Zhongwan, Ren-9 Shuifen, ST-40 Fenglong, SP-6 Sanyinjiao, BL-20 Pishu, ST-36 Zusanli, BL-13 Feishu, Du-14 Dazhui and L.I.-11 Quchi. Reinforce Ren-12, BL-20, and ST-36; reduce all the others. No moxa.

Explanation

- **Du-14** and **L.I.-11** clear Heat.
- All the other points are the same as for Damp-Phlegm and have already been explained.

Herbal treatment

Prescription

QING JIN HUA TAN TANG
Clearing Metal and Resolving Phlegm Decoction
Huang Qin *Radix Scutellariae baicalensis* 9 g
Zhi Zi *Fructus Gardeniae jasminoidis* 6 g
Zhi Mu *Radix Anemarrhenae asphodeloidis* 6 g
Zhe Bei Mu *Bulbus Fritillariae thunbergii* 6 g
Gua Lou *Semen Trichosanthis* 9 g
Sang Bai Pi *Cortex Mori albae radicis* 6 g
Chen Pi *Pericarpium Citri reticulatae* 4.5 g
Fu Ling *Sclerotium Poriae cocos* 6 g
Jie Geng *Radix Platycodi grandiflori* 4.5 g
Mai Men Dong *Tuber Ophiopogonis japonici* 6 g
Gan Cao *Radix Glycyrrhizae uralensis* 3 g

Explanation

- **Huang Qin**, **Zhi Zi** and **Zhi Mu** clear Lung-Heat.
- **Bei Mu**, **Gua Lou** and **Sang Bai Pi** resolve Phlegm-Heat in the Lungs and restore the descending of Lung-Qi.
- **Chen Pi** and **Fu Ling** resolve Dampness which helps to resolve Phlegm.
- **Jie Geng** restores the descending of Lung-Qi and stops cough.

- **Mai Dong** nourishes Lung-Yin, to prevent injury of Lung-fluids from Heat.
- **Gan Cao** harmonizes.

Variations

- As there is nearly always a Spleen deficiency which produces Phlegm, add Bai Zhu *Rhizoma Atractylodis macrocephalae* and Dang Shen *Radix Codonopsis pilosulae*.
- If there is purulent sputum add Dan Nan Xing *Rhizoma Arisaematis praeparata*, Yi Yi Ren *Semen Coicis lachryma jobi* and Dong Gua Ren *Semen Benincasae hispidae*.
- If there is a pronounced feeling of oppression in the chest and constipation add Da Huang *Rhizoma Rhei*.
- If the Heat part of Phlegm-Heat has begun to injure fluids add Nan Sha Shen *Radix Adenophorae*, Tian Men Dong *Tuber Asparagi cochinchinensis* and Tian Hua Fen *Radix Trichosanthis*.

Case history

An 80-year-old woman had been suffering from a persistent cough for 5 years. The cough was productive of scanty-sticky yellow sputum and she experienced a sensation of oppression of the chest. Her health was otherwise very good: she was a keen practitioner and teacher of Yoga. Her body was thin and her skin was dry. Her pulse was slightly Floating-Empty in general and slightly Slippery on the Lung position. Her tongue was Red, dry, and without coating in the front part (Plate 8.1).

Diagnosis
This is a case of retention of Phlegm-Heat in the Lungs on a background of Lung-Yin deficiency. The Phlegm-Heat is indicated by the sticky-yellow sputum and Slippery pulse quality on the Lung position, while the Lung-Yin deficiency is apparent from the thin body, the dry skin, the Floating-Empty pulse and the Red tongue without coating in the front part (Lung area).

Treatment
The treatment principle adopted was to resolve Phlegm, clear Heat, nourish Lung-Yin and clear Lung Empty-Heat. She was treated with herbs only and the decoction used was a variation of Qing Jin Hua Tan Tang *Clearing Metal and Resolving Phlegm Decoction*:

Huang Qin *Radix Scutellariae baicalensis* 6 g
Zhi Zi *Fructus Gardeniae jasminoidis* 4 g
Zhi Mu *Radix Anemarrhenae asphodeloidis* 6 g
Zhe Bei Mu *Bulbus Fritillariae thunbergii* 6 g

Gua Lou *Semen Trichosanthis* 9 g
Sang Bai Pi *Cortex Mori albae radicis* 4 g
Chen Pi *Pericarpium Citri reticulatae* 4.5 g
Fu Ling *Sclerotium Poriae cocos* 6 g
Jie Geng *Radix Platycodi grandiflori* 4.5 g
Mai Men Dong *Tuber Ophiopogonis japonici* 6 g
Gan Cao *Radix Glycyrrhizae uralensis* 3 g
Tian Men Dong *Tuber Asparagi cochinchinensis* 6 g
Kuan Dong Hua (honey-treated) *Flos Tussilaginis farfarae* 9 g
Di Gu Pi *Cortex Lycii chinensis radicis* 4 g

Explanation

The original formula was used as a whole since it corresponds well to the treatment aim of resolving Phlegm, clearing Heat and restoring the descending of Lung-Qi.

– **Tian Men Dong** was added to nourish Lung-Yin.
– **Kuan Dong Hua** was added to restore the descending of Lung-Qi and stop cough.
– **Di Gu Pi** was added to clear Lung Empty-Heat.

This patient made a complete recovery after 3 months of taking herbal decoctions along similar lines as the one above.

(i) Patent remedy

QING QI HUA TAN WAN
Clearing Qi and Resolving Phlegm Pill
Dan Nan Xing *Rhizoma Arisaematis praeparata*
Gua Lou *Semen Trichosanthis*
Huang Qin *Radix Scutellariae baicalensis*
Zhi Shi *Fructus Citri aurantii immaturus*
Chen Pi *Pericarpium Citri reticulatae*
Fu Ling *Sclerotium Poriae cocos*
Xing Ren *Semen Pruni armeniacae*
Ban Xia *Rhizoma Pinelliae ternatae*

Explanation

This pill, which has already been explained under acute cough from Phlegm-Heat, may be used also for a chronic cough from the same cause.

This pill deals only with the Manifestation (Phlegm-Heat) and not the Root which is Spleen-Qi deficiency.

The tongue presentation appropriate to this remedy is a Red body with a sticky-yellow coating.

(ii) Patent remedy

CHUAN BEI PI PA GAO
Fritillaria-Eriobotrya Syrup

Pi Pa Ye *Folium Eriobotryae japonicae*
Chuan Bei Mu *Bulbus Fritillariae cirrhosae*
Nan Sha Shen *Radix Adenophorae*
Wu Wei Zi *Fructus Schisandrae chinensis*
Chen Pi *Pericarpium Citri reticulatae*
Jie Geng *Radix Platycodi grandiflori*
Ban Xia *Rhizoma Pinelliae ternatae*
Bo He *Herba Menthae*
Kuan Dong Hua *Flos Tussilaginis farfarae*
Xing Ren *Semen Pruni armeniacae*
Feng Mi *Mel*

Explanation

This syrup may be used for chronic cough from Phlegm-Heat. It is sweet-tasting and readily accepted by children.

(iii) Patent remedy

QI GUAN YAN KE SOU TAN CHUAN WAN
Bronchial Cough, Phlegm and Dyspnoea Pill
Qian Hu *Radix Peucedani*
Xing Ren *Semen Pruni armeniacae*
Yuan Zhi *Radix Polygalae tenuifoliae*
Sang Ye *Folium Mori albae*
Chuan Bei Mu *Bulbus Fritillariae cirrhosae*
Chen Pi *Pericarpium Citri reticulatae*
Pi Pa Ye *Folium Eriobotryae japonicae*
Kuan Dong Hua *Flos Tussilaginis farfarae*
Dang Shen *Radix Codonopsis pilosulae*
Ma Dou Ling *Fructus Aristolochiae*
Wu Wei Zi *Fructus Schisandrae chinensis*
Sheng Jiang *Rhizoma Zingiberis officinalis recens*
Da Zao *Fructus Ziziphi jujubae*

Explanation

This pill also treats chronic cough from Phlegm-Heat and is suitable for a more chronic condition.

3. PHLEGM-FLUIDS IN THE LUNGS

Clinical manifestations

Cough with a low sound and expectoration of white-watery-dilute sputum, a feeling of cold, a sensation of oppression in the chest, tiredness, poor appetite and low spirits.

Tongue: Pale with a sticky-white coating.
Pulse: Weak-Floating and slightly Slippery.

Treatment principle

Drain Dampness, resolve Phlegm, scatter Cold, tonify the Spleen and Kidneys and stop cough.

Acupuncture

LU-5 Chize, Ren-12 Zhongwan, Ren-9 Shuifen, ST-40 Fenglong, SP-6 Sanyinjiao, BL-20 Pishu, ST-36 Zusanli, BL-13 Feishu, Du-4 Mingmen, BL-23 Shenshu, BL-22 Sanjiaoshu. Reinforcing method on ST-36, Ren-12, BL-20, Du-4 and BL-23, reducing method on the others. Moxa is applicable.

Explanation

With acupuncture, the treatment of Phlegm-Fluids is not very different from that of Damp-Phlegm outlined above.

- **Du-4** and **BL-23** are reinforced with moxa if there is a Kidney-Yang deficiency.
- **BL-22** is reduced to promote the transformation of fluids and therefore resolve Phlegm.
- All the other points have been explained under Damp-Phlegm.

Herbal treatment

Prescription

LING GAN WU WEI JIANG XIN TANG
Poria-Glycyrrhiza-Schisandra-Zingiber-Asarum Decoction
Fu Ling *Sclerotium Poriae cocos* 12 g
Gan Jiang *Rhizoma Zingiberis officinalis* 9 g
Xi Xin *Herba Asari cum radice* 6 g
Wu Wei Zi *Fructus Schisandrae chinensis* 6 g
Gan Cao *Radix Glycyrrhizae uralensis* 3 g

Explanation

- **Fu Ling**, **Gan Jiang** and **Xi Xin** resolve Cold Phlegm and Phlegm-Fluids.
- **Wu Wei Zi** is sour and absorbing and

moderates the scattering effect of Gan Jiang and Xi Xin.
- **Gan Cao** harmonizes and also moderates the scattering effect of Gan Jiang and Xi Xin.

Variations

- This condition is very chronic and occurs on a background of Spleen-Yang deficiency and often Kidney-Yang deficiency. In such cases one should add herbs to tonify Spleen- and Kidney-Yang such as Bai Zhu *Rhizoma Atractylodis macrocephalae*, Huang Qi *Radix Astragali membranacei*, Yin Yang Huo *Herba Epimedii* and Du Zhong *Cortex Eucommiae ulmoidis*.
- If there are very pronounced symptoms of Cold add Fu Zi *Radix Aconiti carmichaeli praeparata*. However, in such a case, one must be absolutely sure that there is no Heat anywhere in the body as the three herbs Gan Jiang, Xi Xin and Fu Zi are very hot, pungent and scattering.
- To enhance the antitussive effect add Su Zi *Fructus Perillae frutescentis*, Xuan Fu Hua *Flos Inulae* and Xing Ren *Semen Pruni armeniacae*.

4. LIVER-FIRE INSULTING THE LUNGS

Clinical manifestations

Sudden bouts of cough with a red face often elicited by emotional stress, dry throat, a feeling of phlegm in the throat, expectoration of scanty phlegm, hypochondrial pain and distension, pain on coughing, bitter taste, dark urine, dry stools, irritability and a dry mouth.
Tongue: Red with redder sides, dry-yellow coating.
Pulse: Wiry and Rapid.

Treatment principle

Clear the Lungs, clear Liver-Fire, restore the descending of Lung-Qi and stop cough.

Acupuncture

LIV-2 Xingjian, G.B.-34 Yanglingquan, L.I.-11

Quchi, LU-5 Chize, LU-1 Zhongfu, Ren-17 Shanzhong, G.B.-21 Jianjing.

Explanation

- **LIV-2** clears Liver-Fire.
- **G.B.-34** pacifies the Liver and eliminates stagnation from the hypochondrial region and chest.
- **L.I.-11** clears Heat.
- **LU-5** and **LU-1** clear Lung-Heat and restore the descending of Lung-Qi.
- **Ren-17** subdues rebellious Qi in the chest and restores the descending of Lung-Qi.
- **G.B.-21** subdues rebellious Qi and makes Qi descend.

Herbal treatment

Prescription

XIE BAI SAN Variation and DAI GE SAN
Draining Whiteness Powder and *Indigo-Concha Cyclinae Powder*
Sang Bai Pi *Cortex Mori albae radicis* 9 g
Di Gu Pi *Cortex Lycii chinensis radicis* 6 g
Zhi Mu *Radix Anemarrhenae asphodeloidis* 6 g
Huang Qin *Radix Scutellariae baicalensis* 6 g
Gan Cao *Radix Glycyrrhizae uralensis* 3 g
Jie Geng *Radix Platycodi grandiflori* 4.5 g
Qing Pi *Pericarpium Citri reticulatae viridae* 4.5 g
Chen Pi *Pericarpium Citri reticulatae* 4.5 g
Qing Dai *Indigo naturalis* 6 g
Hai Ge Ke *Concha Cyclinae sinensis* 12 g
Long Dan Cao *Radix Gentianae scabrae* 6 g

Explanation

- **Sang Bai Pi**, **Di Gu Pi**, **Zhi Mu**, **Huang Qin**, and **Gan Cao** clear Lung-Heat, restore the descending of Lung-Qi and stop cough.
- **Jie Geng**, **Qing Pi** and **Chen Pi** resolve Phlegm and subdue rebellious Qi.
- **Qing Dai**, **Hai Ge Ke** and **Long Dan Cao** resolve Phlegm-Heat and clear Liver-Fire.

Variations

- If symptoms of Heat are pronounced add Zhi Zi *Fructus Gardeniae jasminoidis* and Mu Dan Pi *Cortex Moutan radicis*.
- If there is a lot of Phlegm and severe cough add Zhu Ru *Caulis Bambusae in Taeniis*, Su Zi *Fructus Perillae frutescentis* and Pi Pa Ye *Folium Eriobotryae japonicae*.
- If there is severe cough and other symptoms of rebellious Qi (such as fullness of the chest) add Zhi Shi *Fructus Citri aurantii immaturus* and Xuan Fu Hua *Flos Inulae*.
- If there is chest pain add Yu Jin *Tuber Curcumae*.
- If Fire has begun to injure fluids add Nan Sha Shen *Radix Adenophorae*, Mai Men Dong *Tuber Ophiopogonis japonici* and Tian Hua Fen *Radix Trichosanthis*.

(i) Patent remedy

QING FEI YI HUO PIAN
Clearing the Lungs and Eliminating Fire Tablet
Huang Qin *Radix Scutellariae baicalensis*
Shan Zhi Zi *Fructus Gardeniae jasminoidis*
Da Huang *Rhizoma Rhei*
Qian Hu *Radix Peucedani*
Ku Shen *Radix Sophorae flavescentis*
Tian Hua Fen *Radix Trichosanthis*
Jie Geng *Radix Platycodi grandiflori*
Zhi Mu *Radix Anemarrhenae asphodeloidis*

Explanation

This tablet, already explained under Lung-Fire, can be used for chronic cough from Liver-Fire insulting the Lungs as some of the herbs it contains enter the Liver.

It should be remembered that it can be used only for Lung-Fire (not Lung-Heat) with such symptoms as a very dry-yellow tongue coating, dry stools or constipation, intense thirst, dark urine and a Deep-Full and Rapid pulse.

(ii) Patent remedy

LONG DAN XIE GAN WAN
Gentiana Draining the Liver Pill
Long Dan Cao *Radix Gentianae scabrae*
Huang Qin *Radix Scutellariae baicalensis*
Shan Zhi Zi *Fructus Gardeniae jasminoidis*

Ze Xie *Rhizoma Alismatis orientalis*
Mu Tong *Caulis Akebiae*
Che Qian Zi *Semen Plantaginis*
Sheng Di Huang *Radix Rehmanniae glutinosae praeparata*
Dang Gui *Radix Angelicae sinensis*
Chai Hu *Radix Bupleuri*
Gan Cao *Radix Glycyrrhizae uralensis*

Explanation

This pill can be used for chronic cough from Liver-Fire insulting the Lungs, but it should be noted that it deals only with one part of the condition, i.e. Liver-Fire and it does not contain any herb that restores the descending of Lung-Qi or stops cough.

The tongue presentation appropriate to this remedy is a Red body with redder and swollen sides and a sticky-yellow coating. The sides may also have red points.

DEFICIENCY TYPE

1. LUNG-QI DEFICIENCY

Clinical manifestations

Slight cough with low sound, no phlegm, spontaneous sweating, propensity to catching cold, weak voice, tiredness and pale face.
Tongue: Pale.
Pulse: Empty.

Treatment principle

Tonify Lung-Qi and restore the descending of Lung-Qi.

Acupuncture

LU-9 Taiyuan, BL-13 Feishu, BL-43 Gaohuangshu, Ren-12 Zhongwan, ST-36 Zusanli, SP-6 Sanyinjiao. Reinforcing method, moxa is applicable.

Explanation

- **LU-9** and **BL-13** tonify Lung-Qi and stop cough.

- **BL-43** nourishes Lung-Yin and is specific for chronic Lung problems.
- **Ren-12**, **ST-36** and **SP-6** tonify both Stomach and Lungs (since the Lung channel starts in the Middle Burner).

Herbal treatment

Prescription

BU FEI TANG
Tonifying the Lungs Decoction
Ren Shen *Radix Ginseng* 9 g
Huang Qi *Radix Astragali membranacei* 12 g
Shu Di Huang *Radix Rehmanniae glutinosae praeparata* 12 g
Wu Wei Zi *Fructus Schisandrae chinensis* 6 g
Zi Wan *Radix Asteris tatarici* 9 g
Sang Bai Pi *Cortex Mori albae radicis* 6 g

Explanation

- **Ren Shen**, **Huang Qi**, **Shu Di Huang** and **Wu Wei Zi** tonify Lung-Qi.
- **Zi Wan** and **Sang Bai Pi** restore the descending of Lung-Qi and stop cough.

Patent remedy

PING CHUAN WAN
Calming Breathlessness Pill
Dang Shen *Radix Codonopsis pilosulae*
Dong Chong Xia Cao *Sclerotium Cordicipitis chinensis*
Ge Jie *Gecko*
Xing Ren *Semen Pruni armeniacae*
Chen Pi *Pericarpium Citri reticulatae*
Gan Cao *Radix Glycyrrhizae uralensis*
Sang Bai Pi *Cortex Mori albae radicis*
Bai Qian *Radix et Rhizoma Cynanchii stautoni*
Meng Shi *Lapis Chloritis*
Wu Zhi Mao Tao *Radix Fici simplicissimae*
Man Hu Tui Zi *Semen Elaeagni glabrae thunbergii*

Explanation

This pill tonifies Lung- and Spleen-Qi and Kidney-Yang and restores the descending of Lung-Qi.

It can therefore be used as a long-term treatment for chronic cough from Lung- and Spleen-Qi deficiency. It should be used for several months. If there is Phlegm, it can be combined with the Er Chen Wan *Two Old Pill*.

2. *LUNG-YIN DEFICIENCY*

Clinical manifestations

Dry cough in short bursts and with a low sound, no phlegm or scanty phlegm, blood-flecked sputum, dry throat, feeling of heat in the evening, 5-palm heat, night sweating, thin body, extreme tiredness.
Tongue: Red without coating, dry, Lung cracks.
Pulse: Floating-Empty.

Treatment principle

Nourish Lung-Yin, moisten the Lungs, clear Empty-Heat if necessary, restore the descending of Lung-Qi and stop cough.

Acupuncture

LU-9 Taiyuan, LU-10 Yuji, Ren-12 Zhongwan, LU-1 Zhongfu, ST-36 Zusanli, SP-6 Sanyinjiao, LU-7 Lieque and KI-6 Zhaohai. All with reinforcing method except for LU-10 which should be reduced. No moxa.

Explanation

- **LU-9** and **LU-1** nourish Lung-Yin.
- **LU-10** clears Lung Empty-Heat.
- **Ren-12**, **ST-36** and **SP-6** tonify the Spleen to nourish the Lungs.
- **LU-7** and **KI-6** in combination open the Directing Vessel, benefit the throat, nourish Lung-Yin, restore the descending of Lung-Qi and stop cough from Lung-Yin deficiency.

Herbal treatment

Prescription

SHA SHEN MAI DONG TANG
Glehnia-Ophiopogon Decoction
Bei Sha Shen *Radix Glehniae littoralis* 9 g

Mai Men Dong *Tuber Ophiopogonis japonici* 9 g
Yu Zhu *Rhizoma Polygonati odorati* 6 g
Tian Hua Fen *Radix Trichosanthis* 4.5 g
Sang Ye *Folium Mori albae* 4.5 g
Bian Dou *Semen Dolichoris lablab* 4.5 g
Gan Cao *Radix Glycyrrhizae uralensis* 3 g

Explanation

- **Bei Sha Shen** and **Mai Men Dong** nourish Lung-Yin.
- **Yu Zhu** and **Tian Hua Fen** nourish fluids and clear Empty-Heat.
- **Sang Ye** benefits the throat, restores the descending of Lung-Qi and stops cough.
- **Bian Dou** tonifies Spleen-Yin to tonify Lung-Yin (strengthens Earth to tonify Metal).
- **Gan Cao** harmonizes.

Variations

- To enhance the antitussive effect add Zhe Bei Mu *Bulbus Fritillariae thunbergii* and Xing Ren *Semen Pruni armeniacae*.
- If there are pronounced symptoms of Empty-Heat in the Lungs add Di Gu Pi *Cortex Lycii chinensis radicis* and Qing Hao *Herba Artemisiae apiaceae*.
- If there is sweating at night add Wu Mei *Fructus Pruni mume* and Fu Xiao Mai *Semen Tritici aestivi levis*.
- If there is some scanty yellow sputum add Hai Ge Ke *Concha Cyclinae sinensis* and Huang Qin *Radix Scutellariae baicalensis*.
- If there is blood in the sputum add charred Zhi Zi *Fructus Gardeniae jasminoidis*, Mu Dan Pi *Cortex Moutan radicis* and Bai Mao Gen *Rhizoma Imperatae cylindricae*.

(i) *Patent remedy*

LI FEI WAN
Benefiting the Lungs Pill
Dong Chong Xia Cao *Sclerotium Cordicipitis chinensis*
Ge Jie *Gecko*
Bai He *Bulbus Lilii*
Wu Wei Zi *Fructus Schisandrae chinensis*
Bai Ji *Rhizoma Bletillae striatae*

Bai Bu *Radix Stemonae*
Mu Li *Concha Ostreae*
Pi Pa Ye *Folium Eriobotryae japonicae*
Gan Cao *Radix Glycyrrhizae uralensis*

Explanation

This pill tonifies Lung-Yin and Lung-Qi and stimulates the Kidney's grasping of Qi. It is suitable for chronic cough from Lung-Yin deficiency when the Kidneys are also deficient and fail to grasp Qi.

The tongue presentation for the use of this remedy is a slightly Red body in the front part, but with coating.

(ii) Patent remedy

YANG YIN QING FEI TANG JIANG
Nourishing Yin and Clearing the Lungs Syrup
Mu Dan Pi *Cortex Moutan radicis*
Zhe Bei Mu *Bulbus Fritillariae thunbergii*
Bai Shao *Radix Paeoniae albae*
Xuan Shen *Radix Scrophulariae ningpoensis*
Sheng Di Huang *Radix Rehmanniae glutinosae*
Mai Men Dong *Tuber Ophiopogonis japonici*
Gan Cao *Radix Glycyrrhizae uralensis*
Bo He *Herba Menthae*

Explanation

This syrup is more Yin-nourishing than the previous remedy. This remedy nourishes Lung-Yin and clears Lung Empty-Heat. The main sign pointing to the use of this remedy, apart from a chronic cough from Lung-Yin deficiency and Empty-Heat, is a tongue which is Red, dry and without coating in the front part.

(iii) Patent remedy

BA XIAN CHANG SHOU WAN
Eight Immortals Longevity Pill
Mai Men Dong *Tuber Ophiopogonis japonici*
Wu Wei Zi *Fructus Schisandrae chinensis*
Shu Di Huang *Radix Rehmanniae glutinosae praeparata*
Shan Yao *Radix Dioscoreae oppositae*
Shan Zhu Yu *Fructus Corni officinalis*
Ze Xie *Rhizoma Alismatis orientalis*

Fu Ling *Sclerotium Poriae cocos*
Mu Dan Pi *Cortex Moutan radicis*

Explanation

This well-known pill nourishes Lung- and Kidney-Yin. It is therefore suitable for chronic cough from deficiency of both Lung- and Kidney-Yin, especially in old people. The tongue presentation is a Red body which is dry, cracked and without coating.

3. LUNG-DRYNESS

Clinical manifestations

Dry cough with a low sound, dry throat and mouth.
Tongue: Dry.
Pulse: Floating-Empty.

This is a condition of Dryness of the Lungs but without all the symptoms of Yin deficiency. It is a state that often precedes Yin deficiency. It often occurs in people with a predisposition to Lung deficiency who, through their work, need to use their voice a lot (such as teachers). In such cases it is usually associated with a deficiency of Stomach-Yin as the Stomach is the origin of fluids.

This pattern may also arise following an invasion of Wind-Heat when this dries the Lung-fluids and leads to Dryness with some residual Heat or Phlegm-Heat in the Lungs. It is manifested with a very dry and ticklish cough immediately following an invasion of Wind-Heat. The cough is very persistent and is worse at night.

Treatment principle

Moisten the Lungs, restore the descending of Lung-Qi and stop cough.

Acupuncture

LU-9 Taiyuan, LU-10 Yuji, Ren-12 Zhongwan, LU-1 Zhongfu, ST-36 Zusanli, SP-6 Sanyinjiao, LU-7 Lieque and KI-6 Zhaohai. All with reinforcing method except for LU-10 which should be reduced. No moxa.

Explanation

These points are the same as for Lung-Yin deficiency and have already been explained above.

Herbal treatment

(a) Prescription

SHA SHEN MAI DONG TANG
Glehnia-Ophiopogon Decoction

Explanation

This formula has already been explained above.

(b) Prescription

SHENG MAI SAN
Generating the Pulse Powder
Ren Shen *Radix Ginseng* 9 g
Mai Men Dong *Tuber Ophiopogonis japonici* 9 g
Wu Wei Zi *Fructus Schisandrae chinensis* 3 g

Explanation

This formula is for Qi and Yin deficiency of the Lungs.

- **Ren Shen** tonifies Lung-Qi and generates fluids.
- **Mai Men Dong** and **Wu Wei Zi** nourish Lung-Yin and promote fluids.

Variations

- To enhance the antitussive effect add Sang Bai Pi *Cortex Mori albae radicis* and Zi Wan *Radix Asteris tatarici*.

(c) Prescription

QING ZAO JIU FEI TANG
Clearing Dryness and Rescuing the Lungs Decoction
Sang Ye *Folium Mori albae* 9 g
Shi Gao *Gypsum fibrosum* 7.5 g
Mai Men Dong *Tuber Ophiopogonis japonici* 3.6 g
Ren Shen *Radix Ginseng* 2 g
Hu Ma Ren (Hei Zhi Ma) *Semen Sesami indici* 3 g
E Jiao *Gelatinum Asini* 2.4 g
Xing Ren *Semen Pruni armeniacae* 2 g

Pi Pa Ye *Folium Eriobotryae japonicae* 3 g
Gan Cao *Radix Glycyrrhizae uralensis* 3 g

Explanation

- **Sang Ye** restores the descending of Lung-Qi and stops cough.
- **Shi Gao** clears any residual Lung-Heat.
- **Mai Dong** nourishes and moistens Lung-Yin. These first three herbs "clear within descending"(i.e. Shi Gao and Sang Ye) and "moisten within clearing" (i.e. Mai Dong and Shi Gao).
- **Ren Shen** tonifies Lung-Qi and promotes fluids.
- **Hei Zhi Ma** and **E Jiao** help Mai Dong to moisten Dryness.
- **Xing Ren** and **Pi Pa Ye** help Sang Ye to restore the descending of Lung-Qi. Pi Pa Ye also clears any residual Lung-Heat.
- **Gan Cao** harmonizes.

This formula is for Dryness and residual Heat in the Lungs following an invasion of Wind-Heat. The cough is completely dry, without phlegm.

(d) Prescription

BEI MU GUA LOU SAN
Fritillaria-Trichosanthes Powder
Chuan Bei Mu *Bulbus Fritillariae cirrhosae* 5 g
Gua Lou *Semen Trichosanthis* 3 g
Tian Hua Fen *Radix Trichosanthis* 2.5 g
Fu Ling *Sclerotium Poriae cocos* 2.5 g
Chen Pi *Pericarpium Citri reticulatae* 2.5 g
Jie Geng *Radix Platycodi grandiflori* 2.5 g

Explanation

- **Chuan Bei Mu** restores the descending of Lung-Qi, stops cough and resolves Phlegm-Heat.
- **Gua Lou** resolves Phlegm-Heat and relieves fullness in the chest.
- **Tian Hua Fen** promotes fluids and moistens dryness.
- **Fu Ling** and **Chen Pi** help to resolve Phlegm.
- **Jie Geng** restores the descending of Lung-Qi and stops cough.

This formula is also for Dryness and residual Heat in the Lungs following an invasion of Wind-Heat, but with the addition of some Phlegm. The cough is therefore dry but with some scanty and sticky phlegm which is difficult to expectorate. This situation arises because Wind-Heat may, on the one hand, dry fluids and lead to Dryness and, on the other hand, it condenses fluids into Phlegm.

Patent remedy

QIU LI GAO
Autumn Pear Syrup
Qiu Li *Fructus Pyri*
Mai Men Dong *Tuber Ophiopogonis japonici*
Zhe Bei Mu *Bulbus Fritillariae thunbergii*
Ou Jie *Nodus Nelumbinis neciferae rhizomatis*
Qing Luo Bo *Green turnip*

Explanation

This syrup nourishes and moistens the Lungs. It is specific for Lung-Dryness leading to chronic cough. It contains pear juice which moistens the Lungs. Drinking a decoction of (organic) pear skin also moistens the Lungs and soothes a cough from Dryness.

Prognosis

Both acupuncture and Chinese herbs give excellent results in the treatment of cough. Obviously acute cough, whether it is external or internal, is easier and quicker to treat. Coughs from acute respiratory infections can be cleared in a few days at the Defensive-Qi or Qi level, and it is not necessary to take antibiotics which often only lead to residual Heat.

Chronic coughs are also relatively easy to treat: the most difficult one is that from Lung-Yin deficiency which may take some months to clear. Of all the patterns appearing with a chronic cough, Chinese herbs give better results in the patterns of Damp-Phlegm, Phlegm-Heat, Phlegm-Fluids and Lung-Yin deficiency.

Western differentiation

The following are the main causes of cough from the perspective of Western Medicine.

TRACHEITIS

This usually occurs following an invasion of Wind-Heat (upper respiratory infection). The cough is harsh and painful and the throat and trachea feel very raw and sore. It is usually worse at night.

From a Chinese perspective, this broadly corresponds to Lung-Dryness following an invasion of Wind-Heat.

ACUTE BRONCHITIS

This usually follows an upper respiratory infection and the cough is loose with expectoration of yellow, green or purulent sputum. The temperature and pulse are raised.

From the point of view of Chinese medicine, this broadly corresponds to the Qi Level with Phlegm-Heat in the Lungs.

CHRONIC BRONCHITIS

This is usually the consequence of repeated bouts of acute bronchitis. It is more frequent in smokers over 40.

The cough is productive of white, yellow or blood-flecked sputum.

From a Chinese perspective, this corresponds to either Damp-Phlegm or Phlegm-Heat in the Lungs on a background of Spleen deficiency.

WHOOPING COUGH

This occurs in children, mostly under 5. It starts like an ordinary cold with a cough. After a week, the characteristic "whoop" appears. The cough comes in bouts which are worse at night and are very distressing. The coughing bouts often end in vomiting. The child is flushed or cyanosed and looks frightened.

Chinese medicine can alleviate the symptoms and shorten the course of this disease, but it requires very many treatments given every day.

In the beginning stage it corresponds to invasion of Wind-Heat, in the middle stage to Lung-Heat, and in the recovery stage to Stomach- and Lung-Yin deficiency possibly with some residual Heat.

PLEURISY

This consists in inflammation of the pleura, usually occurring after an upper respiratory infection. The cough is unproductive and distressingly painful. There is also chest pain and the temperature is raised.

From the point of view of Chinese medicine it corresponds to Lung Phlegm-Heat at the Qi level.

PNEUMONIA

This consists in inflammation of the lung alveoli. It may begin abruptly with shivering, a headache, a high temperature and breathlessness. The cough is short and unproductive at first. It then develops scanty sputum which is viscid, rust-coloured and blood-flecked. Pneumonia is nearly always accompanied by pleurisy which causes chest pain. The temperature is high, the patient is flushed, the pulse and the breathing are rapid. There may also be moving of the alae nasi.

From the Chinese point of view it corresponds to Lung-Heat at the Qi level.

CARCINOMA OF THE BRONCHI

This is the most common cancer of all. It occurs more in males between 40 and 55. It is characterized by a dry cough, breathlessness and a deep-seated thoracic pain. There may be some scanty, blood-flecked sputum. The patient is weak, debilitated and lacks appetite.

From the Chinese point of view it corresponds, in its late stage, to Lung-Yin deficiency.

TB OF THE LUNGS

This is an uncommon disease but it is on the increase both in the UK and the USA. It is more frequent between the ages of 15 and 45. The cough is dry or with a scanty, blood-flecked sputum. There is also a chest pain, breathlessness and night-sweating. The patient is also very tired and debilitated and may have a low-grade fever in the afternoons.

From the Chinese point of view, this is a typical condition of Lung-Yin deficiency with Empty-Heat.

BRONCHIECTASIS

This consists in permanent dilatation of bronchi and/or bronchioles. The alveoli become distended and filled with mucus.

The cough occurs more in the mornings and is productive of large amounts of sputum which is purulent and has a "fruity" odour. The breath is offensive after a bout of coughing. During acute episodes there is a temperature.

From the point of view of Chinese medicine, it may broadly correspond to the pattern of "Turbid Phlegm in the Lungs" in "Breathlessness" (*Chuan*).

HEART DISEASE

In the elderly, cough may also occur with heart disease. A cough at night which is productive of a very watery, white and frothy sputum may indicate impending left ventricular failure. On the other hand, left ventricular failure may also cause pulmonary embolism manifesting with a sudden, severe chest pain with dyspnoea and followed by a cough with blood-stained sputum.

END NOTES

---

1. Liu Wan Su 1186 A Collection of Life-Saving Pathologies from the Simple Questions (*Su Wen Bing Ji Qi Yi Bao Ming Ji* 素问病机气宜保命集), p. 215
2. 1979 the Yellow Emperor's Classic of Internal Medicine

— Simple Questions (*Huang Ti Nei Jing Su Wen* 黄帝内经素问), People's Health Publishing House, Beijing. First published c. 100 BC, p. 150.

3. Ibid., p. 215.
4. Ibid., pp. 215–16.
5. Ibid., p. 214.
6. Ibid., p. 216.
7. Zhang Jing Yue 1986 Complete Book of Jing Yue (*Jing Yue Quan Shu* 景岳全书), Shanghai Scientific Publishing House, Shanghai, p. 336. First published 1624.
8. Simple Questions, p. 74.
9. He Ren 1981 A New Explanation of the Essential Prescriptions of the Golden Chest (*Jin Gui Yao Lue Xin Jie* 金匮要略新解), Zhejiang Science Publishing House, p. 56. The "Essential Prescriptions of the Golden Chest" itself was written by Zhang Zhong Jing and first published c. AD 220.
10. Complete Book of Jing Yue, p. 336.

Mental-emotional problems 9

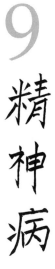

精
神
病

A discussion of the treatment of mental and emotional problems is not possible without first exploring the concept of the mind in Chinese medicine. It is only by understanding the concept of mind and spirit in Chinese culture that we can truly grasp how to treat psychological and emotional problems with acupuncture and Chinese herbs. All too often Chinese concepts of "mind" and "spirit" are mistakenly interpreted in terms of Western (and often Christian) concepts of "mind" and "spirit". The discussion of the treatment of mental-emotional problems will be centred around the following subjects:

– The nature of the Mind in Chinese medicine
– The 5 mental-spiritual aspects of a human being
– The effect of the emotions on the Mind and Spirit
– Aetiology of mental-emotional problems
– Diagnostic signs in mental-emotional problems
– Pathology and treatment of mental-emotional problems
– Prevention of mental-emotional problems.

Nature of the Mind in Chinese medicine

The Mind (*Shen*) is one of the vital substances of the body. It is the most subtle and non-material type of Qi. The word *Shen* is often translated as "spirit" in Western acupuncture books and schools; for reasons which will be clearer as the discussion progresses, I believe "Mind" is a more accurate translation, while what we would call "spirit" in the West is the complex of all five mental-spiritual aspects of a human being, i.e. Ethereal Soul (*Hun*), Corporeal Soul (*Po*), Intellect (*Yi*), Will-Power (*Zhi*) and the Mind (*Shen*) itself.

The word *Shen* is used in the Yellow Emperor's Classic of Internal Medicine with many different meanings. The two main meanings which concern us are the following:

1. *Shen* indicates the activity of thinking, consciousness, insight and memory, all of

which depend on the Heart. I translate this as "Mind".

2. *Shen* indicates the complex of all five mental-spiritual aspects of a human being, i.e. the Mind itself, the Ethereal Soul, the Corporeal Soul, the Intellect and the Will-Power. I translate this as "Spirit".

There is another meaning to the word *Shen* which is frequently mentioned in relation to diagnosis. In this context the word *shen* indicates an undefinable and subtle quality of "life", "flourishing", or "glitter" which can be observed in health. This quality applies to the complexion, the eyes, the tongue and the pulse, as will be explained below.

What is then the Chinese view of the Mind? As explained above, the Mind, like other vital substances, is a form of Qi; in fact, the most subtle and non-material type of Qi. One of the most important characteristics of Chinese medicine is the close integration of body and Mind which is highlighted by the integration of Essence (*Jing*), Qi and Mind, called the "Three Treasures".

The Essence is the origin and biological basis of the Mind. The "Spiritual Axis" in chapter 8 says: *"Life comes about through the Essence; when the two Essences [of mother and father] unite, they form the Mind"*.[1] Zhang Jie Bin says: *"The two Essences, one Yin, one Yang, unite . . . to form life; the Essences of mother and father unite to form the Mind"*.[2]

Therefore the Mind of a newly-conceived being comes from the Pre-natal Essences of its mother and father. After birth, its Pre-natal Essence is stored in the Kidneys and it provides the biological foundation for the Mind. The life and Mind of a newly-born baby, however, also depend on the nourishment from its own Post-natal Essence. The "Spiritual Axis" in chapter 30 says: *"When the Stomach and Intestines are coordinated the 5 Yin organs are peaceful, Blood is harmonized and mental activity is stable. The Mind derives from the refined essence of water and food."*[3] Thus the Mind draws its basis and nourishment from the Pre-natal Essence stored in the Kidneys and the Post-natal Essence produced by Lungs, Stomach and Spleen. Hence the Three Treasures:

MIND   = HEART
QI   = LUNGS-STOMACH-SPLEEN
ESSENCE   = KIDNEYS

These Three Treasures represent three different states of condensation of Qi, the Essence being the densest, Qi the more rarefied, and the Mind the most subtle and non-material. The activity of the Mind relies on the Essence and Qi as its fundamental basis. Hence the Essence is said to be the "foundation of the body and the root of the Mind". Thus if Essence and Qi are strong and flourishing the Mind will be happy, balanced and alert. If Essence and Qi are depleted, the Mind will suffer and may become unhappy, depressed, anxious, or clouded. Zhang Jie Bin says: *"If the Essence is strong, Qi flourishes; if Qi flourishes, the Mind is whole"*.[4]

However, the state of the Mind also affects Qi and Essence. If the Mind is disturbed by emotional stress, becoming unhappy, depressed, anxious, or unstable, it will definitely affect Qi and/or the Essence. In most cases it will affect Qi first since all emotional stress upsets the normal functioning of Qi. Emotional stress will tend to weaken the Essence either when it is combined with overwork and/or excessive sexual activity, or when the Fire generated by long-term emotional tensions injures Yin and Essence.

Of all the organs, the Mind is most closely related to the Heart which is said to be the "residence" of the Mind. The "Simple Questions" in chapter 8 says: *"The Heart is the Monarch and it governs the Mind. . ."*.[5] The "Spiritual Axis" in chapter 71 says: *"The Heart is the Monarch of the 5 Yin organs and 6 Yang organs and it is the residence of the Mind"*.[6]

The "Mind" residing in the Heart or Heart-Mind is responsible for many different mental activities including:

thinking	sleep
memory	intelligence
consciousness	wisdom
insight	ideas
cognition.	

In addition to these, the Heart-Mind is also responsible for hearing, sight, touch, taste and smell. Of course many of the above activities are also carried out by other organs and there often is an overlap between the functions of various organs. For example, although the Heart-Mind is mainly responsible for memory, the Spleen and Kidneys also play a role.

Let us now briefly look at the above functions in more detail.

Thinking depends on the Mind. If the Mind is strong, thinking will be clear. If the Mind is weak or disturbed, thinking will be slow and dull. The Chinese characters for "thought" (*yi*), "to think" (*xiang*) and "pensiveness" (*si*) all have the character for "heart" as their radical.

Memory has two different meanings. On the one hand it indicates the capacity of memorizing data when one is studying or working. On the other hand, it refers to the ability to remember past events. Both of these depend on the Mind and therefore the Heart, although also on the Spleen and Kidneys.

Consciousness indicates the totality of thoughts and perceptions as well as the state of being conscious. In the first sense, the Mind is responsible for the recognition of thoughts, perceptions and feelings. In the latter sense, when the Mind is clear, we are conscious; if the Mind is obfuscated or suddenly depleted, we lose consciousness.

Insight indicates our capacity of self-knowledge and self-recognition. We are subjected to many different emotional stimuli, perceptions, feelings and sensations and all of these are perceived and recognized by the Mind. With regard to emotions, in particular, only the Mind (and therefore the Heart) can "feel" them. Of course emotions definitely affect all the other organs too, but it is only the Mind that actually recognizes and feels them. For example, anger affects the Liver, but the Liver cannot feel it because it does not store the Mind. Only the Heart can feel it because it stores the Mind which is responsible for insight. It is for this reason that all emotions eventually affect the Heart (in addition to other specific organs), and it is in this sense that the Heart is the "emperor" of all the other organs.

Cognition indicates the activity of the Mind in perceiving and conceiving in reaction to stimuli.

Sleep is dependent on the state of the Mind. If the Mind is calm and balanced, a person sleeps well. If the Mind is restless, the person sleeps badly.

Intelligence also depends on the Heart and the Mind. A strong Heart and Mind will make a person intelligent and bright. A weak Heart and Mind will render a person slow and dull. It should be remembered, however, that the Essence, and therefore heredity, plays a role in determining a person's intelligence.

Wisdom derives from a strong Heart and a healthy Mind. As the Mind is responsible for knowing and perceiving, it also gives us the sagacity to apply this knowledge critically and wisely.

Ideas are another function of the Mind. The Heart and Mind are responsible for our ideas, our projects and the dreams which give our lives purpose.

Thus if the Heart is strong and the Mind healthy, a person can think clearly, memory is good, the state of consciousness and insight are sharp, the cognition is clear, sleep is sound, intelligence is bright, ideas flow easily and he or she acts wisely. If the Heart is affected and the Mind weak or disturbed, a person is unable to think clearly, memory is poor, the consciousness is clouded, insight is poor, sleep is restless, intelligence is lacking, ideas are muddled and he or she acts unwisely.

Most of the above functions of the Mind are attributed to the brain in Western medicine. During the course of development of Chinese medicine too there have been doctors who attributed mental functions to the brain rather than the Heart: in particular, Sun Si Miao of the Tang dynasty, Zhao You Qin of the Yuan dynasty, Li Shi Zhen of the Ming dynasty and especially Wang Qing Ren of the Qing dynasty.

As the Heart controls all mental activities of the Mind and is responsible for insight and cognition, which other organs do not have, this is another reason that it is the "emperor" of the organs. For this reason, the Heart is also called the "root of life" as in chapter 9 of the "Simple

Questions": *"The Heart is the root of life and the origin of mental life . . ."*.[7] Apart from the above mental functions, the Mind also plays a role in the senses of sight, hearing, smell, taste and touch.

The eyes and sight are obviously related to the Liver, especially Liver-Blood, and the Ethereal Soul. The book "The Essence of the Convergence between Chinese and Western Medicine" (1892) says: *"When the Ethereal Soul swims to the eyes they can see"*.[8] However, although the eyes rely on the nourishment from Liver-Blood, blood flows to the eyes through blood vessels which are under the control of the Heart. On the other hand, the Mind "gathers" the Ethereal Soul and, in this way, it has an influence on sight. The "Simple Questions" says in chapter 10: *"Blood vessels influence the eyes"*.[9] In fact, the "Simple Questions" also lists excessive use of the eyes as harmful to the blood vessels and Heart. It says in chapter 23: *"Excessive use of the eyes injures Blood [i.e. the Heart]"*.[10] Ren Ying Qiu in "Theories of Chinese Medicine Doctors" says: *"The Heart governs the Mind . . . sight is a manifestation of the activity of the Mind"*.[11] Wang Ken Tang in "Standards of Diagnosis and Treatment" (1602) says: *"The eye is an orifice of the Liver . . . but a function of the Heart"*.[12] From the point of view of channels, both the Heart main and connecting channels flow to the eye.

Hearing depends on the Kidneys but the Heart also has an influence on it in so far as it brings Qi and Blood to the ears. The "Simple Questions" in chapter 4 says: *"The colour of the Southern direction is red, it is related to the Heart which opens into the ears . . ."*.[13] Some types of tinnitus are due to Heart-Qi being deficient and not reaching the ears.

The sense of smell is also dependent on the Heart and Mind besides the Lungs. The "Simple Questions" in chapter 11 says: *"The five odours enter the nose and are stored by Lungs and Heart; if Lungs and Heart are diseased, the nose cannot smell"*.[14] The "Classic of Difficulties" in chapter 14 says: *"The nose pertains to the Lungs but its function depends on the Heart"*.

The sense of taste naturally depends on the Heart and Mind as the tongue is an offshoot of the Heart.

The sense of touch is also dependent on the Heart and Mind as this is responsible for the cognition and organization of external stimuli sensations.

To sum up, all sensations of sight, hearing, smell, taste and touch depend on the Mind in much the same way as they depend on the brain in Western medicine.

The five mental-spiritual aspects

As we have just seen, the Mind, and therefore the Heart, plays a pivotal and leading role in all mental activities. Yu Chang in "Principles of Medical Practice" (1658) says: *"The Mind of the Heart gathers and unites the Ethereal Soul and the Corporeal Soul and it combines the Intellect and the Will-Power"*.[15] However, all other organs also play roles in mental activities, very often overlapping with that of the Heart. In particular, the Yin organs are more directly responsible for mental activities. Each Yin organ "houses" a particular mental-spiritual aspect of a human being. These are:

> Mind (*Shen*) — Heart
> Ethereal Soul (*Hun*) — Liver
> Corporeal Soul (*Po*) — Lungs
> Intellect (*Yi*) — Spleen
> Will-Power (*Zhi*) — Kidneys

The "Simple Questions" in chapter 23 says: *"The Heart houses the Mind, the Lungs house the Corporeal Soul, the Liver houses the Ethereal Soul, the Spleen houses the Intellect and the Kidneys house the Will-Power"*.[16] In chapter 9 it says:

The Heart is the root of life and the origin of the Mind . . . the Lungs are the root of Qi and the dwelling of the Corporeal Soul . . . the Kidneys are the root of sealed storage [Essence] and the dwelling of Will-Power . . . the Liver is the root of harmonization and the residence of the Ethereal Soul . . . .[17]

The commentary to chapter 23 of the "Simple Questions", also based on passages from the "Spiritual Axis", says:

The Mind is a transformation of Essence and Qi:

both Essences [i.e. the Pre-natal and Post-natal Essences] contribute to forming the Mind. The Corporeal Soul is the assistant of the Essence and Qi: it is close to Essence but it moves in and out. The Ethereal Soul complements the Mind and Qi: it is close to the Mind but it comes and goes. The Intellect corresponds to memory: it is the memory which depends on the Heart. The Will-Power is like a purposeful and focused mind: the Kidneys store Essence . . . and through the Will-Power they can fulfil our destiny.[18]

These five aspects together form the "Spirit" which is also called "Shen" or sometimes the "Five Shen" in the old classics. The five Yin organs are the residences of "Shen" i.e. the Spirit, and they are sometimes also called the "Five-Shen residences" as in chapter 9 of the "Simple Questions".[19]

The 5 Yin organs are the physiological basis of the Spirit. The indissoluble relationship between them is well known to any acupuncturist. The state of Qi and Blood of each organ can influence the Mind or Spirit and, conversely, alterations of the Mind or Spirit will affect one or more of the internal organs.

We can now discuss the five mental-spiritual aspects one by one.

THE ETHEREAL SOUL (*HUN*)

The Ethereal Soul broadly corresponds to our Western concept of "soul" or "spirit". According to ancient Chinese beliefs it enters the body shortly after birth. Ethereal in nature, after death it survives the body and flows back to "Heaven" (*Tian*); this is the ancient Chinese concept of "Heaven", i.e. a state of subtle and non-material energies and beings, and has therefore nothing to do with the Western and Christian concept of "Heaven". The Ethereal Soul can be described as *"that part of the Soul [as opposed to Corporeal Soul] which at death leaves the body, carrying with it an appearance of physical form"*.[20]

The Chinese character for Ethereal Soul is as follows:

This is composed of the following parts:

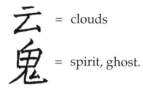

= clouds

= spirit, ghost.

The ancient form of this last radical is:

This is itself composed of two parts:

是 is a head without body

是 is a swirling movement.

This ancient radical therefore depicts the bodiless head of a dead person flowing to Heaven in a swirling movement or swimming in the realm of spirits and ghosts with a swirling movement.

The combination of the two characters for "cloud" and "spirit" in the character for Ethereal Soul conveys the idea of its nature: it is like a spirit but it is Yang and ethereal in nature and essentially harmless, i.e. it is not one of the evil spirits (hence the presence of the "cloud" radical).

There are three types of Ethereal Soul: a vegetative one common to plants, animals and human beings; an animal one common to animals and human beings; and a human one which is present only in human beings.

Zhang Jie Bin in the "Classic of Categories" says: *"The Mind and Ethereal Soul are Yang . . . the Ethereal Soul follows the Mind; if the Mind is unconscious the Ethereal Soul is swept away"*.[21] It also says: *"The Mind corresponds to Yang within Yang, the Ethereal Soul corresponds to Yin within Yang"*.[22] The "Spiritual Axis" in chapter 8 says: *"The Ethereal Soul is the coming and going of the Mind"*.[23] The concept of Ethereal Soul is closely linked to ancient Chinese beliefs in spirits, ghosts and demons. According to these beliefs, spirits, ghosts and demons are spirit-like creatures who preserve a physical appearance and wander in the world of spirit. Some are good and some are evil. In the times prior to the Warring States period (476–221 BC), such spirits were considered to be the main cause of disease. Since the Warring States period, a belief in naturalistic causes of disease (such as weather) gradually came to the fore; however, the belief in spirits has never really disappeared, even to the present day.

What is the Ethereal Soul then and what does it do? It is basically another level of consciousness, different from the Mind but closely related to it. The Ethereal Soul is rooted in the Liver and in particular Liver-Yin (which includes Liver-Blood). If Liver-Yin is depleted, the Ethereal Soul is deprived of its residence and becomes rootless. This can result in insomnia, timidity, fear and a lack of a sense of direction in life. The Ethereal Soul, deprived of its residence, wanders without aim.

The nature and functions of the Ethereal Soul can be summarized under seven headings.

1. SLEEP AND DREAMING

The Ethereal Soul influences sleep and dreaming, including day-dreaming. Zhang Jie Bin says in the "Classic of Categories": *"Absent-mindedness as if in a trance is due to the Ethereal Soul wandering outside its residence"*.[24] Thus if Liver-Blood or Liver-Yin is deficient, the Ethereal Soul wanders off in a day-dream and the person has no sense of purpose or direction in life. On the other hand, the Ethereal Soul is also responsible for "dreaming" in a positive sense, i.e. having a sense of purpose in life and "dreams" in the sense of goals. One of the main features of depression is precisely the lack of direction, purpose and the absence of dreams and goals in one's life.

The length and quality of sleep are also related to the state of the Ethereal Soul. If this is well rooted in the Liver (Liver-Blood or Liver-Yin), sleep is normal and sound and without too many dreams. If Liver-Yin or Liver-Blood is deficient, the Ethereal Soul is deprived of its residence and wanders off at night, causing a restless sleep with many tiring dreams. Tang Zong Hai says: *"At night during sleep the Ethereal Soul returns to the Liver; if the Ethereal Soul is not peaceful there are a lot of dreams"*.[25] In such cases it is necessary to nourish Liver-Yin with sour and

absorbing herbs such as Mu Li *Concha Ostreae*, Long Chi *Dens Draconis*, Suan Zao Ren *Semen Ziziphi spinosae* or Bai Shao *Radix Paeoniae albae*. There is an interesting correlation between the astringent and absorbing quality of such herbs on a physical level and their use in calming the Mind and "absorbing" the Ethereal Soul to draw it back into the Liver.

Of course, the length and quality of sleep also depend on the state of Heart-Blood and there is an overlap between the influence of Heart-Blood and Liver-Blood on sleep.

2. MENTAL ACTIVITIES

The Ethereal Soul assists the Mind in its mental activities. The "Five-Channel Righteousness", a text from the Tang dynasty, says: *"Knowledge is dependent on the sharpness of the Ethereal Soul"*.[26] The Ethereal Soul provides the Mind, which is responsible for rational thinking, with intuition and inspiration. It also gives the Mind "movement" in the sense that it allows the Mind the capacity of self-insight and introspection as well as the ability to project outwards and relate to other people. This capacity for movement and outward projection is closely related to the Liver-Qi quality of quick and free movement.

It will be remembered that the words "movement", "coming and going", "swimming" are often used in connection with the Ethereal Soul. For example, as mentioned above, the Ethereal Soul is the *"coming and going of the Mind"*, or *"when the Ethereal Soul swims to the eyes, they can see"*. It is interesting to compare this quality of the Ethereal Soul, on an ethereal level, with the swirling movement of a spirit depicted in its old character and, on a physical level, with the smooth flow of Liver-Qi.

3. BALANCE OF EMOTIONS

The Ethereal Soul is responsible for maintaining a normal balance between excitation and restraint of the emotional life, under the leadership of the Heart and the Mind. Emotions are a normal part of our mental life: we all experience anger, sadness, worry, or fear on occasion in the course of our life and these do not normally lead to disease. The Ethereal Soul, being responsible for the more intuitive and subconscious part of the Mind, plays a role in keeping an emotional balance and, most of all, prevents the emotions from becoming excessive and therefore turning into causes of disease. This regulatory function of the Ethereal Soul is closely related to the balance between Liver-Blood (the Yin part of the Liver) and Liver-Qi (the Yang part of the Liver). Liver-Blood and Liver-Qi need to be harmonized and Liver-Blood must root Liver-Qi to prevent it from becoming stagnant or rebelling upwards. On a mental-emotional level, Liver-Blood needs to root the Ethereal Soul thus allowing a balanced and happy emotional life. This is one of the meanings, on a mental level, of the Liver being a "regulating and harmonizing" organ. Chapter 9 of the "Simple Questions" says: *"The Liver has a regulating function [lit. is the root of stopping extremes], it houses the Ethereal Soul . . ."*.[27] If Liver-Blood is deficient there will be fear and anxiety; if Liver-Yang is in excess there will be anger. The "Spiritual Axis" in chapter 8 says: *"If the Liver is deficient there will be fear; if it is in excess there will be anger"*.[28] Tang Zong Hai in the "Discussion on Blood Diseases" says: *"If Liver-Blood is deficient Fire agitates the Ethereal Soul resulting in nocturnal emissions with dreams"*.[29]

4. EYES AND SIGHT

The Ethereal Soul is in relation with the eyes and sight. Tang Zong Hai says: *"When the Ethereal Soul wanders to the eyes, they can see"*.[30] This connection with the eyes can be easily related to the rooting of the Ethereal Soul in Liver-Blood. On a mental level, the Ethereal Soul gives us "vision" and insight.

5. COURAGE

The Ethereal Soul is related to courage or cowardice and for this reason the Liver is sometimes called the "resolute organ". Tang Zong Hai says: *"When the Ethereal Soul is not strong, the person*

is timid".[31] The "strength" of the Ethereal Soul in this connection derives mainly from Liver-Blood. If Liver-Blood is abundant, the person is fearless and is able to face up to life's difficulties with an indomitable spirit. Just as in disease Liver-Yang easily flares upwards causing anger, in health the same type of mental energy deriving from Liver-Blood can give a person great creative drive and resoluteness. If Liver-Blood is deficient and the Ethereal Soul is dithering, the person lacks courage and resolve, cannot face up to difficulties or making decisions, and is easily discouraged. A vague feeling of fear at night before falling asleep is also due to a lack of rooting of the Ethereal Soul.

6. PLANNING

The Ethereal Soul influences our capacity for planning our life and giving it a sense of direction. A lack of direction in life and a sense of spiritual confusion may be compared to the wandering of the Ethereal Soul alone in space and time. If the Liver is flourishing the Ethereal Soul is firmly rooted and can help us to plan our life with vision, wisdom and creativity. If Liver-Blood (or Liver-Yin) is deficient, the Ethereal Soul is not rooted and we lack a sense of direction and vision in life. If Liver-Yin is very depleted, at times the Ethereal Soul may even leave the body temporarily at night during or just before sleep. Those who suffer from severe deficiency of Yin may experience a floating sensation in the few moments just before falling asleep: this is said to be due to the "floating" of the Ethereal Soul not rooted in Yin.

7. RELATIONSHIP WITH MIND

It is important to consider the relationship between the Mind and the Ethereal Soul. They are closely connected and both partake in all the mental activities of a human being. We have already seen that the Ethereal Soul is described as the "coming and going" of the Mind. This means that, through the Ethereal Soul, the Mind can project outwards to the external world and to other people and can also turn inwards to receive the intuition, inspiration, dreams and images deriving from the unconscious. Thus if Liver-Blood is abundant and the Ethereal Soul firm, there will be a healthy flow from it to the Mind providing it with inspiration. If, however, the Ethereal Soul is not rooted in the Liver, it may lack movement and inspiration and the person may be depressed, without aim or dreams.

The Mind is also said to "gather" the Ethereal Soul. Thus, on the one hand, the Ethereal Soul brings movement to the Mind, and on the other hand, the Mind provides some stillness and holds the Ethereal Soul together. If the Mind is strong and the Ethereal Soul properly "gathered", there will be harmony between the two and the person has calm vision, insight and wisdom. If the Mind is weak and fails to restrain the Ethereal Soul, this may be too restless and only bring confusion and chaos to the Mind, making the person scattered and unsettled. This can be observed in some people who are always full of ideas, dreams and projects none of which ever comes to fruition because of the chaotic state of the Mind which is therefore unable to restrain the Ethereal Soul.

While the Mind and Ethereal Soul are closely connected, there are some differences between the two. The main difference is that the Ethereal Soul pertains to the world of Image, i.e. non-material existence, to which it returns after death, whilst the Mind is the individual mind of a human being which dies with the person. The role of the Ethereal Soul can be observed in the phenomena of guided day-dreams, coma and sleep-walking.

Guided day-dreams are a technique used in psychotherapy whereby the therapist sets a certain scene for the client who is asked to imagine himself or herself in that scene and to proceed as if in a dream. The aim of this exercise is to by-pass the critical analysis of the Mind and bring forth psychological material from the Ethereal Soul as happens in dreams.

In coma, the Mind is completely devoid of residence and it therefore cannot function at all, and yet the person is not dead. This means that there are other mental aspects at play, and

these are the Ethereal Soul and the Corporeal Soul. Thus, for death to occur, not only must the Mind die, but the Ethereal Soul must leave the body and the Corporeal Soul return to Earth.

Sleep-walking, during which the Mind is inactive but the Ethereal Soul is active, is due to the Ethereal Soul wandering at night as happens in dreams. In fact, the point BL-47 Hunmen (the "Door of the Ethereal Soul") was used for sleep-walking.

Finally, drawing from Buddhist and Jungian ideas, the Mind could be said to be the individual Mind, and the Ethereal Soul the link between the individual and Universal Mind. This can be represented with two diagrams illustrating the same concept in two different ways (Fig. 9.1).

The Universal Mind is the repository of images, archetypes, symbols and ideas belonging to the collective unconscious. These often manifest to our Mind as myths, symbols and dreams. They come into our consciousness (individual Mind) via the Ethereal Soul since this belongs to the world of Image and ideas. Thus the Ethereal Soul is the vehicle through which images, ideas

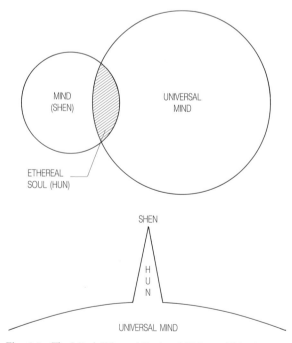

Fig. 9.1　The Mind, Ethereal Soul and Universal Mind

and symbols from the Universal Mind (or collective unconscious) emerge into our individual Mind (conscious). This shows the vital importance of the Ethereal Soul for our mental and spiritual life. Without the Ethereal Soul, our mental and spiritual life would be quite sterile and deprived of images, ideas and dreams. If the Liver is strong and the Ethereal Soul firm and flowing harmoniously, ideas and images from the Universal Mind will flow freely and the mental and spiritual state will be happy, creative and fruitful. If the Ethereal Soul is unsettled, the individual Mind will be cut off from the Universal Mind and will be unhappy, confused, isolated, aimless, sterile and without dreams. On the other hand, if the Mind is disabled, contents breaking through from the Ethereal Soul cannot be integrated by it. It is important for the Mind to assume an integrating position towards the Ethereal Soul so that images, symbols and dreams coming from it can be assimilated. If not, the Mind may be flooded by the contents of the Ethereal Soul with risk of obstruction of the Mind and, in serious cases, psychosis.

According to Jung the unconscious is compensatory to consciousness. He said: *"The psyche is a self-regulating system that maintains itself in equilibrium . . . Every process that goes too far immediately and inevitably calls forth a compensatory activity."*[32] This compensatory relationship between the unconscious and consciousness resembles the balancing relationship between the Ethereal Soul and the Mind.

THE CORPOREAL SOUL

The Corporeal Soul resides in the Lungs and is the physical counterpart of the Ethereal Soul. Its Chinese character is based on the same radical *Gui* which means "spirit" or "ghost"

The character for Corporeal Soul is:

This is composed of the radical *Gui* for spirit or ghost:

and the character for "white":

白

The Corporeal Soul can be defined as *"that part of the Soul [as opposed to the Ethereal Soul] which is indissolubly attached to the body and goes down to Earth with it at death"*.[33] It is closely linked to the body and could be described as the somatic expression of the Soul, or, conversely, the organizational principle of the body. Zhang Jie Bin says:

In the beginning of an individual's life the body is formed; the spirit of the body is the Corporeal Soul. When the Corporeal Soul is in the Interior there is [enough] Yang Qi.[34]

There are seven types of Corporeal Soul: the 5 senses, the limbs and the Corporeal Soul as a whole. The link between the five senses and the Corporeal Soul will be explained shortly. As for movement, the Corporeal Soul gives the body the capacity of movement, agility, balance and coordination of movements.

1. CORPOREAL SOUL AND ESSENCE

The Corporeal Soul is closely linked to the Essence and is described in the "Spiritual Axis" chapter 8 as the *"exiting and entering of Essence"*.[35] It derives from the mother and arises soon after the Pre-natal Essence of a newly-conceived being is formed. It could be described as the manifestation of the Essence in the sphere of sensations and feelings. Just as the Ethereal Soul provides movement to the Mind (*"coming and going of the Mind"*), the Corporeal Soul provides movement to the Essence, i.e. it brings the Essence into play in all physiological processes of the body. Without the Corporeal Soul the Essence would be an inert, albeit precious, vital substance. The Corporeal Soul is the closest to the Essence and is the intermediary between it and the other vital substances of the body. In fact Zhang Jie Bin in the "Classic of Categories" says: *"If the Essence is exhausted the Corporeal Soul declines, Qi is scattered and the Ethereal Soul swims without a residence"*.[36]

The relationship between Corporeal Soul and

Essence also explains the eruption of atopic eczema and asthma in babies. From the Chinese point of view, eczema in babies is due to the surfacing of toxic Heat from the uterus: it is therefore closely linked with the Pre-natal Essence of the baby. Since the Essence is related to the Corporeal Soul which manifests on the skin (with itching and pain), the toxic Heat from the uterus erupts on the baby's skin in the form of eczema. Asthma can be explained in the same way as the deficient Essence of the baby fails to root its Corporeal Soul and therefore its Lungs.

2. INFANCY

The Corporeal Soul, being the closest to the Essence, is responsible for the first physiological processes after birth. Zhang Jie Bin says: *"In the beginning of life ears, eyes and Heart perceive, hands and feet move and breathing starts: all this is due to the sharpness of the Corporeal Soul".*[37]

3. SENSES

Later in life, the Corporeal Soul gives us the capacity of sensation, feeling, hearing and sight. When the Corporeal Soul is flourishing ears and eyes are keen and can register. The decline of hearing and sight in old people is due to a weakening of the Corporeal Soul.

Zhang Jie Bin says: *"The Corporeal Soul can move and do things and [when it is active] pain and itching can be felt"*. This shows that the Corporeal Soul is responsible for sensations and itching and is therefore closely related to the skin through which such sensations are experienced. This explains the somatic expression on the skin of emotional tensions which affect the Corporeal Soul via the Mind and the connection between Corporeal Soul, Lungs and skin. In fact, the Corporeal Soul, being closely related to the body, is the first to be affected when needles are inserted: the almost immediate feeling of relaxation following the insertion of needles is due to the unwinding of the Corporeal Soul. Through it, the Mind, Ethereal Soul, Intellect and Will-Power are all affected.

4. EMOTIONS

The Corporeal Soul is also related to weeping and crying. Just as the Corporeal Soul makes us feel pain on a physical level, it also makes us cry and weep when subject to grief and sadness.

5. PHYSIOLOGICAL ACTIVITIES

Some modern doctors consider the Corporeal Soul the *"basic regulatory activity of all physiological functions of the body"*.[38] In this sense it is the manifestation of the Lung function of regulating all physiological activities.

6. BREATHING

Residing in the Lungs, the Corporeal Soul is closely linked to breathing. Breathing can be seen as the pulsating of the Corporeal Soul. Meditation makes use of the link between breathing and the Corporeal Soul. By concentrating on the breathing, someone who is meditating quietens the Corporeal Soul, the Mind becomes still and empty, and through this the Ethereal Soul becomes open and gets in touch with the universal Mind.

7. CORPOREAL SOUL AND INDIVIDUAL LIFE

The Corporeal Soul is related to our life as individuals while the Ethereal Soul is responsible for our relations with other people. Just as the Lung's Defensive-Qi protects the body from external pathogenic factors on a physical level, on a mental level the Corporeal Soul protects the individual from external psychic influences. Some people are very easily affected by negative influences: this is due to a weakness of the Corporeal Soul.

8. RELATIONSHIP BETWEEN CORPOREAL AND ETHEREAL SOULS

Since the Ethereal Soul and Corporeal Soul

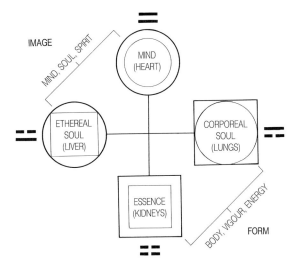

Fig. 9.2 The Ethereal Soul and Corporeal Soul

Restlessness at night with excessive dreaming is due to an unsettled Ethereal Soul; this is Yang and if at night it has no resting place the person is restless and dreams a lot. Restlessness in the daytime and a clouded Mind are due to an unsettled Corporeal Soul; this is Yin and if Yin is deficient in daytime, restlessness and mental confusion result.[40]

The Ethereal Soul pertains to the realm of Image and the Corporeal Soul to that of Form. This can be represented with a diagram (Fig. 9.2).

9. ANUS

Because of the relationship between Corporeal Soul and Lungs and between these and the Large Intestine, the anus is sometimes called *po men*, the "door of the Corporeal Soul" as in chapter 11 of the "Simple Questions": *"The door of the Corporeal Soul [i.e. anus] is the messenger for the five viscera and it drains off water and food without storing them for too long".*[41] In fact, the point BL-42 Pohu (the "Window of the Corporeal Soul") was indicated for incontinence of both urine and faeces from fright.

THE INTELLECT

The Intellect resides in the Spleen and is respon-

are two aspects of the soul, it is interesting to compare and contrast their various characteristics and functions (Table 9.1). Most of these are derived from Zhang Jie Bin's "Classic of Categories".[39]

As can be seen from Table 9.1, the Ethereal Soul is involved in problems occurring at night (although not exclusively), and the Corporeal Soul in problems occurring in daytime. The "Discussion of Blood Diseases" (1884) by Tang Zong Hai says:

Table 9.1 Comparison of Ethereal Soul and Corporeal Soul

Ethereal Soul	Corporeal Soul
Is the "coming and going of the Mind"	Is the "entering and exiting of the Essence"
Pertains to the Mind	Pertains to the body
Is the Qi of the Mind	Is the spirit of the body
Follows the changes of Qi	Follows the changes of the body
Is Yang and moves	Is Yin and is quiescent
Creates action with movement	Creates action without movement
Related to the Mind: when Qi gathers, the Ethereal Soul gathers	Related to the Essence: when this gathers, the Corporeal Soul gathers
At birth the Ethereal Soul joins with the Corporeal Soul	At birth the Corporeal Soul restrains the Ethereal Soul
At death it swims away and returns to Heaven	At death it dissolves and returns to Earth
Is bright and it lights the Corporeal Soul	Is dark and it roots the Ethereal Soul
Is like a fire: the more things you add, the more it burns	Is like a mirror: it shines, but holds only a reflection (of the Ethereal Soul)
Represents the movement of the Mind outwardly	Represents the movement of the Essence inwardly
Is rooted in Blood and Yin	Is connected to Qi and Yang
Disharmony causes problems with sleep at night	Disharmony causes problems in daytime
Disharmony causes lack of direction and inspiration, confusion	Disharmony causes lack of vigour and vitality
It is the link with the universal Mind	It is purely individual
Corresponds to full moon	Corresponds to new moon

sible for applied thinking, studying, memorizing, focusing, concentrating and generating ideas. The Post-natal Qi and Blood are the physiological basis for the Intellect. Thus if the Spleen is strong, thinking will be clear, memory good and the capacity for concentrating, studying and generating ideas will also be good. If the Spleen is weak, the Intellect will be dull and thinking will be slow, memory poor and the capacity for studying, concentrating and focusing will all be weak.

In the sphere of thinking, remembering and memorizing there is considerable overlap between the Intellect (Spleen), the Mind (Heart) and the Will-Power (Kidneys). The main differentiating factor is that the Spleen is specifically responsible for memorizing data in the course of one's work or study. For example, it is not uncommon for someone to have a brilliant memory in his or her field of study or research, and yet be quite forgetful in daily life. The Heart and Kidneys also naturally contribute to this function, but they are also responsible for the memory of past events, whether recent or long-past. In particular, the overlap between the Intellect and the Mind in thinking activity is very close, so much so that the "Spiritual Axis" says in chapter 8: *The Heart function of recollecting is called Intellect*.[42] In turn, the memorizing function of the Intellect is so closely related to the Will-Power that the same chapter continues: *The storing [of data] of the Intellect is called Will-Power [Zhi]*.[43] It should be noted here that I translate the mental aspect of the Kidneys *Zhi* as Will-Power although it also has the meaning of "memory" or "mind".

THE WILL-POWER

The word *Zhi* has at least three meanings:

1. it indicates "memory"
2. it means will power
3. it is sometimes used to indicate the "five *Zhi*", i.e. the five mental aspects Mind, Ethereal Soul, Corporeal Soul, Intellect and Will-Power itself.

So as to avoid confusion between "Mind" (of the Heart), "Intellect" (of the Spleen) and "Memory" (of the Kidneys), I translate "Zhi" as Will-Power, bearing in mind that it also includes the meaning of "memory" and capacity of memorizing and recollecting.

In this sense, the Kidneys influence our capacity for memorizing and storing data. Some of the ancient doctors even said that the Intellect (of the Spleen) and the memory (of the Kidneys) are almost the same thing, except that the Intellect is responsible for memorizing and the memory of the Kidneys is responsible for the storing of data over the long term. Tang Zong Hai says: *Memory [Zhi] indicates Intellect with a capacity for storing [data]*.[44]

In the second sense, the Kidneys house Will-Power which indicates drive, determination, single-mindedness in the pursuit of goals and motivation. Zhang Jie Bin says in the "Classic of Categories": *When one thinks of something, decides on it and then acts on it, this is called Will-Power [Zhi]*.[45]

Thus if the Kidneys are strong, the Will-Power is strong and the person will have drive and determination in the pursuit of goals. If the Kidneys are depleted and the Will-Power weakened, the person will lack drive and initiative, will be easily discouraged and swayed from his or her aims. A deficiency of the Kidneys and Will-Power is an important aspect of chronic depression.

The Will-Power must be coordinated with the Mind, just as, on a physiological level, the Kidneys and Heart must communicate. The Will-Power is the basis for the Mind and the Mind directs the Will-Power. If the Mind is clear in its aims and plans, and the Will-Power is strong, then the person will have the drive to pursue goals. Thus it is necessary for both Will-Power and Mind to be strong. The Mind may be clear in its objectives, but if the Will-Power is weak, the person will have no drive to realize such objectives. Conversely, the Will-Power may be strong, but if the Mind is confused, the force of Will-Power will only become destructive.

The effect of the emotions on the Mind and Spirit

Emotions are mental stimuli which influence our

affective life. Under normal circumstances, they are not a cause of disease. Hardly any human being can avoid being angry, sad, aggrieved, worried, or afraid at some time in his or her life. For example, the death of a relative provokes a very natural feeling of grief. However, we should not identify our mental and spiritual life with our emotional life. It is perfectly possible to be alive and lively without being overburdened by excessive emotions which disturb the mind. The Buddhist practice in seeking enlightenment, for example, is precisely designed to quieten the mind and to render it oblivious to emotional stimuli which only agitate it. But the Buddhist picture of an enlightened being is not that of a boring robot-like person, but rather a vibrant, lively and even jovial person who can mix with people normally.

Emotions become causes of disease only when they are excessive or prolonged or both. For example, hardly anyone can avoid being angry sometimes, but a temporary state of anger does not lead to disease. However, if a person is constantly angry about a certain situation in life for many years, this emotion will definitely disturb the Mind and cause disease.

Although emotions are a definite cause of disease, they also have a healthy counterpart. The same mental energy which produces and "nurtures" excessive emotions, can be used and directed towards creative and fulfilling aims. Thus each emotion (as a cause of disease) is only one side of the coin; the other is a mental energy which pertains to the relevant Yin organ. This, in fact, explains why a certain emotion affects a specific organ: that particular organ already produces a certain mental energy with specific characteristics which, when subject to emotional stimuli, responds to or "resonates" with a particular emotion. Thus emotions are not something that comes from outside the internal organs to attack them; the internal organs already have a positive mental energy which turns into negative emotions only when triggered by certain external circumstances. For example, why does anger affect the Liver? If one considers the Liver's characteristics of free-going, easy and quick movement, its tendency for its Qi to rise, its correspondence to Spring when the powerful

Yang energy bursts upwards and its correspondence to Wood with its expansive movement, it is easy to understand that the Liver would be affected by anger. This emotion, with its quick outbursts, the rising of blood to the head that one feels when very angry, the destructive, expansive quality of rage, mimics, on an affective level, the characteristics of the Liver and Wood outlined above. The same mental and affective qualities of the Liver which may give rise to anger and resentment over many years, could be harnessed and used for very creative mental development. It follows then that the best way of dealing with the emotions (as causes of disease) is neither to ignore them nor suppress them, but to recognize them, look at them and try to use the same mental energy for productive aims. The healthy counterpart of emotions will be further considered when each single emotion is discussed in detail.

In Chinese medicine, emotions (intended as causes of disease) are mental stimuli which disturb the Mind and the Ethereal and Corporeal Souls and, through these, alter the balance of the internal organs and the harmony of Qi and Blood. For this reason, emotional stress is an internal cause of disease which injures the internal organs directly. On the other hand, and this is a very important feature of Chinese medicine, the state of the internal organs affects our emotional state. For example, if Liver-Yin is deficient (perhaps from dietary factors) and causes Liver-Yang to rise, this may cause a person to become irritable all the time. Conversely, if a person is constantly angry about a certain situation or with a particular person, this may cause Liver-Yang to rise. The "Spiritual Axis" in chapter 8 clearly illustrates the reciprocal relationship between the emotions and the internal organs. It says:

The Heart's fear, anxiety and pensiveness injure the Mind . . . the Spleen's worry injures the Intellect . . . the Liver's sadness and shock injure the Ethereal Soul . . . the Lung's excessive joy injures the Corporeal Soul . . . the Kidney's anger injures the Will-Power . . . .[46]

On the other hand, further on it says:

If Liver-Blood is deficient there is fear, if it is in

excess there is anger ... if Heart-Qi is deficient there is sadness, if it is in excess there is manic behaviour ....[47]

These two passages clearly show that on the one hand, emotional stress injures the internal organs and, on the other hand, disharmony of the internal organs causes emotional imbalance.

The emotions taken into consideration in Chinese medicine have varied over the years. From a 5-Element perspective, the Yellow Emperor's Classic considered 5 emotions, each one affecting a specific Yin organ:

Anger affecting the Liver
Joy affecting the Heart
Pensiveness affecting the Spleen
Worry affecting the Lungs
Fear affecting the Kidneys.

However, these are not by any means the only emotions discussed in the Yellow Emperor's Classic. In other passages sadness and shock are added, giving 7 emotions:

Anger affecting the Liver
Joy affecting the Heart
Worry affecting the Lungs and Spleen
Pensiveness affecting the Spleen
Sadness affecting the Lungs and Heart
Fear affecting the Kidneys
Shock affecting the Kidneys and Heart.

Other doctors considered other emotions such as grief, love, hatred and desire. Grief would naturally be akin to sadness. "Love" here means not normal love, such as that of a mother towards her child or that between two lovers, but rather the condition when love becomes an obsession or when it is misdirected, as when a person loves someone who persistently hurts them. Hatred is a common negative emotion which would be akin to anger. "Desire" means excessive craving. The inclusion of this as a cause of disease reflects the Buddhist influence on Chinese medicine which began during the Tang dynasty. The ultimate cause of disease according to Buddhist thought is desire, i.e. clinging to external objects or other people and always wanting more. This excessive craving, which is one aspect of the emotion of "joy" in Chinese medicine, causes the Minister Fire to blaze upwards and harass the Mind.

Finally, there is one last emotion which is not usually mentioned in Chinese medicine, and that is guilt. This is an extremely common and damaging emotion. A feeling of guilt may derive from religious or social taboos or from a person having done something wrong about which he or she feels guilty. Of course, guilt can also arise in those who always tend to blame themselves, even if they have done nothing wrong; for example, someone blaming himself (or herself) unnecessarily for the breakdown of their marriage. This attitude can sometimes be due to patterns established in childhood if a child is never praised and always reprimanded.

In some cases, guilt may also arise from repressed anger. When anger is repressed and not recognized, it may turn inwards and cause an attitude of self-punishment and guilt.

Thus, the list of emotions could be expanded as follows:

Anger (and frustration and resentment) affecting the Liver
Joy affecting the Heart
Worry affecting the Lungs and Spleen
Pensiveness affecting the Spleen
Sadness (and grief) affecting the Lungs
Fear affecting the Kidneys
Shock affecting the Kidneys and Heart
Love affecting the Heart
Hatred affecting the Heart and Liver
Craving affecting the Heart
Guilt affecting the Kidneys and Heart.

The effect of each emotion on a relevant organ should not be interpreted too restrictively. There are passages from the Yellow Emperor's Classic which attribute the effect of emotions to organs other than the ones just mentioned. For example, the "Spiritual Axis" in chapter 28 says: *"Worry and pensiveness agitate the Heart".*[48] The "Simple Questions" in chapter 39 says: *"Sadness agitates the Heart ...".*[49] The effect of an emotion also depends on other circumstances and on whether the emotion is manifested or repressed. For example, anger which is expressed affects the Liver (causing Liver-Yang rising), but anger which is repressed also affects the Heart. If one gets angry at meal-times (as sadly often happens in certain families), the anger will affect the Stomach and this will be manifested with a Wiry quality on the right Middle position of the pulse. The effect of an emotion will also depend on the constitutional traits of a person. For example, if a person has a tendency to a constitutional weakness of the Heart (manifested with a midline crack on the tongue extending all the way to the tip), fear will affect the Heart rather than the Kidneys.

Furthermore, all emotions, besides affecting the relevant organ directly, affect the Heart indirectly because the Heart houses the Mind. It alone, being responsible for consciousness and cognition, can recognize and feel the effect of emotional tension. Fei Bo Xiong (1800–1879) put it very clearly when he said:

The seven emotions injure the 5 Yin organs selectively, but they all affect the Heart. Joy injures the Heart . . . Anger injures the Liver, the Liver cannot recognize anger but the Heart can, hence it affects both Liver and Heart. Worry injures the Lungs, the Lungs cannot recognize it but the Heart can, hence it affects both Lungs and Heart. Pensiveness injures the Spleen, the Spleen cannot recognise it but the Heart can, hence it affects both Spleen and Heart.[50]

Yu Chang in "Principles of Medical Practice" (1658) says:

Worry agitates the Heart and has repercussions on the Lungs; pensiveness agitates the Heart and has repercussions on the Spleen; anger agitates the Heart and has repercussions on the Liver; fear agitates the Heart and has repercussions on the Kidneys. Therefore all the five emotions [including joy] affect the Heart.[51]

Chinese writing clearly bears out the idea that all emotions affect the Heart since the characters for all seven emotions are based on the "heart" radical.

The way that all emotions afflict the Heart also explains why a red tip of the tongue, indicating Heart-Fire, is so commonly seen even in emotional problems related to other organs.

The first effect of emotional stress on the body is to affect the proper circulation and direction of Qi. Qi is non-substantial and the Mind with its mental and emotional energies is the most non-material type of Qi. It is therefore natural that emotional stress affecting the Mind impairs the circulation of Qi first of all.

Each emotion is said to have a particular effect on the circulation of Qi. The "Simple Questions" in chapter 39 says: *"Anger makes Qi rise, joy slows down Qi, sadness dissolves Qi, fear makes Qi descend . . . shock scatters Qi . . . pensiveness knots Qi . . .".*[52] Dr Chen Yan in "A Treatise on the Three Categories of Causes of Diseases" (1174) says: *"Joy scatters, anger arouses, worry makes Qi unsmooth, pensiveness knots, sadness makes Qi tight, fear sinks, shock moves".*[53]

Again, this should not be taken too literally as, in certain cases, emotional pressure may have a different effect on Qi from the one outlined above. For example, fear is said to make Qi descend and it may cause enuresis, incontinence of urine or diarrhoea, since the Kidneys control the two lower orifices (urethra and anus). This is certainly true in cases of extreme and sudden fear which may cause incontinence of urine or diarrhoea, or in the case of children when anxiety about a certain family situation may cause enuresis. However, the effect of fear on Qi depends also on the state of the Heart. If the Heart is strong, it will cause Qi to descend, but if the Heart is weak, it will cause Qi to rise in the form of Empty-Heat. This is more common in old people and in women. In such cases, fear and anxiety may weaken Kidney-Yin and give rise to Empty-Heat of the Heart with such symptoms as palpitations, insomnia, night-sweating, a dry mouth, red face and a Rapid pulse.

Let us now discuss the effects of each emotion individually.

ANGER

The term "anger", perhaps more than any other emotion, should be interpreted very broadly to include several other allied emotional states, such as resentment, repressed anger, feeling aggrieved, frustration, irritation, rage, indignation, animosity, or bitterness.

Any of these emotional states can affect the

Liver, if they persist for a long time, causing stagnation of Liver-Qi or Blood, rising of Liver-Yang or blazing of Liver-Fire. The effect of anger on the Liver depends, on the one hand, on the person's reaction to the emotional stimulus and, on the other hand, on other concurrent factors. If the anger is bottled up it will cause stagnation of Liver-Qi, whereas if it is expressed it will cause Liver-Yang rising or Liver-Fire blazing. In a woman stagnation of Liver-Qi may easily lead to stasis of Liver-Blood. If the person also suffers from some Kidney-Yin deficiency (perhaps from excessive sexual activity), then he or she will develop Liver-Yang rising. If, on the other hand, the person has a tendency to Heat (perhaps from excessive consumption of hot foods), then he or she will tend to develop Liver-Fire blazing.

Anger (intended in the broad sense outlined above) makes Qi rise and many of the symptoms and signs will manifest in the head and neck, such as headaches, tinnitus, dizziness, red blotches on the front part of the neck, a red face, thirst, a Red tongue with red sides and a bitter taste.

The "Simple Questions" in chapter 39 says: *"Anger makes Qi rise and causes vomiting of blood and diarrhoea"*.[54] It causes vomiting of blood because it makes Liver-Qi and Liver-Fire rise and diarrhoea because it induces Liver-Qi to invade the Spleen.

Anger does not always manifest outwardly with outbursts of anger, irritability, shouting, red face, etc. Some individuals may carry anger inside them for years without ever manifesting it. In particular, long-standing depression may be due to repressed anger or resentment. Because the person is very depressed, he or she may look very subdued and pale, walk slowly and speak with a low voice, all signs which one would associate with a depletion of Qi and Blood deriving from sadness or grief. However, when anger rather than sadness is the cause of disease, the pulse and tongue will clearly show it: the pulse will be Full and Wiry and the tongue will be Red with redder sides and with a dry yellow coating. This type of depression is most probably due to long-standing resentment often harboured towards a member of that person's family.

In some cases anger can affect other organs, especially the Stomach. This can be due to stagnant Liver-Qi invading the Stomach. Such a condition is more likely to occur if one gets angry at meal-times, which may happen if family meals become occasions for regular rows. It also happens when there is a pre-existing weakness of the Stomach, in which case the anger may affect only the Stomach without even affecting the Liver.

If one regularly gets angry an hour or two after meals, then the anger will affect the Intestines rather than the Stomach. This happens, for example, when one goes straight back to a stressful and frustrating job after lunch. In this case, stagnant Liver-Qi invades the Intestines and causes abdominal pain, distension and alternation of constipation with diarrhoea.

Finally, anger, like all other emotions, also affects the Heart. This is particularly prone to be affected by anger also because, from a 5-Element perspective, the Liver is the mother of the Heart and often Liver-Fire is transmitted to the Heart giving rise to Heart-Fire. Anger makes the Heart full with blood rushing to it. With time, this leads to Blood-Heat affecting the Heart and therefore the Mind. Anger tends to affect the Heart particularly when the person does a lot of jogging, hurrying or exercising.

Thus, anger may cause either stagnation of Liver-Qi or Liver-Yang rising. When advising patients on how to deal with their anger, we should note that if anger has caused stagnation of Liver-Qi, expressing the anger may be helpful. However, if anger has given rise to Liver-Yang rising, expressing it will not usually help: it is too late and expressing the anger forcefully may only make Liver-Yang rise even more.

In some cases, anger disguises other emotions such as guilt. Some people may harbour guilt inside for many years and may be unable or unwilling to recognize it: they may then use anger as a mask for their guilt. Moreover, there are some families in which every member is perpetually angry: this happens more in Mediterranean countries such as Italy, Spain or Greece. In these families, anger is used as a mask to hide other emotions such as guilt, fear, dislike of being controlled, weakness, or inferiority complex. When this is the case, it is important to be aware of this situation as one needs to treat not the anger, but the underlying psychological and emotional condition.

The counterpart of anger in terms of mental energies is power, dynamism, creativity and generosity. The same energy which is dissipated in outbursts of anger can be harnessed to achieve one's goals in life. It is probably for this reason that the Gall-Bladder (closely related to the Liver) is said to be the source of courage. A strong Gall-Bladder gives one the courage to make decisions and changes in one's life. This aspect of the Gall-Bladder's functions is obviously closely linked to the Liver and the Ethereal Soul. If Liver-Blood is deficient there is fear: therefore if Liver-Blood is abundant the person will be fearless and decisive.

JOY

A normal state of joy is not in itself a cause of disease; on the contrary, it is a beneficial mental state which favours a smooth functioning of the internal organs and their mental faculties. The "Simple Questions" in chapter 39 says: *"Joy makes the Mind peaceful and relaxed, it benefits the Nutritive and Defensive Qi and it makes Qi relax and slow down"*.[55] On the other hand, in chapter 2 the "Simple Questions" says: *"The Heart . . . controls joy, joy injures the Heart, fear counteracts joy"*.[56]

What is meant by "joy" as a cause of disease is obviously not a state of healthy contentment but one of excessive excitement and craving which can injure the Heart. This happens to people who live in a state of continuous mental stimulation (however pleasurable) or excessive excitement: in other words, a life of "hard playing".

As indicated above, inordinate craving is an aspect of the emotion "joy" and it stirs up the Minister Fire which over-stimulates the Mind.

Joy, in the broad sense indicated above, makes the Heart larger. This leads to excessive stimulation of the Heart, which, in time, may lead to Heart-related symptoms and signs. These may deviate somewhat from the classical Heart patterns. The main manifestations would be palpi-tations, over-excitability, insomnia, restlessness, talking a lot and a red tip of the tongue. The pulse would typically be slow, slightly Over-flowing but Empty on the left Front position.

Joy may also be marked out as a cause of disease when it is sudden; this happens, for example, on hearing good news unexpectedly. In this situation, "joy" is akin to shock. Fei Bo Xiong (1800–1879) in "Medical Collection from Four Families from Meng He" says: *"Joy injures the Heart . . . [it causes] Yang Qi to float and the blood vessels to become too open and dilated . . ."*.[57] In these cases of sudden joy and excitement the Heart dilates and slows down and the pulse becomes Slow and slightly Overflowing but Empty. One can understand the effect of sudden joy further if one thinks of situations when a migraine attack is precipitated by the excitement of suddenly hearing good news. Another example of joy as a cause of disease is that of sudden laughter triggering a heart attack; this example also confirms the relationship existing between the Heart and laughter.

WORRY

Worry is one of the most common emotional causes of disease in our society. The extremely rapid and radical social changes that have occurred in Western societies in the past decades have created a climate of such insecurity in all spheres of life that only a handful of Daoist sages are immune to worry! Of course, there are also people who, because of a pre-existing disharmony of the internal organs, are very prone to worry, even about very minor incidents in life. For example, many people appear to be very tense and worry a lot. On close interrogation about their work and family life, often nothing of note emerges. They simply worry excessively about trivial everyday activities and they tend to do everything in a hurry and be pressed for time. This may be due to a constitutional weakness of the Spleen, Heart, or Lungs or a combination of these.

Worry knots Qi, which means that it causes stagnation of Qi, and it affects both Lungs and Spleen: the Lungs because when one is worried breathing is shallow, and the Spleen because this organ is responsible for thinking and ideas. Worry is the pathological counterpart of the Spleen's mental activity in generating ideas. In a few cases, worry may also affect the Liver as a result of the stagnation of the Lungs: in a 5-Element sense that corresponds to Metal insulting Wood. When this happens, the neck and shoulders will tense up and become stiff and painful.

The symptoms and signs caused by worry will vary according to whether they affect the Lungs or the Spleen. If worry affects the Lungs it will cause an uncomfortable feeling of the chest, slight breathlessness, tensing of the shoulders, sometimes a dry cough and a pale complexion. The right Front pulse position (of the Lungs) may feel slightly Tight or Wiry, indicating the knotting action of worry on Qi. When judging the quality of the Lung pulse, one should bear in mind that, in normal circumstances, this should naturally feel relatively soft (in relation to the other pulse positions). Thus a Lung pulse that feels as hard as a (normal) Liver pulse may well be Tight or Wiry.

If worry affects the Spleen it may cause poor appetite, a slight epigastric discomfort, some abdominal pain and distension, tiredness and a pale complexion. The right Middle pulse position (Spleen) will feel slightly Tight but Weak. If worry affects the Stomach as well (which happens if one worries at meal times), the right Middle pulse may be Weak-Floating.

Worry is the emotional counterpart of the Spleen's mental energy which is responsible for concentration and memorization. When the Spleen is healthy we can concentrate and focus on the object of our study or work: the same type of mental energy, when disturbed by worry, leads to constantly thinking, brooding and worrying about certain events of life.

PENSIVENESS

Pensiveness is very similar to worry in its character and effect. It consists in brooding, constantly thinking about certain events or people (even though not worrying), nostalgic hankering after the past and generally thinking intensely about life rather than living it. In extreme cases, pensiveness leads to obsessive thoughts. In a different sense, pensiveness also includes excessive mental work in the process of one's work or study.

Pensiveness affects the Spleen and, like worry, it knots Qi. It will therefore cause similar symptoms as outlined above. The only difference will be that the pulse of the right side will not only feel slightly Tight, but will have no wave. One can feel the normal pulse as a wave under the fingers moving from the Rear towards the Front position. The pulse without wave lacks this flowing movement from Rear to Front position and it is instead felt as if each individual position were separate from the others (Fig. 9.3). In the case of pensiveness, the pulse will lack a wave only on the right Middle position. A pulse without wave in the Front and Middle position indicates Sadness.

The positive mental energy corresponding to pensiveness is obviously quiet contemplation and meditation. The same mental energy which makes us capable of meditation and contemplation will, if excessive and misguided, lead to pensiveness, brooding, or even obsessive thinking.

SADNESS AND GRIEF

Sadness includes the emotion of regret, as when someone regrets a certain action or decision in the past and the Mind is constantly turned towards that time. Sadness and grief affect the Lungs and Heart. In fact, according to the "Simple Questions", sadness affects the Lungs via the Heart. It says in chapter 39: *"Sadness makes the Heart cramped and agitated; this pushes towards the*

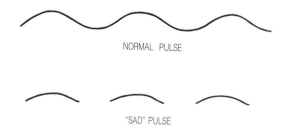

NORMAL PULSE

"SAD" PULSE

Fig. 9.3 Normal pulse and pulse without wave

lungs' lobes, the Upper Burner becomes obstructed, Nutritive and Defensive Qi cannot circulate freely, Heat accumulates and dissolves Qi".[58] According to this passage then, sadness primarily affects the Heart and the Lungs suffer in consequence since they are both situated in the Upper Burner. The Lungs govern Qi and sadness and grief deplete Qi. This is often manifested on the pulse as a Weak quality on both left and right Front positions (Heart and Lungs). In particular, the pulse on both Front positions is Short and has no wave, i.e. it does not flow smoothly towards the thumb. Other manifestations deriving from sadness and grief include a weak voice, tiredness, pale complexion, slight breathlessness, weeping and a feeling of oppression in the chest. In women, deficiency of Lung-Qi from sadness or grief often leads to Blood deficiency and amenorrhoea.

Although sadness and grief deplete Qi and therefore lead to deficiency of Qi, they may also, after a long time, lead to stagnation of Qi, because the deficient Lung- and Heart-Qi fail to circulate properly in the chest.

As mentioned before, each emotion can affect other organs apart from its "specific" one. For example, the "Spiritual Axis" in chapter 8 mentions injury of the Liver from sadness rather than anger: *"When sadness affects the Liver it injures the Ethereal Soul; this causes mental confusion . . . the Yin is damaged, the tendons contract and there is hypochondrial discomfort".*[59] This shows how organs can be affected by emotions other than their "specific" one. In this case, sadness can naturally affect the Ethereal Soul and therefore Liver-Yin. Sadness has a depleting effect on Qi and it therefore, in some cases, depletes Liver-Yin leading to mental confusion, depression, lack of a sense of direction in life and inability to plan one's life.

Case history

A 40-year-old woman was under a great deal of stress due to her divorce which caused her great sadness. She felt often weepy. She felt aimless and questioned her role in her relationships with men; she was at a turning point in her life and did not know what direction to take. She slept badly and her pulse was Choppy.

This is a clear example of sadness affecting the Liver and therefore the Ethereal Soul. She was treated, improving tremendously, with the Yin Linking Vessel points (P-6 Neiguan on the right and SP-4 Gongsun on the left) and BL-23 Shenshu, BL-52 Zhishi and BL-47 Hunmen (see below, p. 228).

Finally, some doctors consider that grief which is unexpressed and borne without tears affects the Kidneys. According to them, when grief is held in without weeping, the fluids cannot come out (in the form of tears) and they upset the fluid metabolism within the Kidneys. This would happen only in situations when grief had been felt for many years.

FEAR

Fear includes both a chronic state of fear and anxiety and a sudden fright. Fear depletes Kidney-Qi and it makes Qi descend. The "Simple Questions" in chapter 39 says: *"Fear depletes the Essence, it blocks the Upper Burner, which makes Qi descend to the Lower Burner".*[60] Examples of Qi descending are nocturnal enuresis in children and incontinence of urine or diarrhoea in adults, following a sudden fright. Situations of chronic anxiety and fear will have different effects on Qi depending on the state of the Heart.

As already mentioned above, if the Heart is strong, it will cause Qi to descend, but if the Heart is weak, it will cause Qi to rise in the form of Empty-Heat. This is more common in old people and in women as fear and anxiety weaken Kidney-Yin and give rise to Empty-Heat of the Heart with such symptoms as palpitations, insomnia, night-sweating, a dry mouth, a malar flush and a Rapid pulse.

There are other causes of fear, not related to the Kidneys. Liver-Blood deficiency and a Gall-Bladder deficiency can also make the person fearful.

The positive counterpart of fear within the mental energies of the Kidneys is flexibility, yielding in the face of adversity and quiet endurance of hardship.

SHOCK

Mental shock scatters Qi and affects Heart and

Kidneys. It causes a sudden depletion of Heart-Qi, makes the Heart smaller and may lead to palpitations, breathlessness and insomnia. It is often reflected in the pulse with a so-called "moving" quality, i.e. a pulse that is short, slippery, shaped like a bean, rapid and gives the impression of vibrating as it pulsates.

Shock also "closes" the Heart or makes the Heart smaller. This can be observed in a bluish tinge on the forehead and a Heart pulse which is Tight and Fine.

Shock also affects the Kidneys because the body draws on the Kidney-Essence to supplement the sudden depletion of Qi. For this reason, shock can cause such symptoms as night sweating, a dry mouth, dizziness, or tinnitus.

LOVE

By "love" is meant here not the normal affection felt by human beings towards one another, such as, for example, the love of parents for their children and vice-versa, or the affection of a loving couple, but rather obsessive love for a particular person. Love also becomes a cause of disease when it is misdirected as happens, for example, when a person loves someone who persistently hurts them, whether physically or mentally. Obsessive jealousy would also fall under this broad category.

"Love" in the sense outlined above affects the Heart and it quickens Qi. This will be felt on the left Front position (Heart) with an Overflowing quality, and the pulse will also be rapid. It may cause such symptoms and signs as palpitations, a red tip of the tongue, a red face, insomnia and mental restlessness.

HATRED

Hatred is quite similar to anger but it differs from it in so far as it indicates a "cold" and calculating malice rather than the uncontrollable and spontaneous outbursts which are typical of anger. When harboured for many years, hatred is a very damaging and destructive emotion. It affects the Heart and Liver and it knots and

slows down Qi. It can be felt on the pulse of the left-hand side with a Wiry but Slow quality. The symptoms and signs caused by hatred include chest pain, hypochondrial pain, insomnia, headache and palpitations. These manifestations include pain in some part of the body as when hatred is felt for many years, it only turns inwards to injure the person himself or herself.

CRAVING

By this is meant a state of constant craving which is never satisfied. This can include craving for material objects or recognition.

Craving affects the Heart and it scatters Qi. Craving also affects the Pericardium by stirring the Minister Fire. In disease, Minister Fire refers to a pathological, excessive Empty-Fire arising from the Kidneys. It arises from the Kidneys and it affects the Pericardium and therefore the Mind.[61] If the Mind is calm, settled and content, the Pericardium follows its direction and there is a happy and balanced life. If the Mind is weak and dissatisfied, the Pericardium follows the demands of the craving and the person constantly desires new objects or new recognition, which, however, even when attained, are never satisfying and leave the person more frustrated. It is for these reasons that both Daoism and Buddhism put the emphasis on reducing craving to prevent the arousal of Minister-Fire which stirs the Mind.

Craving will cause Heart-Fire or Heart Empty-Heat depending on the underlying condition of the person. If there is a tendency to Yin deficiency, which is common in people who tend to overwork, it will lead to Heart Empty-Heat. This will cause palpitations, a malar flush, a dry throat, insomnia and mental restlessness.

GUILT

Guilt is an extremely common emotion and cause of disease in the West. A feeling of guilt may derive from the transgression of social or religious taboos or from having done something wrong which is later regretted. People who are prone to blame themselves for everything that goes wrong may also suffer an unjustified and subjective sense of guilt.

Guilt affects the Heart and Kidneys and it causes Qi to stagnate. It may cause stagnation of Qi in the chest, epigastrium, or abdomen, and its clinical manifestations include an uncomfortable feeling in the chest, epigastric or abdominal pain and distension and a Fine pulse. The tongue will have a red tip and the pulse will be vibrating as it pulsates. The eyes will look unstable and often flap shut while talking.

When guilt results from repressed anger, the pulse will be Wiry.

Aetiology of mental-emotional problems

Emotional problems as discussed above are, of course, the main aetiological factor of mental-emotional problems. There are, however, other factors: specifically constitution, diet, excessive sexual activity, overwork and drugs.

CONSTITUTION

First of all, there is the constitutional make-up of an individual. This is influenced by inborn characteristics or by factors developed *in utero* during pregnancy. In either case, the inherited state of the nervous system plays a role in mental-emotional problems in later life.

For example, shock to the mother during pregnancy may affect the foetus and cause the new-born baby to sleep fitfully, cry during sleep, open and close the eyes slightly during sleep and sometimes develop fevers of unexplained origin. In such cases, the baby often has a bluish colour on the forehead. If not treated, this will have repercussions later in life and affects the Mind and Ethereal Soul.

An inherited weak nervous system is often manifested with a Heart crack on the tongue (Fig. 9.4 and Plates 9.2, 9.3 and 9.9).

This indicates that the person has an inherited weakness of the Heart which, however, may

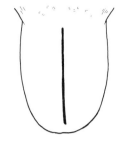

Fig. 9.4 Heart crack

never manifest unless other causative factors intervene later in life.

DIET

Diet plays an important role in contributing to mental-emotional problems. An excessive consumption of hot-energy foods and drinks (including and especially alcohol) leads to Fire which may easily harass the Mind. An excessive consumption of Damp-producing foods leads to the formation of Phlegm which, when combined with Fire, disturbs and obstructs the Mind. This leads to agitation, manic behaviour and insomnia. In such cases the tongue would be Swollen, with a Stomach-Heart crack with a sticky-yellow coating inside it.

EXCESSIVE SEXUAL ACTIVITY AND OVERWORK

Excessive sexual activity and overwork (two causative factors which often occur together) both deplete the Kidneys and the Essence. They can therefore lead to exhaustion and depression from Kidney and Essence deficiency.

DRUGS

Drugs such as cannabis, cocaine, heroine, LSD and others, deeply affect the Mind. Prolonged use of such drugs, even the so-called "light" ones as cannabis, lead to mental confusion and lack of memory and concentration. In combination with other causes of disease, they definitely contribute to mental-emotional problems and clouding of the Mind.

It is usually the overlap of different causative factors, each originating from different times in one's life, that leads to the development of mental-emotional problems.

It is useful to form an idea of the origin of mental-emotional problems in terms of time. To do this, one can divide a person's life into three broad periods, each of which is characterized by its own specific aetiological factors:

1. the period in the womb: constitution
2. childhood, up until about 18: childhood patterns
3. adulthood: diet, sex, overwork, drugs, emotions.

Broadly speaking, inherited traits obviously affect our life in the womb, juvenile development affects our childhood, and emotional problems, diet, sex and overwork affect our adulthood.

Many of the emotional patterns adults fall into are often set during childhood. This may be due to very many different factors such as relations with parents, lack of demonstrative affection from parents, relations with siblings, fighting between parents, emotional strain put on a child by a parent who pours out all his or her troubles to the child, a too strict and rigid upbringing, too many academic demands at school, a parental preference for one child over his or her siblings, pressure on a child to fulfil a parent's failed dreams, a child assuming almost the role of husband or wife after the death of the father or mother respectively, etc.

Thus the three stages of life and their causative factors of mental-emotional problems can be summarized as follows (Table 9.2).

There is of course an interaction among these three periods of life and their respective causes of disease. For example, emotional problems during childhood may also interact with constitutional traits to cause disease later in life. For

instance, if a girl has a constitutional imbalance in the Penetrating and Directing Vessels *and* she is subject to emotional strain at the time of puberty, this will often cause mental illness later in life.

It is important to form an idea of the origin of the problem so that we can give the right advice to the patient.

Diagnosis of mental-emotional problems

The diagnosis of mental-emotional problems follows the same lines as diagnosis of other problems, for the body and Mind are an inseparable unit which, when it is disturbed, gives rise to symptoms and signs in both the physical and mental-emotional spheres.

However, some special diagnostic signs in mental-emotional problems will be discussed below including the following:

- Complexion
- Eyes
- Pulse
- Tongue.

COMPLEXION

All organs can obviously influence the complexion, but, whatever the organ, the complexion shows the state of the Mind and Spirit. Yu Chang in "Principles of Medical Practice" (1658) calls the complexion the "banner of the Mind and Spirit" and he says:

When the Mind and Spirit are flourishing, the complexion is glowing; when the Mind and Spirit are declining, the complexion withers. When the Mind is stable the complexion is florid . . . .[62]

A healthy Mind and Spirit show most of all in a complexion with *shen*. This indicates an indefinable quality of glow, glitter and floridity of the complexion which indicates a good prognosis even if the colour itself is pathological. Shi Pa Nan in "Origin of Medicine" (1861) says:

The shen of the complexion consists in glitter and

Table 9.2   The three periods of life

Inherited or in womb	Childhood	Adult Age
Weak nervous system	Childhood patterns	Emotions, diet, sex, overwork

body. Glitter means that the complexion appears clear and bright from the outside; body means that it is moist and with lustre in the inside.[63]

If a complexion has such attributes, even if the colour is pathological, it indicates that the Mind and Spirit are stable and unaffected and therefore the prognosis is good.

The "Simple Questions" in chapter 17 describes the look of pathological colours with or without *shen*:

A red complexion should look like vermilion covered with white, not like ochre. A white complexion should look like feathers of a goose, not like salt. A blue complexion should look like moistened greyish jade, not like indigo. A yellow complexion should look like realgar covered with gauze, not like loess (the soil in North China along the Yellow River basin). A black complexion should look like dark varnish, not like greyish charcoal.[64]

Dr Chen Shi Duo in "Secret Records of the Stone Room" (1687) goes so far as saying:

If the complexion is dark but with shen, the person will live even if the disease is serious. If the complexion is bright but without shen, the person will die even if there is no disease.[65]

Observation of the complexion must be closely linked to the feeling of the pulse. The pulse shows the state of Qi, while the complexion the state of the Mind and Spirit. If the pulse shows changes but the complexion is normal, it indicates that the problem is recent. If both the pulse and the complexion show pathological changes, it indicates that the problem is old.

The *"shen"* of the complexion should also be checked against the glitter of the eyes. A change in the complexion always indicates a deeper or more long-standing problem. For example, a sustained period of overwork and inadequate sleep may cause the eyes to lack glitter: if the complexion is not changed, this is not too serious and the person can recover easily by resting. If, however, the eyes lack glitter and the complexion is dull, without lustre, or dark, it indicates that the problem is not transient but deeper-rooted.

Various emotions may show on the complexion with specific signs.

Anger usually manifests with a greenish tinge on the cheeks. A greenish tinge on the forehead means that Liver-Qi has invaded the Stomach, a greenish tinge on the tip of the nose that Liver-Qi has invaded the Spleen. A character prone to anger may also manifest with eyebrows that meet in the centre. In some cases, if the anger is bottled up inside as resentment leading to long-standing depression, the complexion may be pale. This is due to the depressing effect of stagnant Liver-Qi on Spleen- or Lung-Qi. In such cases, the Wiry quality of the pulse will betray the existence of anger rather than sadness or grief (indicated by the pale complexion) as a cause of disease.

Excess joy, in the sense outlined above, may manifest with a red colour on the cheek-bones.

Worry causes a greyish complexion and a skin without lustre. Worry knots Lung-Qi and affects the Corporeal Soul which manifests on the skin. For this reason, the skin becomes greyish and lustreless.

Pensiveness may manifest with a sallow complexion because it depletes Spleen-Qi.

Fear shows with a bright-white complexion on the cheeks and forehead. If chronic fear causes deficiency of Kidney-Yin and the rising of Empty-Heat of the Heart, there will be a malar flush, with the underlying colour being bright-white.

Shock also causes a bright-white complexion. Shock early in childhood may manifest with a bluish tinge on the forehead. If there is a bluish tinge on the forehead or around the mouth, it indicates a pre-natal shock (while in the uterus). Hatred often shows with a greenish complexion on the cheeks.

Craving shows with a reddish colour on the cheeks.

Guilt shows with a dark-ruddy complexion.

EYES

Observation of the eyes plays an extremely important role in the diagnosis of emotional and mental problems. The eyes reflect the state of the Mind, Spirit and Essence. The "Spiritual Axis" in chapter 80 says:

The Essence of the five Yin and the six Yang organs ascends to the eyes . . . the essence of bones goes to the pupil, the essence of tendons goes to the iris, the essence of Blood goes to the blood vessels in the eyes, the essence of the Lungs goes to the sclera . . . .[66]

This shows that the essence of all the Yin organs and therefore the Mind, Ethereal Soul, Corporeal Soul, Intellect and Will-Power manifests in the eyes. The same chapter of the "Spiritual Axis" says further on:

The eyes manifest the essence of the 5 Yin and 6 Yang organs, the Nutritive and Defensive Qi and they are the place where the Qi of the Mind is generated . . . the eyes are the messengers of the Heart which houses the Mind. If the Mind and Essence are not coordinated and not transmitted, one has visual hallucinations. The Mind, Ethereal Soul and Corporeal Soul are scattered so that one has bewildering perceptions.[67]

Shi Pa Nan in "Origin of Medicine" (1861) says: *"The Qi of the Mind and Spirit dwells in the eyes".[68]* Zhou Xue Hai in "A Simple Guide to Diagnosis from Body and Colour" (1894) says: *"Even if the illness is serious, if the eyes have good shen, the prognosis is good".[69]*

When looking at the eyes, we need to consider two aspects:

– whether they have glitter or not
– whether they are controlled or not.

If the eyes are clear, have glitter, sparkle or gleam and are brilliant, it shows that the Mind and Spirit are in a good state of vitality. If they are dull as if they were clouded by a mist, it shows that the Mind or Spirit are disturbed.

"Controlled" look means a fixed, sustained and penetrating look: this indicates a stable and integrated personality. "Uncontrolled" means that the look is shifty or too fixed.

If the eyes look uncontrolled it indicates that the person is affected by anger. In terms of personality, an uncontrolled look points to a mercurial character, an unreliable person, a person ridden by guilt, fanatical or possibly destructive.

Sadness, grief and shock make the eyes dull and without glitter.

Joy, in the sense outlined above, makes the eyes uncontrolled and slightly too watery.

Fear makes the eyes bulge out slightly and shift frequently.

Guilt makes the eyes shifty and the eyelids flap shut in rapid movements while talking.

PULSE

The pulse reflects the state of Qi while the eyes directly reflect the state of the Mind and Spirit. Thus, it is only after some years of clinical experience that one can draw conclusions about the relation between certain pulse qualities and mental-emotional problems. For example, sadness and grief can render the eyes dull and without glitter, which definitely indicates a disturbance of the Spirit. The same emotions can make the Lung pulse Weak, but this can be caused by very many other factors too. Thus the pulse, tongue and complexion should always be closely integrated in order to diagnose mental-emotional problems correctly.

Anger makes the pulse Wiry, sometimes only on the left side. A Wiry quality of the pulse is always a reliable pointer to problems from anger when other signs (such as a pale face and weak voice) seem to point to sadness and grief.

If anger occurs at meal-times, it manifests with a Wiry quality on the Stomach position. Repressed anger and resentment make the pulse "stagnant", a quality which is not one of the traditional 28 pulse qualities. A stagnant pulse is somewhat tight, but not so hard as the Tight pulse and it seems to flow reluctantly.

Sadness and grief make the pulse Choppy or Short and it characteristically flows without wave. The pulse without wave seems to flow upwards towards each pulse position separately, rather than flowing smoothly from the rear towards the Front position (see Fig. 9.3).

The sad pulse quality occurs only in the Front or Middle position, never on the Rear position. If only one position is affected (for example, only the Lung position), the sadness has not lasted for over a year. If both the Front and Middle positions of left and right have the sad quality, the sadness is long-standing.

Sometimes these emotions also manifest with a very Weak quality on both Lung and Heart positions. Again, this finding should be checked against others, since such a pulse configuration can also be caused by an accident to the chest.

Excessive joy makes the pulse slow and slightly Hollow or Overflowing-Empty on the Heart position.

Fear and shock render the pulse rapid. In severe cases they can give the pulse a Moving quality, that is, a pulse that is short and shaped like a bean, and which vibrates. Shock also makes the Heart pulse Tight and Fine.

Guilt makes the pulse rapid; the pulse also gives the impression of shaking as it pulsates.

TONGUE

One of the tongue's most reliable indications of emotional problems is a red tip. However, although this is a sure sign of emotional or mental problems, it is not very specific since it can arise from almost any emotional problem. The reason for this is two-fold. Why is the tip of the tongue affected and why is it red? First of all, the tip of the tongue is affected because it corresponds to the Heart and this organ, as mentioned above, is affected by all emotions. This is because the Heart is the seat of insight and feelings and although each emotion affects its relevant organ, it also affects the Heart which alone feels it. Secondly, the tip becomes red because every emotion, after some time, causes some stagnation of Qi and this, in turn, often produces Fire. Hence the Chinese medicine saying: *"All emotions lead to Fire"*. It is important to remember that "tip" here means the very tip of the tongue. If a larger area in the front part of the tongue is red, it usually indicates Lung-Heat.

There are a few other signs on the tongue which show emotional or mental problems. For example, severe mental problems such as manic depression or psychosis can manifest with a grossly abnormal shape of the tongue as in shown in Figure 9.5 and Plate 9.1.

If such a shape is seen in people who do not apparently have any mental problems, it still indicates that they have a tendency to develop such problems if the inner balance is suddenly upset, such as by a shock or by a traumatic childbirth. These people are nearly always sad; even

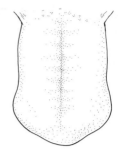

Fig. 9.5 Tongue shape in mental problems

if they do experience happiness, it lasts only a few minutes. If such a tongue is combined with very dull eyes, this is a very bad sign, indicating the possibility of severe mental illness.

Anger very often manifests with red sides of the tongue indicating Liver-Yang rising or Liver-Fire (Fig. 9.6).

If both sides and tip are red, it usually indicates severe emotional problems from anger and frustration affecting both Liver and Heart (Fig. 9.7).

Yet another tongue sign in mental problems is a combined Stomach and Heart crack with a sticky, rough, brush-like yellow coating inside

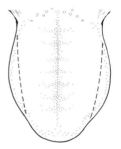

Fig. 9.6 Red sides of the tongue from anger

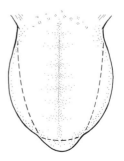

Fig. 9.7 Red sides and tip of the tongue

the crack. Such a crack with sticky coating indicates that Phlegm and Fire obstruct the Stomach and the Heart, misting the Mind. It is often seen in manic-depression (Fig. 9.8).

A midline crack that extends almost to the tip is related to the Heart and its meaning depends on other findings (see Fig. 9.4).

If the tongue-body colour is normal and the crack is not too deep, then it only indicates a constitutional weakness of the Heart. This may never manifest with a Heart problem. However, such a crack does indicate that the person will be more likely to develop emotional-mental problems if he or she is subject to emotional stress in life. Or, in other words, such a person will be less resistant to emotional stress.

If there is such a crack and the tip of the tongue is red, it indicates that the person has already developed some emotional problems. If the whole tongue is Red and the tip redder and with red points, the emotional problems are of a more serious nature.

Pathology and treatment of mental-emotional problems

We can now turn our attention to differentiating the various disease conditions of mental-emotional problems and their treatment. Rather than discussing the treatment of Western-defined mental-emotional diseases such as depression, manic-depression, or schizophrenia, I will discuss the pathology of mental-emotional problems in terms of their effects on Qi, Blood and Yin and classify them in the three broad catego-

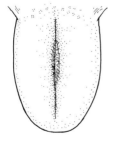

Fig. 9.8 Stomach and Heart crack in mental problems

ries of Mind obstructed, Mind unsettled and Mind weakened (see below).

The effects of the various aetiological factors in mental-emotional problems can be classified into three broad categories:

– effects on Qi
– effects on Blood
– effects on Yin.

Given the indissoluble link between body and mind in Chinese medicine, it should be remembered that, just as emotional problems have an effect on Qi, Blood, or Yin, a disharmony of Qi, Blood, or Yin (from causes other than emotional) will affect the Mind. The following discussion of conditions arising from emotional stress applies equally to mental-emotional problems deriving from a disharmony of Qi, Blood and Yin of the internal organs.

EFFECTS ON QI

The Mind and Spirit are a form of Qi in its subtlest state. Therefore the very first effect of emotional causative factors is to upset the movement and transformation of Qi. As we have seen, each emotion has a certain effect on Qi by raising it, depleting it, knotting it, scattering it, or making it descend. Hence, injury of the Mind or Spirit by emotions causes either Qi-deficiency or rebellious Qi. Rebellious Qi, it will be remembered, indicates a counter-flow movement of Qi, i.e. Qi rising when it should descend (as in the case of Stomach-Qi) or Qi descending when it should rise (as in the case of Spleen-Qi). Ultimately, however, both deficient and rebellious Qi may lead to stagnation of Qi. This happens because, especially in emotional problems, deficient or rebellious Qi impairs the proper circulation and movement of Qi, leading to stagnation. Stagnation of Qi from emotional problems affects various organs but the Liver, Heart and Lungs most of all.

LIVER-QI STAGNATION

This is the most common effect of emotional

stress on the Liver. It derives from anger, especially if it is held in and not manifested.

The main manifestations of Liver-Qi stagnation are distension of the hypochondrium, epigastrium, or abdomen, belching, sighing, nausea, depression, moodiness, feeling wound-up, a feeling of lump in the throat, pre-menstrual tension and irritability with distension of the breasts and a Wiry pulse.

From an emotional perspective the most characteristic and common signs are mental depression, alternation of moods, irritability, "snapping" easily and an intense feeling of frustration. Being due to stagnation of Qi and not affecting Blood, this condition does not affect the Ethereal Soul much and can be ascribed only to the effects of Qi stagnation on the Mind. However, if the stagnation of Qi is severe, it will disturb the Ethereal Soul causing insomnia.

HEART AND LUNG QI STAGNATION

This derives either from worry which knots Qi or from sadness and grief which deplete Qi and lead to Qi-stagnation in the chest after some time.

It is characterized by a feeling of oppression and tightness in the chest, palpitations, sighing, slight breathlessness, a feeling of lump in the throat with difficulty in swallowing, a weak voice, a pale complexion and a pulse which is Weak in both Heart and Lung positions and is without wave. From an emotional point of view, a person will feel very sad and depressed and will tend to weep. This state is due to the constriction of the Corporeal Soul by stagnation of Qi. The person will also be very sensitive to psychic outside influences. Just as the Lungs on a physical level are responsible for protection from exterior pathogenic factors, the Corporeal Soul is responsible for protection from external psychic influences. Such people may, for example, tend to be negatively affected by the problems of people with whom they come into contact.

The effects of emotional causative factors are confined to Qi only in the early stages. After some time, the disruption in the movement and transformation of Qi necessarily leads to the formation of pathogenic factors such as Dampness, Phlegm, stasis of Blood, Fire or Wind, all of which further affect and disturb the Mind and Spirit.

EFFECTS ON BLOOD

The effects of emotional problems on Blood are more important than those on Qi, for it provides the material foundation for the Mind and Spirit. Blood, which is Yin, houses and anchors the Mind and Spirit, which are Yang in nature. It embraces the Mind and Spirit providing the harbour within which they can flourish. The "Simple Questions" in chapter 26 says: *Blood is the Mind of a person*.[70] The "Spiritual Axis" says in chapter 32: *When Blood is harmonized the Mind has a residence*.[71]

Blood is also closely related to Mind and Spirit because of its relation with Heart and Liver. The Heart, which houses the Mind, governs Blood, and the Liver, which houses the Ethereal Soul, stores Blood. Any emotional stress that affects Heart or Liver would influence Heart-Blood or Liver-Blood and therefore the Mind or Ethereal Soul.

The Blood can be affected by emotional problems in three ways: it can become deficient, stagnant, or hot.

BLOOD DEFICIENCY

This is one of the most common consequences of emotional problems. Its manifestations will vary according to whether the Heart or Liver is more affected.

1. HEART-BLOOD DEFICIENCY

If the Heart is affected (as it is by sadness and grief) there will be palpitations, mild anxiety, insomnia (inability to fall asleep), poor memory, mild dizziness, propensity to be startled, a dull-pale complexion, a Pale-Thin tongue and a Choppy pulse. From a mental-emotional point of view, such a person may feel depressed and tired, and the Mind may be confused and lack concentration. This is due to a weakness of the Mind, it being deprived of its residence and therefore failing to direct all the mental activities.

2. LIVER-BLOOD DEFICIENCY

If Liver-Blood is affected (as it is by anger) there will be mild dizziness, numbness of the limbs, insomnia (inability to fall asleep), blurred vision, floaters in eyes, scanty menstruation or amenorrhoea, a dull-pale complexion, muscle cramps, brittle nails, a Pale-Thin tongue and a Choppy pulse. From a mental-emotional viewpoint, the person may also feel depressed and tired, and may lack a sense of direction in life and "vision". He or she may be confused as to what aims in life they should follow. Alternatively, he or she may be fearful of making decisions lest they make the wrong one. This is due to the Ethereal Soul not being rooted in Liver-Blood and therefore failing to provide the Mind with vision, planning, and relating to other people. Both these conditions of Blood deficiency are very much more frequent in women who are more prone to Blood disorders.

BLOOD STASIS

This also affects the Mind albeit in a different way.

1. HEART-BLOOD STASIS

If Blood stasis affects the Heart it will cause chest pain, a feeling of oppression in the chest, anxiety, insomnia, cold hands, cyanosis of lips and nails, a Purple tongue and a Knotted or Choppy pulse. From a mental-emotional point of view this person will feel very anxious with an acute sense of anxiety in the chest, and even up to the throat. The person will be restless and prone to be easily startled. This condition is due to stagnant Blood agitating and confusing the Mind.

In severe cases, the person may lose insight and become psychotic.

2. LIVER-BLOOD STASIS

If Liver-Blood is stagnant there may be vomiting of blood or epistaxis, painful periods with dark and clotted blood, irregular periods, abdominal pain, a feeling of mass in the abdomen, insomnia, a tongue which is Purple on the sides and a Wiry pulse. From a mental-emotional point of view the person will be very anxious, restless and confused about his or her aims in life. He or she will also be very irritable and prone to outbursts of anger. This condition is due to the Ethereal Soul being agitated and confused by the stasis of Blood. In severe cases, this may also lead to psychosis.

BLOOD-HEAT

This is the third possible consequence of emotional problems affecting Blood. It affects the Mind and Spirit by agitating and harassing them. Blood-Heat also mostly affects Heart or Liver.

1. HEART-BLOOD HEAT

If Blood-Heat affects the Heart there will be palpitations, insomnia (inability to stay asleep), anxiety, mental restlessness, thirst, tongue ulcers, a feeling of heat, a red face, dark urine, possibly blood in the urine, a bitter taste, a Red tongue and a Rapid and Overflowing pulse. This person will be extremely anxious and agitated and in some cases may be very impulsive and restless. All these symptoms and signs are due to Blood-Heat agitating the Mind.

2. LIVER-BLOOD HEAT

If Blood-Heat affects the Liver there will be irritability, propensity to outbursts of anger, thirst, a bitter taste, dizziness, tinnitus, insomnia, dream-disturbed sleep, headache, red face and eyes, dark urine, dry stools, a Red tongue which is redder on the sides and a Rapid-Wiry pulse. The person will be very angry and tend to shout at other people a lot; may also be violent and hit people; may also feel angry and frustrated about their life and may tend to be impulsive. All this is due to Blood-Heat disturbing the Ethereal Soul and accentuating too much its essential character of movement towards the outer world and relation with other people.

EFFECTS ON YIN

Blood is part of Yin and the effects of emotional stress on Yin are similar to those on Blood. Affection of Yin may, however, be considered as a deeper level of problem than affection of Blood.

Yin, like Blood, is the residence and anchor of the Mind and Spirit. Emotional problems can affect the Yin of different organs and especially the Heart, Liver, Kidneys, Lungs and Spleen. The effect depends on whether Yin deficiency gives rise to Empty-Heat or not. If there is Yin deficiency only, without Empty-Heat, the Mind and Spirit become weakened and the person feels depressed, tired and dispirited, the Mind is confused and the memory and concentration poor. If Yin deficiency gives rise to Empty-Heat, this unsettles the Mind and Spirit causing anxiety and mental restlessness.

HEART-YIN

Heart-Yin is readily affected by emotional stress since it is the residence of the Mind. Stress deprives the Mind of residence and there will be palpitations, insomnia (inability to stay asleep), propensity to be startled, poor memory, anxiety, mental restlessness, a malar flush, night sweating, a dry mouth, 5-palm heat, a Red tongue (with redder tip) without coating and a Rapid-Thin or Floating-Empty pulse. The person will feel very anxious, particularly in the evening, with a vague and fidgety sense of anxiety, uneasy without knowing why. "Mental restlessness" is a loose translation of a typical Chinese

expression, which always refers to this pattern and literally means "heart feels vexed". The person will also feel dispirited, depressed and tired. Memory and concentration will be poor. The sleep will be disturbed and, typically, the person wakes up frequently during the night. All this is due to the Mind being deprived of its residence.

If there is Empty-Heat as well, the effects on the Mind will be more pronounced; the patient will feel extremely restless and anxious, and the sleep will be very disturbed. On a mental level, the patient may become aggressive and very impatient.

LIVER-YIN

Liver-Yin is the residence of the Ethereal Soul and when emotional stress depletes Liver-Yin it may cause a deep depression, a lack of purpose in life and a confusion about objectives and aims. On a physical level this may cause poor memory, dizziness, dry eyes, skin and hair, scanty periods, insomnia, 5-palm heat, night sweating, a red tongue without coating and a Floating-Empty pulse. The patient may also have a floating sensation immediately before falling asleep.

KIDNEY-YIN

Kidney-Yin is the residence of Will-Power and memory. Emotional stress that affects Kidney-Yin will cause great exhaustion, a lack of will-power and drive and a decrease in mental capacities and memory. On a physical level, it will cause dizziness, tinnitus, night-sweating, 5-palm heat, back-ache, deafness, a Red tongue without coating and a Floating-Empty pulse.

LUNG-YIN

Lung-Yin is the residence of the Corporeal Soul. Emotional problems that affect Lung-Yin will cause tiredness, depression, itching, slight breathlessness, an uncomfortable sensation of the chest, night-sweating, 5-palm heat, a dry throat, a Red tongue without coating and a Floating-Empty pulse. On a mental level, the patient may be prone to be influenced by outside psychic forces, will tend to weep a lot and will feel very dispirited and lonely.

SPLEEN-YIN

Spleen-Yin is the residence of the Intellect and emotional problems affecting Spleen-Yin may cause a dry mouth with no desire to drink, dry lips, dry stools, poor appetite, a slight epigastric pain, a tongue without coating in the centre and a Floating-Empty pulse in the Right-Middle position. From a mental point of view these people will suffer from poor memory and concentration, and will find it very difficult to apply themselves to study. The imbalance may also work in the opposite way and may lead to obsessive ideas.

Thus the effects of emotional stress on the body's vital substances are summarized in Table 9.3 which shows the effects of emotional stress on the vital substances under the column headed "Effect". These conditions themselves become, with time, a cause of further disharmony and the effects are in the column headed "Consequence". For example, Blood-Heat may easily lead to the formation of Phlegm-Fire because Heat condenses the body fluids into Phlegm. Or Qi deficiency of the Spleen, Lungs or Kidneys easily leads to the formation of Phlegm as Qi fails to transform, move and excrete fluids which therefore accumulate into Phlegm. Qi stagnation easily leads to Blood stasis and Yin deficiency may lead to Empty-Heat or internal Wind.

Table 9.3 Effects of emotions on Vital Substances

Vital Substance	Effect	Consequence
Qi	Deficiency Stagnation	Phlegm Blood stasis
Blood	Deficiency Heat Stasis	Phlegm-Fire
Yin	Deficiency	Empty-Heat Internal Wind

All these pathogenic factors, Phlegm, Phlegm-Fire, Empty-Heat and internal Wind, further disturb the Mind. We shall now discuss their effects and symptomatology. Blood stasis has already been discussed above.

PHLEGM

Phlegm obstructs the Mind (the Heart's orifices) and may cause dullness of thought, a fuzzy head, a confused mind and dizziness. In severe cases it may cause mental retardation or even coma. Phlegm obstructs the Mind and thinking but it does not agitate the Mind. Thus the person will not be restless but, on the contrary, tired, subdued, depressed and quiet.

Phlegm always shows with a Swollen tongue body, a sticky coating and a Slippery pulse.

PHLEGM-FIRE

Phlegm-Fire obstructs the Mind but it also agitates it. It therefore makes the person agitated, restless and anxious. In some cases, the person may alternate between periods of depression and confusion (due to Phlegm) and periods of abnormal elation, agitation and manic behaviour (due to Fire). In severe cases this leads to manic-depression. Chinese books always describe this condition as alternation of periods of severe depression (the depressive phase called *Dian*) and periods of manic behaviour (the manic phase called *Kuang*). The manic phase is usually described as shouting, scolding or hitting people, climbing mountains, taking off clothes, crying or laughing uncontrollably. It is important to realize that, in practice, much milder versions of this condition appear fairly frequently and one should not always expect such violent symptomatology in order to diagnose this condition.

Phlegm-Fire manifests with a Slippery and Rapid pulse and a Red-Swollen tongue with a sticky yellow coating and a Heart-crack in the midline.

EMPTY-HEAT

Empty-Heat agitates the Mind and causes severe

anxiety, insomnia, agitation, mental restlessness and fidgetiness. This is sometimes called the rising of Minister-Fire, i.e. Empty-Fire arising from the Kidneys and disturbing the Pericardium and the Mind. It is frequently caused by excess joy, craving, jealousy and excessive love (in the sense outlined before).

It manifests with a Floating-Empty or Fine-Rapid pulse and a Red tongue without coating, possibly with a Heart crack in the midline and a redder tip.

INTERNAL WIND

Internal Wind agitates the Mind and causes nervous tics and tremors.

Thus, the mental effects of emotions and other pathogenic factors may be summarized in three broad types:

- *Mind obstructed*, characterized by confused thinking, clouding of the Mind and, in severe cases, complete loss of insight
- *Mind unsettled*, characterized by agitation, restlessness and anxiety
- *Mind weakened*, characterized by depression, mental exhaustion and melancholy.

The Mind is obstructed by Phlegm or, in mild cases, by stagnation of Qi or Blood. It is important to realize that there are many different degrees of obstruction of the Mind ranging from very mild to full-blown schizophrenia or mania.

The Mind is unsettled by deficiency of Blood or Yin (mild cases), Qi stagnation, Blood stasis, Fire, Empty-Heat, Phlegm-Fire and internal Wind; and it is weakened by Qi, Yang, Blood or Yin deficiency.

Of course there is a considerable degree of overlap among these three conditions as, for example, the Mind may be weakened *and* unsettled.

Case history

A 51-year-old man sought treatment for atopic asthma and eczema. For 10 years from the age of 32 he drank a lot of alcohol and used amphetamines regularly and heavily. His eyes were dull and lacked glitter and he complained of poor memory and concentration. When spoken to he always looked like he was slightly absent and he found it difficult to find words. His tongue was Swollen and had a Stomach-Heart crack with a sticky-yellow coating (Plate 9.2), and his pulse was slightly Slippery.

This is given here as an example of a mild case of obstruction of the Mind, in his case by Phlegm.

The principle of treatment for mental-emotional problems follows the above classification closely and must be based, as usual, on a clear distinction between Deficiency and Excess and between the Root and the Manifestation. Such distinction is very important to choose the correct herbal formula.

The main principles of treatment in mental-emotional problems are five:

1. Nourish the Heart and calm the Mind: this is applicable to Deficiency conditions, i.e. Qi, Blood or Yin deficiency causing Mind Weakened.

2. Clear pathogenic factors and calm the Mind: this is applicable to Excess conditions such as stagnation of Qi or Blood, Phlegm-Fire and Fire, causing Mind Obstructed or Mind Unsettled.

3. Clear pathogenic factors, nourish the Heart and calm the Mind: this is applicable to deficiency of Yin leading to Empty-Heat, causing Mind Unsettled.

4. Resolve Phlegm, open the orifices and calm the Mind: this is applicable to Phlegm or Phlegm-Fire, causing Mind Obstructed.

5. Sink and calm the Mind: this consists in the use of heavy minerals to sink rising Qi and is used as an addition to other methods of treatment to treat the Manifestation when the Mind is very unsettled.

It should be noted that "calm the Mind" is an expression that recurs, as a method of treatment, in all cases of mental-emotional problems. It should be interpreted broadly to include not only the strict sense of calming the Mind (as in anxiety), but also the broader sense of lifting mood (as in depression).

The various pathologies and relevant methods of treatment may be summarized in tabular form (Table 9.4).

Before discussing the acupuncture and herbal treatment of each pattern, it is worth mentioning

Table 9.4   Mind pathologies and methods of treatment

Affliction of Mind	Pathology	Method of treatment
Obstructed	Stagnation of Qi	Move Qi, calm the Mind
	Stasis of Blood	Move Blood, calm the Mind
	Phlegm	Resolve Phlegm, open the orifices, calm the Mind
Unsettled	Blood-Yin Deficiency	Nourish the Heart and calm the Mind
	Yin deficiency with Empty-Heat	Nourish Yin, clear Empty-Heat and calm the Mind
	Qi stagnation	Move Qi and calm the Mind
	Blood stasis	Move Blood and calm the Mind
	Fire	Drain Fire and calm the Mind
	Phlegm-Fire	Drain Fire, resolve Phlegm, open the orifices and calm the Mind
Weakened	Qi deficiency	Tonify Qi, calm and clear the Mind
	Yang deficiency	Tonify Yang, calm and clear the Mind
	Blood deficiency	Nourish Blood and calm the Mind
	Yin deficiency	Nourish Yin and calm the Mind

the action of some of the most frequently used points in mental-emotional problems.

OUTER BLADDER POINTS

These are interesting and intriguing points for mental-emotional problems. They are situated on the outer Bladder line on the back, 3 *cun* from the midline, in correspondence with the Back-Transporting points of the five Yin organs. Their names clearly relate each point to the mental-spiritual aspect of the relevant Yin organ.

BL-42 POHU ("WINDOW OF THE CORPOREAL SOUL")

This point, in correspondence with BL-13 Feishu Back-Transporting point of the Lungs, strengthens and roots the Corporeal Soul in the Lungs. It frees breathing when the Corporeal Soul is constricted by worry, sadness or grief. It calms the Mind and settles the Corporeal Soul to make the person turn inwards and be comfortable with oneself.

From a physical point of view, it also nourishes Lung-Yin in chronic diseases such as Lung-exhaustion.

BL-44 SHENTANG ("HALL OF THE MIND")

This point, in correspondence with BL-15 Xinshu Back-Transporting point of the Heart, strengthens and calms the Mind. It stimulates the Mind's clarity and intelligence. If left in a long time (over 15 minutes) it calms the Mind and clears Heart-Fire.

BL-47 HUNMEN ("THE DOOR OF THE ETHEREAL SOUL")

This point, in correspondence with BL-18 Ganshu Back-Transporting point of the Liver, settles and roots the Ethereal Soul in the Liver. It strengthens the Ethereal Soul's capacity of planning, sense of aim in life, life-dreams, and projects. It is a "door", so this point facilitates the "coming and going" of the Ethereal Soul and Mind, i.e. relationships with other people and the world in general. It has an outward movement which could be compared and contrasted with the inward movement of BL-42 Pohu. As this point facilitates the "coming and going" of the Ethereal Soul, care must be exercised in people whose personality is too open, unstable or vulnerable, as the point could make the Ethereal Soul too mobile and unsettled and make the patient very insecure and shaky. This does not happen if the point is combined with BL-23 Shenshu and BL-52 Zhishi (see below).

The "Explanation of Acupuncture Points" (1654) confirms that, due to this point's nature of "window", the Ethereal Soul goes in and out through it. The text also says that, again this point being a "window", it *stores the 5 Yin organs but these can be seen from the outside.*[72] This confirms the dynamic nature of this point in stimulating the movement of the Ethereal Soul and Mind.

On a physical level, this point is very useful in treating stagnant Liver-Qi insulting the Lungs (as it happens in some types of asthma).

BL-49 YISHE ("HUT OF THE INTELLECT")

This point, in correspondence with BL-20 Pishu Back-Transporting point of the Spleen, strengthens the Intellect, clears the Mind and stimulates memory and concentration. It also relieves the Mind and Intellect of obsessive thoughts, brooding, mentally going round in circles.

On a physical level, this point can be used with direct moxa to dry the Spleen of Dampness and also to tonify the Lungs (according to the principle of strengthening Earth to tonify Metal).

BL-52 ZHISHI ("ROOM OF THE WILL-POWER")

This point, in correspondence with BL-23 Shenshu Back-Transporting point of the Kidneys, strengthens will-power, drive, determination, the capacity of pursuing one's goals with single-mindedness, spirit of initiative and steadfastness. I often use this point, if there is a Kidney deficiency, in combination with one of the above points, as a solid mental-emotional foundation for the other aspects of the psyche. The following are some examples of such combinations:

– BL-23 Shenshu, BL-52 Zhishi and BL-47 Hunmen to strengthen will-power and drive, and to instil a sense of direction and aim in one's life. This combination is excellent to treat the mental exhaustion, lack of drive and aimlessness which is typical of chronic depression.
– BL-23 Shenshu, BL-52 Zhishi and BL-49 Yishe to strengthen will-power and drive and empty the Mind and Intellect of obsessive thoughts, worries and confused thinking.
– BL-23 Shenshu, BL-52 Zhishi and BL-42 Pohu

to strengthen will-power and drive, settle the Corporeal Soul and release emotions constrained in the chest and diaphragm.
– BL-23 Shenshu, BL-52 Zhishi and BL-44 Shentang to strengthen will-power and drive, calm the mind and relieve anxiety, depression, mental restlessness and insomnia. This combination harmonizes Kidneys and Heart (and therefore Will-Power and Mind) on a mental-emotional level.

If we analyze the names of the above five points, we can detect a pattern as the points correspond to a house — an image for the pysche — with the Mind, Will-Power and Intellect corresponding to the hall, room and hut respectively, and the Ethereal Soul and Corporeal Soul corresponding to a door and window. The images of door and window fit well the nature of the Ethereal Soul and Corporeal Soul which provide movement to the pysche, the former providing the "coming and going of the Mind" and the latter the "entering and exiting of the Essence". The correspondence of the Heart to a hall also fits in with old Chinese customs according to which the hall is the most important room of the house as it is the one that gives the first impression to visitors: for this reason, it was always kept scrupulously clean.

HEART CHANNEL

HE-7 Shenmen calms the Mind and nourishes the Heart. It is especially indicated for mental-emotional problems occurring against a background of deficiency of Heart-Blood or Heart-Yin.
HE-6 Yinxi calms the Mind: it is especially used in Excess patterns of the Heart with Empty-Heat.
HE-8 Shaofu and HE-9 Shaochong calm the Mind and are used for severe mental restlessness, anxiety and insomnia from Excess Heart patterns such as Heart-Fire or Heart Phlegm-Fire.

PERICARDIUM

P-7 Daling calms the Mind especially in Excess patterns. It also resolves Phlegm from the Heart and is especially indicated for emotional problems from the breaking of relationships.

P-6 Neiguan calms the Mind, lifts mood, relaxes the chest and is especially indicated for emotional problems associated with stagnation of Qi. The Pericardium channel being related to the Liver channel, P-6 is a very powerful point to calm the Mind and settle the Ethereal Soul when they are affected by stagnation of Liver-Qi deriving from anger, resentment, or frustration. This point is particularly indicated when the emotions are constrained in the chest and the person has a feeling of oppression or tightness of the chest.

To compare and contrast P-6 with P-7, the former has an outward movement, moves Qi, resolves stagnation and "opens" the Mind, whilst the latter has an inward movement and calms the Mind.

P-6 can be combined with:

- SP-4 Gongsun to open the Yin Linking Vessel, nourish Blood, relax the chest, calm the Mind and settle the Ethereal Soul.
- LIV-3 Taichong to strengthen its Qi-moving action in emotional problems from repressed anger.
- Du-20 Baihui to lift mood, clear the Mind and relieve depression.
- Du-26 Renzhong to lift mood, clear the Mind, open the Mind's orifices and relieve depression.
- ST-40 Fenglong to calm the Mind, open the chest to relieve it of constrained emotions, and open the Mind's orifices.

KIDNEY CHANNEL

KI-9 Zhubin calms the Mind, strengthens Will-Power and opens the chest. It is especially indicated to relieve anxiety and depression occurring against a background of Kidney deficiency and with a feeling of oppression of the chest.

SMALL INTESTINE CHANNEL

S.I.-5 Yanggu clears mental confusion and indecision due to difficulty in discriminating choices in life.

S.I.-3 Houxi strengthens the Will-Power, drive and determination. It is an important point to relieve depression occurring against a background of Kidney deficiency.

GALL-BLADDER CHANNEL

G.B.-40 Qiuxu strengthens the Will-Power and the Mind. It bolsters the person's capacity of making decisions.

G.B.-13 Benshen calms the Mind, settles the Ethereal Soul and gathers Essence to the head. It is particularly indicated for severe anxiety and mental restlessness occurring against a background of a Liver disharmony. It is also for jealousy and suspicion. The "Complete Book of Jing Yue" (1624) says that this point is for lack of clarity of the Mind deriving from injury of the Ethereal Soul by sadness.[73]

This point can be combined with:

- Du-24 Shenting to enhance its calming effect: the combination of these two points has a powerful calming effect on the Mind and Ethereal Soul and they are particularly useful in Liver disharmonies.
- HE-7 Shenmen to calm the Mind in severe anxiety occurring against a background of Heart disharmonies.

G.B.-15 Toulinqi calms the Mind and settles the Ethereal Soul. This point is used when the person is subject to emotional fluctuations and obsessive thoughts.

G.B.-17 Zhengying calms and clears the Mind. It stimulates memory and concentration. It is indicated in depression.

G.B.-18 Chengling settles the Ethereal Soul and Corporeal Soul and stops obsessive thoughts. On a physical level, it stimulates the dispersing and descending of Lung-Qi and opens the nose.

LUNG CHANNEL

LU-7 Lieque settles and opens up the Corporeal Soul. This point has a releasing effect on emotions (especially sadness, worry and grief) constraining the Corporeal Soul in the chest.

DIRECTING VESSEL

Ren-15 Jiuwei calms the Mind and settles the Corporeal Soul. It is especially indicated to release emotions constraining the Corporeal Soul in the chest and manifesting with a feeling of oppression or tightness of the chest. It is a very calming point, especially in mental-emotional problems occurring against a background of Deficiency conditions.

This point combines well with Du-19 Houding to calm the Mind and relieve anxiety, insomnia and mental restlessness.

Ren-4 Guanyuan strengthens the Will-Power and calms the Mind. It is a very grounding point which calms the Mind by attracting Qi downwards and rooting it in the Kidneys. It is indicated in anxiety and mental restlessness occurring against a background of Kidney deficiency.

GOVERNING VESSEL

Du-24 Shenting stimulates intelligence and clears the Mind. Its combination with G.B.-13 has been described above.

Du-21 Qianting strengthens the Mind. It is indicated in conditions of Mind Weakened causing slight anxiety, insomnia and depression.

Du-20 Baihui clears the Mind, lifts mood, and stimulates memory and concentration.

Du-19 Houding calms the Mind and strengthens Will-Power. It is indicated in severe anxiety and mental restlessness occurring against a background of Kidney deficiency with Empty-Heat unsettling the Mind.

Du-18 Qiangjian opens the Mind's orifices and calms the Mind. It also regulates Liver-Blood and is therefore indicated for severe mental restlessness, agitation, mental confusion and obsessive thoughts from Mind Obstructed occurring against a background of Blood stasis.

Finally, the following are point combinations used in the Provincial Psychiatric Hospital in Nanjing:

Dreamy state: Du-14 Dazhui, L.I.-11 Quchi, G.B.-34 Yanglingquan, Ren-8 Shenque and Ren-4 Guanyuan.

Forgetting words: Du-20 Baihui, BL-8 Luoque, HE-5 Tongli, KI-4 Dazhong.
Obsessive ideas: Du-18 Qiangjian, S.I.-3 Houxi, G.B.-39 Xuanzhong.
Jealousy: P-7 Daling and G.B.-43 Xiaxi.
Difficulty in concentrating: G.B.-17 Zhengying, P-5 Jianshi, Yintang, ST-40 Fenglong.
Poor memory: Du-20 Baihui, HE-7 Shenmen, KI-3 Taixi, G.B.-18 Chengling.
Lack of will-power: Du-19 Houding, G.B.-6 Xuanli, P-6 Neiguan, SP-10 Xuehai.
Emotionally up and down: G.B.-15 Toulinqi, Du-20 Baihui, P-8 Laogong, KI-1 Yongquan, Du-25 Suliao.

We can now discuss the acupuncture and herbal treatment for each of the patterns discussed above. The discussion of the treatment will be structured as follows:

MIND OBSTRUCTED

STAGNATION OF QI

1. Stagnation of Liver-Qi
2. Stagnation of Heart- and Lung-Qi

BLOOD STASIS

1. Heart-Blood Stasis
2. Liver-Blood Stasis
3. Stasis of Blood in the Lower Burner

PHLEGM MISTING THE MIND

Phlegm-Heat Harassing the Mind

MIND UNSETTLED

BLOOD DEFICIENCY

Heart-Blood Deficiency

YIN DEFICIENCY

1. Heart-Yin Deficiency
2. Liver-Yin Deficiency
3. Kidney-Yin Deficiency

YIN DEFICIENCY WITH EMPTY-HEAT

1. Heart- and Kidney-Yin Deficiency with Heart Empty-Heat
2. Liver-Yin Deficiency with Empty-Heat

QI STAGNATION

BLOOD STASIS

FIRE

1. Heart-Fire
2. Liver-Fire

PHLEGM-FIRE

1. Stomach and Heart Phlegm-Fire

MIND WEAKENED

QI AND BLOOD DEFICIENCY

1. Qi Deficiency
2. Qi and Blood Deficiency

YANG DEFICIENCY

Kidney-Yang Deficiency

BLOOD DEFICIENCY

YIN DEFICIENCY

1. Kidney-Yin Deficiency
2. Lung- and Kidney-Yin Deficiency
3. Kidney- and Liver-Yin Deficiency
4. Kidney-Essence Deficiency

The mental-emotional pattern for each of these syndromes will be mentioned after the relevant herbal prescription: those who use only acupuncture are invited to read the "mental-emotional patterns" for each syndrome as they obviously apply whether one uses acupuncture or herbs. Figure 9.9 clarifies how the discussion of the treatment for each pattern is structured.

MIND OBSTRUCTED

The Mind may be obstructed or "misted" by stagnation of Qi, stasis of Blood or Phlegm. It may also be obstructed by Heat during an acute febrile disease, such as in the pattern "Heat in Pericardium" at the Nutritive Qi level, but this is a special case which does not concern us here.

Obstruction of the Mind causes mental confusion because the obstructing factor impairs the Mind's activity of thinking, memory, concep-

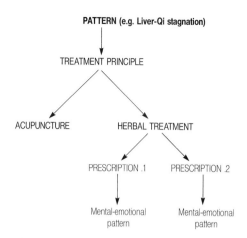

Fig. 9.9 Structure of patterns' treatment discussion

tualization, application and understanding. Thus the person will suffer from mental confusion, poor memory, dizziness, poor concentration, inability to find the right words, and slow thinking. On an emotional level, the person will feel blunted and somewhat numb and will often be unable to express his or her emotions. Obstruction of the Mind can occur in many different degrees ranging from very mild and manifesting with a slight mental confusion, to very severe in which case there may be complete loss of insight in conditions such as manic-depression, psychosis or schizophrenia.

Of course there is a difference of degree in obstruction of the Mind by stagnation of Qi, stasis of Blood, or Phlegm, stagnation of Qi being the mildest, and Phlegm the most severe.

The treatment principle in obstruction of the Mind is to eliminate the pathogenic factors, open the Mind's orifices and calm the Mind.

Herbs to open the orifices in mental-emotional problems include:

Shi Chang Pu *Rhizoma Acori graminei*
Yu Jin *Tuber Curcumae*
Yuan Zhi *Radix Polygalae tenuifoliae*
He Huan Pi *Cortex Albizziae julibrissin*
Su He Xiang *Styrax liquidis*
Hu Po *Succinum*

Acupuncture points that open the Mind's orifices include:

P-5 Jianshi, Du-20 Baihui, Du-26 Renzhong,

ST-40 Fenglong, ST-25 Tianshu, all the Well points, G.B.-18 Chengling, Du-19 Houding, G.B.-13 Benshen.

STAGNATION OF QI

1. STAGNATION OF LIVER-QI

Treatment principle

Move Qi, pacify the Liver, settle the Ethereal Soul and calm the Mind.

Acupuncture

LIV-3 Taichong, L.I.-4 Hegu, LIV-14 Qimen, P-6 Neiguan, P-7 Daling, T.B.-6 Zhigou, Du-24 Shenting, G.B.-13 Benshen.

Explanation

– **LIV-3** is the main point to simultaneously move Liver-Qi and calm the Mind. In combination with L.I.-4 (the "Four Gates"), it has a very powerful calming effect on the Mind.
– **LIV-14**, Front-Collecting point of the Liver, moves Liver-Qi.
– **P-6** and **P-7**, indirectly connected to the Liver via the Terminal Yin channels, move Liver-Qi and calm the Mind. P-6 has more of a moving effect and lifts mood, while P-7 is better at calming the Mind when there is severe mental restlessness.
– **T.B.-6** moves Liver-Qi.
– **Du-24** and **G.B.-13** powerfully calm the Mind in any Liver pattern.

Special formula

ST-30 Qichong, KI-14 Siman, KI-13 Qixue, LIV-3 Taichong, P-6 Neiguan, BL-15 Xinshu, BL-18 Ganshu, SP-6 Sanyinjiao.

Explanation

This formula is used for Liver-Qi stagnating in the lower abdomen and Qi of the Penetrating Vessel rebelling upwards to disturb the Heart.

This condition arises from shock or prolonged worry and pensiveness which cause stagnation of Qi. Combined with other causes of disease (such as, for example, excessive lifting, loss of blood in childbirth, or declining Blood and Yin during the menopause), this may cause stagnation of Liver-Qi and rebellious Qi in the Penetrating Vessel. The Liver channel courses through the lower abdomen, the stomach, diaphragm, lungs and throat; the Kidney channel goes through the liver, diaphragm, lungs and throat. Thus they both go up to the throat where they may cause a feeling of constriction of the throat. They both also go to the chest where, with stagnation of Qi, they may cause a feeling of oppression and tightness of the chest. In the chest, they affect Heart and Lungs and therefore Mind and Corporeal Soul, giving rise to anxiety, palpitations and unhappiness. The "Spiritual Axis" in chapter 65 says: *"The Penetrating and Directing Vessels originate from the uterus, go up through the spine and form the Sea of channels . . . from the abdomen, they go up to the throat."*[74] The "Simple Questions" in chapter 60 says: *"The Penetrating Vessel rises through ST-30 Qichong, follows the Kidney channel to the umbilicus and chest where it scatters."*[75] Thus, rebellious Qi in the Penetrating Vessel affects the Heart causing anxiety, palpitations and mental confusion.

– **ST-30** is an important point of the Penetrating Vessel which emerges at this point coming from the perineum. The point name means "rushing Qi" or "penetrating Qi" and the *"chong"* in its name refers to the *Chong Mai*, i.e. the Penetrating Vessel. This vessel is also related to the Bright Yang and the connection takes place through this point. ST-30 is therefore used to subdue rebellious Qi in the Penetrating Vessel affecting not only lower abdomen, but the whole length of this vessel.
– **KI-14** also subdues rebellious Qi in the Penetrating Vessel when this affects the lower abdomen. The name of this point means "four fullnesses" which may refer to a feeling of fullness of the lower abdomen radiating in all four directions: this feeling of fullness derives from stagnation of Qi in the Penetrating

Vessel. Another meaning of its name is that the point treats four fullnesses deriving from stagnation of Qi, Blood, food, and Dampness.
- **KI-13** is another point along the Penetrating Vessel and it also regulates its Qi by strengthening its root in the lower abdomen.
- **LIV-3** subdues rebellious Qi in the Liver channel and settles the Ethereal Soul.
- **P-6** also subdues rebellious Qi in the Liver channel, relaxes the chest, calms the Mind, settles the Ethereal Soul, and relieves unhappiness.
- **BL-15** and **BL-18** regulate Qi of the Heart and Liver channel, move Qi, calm the Mind, and settle the Ethereal Soul.
- **SP-6** helps to subdue rebellious Qi by strengthening the root, i.e. Liver and Kidneys.

Herbal treatment

Prescription

YUE JU WAN
Gardenia-Ligusticum Pill
Cang Zhu *Rhizoma Atractylodis lanceae* 6 g
Chuan Xiong *Rhizoma Ligustici wallichii* 6 g
Xiang Fu *Rhizoma Cyperi rotundi* 6 g
Zhi Zi *Fructus Gardeniae jasminoidis* 6 g
Shen Qu *Massa Fermentata Medicinalis* 6 g

Explanation

This formula is primarily for Liver-Qi stagnation although it also treats stasis of Blood, retention of Food, stagnation of Phlegm and Dampness and knotted Heat. For this reason it is called the "formula for the six stagnations". It is, however, extremely effective in moving Qi, pacifying the Liver and calming the Mind. It is especially effective in opening the Mind's orifices and lifting mental depression deriving from stagnation of Liver-Qi.

- **Cang Zhu** resolves Dampness and Phlegm.
- **Chuan Xiong** moves Blood.
- **Xiang Fu** moves Liver-Qi.
- **Zhi Zi** clears Heat.
- **Shen Qu** resolves retention of food.

Mental-emotional pattern

This formula addresses the emotional and mental manifestations of stagnation of Liver-Qi when it causes the Mind to be obstructed: moodiness, mental depression, pre-menstrual tension, irritability, frustration, annoyance and impatience. A typical feature of this condition of Mind obstructed is first of all a certain mental confusion deriving from stagnation, and secondly, a strong resistance to any mental or affective change. This formula is extremely effective for mental depression of this type. On a physical level there would be a feeling of distension, sighing, belching, tiredness, hypochondrial pain, a feeling of tightness in the chest, irregular periods, clumsiness, breast distension and a Wiry pulse (which may be Wiry only on the left side). In most cases, the tongue may not change, whilst in severe cases it may be slightly red on the sides.

This formula also harmonizes Liver and Stomach and is particularly suited for stagnant Liver-Qi invading the Stomach deriving from emotional upsets occurring at meal-times.

The three most important signs for the use of this formula are tiredness, depression and a Wiry pulse.

Variations

- For the Mind obstruction of this condition add Shi Chang Pu *Rhizoma Acori graminei* to open the Mind's orifices and Yu Jin *Tuber Curcumae* to open orifices and move Qi. Yu Jin, in particular, is extremely effective for mental depression since its strongly moving nature provides the necessary "push" to unblock the set patterns established by chronic depression.
- If there is pronounced stagnation of Qi increase the dosage of Xiang Fu and, if necessary, add Mu Xiang *Radix Saussureae* and Fu Shou *Fructus Citri sarcodactylis*.
- If there is pronounced depression add He Huan Pi *Cortex Albizziae julibrissin*.
- If Dampness is pronounced increase the dosage of Cang Zhu and, if necessary, add Fu Ling *Sclerotium Poriae cocos*, Ze Xie *Rhizoma*

Alismatis orientalis and Hou Po *Cortex Magnoliae officinalis*.

– If stasis of Blood is pronounced increase the dosage of Chuan Xiong and, if necessary, add Hong Hua *Flos Carthami tinctorii* and Tao Ren *Semen Persicae*.

– If Fire is pronounced increase the dosage of Zhi Zi and, if necessary, add Huang Lian *Rhizoma Coptidis*.

– If Phlegm is pronounced add Ban Xia *Rhizoma Pinelliae ternatae*.

– If retention of food is pronounced increase the dosage of Shen Qu and, if necessary, add Mai Ya *Fructus Hordei vulgaris germinatus*, Shan Zha *Fructus Crataegi* and Sha Ren *Fructus seu Semen Amomi*.

– If there is emotional confusion add Shi Chang Pu *Rhizoma Acori graminei*.

Case history

A 38-year-old woman sought treatment for primary infertility. She had been trying to conceive for 2 years. The gynaecologist had diagnosed endometriosis and adhesions in the fallopian tubes for which she had had laser treatment. Her periods were quite normal and regular, except for being rather scanty (lasting 3 days). She suffered from very pronounced abdominal distension and fullness. She had panic attacks and experienced a feeling of oppression of the chest and palpitations. During such attacks she also had a suffocating feeling in the throat. Her eyes had an unstable look as if she were scared. Her tongue had a Red tip and sides, but apart from that, it was quite normal. Her pulse was Slippery, Short and Moving (the Moving pulse being short, shaped like a bean and vibrating).

During the consultation, on asking her about any shocks she might have had, she said she had been raped when she was 22.

Diagnosis
This is a condition of stagnation of Qi in the Liver channel and the Penetrating Vessel affecting the Heart. Shock affects the Heart, but also the Kidneys: in women, this often causes stagnation of Qi in the Penetrating Vessel and the Liver channel. Rebellious Qi in the lower abdomen rises upwards to harass the Heart and the Mind causing, in her case, palpitations, a feeling of oppression of the chest and anxiety. The stagnation of Qi in the Penetrating Vessel in the lower abdomen caused the feeling of fullness and distension there. Her eyes and her pulse clearly showed the strong possibility of shock in the past, and this was the reason for me asking her about this. The tongue

also showed stagnation in the Liver and Heart. In this case, therefore, infertility was not due to a deficiency, but to stagnation of Qi in the Penetrating and Directing Vessels preventing conception.

Treatment
She was treated with both acupuncture and herbs. The acupuncture treatment was quite infrequent as she lived over 100 miles away. Whenever I saw her I used the special formula indicated above, more or less unchanged, i.e.:

– **ST-30** Qichong, **KI-14** Siman, **KI-13** Qixue, **LIV-3** Taichong, **P-6** Neiguan, **BL-15** Xinshu, **BL-18** Ganshu, and **SP-6** Sanyinjiao.

This formula was explained above under the "Stagnation of Liver-Qi" pattern.
The herbal decoction used was a variation of two formulae together: Yue Ju Wan *Ligusticum-Gardenia Pill* and An Shen Ding Zhi Wan *Calming the Mind and Settling the Will-Power Pill*:

Xiang Fu *Rhizoma Cyperi rotundi* 9 g
Shan Zhi Zi *Fructus Gardeniae jasminoidis* 4 g
Chuan Xiong *Radix Ligustici wallichii* 4 g
Shen Qu *Massa Fermentata Medicinalis* 4 g
Cang Zhu *Rhizoma Atractylodis lanceae* 4 g
Dang Shen *Radix Codonopsis pilosulae* 6 g
Fu Shen *Sclerotium Poriae cocos pararadicis* 6 g
Yuan Zhi *Radix Polygalae tenuifoliae* 6 g
Long Chi *Dens Draconis* 12 g
Shi Chang Pu *Rhizoma Acori graminei* 4 g
Gui Ban *Plastrum Testudinis* 12 g
Dang Gui *Radix Angelicae sinensis* 6 g
Chen Xiang *Lignum Aquilariae* 4 g
Suan Zao Ren *Semen Ziziphi spinosae* 4 g
Bai Zi Ren *Semen Biotae orientalis* 6 g
Zhi Gan Cao *Radix Glycyrrhizae uralensis praeparata* 3 g

Explanation
– The first 5 herbs constitute the Yue Ju Wan *Ligusticum-Gardenia Pill* which pacifies the Liver and eliminates stagnation. The emphasis is on Xiang Fu (hence with a higher dose) to eliminate stagnation and subdue rebellious Qi in the Penetrating Vessel.

– The next 5 herbs make the An Shen Ding Zhi Wan *Calming the Mind and Settling the Will-Power Pill* which tonifies the Heart and calms the Mind, especially after shock.

– **Gui Ban** and **Dang Gui** were added to nourish and root the Penetrating Vessel in the lower abdomen: this will help to root it and subdue rebellious Qi. According to Li Shi Zhen, Gui Ban is the main substance to nourish and root the Penetrating and Directing Vessels.[76]

– **Chen Xiang** was added to subdue rebellious Qi in the Penetrating Vessel, a function attributed to it also by Li Shi Zhen in his book on the Extraordinary Vessels (see note 76).

– **Suan Zao Ren** and **Bai Zi Ren** were added to settle the Ethereal Soul and calm the Mind.

After 6 months of this treatment she conceived but unfortunately, she miscarried in the second month. She re-started the treatment and again she became pregnant after 6 months. This time, I prescribed a decoction to take as soon as she became pregnant to prevent miscarriage:

Tu Si Zi *Semen Cuscutae* 6 g
Du Zhong *Cortex Eucommiae ulmoidis* 6 g
Sha Ren *Fructus seu Semen Amomi* 4 g
Zi Su Ye *Folium Perillae frutescentis* 4 g
Bai Zhu *Rhizoma Atractylodis macrocephalae* 6 g

All these herbs prevent miscarriage and, this time, she was able to continue her pregnancy to full term and give birth to a baby.

2. STAGNATION OF HEART- AND LUNG-QI

Treatment principle

Move Qi, stimulate the descending of Heart- and Lung-Qi and calm the Mind.

Acupuncture

LU-7 Lieque, HE-7 Shenmen, P-6 Neiguan, Ren-15 Jiuwei, Ren-17 Shanzhong, ST-40 Fenglong, L.I.-4 Hegu, S.I.-5 Yanggu. Reducing or even method if the condition is chronic.

Explanation

– **LU-7** stimulates the descending of Lung-Qi and calms the Corporeal Soul. It has a strong mental effect and it relieves stagnation of Qi in the chest. According to "An Explanation of Acupuncture Points" (1654) this point is used when the person is sad and cries a lot.[77]
– **HE-7** stimulates the descending of Heart-Qi and calms the Mind.
– **P-6** stimulates the descending of Heart-Qi, opens the chest, relieves fullness and stagnation and calms the Mind.
– **Ren-15** has a powerful calming effect on the Mind. It also relieves fullness in the chest.
– **Ren-17** stimulates the descending of Lung-Qi and relieves fullness and stagnation in the chest.
– **ST-40** harmonizes the Stomach, opens the chest and calms the Mind.

– **L.I.-4** harmonizes the ascending and descending of Qi in the Middle Burner, relieves fullness and calms the Mind.
– **S.I.-5** opens the Mind's orifices and relieves confusion. It helps the patient to see issues clearly.

Herbal treatment

Prescription

BAN XIA HOU PO TANG
Pinellia-Magnolia Decoction
Ban Xia *Rhizoma Pinelliae ternatae* 12 g
Hou Po *Cortex Magnoliae officinalis* 9 g
Su Ye *Folium Perillae frutescentis* 6 g
Fu Ling *Sclerotium Poriae cocos* 12 g
Sheng Jiang *Rhizoma Zingiberis officinalis recens* 9 g

Explanation

– **Ban Xia** resolves Phlegm, eliminates stagnation, harmonizes the Stomach and subdues rebellious Qi. It is the emperor herb in this formula which treats the plum-stone pattern characterized by the feeling of a lump in the throat.
– **Hou Po** eliminates stagnation, relieves fullness, subdues rebellious Qi and calms the Mind.
– **Su Ye** moves Qi, harmonizes the Stomach, opens the chest and calms the Mind.
– **Fu Ling** helps Ban Xia to resolve Phlegm and calms the Mind.
– **Sheng Jiang** harmonizes the Stomach.

This formula, from the "Discussion of Cold-Induced Diseases", is normally used for the plum-stone pattern characterized by a feeling of obstruction in the throat, mental depression and irritability. In modern times this pattern is related to stagnation of Liver-Qi, for which this formula is used. An analysis of the formula, however, reveals that it contains no herbs that move Liver-Qi or even enter the Liver. The main emphasis of the formula is to move stagnant Heart- and Lung-Qi. Stagnation of Heart- and Lung-Qi derives from sadness and grief over a long period of time. These emotions first deplete

Heart-Qi and Lung-Qi and depress the Mind and Corporeal Soul. The depletion of Lung-Qi from sadness and grief leads to shallow breathing and poor circulation of Qi in the chest and, eventually, to stagnation of Lung-Qi in the chest. The simultaneous weakness and stagnation of Lung-Qi may also lead to Phlegm. The Lung channel influences the throat and its stagnation can cause a feeling of obstruction in the throat. Other manifestations include sighing, difficulty in swallowing, slight breathlessness, tightness of the chest, nausea and vomiting. The pulse will be Weak on both Front positions on the left and right and without wave. The tongue will be Swollen if there is some Phlegm.

Mental-emotional pattern

Stagnation of Heart- and Lung-Qi derives from long-term sadness and grief with the resulting depletion of the Mind and Corporeal Soul. This resides in the Lungs and it therefore affects breathing. The person becomes anxious as well as sad, sighs frequently and has the typical feeling of obstruction in the throat and chest. This is caused by the constriction of the Corporeal Soul in the throat and chest. The chronic stagnation of Heart-Qi obstructs the Mind and causes severe confusion.

This formula is used to literally "get it off one's chest".

Variations

- Similarly as for stagnation of Liver-Qi, Shi Chang Pu *Rhizoma Acori graminei* should be added to open the Mind's orifices.
- If there is a pronounced feeling of oppression of the chest from Qi stagnation (slightly Wiry pulse) add Qing Pi *Pericarpium Citri reticulatae viridae* and Mu Xiang *Radix Saussureae*.
- If there is vomiting increase Ban Xia and Sheng Jiang.
- If there is a feeling of heaviness under the heart add Zhi Shi *Fructus Citri aurantii immaturus*.
- If there is epigastric pain add Sha Ren *Fructus seu Semen Amomi*.
- If there is sour regurgitation with a yellow

tongue coating add Huang Lian *Rhizoma Coptidis*.
- If there is sour regurgitation with a Pale tongue add Wu Zei Gu *Os Sepiae*.
- If there is a bitter taste add Huang Qin *Radix Scutellariae baicalensis*.
- If mental restlessness and irritability are pronounced add He Huan Pi *Cortex Albizziae julibrissin*.

Associated prescription

SI QI TANG
Four-Seven Decoction
This consists of Ban Xia Hou Po Tang plus Da Zao *Fructus Ziziphi jujubae*.

This formula has the same use and indications as Ban Xia Hou Po Tang, except that its effect on the Mind is even stronger. "Seven" in the name of the formula stands for the 7 emotions and "Four" stands for the four seasons, indicating a condition that spans at least four seasons, i.e. a chronic condition.

BLOOD STASIS

1. HEART-BLOOD STASIS

Treatment principle

Move Blood, eliminate stasis, clear the Heart, calm the Mind.

Acupuncture

P-6 Neiguan, Ren-14 Juque, BL-14 Jueyinshu, BL-15 Xinshu, Ren-17 Shanzhong, HE-7 Shenmen, SP-6 Sanyinjiao, BL-17 Geshu, BL-44 Shentang. Reducing or even method if the condition is chronic.

Explanation

- **P-6** moves Heart-Blood, opens the chest and calms the Mind.
- **Ren-14**, Front-Collecting point of the Heart, moves Heart-Blood and calms the Mind.
- **BL-14** and **BL-15**, Back-Transporting points of the Pericardium and Heart respectively, move Blood and calm the Mind.

- **Ren-17** moves Qi in the chest: moving Qi will help to move Blood.
- **HE-7** calms the Mind.
- **SP-6** moves Blood and calms the Mind.
- **BL-17**, Gathering point for Blood, moves Blood (if needled with reducing or even method).
- **BL-44** clears the Heart and calms the Mind.

Herbal treatment

Prescription

XUE FU ZHU YU TANG
Blood-Mansion Eliminating Stasis Decoction
Dang Gui *Radix Angelicae sinensis* 9 g
Sheng Di Huang *Radix Rehmanniae glutinosae* 9 g
Chi Shao *Radix Paeoniae rubrae* 6 g
Chuan Xiong *Rhizoma Ligustici wallichii* 5 g
Tao Ren *Semen Persicae* 12 g
Hong Hua *Flos Carthami tinctorii* 9 g
Chai Hu *Radix Bupleuri* 3 g
Zhi Ke *Fructus Citri aurantii* 6 g
Niu Xi *Radix Cyathulae* 9 g
Jie Geng *Radix Platycodi grandiflori* 5 g
Gan Cao *Radix Glycyrrhizae uralensis* 3 g

Explanation

The first six herbs make up the Tao Hong Si Wu Tang *Persica-Carthamus Four Substances Decoction* which nourishes and moves Blood.

- **Chai Hu** and **Zhi Ke** move Liver-Qi which helps to move Liver-Blood.
- **Niu Xi** and **Jie Geng**, one with a descending movement, the other with a rising movement, are coordinated to move Qi.
- **Gan Cao** harmonizes.

This formula is very widely used for stasis of Blood in the Upper Burner causing chest pain. The tongue is Purple and the pulse is Wiry or Choppy.

Mental-emotional pattern

Since Blood is the residence of the Mind, any Blood pathology can affect the Mind. Blood stasis agitates and obstructs the Mind. It agitates the Mind because Qi and Blood cannot flow smoothly and this is reflected on the mental-emotional level. It obstructs the Mind because the impeded flow of Blood retards the circulation of Blood to the Mind and thus obfuscates its orifices.

Anger, frustration, resentment, excess joy, shock, craving and guilt can all lead to Heart-Blood stasis. This usually occurs only after a long period of time, going through the stage of Qi stagnation first.

When stagnant Blood in the Heart affects the Mind, it may cause depression, palpitations, insomnia, a suffocating sensation in the chest, irritability, mood swings and, in severe cases, psychosis. Sleep is very disturbed, the patient waking up frequently at night, tossing and turning and with nightmares.

Variations

- Shi Chang Pu *Rhizoma Acori graminei* and Yu Jin *Tuber Curcumae* should be added to open the Mind's orifices and move Blood.

2. *LIVER-BLOOD STASIS*

Treatment principle

Move Blood, pacify the Liver, calm the Mind and settle the Ethereal Soul.

Acupuncture

LIV-3 Taichong, LIV-14 Qimen, BL-18 Ganshu, BL-17 Geshu, BL-47 Hunmen, P-6 Neiguan, P-7 Daling, SP-6 Sanyinjiao, Du-24 Shenting and G.B.-13 Benshen. Reducing or even method if the condition is chronic, except for BL-47 which should be reinforced.

Explanation

- **LIV-3** moves Liver-Blood and calms the Mind and Ethereal Soul.
- **LIV-14** and **BL-18**, Front-Collecting and Back-Transporting point respectively, move Liver-Blood.
- **BL-17** moves Blood.
- **BL-47** settles the Ethereal Soul.
- **P-6** moves Blood, pacifies the Liver and calms the Mind.

- **P-7** moves Blood, opens the Mind orifices and calms the Mind.
- **SP-6** moves Blood and calms the Mind.
- **Du-24** and **G.B.-13** calm the Mind in any Liver pattern.

Herbal treatment

Prescription

YUE JU WAN
Gardenia-Ligusticum Pill
Cang Zhu *Rhizoma Atractylodis lanceae* 6 g
Chuan Xiong *Rhizoma Ligustici wallichii* 6 g
Xiang Fu *Rhizoma Cyperi rotundi* 6 g
Zhi Zi *Fructus Gardeniae jasminoidis* 6 g
Shen Qu *Massa Fermentata Medicinalis* 6 g

Explanation

This formula has already been discussed under Liver-Qi stagnation. It can be adapted to treat Liver-Blood stasis by increasing the dosage of Chuan Xiong.

Mental-emotional pattern

Anger, resentment, frustration, jealousy and hatred may all lead to Liver-Blood stasis. This will cause extreme depression, severe mood swings, intense irritability, propensity to violent outbursts of anger, obsessive jealousy and, in severe cases, manic-depression.

Variations

- Yu Jin *Tuber Curcumae* should be added to move Liver-Blood, open the Mind's orifices and relieve depression.
- In cases of severe depression add He Huan Pi *Cortex Albizziae julibrissin*.
- In cases of violent outbursts of anger add Suan Zao Ren *Semen Ziziphi spinosae* and Long Chi *Dens Draconis*.

3. STASIS OF BLOOD IN THE LOWER BURNER

Treatment principle

Move Blood, harmonize the Penetrating and Directing vessels, eliminate stasis and calm the Mind.

Acupuncture

SP-10 Xuehai, SP-6 Sanyinjiao, SP-4 Gongsun and P-6 Neiguan, Ren-6 Qihai, ST-29 Guilai, BL-18 Ganshu, BL-17 Geshu, SP-1 Yinbai, Du-18 Qiangjian. Reducing method.

Explanation

- **SP-10** moves Blood in the uterus.
- **SP-6** moves Blood and calms the Mind.
- **SP-4** and **P-6** in combination open the Penetrating vessel and move Blood.
- **Ren-6** moves Qi in order to move Blood.
- **ST-29** moves Blood in the uterus.
- **BL-18** and **BL-17** in combination move Blood.
- **SP-1** moves Blood in the uterus and calms the Mind.
- **Du-18** opens the Mind orifices, calms the Mind and regulates Liver-Blood. It is a strong head point for mental restlessness, manic behaviour and agitation.

Herbal treatment

Prescription

TAO HE CHENG QI TANG
Persica Conducting Qi Decoction
Tao Ren *Semen Persicae* 12 g
Da Huang *Rhizoma Rhei* 12 g
Gui Zhi *Ramulus Cinnamomi cassiae* 6 g
Mang Xiao *Mirabilitum* 6 g
Zhi Gan Cao *Radix Glycyrrhizae uralensis praeparata* 6 g

Explanation

- **Tao Ren** strongly moves Blood and eliminates stasis. It enters the Heart and opens the Heart orifices.
- **Da Huang** eliminates stasis of Blood by moving downward and clears Fire.
- **Gui Zhi** helps Tao Ren to eliminate stasis of Blood because it enters the blood vessels.
- **Mang Xiao** clears Heat, softens hardness and helps Da Huang to move downwards.

– **Zhi Gan Cao** harmonizes and moderates the strong action of the other herbs.

Mental-emotional pattern

This prescription is from the "Discussion of Cold-induced Diseases" and it refers to the Greater Yang-organ pattern from accumulation of Blood. This consists in accumulation of Blood in the hypogastrium following an invasion of Cold. It manifests with fever at night, delirium, severe lower abdominal pain, mental restlessness and manic behaviour. This is the original use of the formula. It can be used for mental-emotional problems deriving from (or causing) stasis of Blood in the Lower Burner.

Anger, frustration, hatred, resentment and guilt may all lead to this condition over a long period of time. Why do these emotions in this case lead to stasis of Blood in the Lower Burner and not somewhere else? First of all, it is obviously more common in women who are prone to stasis of Blood in the uterus. However, it may also be due to other concurrent causes of disease such as excessive lifting which leads to stagnation in the Lower Burner.

Guilt frequently leads to stasis of Blood in the Lower Burner especially in women. This happens especially if the guilt is centred around sexual behaviour.

A special use of this formula is for psychosis from stasis of Blood in the uterus following childbirth.

PHLEGM MISTING THE MIND

PHLEGM-HEAT HARASSING THE MIND

Treatment principle

Resolve Phlegm, open the orifices and calm the Mind.

Acupuncture

ST-40 Fenglong, P-7 Daling, P-6 Neiguan, P-5 Jianshi, Du-14 Dazhui, BL-15 Xinshu, BL-44 Shentang, Du-20 Baihui, L.I.-4 Hegu, LU-7 Lieque, Ren-12 Zhongwan, ST-36 Zusanli, BL-20

Pishu, L.I.-7 Wenliu, ST-25 Tianshu. Reducing or even method, except for Du-14, Du-20, Ren-12, ST-36, BL-20, BL-15 and BL-44 which should be reinforced.

Explanation

– **ST-40** resolves Phlegm.
– **P-7** resolves Phlegm from the Heart and calms the Mind.
– **P-6** opens the Mind's orifices.
– **P-5** resolves Phlegm from the Heart.
– **Du-14,** with reinforcing method and moxa, tonifies the Heart and clears the Mind.
– **BL-15** and **BL-44** tonify the Heart and clear the Mind.
– **Du-20** clears the Mind.
– **L.I.-4** and **LU-7** regulate the ascending of clear Qi and descending of turbid Qi in the head, thus clearing the Mind.
– **Ren-12**, **ST-36** and **BL-20** tonify the Spleen to resolve Phlegm.
– **L.I.-7** opens the Mind's orifices. The book "An Explanation of Acupuncture Points" (1654) says this point is for *"madness and seeing ghosts"*.[78]
– **ST-25** is an important point for mental-emotional problems from Phlegm misting the Mind. It regulates the Stomach and opens the Mind's orifices. The book "An Explanation of Acupuncture Points" says this points is used when *"Ethereal Soul and Corporeal Soul have no residence"*.[79]

Herbal treatment

1. Prescription

BAN XIA BAI ZHU TIAN MA TANG
Pinellia-Atractylodes-Gastrodia Decoction
Ban Xia *Rhizoma Pinelliae ternatae* 9 g
Tian Ma *Rhizoma Gastrodiae elatae* 6 g
Bai Zhu *Rhizoma Atractylodis macrocephalae* 15 g
Fu Ling *Sclerotium Poriae cocos* 6 g
Chen Pi *Pericarpium Citri reticulatae* 6 g
Gan Cao *Rhizoma Glycyrrhizae uralensis* 4 g
Sheng Jiang *Rhizoma Zingiberis officinalis recens* 1 slice
Da Zao *Fructus Ziziphi jujubae* 2 pieces

Explanation

- **Ban Xia**, **Fu Ling**, **Chen Pi**, **Sheng Jiang**, **Da Zao** and **Gan Cao** form the Er Chen Tang *Two Old Decoction* which resolves Phlegm.
- **Tian Ma** subdues Wind from the head and relieves headache.
- **Bai Zhu** tonifies the Spleen and resolves Dampness.

This formula is used for Wind-Phlegm, i.e. when Phlegm is combined with internal Wind, as it so often is in old people. In this case, by making use of Tian Ma which treats the head, it can be used to resolve Phlegm from the head misting the Mind.

The main manifestations on a physical level would be dizziness, a dull headache, a feeling of heaviness of the head and body, nausea, a desire to lie down, a feeling of oppression of the chest, poor appetite, tiredness, a Swollen tongue with a sticky coating and a Slippery-Wiry pulse.

Mental-emotional pattern

Worry and pensiveness affect Lungs and Spleen and may easily cause these two organs not to transform and move fluids properly. This often leads to Phlegm which mists the Mind. The reverse process is of course possible: any cause that might lead to Phlegm (such as irregular diet or congenital weakness of the Spleen) may induce this condition.

The main manifestations would be mental confusion, poor memory and concentration, depression, weeping and lack of mental clarity.

Phlegm obstructs the Mind and Fire harasses it.

Variations

- Shi Chang Pu *Rhizoma Acori graminei* would be an essential addition to this formula in order to open the Mind's orifices and clear the Mind.
- If there is depression add Yu Jin *Tuber Curcumae* to open the orifices and relieve depression, and He Huan Pi *Cortex Albizziae julibrissin* to move Qi and Blood and relieve depression.

2. *Prescription*

WEN DAN TANG
Warming the Gall-Bladder Decoction
Ban Xia *Rhizoma Pinelliae ternatae* 6 g
Fu Ling *Sclerotium Poriae cocos* 5 g
Chen Pi *Pericarpium Citri reticulatae* 9 g
Zhu Ru *Caulis Bambusae in Taeniis* 6 g
Zhi Shi *Fructus Citri aurantii immaturus* 6 g
Zhi Gan Cao *Radix Glycyrrhizae uralensis prae-parata* 3 g
Sheng Jiang *Rhizoma Zingiberis officinalis recens* 5 slices
Da Zao *Fructus Ziziphi jujubae* one date

Explanation

- **Ban Xia**, **Fu Ling** and **Chen Pi** constitute the Er Chen Tang *Two Old Decoction* and they resolve Phlegm and Dampness.
- **Zhu Ru** resolves Phlegm-Heat and calms the Mind.
- **Zhi Shi** moves Qi in the chest and helps to resolve Phlegm.
- **Gan Cao**, **Sheng Jiang** and **Da Zao** harmonize.

This interesting formula (dating from 1174) has two main interpretations. Originally it was used for a Gall-Bladder deficiency following a severe acute disease, the Gall-Bladder deficiency manifesting with timidity, jumpiness, insomnia (waking up early in the morning) and mental restlessness. In more recent times, it is more frequently used for Phlegm-Fire affecting Stomach, Heart, or Lungs. The main manifestations for which it is used in this context are mental restlessness, jumpiness, insomnia, a bitter and sticky taste, a flustered feeling in the heart region, nausea, vomiting, palpitations, dizziness, a Swollen tongue with a sticky-yellow coating and a Wiry or Slippery pulse.

Two characteristic pulse and tongue configurations strongly indicate the use of this formula. One is a tongue which is Swollen and has a combination of Heart and Stomach crack with a rough, brush-like yellow coating inside the Stomach crack. A combined Heart and Stomach crack extends all the way to the tip, as a Heart crack would do, but it is wide and shallow in the centre, as a Stomach crack would be (see Fig. 9.8).

The other sign is a pulse which is Big, Slippery and Wiry on both Middle positions of left and right.

Mental-emotional pattern

Phlegm-Heat disturbs the Mind in two ways: Phlegm obstructs the Mind's orifices and Heat agitates the Mind. The combination of these two factors will cause mental restlessness, manic behaviour alternated with severe depression, crying or laughing without reason and insomnia. In severe cases this corresponds to manic-depressive illness or schizophrenia.

3. Prescription

GUI SHEN TANG
Restoring the Mind Decoction
Ren Shen *Radix Ginseng* 15 g
Bai Zhu *Rhizoma Atractylodis macrocephalae* 30 g
Ba Ji Tian *Radix Morindae officinalis* 30 g
Fu Shen *Sclerotium Poriae cocos pararadicis* 15 g
Zi He Che *Placenta hominis* 6 g
Ban Xia *Rhizoma Pinelliae ternatae* 9 g
Chen Pi *Pericarpium Citri reticulatae* 3 g
Bai Jie Zi *Semen Sinapis albae* 9 g
Shi Chang Pu *Rhizoma Acori graminei* 3 g
Zhu Sha *Cinnabaris* 3 g
Mai Men Dong *Tuber Ophiopogonis japonici* 6 g
Bai Zi Ren *Semen Biotae orientalis* 6 g
Zhi Gan Cao *Radix Glycyrrhizae uralensis praeparata* 3 g

Explanation

- **Ren Shen**, **Bai Zhu**, **Ba Ji Tian** and **Fu Shen** tonify Spleen and Kidneys.
- **Zi He Che**: interestingly, the original text explains the inclusion of placenta by saying that it is the "mother of the Pre-Natal Qi" and therefore restores the Mind.
- **Ban Xia**, **Chen Pi** and **Bai Jie Zi** resolve Cold Phlegm.
- **Chang Pu** and **Zhu Sha** open the orifices. If Zhu Sha is not used (as it is toxic) the dosage of Chang Pu can be increased to at least 9 g.

- **Mai Dong** and **Bai Zi Ren** nourish Heart-Blood and calm the Mind.
- **Zhi Gan Cao** harmonizes.

Mental-emotional pattern

This formula combines opening the Mind's orifices and resolving Phlegm with tonifying the Spleen, Heart and Kidneys. It is therefore suitable in chronic conditions when Phlegm mists the Mind on a background of Qi and Yang deficiency.

From a mental-emotional viewpoint, the patient will be calmer than in the previous two cases. He or she will feel very confused mentally, exhausted and depressed. The obstruction of the Mind by Phlegm, combined with the deficient Heart and Kidneys not nourishing the Mind, will make this person very forgetful and disorientated. In severe cases, the depression may be such that the patient feels suicidal.

Case history

A 39-year-old man had been suffering from what was labelled as "phobic anxiety" for 8 years. His history was quite complex and many factors contributed to his problem, so, rather than starting from his presenting symptoms, it might be better to describe his history from the beginning. His childhood had been very troubled, most of all because his mother was very unloving towards him and she constantly reproached him. At the age of 28 he worked in Belfast at the time of a very tense political and military situation which caused a great deal of anxiety to him. He suffered a shock when he found a bomb under his car. When he was 30 he had a car accident and had concussion. Nine months after that he contracted an extremely severe case of influenza which was nearly fatal. He was in bed for a month with a constant temperature. A few months after that he collapsed crying hysterically, he was unable to speak, could not move and could not bear to look at the light. His GP thought he had a brain haemorrhage but this was not the case. After that collapse he continued to be extremely anxious, lost all confidence in himself, lacked self-esteem, felt extremely insecure and was prone to bouts of crying. At this time he started seeing a psychotherapist and then a psychiatrist who prescribed tranquillizers (diazepam and temazepam) and anti-depressants of the MAOI kind.

He started having acupuncture with a colleague who referred him to me for herbal treatment.

His main symptoms when he came to me were

epigastric pain, alternation of constipation and diarrhoea, ache in the joints, burning eyes and a hot feeling at the back of the head.

On a mental level his main manifestations were severe anxiety, insomnia, bouts of crying, poor memory and concentration, depression and a lack of confidence and self-esteem.

His eyes lacked glitter and looked scared, his body was overweight and his complexion was very dull and sallow.

His tongue was dark-Red, Swollen, with a Heart-crack, without coating and dry. The tip of the tongue was redder and the root had no spirit (Plate 9.3). His pulse, however, was slightly Rapid, quite Full and Slippery.

Diagnosis
This is an extremely complex condition. As far as patterns are concerned there are basically two main patterns: severe Yin deficiency of the Heart and Kidneys (Red-peeled tongue with red tip and root without spirit, mental restlessness, anxiety, insomnia, burning eyes, a hot feeling on the occiput, lack of confidence and self-esteem) and Phlegm-Heat misting the Mind (crying without reason, poor memory and concentration). There are a few other patterns but these can be considered secondary. For example, there is Stomach-Yin deficiency causing the epigastric pain, Damp-Heat causing the joint pain, some stagnation of Liver-Qi causing the alternation of constipation and diarrhoea and some Spleen deficiency causing him to be overweight and generally tired. It is this underlying Spleen deficiency which, over the years, led to the formation of Phlegm, later transformed into Phlegm-Heat.

If there is Phlegm, why does the tongue not have a thick-sticky coating? This is because there is an underlying severe deficiency of Yin which caused the coating to fall off. Thus, although not shown on the tongue-body colour, Phlegm does manifest in the swelling of tongue body (which in such a severe case of Yin deficiency should have been Thin) and in the symptoms and the pulse which is Full and Slippery.

The Yin deficiency obviously derived from the time of his severe influenza. A constant temperature for a month burned the body fluids and injured Yin. The deficiency of Yin over the years led to the formation of Empty-Heat which harasses the Mind. On the other hand, the deficiency of Yin itself deprives the Mind and Ethereal Soul of their root and causes lack of confidence and self-esteem. Phlegm-Heat, conversely, obstructs the Mind and causes the bouts of crying.

Obviously all this is affected by his childhood experiences which formed the basis for the development of his condition later on in life especially causing his lack of confidence and self-esteem having never received love from his mother. Other aetiological factors also played a role. The concussion suffered following the car accident could have

affected his brain and therefore contributed to his illness.

Thus we can summarize his causes of disease in three stages (Fig. 9.10):

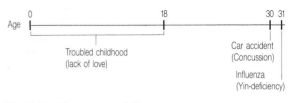

Fig. 9.10   Three causes of disease

Treatment principle
Treatment was focused on the two main patterns of Yin deficiency and Phlegm-Heat: to nourish Heart- and Kidney-Yin, clear Empty-Heat, open the Mind's orifices, calm the Mind, root the Ethereal Soul and Corporeal Soul and strengthen Will-Power.

Herbal treatment
This patient was treated for 4 years and is still under treatment; therefore the formula used was obviously modified very many times. The formula used most frequently was a variation of three prescriptions:

- Wen Dan Tang *Warming the Gall-Bladder Decoction*
- Tian Wang Bu Xin Dan *Heavenly Emperor's Tonifying the Heart Pill*
- Gan Mai Da Zao Tang *Glycyrrhiza-Triticum-Ziziphus Decoction*

An example of a formula used is:

Zhu Ru *Caulis Bambusae in Taeniis* 6 g
Zhi Shi *Fructus Citri aurantii immaturus* 4 g
Ban Xia *Rhizoma Pinelliae ternatae* 6 g
Fu Ling *Sclerotium Poriae cocos* 6 g
Chen Pi *Pericarpium Citri reticulatae* 3 g
Sheng Di Huang *Radix Rehmanniae glutinosae* 9 g
Mai Men Dong *Tuber Ophiopogonis japonici* 6 g
Xuan Shen *Radix Scrophulariae ningpoensis* 4 g
Ren Shen *Radix Ginseng* 6 g
Bai Zi Ren *Semen Biotae orientalis* 6 g
Suan Zao Ren *Semen Ziziphi spinosae* 6 g
Wu Wei Zi *Fructus Schisandrae chinensis* 4 g
Yuan Zhi *Radix Polygalae tenuifoliae* 9 g
Shi Chang Pu *Rhizoma Acori graminei* 4 g
Yu Jin *Tuber Curcumae* 4 g
Fu Xiao Mai *Semen Tritici aestivi levis* 6 g
Zhi Gan Cao *Radix Glycyrrhizae uralensis praeparata* 9 g
Da Zao *Fructus Ziziphi jujubae* 10 dates

Explanation
This is a variation of the three formulae listed above. The main additions are:

- **Chang Pu** and **Yu Jin** to open the Mind's orifices. These two herbs were not used every time as they are pungent and therefore injure Yin.

Variations
Variations used at different times according to the patient's condition were:

– **Du Zhong** *Cortex Eucommiae ulmoidis* to strengthen the Kidneys, the Will-Power and his sense of self-confidence and self-esteem. Although this herb tonifies Kidney-Yang it can be added to the prescription in combination with the many herbs which nourish Yin.
– **He Huan Pi** *Cortex Albizziae julibrissin* to open the Mind's orifices and lift depression.
– **Bai He** *Bulbus Lilii* to nourish Lung-Yin and relieve sadness and crying.
– **Ju Hua** *Flos Chrysanthemi morifolii* to relieve burning eyes.
– **Ye Jiao Teng** *Caulis Polygoni multiflori* to promote sleep.
– **Mu Xiang** *Radix Saussureae* to move Qi to help to resolve Phlegm.
– **Tai Zi Shen** *Radix Pseudostellariae heterophyllae* and **Shan Yao** *Radix Dioscoreae oppositae* to nourish Stomach-Yin.
– **Long Chi** *Dens Draconis* and **Zhen Zhu Mu** *Concha margaritiferae* to sink Qi and calm the Mind.

Recently this patient had a consultation with Professor Zhou Zhong Ying, one of my teachers from Nanjing, and he confirmed the diagnosis of Phlegm-Heat misting the Mind and Yin deficiency. He suggested a prescription which incorporates the formula Bai He Zhi Mu Tang *Lilium-Anemarrhena Decoction* from the "Essential Prescriptions from the Golden Chest".[80] A mental condition similar to this patient's was described in this old classic and was called "Lilium syndrome". The book says: *"Symptoms and signs [of the Lilium syndrome] include: the patient wants to eat but he cannot swallow and cannot speak. He wants to lie in bed yet he cannot lie quietly as he is restless. He wants to walk but soon becomes tired. Sometimes he likes eating, at other times he cannot tolerate the smell of food. He feels sometimes hot and sometimes cold, but without fever or chill. He has a bitter taste and the urine is dark. The patient looks as if he was possessed and his pulse is rapid".*[81]

The treatment suggested for this condition is a decoction of Bai He *Bulbus Lilii* and Zhi Mu *Radix Anemarrhenae asphodeloidis*.

Thus the formula suggested by Professor Zhou was:

Huang Lian *Rhizoma Coptidis* 4 g
Ban Xia *Rhizoma Pinelliae ternatae* 6 g
Dan Nan Xing *Rhizoma Arisaematis praeparata* 4 g
Fu Ling *Sclerotium Poriae cocos* 9 g
Zhi Gan Cao *Radix Glycyrrhizae uralensis praeparata* 3 g
Chen Pi *Pericarpium Citri reticulatae* 4 g
Zhu Ru *Caulis Bambusae in Taeniis* 6 g
Dan Shen *Radix Salviae miltiorrhizae* 6 g

Mai Men Dong *Tuber Ophiopogonis japonici* 9 g
Zhi Mu *Radix Anemarrhenae asphodeloidis* 9 g
Bai He *Bulbus Lilii* 9 g
Mu Li *Concha Ostreae* 15 g

Explanation
– The first seven herbs are a variation of Wen Dan Tang *Warming the Gall-Bladder Decoction* eliminating Zhi Shi *Fructus Citri aurantii immaturus* and adding Huang Lian and Nan Xing to resolve Phlegm-Heat.
– **Dan Shen** enters the Heart and calms the Mind.
– **Mai Dong** nourishes Heart-Yin.
– **Zhi Mu** nourishes Yin and clears Empty-Heat.
– **Bai He** nourishes Yin and relieves sadness and crying.
– **Mu Li** nourish Yin.

After four years of treatment this patient has improved considerably although there is still a way to go. On a physical level, he has lost all his symptoms and his tongue is considerably less Red and has now a thin coating. On a mental level, his memory and concentration have improved and his self-confidence and self-esteem are much better. He is less anxious and is off all medication.

MIND UNSETTLED

The Mind, Ethereal Soul and Corporeal Soul may be unsettled either because of a deficiency of Blood-Yin or because of the presence of a pathogenic factor which disturbs the Mind. Such pathogenic factors may be stagnation of Qi, stasis of Blood, Fire, Phlegm-Fire or Empty-Heat. The manifestations will be similar in both cases except that they will be milder if they are due purely to a deficiency, without a pathogenic factor.

The main manifestations of unsettled Mind are anxiety, mental restlessness, insomnia in the sense of waking up at night and agitation. In case of unsettled Ethereal Soul there will be in addition, nightmares, irritability, absent-mindedness, depression and inability to plan one's life. In cases of unsettled Corporeal Soul there will be anxiety with breathlessness and a feeling of tightness of the chest, worrying a lot and some somatization of the emotions on the skin such as itchy rashes.

The treatment principle for an unsettled Mind is to nourish Blood or Yin, eliminate pathogenic factors and calm the Mind.

BLOOD DEFICIENCY

HEART-BLOOD DEFICIENCY

Treatment principle

Tonify the Heart, nourish Blood and calm the Mind.

Acupuncture

BL-15 Xinshu, BL-44 Shentang, Ren-14 Juque, HE-7 Shenmen, P-7 Daling, Ren-4 Guanyuan, ST-36 Zusanli, SP-6 Sanyinjiao, P-6 Neiguan and SP-4 Gongsun. Reinforcing method, moxa may be applied.

Explanation

– **BL-15,** Back-Transporting point of the Heart, tonifies the Heart. It can be used with direct moxa cones only.
– **BL-44** tonifies the Heart and calms the Mind.
– **Ren-14,** Front-Collecting point of the Heart, and **HE-7** calm the Mind.
– **P-7** strongly calms the Mind and would be needled in a case of severe anxiety.
– **Ren-4** nourishes Blood and calms the Mind.
– **ST-36** nourishes Blood.
– **SP-6** nourishes Blood and calms the Mind. It is effective for insomnia from Blood deficiency.
– **P-6** and **SP-4** open the Yin Linking vessel which nourishes Blood and calms the Mind.

Herbal treatment

Prescription

YANG XIN TANG
Nourishing the Heart Decoction
Ren Shen *Radix Ginseng* (or **Dang Shen** *Radix Codonopsis pilosulae)* 6 g
Huang Qi *Radix Astragali membranacei* 9 g
Dang Gui *Radix Angelicae sinensis* 6 g
Chuan Xiong *Radix Ligustici wallichii* 4.5 g
Fu Ling *Sclerotium Poriae cocos* 6 g
Bai Zi Ren *Semen Biotae orientalis* 6 g
Suan Zao Ren *Semen Ziziphi spinosae* 4.5 g
Yuan Zhi *Radix Polygalae tenuifoliae* 6 g
Wu Wei Zi *Fructus Schisandrae chinensis* 4.5 g

Ban Xia *Rhizoma Pinelliae ternatae* 4.5 g
Rou Gui *Cortex Cinnamomi cassiae* 1.5 g
Zhi Gan Cao *Radix Glycyrrhizae uralensis praeparata* 4.5 g

Explanation

– **Dang Shen** and **Huang Qi** tonify Qi in order to tonify Blood.
– **Dang Gui** and **Chuan Xiong** nourish and harmonize Blood.
– **Fu Ling**, **Bai Zi Ren, Suan Zao Ren** and **Yuan Zhi** nourish the Heart and calm the Mind.
– **Wu Wei Zi** nourishes Yin in order to nourish Blood and, being sour in taste, it "absorbs" and roots the Mind in Blood and Yin.
– **Ban Xia** is added to resolve Phlegm which might derive from Qi deficiency. In this respect it is coordinated with Fu Ling. Ban Xia also resolves any Phlegm that might mist the Mind: in this respect it is coordinated with Yuan Zhi which also opens the Mind's orifices.
– **Rou Gui** is here to stimulate the production of Qi and Blood, which is one of its functions. It is added also to attract any Empty-Heat that there might be downwards towards its source, i.e. towards the Kidneys.
– **Gan Cao** harmonizes.

This formula is specific to treat any mental and emotional effect of Heart-Blood deficiency, such as insomnia (difficulty in falling asleep), palpitations, mild anxiety and poor memory. Other manifestations would include a dull-pale complexion, a Pale-Thin tongue and a Choppy pulse.

Mental-emotional pattern

Fear and worry may weaken Heart-Blood and cause this condition. This person would be pale with a dull complexion, the eyes would look anxious and rather dull and he or she would be fearful, mildly anxious and vaguely depressed. In this case, the manifestations of an unsettled Mind (anxiety and agitation) would be rather mild as there is only deficiency of Blood with no Empty-Heat. He or she would also be very eager to please other people and members of his or her family. Due to women's propensity for Blood deficiency, this condition is much more common in women. In fact, it may also arise from loss of Blood in childbirth. The loss of Blood from the Directing and Penetrating vessels during childbirth may affect the Heart, also due to its connection with the uterus via the Uterus-Vessel (*Bao-Mai*). When Heart-Blood is weakened the Mind is deprived of its residence and becomes fearful and anxious.

Variations

- If there is severe insomnia add Long Yan Rou *Arillus Euphoriae longanae* which nourishes Heart-Blood and calms the Mind.

(i) Patent remedy

BAI ZI YANG XIN WAN
Biota Nourishing the Heart Pill
This pill has the same ingredients as the above decoction with the addition of Zhu Sha *Cinnabaris*. It tonifies Spleen-Qi, nourishes Heart-Blood and calms the Mind. When the Mind is restless from a deficiency of Spleen and Heart, this is an excellent remedy.

Please note that, although this remedy shares the same name as the following formula (p. 246), it has different ingredients and indications. This remedy, in fact, nourishes Heart-Blood while the formula of the same name nourishes Heart-Yin.

YIN DEFICIENCY

1. HEART-YIN DEFICIENCY

Treatment principle

Tonify the Heart, nourish Yin and calm the Mind.

Acupuncture

BL-15 Xinshu, BL-44 Shentang, Ren-14 Juque, HE-7 Shenmen, HE-6 Yinxi, P-7 Daling, Ren-15 Jiuwei, Ren-4 Guanyuan, ST-36 Zusanli, SP-6 Sanyinjiao. Reinforcing method, no moxa.

Explanation

- **BL-15**, Back-Transporting point of the Heart, tonifies the Heart.
- **BL-44** tonifies the Heart and calms the Mind.
- **Ren-14**, Front-Collecting point of the Heart, and **HE-7** calm the Mind.
- **HE-6** nourishes Heart-Yin.
- **P-7** strongly calms the Mind and would be needled in cases of severe anxiety.
- **Ren-15** strongly calms the Mind and relieves anxiety.
- **Ren-4** nourishes Yin and calms the Mind. It nourishes Kidney-Yin which is often at the basis of Heart-Yin deficiency.
- **ST-36** nourishes Stomach-Yin.
- **SP-6** nourishes Yin and calms the Mind.

Herbal treatment

Prescription

BAI ZI YANG XIN WAN
Biota Nourishing the Heart Pill
Bai Zi Ren *Semen Biotae orientalis* 120 g
Fu Shen *Sclerotium Poriae Cocos pararadicis* 30 g
Gou Qi Zi *Fructus Lycii chinensis* 90 g
Shu Di Huang *Radix Rehmanniae glutinosae praeparata* 60 g
Dang Gui *Radix Angelicae sinensis* 30 g
Xuan Shen *Radix Scrophulariae ningpoensis* 60 g
Mai Men Dong *Tuber Ophiopogonis japonici* 30 g
Shi Chang Pu *Rhizoma Acori graminei* 30 g
Gan Cao *Radix Glycyrrhizae uralensis* 15 g

Explanation

- **Bai Zi Ren** and **Fu Shen** nourish the Heart and calm the Mind.
- **Gou Qi Zi**, **Shu Di Huang** and **Dang Gui** nourish Blood and Yin. Dang Gui and Shu Di enter the Heart.
- **Xuan Shen** and **Mai Men Dong** nourish Yin. Mai Dong enters the Heart.
- **Shi Cang Pu** opens the Mind's orifices.
- **Gan Cao** harmonizes.

This formula is similar to the previous one as it also nourishes Heart-Blood; it differs from it in so far as it nourishes Heart-Yin. The configuration of symptoms and signs would therefore be different as there would be more Yin-deficiency manifestations; insomnia (waking up at night frequently), a feeling of heat in the evening, a dry mouth and throat, night-sweating, more pronounced anxiety and mental restlessness, a malar flush, palpitations, a Red tongue without coating with a redder tip and a Floating-Empty pulse.

Mental-emotional pattern

Fear and worry, combined with overwork over many years may lead to Heart-Yin deficiency. Yin deficiency is a deeper level of deficiency than Blood deficiency, and when it affects the Heart, the Mind is deprived of its residence. This makes the person fearful, very anxious and restless. These symptoms would be more severe than in Heart-Blood deficiency. Another difference is that they would be more pronounced in the evening. Thus Yin deficiency makes the Mind unsettled even without Empty-Heat.

A person suffering from this condition would tend to be depressed and dispirited, lacking willpower and drive, and the body would probably be thin.

Patent remedy

BU NAO WAN
Tonifying the Brain Pill
Dang Gui *Radix Angelicae sinensis*
Suan Zao Ren *Semen Ziziphi spinosae*
Rou Cong Rong *Herba Cistanchis*
Bai Zi Ren *Semen Biotae orientalis*
Yuan Zhi *Radix Polygalae tenuifoliae*
Tao Ren *Semen Persicae*
Tian Nan Xing *Rhizoma Arisaematis*
Shi Chang Pu *Rhizoma Acori graminei*
Gou Qi Zi *Fructus Lycii chinensis*
Hu Po *Succinum*
Long Chi *Dens Draconis*
Wu Wei Zi *Fructus Schisandrae chinensis*

Explanation

Like many of the commercial preparations, this pill "hedges its bets" by covering several different conditions. In fact, it contains herbs which

nourish the Heart, tonify the Kidneys, move Blood, open the Mind's orifices and have a sinking movement. However, the main thrust of the pill is to nourish Heart-Yin and calm the Mind.

Case history

A 28-year-old man complained of nervousness with shaking of the hands. He said he felt nearly always very nervous especially at work and found the shaking of his hands very distressing. He also complained of dryness of the mouth, sweating, shortness of breath and insomnia (waking up during the night). He also lacked confidence and felt insecure, worried and anxious most of the time.

His tongue was unremarkable being only slightly Swollen. His pulse was Moving: this is a pulse which is Rapid, Short, shaped like a bean and giving the impression of vibrating rather than pulsating.

Diagnosis
This man's symptoms fall somewhat outside the scope of regular patterns. Some of the symptoms seem to point to Yin deficiency (waking up at night and feeling hot) but they are not severe enough to warrant such a diagnosis and the tongue does not show any Yin deficiency. There are, on the other hand, some signs of Qi deficiency (sweating, shortness of breath).

This is a problem caused by fear and worry over many years: fear affected the Heart and the Mind and worry affected the Lungs and Corporeal Soul. Affliction of the Mind caused the insomnia and affliction of the Corporeal Soul caused the breathlessness, sweating and shaking of the hands.

When asked about his childhood he said that it was quite troubled and insecure due to his father's open preference for his sister. His father constantly praised his sister for being quite brilliant at school and blamed him for not being up to his sister's standards. The unyielding censure by his father over several years of childhood development instilled a deep feeling of insecurity in him which led to fear and worry.

Treatment principle
Tonify Qi and Yin of Lungs and Heart, nourish and calm the Mind and settle the Corporeal Soul.

Acupuncture
The following points were reinforced:

– **HE-7** Shenmen, **SP-6** Sanyinjiao, **BL-15** Xinshu, **BL-39** Shentang and **Ren-15** Jiuwei nourish the Heart and calm the Mind.
– **LU-9** Taiyuan, **BL-13** Feishu and **BL-37** Pohu tonify the Lungs and settle the Corporeal Soul.

After six months of weekly treatments all his symptoms disappeared and his hands stopped shaking. In conjunction with counselling which I recommended, he explored the behavioural patterns developed in his childhood and gained much self-confidence and self-assurance.

2. LIVER-YIN DEFICIENCY

Treatment principle

Tonify the Liver, nourish Yin, calm the Mind and settle the Ethereal Soul.

Acupuncture

LIV-8 Ququan, SP-6 Sanyinjiao, KI-3 Taixi, Ren-4 Guanyuan, Du-24 Shenting, G.B.-13 Benshen, BL-18 Ganshu, BL-47 Hunmen. Reinforcing method, no moxa.

Explanation

- **LIV-8** nourishes Liver-Yin.
- **SP-6** nourishes Yin and strengthens Liver, Spleen and Kidneys.
- **KI-3** and **Ren-4** nourish Kidney-Yin. As this is the mother of Liver-Yin, it will indirectly nourish Liver-Yin. Ren-4 has also a strong grounding effect and it calms the Mind and settles the Ethereal Soul.
- **Du-24** and **G.B.-13** calm the Mind, especially in Liver disharmonies.
- **BL-18** and **BL-47** root the Ethereal Soul.

Herbal treatment

(a) Prescription

HUANG LIAN E JIAO TANG
Coptis-Gelatinum Corii Asini Decoction
Huang Lian *Rhizoma Coptidis* 3 g
Huang Qin *Radix Scutellariae baicalensis* 9 g
Bai Shao *Radix Paeoniae albae* 9 g
Ji Zi Huang *Egg yolk* 2 yolks
E Jiao *Gelatinum Corii Asini* 9 g

Explanation

- **Huang Lian** and **Huang Qin** clear Heat and calm irritability.
- **Bai Shao** and **Ji Zi Huang** nourish Liver-Yin.

Bai Shao calms the Mind and "absorbs" the Ethereal Soul into Liver-Yin. It is coordinated with Huang Lian: this clears Heat and prevents injury of Yin by Heat, whilst Bai Shao nourishes Yin and prevents this from harbouring Empty-Heat.
- **E Jiao** nourishes Liver-Blood and Liver-Yin.

This prescription therefore nourishes Liver-Yin, clears any Empty-Heat that there might be, calms the Mind and settles the Ethereal Soul. The main manifestations would be a feeling of heat in the evening, poor memory, insomnia (waking up at night), a dry throat, dry hair, a Red tongue without coating and a Floating-Empty pulse.

Mental-emotional pattern

Anger, frustration and resentment combined with overwork and/or excessive sexual activity over many years may lead to this condition. In women, a contributory factor is excessive loss of blood at childbirth or a prolonged, excessive loss of blood if the periods are heavy.

Liver-Yin deficiency deprives the Ethereal Soul of its residence and it necessarily affects the Mind as well since Liver-Yin is the mother of Heart-Yin. Those suffering from this condition will feel depressed, lack a sense of direction in life and be mentally restless. Their sleep will be broken and they may wake up frequently during the night. They may also have restless dreams due to the wandering of the unrooted Ethereal Soul at night.

The formula Suan Zao Ren Tang *Ziziphus Decoction* may also be used for this pattern (see below, p. 254 under "Liver-Yin Deficiency with Empty-Heat").

(b) Prescription

ZHEN ZHU MU WAN
Concha margaritiferae Pill
Zhen Zhu Mu *Concha margaritiferae* 30 g
Long Chi *Dens Draconis* 18 g
Chen Xiang *Lignum Aquilariae* 3 g
Zhu Sha *Cinnabaris* 1.5 g
Shu Di Huang *Radix Rehmanniae glutinosae prae-parata* 12 g

Dang Gui *Radix Angelicae sinensis* 6 g
Ren Shen *Radix Ginseng* 6 g
Suan Zao Ren *Semen Ziziphi spinosae* 6 g
Bai Zi Ren *Semen Biotae orientalis* 6 g
Fu Shen *Sclerotium Poriae cocos pararadicis* 6 g
Shui Niu Jiao *Cornu Bufali* 6 g

Explanation

- **Zhen Zhu Mu, Long Chi, Chen Xiang** and **Zhu Sha** sink Liver-Yang, calm the Mind and settle the Ethereal Soul. Zhu Sha is a toxic substance and should be used for short periods only (a few weeks).
- **Shu Di Huang** and **Dang Gui** nourish the Liver.
- **Ren Shen** tonifies Qi.
- **Suan Zao Ren, Bai Zi Ren** and **Fu Shen** nourish the Heart and Liver, calm the Mind and settle the Ethereal Soul.
- **Shui Niu Jiao** opens the Mind's orifices and subdues Wind. This herb may be omitted; it is included here to deal with the Blood level in the context of the Four Levels.

This formula, originally for the pattern of Liver-Wind at the Blood level of the Four Levels, nourishes Liver-Yin, subdues Liver-Yang, calms the Mind and settles the Ethereal Soul. It has a similar action to the previous one, but it differs in so far as the emphasis is on subduing Liver-Yang and calming the Mind, whereas in the previous one the emphasis was more on nourishing Yin and clearing Heat.

The main manifestations leading to the use of this prescription are dizziness, tinnitus, headache, insomnia, propensity to outbursts of anger, poor memory, dry hair and eyes, numbness of the limbs, a tongue with red sides and a Wiry-Fine pulse.

Mental-emotional pattern

Anger, frustration, resentment and hatred can cause this condition. In particular, anger will cause Liver-Yang or Liver-Wind to rise, for which condition this prescription is indicated. This person would therefore be very angry and be prone to outbursts of anger. His or her sleep would be very restless and filled with unpleasant dreams.

(c) Prescription

YIN MEI TANG
Attracting Sleep Decoction
Bai Shao *Radix Paeoniae albae* 30 g
Dang Gui *Radix Angelicae sinensis* 15 g
Long Chi *Dens Draconis* 6 g
Tu Si Zi *Semen Cuscutae* 9 g
Mai Men Dong *Tuber Ophiopogonis japonici* 15 g
Bai Zi Ren *Semen Biotae orientalis* 6 g
Suan Zao Ren *Semen Ziziphi spinosae* 9 g
Fu Shen *Sclerotium Poriae cocos pararadicis* 9 g

Explanation

This formula restores Liver-Blood and Liver-Yin to allow the Ethereal Soul to settle and the person to sleep peacefully. When Liver-Yin is deficient the Ethereal Soul has no residence and there is insomnia. This formula makes the Ethereal Soul peaceful so that it does not wander. It tonifies Liver- and Heart-Yin, calms the Mind and settles the Ethereal Soul. The tongue presentation appropriate to this formula is a Red body without coating.

The original text says that this formula makes the Ethereal Soul peaceful so that it cannot "jump over".

- **Bai Shao** and **Dang Gui** nourish Liver-Blood and Liver-Yin.
- **Long Chi** sinks Yang and calms the Mind. It enters the Liver and is absorbing, drawing the Ethereal Soul back into Liver-Yin. In insomnia there is excessive movement of Mind and Ethereal Soul; Long Chi calms this movement and absorbs the Ethereal Soul. The original text states that the ancients believed that a restless Corporeal Soul is treated by tiger's eyeballs and a restless Ethereal Soul by dragon's teeth (Long Chi). This is because the tiger pertains to Yin and corresponds to Metal (hence the Lungs and Corporeal Soul) and the dragon pertains to Yang and corresponds to Wood (hence the Liver and Ethereal Soul). In order to treat a restless Ethereal Soul one needs to use Long Chi which pacifies the

Liver. This substance can "calm movement", and in insomnia and anxiety there is excessive movement of the Ethereal Soul and therefore Mind. Long Chi calms this movement and absorbs the Ethereal Soul into the Liver.

- **Tu Si Zi** nourishes the Kidneys: this helps to nourish the Liver and these two organs have a common root.
- **Mai Dong**, **Bai Zi Ren** and **Fu Shen** nourish the Heart and calm the Mind.
- **Suan Zao Ren** nourishes Liver-Yin and settles the Ethereal Soul.

Mental-emotional pattern

Frustration, resentment, old grudges and sometimes sadness, can cause Liver-Yin to become deficient. This person's Liver-Yin would have been consumed by repressed anger over many years: he or she would feel very tense, anxious and sleep very badly with the sleep being disturbed by unpleasant dreams. The pulse would be Fine but also slightly Wiry on the left side.

In some cases, sadness depletes Liver-Yin: in this case the person would feel very depressed and sad and also sleep badly, but without too many dreams. The pulse would be Choppy or Fine.

Patent remedy

AN SHEN BU XIN PIAN
Calming the Mind and Tonifying the Heart Tablet
Zhen Zhu Mu *Concha margaritiferae*
Ye Jiao Teng *Caulis Polygoni multiflori*
Nu Zhen Zi *Fructus Ligustri lucidi*
Han Lian Cao *Herba Ecliptae prostratae*
He Huan Pi *Cortex Albizziae julibrissin*
Dan Shen *Radix Salviae miltiorrhizae*
Sheng Di Huang *Radix Rehmanniae glutinosae*
Shu Di Huang *Radix Rehmanniae glutinosae praeparata*
Wu Wei Zi *Fructus Schisandrae chinensis*
Shi Chang Pu *Rhizoma Acori graminei*

Explanation

This remedy is for insomnia, mental restlessness,

depression and lack of will-power deriving from Liver- and Heart-Yin deficiency.

Besides nourishing Liver- and Heart-Yin it also moves Liver-Qi and is therefore ideal for mental-emotional problems from stagnation of Liver-Qi when this is secondary to a deficiency of Liver-Yin, a situation which is very common in women.

3. KIDNEY-YIN DEFICIENCY

Treatment principle

Tonify the Kidneys, nourish Yin, calm the Mind and strengthen the Will-Power.

Acupuncture

KI-3 Taixi, KI-6 Zhaohai, Ren-4 Guanyuan, BL-23 Shenshu, BL-52 Zhishi, HE-6 Yinxi, P-7 Daling, Ren-15 Jiuwei. Reinforcing method except for HE-6, P-7 and Ren-15 which are either reduced or needled with even method according to how chronic the condition is.

Explanation

- **KI-3** and **KI-6** nourish Kidney-Yin.
- **Ren-4** nourishes Kidney-Yin and calms the Mind.
- **BL-23** strengthens the Kidneys.
- **BL-52** strengthens the Will-Power.
- **HE-6** clears Heart Empty-Heat.
- **P-7** and **Ren-15** calm the Mind.

Herbal treatment

(a) Prescription

GUI ZHI GAN CAO LONG GU MU LI TANG
Ramulus Cinnamomi-Glycyrrhiza-Os Draconis-Ostrea Decoction
Gui Zhi *Ramulus Cinnamomi cassiae* 9 g
Zhi Gan Cao *Radix Glycyrrhizae uralensis praeparata* 18 g
Long Gu *Os Draconis* 30 g
Mu Li *Concha Ostreae* 30 g

Explanation

- **Gui Zhi** and **Gan Cao** warm and tonify the

Heart. Gan Cao in a high dose such as this strengthens the Middle Burner and harmonizes the ascending of Yang and descending of Yin in the Middle Burner.
- **Long Gu** and **Mu Li** sink and calm the Mind. Mu Li also nourishes Kidney-Yin and strengthens Will-Power. These two substances also help timidity. Being astringent, on a physical level they stop sweating, whilst on a mental level they "absorb" the Mind and the Ethereal Soul into the Yin.

This formula nourishes the Kidneys, strengthens the Heart, calms the Mind, settles the Ethereal Soul and bolsters Will-Power. The main manifestations are palpitations, mental restlessness, propensity to be startled, sweating, cold limbs and a Pale tongue.

Although it contains Mu Li which primarily strengthens Kidney-Yin, this formula can be adapted to treat both Kidney-Yin and Kidney-Yang deficiency. In fact, its primary aim is to strengthen Heart-Yang with Gui Zhi and Zhi Gan Cao (hence the Pale tongue) and calm the Mind with the sinking substances Long Gu and Mu Li.

Mental-emotional pattern

This formula is suitable, with adaptations, to treat the mental restlessness deriving from Kidney-Yin deficiency and Heart deficiency. Fear, guilt and shock, perhaps combined with overwork and/or excessive sexual activity, may lead to this condition, which guilt is especially liable to cause. This emotion, when suffered for a long time, weakens the Kidneys and the Will-Power and it gnaws away at the Mind, thus depleting the Heart. Such patients are very anxious and mentally restless, and they sleep fitfully. They tend to be thin (indicating Yin deficiency), are tired, depressed, and lack will-power.

(b) Prescription

ZHEN ZHONG DAN
Bedside Pill
Gui Ban *Plastrum Testudinis* 10 g
Long Gu *Os Draconis* 10 g

Yuan Zhi *Radix Polygalae tenuifoliae* 10 g
Shi Chang Pu *Rhizoma Acori graminei* 10 g

Explanation

- **Gui Ban** nourishes Kidney-Yin and clears Empty-Heat.
- **Long Gu** calms the Mind.
- **Yuan Zhi** and **Chang Pu** open the Mind's orifices, calm the Mind and benefit intelligence and wisdom. These two herbs, combined with Gui Ban and Long Gu, harmonize Heart and Kidneys and calm the Mind.

This formula nourishes Kidney-Yin, strengthens Will-Power and intelligence and calms the Mind. It differs from the previous one in so far as it is slightly more directed at opening the Mind's orifices and clearing the Heart, whilst the previous one tonifies the Heart.

On a physical level, the manifestations corresponding to this prescription would include insomnia, anxiety, back-ache, night-sweating, dizziness, tinnitus, poor memory, a Red tongue without coating and a Floating-Empty pulse.

Mental-emotional pattern

A person with this condition would suffer from a confused Mind and would be unable to see clearly what needs to be done. He or she would also be anxious, depressed and lack will power, and would sleep badly and sweat at night. This condition would also be caused by fear or guilt.

YIN DEFICIENCY WITH EMPTY-HEAT

1. HEART- AND KIDNEY-YIN DEFICIENCY WITH HEART EMPTY-HEAT

Treatment principle

Nourish Heart- and Kidney-Yin, strengthen the Will-Power and calm the Mind.

Acupuncture

HE-7 Shenmen, HE-6 Yinxi, P-7 Daling, Yintang, Ren-15 Jiuwei, Du-19 Houding, KI-3 Taixi, KI-6

Zhaohai, KI-10 Yingu, KI-9 Zhubin, Ren-4 Guanyuan, SP-6 Sanyinjiao. The first three with reducing or even method; Yintang, Ren-15 and Du-19 with even method; all the others with reinforcing method. No moxa.

Explanation

- **HE-7**, **HE-6** and **P-7** can all calm the Mind. HE-6 also stops night-sweating in combination with KI-7 Fuliu.
- **Yintang**, **Ren-15** and **Du-19** calm the Mind.
- **KI-3**, Source point, nourishes the Kidneys.
- **KI-6** nourishes Kidney-Yin, benefits the throat, promotes fluids and helps sleep.
- **KI-10** nourishes Kidney-Yin.
- **KI-9** tonifies the Kidneys, calms the Mind and opens the chest.
- **Ren-4** nourishes Kidney-Yin and roots the Mind.
- **SP-6** nourishes Yin, calms the Mind and promotes sleep.

Herbal treatment

(a) Prescription

TIAN WANG BU XIN DAN
Heavenly Emperor Tonifying the Heart Pill
Sheng Di Huang *Radix Rehmanniae glutinosae* 12 g
Xuan Shen *Radix Scrophulariae ningpoensis* 6 g
Mai Men Dong *Tuber Ophiopogonis japonici* 6 g
Tian Men Dong *Tuber Asparagi cochinchinensis* 6 g
Ren Shen *Radix Ginseng* 6 g
Fu Ling *Sclerotium Poriae cocos* 6 g
Wu Wei Zi *Fructus Schisandrae chinensis* 6 g
Dang Gui *Radix Angelicae sinensis* 6 g
Dan Shen *Radix Salviae miltiorrhizae* 6 g
Bai Zi Ren *Semen Biotae orientalis* 6 g
Suan Zao Ren *Semen Ziziphi spinosae* 6 g
Yuan Zhi *Radix Polygalae tenuifoliae* 6 g
Jie Geng *Radix Platycodi grandiflori* 3 g

Explanation

- **Sheng Di Huang** and **Xuan Shen** nourish Kidney-Yin, cool Blood and clear Empty-Heat.
- **Mai Men Dong** and **Tian Men Dong** nourish Yin.

- **Ren Shen** and **Fu Ling** tonify Qi to strengthen the Heart. Fu Ling also calms the Mind.
- **Wu Wei Zi** is astringent and helps to nourish Yin. It also stops sweating.
- **Dang Gui** and **Dan Shen** nourish and harmonize Blood. They both enter the Heart and Dan Shen calms the Mind.
- **Bai Zi Ren**, **Suan Zao Ren** and **Yuan Zhi** nourish the Heart and calm the Mind. Suan Zao Ren also stops sweating.
- **Jie Geng** is used as a messenger to direct the herbs upwards.

This is the most widely-used formula to nourish Heart- and Kidney-Yin (also called "harmonizing Heart and Kidneys"), clear Empty-Heat and calm the Mind. The main manifestations are night-sweating, back-ache, dizziness, tinnitus, a malar flush, feeling of heat in the evening, palpitations, insomnia, restless sleep, dry mouth and throat, poor memory, dry stools, a Red tongue without coating with a redder tip and a Rapid-Fire pulse. Such a condition is common in menopause.

Mental-emotional pattern

Fear, guilt and shock can all cause this condition. Since there is a definite deficiency of Kidney-Yin there usually are concurrent causes of disease such as overwork, irregular diet and excessive sexual activity. It is also a common pattern appearing in menopausal problems.

This person would be very anxious especially in the evening, and he or she would sleep very badly waking up at night several times. There might be dreams of fires or flying. He or she would be totally unable to relax and there would be palpitations.

Variations

- If there is severe mental restlessness and insomnia add Long Chi *Dens Draconis* to sink and calm the Mind.

(b) Prescription

LIU WEI DI HUANG WAN Variation
Six-Ingredient Rehmannia Pill

Shu Di Huang *Radix Rehmanniae glutinosae prae-parata* 30 g
Shan Zhu Yu *Fructus Corni officinalis* 12 g
Shan Yao *Radix Dioscoreae oppositae* 12 g
Ze Xie *Rhizoma Alismatis orientalis* 9 g
Mu Dan Pi *Cortex Moutan radicis* 9 g
Fu Ling *Sclerotium Poriae cocos* 9 g
Bai Shao *Radix Paeoniae albae* 15 g
Chai Hu *Radix Bupleuri* 1.5 g
Mai Men Dong *Tuber Ophiopogonis japonici* 15 g
Wu Wei Zi *Fructus Schisandrae chinensis* 3 g
Suan Zao Ren *Semen Ziziphi spinosae* 15 g
Ju Hua *Flos Chrysanthemi morifolii* 9 g

Explanation

This formula is used for mental restlessness and insomnia from Yin deficiency and Empty-Heat especially in the elderly. It is specific to restore the connection between Heart-Fire and Kidney-Water: the Heart-fluids rely on the nourishment of the Kidney-Essence. Thus one needs to nourish Kidney-Water in order to subdue Heart Empty-Heat.

- The first six herbs constitute the Liu Wei Di Huang Wan which nourishes Kidney-Water.
- **Bai Shao** and **Chai Hu** are included to regulate and pacify the Liver. The original text says that when the Liver is pacified the Minister-Fire (which produces Empty-Heat in the Heart) is subdued and cannot agitate the Fire of the Pericardium. Thus, acting on the Liver with these two herbs will help the Pericardium to which the Liver is related within the Terminal Yin. Please note the minute dosage of Chai Hu (1.5g).
- **Mai Dong** and **Wu Wei Zi** nourish and transform the Original Qi and nourish Yin.
- **Suan Zao Ren** and **Ju Hua** comfort Heart-Qi and make it communicate with Kidney-Water. Both these herbs are moistening and nourishing and they relieve dryness and "bitterness". "Bitterness" is intended here on two levels: on a physical level, they will relieve the bitter taste associated with Heat, and on a mental level, they will soothe the Mind when it is embittered by emotional strain.

Mental-emotional pattern

This is almost the same as for the previous formula, except that the emphasis is on Yin deficiency with the consequent depression and lack of will-power. Also, because of its emphasis on the Liver, it is suitable for mental-emotional problems deriving from resentment and bitterness harboured for many years.

Patent remedy

TIAN WANG BU XIN DAN
Heavenly Emperor's Tonifying the Heart Pill
This very well-known patent remedy has the same ingredients and indications as the prescription of the same name. It should be noted that some of the pills on sale are coated with cinnabar (Zhu Sha) which is toxic and should be used only for a few weeks; pills which are of a reddish colour have most probably been coated with cinnabar.

Case history

A 52-year-old woman sought treatment for persistent night sweating and hot flushes. She also complained of abdominal distension and water retention. Her periods had stopped the year before and she had been worse since then. Apart from the above symptoms, she often felt anxious in the evening and experienced palpitations. Her sleep was disturbed by the hot flushes and she felt mentally restless. She was overweight, her cheek-bones were slightly red and her eyes had no glitter and looked scared.

Her tongue was slightly Red, Swollen on the sides (Spleen-type of swelling), cracked and with a rootless coating; it also had a Heart crack in the middle (Plate 9.4). Her pulse was Weak on both Rear positions, the Heart position was Weak and Short and the whole pulse had no wave.

She had been treated with acupuncture elsewhere (tonifying Spleen and resolving Dampness) without much result. Her acupuncturist referred her to me.

Diagnosis
This lady obviously has a Spleen deficiency manifesting with being overweight, water retention and a swelling on the sides of the tongue. However, there are other factors involved. The hot flushes, red cheek-bones, insomnia, mental restlessness, Red tongue with rootless coating and Weak pulse on both Kidney positions clearly indicate Kidney-Yin deficiency. Besides this, there is also a Heart

deficiency as evidenced by the palpitations and the eyes without glitter indicating that the Mind is disturbed.

When asked about it, she confirmed that she had been under tremendous strain when she lived in East Africa having to manage a large farm for two years after being widowed suddenly. Thus the main causes of disease were sadness and shock (from bereavement) and fear. The sadness showed in her eyes' lack of glitter and the fear in their scared look.

Treatment principle
Nourish Kidney-Yin and Heart-Yin, subdue Empty-Heat, calm the Mind and strengthen Will-Power.

Herbal treatment
She was treated with herbs only. The main formula used was a variation of Tian Wang Bu Xin Dan *Heavenly Emperor Tonifying the Heart Pill*:

Sheng Di Huang *Radix Rehmanniae glutinosae* 12 g
Mai Men Dong *Tuber Ophiopogonis japonici* 6 g
Tian Men Dong *Tuber Asparagi cochinchinensis* 6 g
Ren Shen *Radix Ginseng* 6 g
Fu Ling *Sclerotium Poriae cocos* 6 g
Wu Wei Zi *Fructus Schisandrae chinensis* 6 g
Dang Gui *Radix Angelicae sinensis* 6 g
Dan Shen *Radix Salviae miltiorrhizae* 6 g
Bai Zi Ren *Semen Biotae orientalis* 6 g
Suan Zao Ren *Semen Ziziphi spinosae* 6 g
Yuan Zhi *Radix Polygalae tenuifoliae* 6 g
Jie Geng *Radix Platycodi grandiflori* 3 g
Ze Xie *Rhizoma Alismatis orientalis* 4 g
Qing Hao *Herba Artemisiae apiaceae* 3 g
Qin Jiao *Radix Gentianae macrophyllae* 3 g
Zhi Gan Cao *Radix Glycyrrhizae uralensis praeparata* 3 g

Explanation
The first twelve herbs constitute the original formula which nourishes Kidney-Yin and Heart-Yin, clears Empty-Heat and calms the Mind. Xuan Shen was eliminated from the formula as Yin deficiency is not too pronounced yet.

- Ze Xie, Qing Hao and Qin Jiao were added to clear Empty-Heat and treat the hot flushes.
- Gan Cao harmonizes.

This formula, repeated several times, produced a dramatic improvement in her mental state from the beginning, feeling much more relaxed, calmer and happier. Her eyes gradually changed too, acquiring more glitter.

2. LIVER-YIN DEFICIENCY WITH EMPTY-HEAT

Treatment principle

Nourish Liver-Yin, clear Empty-Heat, calm the Mind and settle the Ethereal Soul.

Acupuncture

LIV-8 Ququan, SP-6 Sanyinjiao, KI-3 Taixi, Ren-4 Guanyuan, Du-24 Shenting, G.B.-13 Benshen, Du-18 Qiangjian, BL-18 Ganshu, BL-47 Hunmen, KI-2 Rangu and LIV-3 Taichong. Reinforcing method, except for the last two points which should be reduced.

Explanation

- **LIV-8** nourishes Liver-Yin.
- **SP-6** nourishes Yin and strengthens Liver, Spleen and Kidneys.
- **KI-3** and **Ren-4** nourish Kidney-Yin. As this is the mother of Liver-Yin, it will indirectly nourish Liver-Yin. Ren-4 has also a strong grounding effect and it calms the Mind.
- **Du-24** and **G.B.-13** calm the Mind, especially in Liver disharmonies.
- **Du-18** calms the Mind and settles the Ethereal Soul. It is indicated for mental restlessness, agitation and manic behaviour.
- **BL-18** and **BL-47** root the Ethereal Soul.
- **KI-2** and **LIV-3** would be used only if there is Empty-Heat.

Herbal treatment

Prescription

SUAN ZAO REN TANG
Ziziphus Decoction
Suan Zao Ren *Semen Ziziphi spinosae* 18 g
Chuan Xiong *Radix Ligustici wallichii* 6 g
Fu Ling *Sclerotium Poriae cocos* 12 g
Zhi Mu *Rhizoma Anemarrhenae asphodeloidis* 9 g
Gan Cao *Radix Glycyrrhizae uralensis* 3 g

Explanation

- **Suan Zao Ren** is the emperor herb to nourish Liver-Yin. It tonifies the Liver and calms the Mind. It is sour and just as the sour taste is astringent on a physical level, on a mental level it "absorbs" and roots the Ethereal Soul in Yin. It performs the function of "tonification by sour taste".
- **Chuan Xiong** is pungent and warm and it moves and scatters. It enters the Liver and

moves Qi and Blood. It is coordinated with Suan Zao Ren: while this is sour and absorbing, Chuan Xiong is pungent and scattering. Together they harmonize the Liver. Chuan Xiong performs the function of "tonification by pungent taste". It attracts and draws Zhi Mu and Fu Ling to eliminate pathogenic factors (in this case Empty-Heat).

- **Fu Ling** strengthens the Spleen and calms the Mind: it helps Suan Zao Ren to calm the Mind and root the Ethereal Soul.
- **Zhi Mu** nourishes Yin and clears Empty-Heat. It moistens and relieves mental restlessness. It moderates Chuan Xiong's pungent and scattering effect. Zhi Mu is also coordinated with Fu Ling: the former nourishes Yin-Water and clears Empty-Heat, while the latter benefits Yang-Water and levels Yin. Together they nourish Water and therefore create the basis for the Ethereal Soul and, by clearing Empty-Heat, they calm the Mind.
- **Gan Cao** is sweet and, together with Suan Zao Ren which is sour, it pacifies the Liver and calms irritability. It also prevents Chuan Xiong from moving too much.

Mental-emotional pattern

This formula is specific for Liver-Yin deficiency with its associated symptoms and signs such as insomnia, waking up frequently at night, dry throat, blurred vision, dry eyes, mental restlessness, night sweating, a Red tongue without coating and a Floating-Empty pulse.

This situation can arise in two ways. Emotional stress, such as anger, resentment, or frustration, may lead to the rising of Minister Fire which agitates the Heart and the Liver. Fire injures Yin so that the Ethereal Soul is deprived of its residence. Alternatively, it may start with a reverse process: overwork combined with irregular diet and excessive sexual activity (and in women too many childbirths) may deplete Liver-Yin and therefore deprive the Ethereal Soul of its residence. No matter how this situation arises, the end-result is a condition characterized most of all by insomnia. The person may also be depressed and lack any sense of vision in life. The mental restlessness in this condition derives from Yin deficiency and typically manifests with a vague feeling of anxiety, restlessness and fidgetiness which is worse in the evening.

The Liver is a harmonizing organ and its harmony derives from a proper balance between its Yang (the free flow of Liver-Qi) and its Yin aspect (Blood and Yin). Mental irritation from emotional stress stirs up Liver-Yang and injures Liver-Yin and thus alters the balance of Yin and Yang within the Liver.

This formula is also applicable to some women's problems such as pre-menstrual tension with breast distension or breast lumps from stagnation of Liver-Qi on a background of Liver-Yin deficiency. In women, Liver-Yin deficiency is even more likely to happen due to the monthly loss of menstrual blood which depletes Liver-Blood. In these cases, stagnation of Liver-Qi, with its associated emotional consequences, is very often secondary to a deficiency of Liver-Yin. The Yin and Yang aspects of the Liver need to be harmonized and coordinated. If Liver-Yin is deficient, the Yang aspect of the Liver gets out of control and this may lead to both stagnation of Liver-Qi and Liver-Yang rising. Thus, this formula can be used for pre-menstrual tension if it presents with the above configuration.

Finally, although this formula is specific for Liver-Yin deficiency with Empty-Heat, it can also be used for Liver-Yin deficiency without Empty-Heat. It is therefore applicable also to Mind Unsettled or Mind Weakened from Yin deficiency.

Variations

- If Empty-Heat manifestations are severe (malar flush and feeling of heat) decrease the amount of Chuan Xiong and add Sheng Di Huang *Radix Rehmanniae glutinosae*, Nu Zhen Zi *Fructus Ligustri lucidi* and Han Lian Cao *Herba Ecliptae prostratae*.
- If night-sweating is profuse add Di Gu Pi *Cortex Lycii chinensis radicis* and Wu Wei Zi *Fructus Schisandrae chinensis*.
- If insomnia is difficult to treat add Ye Jiao Teng *Caulis Polygoni multiflori*.
- If the person is very depressed add He Huan Pi *Cortex Albizziae julibrissin*.

(i) Patent remedy

SUAN ZAO REN TANG PIAN
Tablet of Ziziphus Decoction
This very well-known pill has the same ingredients and indications as the formula of the same name.

It is indicated for insomnia and mental restlessness deriving from Liver-Yin deficiency and Empty-Heat.

(ii) Patent remedy

AN SHEN BU NAO PIAN
Calming the Mind and Tonifying the Brain Tablet
Huang Jing *Rhizoma Polygonati*
Nu Zhen Zi *Fructus Ligustri lucidi*
Dang Gui *Radix Angelicae sinensis*
He Huan Pi *Cortex Albizziae julibrissin*
Han Lian Cao *Herba Ecliptae prostratae*
Suan Zao Ren *Semen Ziziphi spinosae*
Fu Ling *Sclerotium Poriae cocos*
Shou Wu *Radix Polygoni multiflori*
Yuan Zhi *Radix Polygalae tenuifoliae*
Zhu Sha *Cinnabaris*

Explanation

This remedy nourishes Liver- and Heart-Yin and clears Empty-Heat. It is therefore suitable for Liver-Yin deficiency and Empty-Heat causing insomnia, anxiety, mental restlessness, a feeling of heat in the evening, blurred vision, irregular periods and a dry throat. It differs from Suan Zao Ren Tang Pian in so far as it is more nourishing.

(iii) Patent remedy

AN MIAN PIAN
Peaceful Sleep Tablet
Suan Zao Ren *Semen Ziziphi spinosae*
Yuan Zhi *Radix Polygalae tenuifoliae*
Fu Ling *Sclerotium Poriae cocos*
Shan Zhi Zi *Fructus Gardeniae jasminoidis jasminoidis*
Shen Qu *Massa Fermentata Medicinalis*
Quan Xie *Buthus Martensi*
Gan Cao *Radix Glycyrrhizae uralensis*

Explanation

This tablet is for insomnia and mental restlessness deriving from Liver-Yin deficiency and Empty-Heat. It also addresses the condition of Liver-Yang or Liver-Wind rising which might arise from Liver-Yin deficiency; this is the main difference from the previous two remedies.

It is especially suited for old people with Liver-Yin deficiency, Empty-Heat and some Liver-Yang or Liver-Wind manifesting with tremors, giddiness and possibly hypertension.

(iv) Patent remedy

HU PO DUO MEI WAN
Succinum Good Sleep Pill
Hu Po *Succinum*
Yuan Zhi *Radix Polygalae tenuifoliae*
Fu Ling *Sclerotium Poriae cocos*
Dang Shen *Radix Codonopsis pilosulae*
Gan Cao *Radix Glycyrrhizae uralensis*
Ling Yang Jiao *Cornu Antelopis*

Explanation

This pill is for insomnia and mental restlessness deriving from Liver-Yang rising. It subdues Liver-Yang and calms the Mind and Ethereal Soul.

It differs from the previous three remedies in so far as it is specific for mental-emotional problems deriving from Liver-Yang rising and it is not as nourishing as the others.

Case history

A 63-year-old woman sought treatment for hypertension. The systolic blood pressure which oscillated between 200 and 150, was more of a problem than the diastolic one, which was always 95. Her main physical symptoms included a stiff neck, a feeling of pressure in the head, throbbing headaches on the vertex, dizziness, tinnitus, blurred vision, dry eyes, insomnia (waking up frequently during the night) and a feeling of heat in the evening.

Her complexion was dull with red patches on both cheek-bones and her eyes were rather dull and without glitter.

Her tongue was Red, redder on the sides, slightly Stiff and the coating was too thin. Her pulse was Wiry but Fine.

Diagnosis
The blurred vision, dry eyes, insomnia, Fine pulse and Stiff tongue with insufficient tongue-coating indicate Liver-Yin deficiency while the feeling of heat in the evening, red cheek-bones and Red tongue with insufficient coating denote Empty-Heat.

Due to the deficiency of Liver-Yin, there was also Liver-Yang rising as manifested by the stiff neck, throbbing vertical headaches, dizziness, tinnitus, a feeling of pressure in the head and a Wiry pulse.

Her hypertension, which was the reason for seeking treatment, was due to the rising of Liver-Yang. When the systolic pressure is high while the diastolic one is near to normal, it usually indicates the rising of Liver-Yang. Furthermore, when the systolic reading oscillates considerably from day to day, it indicates that nervous stress, rather than a hardening of the arteries, is the cause of the problem. This is usually due to emotional strain affecting the Liver. In this patient's case, this was very obvious from the dullness of her complexion (lack of *shen*) and eyes which indicate long-standing affliction of the Mind and/or Ethereal Soul by emotional strain.

When asked about emotional strain, she confirmed that she had been under great stress about her daughter's marital problems. Due to financial problems, her daughter was trapped in a marriage to a very cruel husband and suffered a great deal: this made her mother very angry towards her son-in-law and, over the years, caused the rising of Liver-Yang and deficiency of Liver-Yin.

Treatment principle
Nourish Liver-Yin, clear Empty-Heat, subdue Liver-Yang, calm the Mind and root the Ethereal Soul.

Acupuncture
Reinforce: LIV-8 Ququan, Ren-4 Guanyuan, SP-6 Sanyinjiao, KI-3 Taixi. Even method: LIV-3 Taichong, KI-2 Rangu, Du-24 Shenting, G.B.-13 Benshen, P-7 Daling.

Explanation
- **LIV-8**, **Ren-4**, **SP-6** and **KI-3** nourish Liver-Yin.
- **LIV-3** subdues Liver-Yang.
- **KI-2**, in combination with LIV-3, clears Empty-Heat from Liver-Yin deficiency.
- **Du-24** and **G.B.-13** calm the Mind and root the Ethereal Soul.
- **P-7** calms the Mind and indirectly subdues Liver-Yang.

Herbal treatment
No herbs were prescribed but only the patent remedy Suan Zao Ren Tang Pian *Tablet of Ziziphus Decoction* which fitted her symptoms quite well.

After 20 weekly treatments most of her symptoms had cleared up or decreased in intensity and she was able to react more calmly to her daughter's plight and not to allow her anger to dominate her life.

QI STAGNATION

This has already been discussed under "Mind obstructed" above (p. 233). The manifestations of Qi stagnation when it causes the Mind to be unsettled are similar. The main difference is that, instead of mental confusion, the predominant manifestations will be anxiety and mental restlessness.

TREATMENT PRINCIPLE

Move Qi, eliminate stagnation and calm the Mind.

The same prescriptions and acupuncture points indicated for stagnation of Qi under "Mind obstructed" are applicable.

BLOOD STASIS

Again, the manifestations of this condition are similar to those discussed under "Mind obstructed" from Blood stasis (p. 237). The main difference is that, when stasis of Blood causes the Mind to become unsettled, there will be severe anxiety and mental restlessness.

TREATMENT PRINCIPLE

Move Blood, eliminate stasis and calm the Mind.

The same prescriptions and acupuncture points indicated under "Mind obstructed" from Blood stasis are applicable.

FIRE

1. HEART-FIRE

Treatment principle

Clear the Heart, drain fire and calm the Mind.

Acupuncture

HE-8 Shaofu, HE-7 Shenmen, P-7 Daling, Ren-15 Jiuwei, SP-6 Sanyinjiao, G.B.-15 Toulinqi.

Explanation

- **HE-8** clears Heart-Fire and calms the Mind.
- **HE-7** calms the Mind.
- **P-7** strongly calms the Mind.
- **Ren-15** calms the Mind.
- **SP-6** nourishes Yin which helps to cool Fire and it calms the Mind.
- **G.B.-15** clears Heat and calms the Mind. It balances moods when they oscillate violently. It is particularly indicated if the eyes are red.

Herbal treatment

Prescription

DAO CHI SAN
Eliminating Redness Powder
Sheng Di Huang *Radix Rehmanniae glutinosae* 15 g
Mu Tong *Caulis Akebiae* 3 g
Zhu Ye *Herba Lophatheri gracilis* 3 g
Gan Cao *Radix Glycyrrhizae uralensis* 6 g

Explanation

- **Sheng Di Huang** clears Heat and cools Blood. It enters the Heart.
- **Mu Tong** and **Zhu Ye** clear Heart-Fire. They conduct Fire downwards via urination.
- **Gan Cao** clears Fire and detoxifies.

This formula clears Heart-Fire causing such symptoms as a sensation of heat in the chest, thirst, red face, tongue ulcers, mental restlessness, red eyes, scanty-dark urine, burning on urination, a Red tongue with a redder tip and yellow coating and an Overflowing pulse.

Mental-emotional pattern

Excess joy, worry and craving may lead to this pattern. These emotions agitate the Mind and create an implosion of Qi which leads to Fire. Fire agitates the Mind and the person will be very agitated, restless, impatient and unable to sleep well. The sleep will be very restless and disturbed by violent dreams, which may involve flying, fires and killings. The mental restlessness deriving from Fire is quite different from that deriving from Empty-Heat. A person with Empty-Heat will feel restless and anxious, especially in the evening, but will by and large endure it in silence. A person with Fire will feel restless all the time and will project it outwards towards other people or always doing something in a compulsive way. These people may be quite creative and artistic.

Variations

- In case of severe anxiety add Bai Zi Ren *Semen Biotae orientalis*, Suan Zao Ren *Semen Ziziphi spinosae* and Yuan Zhi *Radix Polygalae tenuifoliae*.

Case history

A 33-year-old woman sought treatment for infertility. She had been trying to become pregnant for 8 years and there was no abnormality in her hormone levels or fallopian tubes. Her periods were always late (from a 32- to a 44-day cycle), the menstrual blood was bright-red but with dark clots and the periods were painful. She also felt cold during the period and liked to have a hot-water bottle on her abdomen.

She suffered from lower back-ache, loose stools and general exhaustion. The back-ache started after a fall 10 years before. Her memory was poor and she dreamt a lot every night. Her dreams were always unpleasant and she regularly dreamed of burning buildings, often waking up crying or laughing. She occasionally experienced palpitations.

In her teenage years, from 13 to 18, she had been very nervous, frequently had palpitations and often fainted.

Facial diagnosis revealed an uneven, blemished surface on the forehead in the area corresponding to the teenage years between 16 and 19 (Fig. 9.11) and rather dull eyes.

Her tongue was Pale but with a Red tip. Her pulse was Weak on the right side and on both Rear positions and the Heart pulse was relatively Overflowing and very slightly Moving, i.e. it was Overflowing in relation to all the other pulse positions which were Weak.

Diagnosis
At first observation, all her symptoms would seem to point to Spleen- and Kidney-Yang deficiency. Whilst there certainly was a Spleen-Yang deficiency (tiredness, loose stools, Pale tongue and pulse Weak on the right side), there was not much Kidney-Yang deficiency. The symptoms which would seem to point to Kidney-Yang deficiency are a late menstrual cycle, feeling cold during the period, infertility, back-ache and poor memory. However, on closer analysis,

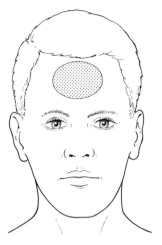

Fig. 9.11 Area corresponding to parents' influence and years from 16 to 19

although there was some Kidney-Yang deficiency some of these symptoms could be explained differently. First of all, the back-ache started only after the fall and was therefore due to a structural rather than an energetic Kidney problem.

As for the other symptoms, they are also partially due to the Heart's influence on the Kidneys. The Fire of the Heart (in a 5-Element sense) needs to communicate with Kidney-Water: Kidney-Water needs to flow upwards to nourish Heart-Yin, while the Fire of the Heart needs to flow downwards to the Kidneys and the Lower Burner. In this case, this patient had been affected by deep emotional problems during her teenage years. This was probably a mixture of shock and sadness which caused Heart-Fire (in a pathological sense). This was deduced from the Heart-pulse's Overflowing and Moving quality, from the blemished area on her forehead, dull eyes and her dreams. The shock and sadness had obviously affected the Heart (causing dreams of fire and waking up laughing) and Lungs (causing dreams of buildings and waking up crying). When asked about it, she confirmed this was true but she did not wish to discuss it further. Thus, Heart-Fire was blocked upwards, unable to communicate downwards with the Kidneys and Lower Burner which became cold. This was the cause of the infertility, delayed menstrual cycle, blood clots and cold feeling.

Treatment principle
The main treatment principle adopted was to calm the Mind, and conduct Heart-Fire downwards to communicate with the Kidneys. In this case, it was not a matter of "clearing" Heart-Fire so much as to establish a communication between the Fire of the Heart and the Kidneys. Shock "closes" the Heart and makes it smaller while sadness depletes Heart- and

Lung-Qi. The formula therefore needs some herbs with a pungent taste to open the Heart's orifices, some with a sour taste to nourish the Heart and calm the Mind and some sinking substances to calm the Mind and make Heart-Qi descend to the Lower Burner.

Herbal treatment
She was already receiving acupuncture from another practitioner who referred to me for herbal treatment. The prescription used was not a classical one but one I formulated for this particular case. This was:

Dang Shen *Radix Codonopsis pilosulae* 9 g
Fu Shen *Sclerotium Poriae cocos pararadicis* 6 g
Yuan Zhi *Radix Polygalae tenuifoliae* 9 g
Bai Zi Ren *Semen Biotae orientalis* 6 g
Suan Zao Ren *Semen Ziziphi spinosae* 3 g
Long Chi *Dens Draconis* 12 g
Bai He *Bulbus Lilii* 6 g
Shi Chang Pu *Rhizoma Acori graminei* 4 g
Huang Qin *Radix Scutellariae baicalensis* 3 g
Rou Gui *Cortex Cinnamomi cassiae* 1.5 g
Zhi Gan Cao *Radix Glycyrrhizae uralensis praeparata* 2 g
Hong Zao *Fructus Ziziphi jujubae* 3 dates

Explanation
- **Dang Shen** and **Fu Shen** tonify the Spleen. Fu Shen also calms the Mind.
- **Yuan Zhi**, **Bai Zi Ren** and **Suan Zao Ren** calm the Mind and nourish the Heart. Yuan Zhi is pungent and opens the Heart's orifices while Bai Zi Ren and Suan Zao Ren are sweet and sour respectively and therefore nourish the Heart and calm the Mind.
- **Long Chi** is a sinking substance to calm the Mind.
- **Bai He** nourishes the Lungs especially when they are affected by sadness.
- **Chang Pu** opens the Mind's orifices and counteracts the effects of shock.
- **Huang Qin** clears Heart-Heat and calms the Mind. It is used in a very small dose more to enter the Heart than to clear it.
- **Rou Gui** was used to warm the Fire of the Gate of Vitality, attract the Fire of the Heart downwards and re-establish the communication between Kidneys and Heart.
- **Zhi Gan Cao** and **Hong Zao** harmonize.

This formula was repeated with minor variations over a period of 4 months producing a marked improvement in the mental state of this patient. Her dreams of fire stopped and the menstrual blood became normal.

2. LIVER-FIRE

Treatment principle

Drain Liver-Fire, calm the Mind and settle the Ethereal Soul.

Acupuncture

LIV-2 Xingjian, LIV-3 Taichong, L.I.-4 Hegu, BL-18 Ganshu, SP-6 Sanyinjiao, Du-18 Qiangjian, Du-24 Shenting, G.B.-13 Benshen, G.B.-15 Toulinqi, HE-7 Shenmen, P-7 Daling, LU-3 Tianfu.

Explanation

- **LIV-2** clears Liver-Fire.
- **LIV-3** pacifies the Liver and calms the Mind. In combination with **L.I.-4** it strongly calms the Mind and settles the Ethereal Soul.
- **BL-18**, Back-Transporting point of the Liver, clears Liver-Fire.
- **SP-6** nourishes Yin and calms the Mind.
- **Du-18** calms the Mind, regulates the Liver and settles the Ethereal Soul.
- **Du-24** and **G.B.-13** calm the Mind and settle the Ethereal Soul in Liver disharmonies. G.B.-13 also treats jealousy and suspicion.
- **G.B.-15** clears Heat, brightens the eyes and settles the Ethereal Soul.
- **HE-7** and **P-7** calm the Mind. P-7 is related to the Liver via the Terminal Yin channels.
- **LU-3** harmonizes Liver and Lungs and, according to "An Explanation of Acupuncture Points" (1654), is particularly indicated when Liver-Fire obstructs the Lungs causing forgetfulness. The book also says this point is indicated when the person *"talks to ghosts"*.[82]

Herbal treatment

Prescription

XIE GAN AN SHEN WAN
Draining the Liver-Calming the Mind Pill
Long Dan Cao *Radix Gentianae scabrae* 9 g
Shan Zhi Zi *Fructus Gardeniae jasminoidis* 6 g
Huang Qin *Radix Scutellariae baicalensis* 6 g
Bai Ji Li *Fructus Tribuli terrestris* 4 g
Shi Jue Ming *Concha Haliotidis* 12 g
Ze Xie *Rhizoma Alismatis orientalis* 6 g
Che Qian Zi *Semen Plantaginis* 6 g
Dang Gui *Radix Angelicae sinensis* 6 g
Sheng Di Huang *Radix Rehmanniae glutinosae* 9 g
Mai Men Dong *Tuber Ophiopogonis japonici* 6 g
Zhen Zhu Mu *Concha margaritiferae* 12 g
Long Gu *Os Draconis* 12 g
Mu Li *Concha Ostreae* 12 g
Fu Shen *Sclerotium Poriae cocos pararadicis* 6 g
Yuan Zhi *Radix Polygalae tenuifoliae* 6 g
Bai Zi Ren *Semen Biotae orientalis* 6 g
Suan Zao Ren *Semen Ziziphi spinosae* 6 g
Gan Cao *Radix Glycyrrhizae uralensis* 3 g

Explanation

- **Long Dan Cao** is the emperor herb to clear Liver-Fire.
- **Zhi Zi** and **Huang Qin** help the emperor herb to clear Liver-Fire.
- **Bai Ji Li** and **Shi Jue Ming** subdue Liver-Wind and Liver-Yang. Shi Jue Ming also clears Liver-Fire.
- **Ze Xie** and **Che Qian Zi** help to clear Fire via urination.
- **Dang Gui** nourishes Liver-Blood and harmonizes the Liver.
- **Sheng Di Huang** and **Mai Men Dong** nourish Yin. Sheng Di nourishes Liver-Yin and cools Blood.
- **Zhen Zhu Mu**, **Long Gu** and **Mu Li** sink and calm the Mind and settle the Ethereal Soul.
- **Fu Shen** and **Yuan Zhi** calm the Mind.
- **Suan Zao Ren** and **Bai Zi Ren** nourish the Liver, calm the Mind and settle the Ethereal Soul.
- **Gan Cao** harmonizes.

This formula (a variation of Long Dan Xie Gan Tang *Gentiana Draining the Liver Decoction*) specifically drains Liver-Fire and calms the Mind. It addresses the mental restlessness and irritability deriving from Liver-Fire. The main manifestations are dizziness, tinnitus, red face and eyes, thirst, scanty-dark urine, dry stools, insomnia, dream-disturbed sleep, propensity to outbursts of anger, headache, a Red tongue with redder sides and yellow coating and a Wiry and Rapid pulse.

Mental-emotional pattern

Anger, frustration, resentment and hatred can all cause rising of Liver-Yang and, over a long period of time, Liver-Fire. This especially happens if the person eats very greasy food and drinks alcohol. These people would be very angry, prone to outbursts of anger, impatient, mentally restless and irritable and their sleep would be very disturbed by violent dreams of fights. In this condition, Fire harasses the Ethereal Soul and makes the person destructive and restless.

At times, this situation may lead to depression especially if the anger (usually towards a member of the family) is harboured inside for many years. In these cases, the appearance of the person, depressed, subdued and speaking in a low voice, may disguise the true origin of the problem and look as if sadness and grief were the cause of the disease. However, the Red tongue with redder sides and the Wiry and Rapid pulse clearly point to the true origin of the problem, i.e. anger.

Case history

A 40-year-old woman complained of asthma which had started in her early 20s from "emotional trauma" as she herself described it. She used Ventolin and Becotide inhalers every day as well as tablets of Prednisolone. Her attacks were clearly elicited by emotional strain and the asthma did not have an allergic basis.

She felt very tense and irritable and often had a pain under the right rib-cage. She also suffered from pre-menstrual tension.

Her tongue was Red, redder on the sides, with a yellow coating (Plate 9.5). Her pulse was Weak on the right and Wiry on the left.

Diagnosis
The main problem in this case is Liver-Qi stagnation leading to Liver-Fire. Prolonged stagnation of Qi over many years often leads to Fire. Liver-Fire can overflow into the chest and obstruct the descending of Lung-Qi causing asthma. This type of asthma starts later in life (i.e. not during childhood) and is clearly related to emotional strain as it is in this case. Liver-Fire is evident from the Red sides of the tongue but not many other symptoms: this is because it did not arise independently but from stagnation of Liver-Qi. Hence the symptoms of stagnation of Liver-Qi such as the hypochondrial pain, the irritability, the pre-menstrual tension and the Wiry pulse on the left.

Treatment principle
When Liver-Fire develops from Liver-Qi stagnation it does not require draining with bitter-cold herbs or purging, but only clearing with a combination of pungent herbs to open and move Qi and some light-bitter herbs to clear.

Hence the treatment principle is to move Qi, clear Liver-Fire, restore the descending of Lung-Qi, calm the Mind and settle the Ethereal Soul.

Acupuncture
LU-7 Lieque, LU-1 Zhongfu, G.B.-34 Yanglingquan, LIV-3 Taichong, LIV-14 Qimen, P-7 Daling, P-6 Neiguan, ST-40 Fenglong. All with even method.

Explanation
- **LU-7** and **LU-1** restore the descending of Lung-Qi.
- **G.B.-34**, **LIV-3** and **LIV-14** move Liver-Qi. LIV-14, in particular, will move Liver-Qi in the chest.
- **P-7** and **P-6** calm the Mind, settle the Ethereal Soul, indirectly move Liver-Qi, restore the descending of Lung-Qi and open the chest.
- **ST-40**, especially in combination with P-6, opens the chest and eases breathing.

Herbal treatment
The formula used was a variation of Si Ni San *Four Rebellious Powder*:

Chai Hu *Radix Bupleuri* 6 g
Bai Shao *Radix Paeoniae albae* 9 g
Zhi Shi *Fructus Citri aurantii immaturus* 6 g
Zhi Gan Cao *Radix Glycyrrhizae uralensis praeparata* 6 g
Huang Qin *Radix Scutellariae baicalensis* 3 g
Shan Zhi Zi *Fructus Gardeniae jasminoidis* 3 g
Xing Ren *Semen Pruni armeniacae* 6 g
Su Zi *Fructus Perillae frutescentis* 6 g
Suan Zao Ren *Semen Ziziphi spinosae* 4 g
He Huan Pi *Cortex Albizziae julibrissin* 6 g

Explanation
The first four herbs constitute the Si Ni San.

- **Huang Qin** and **Zhi Zi** lightly clear Heat. In combination with the pungent herbs to move Qi, they clear Liver-Fire from stagnation of Liver-Qi.
- **Xing Ren** and **Su Zi** restore the descending of Lung-Qi and ease asthma.
- **Suan Zao Ren** and **He Huan Pi** calm the Mind and settle the Ethereal Soul.

This patient was off all medication after 6 months of treatment and felt much less irritable and depressed.

PHLEGM-FIRE

STOMACH AND HEART PHLEGM-FIRE

Treatment principle

Resolve Phlegm, harmonize the Stomach, open the Mind's orifices, clear the Heart and calm the Mind.

Acupuncture

ST-40 Fenglong, Ren-12 Zhongwan, Ren-9

Shuifen, ST-25 Tianshu, G.B.-13 Benshen, ST-8 Touwei, G.B.-18 Chengling, G.B.-15 Toulinqi, G.B.-17 Zhengying, BL-20 Pishu, BL-49 Yishe, P-7 Daling, Du-20 Baihui. ST-40 and P-7 with reducing method, Ren-12, BL-20 and BL-49 with reinforcing method and all the others with even method.

Explanation

- **ST-40** resolves Phlegm, harmonizes the Stomach and calms the Mind.
- **Ren-12** and **Ren-9** tonify the Spleen to resolve Phlegm.
- **ST-25** calms the Mind, opens the Mind's orifices and settles the Ethereal Soul and Corporeal Soul. It is an important point for mental-emotional problems occurring against a background of Stomach-Fire or Stomach Phlegm-Fire.
- **G.B.-13** clears the Mind's orifices and calms mental restlessness.
- **ST-8** is a local point to resolve Phlegm affecting the head.
- **G.B.-18** calms the Mind, stops obsessive ideas and relieves dizziness.
- **G.B.-15** calms the Mind, settles the Ethereal Soul and clears Heat.
- **G.B.-17** calms the Mind and stimulates concentration. It combines with ST-40 to clear Phlegm from the head and clear the Mind.
- **BL-20** tonifies the Spleen to resolve Phlegm.
- **BL-49** strengthens the Intellect and clears the Mind.
- **P-7** calms the Mind and resolves Phlegm-Fire from the Heart.
- **Du-20** clears the Mind.

Herbal treatment

Prescription

WEN DAN TANG
Warming the Gall-Bladder Decoction
Ban Xia *Rhizoma Pinelliae ternatae* 6 g
Fu Ling *Sclerotium Poriae cocos* 5 g
Chen Pi *Pericarpium Citri reticulatae* 9 g
Zhu Ru *Caulis Bambusae in Taeniis* 6 g
Zhi Shi *Fructus Citri aurantii immaturus* 6 g

Zhi Gan Cao *Radix Glycyrrhizae uralensis praeparata* 3 g
Sheng Jiang *Rhizoma Zingiberis officinalis recens* 5 slices
Da Zao *Fructus Ziziphi jujubae* one date

Explanation

- **Ban Xia**, **Chen Pi** and **Fu Ling** form the Er Chen Tang *Two Old Decoction* which resolves Phlegm.
- **Zhu Ru** resolves hot Phlegm and calms the Mind. It calms irritability deriving from Fire.
- **Zhi Shi** helps to resolve Phlegm by moving Qi and making Qi descend.
- **Sheng Jiang** and **Da Zao** harmonize the Stomach.
- **Gan Cao** harmonizes.

This formula, already discussed above under "Mind Obstructed" (p. 241) resolves Phlegm-Heat from the Stomach and Heart.

Mental-emotional pattern

Worry and pensiveness knot Qi and, after a long time, the impaired Qi movement leads to the formation of Phlegm. On the other hand, knotted Qi easily turns into Fire after a long time. Fire, in turn, may lead to the formation of more Phlegm as it burns and condenses fluids.

Phlegm-Fire both mists and agitates the Mind. The Phlegm aspect of it causes mental confusion, poor memory, dizziness and, in severe cases, total mental confusion with loss of insight. The Fire aspect of it causes agitation, mental restlessness, insomnia, a flustered feeling in the chest, anxiety and, in severe cases, manic behaviour. Nowadays this formula is widely used for manic-depression.

Phlegm-Fire in this case affects Stomach, Heart and Gall-Bladder. In the Heart, it mists the Mind and causes mental confusion. In the Gall-Bladder, it prevents the Ethereal Soul from returning to the Liver at night, hence the insomnia. Disturbance of the Ethereal Soul also causes depression and a lack of direction in life.

Obviously, irregular eating plays an important role in the development of this pattern. These people are often busy executives who eat at irregular times, or in a hurry while working or late at night.

Variations

- If Heart-Fire is evident add Huang Lian *Rhizoma Coptidis*.
- If obstruction of the Mind by Phlegm is pronounced add Shi Chang Pu *Rhizoma Acori graminei* and Yuan Zhi *Radix Polygalae tenuifoliae*.
- If there is pronounced mental restlessness and anxiety add Suan Zao Ren *Semen Ziziphi spinosae* and Zhen Zhu Mu *Concha margaritiferae*.
- If insomnia is pronounced add Ye Jiao Teng *Caulis Polygoni multiflori*.

Case history

A 54-year-old woman complained of long-standing depression and anxiety since she was 10. She had had a very unhappy childhood and harboured deep feelings of resentment towards her father. She had been on anti-depressants (tri-cyclic type) for several years and she had just recently come off tranquillizers (Valium). Inspite of the anti-depressants she still felt very depressed and she described her condition as a "black cloud hanging over her". She felt also extremely anxious and her sleep was very restless. She also suffered from severe, stabbing headaches on the forehead and was prone to a lot of catarrh. Her tongue was Reddish-Purple, Stiff, Swollen, with a Stomach crack in the centre, and a thick-sticky-yellow coating (Plate 9.6). Her pulse was Wiry, Slippery and Full.

Diagnosis
This patient suffered from two main conditions: Phlegm-Fire affecting Stomach and Heart and stasis of Blood. Both Phlegm-Fire and stasis of Blood agitate the Mind and the Ethereal Soul leading to depression and anxiety.

Treatment
The principle of treatment adopted was to resolve Phlegm, drain Fire, move Blood, calm the Mind, and settle the Ethereal Soul. She was treated with herbs only and the formula used was a variation of Wen Dan Tang *Warming the Gall-Bladder Decoction*:

Ban Xia *Rhizoma Pinelliae ternatae* 6 g
Fu Ling *Sclerotium Poriae cocos* 5 g
Chen Pi *Pericarpium Citri reticulatae* 9 g
Zhu Ru *Caulis Bambusae in Taeniis* 6 g

Zhi Shi *Fructus Citri aurantii immaturus* 6 g
Zhi Gan Cao *Radix Glycyrrhizae uralensis praeparata* 3 g
Sheng Jiang *Rhizoma Zingiberis officinalis recens* 5 slices
Da Zao *Fructus Ziziphi jujubae* one date
Yuan Zhi *Radix Polygalae tenuifoliae* 6 g
Suan Zao Ren *Semen Ziziphi spinosae* 4 g
He Huan Pi *Cortex Albizziae julibrissin* 6 g
Yu Jin *Tuber Curcumae* 6 g

Explanation
- The first 8 herbs constitute the root formula which resolves Phlegm-Heat from the Stomach and Heart.
- **Yuan Zhi** and **Suan Zao Ren** calm the Mind and open the Mind's orifices. These two herbs blend particularly well together as one is pungent and the other sour.
- **He Huan Pi** and **Yu Jin** move Blood, open the Mind's orifices and lift depression.

She was treated with variations of the above prescription for 9 months after which she felt a lot better in herself and was able to come off the anti-depressants completely.

MIND WEAKENED

This is characterized by physical and mental exhaustion, depression, lack of will-power and initiative, insomnia (waking up early), mild anxiety, poor memory, dislike to speak and pessimism.

More than the conditions associated with unsettled Mind and obstructed Mind, the conditions of weakened Mind are often the result rather than the cause of a disharmony of the internal organs and of Qi and Blood. For example, the Mind can easily become weakened after a long chronic disease, after many childbirths too close together or after a life-time of overwork which has severely depleted Qi and Essence.

The conditions causing a weakened Mind are Qi deficiency, Blood deficiency, or Yin deficiency.

The treatment of principle for weakened Mind is to nourish Qi, Yang, Blood, or Yin, calm the Mind and strengthen Will-Power.

QI AND BLOOD DEFICIENCY

1. *QI DEFICIENCY*

Treatment principle

Tonify Qi, strengthen the Mind.

Acupuncture

ST-36 Zusanli, SP-3 Taibai, Ren-6 Qihai, BL-20 Pishu, BL-21 Weishu, Du-20 Baihui, HE-7 Shenmen, LU-3 Tianfu, BL-15 Xinshu, BL-13 Feishu, BL-44 Shentang and BL-42 Pohu. All with reinforcing method. Moxa is applicable.

Explanation

- **ST-36, SP-3, BL-20** and **BL-21** tonify Stomach- and Spleen-Qi. As the Stomach and Spleen are the source of the Post-natal Qi, they should always be tonified in Qi deficiency.
- **Ren-6** tonifies Original Qi.
- **Du-20** clears the Mind and lifts mood.
- **HE-7** calms the Mind.
- **BL-15** with direct moxa, tonifies Heart-Qi, clears the Mind and lifts mood.
- **BL-13** tonifies Lung-Qi and is selected if there is Lung deficiency as there would be when sadness is the cause of this pattern.
- **BL-44** tonifies the Heart and calms and clears the Mind.
- **BL-42** tonifies the Lungs and settles the Corporeal Soul which suffers from sadness and grief.

Herbal treatment

(a) Prescription

AN SHEN DING ZHI WAN
Calming the Mind and Settling the Will-Power Pill
Ren Shen *Radix Ginseng* 9 g
Fu Ling *Sclerotium Poriae cocos* 12 g
Fu Shen *Sclerotium Poriae cocos pararadicis* 9 g
Long Chi *Dens Draconis* 15 g
Yuan Zhi *Radix Polygalae tenuifoliae* 6 g
Shi Chang Pu *Rhizoma Acori graminei* 8 g

Explanation

- **Ren Shen** tonifies Qi and the Original Qi.
- **Fu Ling** combines with Ren Shen to tonify Qi and prevent Dampness. It also calms the Mind.
- **Fu Shen** calms the Mind.
- **Long Chi** sinks and calms the Mind and settles the Ethereal Soul.
- **Yuan Zhi** nourishes the Heart and calms the Mind.

- **Shi Chang Pu** opens the Mind's orifices and clears the Mind.

This formula tonifies Qi, strengthens the Original Qi, calms and clears the Mind and lifts mood. It is used for chronic Qi deficiency affecting the Mind making it on the one hand restless and, on the other hand, confused and depressed. The main manifestations would be extreme tiredness, dislike to speak, slight breathlessness, no appetite, restless sleep with unpleasant dreams, palpitations, a weak voice, a Pale tongue and an Empty or Weak pulse.

Mental-emotional pattern

This pattern either arises from a depletion of Qi consequent on a chronic disease, or from emotional problems affecting Qi. Sadness, grief and regret are the most likely causes of this condition. They deplete Qi of the Lungs and Heart. This person would feel very tired, be depressed and not sleep well. He or she would also lack motivation.

(b) Prescription

DING ZHI WAN
Settling the Will-Power Pill
Ren Shen *Radix Ginseng* 9 g
Fu Ling *Sclerotium Poriae cocos* 6 g
Shi Chang Pu *Rhizoma Acori graminei* 6 g
Yuan Zhi *Radix Polygalae tenuifoliae* 6 g

Explanation

- **Ren Shen** tonifies Qi and the Original Qi.
- **Fu Ling** combines with Ren Shen to tonify Qi and prevent Dampness. It also calms the Mind.
- **Chang Pu** calms the Mind, opens the Mind's orifices and clears the Mind.
- **Yuan Zhi** calms the Mind and opens the Mind's orifices.

This formula is very similar to the previous one. It differs from it in so far as it does not have as strong a calming effect on the Mind due to the omission of Long Chi *Dens Draconis*. This formula tonifies Qi, strengthens the Original Qi, calms and clears the Mind and lifts mood. It is used for chronic Qi deficiency affecting the Mind making it confused and depressed. The main manifestations would be extreme tiredness, dislike to speak, slight breathlessness, no appetite, palpitations, a weak voice, a Pale tongue and an Empty or Weak pulse.

Mental-emotional pattern

As in the previous case, this pattern arises either from a depletion of Qi consequent on a chronic disease, or from emotional problems affecting Qi. Sadness, grief and regret are the most likely causes of this condition. They deplete Qi of the Lungs and Heart. This person would feel very tired and depressed. He or she would also lack motivation.

Case history

A 41-year-old woman suffered from abdominal distension, belching, constipation and hypochondrial pain. Her periods started hesitantly and were painful. The menstrual blood was dark with some clots. She also complained of pre-menstrual tension and irritability.

   She had a feeling of vague anxiety at night with a sensation of tightness of the chest. Some years before she had gone through a difficult period emotionally and experienced great sadness. Her complexion was pale and her eyes were slightly dull. Her tongue-body colour was normal with teethmarks. Her pulse was very Weak and Fine on the Lung position and slightly Wiry on the left side.

Diagnosis
Most of the symptoms and signs point to stagnation of Liver-Qi and Liver-Blood: abdominal distension, belching, hypochondrial pain, painful periods with dark blood and pre-menstrual tension. However, the very Fine Lung pulse, the feeling of anxiety at night, the pale complexion and the teethmarks on the tongue point to Lung-Qi deficiency. This, combined with the absence of a Red colour on the sides of the tongue, indicated that the main problem lay in deficient Lung-Qi not controlling the Liver (Metal insulting Wood from a 5-Element perspective) and leading to stagnation of Liver-Qi. The feeling of vague anxiety at night was due to agitation of the Corporeal Soul from Lung-Qi deficiency. The deficiency of Lung-Qi was obviously due to the period of great sadness years before.

Treatment principle
Tonify Lung-Qi, settle the Corporeal Soul and Ethereal Soul and move Liver-Qi.

Herbal treatment
The prescription used was not a classical one but one I formulated for this patient:

Bai He *Bulbus Lilii* 9 g
Mai Men Dong *Tuber Ophiopogonis japonici* 6 g
Bei Sha Shen *Radix Glehniae littoralis* 6 g
Huang Qi *Radix Astragali membranacei* 6 g
Dang Shen *Radix Codonopsis pilosulae* 9 g
Wu Wei Zi *Fructus Schisandrae chinensis* 4 g
Shu Di Huang *Radix Rehmanniae glutinosae praeparata* 9 g
Bai Shao *Radix Paeoniae albae* 9 g
Yi Mu Cao *Herba Leonori heterophylli* 4 g
Yu Jin *Tuber Curcumae* 6 g
Zhi Gan Cao *Radix Glycyrrhizae uralensis praeparata* 6 g

Explanation
- **Bai He**, **Mai Men Dong** and **Bei Sha Shen** nourish Lung-Yin. Although she does not suffer from Lung-Yin deficiency, these herbs are used to nourish and settle the Corporeal Soul and relieve sadness.
- **Huang Qi** and **Dang Shen** tonify Lung- and Spleen-Qi. It is necessary to tonify Spleen-Qi according to the principle of reinforcing Earth to strengthen Metal.
- **Wu Wei Zi** tonifies Lung-Qi and Lung-Yin and settles the Corporeal Soul.
- **Shu Di**, **Bai Shao** and **Yi Mu Cao** harmonize Liver-Blood. Bai Shao is sour and absorbing and, in combination with Gan Cao, it stops pain, calms the Mind and moderates urgency.
- **Yu Jin** moves Liver-Blood, opens the Mind's orifices and lifts depression.
- **Zhi Gan Cao**, in a larger dose than normal, is combined with Bai Shao as indicated above.

After taking this prescription for 2 weeks she experienced less abdominal distension, less belching and no constipation. She felt calmer in the evening and brighter in herself but also more moody and more up and down emotionally. I attributed this to Yu Jin *Tuber Curcumae* within the prescription: this herb is pungent and hot and powerfully moves Liver-Qi and Liver-Blood. The second prescription was:

Bai He *Bulbus Lilii* 9 g
Bei Sha Shen *Radix Glehniae littoralis* 6 g
Mai Men Dong *Tuber Ophiopogonis japonici* 6 g
Dang Shen *Radix Codonopsis pilosulae* 6 g
Hou Po *Cortex Magnoliae officinalis* 6 g
Ban Xia *Rhizoma Pinelliae ternatae* 6 g
Su Ye *Folium Perillae frutescentis* 6 g
Fu Ling *Sclerotium Poriae cocos* 4 g
Xiang Fu *Rhizoma Cyperi rotundi* 4 g
Suan Zao Ren *Semen Ziziphi spinosae* 3 g
Zhi Gan Cao *Radix Glycyrrhizae uralensis praeparata* 6 g
Bai Shao *Radix Paeoniae albae* 6 g
Da Zao *Fructus Ziziphi jujubae* 5 dates

Explanation
- The first four herbs have already been discussed above.
- **Hou Po**, **Ban Xia**, **Su Ye**, and **Fu Ling** constitute Ban Xia Hou Po Tang *Pinellia-Magnolia Decoction* which moves Liver-Qi in the chest and makes Lung-Qi and Stomach-Qi descend. It particularly relieves depression, moodiness and sadness associated with the Lungs.
- **Xiang Fu** and **Suan Zao Ren** move Liver-Qi and settle the Ethereal Soul. They are coordinated as one is pungent and moves, the other is sour and absorbs.
- **Zhi Gan Cao** and **Bai Shao** stop pain, harmonize the Liver and moderate urgency.
- **Da Zao** harmonizes.

After repeating this prescription three times she was much better all round and her periods became painless.

2. QI AND BLOOD DEFICIENCY

Treatment principle

Tonify Qi, nourish Blood and calm the Mind.

Acupuncture

ST-36 Zusanli, SP-6 Sanyinjiao, Ren-4 Guanyuan, BL-20 Pishu, BL-21 Weishu, Du-20 Baihui, HE-7 Shenmen, Ren-15 Jiuwei, BL-15 Xinshu, and BL-44 Shentang. All with reinforcing method. Moxa is applicable.

Explanation

- **ST-36**, **SP-6**, **BL-20** and **BL-21** tonify Stomach- and Spleen-Qi. As the Stomach and Spleen are the source of the Post-natal Qi, they should always be tonified in Qi deficiency. SP-6 also nourishes Blood, calms the Mind and promotes sleep.
- **Ren-4** tonifies Original Qi and nourishes Blood.
- **Du-20** clears the Mind and lifts mood.
- **HE-7** calms the Mind.
- **Ren-15** calms the Mind and nourishes Heart-Blood.
- **BL-15** with direct moxa, tonifies Heart-Qi, clears the Mind and lifts mood.
- **BL-44** tonifies the Heart and calms and clears the Mind.

Herbal treatment

(a) Prescription

GUI PI TANG
Tonifying the Spleen Decoction
Ren Shen *Radix Ginseng* 6 g (**Dang Shen** *Radix Codonopsis pilosulae* 12 g)
Huang Qi *Radix Astragali membranacei* 15 g
Bai Zhu *Rhizoma Atractylodis macrocephalae* 12 g
Dang Gui *Radix Angelicae sinensis* 6 g
Fu Shen *Sclerotium Poriae cocos pararadicis* 9 g
Suan Zao Ren *Semen Ziziphi spinosae* 9 g
Long Yan Rou *Arillus Euphoriae longanae* 12 g
Yuan Zhi *Radix Polygalae tenuifoliae* 9 g
Mu Xiang *Radix Saussureae* 6 g
Zhi Gan Cao *Radix Glycyrrhizae uralensis praeparata* 4 g
Sheng Jiang *Rhizoma Zingiberis officinalis recens* 3 slices
Hong Zao *Fructus Ziziphi jujubae* 5 dates

Explanation

- **Ren Shen**, **Huang Qi** and **Bai Zhu** tonify Qi.
- **Dang Gui** nourishes Blood.
- **Fu Shen** combines with the Qi tonics to prevent Dampness. It also calms the Mind.
- **Suan Zao Ren**, **Long Yan Rou** and **Yuan Zhi** nourish the Heart and calm the Mind.
- **Mu Xiang** moves Qi and is used to counterbalance the cloying nature of the Qi and Blood tonics.
- **Zhi Gan Cao** helps the Qi tonics to tonify Qi and harmonizes.
- **Sheng Jiang** and **Hong Zao** harmonize the formula, harmonize Defensive and Nutritive Qi and help to tonify Spleen-Qi.

This well-tested prescription is excellent to tonify Spleen-Qi and Heart-Blood and calm the Mind. Besides calming the Mind it also clears and stimulates it, helping memory, thinking and concentration. The main manifestations are palpitations, tiredness, a pale complexion, insomnia (difficulty in falling asleep), poor memory, poor appetite, menorrhagia in women (from Spleen-Qi not holding Blood), a Pale tongue and a Weak or Choppy pulse.

Mental-emotional pattern

Worry and pensiveness over a long period of time injure the Spleen and Heart and lead to Spleen-Qi deficiency and Heart-Blood deficiency. This weakens the Mind which is deprived of its residence. Thus the patient becomes tired and depressed and finds sleep difficult. The Mind controls memory and thinking and there is therefore a poor memory, poor concentration and slow thinking. Another feature of this pattern is obsessive thinking or phobias which are due to Spleen and Blood deficiency. The Spleen controls thinking, intelligence and concentration and, when in disharmony, these same qualities may generate obsessive thinking or phobias.

Variations

– If Blood deficiency is pronounced add Shu Di Huang *Radix Rehmanniae glutinosae praeparata*. With the addition of this herb, this formula is called Hei Gui Pi Tang *Black Tonifying the Spleen Decoction*.

(b) Prescription

SHI WEI WEN DAN TANG
Ten-Ingredient Warming the Gall-Bladder Decoction
Ban Xia *Rhizoma Pinelliae ternatae* 6 g
Chen Pi *Pericarpium Citri reticulatae* 6 g
Fu Ling *Sclerotium Poriae cocos* 4.5 g
Zhi Shi *Fructus Citri aurantii immaturus* 6 g
Ren Shen *Radix Ginseng* 3 g (**Dang Shen** *Radix Codonopsis pilosulae* 9 g)
Shu Di Huang *Radix Rehmanniae glutinosae praeparata* 9 g
Suan Zao Ren *Semen Ziziphi spinosae* 3 g
Yuan Zhi *Radix Polygalae tenuifoliae* 3 g
Wu Wei Zi *Fructus Schisandrae chinensis* 3 g
Zhi Gan Cao *Radix Glycyrrhizae uralensis praeparata* 1.5 g
Sheng Jiang *Rhizoma Zingiberis officinalis recens* 5 slices
Hong Zao *Fructus Ziziphi jujubae* 1 date

Explanation

– **Ban Xia**, **Chen Pi** and **Fu Ling** resolve Phlegm.

– **Zhi Shi** moves Qi to help to resolve Phlegm.
– **Ren Shen** tonifies Qi and Original Qi.
– **Shu Di Huang** nourishes Blood.
– **Suan Zao Ren** and **Yuan Zhi** calm the Mind and open the Mind's orifices.
– **Wu Wei Zi** calms the Mind, being sour it "absorbs" the Mind into the Heart, and, being astringent, it stops sweating.
– **Zhi Gan Cao** harmonizes and helps to tonify Qi.
– **Sheng Jiang** and **Hong Zao** harmonize.

This formula is a variation of Wen Dan Tang *Warming the Gall-Bladder Decoction*. Of the latter prescription, it preserves the element of resolving Phlegm, but, contrary to it, it does not clear Heat. In addition, this formula tonifies Qi and Blood. The main manifestations are tiredness, poor appetite, poor memory, timidity, insomnia, palpitations, mild anxiety, propensity to be startled, a Pale tongue and a Weak or Choppy pulse.

This formula, contrary to the previous one, also addresses any sweating that may derive from some Empty-Heat developing from Blood deficiency. This is quite possible and it happens more frequently in women. In the prescription, Wu Wei Zi and Suan Zao Ren have this function.

Another important difference from the previous formula, is that this one resolves Phlegm as well. It is therefore suited to treat mental confusion as well as anxiety and restlessness.

Mental-emotional pattern

Worry and pensiveness deplete the Spleen and the Heart and this leads to deficiency of Qi and Blood. The Mind is deprived of its residence and the person feels exhausted, depressed and anxious. The Spleen-Qi deficiency leads to the formation of Phlegm which mists the Mind causing confused thinking and obsessive thoughts. The Blood deficiency causes insomnia, poor memory, timidity and propensity to be startled.

(c) Prescription

GAN MAI DA ZAO TANG
Glycyrrhiza-Triticum-Ziziphus Decoction
Fu Xiao Mai *Semen Tritici aestivi levis* 15 g

Gan Cao *Radix Glycyrrhizae uralensis* 9 g
Da Zao *Fructus Ziziphi jujubae* 7 dates

Explanation

- **Fu Xiao Mai** tonifies Heart-Qi and calms the Mind. It is astringent and it therefore can "absorb" the restless Mind back into the Heart.
- **Gan Cao** tonifies Qi, harmonizes the Middle Burner and nourishes the Heart.
- **Da Zao** tonifies Qi and harmonizes.

This interesting formula has been the subject of much speculation and different interpretations. Essentially, it tonifies Heart-Qi and calms the Mind. It can also be used for deficiency of Heart-Yin with Empty-Heat, only when, however, the Empty-Heat is not such that it requires the use of bitter-cold herbs because these would further injure Qi. On the other hand, the deficiency of Qi is not such that it requires strong tonifying herbs, hence the gentle tonification of these three herbs. The hallmark of this prescription, then, is that it provides enough tonification but not so much that it would make any Empty-Heat worse. All the herbs in it are sweet and this taste soothes the Liver. For this reason, this formula is also said to treat Liver-Qi stagnation which may be associated with Heart-Qi deficiency.

Mental-emotional pattern

All the manifestations normally relevant to this formula are of mental or emotional character. Worry, excess joy, craving, love and pensiveness may all injure Heart-Qi and lead to this condition. The main manifestations are worrying, anxiety, sadness, weeping, insomnia, depression, inability to control oneself, yawning, moaning, speaking to oneself, disorientation, a Weak pulse and a Pale tongue. The tongue may be Red without coating if there is Heart-Yin deficiency.

In severe cases, this corresponds to the depressive phase of manic-depression.

This formula is often added as a whole to other prescriptions to treat the above manifestations.

(i) Patent remedy

DING XIN WAN
Settling the Heart Pill
Dang Shen *Radix Codonopsis pilosulae*
Dang Gui *Radix Angelicae sinensis*
Fu Shen *Sclerotium Poriae cocos pararadicis*
Yuan Zhi *Radix Polygalae tenuifoliae*
Suan Zao Ren *Semen Ziziphi spinosae*
Bai Zi Ren *Semen Biotae orientalis*
Mai Men Dong *Tuber Ophiopogonis japonici*
Hu Po *Succinum*

Explanation

This remedy tonifies the Heart (Qi, Blood and Yin), and calms and strengthens the Mind: it can be used for depression and insomnia from Heart deficiency.

Although it tonifies Qi, Blood and Yin, the emphasis is on Heart-Qi deficiency and the tongue presentation appropriate to this remedy is therefore a Pale body with a Heart crack.

(ii) Patent remedy

LING ZHI PIAN
Ganoderma Tablet
Ling Zhi *Fructus Ganodermae lucidi*

Explanation

This tablet contains only Ling Zhi which tonifies Qi, Blood and Yin and calms the Mind. It is used for insomnia and depression from Qi and Blood deficiency.

YANG DEFICIENCY

KIDNEY-YANG DEFICIENCY

Treatment principle

Tonify and warm Yang, strengthen the Kidneys, calm the Mind and lift mood.

Acupuncture

BL-23 Shenshu, BL-52 Zhishi, Du-4 Mingmen, Du-14 Dazhui, Ren-4 Guanyuan, KI-3 Taixi, KI-7

Fuliu, ST-36 Zusanli, SP-6 Sanyinjiao, Du-20 Baihui, BL-8 Luoque, BL-10 Tianzhu. All with re-inforcing method except for the points in the head which are usually needled with even method. Moxa should be used.

Explanation

- **BL-23** tonifies Kidney-Yang.
- **BL-52** tonifies the Kidneys and strengthens the Will-Power.
- **Du-4,** with direct moxa, strongly tonifies the Fire of the Gate of Vitality and it lifts mood.
- **Du-14**, with direct moxa, tonifies Yang and lifts mood.
- **Ren-4** nourishes the Kidneys and calms the Mind.
- **KI-3** and **KI-7** tonify Kidney-Yang. KI-7 in particular, would resolve oedema, a possible consequence of Kidney-Yang deficiency.
- **ST-36** and **SP-6** tonify the Stomach and Spleen to raise vitality in general. In particular, SP-6 also nourishes Yin and is therefore indicated in complicated cases of deficiency of both Yang and Yin of the Kidneys.
- **Du-20** raises Yang, improves memory and concentration and lifts mood.
- **BL-8** calms the Mind, lifts mood and strengthens memory.
- **BL-10** clears the Mind.

Herbal treatment

Prescription

YOU GUI WAN
Restoring the Right [Kidney] Pill
Fu Zi *Radix Aconiti carmichaeli praeparata* 3 g
Rou Gui *Cortex Cinnamomi cassiae* 3 g
Du Zhong *Cortex Eucommiae ulmoidis* 6 g
Tu Si Zi *Semen Cuscutae* 6 g
Lu Jiao Jiao *Colla Cornu Cervi* 6 g
Shu Di Huang *Radix Rehmanniae glutinosae prae-parata* 12 g
Shan Yao *Radix Dioscoreae oppositae* 6 g
Shan Zhu Yu *Fructus Corni officinalis* 4.5 g
Gou Qi Zi *Fructus Lycii chinensis* 6 g
Dang Gui *Radix Angelicae sinensis* 4.5 g

Explanation

- **Rou Gui** and **Fu Zi** tonify and warm Kidney-Yang and stoke-up the Fire of the Gate of Vitality.
- **Du Zhong**, **Tu Si Zi** and **Lu Jiao Jiao** tonify and warm Kidney-Yang and strengthen the Will-Power.
- **Shu Di Huang**, **Shan Yao** and **Shan Zhu Yu** tonify the Kidneys, Stomach and Liver. They are a contracted variation (without the three draining herbs Ze Xie *Rhizoma Alismatis orientalis*, Fu Ling *Sclerotium Poriae cocos* and Mu Dan Pi *Cortex Moutan radicis*) of the Liu Wei Di Huang Wan *Six-Ingredient Rehmannia Pill*.
- **Gou Qi Zi** and **Dang Gui** nourish Blood.

This formula is excellent to tonify Kidney-Yang and the Fire of the Gate of Vitality with its associated mental manifestations. The main physical manifestations are back-ache, weak knees, poor memory, exhaustion, cold legs and back, frequent-pale urination, a Pale and Swollen tongue and a Weak-Deep pulse. This formula is preferable to the Jin Gui Shen Qi Wan *Golden Chest Kidney-Qi Pill* for two reasons: first of all, it also nourishes Blood which makes it more suitable for women (due to the inclusion of Gou Qi Zi *Fructus Lycii chinensis* and Dang Gui *Radix Angelicae sinensis*), and secondly, because it is better for the mental aspects of Kidney-Yang deficiency (due to the inclusion of Du Zhong *Cortex Eucommiae ulmoidis* and Lu Jiao Jiao *Colla Cornu Cervi*).

Mental-emotional pattern

Fear, shock and guilt may injure the Kidneys and cause this condition. However, it is also often the result rather than the cause of Kidney-Yang deficiency. Kidney-Yang may be depleted by a chronic disease, overwork, excessive physical work and lifting and excessive sexual activity.

This person will feel mentally and physically exhausted, will be depressed and will lack will-power and spirit of initiative. He or she will have almost given up any hope of getting better or of starting or changing anything in life. Everything is too much effort.

This condition is characterized not only by

Kidney-Yang deficiency but also by Essence depletion. The Kidney-Essence is the material basis for all the Kidney's physiological activities. The Essence has a Yin and a Yang aspect and, in this case, its Yang aspect is deficient. Because the Essence is the foundation for the Three Treasures, the Essence, Qi and Mind, a deficiency of its Yang aspect causes extreme exhaustion and low spirits.

Variations

– In cases of severe depression and exhaustion replace Lu Jiao Jiao with the stronger Lu Rong *Cornu Cervi parvum*.
– In cases of mixed Yin and Yang deficiency symptoms of the Kidneys (a very frequent occurrence) halve the dosage of Fu Zi and Rou Gui to 1.5 g each, and replace Shu Di Huang with Sheng Di Huang *Radix Rehmanniae glutinosae*.

Case history

A 46-year-old woman complained of nocturia: she had to get up to urinate up to seven times a night. Her urine was generally pale and she experienced a dry mouth at night when she woke up. She had a lower back-ache and felt generally cold although she occasionally also felt hot in the face.

Her tongue was slightly Pale with a Red tip with red points (Plate 9.7). Her pulse was Weak on both Kidney positions of left and right.

Diagnosis
This is a clear pattern of Kidney-Yang deficiency. Although this is the predominant condition, there is also the very beginning of some Kidney-Yin deficiency manifesting with a dry mouth at night and the occasional hot flush.

When asked about her earlier life and how the condition might have developed she said that as a child she was evacuated during the war to stay with a family who did not treat her well. She was with them from the age of 4 to 8. She was intimidated by her foster parents and was often scared. At that time she developed nocturnal enuresis which did not disappear until she was 13. This is a very clear example of the effect of fear on the Kidneys in children, producing a deficiency of Kidney-Yang which persisted throughout her life.

Treatment principle
Tonify Kidney-Yang, astringe the Essence, strengthen Will-Power and calm the Mind.

Acupuncture
The following points were reinforced:

– **BL-23** Shenshu, **Du-4** Mingmen (with moxa), **Ren-4** Guanyuan (moxa) and **KI-3** to tonify Kidney-Yang and strengthen Will-Power.
– **P-7** Daling and **Ren-15** to calm the Mind.

Herbal treatment
No herbs were used but only the patent remedy Jin Suo Gu Jing Wan *Golden Lock Consolidating the Essence Pill*:

Qian Shi *Semen Euryales ferocis*
Lian Xu *Stamen Nelumbinis nuciferae*
Long Gu *Os Draconis* (calcined)
Mu Li *Concha Ostreae* (calcined)
Lian Zi *Semen Nelumbinis nuciferae*
Sha Yuan Ji Li *Semen Astragali membranacei*

This remedy is mostly astringent rather than tonifying. It treats the Manifestation by astringing the urine but not the Root, i.e. Kidney-Yang deficiency. It is therefore suitable to be used in conjunction with the acupuncture treatment which is aimed at treating the Root.

BLOOD DEFICIENCY

Treatment principle

Nourish Blood and calm the Mind.

Acupuncture

The same points used for Blood deficiency under Mind Unsettled are applicable here.

Herbal treatment

The same prescriptions used for Blood deficiency under Mind Unsettled are applicable here.

YIN DEFICIENCY

1. KIDNEY-YIN DEFICIENCY

Treatment principle

Nourish Yin, calm the Mind and lift mood.

Acupuncture

KI-3 Taixi, KI-6 Zhaohai, SP-6 Sanyinjiao, Ren-4 Guanyuan, BL-23 Shenshu, BL-52 Zhishi, Du-20 Baihui. Reinforcing method.

Explanation

- **KI-3**, **KI-6**, **SP-6** and **Ren-4** nourish Kidney-Yin and calm the Mind.
- **BL-23** and **BL-52** tonify the Kidneys and strengthen Will-Power. Although BL-23 is better to tonify Kidney-Yang, it is added here for its mental effect in lifting mood.
- **Du-20** lifts mood and relieves depression.

Herbal treatment

All the prescriptions mentioned for Yin deficiency causing unsettled Mind are applicable here. However, the emphasis of those prescriptions was on calming the Mind, whilst in the case of weakened Mind, the emphasis should be on clearing the Mind and lifting mood. They should therefore be suitably adapted by the addition of more Yin-nourishing herbs such as Sheng Di Huang *Radix Rehmanniae glutinosae*, Mai Men Dong *Tuber Ophiopogonis japonici* or Tian Men Dong *Tuber Asparagi cochinchinensis*.

The following are formulae which nourish Yin with the emphasis on lifting mood rather than calming the Mind.

Prescription

LIU WEI DI HUANG WAN
Six-Ingredient Rehmannia Pill
Shu Di Huang *Radix Rehmanniae glutinosae praeparata* 24 g
Shan Zhu Yu *Fructus Corni officinalis* 12 g
Shan Yao *Rhizoma Dioscoreae oppositae* 12 g
Ze Xie *Rhizoma Alismatis orientalis* 9 g
Mu Dan Pi *Cortex Moutan radicis* 9 g
Fu Ling *Sclerotium Poriae cocos* 9 g

Explanation

This is the most famous Yin-nourishing formula. Fear, guilt and shock can deplete the Kidneys. A feeling of guilt, especially when harboured for many years, is very destructive and may lead to Kidney deficiency. The main manifestations that apply to this formula are dizziness, tinnitus, back-ache, night-sweating, a dry mouth, 5-palm heat, exhaustion, a dark complexion, a thin body, dry hair, a Red tongue without coating and a Floating-Empty pulse.

Mental-emotional pattern

Again, this condition can arise either as a consequence of emotional problems due to shock, fear, or guilt, or, vice versa, as a result of depletion of Kidney-Yin and Kidney Essence.

This person will feel very exhausted and depressed, lacking in will-power and spirit of initiative. Unlike those who suffer from Kidney-Yang deficiency with similar mental characteristics, those who suffer from Kidney-Yin deficiency are slightly more restless, uneasy and fidgety. They may also tend to complain more.

The Essence is the foundation of the Three Treasures, Essence, Qi and Mind, and when it is depleted, the Mind and the Will-Power suffer causing exhaustion, depression and despair.

2. LUNG- AND KIDNEY-YIN DEFICIENCY

Treatment principle

Nourish Lung- and Kidney-Yin, strengthen Will-Power and settle the Corporeal Soul.

Acupuncture

LU-9 Taiyuan, LU-5 Chize, KI-3 Taixi, Ren-4 Guanyuan, LU-7 Lieque and KI-6 Zhaohai, BL-23 Shenshu, BL-52 Zhishi, BL-42 Pohu. Reinforcing method.

Explanation

- **LU-9** tonifies Lung-Yin.
- **LU-5** nourishes the Water of the Lungs and, according to the book "An Explanation of Acupuncture Points" (1654) when sadness has affected the Lungs causing dryness of this organ and the person cries a lot.[83]
- **KI-3** and **Ren-4** nourish Kidney-Yin and calm the Mind.
- **LU-7** and **KI-6** open the Directing Vessel, nourish Lung- and Kidney-Yin and benefit the throat.

- **BL-23** and **BL-52** tonify the Kidneys and strengthen Will-Power.
- **BL-42** tonifies the Lungs and settles the Corporeal Soul.

Herbal treatment

(a) Prescription

MAI WEI DI HUANG WAN
Ophiopogon-Schisandra-Rehmannia Pill
Shu Di Huang *Radix Rehmanniae glutinosae praeparata* 24 g
Shan Zhu Yu *Fructus Corni officinalis* 12 g
Shan Yao *Radix Dioscoreae oppositae* 12 g
Ze Xie *Rhizoma Alismatis orientalis* 9 g
Mu Dan Pi *Cortex Moutan radicis* 9 g
Fu Ling *Sclerotium Poriae cocos* 9 g
Mai Men Dong *Tuber Ophiopogonis japonici* 6 g
Wu Wei Zi *Fructus Schisandrae chinensis* 6 g

Explanation

This is a variation of the previous formula with the addition of Mai Men Dong and Wu Wei Zi which nourish Lung-Yin. The main physical manifestations, in addition to those of Liu Wei Di Huang Wan, are therefore a dry cough, a dry throat, slight breathlessness and possibly blood-flecked sputum.

Mental-emotional pattern

All the mental-emotional characteristics of the previous case apply here. The main difference is that, in this case, the Corporeal Soul is affected and this condition may be caused by emotions which injure the Lungs such as sadness, worry and grief.

In terms of mental-emotional manifestations, this person will probably somatize the emotions on the skin which will be dry with skin rashes.

This person will also tend to be more melancholic, sad and apt to hanker nostalgically after the past.

(b) Prescription

DI PO TANG
Earth Corporeal Soul Decoction
Mai Men Dong *Tuber Ophiopogonis japonici* 9 g

Wu Wei Zi *Fructus Schisandrae chinensis* 3 g
Xuan Shen *Radix Scrophulariae ningpoensis* 9 g
Bai Shao *Radix Paeoniae albae* 9 g
Mu Li *Concha Ostreae* 9 g
Ban Xia *Rhizoma Pinelliae ternatae* 9 g
Gan Cao *Radix Glycyrrhizae uralensis* 3 g

Explanation

- **Mai Dong**, **Wu Wei Zi** and **Xuan Shen** nourish Lung-Yin.
- **Bai Shao** and **Mu Li** are both absorbing and help to nourish Yin. Being astringent they help to root the Corporeal Soul into the Lungs.
- **Ban Xia** subdues rebellious Lung-Qi.
- **Gan Cao** harmonizes.

Mental-emotional pattern

This formula is from the "Discussion on Blood Diseases" (1884) and is for mental confusion and restlessness resulting from an unsettled Corporeal Soul.

The patient is mildly restless, depressed, slightly confused, and has palpitations, symptoms occurring against a background of deficient Lung-Yin not rooting the Corporeal Soul.

Case history

A 35-year-old man presented with insomnia (waking up during the night), slight anxiety, depression, lack of concentration, numbness of the hands at night, a dry mouth, a feeling of heat in the evening and palpitations.

His eyes lacked glitter and were unstable, his tongue was Red, with a Heart crack and without enough coating (Plate 9.8), and his pulse was Rapid and Moving.

Diagnosis
The pattern is Heart-Yin deficiency and his eyes and pulse (Moving quality) clearly point to shock as the cause of the disease. When asked about it, he confirmed that he had suffered a tremendous shock when his brother was murdered a few years before.

Treatment principle
Nourish the Heart, tonify Yin, open the Heart's orifices and calm the Mind. It is necessary to open the Heart's orifices as shock "closes" the Heart.

Acupuncture
The main points used (with reinforcing method) were:

– **HE-7** Shenmen, **SP-6** Sanyinjiao and **Ren-14** Juque to nourish the Heart and calm the Mind.
– **Ren-15** Jiuwei and **BL-15** Xinshu to open the Heart's orifices.
– **Ren-4** Guanyuan to nourish Yin and root the Mind.

Herbal treatment
The formula used was a variation of Mai Wei Di Huang Wan
Ophiopogon-Schisandra-Rehmannia Pill:

Shu Di Huang *Radix Rehmanniae glutinosae praeparata* 12 g
Ren Shen *Radix Ginseng* 6 g
Ze Xie *Rhizoma Alismatis orientalis* 6 g
Fu Shen *Sclerotium Poriae cocos pararadicis* 6 g
Mai Men Dong *Tuber Ophiopogonis japonici* 9 g
Wu Wei Zi *Fructus Schisandrae chinensis* 6 g
Yuan Zhi *Radix Polygalae tenuifoliae* 6 g
Shi Chang Pu *Rhizoma Acori graminei* 6 g
Zhi Gan Cao *Radix Glycyrrhizae uralensis praeparata* 3 g

Explanation
The original formula nourishes Lung- and Kidney-Yin but, modified as above, it can nourish Heart-Yin and calm the Mind.

– **Shu Di**, besides tonifying the Kidneys also enters the Heart and therefore settles the Mind.
– **Shan Zhu Yu** and **Mu Dan Pi** were eliminated; they are in the original formula to nourish the Liver which is not deficient in this case.
– **Shan Yao** was replaced by **Ren Shen** as this enters the Heart. Also, in combination with Wu Wei Zi and Mai Men Dong (see below) it makes the Sheng Mai Tang which nourishes Qi and Yin of the Heart.
– **Ze Xie** combines with Shu Di Huang to clear any Empty-Heat.
– **Fu Ling** was replaced with **Fu Shen** to calm the Mind.
– **Mai Dong** and **Wu Wei Zi** are part of the original prescription and they both enter the Heart.
– **Yuan Zhi** and **Chang Pu** open the Heart's orifices. They are both pungent and therefore scattering and are coordinated with Wu Wei Zi which is sour and absorbing.
– **Zhi Gan Cao** harmonizes.

This patient was treated for 9 months producing an all-round improvement in his physical and mental symptoms.

3. KIDNEY- AND LIVER-YIN DEFICIENCY

Treatment principle

Nourish Kidney- and Liver-Yin, strengthen the Will-Power and settle the Ethereal Soul.

Acupuncture

KI-3 Taixi, KI-6 Zhaohai, SP-6 Sanyinjiao, Ren-4 Guanyuan, LIV-8 Ququan, BL-23 Shenshu, BL-52 Zhishi, BL-47 Hunmen. Reinforcing method.

Explanation

– **KI-3**, **KI-6**, **SP-6**, **Ren-4** and **LIV-8** Ququan nourish Kidney- and Liver-Yin.
– **BL-23** and **BL-52** strengthen the Kidneys and Will-Power.
– **BL-47** settles the Ethereal Soul. The combination of BL-47, BL-23 and BL-52 is excellent to relieve mental depression deriving from a deficiency of Liver and Kidneys.

Herbal treatment

(a) Prescription

DA BU YIN JIAN
Great Tonifying Yin Decoction
Shu Di Huang *Radix Rehmanniae glutinosae praeparata* 15 g
Shan Yao *Radix Dioscoreae oppositae* 12 g
Shan Zhu Yu *Fructus Corni officinalis* 9 g
Gou Qi Zi *Fructus Lycii chinensis* 12 g
Dang Gui *Radix Angelicae sinensis* 9 g
Dang Shen *Radix Codonopsis pilosulae* 12 g
Du Zhong *Cortex Eucommiae ulmoidis* 9 g
Zhi Gan Cao *Radix Glycyrrhizae uralensis praeparata* 6 g

Explanation

– **Shu Di Huang**, **Shan Yao** and **Shan Zhu Yu** nourish the Yin of Kidneys, Stomach and Liver. They are a contracted version of the Liu Wei Di Huang Wan without the three draining herbs.
– **Gou Qi Zi** and **Dang Gui** nourish Liver-Yin and Liver-Blood.
– **Dang Shen** tonifies Qi.
– **Du Zhong** tonifies Kidney-Yang.
– **Zhi Gan Cao** harmonizes.

This formula is for deficiency of Kidney- and Liver-Yin. The main manifestations are dizziness, tinnitus, backache, weak knees, blurred vision, dry eyes, night-sweating, 5-palm heat, headache, a Red tongue without coating and a Floating-Empty pulse.

Mental-emotional pattern

Fear, shock and guilt may cause a deficiency of Kidney and Liver-Yin in the same way as mentioned above. In this case, the Mind, the Ethereal Soul and the Will-Power are all three affected.

This person will feel exhausted and depressed and will lack will-power. As the Ethereal Soul is deprived of its residence, he or she will also feel aimless and sleep badly.

(b) Prescription

ZUO GUI WAN
Restoring the Left [Kidney] Pill
Shu Di Huang *Radix Rehmanniae glutinosae praeparata* 15 g
Shan Yao *Radix Dioscoreae oppositae* 9 g
Shan Zhu Yu *Fructus Corni officinalis* 9 g
Gou Qi Zi *Fructus Lycii chinensis* 9 g
Chuan Niu Xi *Radix Cyathulae* 6 g
Tu Si Zi *Semen Cuscutae* 9 g
Lu Jiao Jiao *Colla Cornu Cervi* 9 g
Gui Ban Jiao *Colla Plastri Testudinis* 9 g

Explanation

– **Shu Di Huang**, **Shan Yao** and **Shan Zhu Yu** nourish the Yin of Kidneys, Stomach and Liver.
– **Gou Qi Zi** nourishes Liver-Yin.
– **Chuan Niu Xi** nourishes Kidneys and Liver and strengthens tendons and bones.
– **Tu Si Zi** and **Lu Jiao Jiao** strengthen Kidney-Yang.
– **Gui Ban Jiao** nourishes Kidney-Yin and subdues rebellious Yang.

This formula nourishes Liver- and Kidney-Yin. Its emphasis is on strengthening the tendons and bones, tissues related to Liver and Kidneys respectively. Niu Xi and Lu Jiao have this function in the prescription. There is a correlation between the physical aspect of strengthening tendons and bones with herbs which act

on the Liver and Kidneys and the strengthening of the Ethereal Soul and Will-Power related to these organs.

The main physical manifestations for this formula are, apart from other Yin-deficiency symptoms as above, weakness, stiffness and ache of the lower back and knees, a cold sensation of legs, knees and lower back, dizziness and a headache with a feeling of emptiness of the head.

Mental-emotional pattern

The same emotions mentioned for the previous two formulae may lead to this condition. Alternatively, a weakness of the Liver and Kidneys from overwork and excessive sexual activity or simply from old age, may cause this condition.

This person will feel exhausted, depressed and will lack will-power. In the same way that there is physical stiffness in the back, this person may tend to be rather rigid in his or her mental attitude.

Case history

A 39-year-old woman complained of an irregular menstrual cycle (being always late) with some premenstrual tension, a lack of will-power and insomnia (waking up during the night). Her eyes felt often very dry. She also felt generally very tired both physically and mentally. She had had a lot of stress in the past due to a difficult divorce and she now felt aimless, was undecided about her current relationship and did not know what direction to take in her life.

Her tongue was Red, with a Heart crack, almost entirely without coating (Plate 9.9), and her pulse was Empty on the deep level on the left side and Choppy on the right. The pulse also completely lacked any wave.

Diagnosis
This is a clear pattern of Liver-Yin deficiency even though there are not many symptoms. However, the pulse and tongue clearly indicate Yin deficiency and the insomnia, late menstrual cycle and dry eyes allow us to locate the Yin deficiency in the Liver. Most of all, the feeling of being aimless, the indecision and lack of direction in life clearly point to the Ethereal Soul being deprived of its root in Liver-Yin. Secondary to Liver-Yin deficiency, there was some Liver-Qi stagnation manifested in the pre-menstrual tension.

The lack of wave in the pulse, as described before

in this chapter, points to sadness as the emotion at the root of the problem. Different individuals react in different ways to the stresses of life. When going through a painful and stressful divorce, some may feel angry, some worried, some discouraged, etc. This woman reacted by feeling very sad about the breaking-up of her marriage and sadness weakened Liver-Blood and Liver-Yin.

Treatment principle
Nourish Yin, strengthen the Liver and root the Ethereal Soul.

Acupuncture
This patient was treated only four times with very good results.

The first treatment consisted only in the opening points of the Yin Linking Vessel, i.e. P-6 Neiguan on the right and SP-4 Gongsun on the left. This extraordinary vessel nourishes Yin and roots the Ethereal Soul.

In the second treatment the opening points of the Yin Linking Vessel were repeated with the addition of SP-6 Sanyinjiao and Ren-15 Jiuwei (both reinforced) to help to nourish Yin and root the Ethereal Soul. In the third and fourth treatments the above points were needled again with the addition of the following points:

- **ST-36** Zusanli and **LIV-8** Ququan to nourish the Liver.
- **BL-23** Shenshu, **BL-52** Zhishi and **BL-47** Hunmen to nourish the Kidneys and Liver and root the Ethereal Soul. The Kidneys were treated not because there was any Kidney deficiency but because Liver and Kidneys share a common root and the points BL-52 and BL-47, combined with BL-23, strengthen the Will-Power, root the Ethereal Soul and help a person find a sense of direction.

After these four treatments she felt much better and more positive and decisive, so much so that she decided to break off her current troubled relationship, which she felt very good about.

Case history

A 32-year-old woman complained of fatigue, hypochondrial pain, a feeling of oppression of the chest and an ache behind the eyes. Her periods were always late and painful and the menstrual blood was dark with clots. Her sleep was restless and disturbed by many dreams, she felt hot in the evenings and her vision was sometimes blurred.

She felt aimless and lacked a sense of direction in her life. She was at a crossroads in both her work and a personal relationship and she often felt that she "did not see the point of it all". Her tongue was Red and without coating. Her pulse was Floating-Empty and Fine but also slightly Wiry on the left side.

Diagnosis
This is another clear example of Liver-Yin deficiency as in the previous patient. In this case, however, there is a much more pronounced stagnation of Liver-Qi and Liver-Blood (hypochondrial pain, feeling of oppression of the chest, painful period with dark blood). In this case too, stagnation of Liver-Qi is secondary to Liver-Yin deficiency.

The deficient Liver-Yin fails to root the Ethereal Soul and this causes the feeling of aimlessness in her life and dream-disturbed sleep.

Treatment principle
Nourish Liver-Yin, move Liver-Qi and Liver-Blood and root the Ethereal Soul.

Acupuncture
The main points used were:

- **LIV-8** Ququan, **ST-36** Zusanli, **Ren-4** Guanyuan and **SP-6** Sanyinjiao, reinforced, to nourish Liver-Yin.
- **LIV-3** Taichong and **G.B.-34** Yanglingquan, with even method, to move Liver-Qi and Liver-Blood.
- **Ren-15** Jiuwei and **BL-47** Hunmen to root the Ethereal Soul.

Herbal treatment
The formula used was a variation of Da Bu Yin Jian *Great Tonifying Yin Decoction*:

Shu Di Huang *Radix Rehmanniae glutinosae praeparata* 12 g
Shan Yao *Radix Dioscoreae oppositae* 9 g
Shan Zhu Yu *Fructus Corni officinalis* 4 g
Gou Qi Zi *Fructus Lycii chinensis* 9 g
Dang Gui *Radix Angelicae sinensis* 6 g
Dang Shen *Radix Codonopsis pilosulae* 6 g
Du Zhong *Cortex Eucommiae ulmoidis* 6 g
Zhi Gan Cao *Radix Glycyrrhizae uralensis praeparata* 3 g
Chuan Lian Zi *Fructus Meliae toosendan* 4 g
Mei Gui Hua *Flos Rosae rugosae* 3 g
Yi Mu Cao *Herba Leonori heterophylli* 4 g
Suan Zao Ren *Semen Ziziphi spinosae* 4 g

Explanation
The formula was left unchanged apart from the dosages which were reduced. Du Zhong could have been eliminated as there is no Kidney deficiency, but it was left in for its mental effect of strengthening the Will-Power and providing a strong basis for the Ethereal Soul.

- **Chuan Lian Zi** and **Mei Gui Hua** move Liver-Qi without injuring Yin.
- **Yi Mu Cao** moves Liver-Blood.
- **Suan Zao Ren**, sour and astringent, roots the Ethereal Soul and calms the Mind.

Apart from an improvement in her menstrual cycle, this patient felt a lot stronger, more focused and determined after 3 months' treatment.

4. KIDNEY-ESSENCE DEFICIENCY

Treatment principle

Nourish the Kidneys, tonify the Essence and strengthen Will-Power.

Acupuncture

Ren-4 Guanyuan, Ren-7 Yinjiao, BL-23 Shenshu, BL-52 Zhishi, KI-3 Taixi, SP-6 Sanyinjiao, G.B.-13 Benshen, Du-20 Baihui. Reinforcing method. These points are suitable to treat both Kidney-Yang and Kidney-Yin deficiency, depending on whether one uses moxa or not.

Explanation

- **Ren-4** and **Ren-7** nourish the Essence.
- **BL-23** and **BL-52** tonify the Kidneys and strengthen Will-Power.
- **KI-3** and **SP-6** nourish Kidney-Yin.
- **G.B.-13** gathers Essence to the brain.
- **Du-20** raises clear Qi and lifts depression.

Herbal treatment

Prescription

HE CHE DA ZAO WAN
Placenta Great Fortifying Pill
Zi He Che *Placenta hominis* 1 placenta
Shu Di Huang *Radix Rehmanniae glutinosae praeparata* 60 g
Sheng Di Huang *Radix Rehmanniae glutinosae* 45 g
Gou Qi Zi *Fructus Lycii chinensis* 45 g
Tian Men Dong *Tuber Asparagi cochinchinensis* 20 g
Wu Wei Zi *Fructus Schisandrae chinensis* 20 g
Dang Gui *Radix Angelicae sinensis* 20 g
Niu Xi *Radix Achyranthis bidentatae seu Cyathulae* 20 g
Du Zhong *Cortex Eucommiae ulmoidis* 30 g
Suo Yang *Herba Cynomorii songarici* 20 g
Rou Cong Rong *Herba Cistanchis* 20 g
Huang Bo *Cortex Phellodendri* 20 g

Explanation

- **Zi He Che, Shu Di Huang, Sheng Di Huang,**
Gou Qi Zi and **Tian Men Dong** nourish Yin, strengthen the Kidneys and Liver and benefit Essence.
- **Wu Wei Zi** is astringent and helps to nourish Yin. It also calms the Mind and settles the Corporeal Soul.
- **Dang Gui** and **Niu Xi** nourish Blood and strengthen tendons and bones.
- **Du Zhong**, **Suo Yang** and **Rou Cong Rong** tonify Kidney-Yang. Du Zhong also strengthens the back and Suo Yang benefits the Essence.
- **Huang Bo** clears any Empty-Heat that there might be or that might be induced by the Yang tonics.

This formula's emphasis is on tonification of the Essence. Zi He Che, Wu Wei Zi, Gou Qi Zi and Suo Yang all benefit the Essence. Its secondary therapeutic aim is also to tonify Kidney-Yang. This formula is therefore well adapted to treat complicated cases of deficiency of all aspects of the Kidneys: Yin, Essence and Yang.

It should be noted that the above doses are to make a quantity of pills, not for individual daily decoctions. The daily dosages of a decoction can be adapted according to proportions. As for Zi He Che (placenta), due to the obvious difficulty of obtaining one, this can be replaced by placenta pills which could be swallowed with the rest of the decoction.

The main manifestations for this prescription would be exhaustion, depression, weak back and knees, weak sexual function (lack of desire or impotence), nocturnal emissions, weak teeth, prematurely grey or falling hair, dizziness, tinnitus, night-sweating, a thin body, a Red tongue without coating and a Floating-Empty pulse.

Mental-emotional pattern

Fear, shock and guilt may cause a deficiency of Kidney-Yin and Kidney-Essence, or vice versa; this may be the result of overwork and excessive sexual activity. In women it may result from too many childbirths or prolonged loss of blood with the periods over many years.

This person will feel mentally and physically exhausted and depressed and will lack will-power and initiative. He or she may also suffer from some deficiency in the sexual function such as lack of desire or impotence.

Variations

The following are variations which apply to all four above formulae. It should, first of all, be noted that, when nourishing Kidney-Yin in mental-emotional problems, it is advisable to add one or two Kidney-Yang tonics in a small dosage. This is necessary to make the formula more moving and dynamic and thus affect the Mind and Will-Power more readily. In chronic depression especially, one of the clear features of the condition is the way the patient is "stuck" in a mental-emotional pattern from which it is very difficult to break out. A certain resistance to treatment, hopelessness and despair are typical of chronic depression. In such cases, assuming they present with a configuration of Yin deficiency, it is important to add some Kidney-Yang tonics to invigorate Yang and provide movement to the prescription. In particular, one would choose those Kidney-Yang tonics which are pungent in taste as this taste moves and invigorates. Two examples are Du Zhong *Cortex Eucommiae ulmoidis* and Ba Ji Tian *Radix Morindae officinalis*. Of course, some of the above four prescriptions already contain some Kidney-Yang tonics.

Another frequent addition to the above Yin-nourishing prescriptions is Shi Chang Pu *Rhizoma Acori graminei* to open the Mind's orifices, clear the Mind and lift mood. This would be an essential addition to all four previous prescriptions. It is also pungent in taste and would therefore also have a beneficial moving effect as the Yang tonics mentioned above.

Finally, if there is deep depression and exhaustion, Lu Rong *Cornu Cervi parvum* should be added even though it is a Yang tonic. It tonifies Kidney-Yang without drying, stokes up the Fire of the Gate of Vitality without creating Empty-Heat, benefits the Essence and powerfully lifts mood.

NOTE

As will be remembered, the main treatment methods used in mental-emotional problems were five:

1. Nourish the Heart and calm the Mind
2. Clear pathogenic factors and calm the Mind
3. Clear pathogenic factors, nourish the Heart and calm the Mind
4. Resolve Phlegm, open the orifices and calm the Mind
5. Sink and calm the Mind.

The first four have all been discussed when dealing with the various patterns of mental-emotional problems. We should now discuss the fifth method of treatment and that is to sink and calm the Mind. This consists in the use of minerals and shells which have a high density and are heavy. The traditional idea is that they weigh upon the Heart to sink the Mind, thus relieving anxiety, agitation and insomnia when these are caused by rebellious Qi. This is usually either Liver-Yang or Liver-Wind rising or Heart Empty-Heat.

These substances may be added to any of the formulae we discussed to treat the Manifestation whenever the symptoms are severe, i.e. very severe agitation, intractable insomnia, intense anxiety and, in serious cases, violent behaviour.

All these substances have side-effects because they are indigestible and therefore their prolonged use may injure the Stomach and Spleen. For this reason they are usually combined with digestive herbs. Some of the sinking substances are toxic and should be used with great caution and, in any case, for short periods only (a few weeks). An example of this is Zhu Sha *Cinnabaris*.

The main sinking substances that calm the Mind are:

Long Gu *Os Draconis*
Long Chi *Dens Draconis*
Mu Li *Concha Ostreae*
Ci Shi *Magnetitum*
Zhu Sha *Cinnabaris*
Zhen Zhu Mu *Concha margaritiferae*
Hu Po *Succinum*

Long Chi, Long Gu and Mu Li are all astringent and therefore also nourish Yin. Mu Li is especially good at nourishing Yin while Long

Chi is the best of the three to sink and calm the Mind.

Ci Shi and Zhen Zhu Mu both sink Liver-Yang and Liver-Wind while Zhu Sha specifically enters the Heart and calms the Mind. It also opens the Heart's orifices.

Hu Po, besides sinking and calming the Mind, also moves Blood and enters the Liver: this makes it useful to treat depression and anxiety from Liver-Qi or Liver-Blood stagnation.

As for sinking and calming the Mind prescriptions, these have not been mentioned because many of them contain many indigestible and often toxic minerals. Their use is not often necessary. Most mental-emotional problems can be treated by the prescriptions discussed above with the addition of one or two sinking substances if the manifestations call for it.

The main sinking formulae are listed here with a brief description of their therapeutic application:

1. ZHU SHA AN SHEN WAN

Cinnabar Calming the Mind Pill
Huang Lian *Rhizoma Coptidis* 3 g
Sheng Di Huang *Radix Rehmanniae glutinosae* 12 g
Dang Giu *Radix Angelicae sinensis* 6 g
Fu Ling *Sclerotium Poriae cocos* 6 g
Suan Zao Ren *Semen Ziziphi spinosae* 6 g
Zhu Sha *Cinnabaris* 3 g
Yuan Zhi *Radix Polygalae tenuifoliae* 6 g
Gan Cao *Radix Glycyrrhizae uralensis* 3 g

This formula clears Heart Empty-Heat and sinks and calms the Mind.

2. CI ZHU WAN

Magnetitum-Cinnabar Pill
Ci Shi *Magnetitum* 6 g
Zhu Sha *Cinnabaris* 3 g
Shen Qu *Massa Fermentata Medicinalis* 9 g

This formula is purely sinking and can be added to any other prescription to sink and calm the Mind.

3. SHENG TIE LUO YIN

Frusta Ferri Decoction
Sheng Tie Luo *Frusta Ferri* 60 g
Dan Nan Xing *Rhizoma Arisaematis praeparata* 9 g
Zhe Bei Mu *Bulbus Fritillariae thunbergii* 9 g
Xuan Shen *Radix Scrophulariae ningpoensis* 9 g
Tian Men Dong *Tuber Asparagi cochinchinensis* 9 g
Mai Men Dong *Tuber Ophiopogonis japonici* 9 g
Lian Qiao *Fructus Forsythiae suspensae* 9 g
Dan Shen *Radix Salviae miltiorrhizae* 12 g
Fu Ling *Sclerotium Poriae cocos* 12 g
Chen Pi *Pericarpium Citri reticulatae* 6 g
Shi Chang Pu *Rhizoma Acori graminei* 6 g
Yuan Zhi *Radix Polygalae tenuifoliae* 6 g
Zhu Sha *Cinnabaris* 1.8 g

This formula clears Phlegm-Fire from the Heart and sinks and calms the Mind. It can be used for unsettled Mind from Phlegm-Fire obstructing the Heart and Mind.

Prevention of mental-emotional problems

Mental activity is the most important aspect of the Mind and this is affected by either excessive thinking or excessive emotional strain. It follows then that the most important measures one can take to prevent mental-emotional problems are to restrain one's mental activity and avoid emotional strain. "To restrain one's mental activity" means not only avoiding excessive mental work, but also avoiding thinking too much altogether. These concepts are heavily influenced by Daoist ideas of "nourishing life" by calming the Mind and preventing distracting thoughts. The very first chapter of the "Simple Questions" says:

. . . one should live a quiet life with few desires so that one can preserve one's Qi and guard one's Mind in order to avoid disease. Thus if emotions are absent and craving is curbed, the Heart is peaceful and there is no fear.[84]

Thus, in order to attain a tranquil Mind the

ancient Daoist sages advocated three basic attitudes:

1. Avoid excessive thinking
2. Avoid excessive craving
3. Avoid distracting thoughts.

Restraining craving is particularly applicable to Western industrialized societies where consumerism is rampant and the pressures of advertising contribute to creating ever new "needs". Restraining craving and desire is very important to achieve mental tranquillity as excessive craving stirs up the Minister Fire which harasses the Heart and Pericardium.

This Daoist ideal is of course terribly difficult to attain but even just barely striving towards parts of it is a step in the right direction.

In the past, some Daoist doctors even formulated "prescriptions", mimicking herbal prescriptions, to calm the Mind, restrain thinking and curb emotions. Two of them will be presented here as examples.

1. XIANG SUI WAN

"Pill" to the Likeness of Marrow

- NOT THINKING TOO MUCH = nourishes the Heart (emperor ingredient)
- RESTRAINING ANGER = nourishes the Liver
- RESTRAINING SEXUAL DESIRE = nourishes the Kidneys
- CAREFUL TALKING = nourishes the Lungs
- REGULATING DIET = nourishes the Spleen.

2. ZHEN REN YANG ZANG GAO

The Sage's "Paste" to Nourish the Internal Organs

- REMAIN INDIFFERENT WHETHER GRANTED FAVOURS OR SUBJECTED TO HUMILIATION = makes the Liver balanced
- BE INDIFFERENT WHETHER MOVING OR STILL = calms Heart-Fire
- REGULATE DIET = does not over-burden the Spleen
- REGULATE BREATHING AND MODERATE TALKING = makes Lungs healthy
- CALM THE MIND AND PREVENT DISTRACTING THOUGHTS = replenishes the Kidneys.

END NOTES

1. 1981 Spiritual Axis (*Ling Shu Jing* 灵枢经), People's Health Publishing House, Beijing. First published *c.* 100 BC, p. 23.
2. Zhang Jie Bin 1982 Classic of Categories (*Lei Jing* 类经), People's Health Publishing House, Beijing, p. 49. First published in 1624.
3. Spiritual Axis, p. 71.
4. Classic of Categories, p. 63.
5. 1979 The Yellow Emperor's Classic of Internal Medicine Simple Questions, (*Huang Ti Nei Jing Su Wen* 黄帝内经素问), People's Health Publishing House, Beijing. First published *c.* 100 BC, p. 58.
6. Spiritual Axis, p. 128.
7. Simple Questions, p. 67.
8. Tang Zong Hai 1892 The Essence of Medical Classics on the Convergence of Chinese and Western Medicine (*Zhong Xi Hui Tong Yi Jing Jing Yi* 中西汇通医经精), cited in Wang Ke Qin 1988 Theory of the Mind in Chinese Medicine (*Zhong Yi Shen Zhu Xue Shuo* 中医神主学说), Ancient Chinese Medical Texts Publishing House, p. 22.
9. Simple Questions, p. 72.
10. Ibid., p. 154.
11. Ren Ying Qiu 1985 Theories of Chinese Medicine Doctors cited in Theory of the Mind in Chinese Medicine, p. 22.
12. Wang Keng Tang 1602 Standards of Diagnosis and Treatment (*Zheng Zhi Zhun Sheng* 证治准绳), cited in Theory of the Mind in Chinese Medicine, p. 22.
13. Simple Questions, p. 26.
14. Ibid., p. 78.
15. Yu Chang 1658 Principles of Medical Practice (*Yi Men Fa Lu* 医门法律), cited in Theory of the Mind in Chinese Medicine, p. 39.
16. Simple Questions, p. 153.
17. Ibid., pp. 67–8.
18. Ibid., p. 153.
19. Ibid., p. 63.
20. Giles H 1912 Chinese-English Dictionary, Kelly & Walsh, Shanghai, p. 650.
21. Classic of Categories, p. 50.
22. Ibid, p. 50.
23. Spiritual Axis, p. 23.
24. Classic of Categories, p. 50.
25. The Essence of Medical Classics on the Convergence of Chinese and Western Medicine, cited in Theory of the Mind in Chinese Medicine, p. 36.
26. Kong Ying Da Five-Channel Righteousnes (*Wu Jing Zheng Yi* 五经正义), cited in Theory of the Mind in Chinese Medicine, p. 37.

27. Simple Questions, p. 68.
28. Spiritual Axis, p. 24.
29. Tang Zong Hai 1884 Discussion on Blood Diseases (*Xue Zheng Lun* 血证论), edited by Pei Zheng Xue and Yin Xin Min, People's Health Publishing House, 1979, p. 29.
30. The Essence of the Convergence between Chinese and Western Medicine, cited in Theory of the Mind in Chinese Medicine, p. 36.
31. Ibid., p. 36.
32. Jung C G 1961 Modern Man in Search of a Soul, Routledge & Kegan Paul, London.
33. Giles H 1912 Chinese-English Dictionary, p. 1144.
34. Classic of Categories, p. 63.
35. Spiritual Axis, p. 23.
36 Classic of Categories, p. 63.
37. Ibid., p. 63.
38. Zhao You Chen 1979 Chinese Medicine of Liao Ning (*Liao Ning Zhong Yi* 辽宁中医) no. 5, p. 24.
39. Classic of Categories, pp. 63–4.
40. Discussion on Blood Diseases, p. 236.
41. Simple Questions, p. 77.
42. Spiritual Axis, p. 23.
43. Ibid, p. 23.
44. The Essence of Medical Classics on the Convergence of Chinese and Western Medicine cited in the Theory of the Mind in Chinese Medicine, p. 38.
45. Classic of Categories, p. 50.
46. Spiritual Axis, p. 24.
47. Ibid, p. 24.
48. Ibid., p. 67.
49. Simple Questions, p. 221.
50. Fei Bo Xiong et al 1985 Medical Collection from Four Families from Meng He (*Meng He Si Jia Yi Ji* 孟河四家医集), Jiangsu Science Publishing House, p. 40.
51. Principles of Medical Practice, cited in Theory of the Mind in Chinese Medicine, p. 34.
52. Simple Questions, p. 221.
53. Chen Yan 1174 A Treatise on the Three Categories of Causes of Disease (*San Yin Ji Yi Bing Zheng Fang Lun* 三因极一病证方论), cited in Theory of the Mind in Chinese Medicine, p. 55.
54. Simple Questions, p. 221.
55. Ibid., p. 221
56. Ibid., p. 38.
57. Medical Collection from Four Families from Meng He, p. 40.
58. Simple Questions, p. 221.
59. Spiritual Axis, p. 24.
60. Simple Questions, p. 222.
61. For this reason "Minister Fire" refers both to the physiological or pathological Fire of the Kidneys and to the Pericardium. This accounts for the assignment of the Right-Rear position on the pulse either to the Kidney-Yang by some doctors, or to the Pericardium by others.
62. Principles of Medical Practice, cited in Theory of the Mind in Chinese Medicine, p. 56.
63. Shi Pa Nan 1861 Origin of Medicine (*Yi Yuan* 医原), cited in Theory of the Mind in Chinese Medicine, p. 55.
64. Simple Questions, p. 99.
65. Chen Shi Duo 1687 Secret Records of the Stone Room (*Shi Shi Mi Lu* 石室秘录), cited in Theory of the Mind in Chinese Medicine, p. 56.
66. Spiritual Axis, pp. 151–2.
67. Ibid, pp. 151–2.
68. Shi Pa Nan 1861 Origin of Medicine, cited in Guo Zhen Qiu 1985 Diagnosis in Chinese Medicine (*Zhong Yi Zhen Duan Xue* 中医诊断学), Hunan Science Publications, p. 33.
69. Zhou Xue Hai 1894 A Simple Guide to Diagnosis from Body and Colour (*Xing Se Wai Zhen Jian Mo* 形色外诊简摩), cited in Diagnosis in Chinese Medicine, p. 33.
70. Simple Questions, p. 168.
71. Spiritual Axis, p. 72.
72. Yue Han Zhen 1654 An Explanation of Acupuncture Points (*Jing Xue Jie* 经穴解), People's Health Publishing House, Beijing (1990), p. 211.
73. Zhang Jie Bin 1986 The Complete Book of Jing Yue (*Jing Yue Quan Shu* 景岳全书), Shanghai Science Publishing House, Shanghai, p. 573. First published in 1624.
74. Spiritual Axis, p. 120.
75. Simple Questions, p. 319.
76. Wang Luo Zhen 1985 A Compilation of a "Study of the Eight Extraordinary Vessels" (*Qi Jing Ba Mai Kao Jiao Zhu* 奇经八脉考校注), Shanghai Science Publishing House, Shanghai, p. 75. The "Study of the Eight Extraordinary Vessels" itself was written by Li Shi Zhen and published in 1578.
77. An Explanation of Acupuncture Points, p. 31.
78. Ibid, p. 45.
79. Ibid., p. 88.
80. He Ren 1981 A New Explanation of the Essential Prescriptions of the Golden Chest (*Jin Gui Yao Lue Xin Jie* 金匮要略新解), Zhejiang Scientific Publishing House, p. 24. The "Essential Prescriptions of the Golden Chest" itself was written by Zhang Zhong Jing and first published *c.* AD 220.
81. Ibid, p. 24.
82. An Explanation of Acupuncture Points, pp. 26–27.
83. Ibid, p. 28.
84. Simple Questions, p. 3.

Insomnia (somnolence, poor memory) 10 不寐

The term "insomnia" covers a number of different problems such as inability to fall asleep easily, waking up during the night, sleeping restlessly, waking up early in the morning and dream-disturbed sleep.

The amount and quality of sleep depend of course on the state of the Mind (*Shen*). The Mind is rooted in the Heart and specifically in Heart-Blood and Heart-Yin. If the Heart is healthy and the Blood abundant, the Mind is properly rooted and sleep will be sound. If the Heart is deficient or if it is agitated by pathogenic factors such as Fire, the Mind is not properly rooted and sleep will be affected.

As always in Chinese medicine, there is an interrelationship between body and Mind. On the one hand, a deficiency of Blood or a pathogenic factor such as Fire may affect the Mind; on the other hand, emotional stress affecting the Mind may cause a disharmony of the internal organs. In fact, any disharmony of the internal organs, whether it is due to a Deficiency or an Excess, affects Blood and Essence. Since the Essence and Qi are the root of the Mind (the "Three Treasures"), the Mind has then no residence and insomnia may result. The "Simple Questions" in chapter 46 says: *"When a person lies down and cannot sleep, [it means] the Yin organs are injured [so that] the Essence has no residence and is not quiet and the person cannot sleep".*[1]

As far as sleep is concerned the Mind is not the only mental-spiritual faculty involved. The Ethereal Soul (*Hun*) also plays an important role in the physiology and pathology of sleep and the length and quality of sleep are related to its state (see ch. 9). If the Ethereal Soul is well rooted in the Liver (Liver-Blood or Liver-Yin), sleep is normal, sound and without too many dreams. If Liver-Yin or Liver-Blood is deficient, the Ethereal Soul is deprived of its residence and wanders off at night, causing a restless sleep with many tiring dreams. Tang Zong Hai says: *"At night during sleep the Ethereal Soul returns to the Liver; if the Ethereal Soul is not peaceful there are a lot of dreams".*[2]

The Ethereal Soul is affected not only by a deficiency of the Liver, but also by any pathogenic factor (such as Fire or Wind) agitating the Liver. The "Complete Book of Jing Yue" (1624) by Zhang Jing Yue says: *"Overexertion, worrying and excessive thinking injure Blood and fluids so that the Mind and Ethereal Soul are deprived of residence and insomnia results".*[3] It also says: *"Worrying and excessive thinking injure the Spleen so that it cannot make Blood and insomnia results".*[4]

When a patient complains of poor sleep we must ascertain that the condition is true insomnia and not an inability to sleep well due to other external or temporary causes. For example, a sudden change in weather, a bedroom which is too hot or too cold, drinking a lot of tea or coffee, an emotional upset or worrying about something specific may all cause a person to sleep badly but cannot be defined as "insomnia". In fact, once the above causes are removed, the person sleeps well. Also, one cannot diagnose insomnia when sleep is disturbed by other conditions such as asthma, a pain (e.g. shoulder, hip or back pain) or itching from a skin disease; in such cases, sleep is restored once the relevant disease is treated successfully.

Finally, according to traditional Chinese views, the best sleeping position is lying on the right side, with the legs slightly bent, the right arm bent and resting in front of the pillow, and the left arm resting on the left thigh. According to these views, with this position the heart is in a high position so that Blood can circulate freely, the liver is in a low position so that Blood can collect there and root the Ethereal Soul to promote sleep, and the stomach and duodenum are in such a position that facilitates the downward movement of food.

Aetiology and pathology

1. OVEREXERTION AND WORRY

Worrying a lot and overexertion injure the Spleen, Lungs and Heart. When the Spleen is deficient, it cannot produce enough Blood and this deficiency affects the Heart and the Mind. Moreover, Heart-Blood is directly weakened by worry and this also leads to the Mind's being deprived of its residence and therefore to insomnia.

In some people worry, anxiety and pensiveness lead not to Heart-Blood deficiency, but to Heart-Fire. This is also due to a constitutional tendency to Yang Excess. Heart-Fire flares upwards to agitate the Mind, and insomnia results.

2. OVERWORK

Mental overwork, working long hours without adequate rest, working under conditions of severe stress combined with irregular diet and excessive sexual activity, all weaken Kidney-Yin. When Kidney-Yin is deficient over a long period of time, it fails to nourish Heart-Yin so that Heart Empty-Heat develops. This especially happens when the person worries a lot. This pattern is also called "Heart and Kidneys not harmonized".

The same pattern may be the result of the reverse process. Severe emotional strain over a long period of time may lead to the formation of Heart-Fire, which flares upwards and fails to communicate downwards with the Kidneys. On the other hand, excessive Fire injures the Yin and may lead to Kidney-Yin deficiency. The end result is a similar condition: Heart and Kidneys are not harmonized. This is a common cause of insomnia in the elderly.

3. ANGER

Anger, intended in a broad sense including frustration, resentment and irritation, leads to either Liver-Yang rising or Liver-Fire. Both of these may cause insomnia, especially in young or middle-aged people.

4. "GALL-BLADDER TIMID"

A constitutional weakness of both Heart and Gall-Bladder may give rise to a timid character. The Gall-Bladder is the mother of the Heart and a person whose Gall-Bladder is weak will be timid, fearful and indecisive and will lack self-assertiveness. Chinese language bears out this connection between the Gall-Bladder and timidity: "big gall-bladder" means "courageous", while "small gall-bladder" means "timid" or "cowardly".

This constitutional deficiency of Heart and Gall-Bladder causes insomnia, especially waking up early.

5. IRREGULAR DIET

Irregular diet, over-eating or eating too much

greasy and hot food may lead to the formation of Phlegm-Heat in the Stomach which harasses the Mind leading to insomnia.

6. CHILDBIRTH

A large loss of blood during childbirth may induce a deficiency of Blood of the Liver. This may also happen not because the loss of blood is substantial but because of a pre-existing condition of deficiency of Blood. In either case, it causes a fairly sudden and severe deficiency of Liver-Blood. Deprived of its residence, the Ethereal Soul floats at night, causing insomnia and excessive dreaming.

7. RESIDUAL HEAT

During an invasion of Wind-Heat, the pathogenic factor may progress into the Interior and give rise to interior Heat. If this is not cleared properly, the person may make an apparent recovery but residual Heat is left in the body. This is said to lodge in the diaphragm where it harasses the Heart and may lead to insomnia.

Thus the pathology of insomnia boils down to two possible conditions: either a deficiency of Blood/Yin which deprives the Mind and/or Ethereal Soul of their residence, or a pathogenic factor (Full condition) agitating the Mind and/or the Ethereal Soul. The various aetiological factors and pathologies may be summarized in a diagram (Fig. 10.1).

As can be seen from Figure 10.1, the Deficiency conditions causing insomnia occur mostly in Heart, Spleen, Liver and Kidneys, whilst the Excess conditions occur in the Liver and Stomach.

ACUPUNCTURE

From the perspective of the channel system, insomnia is due to a breakdown of the interconnection of Yin and Yang. Yang-Qi and Yin-Qi have to be harmonized and flow into one another in a daily cycle.

Defensive Qi flows in the Yang during the day and in the Yin during the night. If it remains in the Yang by night as well as by day, the person cannot sleep. The "Spiritual Axis" in chapter 80 says: "*If Defensive Qi does not enter into the Yin at night and remains in the Yang, Yang-Qi becomes Full and the Yang Heel Vessel in Excess, Yin becomes deficient and the eyes cannot close*".[5] For this reason, the beginning points of the Yang and Yin Heel Vessels (BL-62 Shenmai and KI-6 Zhaohai respectively) can be used, together with BL-1 Jingming, for insomnia (see below).

Diagnosis

When questioning a patient about insomnia it

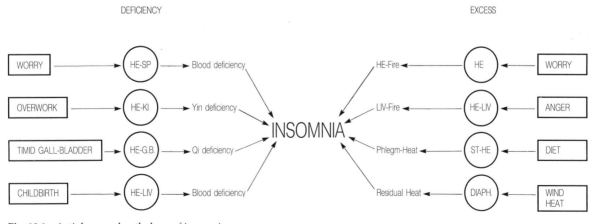

Fig. 10.1 Aetiology and pathology of insomnia

is important to establish clearly what the main problem is.

Difficulty in falling asleep usually indicates deficiency of Blood, whilst falling asleep easily but waking up frequently during the night denotes Yin deficiency. This is not, however, an absolute rule. Of course the two conditions may coexist in which case the person has difficulty in falling asleep and wakes up during the night.

Waking up early in the morning indicates Heart and Gall-Bladder deficiency.

As for dreams, they are due to the wandering of the Mind and/or Ethereal Soul at night. A certain amount of dreaming is therefore normal. The old classics described various types of unpleasant dreams such as nightmares, waking up screaming, sleep-walking and talking in one's sleep. They related dreaming to the wandering of the Ethereal Soul at night.

When a person's physical body receives something it is real; when the Mind receives something it produces dreams. When the Mind is slave to objects [i.e. pursues objects] the Ethereal Soul and the Corporeal Soul become restless, they fly around and, gathering at the eyes, they produce dreams. Grasping [i.e. excessive craving] in daytime produces dreaming at night.

"Excessive" dreaming may be defined as dreaming which causes restless sleep or nightmares, resulting in the person feeling very tired the following morning. Dreaming which does not make the sleep restless, is not frightening, does not disturb the Mind the morning after, and does not leave the person very tired in the morning, can be described as normal and is not a pathological condition.

Excessive dreaming may be due to deficiency of Blood or Yin. Frightening dreams which wake one up denote a deficiency of Gall-Bladder and Heart. Restless dreams are often due to Phlegm-Heat affecting Stomach and Heart. The following is a list of dreams from the "Simple Questions" and "Spiritual Axis":

- Flying: Emptiness in the Lower Burner[6]
- Falling: Fullness in the Lower Burner[7]
- Floods and fear: Excess of Yin[8]
- Fire: Excess of Yang[9]
- Killing and destruction: Yin and Yang both in Excess[10]
- Giving away things: Excess condition[11]
- Receiving things: Deficiency condition[12]
- Being angry: Liver in Excess[13]
- Crying, weeping: Lungs in Excess[14]
- Crowds: round worms in the intestines[15]
- Attack and destruction: tape-worms in the intestines[16]
- Fires: Heart deficiency[17]
- Volcanic eruptions (if the dream takes place in summertime): Heart deficiency[18]
- Laughing: Heart in Excess[19]
- Mountains, fire and smoke: Heart deficiency[20]
- Very fragrant mushrooms: Liver deficiency[21]
- Lying under a tree being unable to get up (if the dream takes place in springtime): Liver deficiency[22]
- Forests on mountains: Liver deficiency[23]
- White objects or bloody killings: Lung deficiency[24]
- Battles and war (dream taking place in the autumn): Lung deficiency[25]
- Worry, fear, crying, flying: Lungs in Excess[26]
- Flying and seeing strange objects made of gold or iron: Lung deficiency[27]
- Being hungry: Spleen deficiency[28]
- Building a house (dream taking place in late summer): Spleen deficiency[29]
- Singing and feeling very heavy: Spleen in Excess[30]
- Abysses in mountains and marshes: Spleen deficiency[31]
- Swimming after a shipwreck: Kidney deficiency[32]
- Plunging into water and being scared (dream taking place in wintertime): Kidney deficiency[33]
- Spine being detached from the body: Kidneys in Excess (i.e. Dampness in Kidneys)[34]
- Being immersed in water: Kidney deficiency[35]
- Having a large meal: Stomach deficiency[36]
- Large cities: Small Intestine deficiency[37]
- Open fields: Large Intestine deficiency[38]
- Fights, trials, suicide: Gall-Bladder deficiency[39]

– Voyages: Bladder deficiency[40]
– Crossing the sea and being scared: Excess of Yin.[41]

SLEEPING POSITIONS

If a person is unable to sleep supine (lying on the back), it indicates an Excess condition, often of the Lungs or Heart. The "Simple Questions" in chapter 46 says: *The Lung is the 'lid' of the other organs, when Lung-Qi is in Excess [i.e. obstructed by a pathogenic factor] the channels and blood vessels are full and the person cannot lie on the back*.[42] This often occurs in asthma, for example, when the Lungs are obstructed by Phlegm.

If a person can only sleep on the back with the arms outstretched, it indicates a Hot condition. If a person always sleeps in a prone position, it indicates a Deficiency condition often of the Stomach.

If a person can *only* sleep on one side it indicates that there is either a deficiency of Qi-Blood on that side of the body or an Excess on the opposite side. This especially applies to Heart or Lungs and can be checked on the pulse. By rolling the finger medially and laterally on the Lung pulse one can feel the state of Qi in right (laterally) and left (medially) lung. If an imbalance is felt, the patient is only able to sleep on the deficient side.

SNORING

Snoring is usually due to Phlegm affecting the Stomach channel and to rebellious Qi in the three Yang channels of the leg. Chapter 34 of the "Simple Questions" says:

Those who suffer from rebellious Qi cannot sleep well and have noisy breathing [snoring], this is due to rebellious Qi in the Bright Yang channels. When the Qi of the three Yang channels of the leg cannot flow down and rebels upwards it causes insomnia and snoring.[43]

Differentiation and treatment

The most important distinction is that between Full- and Empty-type of insomnia. The main patterns are:

EXCESS-TYPE

Liver-Fire blazing
Heart-Fire blazing
Phlegm-Heat harassing the Mind
Residual Heat in the diaphragm

DEFICIENCY-TYPE

Heart and Spleen Blood Deficiency
Heart-Yin Deficiency
Heart and Kidneys not harmonized
Heart and Gall-Bladder Deficiency
Liver-Yin Deficiency

EXCESS

1. LIVER-FIRE BLAZING

CLINICAL MANIFESTATIONS

Restless sleep, unpleasant dreams, nightmares, dreaming of fires, irritability, bitter taste, headache, thirst, dark urine, dry stools and dizziness. Tongue: Red, redder on the sides with a dry-yellow coating. Pulse: Wiry and Rapid.

TREATMENT PRINCIPLE

Drain Liver-Fire, calm the Mind and settle the Ethereal Soul.

ACUPUNCTURE

LIV-2 Xingjian, LIV-3 Taichong, G.B.-44 Qiaoyin, G.B.-12 Wangu, G.B.-20 Fengchi, SP-6 Sanyinjiao, BL-18 Ganshu, Du-24 Shenting, G.B.-13 Benshen, G.B.-15 Toulinqi, BL-47 Hunmen, BL-62 Shenmai (reduced), BL-1 Jingming (even) and KI-6 Zhaohai (reinforced). Reducing method, no moxa.

Explanation

– **LIV-2** is the main point to drain Liver-Fire.

- **LIV-3** is added because it has a better Mind-calming effect than LIV-2.
- **G.B.-44** clears Liver and Gall-Bladder Heat and is specific for dream-disturbed sleep.
- **G.B.-12** and **G.B.-20** subdue rebellious Liver-Qi and promote sleep.
- **SP-6** cools Blood and calms the Mind.
- **BL-18** regulates the Liver and clears Liver-Fire.
- **Du-24** and **G.B.-13** in combination have a strong effect in calming the Mind and settling the Ethereal Soul in Liver patterns.
- **G.B.-15** is used instead of G.B.-13 if the Mind is very overactive and the person cannot stop thinking obsessively.
- **BL-47** roots the Ethereal Soul into Liver-Yin at night, thus promoting sleep.
- **BL-62** (reduced), **BL-1** (even) and **KI-6** (in combination) harmonize the flow of the Yin and Yang Heel Vessels to the eyes and promote sleep. The Yin Heel Vessel carries Yin-Qi and the Yang Heel Vessel Yang-Qi, to the eyes. If Yang is in Excess, Yang-Qi cannot flow back into the Yin at night, the eyes stay open at night and insomnia results. The opposite would cause somnolence. The "Spiritual Axis" in chapter 21 says: *"The Yin and Yang of the Yin and Yang Heel Vessels interconnect: Yang enters Yin and Yin exits towards Yang and the two meet at the corner of the eyes. When Yang-Qi is in Excess the eyes stay open; when Yin-Qi is in Excess, they stay closed".*[44]

These points may be used for any of the other Full types of insomnia.

HERBAL TREATMENT

Prescription

LONG DAN XIE GAN TANG Variation
Gentiana Draining the Liver Decoction
Long Dan Cao *Radix Gentianae scabrae* 6 g
Huang Qin *Radix Scutellariae baicalensis* 9 g
Shan Zhi Zi *Fructus Gardeniae jasminoidis* 9 g
Ze Xie *Rhizoma Alismae orientalis* 9 g
Mu Tong *Caulis Akebiae* 9 g
Che Qian Zi *Semen Plantaginis* 9 g
Sheng Di Huang *Radix Rehmanniae glutinosae praeparata* 12 g

Dang Gui *Radix Angelicae sinensis* 9 g
Chai Hu *Radix Bupleuri* 9 g
Gan Cao *Radix Glycyrrhizae uralensis* 3 g
Zhen Zhu Mu *Concha margaritiferae* 15 g
Suan Zao Ren *Semen Ziziphi spinosae* 6 g

Explanation

- **Long Dan Cao** is the emperor herb to drain Liver-Fire.
- **Huang Qin** and **Zhi Zi** are minister herbs which help the emperor herb in draining Fire.
- **Ze Xie**, **Mu Tong** and **Che Qian Zi** are assistant herbs which help to drain Fire via urination.
- **Sheng Di Huang** and **Dang Gui** enter the Liver and harmonize Liver-Blood and Liver-Yin. Sheng Di also cools Blood and helps to drain Fire.
- **Chai Hu** is a messenger herb to enter the Liver channel.
- **Gan Cao** harmonizes.
- **Zhen Zhu Mu** calms the Mind and settles the Ethereal Soul.
- **Suan Zao Ren** nourishes the Liver and settles the Ethereal Soul.

Variations

- To strengthen the Mind-calming effect and promote sleep add Fu Shen *Sclerotium Poriae cocos pararadicis*, Ye Jiao Teng *Caulis Polygoni multiflori* and Long Chi *Dens Draconis*.
- If the symptoms and signs of Fire are not too evident (no thirst, no bitter taste, urine not dark, stools not dry), omit Huang Qin and Zhi Zi.
- If there are symptoms of Liver-Yang rising (frequent headaches, dizziness, tinnitus) add Tian Ma *Rhizoma Gastrodiae elatae*.

Patent remedy

AN MIAN PIAN
Peaceful Sleep Tablet
Suan Zao Ren *Semen Ziziphi spinosae*
Yuan Zhi *Radix Polygalae tenuifoliae*
Fu Ling *Sclerotium Poriae cocos*
Shan Zhi Zi *Fructus Gardeniae jasminoidis*

Shen Qu *Massa Fermentata Medicinalis*
Quan Xie *Buthus Martensi*
Gan Cao *Radix Glycyrrhizae uralensis*

Explanation

Although not specific for Liver-Fire, this tablet can be used for this pattern due to the inclusion of Zhi Zi.

The tongue presentation appropriate to this remedy is a Red tongue body, with redder sides, and a yellow coating.

2. HEART FIRE BLAZING

CLINICAL MANIFESTATIONS

Waking up during the night, nightmares, dreams of flying, mental restlessness, bitter taste, thirst, tongue ulcers and palpitations.
Tongue: Red, redder tip with red points, yellow coating.
Pulse: Rapid and Overflowing on the left Front position.

TREATMENT PRINCIPLE

Drain Heart-Fire, calm the Mind.

ACUPUNCTURE

HE-8 Shaofu, HE-7 Shenmen, SP-6 Sanyinjiao, L.I.-11 Quchi, Ren-15 Jiuwei, Du-19 Houding, BL-15 Xinshu, BL-44 Shentang. Reducing method. No moxa.

Explanation

- **HE-8** drains Heart-Fire.
- **HE-7** calms the Mind and promotes sleep.
- **SP-6** cools Blood and calms the Mind.
- **L.I.-11** is used if there are pronounced general signs of Fire.
- **Ren-15** clears the Heart, calms the Mind and promotes sleep.
- **Du-19** in combination with Ren-15 calms the Mind and promotes sleep.

- **BL-15** drains Heart-Fire.
- **BL-44** calms the Mind and promotes sleep.

HERBAL TREATMENT

(a) Prescription

XIE XIN TANG
Draining the Heart Decoction
Da Huang *Rhizoma Rhei* 9 g
Huang Lian *Rhizoma Coptidis* 6 g
Huang Qin *Radix Scutellariae baicalensis* 9 g

Explanation

This formula drains Heart-Fire by moving downwards. It is applicable only if there is Full-Fire without any signs of Yin deficiency. An important condition for the use of this formula is that the tongue should have a thick, dry and yellow coating.

- **Da Huang** drains Fire by moving downwards.
- **Huang Lian** and **Huang Qin** drain Heart-Fire.

(b) Prescription

DAO CHI SAN
Eliminating Redness Powder
Sheng Di Huang *Radix Rehmanniae glutinosae* 15 g
Mu Tong *Caulis Akebiae* 3 g
Sheng Can Cao *Radix Glycyrrhizae uralensis* 6 g
Zhu Ye *Herba Lophatheri gracilis* 3 g

Explanation

This formula differs from the previous one in so far as in addition to draining Heart-Fire it also cools Blood and nourishes Yin (because of the inclusion of Sheng Di Huang). It is therefore suitable for cases when Fire has begun to injure the Yin. The tongue would therefore be Red with a yellow coating, though this coating might be rootless or missing in places.

- **Sheng Di** clears Heat and cools Blood.
- **Mu Tong** drains Heart-Fire.

- **Gan Cao** resolves Fire-Poison.
- **Zhu Ye** clears Heart-Fire.

Variations

- Other versions of this formula include Deng Xin Cao *Medulla Junci effusi* to clear Heart-Heat and calm the Mind.
- To enhance the sleep-promoting effect of both this formula and the previous one, add Ye Jiao Teng *Caulis Polygoni multiflori*, Fu Shen *Sclerotium Poriae cocos pararadicis* and Yuan Zhi *Radix Polygalae tenuifoliae*.

Patent remedy

ZHU SHA AN SHEN WAN
Cinnabar Calming the Mind Pill
Dang Gui *Radix Angelicae sinensis*
Sheng Di Huang *Radix Rehmanniae glutinosae*
Zhu Sha *Cinnabaris*
Huang Lian *Rhizoma Coptidis*
Gan Cao *Radix Glycyrrhizae uralensis*

Explanation

Although not specific for Heart-Fire, this pill can be used for this pattern as Huang Lian drains Heart-Fire and both Dang Gui and Sheng Di enter the Heart.

The tongue presentation appropriate to this remedy is a Red tongue body with a redder tip and a yellow coating.

Please note that this pill contains Zhu Sha which is a toxic substance and should therefore only be taken for a few weeks at a time.

3. PHLEGM-HEAT HARASSING THE MIND

CLINICAL MANIFESTATIONS

Restless sleep, tossing and turning, unpleasant dreams, a feeling of heaviness, dizziness, a feeling of oppression of the chest, nausea, no appetite, palpitations, mental restlessness and a sticky taste.
Tongue: Red with a sticky-yellow coating. Stomach-crack with sticky-rough yellow coating inside it.
Pulse: Slippery and Rapid.

This pattern is due to Phlegm-Heat in the Stomach and Stomach-Qi rebelling upwards. When Phlegm is present, Stomach-Qi rebelling upwards will carry Phlegm and Heat to the Upper Burner to harass the Heart and Mind, thus causing insomnia. In severe cases this causes mental illness. The "Simple Questions" in chapter 34 says: *"The Stomach is the Sea of the 5 Yin and 6 Yang organs, its Qi must go downwards, when Stomach-Qi rebels upwards . . . one cannot sleep"*.[45]

TREATMENT PRINCIPLE

Clear Heat, resolve Phlegm and calm the Mind.

ACUPUNCTURE

ST-40 Fenglong, Ren-12 Zhongwan, Ren-9 Shuifen, SP-9 Yinlingquan, BL-20 Pishu, L.I.-11 Quchi, ST-8 Touwei, G.B.-12 Wangu, SP-6 Sanyinjiao, ST-45 Lidui, SP-1 Yinbai. Reducing method except for Ren-12 and BL-20 which should be reinforced. No moxa, except for ST-45 (see below).

Explanation

- **ST-40** resolves Phlegm and calms the Mind.
- **Ren-12**, **Ren-9** and **BL-20** tonify the Spleen to resolve Phlegm.
- **SP-9** and **SP-6** resolve Dampness which helps to resolve Phlegm. SP-6 also calms the Mind.
- **L.I.-11** resolves Phlegm and clears Heat.
- **ST-8** is the main local point to resolve Phlegm from the head and it promotes sleep.
- **G.B.-12** promotes sleep.
- **ST-45** relieves retention of food, calms the Mind and promotes sleep. Very small moxa cones can be used after needling to conduct Fire downwards. This is one of the few cases when moxa is used to counteract Heat.
- **SP-1**, often combined with ST-44, clears Heat in the Stomach and Spleen, calms the Mind and promotes sleep. The points ST-44 and SP-1 are also specific for excessive and unpleasant dreaming.

HERBAL TREATMENT

(a) Prescription

SHI WEI WEN DAN TANG
Ten-Ingredient Warming the Gall-Bladder Decoction
Ban Xia *Rhizoma Pinelliae ternatae* 6 g
Chen Pi *Pericarpium Citri reticulatae* 6 g
Fu Ling *Sclerotium Poriae cocos* 4.5 g
Zhi Shi *Fructus Citri aurantii immaturus* 6 g
Ren Shen *Radix Ginseng* 3 g (**Dang Shen** *Radix Codonopsis pilosulae* 9 g)
Shu Di Huang *Radix Rehmanniae glutinosae praeparata* 9 g
Suan Zao Ren *Semen Ziziphi spinosae* 3 g
Yuan Zhi *Radix Polygalae tenuifoliae* 3 g
Zhi Gan Cao *Radix Glycyrrhizae uralensis praeparata* 1.5 g
Sheng Jiang *Rhizoma Zingiberis officinalis recens* 5 slices
Hong Zao *Fructus Ziziphi jujubae* one date

Explanation

This prescription is used if there is Phlegm-Heat in the Stomach and Heart together with some deficiency of Qi and Blood, which is a very common situation.

- **Ban Xia**, **Chen Pi**, **Fu Ling** and **Zhi Shi** are a contracted form of Wen Dan Tang *Warming the Gall-Bladder Decoction* (without Zhu Ru) to resolve Phlegm.
- **Ren Shen** and **Shu Di** tonify Qi and Blood.
- **Suan Zao Ren** and **Yuan Zhi** calm the Mind and promote sleep.
- **Gan Cao**, **Sheng Jiang** and **Hong Zao** harmonize.

(b) Prescription

HUANG LIAN WEN DAN TANG
Coptis Warming the Gall-Bladder Decoction
Huang Lian *Rhizoma Coptidis* 4.5 g
Ban Xia *Rhizoma Pinelliae ternatae* 6 g
Fu Ling *Sclerotium Poriae cocos* 5 g
Chen Pi *Pericarpium Citri reticulatae* 9 g
Zhu Ru *Caulis Bambusae in Taeniis* 6 g
Zhi Shi *Fructus Citri aurantii immaturus* 6 g
Zhi Gan Cao *Radix Glycyrrhizae uralensis praeparata* 3 g
Sheng Jiang *Rhizoma Zingiberis officinalis recens* 5 slices
Da Zao *Fructus Ziziphi jujubae* one date

Explanation

This formula is used in preference to the previous one if symptoms and signs of Heat are more pronounced and the tongue is definitely Red with a thick-yellow coating.

- **Huang Lian** clears Heart-Fire and calms the Mind.
- All the other herbs constitute Wen Dan Tang *Warming the Gall-Bladder Decoction* which resolves Phlegm-Heat and calms the Mind.

Variations

These formulae have a powerful effect in calming the Mind and promoting sleep and may need little variation or addition.

- To enhance the sleep-promoting effect add Ye Jiao Teng *Caulis Polygoni multiflori* and Yuan Zhi *Radix Polygalae tenuifoliae*.
- If there are symptoms of retention of food add Shen Qu *Massa Fermentata Medicinalis* and Lai Fu Zi *Semen Raphani sativi*.
- If there are more symptoms of retention of food rather than those of Phlegm-Heat, use Bao He Wan *Preserving and Harmonizing Pill* instead.
- If there is constipation add Da Huang *Rhizoma Rhei*.

Patent remedy

AN SHEN BU XIN WAN
Calming the Mind and Tonifying the Heart Pill
Zhen Zhu Mu *Concha margaritiferae*
Shou Wu *Radix Polygoni multiflori*
Nu Zhen Zi *Fructus Ligustri lucidi*
Han Lian Cao *Herba Ecliptae prostratae*
Dan Shen *Radix Salviae miltiorrhizae*
He Huan Pi *Cortex Albizziae julibrissin*
Tu Si Zi *Semen Cuscutae*
Wu Wei Zi *Fructus Schisandrae chinensis*
Shi Chang Pu *Rhizoma Acori graminei*

Explanation

Although not specific for Phlegm-Fire, this pill can be used for this pattern as it contains He Huan Pi and Shi Chang Pu which open the Mind's orifices. Other ingredients are mostly tonifying and nourishing and this patent remedy is only indicated when combined with an acupuncture strategy aimed at draining Fire and resolving Phlegm.

4. RESIDUAL HEAT IN THE DIAPHRAGM

CLINICAL MANIFESTATIONS

Restless sleep, waking up during the night, mental restlessness, cannot lie down or sit, a feeling of stuffiness of the chest, epigastric discomfort and sour regurgitation.
Tongue: Red in the front part or red points around the centre.
Pulse: Deep and slightly Rapid.

This condition arises after an invasion of Wind-Heat which has turned into Interior Heat and has not been cleared properly, often through wrong use of antibiotics: some residual Heat remains in the body and settles in the diaphragm area. From here it rebels upwards to disturb the Heart and Mind.

TREATMENT PRINCIPLE

Clear residual Heat, calm irritability and calm the Mind.

ACUPUNCTURE

LU-10 Yuji, HE-8 Shaofu, BL-17 Geshu, ST-40 Fenglong, L.I.-11 Quchi, SP-6 Sanyinjiao, Ren-15 Jiuwei. Reducing method, no moxa.

Explanation

- **LU-10** and **HE-8** clear Lung-Heat and Heart-Heat respectively. They are chosen because, from the point of view of channels, residual Heat in the diaphragm is located in Lungs and Heart. Besides this, HE-8 also calms the Mind.

- **BL-17** relaxes the diaphragm.
- **ST-40** relaxes the diaphragm, subdues rebellious Qi and calms the Mind.
- **L.I.-11** clears Heat.
- **SP-6** calms the Mind and protects Yin from injury from Heat.
- **Ren-15** relaxes the diaphragm, clears the Heart and calms the Mind.

HERBAL TREATMENT

(a) Prescription

ZHU YE SHI GAO TANG
Zhu Ye *Herba Lophatheri gracilis* 15 g
Shi Gao *Gypsum fibrosum* 30 g
Ban Xia *Rhizoma Pinelliae ternatae* 9 g
Mai Men Dong *Tuber Ophiopogonis japonici* 15 g
Ren Shen *Radix Ginseng* 5 g
Gan Cao *Radix Glycyrrhizae uralensis* 3 g
Geng Mi *Semen Oryzae sativae* 15 g

Explanation

This is one of the formulae for clearing residual Heat, especially from the diaphragm area.

- **Zhu Ye** and **Shi Gao** are pungent and cold and clear Heat by pushing it outwards.
- **Ban Xia** harmonizes the Stomach, subdues rebellious Qi in the diaphragm and stops nausea.
- **Mai Dong** and **Ren Shen**, tonify Qi and Yin since Qi is weakened by an external invasion and Yin is injured by Heat.
- **Gan Cao** and **Geng Mi** harmonize the Stomach.

(b) Prescription

ZHI ZI CHI TANG
Gardenia-Soja Decoction
Zhi Zi *Fructus Gardeniae jasminoidis* 9 g
Dan Dou Chi *Semen Sojae praeparatum* 9 g

Explanation

This formula lightly clears Heat and is often used to clear residual Heat.

- **Zhi Zi** clears Heat.
- **Dan Dou Chi** clears Heat and stops irritability.

Variations

- To enhance the sleep-promoting effect add Fu Shen *Sclerotium Poriae cocos pararadicis*, Deng Xin Cao *Medulla Junci effusi* and Ye Jiao Teng *Caulis Polygoni multiflori*.

DEFICIENCY

1. HEART AND SPLEEN BLOOD DEFICIENCY

CLINICAL MANIFESTATIONS

Difficulty in falling asleep, palpitations, tiredness, poor appetite, slight anxiety, blurred vision, dizziness, poor memory, pale face.
Tongue: Pale.
Pulse: Choppy.

This is a very common type of insomnia, due to deficiency of Blood. Since Blood is deficient, the person cannot fall asleep easily but once asleep, because Yin is sufficient, he or she stays asleep. It should be remembered that because in old people there is a physiological decline of Qi and Blood, they normally need less sleep than younger people. Chapter 18 of the "Spiritual Axis" says:

Young people have abundant Qi and Blood . . . [so that] they are energetic in the daytime and sleep well at night. Old people have declining Qi and Blood . . . [so that] they are less active in daytime and cannot sleep at night.[46]

TREATMENT PRINCIPLE

Tonify the Spleen, nourish Blood, tonify the Heart and calm the Mind.

ACUPUNCTURE

ST-36 Zusanli, SP-6 Sanyinjiao, HE-7 Shenmen, Ren-14 Juque, BL-20 Pishu, BL-15 Xinshu, Yintang. Reinforcing method; moxa may be used.

Explanation

- **ST-36**, **SP-6** and **BL-20** tonify the Spleen to produce Blood. SP-6 also calms the Mind.
- **HE-7** and **Ren-14** nourish Heart-Blood and calm the Mind.
- **BL-15** nourishes Heart-Blood and calms the Mind.
- **Yintang** calms the Mind and promotes sleep, especially in Empty conditions. The patient may also be advised to apply gentle moxibustion to this point with a moxa stick every night.

HERBAL TREATMENT

Prescription

GUI PI TANG
Tonifying the Spleen Decoction
Ren Shen *Radix Ginseng* 6 g (**Dang Shen** *Radix Codonopsis pilosulae* 12 g)
Huang Qi *Radix Astragali membranacei* 15 g
Bai Zhu *Rhizoma Atractylodis macrocephalae* 12 g
Dang Gui *Radix Angelicae sinensis* 3 g
Fu Shen *Sclerotium Poriae cocos pararadicis* 9 g
Suan Zao Ren *Semen Ziziphi spinosae* 9 g
Long Yan Rou *Arillus Euphoriae longanae* 12 g
Yuan Zhi *Radix Polygalae tenuifoliae* 9 g
Mu Xiang *Radix Saussureae* 6 g
Zhi Gan Cao *Radix Glycyrrhizae uralensis praeparata* 4 g
Sheng Jiang *Rhizoma Zingiberis officinalis recens* 3 slices
Hong Zao *Fructus Ziziphi jujubae* 5 dates

Explanation

This formula tonifies Spleen-Qi and Heart-Qi, nourishes Heart-Blood and calms the Mind.

- **Ren Shen**, **Huang Qi** and **Bai Zhu** tonify Heart-Qi.
- **Dang Gui** nourishes Blood.
- **Fu Shen**, **Suan Zao Ren**, **Long Yan Rou** and

Yuan Zhi calm the Mind and promote sleep. Long Yan Rou also nourishes Blood.
– **Mu Xiang** moves Qi and is added to counteract the possible stickiness of the Qi and Blood tonics.
– **Gan Cao**, **Sheng Jiang** and **Hong Zao** harmonize and tonify Qi and Blood.

Variations

This formula is very specific for this pattern and it promotes sleep; therefore no variations are needed.

(a) Patent remedy

GUI PI WAN
Tonifying the Spleen Pill

Explanation

This pill has the same ingredients and indications as the homonymous prescription above.
The tongue presentation appropriate to this remedy is a Pale body.

(b) Patent remedy

BAI ZI YANG XIN WAN
Biota Nourishing the Heart Pill
Ren Shen *Radix Ginseng* (or Dang Shen *Radix Codonopsis pilosulae*)
Huang Qi *Radix Astragali membranacei*
Dang Gui *Radix Angelicae sinensis*
Chuan Xiong *Radix Ligustici wallichii*
Fu Ling *Sclerotium Poriae cocos*
Bai Zi Ren *Semen Biotae orientalis*
Suan Zao Ren *Semen Ziziphi spinosae*
Yuan Zhi *Radix Polygalae tenuifoliae*
Wu Wei Zi *Fructus Schisandrae chinensis*
Ban Xia *Rhizoma Pinelliae ternatae*
Rou Gui *Cortex Cinnamomi cassiae*
Zhi Gan Cao *Radix Glycyrrhizae uralensis praeparata*

Explanation

This remedy is for insomnia from Spleen- and Heart-Blood deficiency: it tonifies Qi, nourishes Blood and calms the Mind.

The tongue and pulse presentation appropriate to this remedy is a Pale and Thin tongue and a Choppy pulse.

2. HEART-YIN DEFICIENCY

CLINICAL MANIFESTATIONS

Waking up frequently at night, dry throat, mental restlessness, palpitations, night-sweating, poor memory, 5-palm heat.
Tongue: Red without coating, Heart-crack, tip redder.
Pulse: Floating-Empty.

TREATMENT PRINCIPLE

Nourish Heart-Yin and calm the Mind.

ACUPUNCTURE

HE-7 Shenmen, BL-15 Xinshu, Ren-14 Juque, SP-6 Sanyinjiao, ST-36 Zusanli, Ren-4 Guanyuan. Reinforcing method.

Explanation

– **HE-7** nourishes the Heart, calms the Mind and promotes sleep.
– **BL-15** and **Ren-14**, Back-Transporting points and Front-Collecting point of the Heart, nourish the Heart and calm the Mind.
– **SP-6** and **ST-36** nourish Qi and Yin in general.
– **Ren-4** nourishes Yin in general and calms the Mind.

HERBAL TREATMENT

Prescription

YANG XIN TANG (II)
Nourishing the Heart Decoction
Huang Qi *Radix Astragali membranacei* 6 g
Ren Shen *Radix Ginseng* 6 g
Bai Zi Ren *Semen Biotae orientalis* 9 g

Fu Shen *Sclerotium Poriae cocos pararadicis* 6 g
Chuan Xiong *Radix Ligustici wallichii* 3 g
Yuang Zhi *Radix Polygalae tenuifoliae* 6 g
Mai Men Dong *Tuber Ophiopogonis japonici* 6 g
Wu Wei Zi *Fructus Schisandrae chinensis* 6 g
Zhi Gan Cao *Radix Glycyrrhizae uralensis prae-parata* 3 g
Sheng Jiang *Rhizoma Zingiberis officinalis recens* 1 slice

Explanation

This formula tonifies Heart-Qi, Heart-Blood and Heart-Yin. It shares the same name as another formula (Yang Xin Tang I) which tonifies Heart-Qi and Heart-Blood. When used for Heart-Yin, it can be modified by reducing the dosage of the Qi tonics and increasing that of the Yin tonics.

- **Huang Qi** and **Ren Shen** tonify Heart-Qi.
- **Bai Zi Ren** nourishes Heart-Blood, calms the Mind and promotes sleep.
- **Fu Shen** calms the Mind and promotes sleep.
- **Chuan Xiong** harmonizes Blood and directs the herbs upwards to the Mind.
- **Yuan Zhi** calms the Mind.
- **Mai Dong** and **Wu Wei Zi** nourish Heart-Yin and calm the Mind.
- **Gan Cao** and **Sheng Jiang** harmonize.

Variations

- If the symptoms of Yin deficiency are pronounced add Tian Men Dong *Tuber Asparagi cochinchinensis* and Sheng Di Huang *Radix Rehmanniae glutinosae*.
- If there are pronounced symptoms of Empty-Heat add Qing Hao *Herba Artemisiae apiaceae* and Mu Li *Concha Ostreae*.

(a) Patent remedy

DING XIN WAN
Settling the Heart Pill
Dang Shen *Radix Codonopsis pilosulae*
Dang Gui *Radix Angelicae sinensis*
Fu Shen *Sclerotium Poriae cocos pararadicis*
Yuan Zhi *Radix Polygalae tenuifoliae*
Suan Zao Ren *Semen Ziziphi spinosae*

Bai Zi Ren *Semen Biotae orientalis*
Mai Men Dong *Tuber Ophiopogonis japonicis*
Hu Po *Succinum*

Explanation

This pill nourishes both Heart-Blood and Heart-Yin. For this reason, the tongue presentation appropriate to this remedy may be either a Pale and Thin body or a Red body with rootless coating.

(b) Patent remedy

AN SHEN BU NAO PIAN
Calming the Mind and Tonifying the Brain Tablet
Huang Jing *Rhizoma Polygonati*
Nu Zhen Zi *Fructus Ligustri lucidi*
Dang Gui *Radix Angelicae sinensis*
He Huan Pi *Cortex Albizziae julibrissin*
Han Lian Cao *Herba Ecliptae prostratae*
Suan Zao Ren *Semen Ziziphi spinosae*
Fu Ling *Sclerotium Poriae cocos*
Shou Wu *Radix Polygoni multiflori*
Yuan Zhi *Radix Polygalae tenuifoliae*
Zhu Sha *Cinnabaris*

Explanation

This tablet nourishes Heart-Yin and calms the Mind. It has a more pronounced Yin-nourishing effect than the previous remedy and the tongue presentation appropriate to this remedy is therefore a Red tongue without coating and with a Heart-crack.

3. HEART AND KIDNEYS NOT HARMONIZED ≈ HT+K1 Yin↓

CLINICAL MANIFESTATIONS

Waking up frequently during the night, difficulty in falling asleep, dry throat, night-sweating, 5-palm heat, poor memory, palpitations, dizziness, mental restlessness, tinnitus, backache.
Tongue: Red without coating, tip redder, Heart-crack, dry.
Pulse: Floating-Empty and slightly Rapid.

This pattern consists in deficiency of Kidney-Yin, deficiency of Heart-Yin and Heart Empty-Heat.

TREATMENT PRINCIPLE

Nourish Yin, tonify Kidneys and Heart, clear Empty-Heat and calm the Mind.

ACUPUNCTURE

HE-7 Shenmen, HE-6 Yinxi, P-7 Daling, Ren-4 Guanyuan, SP-6 Sanyinjiao, KI-3 Taixi, KI-6 Zhaohai, Ren-15 Jiuwei, BL-15 Xinshu, BL-23 Shenshu, BL-44 Shentang, BL-52 Zhishi. Reinforcing method on all points except HE-6 which should be reduced.

Explanation

– **HE-7** calms the Mind and promotes sleep.
– **HE-6** clears Heart Empty-Heat.
– **P-7** calms the Mind.
– **Ren-4** nourishes Kidney-Yin and calms the Mind.
– **SP-6**, **KI-3** and **KI-6** nourish Kidney-Yin.
– **Ren-15** nourishes the Heart and calms the Mind.
– **BL-15** and **BL-23** harmonize Heart and Kidneys.
– **BL-44** and **BL-52** harmonize the Mind and Will-Power.

HERBAL TREATMENT

Prescription

TIAN WANG BU XIN DAN
Heavenly Emperor Tonifying the Heart Pill
Sheng Di Huang *Radix Rehmanniae glutinosae* 12 g
Xuan Shen *Radix Scrophulariae ningpoensis* 6 g
Mai Men Dong *Tuber Ophiopogonis japonici* 6 g
Tian Men Dong *Tuber Asparagi cochinchinensis* 6 g
Ren Shen *Radix Ginseng* 6 g
Fu Ling *Sclerotium Poriae cocos* 6 g
Wu Wei Zi *Fructus Schisandrae chinensis* 6 g

Dang Gui *Radix Angelicae sinensis* 6 g
Dan Shen *Radix Salviae miltiorrhizae* 6 g
Bai Zi Ren *Semen Biotae orientalis* 6 g
Suan Zao Ren *Semen Ziziphi spinosae* 6 g
Yuan Zhi *Radix Polygalae tenuifoliae* 6 g
Jie Geng *Radix Platycodi grandiflori* 3 g

Explanation

This prescription nourishes Kidney- and Heart-Yin.

– **Sheng Di**, **Xuan Shen**, **Mai Dong** and **Tian Dong** nourish Kidney- and Heart-Yin.
– **Ren Shen** and **Fu Ling** tonify Heart-Qi to help to nourish Heart-Yin. Fu Ling also calms the Mind.
– **Wu Wei Zi** is sour and absorbing and it helps to nourish Yin. It also calms the Mind.
– **Dang Gui** and **Dan Shen** harmonize Heart-Blood to help to nourish Yin. Dan Shen is also used as a messenger to enter the Heart channel.
– **Bai Zi Ren**, **Suan Zao Ren** and **Yuan Zhi** nourish the Heart and calm the Mind. Suan Zao Ren and Yuan Zhi combine well as the former is sour and absorbing while the latter is pungent and scattering. The combination of these two tastes and actions harmonizes the Heart and calms the Mind.
– **Jie Geng** is used as a messenger to direct the herbs to the Upper Burner.

Variations

– To enhance the sleep-promoting effect add Ye Jiao Teng *Caulis Polygoni multiflori*.
– If there are pronounced symptoms of Empty-Heat add Mu Li *Concha Ostreae* and Qing Hao *Herba Artemisiae apiaceae*.

Patent remedy

TIAN WAN BU XIN DAN
Heavenly Emperor Tonifying the Heart Pill

Explanation

This remedy has the same ingredients and indications as the above homonymous prescription.

The tongue presentation appropriate to this remedy is a Red body, without coating and a Heart crack.

Case history

A 58-year-old man had been suffering from insomnia for 2 years. He fell asleep easily but woke up several times during the night with a feeling of dryness of the throat. He had also been suffering from impotence for 3 years.

His tongue was Red, the coating was too thin and it had a Heart-crack. His pulse was Empty at the deep level and extremely Weak and Fine on the left Rear and Middle positions.

He was born with one kidney.

Diagnosis
The insomnia in this case was due to Kidney-Yin deficiency and Kidney and Heart not harmonized. Although he had comparatively few symptoms, judging from the pulse, the Kidney deficiency was very severe and this obviously also had something to do with his congenital anatomical abnormality.

Treatment principle
Nourish Kidney-Yin and Heart-Yin and calm the Mind.

Acupuncture
The main points used were:

– **S.I.-3** Houxi and **BL-62** Shenmai to open the Governing Vessel and strengthen the Kidneys. Although this combination strengthens Kidney-Yang more than Kidney-Yin, it was used to help his impotence which was worrying him more than the insomnia.
– **Ren-4** Guanyuan, **SP-6** Sanyinjiao and **KI-3** Taixi nourish Kidney-Yin.
– **BL-23** Shenshu to strengthen the Kidneys.
– **HE-7** Shenmen, **Ren-15** Jiuwei and **Du-19** Houding to calm the Mind.
– **G.B.-12** Wangu and **Yintang** to promote sleep.

Herbal treatment
No herbs were prescribed but only the patent remedy Tian Wang Bu Xin Dan *Heavenly Emperor's Tonifying the Heart Pill* to nourish Kidney- and Heart-Yin and calm the Mind.

His sleep became normal after six months of treatment while his impotence improved by about 50%.

4. HEART AND GALL-BLADDER DEFICIENCY

CLINICAL MANIFESTATIONS

Waking up very early in the morning and being unable to fall asleep again, light sleep, dreaming a lot, propensity to being easily startled, timidity, lack of initiative and assertiveness, palpitations, breathlessness, tiredness.

Tongue: Pale, Heart-crack.
Pulse: Empty.

More than a pattern, this describes a certain character type of a person. Such character may be constitutional or may arise as a consequence of a protracted illness; for example glandular fever (mononucleosis). Originally, the formula Wen Dan Tang *Warming the Gall-Bladder Decoction* was used for this condition, but nowadays it is more often used for Phlegm-Heat.

TREATMENT PRINCIPLE

Tonify Heart and Gall-Bladder, calm the Mind.

ACUPUNCTURE

HE-7 Shenmen, G.B.-40 Qiuxu.

Explanation

– **HE-7** and **G.B.-40**, both Source points, tonify Heart and Gall-Bladder, calm the Mind and stimulate the person's drive and assertiveness.

HERBAL TREATMENT

Prescription

AN SHEN DING ZHI WAN
Calming the Mind and Settling the Will-Power Pill
Ren Shen *Radix Ginseng* 9 g
Fu Ling *Sclerotium Poriae cocos* 12 g
Fu Shen *Sclerotium Poriae cocos pararadicis* 9 g
Long Chi *Dens Draconis* 15 g
Yuan Zhi *Radix Polygalae tenuifoliae* 6 g
Shi Chang Pu *Rhizoma Acori graminei* 8 g

Explanation

– **Ren Shen**, **Fu Ling** and **Fu Shen** tonify Heart-Qi. Fu Ling and Fu Shen also calm the Mind.

– **Long Chi** sinks, calms the Mind and settles the Spirit.
– **Yuan Zhi** and **Chang Pu** open the Heart-orifices and calm the Mind.

5. LIVER-YIN DEFICIENCY

CLINICAL MANIFESTATIONS

Waking up during the night, dreaming a lot, talking in one's sleep, in severe cases sleep-walking, dry throat, irritability, blurred vision, feeling of heat, sore and dry eyes, dry skin and hair, dizziness.
Tongue: Red without coating.
Pulse: Floating-Empty, especially on the left side.
   The deficiency of Liver-Yin causes the Ethereal Soul to be deprived of its root and to "wander" at night during sleep. This causes insomnia and excessive dreaming.

TREATMENT PRINCIPLE

Nourish Liver-Yin, root the Ethereal Soul and calm the Mind.

ACUPUNCTURE

LIV-8 Ququan, Ren-4 Guanyuan, SP-6 Sanyinjiao, P-7 Daling, Du-24 Shenting and G.B.-15 Toulinqi, BL-47 Hunmen, Anmien. Reinforcing method. No moxa.

Explanation

– **LIV-8** nourishes Liver-Blood and Liver-Yin.
– **Ren-4** nourishes Liver- and Kidney-Yin and calms the Mind.
– **SP-6** nourishes Liver-Yin and calms the Mind.
– **P-7** harmonizes the Liver (due to the relationship between Pericardium and Liver within the Terminal Yin), calms the Mind and settles the Ethereal Soul.
– **Du-24** and **G.B.-15** calm the Mind especially in Liver patterns.

– **BL-47**, called the "Door of the Ethereal Soul", settles the Ethereal Soul into the Liver at night. Some old books give sleep-walking as an indication for this point.
– **Anmien** calms the Ethereal Soul and the Mind and promotes sleep in Liver patterns.

HERBAL TREATMENT

(a) Prescription

SUAN ZAO REN TANG
Ziziphus Decoction
Suan Zao Ren *Semen Ziziphi spinosae* 18 g
Chuan Xiong *Radix Ligustici wallichii* 6 g
Fu Ling *Sclerotium Poriae cocos* 12 g
Zhi Mu *Rhizoma Anemarrhenae asphodeloidis* 9 g
Gan Cao *Radix Glycyrrhizae uralensis* 3 g

Explanation

This is an excellent formula for this condition and it is very reliable in its sleep-promoting effect.

– **Suan Zao Ren** is the main herb. It enters the Liver, is sour and absorbing, nourishes Yin and, by virtue of its taste, it "absorbs" the Ethereal Soul back into Liver-Yin, thus promoting sleep.
– **Chuan Xiong** and **Zhi Mu** are coordinated: one is pungent and warm, the other sweet and cold. One scatters, the other nourishes (Yin). Chuan Xiong is also coordinated with Suan Zao Ren: the former is pungent, the latter sour and both enter the Liver. Together they harmonize the Liver.
– **Fu Ling** calms the Mind.
– **Gan Cao** is sweet and together with Suan Zao Ren which is sour, nourishes Yin and moistens.

Variations

– If there is Empty-Heat arising from Liver-Yin deficiency add Han Lian Cao *Herba Ecliptae prostratae* and Mu Li *Concha Ostreae*.
– If there are symptoms of Liver-Yang rising add Tian Ma *Rhizoma Gastrodiae elatae* and Gou Teng *Ramulus Uncariae*.

(b) Prescription

YIN MEI TANG
Attracting Sleep Decoction
Bai Shao *Radix Paeoniae albae* 30 g
Dang Gui *Radix Angelicae sinensis* 15 g
Long Chi *Dens Draconis* 6 g
Tu Si Zi *Semen Cuscutae* 9 g
Mai Men Dong *Tuber Ophiopogonis japonici* 15 g
Bai Zi Ren *Semen Biotae orientalis* 6 g
Suan Zao Ren *Semen Ziziphi spinosae* 9 g
Fu Shen *Sclerotium Poriae cocos pararadicis* 9 g

Explanation

This formula, already explained in chapter 9, is specific to nourish Liver-Yin and promote sleep by rooting the Ethereal Soul in the Liver. Compared to the previous formula, it is used when the person has many unpleasant dreams.

Patent remedy

SUAN ZAO REN TANG PIAN
Ziziphus Decoction Tablet

Explanation

This tablet has the same ingredients and indications as the above homonymous prescription.

The tongue presentation appropriate to this remedy is a Red body without coating or with rootless coating.

Case history

A 61-year-old man had been suffering from insomnia ever since his wife died 2 years previously. He found it difficult to fall asleep and also woke up frequently during the night. He was extremely sad about his wife's death and found it very difficult to come to terms with it.

His vision was sometimes blurred and his memory was affected. His tongue was Red, dry, Flabby, and its coating was too thin (Plate 10.1). His pulse was Floating-Empty and very slightly Wiry on the left side.

Diagnosis
In this case sadness affected the Liver and Heart rather than the Lungs and Heart. In particular, sadness weakened Liver-Yin so that the Ethereal Soul was deprived of its root. When this happens it wanders at night causing insomnia.

The "Spiritual Axis" in chapter 8 clearly states that sadness can affect the Liver: "*. . . The Liver's sadness and shock injure the Ethereal Soul . . .*" and "*When sadness affects the Liver it injures the Ethereal Soul; this causes mental confusion . . . the Yin is damaged, the tendons contract and there is hypochondrial discomfort*".[47] This quotation clearly indicates that Liver-Yin may be damaged by sadness.

The blurred vision confirms the deficiency of Liver-Yin.

Treatment principle
Nourish Liver-Yin, root the Ethereal Soul and calm the Mind.

Acupuncture
The points used were:

- **LIV-8** Ququan, **SP-6** Sanyinjiao and **Ren-4** Guanyuan to nourish Liver-Yin.
- **HE-7** Shenmen and **Ren-15** Jiuwei to calm the Mind.
- **Du-24** Shenting and **G.B.-13** Benshen to calm the Mind and root the Ethereal Soul.

Herbal treatment
No herbs were prescribed but only the patent remedy Suan Zao Ren Tang Pian *Tablet of the Ziziphus Decoction* which specifically treats insomnia from Liver-Yin deficiency.

This patient's sleep pattern first improved by being able to fall asleep easily although he still woke up during the night. Presumably this is because Liver-Blood (responsible for not falling asleep) was helped before Liver-Yin. After about 6 months of fortnightly treatments he started sleeping through the night.

Appendix I

SOMNOLENCE

Somnolence indicates the tendency to be always rather sleepy and lethargic. Like insomnia, this is also due either to a pathogenic factor obstructing the Mind or to deficient Qi and Blood reaching the Mind.

1. DAMPNESS AND/OR PHLEGM MISTING THE MIND

CLINICAL MANIFESTATIONS

Sleepiness after lunch, a feeling of heaviness, a feeling of muzziness of the head as if it were full

of cotton-wool, a feeling of oppression of the chest, dizziness (if there is Phlegm).
Tongue: Pale, Swollen and with a sticky coating.
Pulse: Slippery or Weak-Floating and slightly Slippery.

This pattern is due to Dampness obstructing the head and preventing the clear Qi from rising upwards to brighten the upper orifices. Another explanation of somnolence deriving from Damp-ness and/or Phlegm is that Dampness obstructs the space between the skin and muscles where the Defensive Qi flows. Because this space is obstructed, the Defensive Qi, Yang in nature, cannot flow there, so it stays in the Yin and the patient feels always sleepy. Chapter 80 of the "Spiritual Axis" says:

Defensive Qi flows in the Yang during the day and in the Yin at night, when Yang slows down one is sleepy, when Yin slows down one is awake. When Stomach and Intestines are big, Defensive Qi stays there for a long time, the skin is obstructed by Dampness . . . Defensive Qi slows down, it stays in the Yin for a long time, Qi is not clear and somnolence results.[48]

TREATMENT PRINCIPLE

Resolve Dampness and/or Phlegm and tonify the Spleen.

ACUPUNCTURE

Ren-12 Zhongwan, Ren-9 Shuifen, BL-20 Pishu, ST-36 Zusanli, ST-40 Fenglong, SP-6 Sanyinjiao, BL-22 Sanjiaoshu, LU-7 Lieque, ST-8 Touwei, Du-20 Baihui, Du-24 Shenting. Reinforcing method on Ren-12, BL-20 and ST-36. Reducing method on Ren-9, ST-40, SP-6 and BL-22. Even method on LU-7, ST-8, Du-20 and Du-24.

Explanation

- **Ren-12**, **BL-20** and **ST-36** tonify the Spleen to resolve Dampness.
- **Ren-9**, **SP-6** and **BL-22** drain Dampness.
- **ST-40** resolves Phlegm.

- **LU-7** removes obstruction from the channels in the head and favours the ascending of clear Qi to the head.
- **ST-8** and **Du-20** are local points to expel Dampness from the head and facilitate the rising of clear Yang to the head.
- **Du-24** clears the brain.

HERBAL TREATMENT

Prescription

PING WEI SAN Variation
Balancing the Stomach Powder
Cang Zhu *Rhizoma Atractylodis lanceae* 9 g
Chen Pi *Pericarpium Citri reticulatae* 6 g
Hou Po *Cortex Magnoliae officinalis* 6 g
Zhi Gan Cao *Radix Glycyrrhizae uralensis prae-parata* 3 g
Sheng Jiang *Rhizoma Zingiberis officinalis recens* 3 g
Da Zao *Fructus Ziziphi jujubae* 3 dates
Huo Xiang *Herba Agastachis* 4.5 g
Pei Lan *Herba Eupatorii fortunei* 4.5 g
Yi Yi Ren *Semen Coicis lachryma jobi* 15 g

Explanation

- The first six herbs constitute the Ping Wei San which drains Dampness from the Middle Burner.
- **Huo Xiang** and **Pei Lan** are both aromatic herbs which fragrantly expel Dampness. They would specifically affect the head to relieve the sleepy and muzzy feeling.
- **Yi Yi Ren** drains Dampness by urination. It is combined with the previous two herbs to resolve Dampness by sweating and urination.

Variations

- If there is Phlegm add Ban Xia *Rhizoma Pinelliae ternatae* and Dan Nan Xing *Rhizoma Arisaematis praeparata*.
- To relieve the muzzy feeling of the head add Shi Chang Pu *Rhizoma Acori graminei*.
- If there are signs of Spleen deficiency add Bai Zhu *Rhizoma Atractylodis macrocephalae* and Huang Qi *Radix Astragali membranacei*.

2. SPLEEN DEFICIENCY

CLINICAL MANIFESTATIONS

Somnolence, lethargy, tiredness, feeling of heaviness, slight abdominal distension, poor appetite, loose stools.
Tongue: Pale and Swollen.
Pulse: Weak and slightly Slippery.
Although this pattern is primarily one of deficiency, there is also some Dampness.

TREATMENT PRINCIPLE

Tonify the Spleen and resolve Dampness.

ACUPUNCTURE

ST-36 Zusanli, SP-3 Taibai, Ren-12 Zhongwan, BL-20 Pishu, SP-6 Sanyinjiao, BL-22 Sanyinjiao, ST-8 Touwei, Du-20 Baihui. Reinforcing method on the first four points and even method on the others. Moxa can be used.

Explanation

- **ST-36**, **SP-3**, **Ren-12** and **BL-20** tonify the Spleen.
- **SP-6** and **BL-22** resolve Dampness.
- **ST-8** and **Du-20** drain Dampness from the head and facilitate the rising of clear Yang to the head.

HERBAL TREATMENT

(a) Prescription

LIU JUN ZI TANG Variation
Six Gentlemen Decoction
Ren Shen *Radix Ginseng* 10 g
Bai Zhu *Rhizoma Atractylodis macrocephalae* 9 g
Fu Ling *Sclerotium Poriae cocos* 9 g
Zhi Gan Cao *Radix Glycyrrhizae uralensis praeparata* 6 g
Chen Pi *Pericarpium Citri reticulatae* 9 g
Ban Xia *Rhizoma Pinelliae ternatae* 12 g
Mai Ya *Fructus Hordei vulgaris germinatus* 9 g
Shen Qu *Massa Fermentata Medicinalis* 9 g
Shan Zha *Fructus Crataegi* 6 g
Shi Chang Pu *Rhizoma Acori graminei* 6 g

Explanation

- The first six herbs constitute the Liu Jun Zi Tang which tonifies the Spleen and resolves Dampness.
- **Mai Ya**, **Shen Qu** and **Shan Zha** are digestives which help to resolve Dampness and facilitate the proper separation of pure and impure in the digestive system so that the clear Yang can ascend to the head.
- **Shi Chang Pu** opens the orifices and facilitates the draining of Dampness from the head and the rising of clear Yang to it.

(b) Prescription

BU ZHONG YI QI TANG Variation
Tonifying the Centre and Benefiting Qi Decoction
Huang Qi *Radix Astragali membranacei* 12 g
Ren Shen *Radix Ginseng* 9 g
Bai Zhu *Rhizoma Atractylodis macrocephalae* 9 g
Dang Gui *Radix Angelicae sinensis* 6 g
Chen Pi *Pericarpium Citri reticulatae* 6 g
Sheng Ma *Rhizoma Cimicifugae* 3 g
Chai Ma *Radix Bupleuri* 3 g
Zhi Gan Cao *Radix Glycyrrhizae uralensis praeparata* 3 g
Gan Jiang *Rhizoma Zingiberis officinalis* 3 g

Explanation

This formula is used if there is Spleen-Yang deficiency. The original formula tonifies the Spleen and raises Qi.

3. KIDNEY-YANG DEFICIENCY (DEFICIENCY OF SEA OF MARROW)

CLINICAL MANIFESTATIONS

Lethargy, tiredness, apathy, lack of will power, lack of initiative, depression, chilliness.
Tongue: Pale
Pulse: Deep and Weak.

TREATMENT PRINCIPLE

Tonify Kidney-Yang, nourish the Sea of Marrow and stimulate the rising of Qi.

ACUPUNCTURE

KI-3 Taixi, BL-23 Shenshu, BL-52 Zhishi, Du-20 Baihui, Du-24 Shenting, Ren-6 Qihai, Du-16 Fengfu.

Explanation

- **KI-3**, **BL-23** and **BL-52** tonify the Kidneys, strengthen Will-Power and nourish Marrow.
- **Du-20** and **Du-24** facilitate the rising of clear Yang to the head.
- **Ren-6** with direct moxa tonifies Yang.
- **Du-16**, point of the Sea of Marrow, nourishes Marrow.

HERBAL TREATMENT

Prescription

SHI BU WAN
Fu Zi *Radix Aconiti carmichaeli praeparata* 3 g
Gui Zhi *Ramulus Cinnamomi cassiae* 3 g
Shu Di Huang *Radix Rehmanniae glutinosae praeparata* 24 g
Shan Zhu Yu *Fructus Corni officinalis* 12 g
Shan Yao *Radix Dioscoreae oppositae* 12 g
Ze Xie *Rhizoma Alismatis orientalis* 9 g
Mu Dan Pi *Cortex Moutan radicis* 9 g
Fu Ling *Sclerotium Poriae cocos* 9 g
Lu Rong *Cornu Cervi parvum* 6 g
Wu Wei Zi *Fructus Schisandrae chinensis* 6 g

Explanation

- The first eight herbs constitute the Jin Gui Shen Qi Wan *Golden Chest Kidney-Qi Pill* which tonifies Kidney-Yang.
- **Lu Rong** tonifies Kidney-Yang, benefits the Essence, nourishes Marrow and strengthens the Governing Vessel.
- **Wu Wei Zi** nourishes the Essence.

Appendix II

POOR MEMORY

In Chinese medicine, memory depends on the state of the Spleen, Kidneys and Heart and there is a considerable overlap among these three organs' functions.

The Spleen houses Intellect and influences memory in the sense of memorization, studying and concentrating. Its corresponding pathological aspect is excessive thinking and pensiveness.

The Kidneys house Will-Power and influence the brain since the Kidney-Essence produces Marrow which nourishes the brain. The Kidneys are responsible for memory in the sense of memorization of everyday events, names, faces, etc. It will be remembered (see chapter 9 on mental-emotional problems) that *Zhi* of the Kidneys, apart from "will-power", also means "memory".

The Heart controls memory because it houses the Mind. There is a considerable overlap between the Kidneys and Heart with regard to memory, but the Heart is responsible more for the memory of long-past events rather than of everyday things like the Kidneys.

AETIOLOGY

1. WORRY AND PENSIVENESS

Worry and pensiveness affect Lungs, Spleen and Heart and they influence memory simply because the Spleen and Heart's mental capacity is employed in worrying and obsessive thinking and cannot therefore be used for memorization.

2. OVERWORK AND EXCESSIVE SEXUAL ACTIVITY

Overwork and excessive sexual activity weaken Kidney-Yin and Kidney-Essence which decreases mental power and memory.

3. CHILDBIRTH

Excessive bleeding at childbirth weakens Blood

and affects the Heart. Deficient Heart-Blood is unable to nourish the brain and the Mind, and poor memory results.

4. SADNESS

Sadness depletes Heart-Qi so that this cannot brighten the Mind and poor memory results.

5. "RECREATIONAL" DRUGS

Prolonged and continued use of cannabis and other drugs is an important cause of poor memory and concentration. It would appear that the conversion of short-term to long-term memory is impaired by prolonged use of cannabis due to interference by a flow of sensory impressions.[49] Moreover, there have also been reports of loss of brain substance in heavy users of cannabis.[50] I have certainly verified the relationship between heavy, long-term use of cannabis and poor memory in my clinical practice.

DIFFERENTIATION AND TREATMENT

1. SPLEEN DEFICIENCY

Clinical manifestations

Inability to concentrate and study, poor memory, tiredness, poor appetite.
Tongue: Pale.
Pulse: Weak.

Treatment principle

Tonify the Spleen and strengthen the Intellect.

Acupuncture

ST-36 Zusanli, SP-3 Taibai, Du-20 Baihui, BL-15 Xinshu, Du-14 Dazhui with moxa, BL-20 Pishu, BL-49 Yishe. Reinforcing method.

Explanation

- **ST-36** and **SP-3** tonify the Spleen and strengthen the Intellect.
- **Du-20** raises clear Yang to the head to brighten the Mind and Intellect.

- **BL-15**, Back-Transporting point of the Heart, strengthens the Mind and the Intellect.
- **Du-14** with moxa also facilitates the rising of clear Yang to the brain.
- **BL-20** and **BL-49** tonify the Spleen and strengthen the Intellect and memory.

Herbal treatment

Prescription

GUI PI TANG
Tonifying the Spleen Decoction
Ren Shen *Radix Ginseng* 6 g (**Dang Shen** *Radix Codonopsis pilosulae* 12 g)
Huang Qi *Radix Astragali membranacei* 15 g
Bai Zhu *Rhizoma Atractylodis macrocephalae* 12 g
Dang Gui *Radix Angelicae sinensis* 3 g
Fu Shen *Sclerotium Poriae cocos pararadicis* 9 g
Suan Zao Ren *Semen Ziziphi spinosae* 9 g
Long Yan Rou *Arillus Euphoriae longanae* 12 g
Yuan Zhi *Radix Polygalae tenuifoliae* 9 g
Mu Xiang *Radix Saussureae* 6 g
Zhi Gan Cao *Radix Glycyrrhizae uralensis praeparata* 4 g
Sheng Jiang *Rhizoma Zingiberis officinalis recens* 3 slices
Hong Zao *Fructus Ziziphi jujubae* 5 dates

Explanation

This formula, which has already been explained in this chapter and chapter 9, tonifies Heart-Qi and Heart-Blood and therefore strengthens the Mind and memory.

2. KIDNEY-ESSENCE DEFICIENCY

Clinical manifestations

Poor everyday memory, dizziness, tinnitus, weak knees and back.
Tongue: Pale or Red according to whether there is Kidney-Yang or Kidney-Yin deficiency.
Pulse: Deep and Fine.

Treatment principle

Tonify the Kidneys, nourish Essence and Marrow and strengthen memory.

Acupuncture

KI-3 Taixi, Ren-4 Guanyuan, BL-23 Shenshu, BL-52 Zhishi, BL-15 Xinshu, Du-20 Baihui. Reinforcing method.

Explanation

- **KI-3**, **Ren-4** and **BL-23** tonify the Kidneys.
- **BL-52** strengthens the Will Power and memory.
- **BL-15** strengthens the Mind and memory.
- **Du-20** facilitates the rising of clear Yang to the head.

Herbal treatment

Prescription

LIU WEI DI HUANG WAN Variation
Six-Ingredient Rehmannia Pill
Shu Di Huang *Radix Rehmanniae glutinosae praeparata* 24 g
Shan Zhu Yu *Fructus Corni officinalis* 12 g
Shan Yao *Radix Dioscoreae oppositae* 12 g
Ze Xie *Rhizoma Alismatis orientalis* 9 g
Mu Dan Pi *Cortex Moutan radicis* 9 g
Fu Ling *Sclerotium Poriae cocos* 9 g
Suan Zao Ren *Semen Ziziphi spinosae* 4.5 g
Wu Wei Zi *Fructus Schisandrae chinensis* 4.5 g
Yuan Zhi *Radix Polygalae tenuifoliae* 6 g
Shi Chang Pu *Rhizoma Acori graminei* 6 g

Explanation

- The first six herbs contitute the Liu Wei Di Huang Wan which nourishes Kidney-Yin.
- **Suan Zao Ren**, **Wu Wei Zi** and **Yuan Zhi** are added to enter the Heart and strengthen the Mind and memory.
- **Chang Pu** opens the Mind's orifices and improves memory by facilitating the rising of clear Qi to the head.

Variations

- If there is both Yin and Yang deficiency add Lu Jiao Jiao *Colla Cornu Cervi*, Ba Ji Tian *Radix Morindae officinalis* and Zi He Che *Placenta hominis*.

3. HEART DEFICIENCY

Clinical manifestations

Poor memory of past events, forgetting names, absent-mindedness, palpitations, slight breathlessness on exertion, tiredness.
Tongue: Heart-crack. Pale or Red, depending whether there is Yang or Yin deficiency.
Pulse: Weak.

Treatment principle

Tonify the Heart, strengthen the Mind and memory.

Acupuncture

HE-5 Tongli, BL-15 Xinshu, BL-44 Shentang, Ren-6 Qihai, Du-14 Dazhui, with reinforcing method.

If Phlegm obstructs the Heart, use ST-40 Fenglong and Ren-14 Juque with reducing method.

Explanation

- **HE-5** and **BL-15** tonify Heart-Qi and strengthen the Mind.
- **BL-44** strengthens the Mind and memory.
- **Ren-6** with moxa tonifies Qi in general.
- **Du-14** with moxa tonifies the Heart and brightens the Mind. It is coordinated with Ren-6: one is on the Directing Vessel, the other on the Governing Vessel, both of which flow through the Heart.
- **ST-40** and **Ren-14** resolve Phlegm from the Heart.

Herbal treatment

Prescription

ZHEN ZHONG DAN
Bedside Pill
Gui Ban *Plastrum Testudinis* 10 g
Long Gu *Os Draconis* 10 g
Yuan Zhi *Radix Polygalae tenuifoliae* 10 g
Shi Chang Pu *Rhizoma Acori graminei* 10 g

Explanation

- **Gui Ban** and **Long Gu** are absorbing and sinking substances. They pacify the Mind by sinking Qi and restoring the Mind to its residence, i.e. the Heart.

- **Yuan Zhi** and **Chang Pu** open the Heart's orifices and brighten the Mind.

This formula could also be used for poor memory from other Heart patterns such as Heart Empty-Heat.

END NOTES

1. 1979 The Yellow Emperor's Classic of Internal Medicine — Simple Questions (*Huang Ti Nei Jing Su Wen* 黄帝内经素问), People's Health Publishing House, Beijing. First published *c.* 100 BC, p. 256.
2. Tang Zong Hai 1892 The Essence of the Convergence between Chinese and Western Medicine (*Zhong Xi Hui Tong Yi Jing Jing Yi* 中西汇通医经精), cited in Theory of the Mind in Chinese Medicine, p. 36.
3. Zhang Jing Yue 1986 The Complete Book of Jing Yue (*Jing Yue Quan Shu* 景岳全书), Shanghai Science Publishing House, Shanghai. First published 1624, p. 329.
4 Ibid., p. 329.
5. Spiritual Axis, p. 152.
6. Simple Questions, p. 102.
7. Ibid., p. 102.
8. Ibid., p. 102.
9. Ibid., p. 102.
10. Ibid., p. 102.
11. Ibid., p. 102.
12. Ibid., p. 102.
13. Ibid., p. 102.
14. Ibid., p. 102.
15. Ibid., p. 102.
16. Ibid., p. 103.
17. Ibid., p. 569.
18. Ibid., p. 569.
19. 1981 Spiritual Axis (*Ling Shu Jing* 灵枢经), People's Health Publishing House, Beijing. First published *c.* 100 BC, p. 84.
20. Ibid., p. 84.
21. Simple Questions, p. 569.
22. Ibid., p. 569.
23. Spiritual Axis, p. 85.
24. Simple Questions, p. 569.
25. Ibid., p. 569.
26. Spiritual Axis, p. 85.
27. Ibid., p. 85.
28. Simple Questions, p. 569.
29. Ibid., p. 569.
30. Spiritual Axis, p. 85.
31. Ibid., p. 85.
32. Simple Questions, p. 569.
33. Ibid., p. 569.
34. Spiritual Axis, p. 85.
35. Ibid., p. 85.
36. Ibid., p. 85.
37. Ibid., p. 85.
38. Ibid., p. 85.
39. Ibid., p. 85.
40. Ibid., p. 85.
41. Ibid., p. 85.
42. Simple Questions, p. 256.
43. Ibid., p. 199.
44. Spiritual Axis, p. 56.
45. Simple Questions, p. 199.
46. Spiritual Axis, p. 51.
47. Ibid., p. 24.
48. Spiritual Axis, p. 152.
49. D. R. Laurence 1973 Clinical Pharmacology, Churchill Livingstone, Edinburgh, p. 14.29.
50. Ibid., p. 14.30.

Tinnitus 11

耳

鳴

Tinnitus indicates the subjective sensation experienced on hearing a noise in one or both ears. The noise may be constant or coming in bouts and may vary in intensity and character. It may sound like a high-pitched whistle, like bells, like an engine running, or like rushing water.

Although the Kidneys open into the ears, many other organs also influence the ears and may be involved in causing tinnitus. The Gall-Bladder channel, for example, flows through the ear and is very much involved in ear problems, especially those of an Excess nature.

Aetiology and pathology

1. EMOTIONAL STRAIN

Emotional problems such as anger, frustration, resentment, or hatred cause Liver-Qi stagnation and, in the long run, Liver-Fire which may rise upwards to disturb the ears. This may cause tinnitus with a sudden onset and a loud noise.

Emotions such as sadness, grief and worry which weaken Lungs and Heart may also lead to tinnitus. This occurs when deficient Heart- and Lung-Qi fail to rise to the head to brighten the ear orifices.

2. EXCESSIVE SEXUAL ACTIVITY AND OVERWORK

These weaken the Kidneys so that they cannot nourish the ear and tinnitus may result. This type of tinnitus is of gradual onset and the noise is of low pitch. This is the most common cause of tinnitus.

3. OLD AGE

Kidney-Essence declines naturally as we grow older and, in old people, it may fail to nourish the ears and brain leading to tinnitus. This does not mean, of course, that every old person will inevitably suffer from tinnitus. This type of tinnitus would also have a very gradual onset and a low sound.

4. DIET

Excessive consumption of dairy products and greasy foods, together with irregular eating habits, may lead to the formation of Phlegm which may rise to the head. Here it prevents the rising of clear Qi to the head to brighten its orifices (which include the ears), and the descending of turbid Qi from the head, resulting in tinnitus and dizziness.

5. EXPOSURE TO LOUD SOUNDS

Long-term exposure to very loud sounds such as may occur in certain factories or in discotheques where loud rock music is played may also cause tinnitus.

Thus, as always, the most important differentiation is that between Full and Empty types of tinnitus. Full types of tinnitus are caused by the flaring up of some pathogenic factors disturbing the ear. These are usually Fire, Wind, Yang, Phlegm, or Phlegm-Fire. The tinnitus deriving from exposure to loud sounds is also considered to be of the Full type and is treated as such. Empty types of tinnitus are due to not enough Qi (intended in a broad sense) reaching the head and ears. This may be Kidney-Qi, Kidney-Essence, Lung-Qi or Heart-Blood.

From a diagnostic point of view, tinnitus with a sudden onset and a loud sound is of the Full type. It is also aggravated by cupping one's hands over the ears. Tinnitus with a gradual onset and a low sound is of the Empty type. It is improved by cupping one's hands over the ears.

Differentiation and treatment

The patterns discussed will be:

EXCESS TYPE

Rising of Liver and Gall-Bladder Fire
Phlegm-Fire Flaring Upwards

DEFICIENCY TYPE

Kidney-Essence Deficiency
Upper Burner Qi Weak
Heart-Blood Deficiency

EXCESS

1. RISING OF LIVER AND GALL-BLADDER FIRE

CLINICAL MANIFESTATIONS

Tinnitus with a sudden onset and loud sound and clearly related to emotional strain, headache, irritability, a bitter taste, thirst, red face, dizziness, constipation.
Tongue: Red with redder sides, yellow coating.
Pulse: Wiry and Rapid.

TREATMENT PRINCIPLE

Drain Liver-Fire, ease the ears, calm the Mind and settle the Ethereal Soul.

ACUPUNCTURE

LIV-2 Xingjian, T.B.-17 Yifeng, T.B.-5 Waiguan, T.B.-3 Zhongzhu, G.B.-43 Xiaxi, G.B.-20 Fengchi, G.B.-8 Shuaigu. Reducing method.

Explanation

- **LIV-2** drains Liver-Fire.
- **T.B.-17** is the main local point for this type of tinnitus. The needle should be inserted to a depth of 1 *cun* and the needling sensation should be very strong.
- **T.B.-5** subdues Liver-Yang.
- **T.B.-3** subdues Liver-Yang and eases the ears.
- **G.B.-43** drains Gall-Bladder Fire and affects the ears.

- **G.B.-20** subdues Liver-Yang and eases the ear if needled with the tip of the needle pointing towards the area between eye and ear on the same side. In other words, the needle is oblique towards the front of the face.
- **G.B.-8** is an adjacent point which eases the ear and subdues Liver-Yang.

HERBAL TREATMENT

Prescription

LONG DAN XIE GAN TANG
Gentiana Draining the Liver Decoction
Long Dan Cao *Radix Gentianae scabrae* 6 g
Huang Qin *Radix Scutellariae baicalensis* 9 g
Shan Zhi Zi *Fructus Gardeniae jasminoidis* 9 g
Ze Xie *Rhizoma Alismatis orientalis* 9 g
Mu Tong *Caulis Akebiae* 9 g
Che Qian Zi *Semen Plantaginis* 9 g
Sheng Di Huang *Radix Rehmanniae glutinosae* 12 g
Dang Gui *Radix Angelicae sinensis* 9 g
Chai Hu *Radix Bupleuri* 9 g
Gan Cao *Radix Glycyrrhizae uralensis* 3 g

Explanation

This formula, which has already been explained in chapters 1 and 10, is suitable to treat tinnitus without modifications.

Variations

- To direct the prescription to the ears add Ci Shi *Magnetitum*. Especially in combination with Chai Hu, this herb directs other herbs to the ear.
- If there are symptoms of Liver-Yang or Liver-Wind rising add Tian Ma *Rhizoma Gastrodiae elatae*, Gou Teng *Ramulus Uncariae* and Shi Jue Ming *Concha Haliotidis*.
- If there is constipation and a very thick and dry tongue coating add Da Huang *Rhizoma Rhei*.

(i) Patent remedy

JI GU CAO WAN
Abrum Pill

Ji Gu Cao *Fructus Abri*
She Dan *Snake's bile*
Zhen Zhu *Margarita*
Niu Huang *Calculus Bovis*
Dang Gui *Radix Angelicae sinensis*
Gou Qi Zi *Fructus Lycii chinensis*
Dan Shen *Radix Salviae miltiorrhizae*

This pill is suitable for tinnitus from Liver-Fire or Liver-Yang rising.

The tongue presentation appropriate to this remedy is a Red body with a dirty-sticky coating.

(ii) Patent remedy

LONG DAN XIE GAN WAN
Gentiana Draining the Liver Pill
This remedy has the same ingredients and indications as the decoction above.

This pill is also suitable for tinnitus from Liver-Fire and more widely used than the previous one.

The tongue presentation appropriate to this remedy is a Red body with redder sides and a yellow coating.

Case history

A 39-year-old man had been suffering from tinnitus for one year. It had started fairly suddenly and was of a high pitch. It was better with rest and worse when under stress. He did not have any other symptom.

His tongue was Red, redder on the sides, with a yellow coating. His pulse was very Full and Wiry and slightly Rapid and slightly Weak on both Rear positions.

Diagnosis
His tinnitus was due primarily to Liver and Gall-Bladder Fire blazing upwards. Although he did not have many symptoms, the high pitch of the tinnitus, its aggravation under stress and, most of all, the tongue indicated Liver-Fire. However, there was also an underlying slight deficiency of Kidney-Yin as shown by the pulse being Weak on both Rear positions and also by the fact that the tinnitus improved with rest. This is probably the reason why the tinnitus started at an age when Kidney-Qi is just beginning to decline.

Treatment principle
Clear the Liver and Gall-Bladder, drain Fire, benefit the ears and nourish Kidney-Yin.

Acupuncture
T.B.-2 Yemen, L.I.-4 Hegu, LIV-2 Xingjian, G.B.-43
Xiaxi, T.B.-17 Yifeng, G.B.-2 Tinghui, SP-6 Sanyinjiao
and KI-3 Taixi. The first six points were reduced
while the last two were reinforced.

Explanation
- **T.B.-2** indirectly subdues Liver-Fire and benefits
  the ear. It is an important distal point for tinnitus of
  the Excess type.
- **L.I.-4** was used as a distal point to affect the ear and
  also to calm the Mind.
- **LIV-2** and **G.B.-43** clear Liver-Fire and Gall-
  Bladder-Fire respectively. G.B.-43 also affects the
  ear.
- **T.B.-17** and **G.B.-2** are the main local points for
  tinnitus of the Excess type.
- **SP-6** and **KI-3** nourish Kidney-Yin.

Herbal treatment
No herbs were prescribed but two patent remedies
were used: Long Dan Xie Gan Wan *Gentiana Draining
the Liver Pill* (8 pills twice a day) to drain Liver and
Gall-Bladder Fire and Er Ming Zuo Ci Wan *Tinnitus
Pill that is Kind to the Left [Kidney]* (a small dose of 6
pills a day in the evening) to nourish Kidney-Yin.

2. PHLEGM-FIRE FLARING UPWARDS

CLINICAL MANIFESTATIONS

Tinnitus sound like cicadas or crickets, impaired
hearing, a feeling of oppression of the chest, expectoration of sputum, thirst, a feeling of muzziness in the head and dizziness.
Tongue: Red, Swollen, sticky-yellow coating.
Pulse: Slippery and Rapid.

TREATMENT PRINCIPLE

Resolve Phlegm, drain Fire, subdue Liver-Yang,
regulate the ascending of clear Qi and descending of turbid Qi, tonify the Spleen.

ACUPUNCTURE

T.B.-21 Ermen, S.I.-19 Tinggong, G.B.-2 Tinghui,
T.B.-5 Waiguan, T.B.-3 Zhongzhu, L.I.-4 Hegu,
Ren-9 Shuifen, ST-40 Fenglong, SP-9 Yinling-
quan, G.B.-20 Fengchi, Ren-12 Zhongwan, BL-20
Pishu. Reducing method on all points except the
last two which should be reinforced.

Explanation

- **T.B.-21** is the main local point for this type of
  tinnitus.
- **T.B.-21**, **S.I.-19** and **G.B.-2** can regulate the
  ascending of clear Qi to the ear and
  descending of turbid Qi away from the ear.
  Some doctors recommend needling these
  three points, for 5 consecutive treatments,
  simultaneously horizontally from top to
  bottom, i.e. from T.B.-21 to G.B.-2: this makes
  the turbid Qi descend from the ear. Then
  needle the same three points, for another 5
  consecutive treatments, horizontally
  upwards, i.e. from G.B.-2 to T.B.-21: this
  makes the clear Qi ascend to the ear.
- **T.B.-5** and **T.B.-3** subdue Liver-Yang and ease
  the ear.
- **L.I.-4** regulates the ascending of clear Qi and
  descending of turbid Qi in the head.
- **Ren-9**, **ST-40** and **SP-9** resolve Phlegm.
- **G.B.-20** subdues Liver-Yang and eases the ear
  if needled as explained for the previous
  pattern.
- **Ren-12** and **BL-20** tonify the Spleen to resolve
  Phlegm.

HERBAL TREATMENT

Prescription

WEN DAN TANG
Warming the Gall-Bladder Decoction
Ban Xia *Rhizoma Pinelliae ternatae* 6 g
Fu Ling *Sclerotium Poriae cocos* 5 g
Chen Pi *Pericarpium Citri reticulatae* 9 g
Zhu Ru *Caulis Bambusae in Taenis* 6 g
Zhi Shi *Fructus Citri aurantii immaturus* 6 g
Zhi Gan Cao *Radix Glycyrrhizae uralensis prae-
parata* 3 g
Sheng Jiang *Rhizoma Zingiberis officinalis recens*
5 slices
Da Zao *Fructus Ziziphi jujubae* one date

Explanation

This formula, which has already been explained
in chapter 9, resolves Phlegm-Heat mostly from
the chest.

Variations

- To direct the prescription to the ears add Chai Hu *Radix Bupleuri* and Ci Shi *Magnetitum*.
- If Phlegm is abundant add Dan Nan Xing *Rhizoma Arisaemae* and Hai Fu Shi *Pumice*.

Case history

A 39-year-old man had been suffering from tinnitus for the previous 11 years. The tinnitus had started gradually and he said it sounded like a jet engine. He also suffered from lower back-ache, dizziness, a slight loss of hearing and slight impotence with an occasional discharge of mucus-like substance from the penis.

He also complained of diarrhoea or loose stools, a problem he had had since his teenage years. His stools were often mixed with some mucus. He slept badly, waking up frequently with a dry throat.

He had some soft swellings under the skin on the limbs which had been diagnosed as ganglioneuromas. Finally, he also complained of constant mucus on his chest and dryness of the mouth.

His tongue and pulse were rather complex. His tongue was slightly Red, Swollen with swollen sides (of the Spleen type). The coating was rootless and missing in places. There was a deep Heart-crack. His pulse was Fine on the right, slightly Slippery and Full on the left, with the left Front position (Heart) very slightly Overflowing but Empty and somewhat pointed in shape.

Diagnosis

There are three main problems, the longest standing being Spleen deficiency leading to Phlegm. The Spleen deficiency causes diarrhoea and loose stools and a Fine pulse on the right side. Phlegm is reflected by the Slippery pulse, the presence of mucus in the stools, the discharge from the penis, the ganglioneuromas and the swelling of the tongue. The second problem is a Kidney-Yin deficiency reflected in the dizziness, loss of hearing, insomnia with dry throat at night and impotence. Finally, there is also some Stomach-Yin deficiency which most probably preceded the Kidney-Yin deficiency. The Stomach-Yin deficiency is mirrored in the coating being rootless and missing in places and in the dryness of the mouth. Underlying all of this, there was also a certain deficiency of Heart-Qi from emotional problems obviously dating back to childhood or teenage years. One can tell this from the Heart-crack on the tongue and the Heart pulse being slightly Overflowing but Empty. These two findings often indicate that the Heart is affected by emotional problems. That these date back to the patient's early years is indicated by the depth of the crack: the deeper it is, the older the emotional problems that caused it.

As for the tinnitus, this is caused by both an Excess and a Deficiency: Excess in the form of Phlegm obstructing the head's orifices (in this case the ears) and Deficiency in the form of Kidney-Yin deficiency.

Treatment principle

Tonify the Spleen, resolve Phlegm, nourish Kidney-Yin and calm the Mind.

Acupuncture

Many different points were used at different times, but the main ones were:
- **ST-36** Zusanli, **Ren-12** Zhongwan and **ST-40** Fenglong to tonify the Spleen and resolve Phlegm.
- **ST-25** Tianshu to stop diarrhoea.
- **KI-3** Taixi and **Ren-4** Guanyuan to nourish Kidney-Yin.
- **HE-5** Tongli and **HE-7** Shenmen to calm the Mind.
- **S.I.-19** Tinggong and **T.B.-17** Yifeng as local points for the tinnitus.

Herbal treatment

No decoctions were used but herbal powders were. The formulae used were Shen Ling Bai Zhu San *Ginseng-Poria-Atractylodes Powder* to tonify Spleen-Qi and Stomach-Yin and Ban Xia Bai Zhu Tian Ma Tang *Pinellia-Atractylodes-Gastrodia Decoction* to resolve Phlegm from the head.

This patient is gradually improving and is still being treated at the time of writing.

DEFICIENCY

1. KIDNEY-ESSENCE DEFICIENCY

CLINICAL MANIFESTATIONS

Tinnitus with gradual onset and low sound sometimes like rushing water and coming in bouts, slight dizziness, a feeling of emptiness of the head, poor memory, blurred vision, sore back and knees, diminished sexual desire or performance.

Tongue: Pale or Red without coating depending on whether there is a deficiency of Kidney-Yang or Kidney-Yin.

Pulse: Deep and Weak if there is Kidney-Yang deficiency and Floating-Empty in case of Kidney-Yin deficiency.

- If the Kidneys and Heart are not harmonized there will also be palpitations, insomnia, mental restlessness and a dry throat.
- If there is Liver-Yang rising from Kidney-Yin deficiency there will also be dizziness, irritability and headaches.

This corresponds to deficiency of the Sea of Marrow and brain. The deficient Kidney-Essence fails to nourish the Sea of Marrow and brain and ears resulting in tinnitus, dizziness and poor memory. The Kidney-Essence has a Yang and a Yin aspect and its deficiency can therefore manifest with symptoms of deficiency of either.

The Kidneys and Heart communicate with each other, Kidney-Water flowing upwards to the Heart and Heart-Fire flowing downwards to the Kidneys. If Heart-Fire fails to reach down to the Kidneys, the tinnitus will be worse and there will be the additional symptoms outlined above.

If Kidney-Yin is deficient it may cause Liver-Yang to rise: in this case the tinnitus may present with contradictory signs as it is caused both by the deficiency of Kidney-Yin and the rising of Liver-Yang. For example, tinnitus with a loud sound and a high pitch (which indicates an Excess condition, in this case Liver-Yang rising) may have a gradual onset (which indicates a Deficiency condition, in this case Kidney-Yin deficiency).

TREATMENT PRINCIPLE

Nourish the Essence, benefit the Sea of Marrow, tonify Kidney-Yang or nourish Kidney-Yin. If necessary, harmonize Heart and Kidneys and subdue Liver-Yang.

ACUPUNCTURE

G.B.-2 Tinghui, KI-3 Taixi, Ren-4 Guanyuan, BL-23 Shenshu, KI-7 Fuliu, Du-4 Mingmen, SP-6 Sanyinjiao, HE-6 Yinxi, LIV-3 Taichong. Reinforcing method on all points except for the last two which should be needled with even method. Use moxa in Kidney-Yang deficiency.

Explanation

- **G.B.-2** is the main local point for this type of tinnitus.
- **KI-3**, **Ren-4**, **BL-23** and **KI-7** tonify the Kidneys and the Essence.
- **Du-4**, with moxa, is used only if there is a Kidney-Yang deficiency.

- **SP-6** helps to nourish the Kidneys.
- **HE-6**, in combination with KI-7, harmonizes Heart and Kidneys.
- **LIV-3** subdues Liver-Yang.

HERBAL TREATMENT

(a) Prescription

ER LONG ZUO CI WAN
Pill for Deafness that is Kind to the Left [Kidney]
Shu Di Huang *Radix Rehmanniae glutinosae praeparata* 24 g
Shan Zhu Yu *Fructus Corni officinalis* 12 g
Shan Yao *Radix Dioscoreae oppositae* 12 g
Ze Xie *Rhizoma Alismatis orientalis* 9 g
Mu Dan Pi *Cortex Moutan radicis* 9 g
Fu Ling *Sclerotium Poriae cocos* 9 g
Ci Shi *Magnetitum* 24 g
Shi Chang Pu *Rhizoma Acori graminei* 9 g
Wu Wei Zi *Fructus Schisandrae chinensis* 6 g

Explanation

This formula is selected if the deficiency of Kidney-Essence presents with symptoms and signs of Kidney-Yin deficiency.

- The first six herbs constitute the Liu Wei Di Huang Wan to nourish Kidney-Yin.
- **Ci Shi** sinks Liver-Yang and treats tinnitus and deafness.
- **Chang Pu** opens the orifices and therefore opens the ears.
- **Wu Wei Zi** nourishes Yin and, being sour, moderates the pungency of Chang Pu.

Variations

- If the symptoms of Yin deficiency are pronounced add Gui Ban *Plastrum Testudinis*, Mu Li *Concha Ostreae* and Nu Zhen Zi *Fructus Ligustri lucidi*.

(b) Prescription

YOU GUI WAN
Restoring the Right [Kidney] Pill
Fu Zi *Radix Aconiti carmichaeli praeparata* 3 g
Rou Gui *Cortex Cinnamomi cassiae* 3 g

Du Zhong *Cortex Eucommiae ulmoidis* 6 g
Shan Zhu Yu *Fructus Corni officinalis* 4.5 g
Tu Si Zi *Semen Cuscutae* 6 g
Lu Jiao Jiao *Colla Cornu Cervi* 6 g
Shu Di Huang *Radix Rehmanniae glutinosae prae-parata* 12 g
Shan Yao *Rhizoma Dioscoreae oppositae* 6 g
Gou Qi Zi *Fructus Lycii chinensis* 6 g
Dang Gui *Radix Angelicae sinensis* 4.5 g

Explanation

This formula, which has already been explained in chapter 1, tonifies Kidney-Yang. It is suitable for tinnitus from Kidney-Essence deficiency because it contains also Lu Jiao Jiao and Gou Qi Zi which nourish the Essence.

Variations

– To direct the formula to the ear and treat tinnitus add Chai Hu *Radix Bupleuri* and Ci Shi *Magnetitum*.

(c) Prescription

TIAN WANG BU XIN DAN
Heavenly Emperor Tonifying the Heart Pill
Sheng Di Huang *Radix Rehmanniae glutinosae* 12 g
Xuan Shen *Radix Scrophulariae ningpoensis* 6 g
Mai Men Dong *Tuber Ophiopogonis japonici* 6 g
Tian Men Dong *Tuber Asparagi cochinchinensis* 6 g
Ren Shen *Radix Ginseng* 6 g
Fu Ling *Sclerotium Poriae cocos* 6 g
Wu Wei Zi *Fructus Schisandrae chinensis* 6 g
Dang Gui *Radix Angelicae sinensis* 6 g
Dan Shen *Radix Salviae miltiorrhizae* 6 g
Bai Zi Ren *Semen Biotae orientalis* 6 g
Suan Zao Ren *Semen Ziziphi spinosae* 6 g
Yuan Zhi *Radix Polygalae tenuifoliae* 6 g
Jie Geng *Radix Platycodi grandiflori* 3 g

Explanation

This formula, which has already been explained in chapter 9, is selected if there is deficiency of both Kidney- and Heart-Yin.

(i) Patent remedy

ER MING ZUO CI WAN
Tinnitus Pill that is Kind to the Left [Kidney]
Shu Di Huang *Radix Rehmanniae glutinosae praeparata*
Shan Yao *Rhizoma Dioscoreae oppositae*
Shan Zhu Yu *Fructus Corni officinalis*
Ze Xie *Rhizoma Alismatis orientalis*
Fu Ling *Sclerotium Poriae cocos*
Mu Dan Pi *Cortex Moutan radicis*
Ci Shi *Magnetitum*
Chai Hu *Radix Bupleuri*

This remedy nourishes Kidney-Yin, subdues Liver-Yang and benefits the ear. It is specific for tinnitus. If a patient suffers from Kidney-Yang deficiency, this remedy may still be given in the evening (about 10 pills) supplemented by 10 pills of Jin Gui Shen Qi Wan *Golden Chest Kidney-Qi Pill* in the morning.

The tongue presentation appropriate to this remedy is a Red body without coating.

(ii) Patent remedy

GE JIE DA BU WAN
Gecko Big Tonifying Pill
Ge Jie *Gecko*
Dang Sheng *Radix Codonopsis pilosulae*
Huang Qi *Radix Astragali membranacei*
Gou Qi Zi *Fructus Lycii chinensis*
Dang Gui *Radix Angelicae sinensis*
Fu Ling *Sclerotium Poriae cocos*
Shu Di Huang *Radix Rehmanniae glutinosae praeparata*
Nu Zhen Zi *Fructus Ligustri lucidi*
Gan Cao *Radix Glycyrrhizae uralensis*
Shan Yao *Radix Dioscoreae oppositae*
Mu Gua *Fructus Chaenomelis lagenariae*
Ba Ji Tian *Radix Morindae officinalis*
Bai Zhi *Radix Angelicae dahuricae*
Xu Duan *Radix Dipsaci*
Du Zhong *Cortex Eucommiae ulmoidis*
Huang Jing *Rhizoma Polygonati*
Gu Sui Bu *Rhizoma Gusuibu*

This remedy is suitable for tinnitus from Kidney-Yang deficiency.

The tongue presentation appropriate to this remedy is a Pale and wet body.

(iii) Patent remedy

JIAN NAO WAN
Strengthening the Brain Pill
Suan Zao Ren *Semen Ziziphi spinosae*
Shan Yao *Radix Dioscoreae oppositae*
Rou Cong Rong *Herba Cistanchis*
Wu Wei Zi *Fructus Schisandrae chinensis*
Hu Po *Succinum*
Long Chi *Dens Draconis*
Tian Ma *Rhizoma Gastrodiae elatae*
Ren Shen *Radix Ginseng*
Dang Gui *Radix Angelicae sinensis*
Gou Qi Zi *Fructus Lycii chinensis*
Yi Zhi Ren *Fructus Alpiniae oxyphyllae*
Tian Zhu Huang *Concretio Silicea Bambusae*
Jiu Jie Chang Pu *Rhizoma Anemonis altaicae*
Zhu Sha *Cinnabaris*
Bai Zi Ren *Semen Biotae orientalis*

This pill is suitable for tinnitus from both Kidney-Yin or Kidney-Yang deficiency. It should be noted that it contains cinnabar which is toxic and should therefore be used only for short periods (a few weeks) at a time.

(iv) Patent remedy

TIAN WANG BU XIN DAN
Heavenly Emperor Tonifying the Heart Pill
Same ingredients as decoction of the same name.

This pill is for tinnitus from Kidney and Heart not harmonized, i.e. deficiency of Kidney-Yin and Heart-Yin with Heart Empty-Heat.

It should be noted that this pill is often coated with cinnabar in which case it should only be used for short periods (a few weeks) at a time. Not all manufacturers, however, coat the pills with cinnabar. The pills are reddish in colour if coated in cinnabar, black, if not.

Case history

A 36-year-old man had complained of tinnitus for the past 10 years. The tinnitus started gradually over several years and other symptoms included lower back-ache, dizziness, sweating at night and general tiredness. He also slept badly, waking up frequently with a dry mouth.

His tongue was Red with a coating which was too thin although not entirely missing. His pulse was weak on both Rear positions.

Diagnosis
This is a very clear case of Kidney-Yin deficiency as indicated by the symptoms and the tongue. The tongue still has a coating, albeit too thin, as he is still young. If the condition were allowed to deteriorate without treatment, the tongue would gradually lose its coating completely over the next few years.

Treatment principle
Nourish Kidney-Yin and benefit the ears.

Acupuncture
The main points used were:

- **KI-3** Taixi and **Ren-4** Guanyuan to strengthen the Kidneys.
- **ST-36** Zusanli and **SP-6** Sanyinjiao to tonify Qi and Blood which will help to nourish the Kidney-Essence.
- **T.B.-17** Yifeng and **S.I.-19** Tinggong as local points.

Herbal treatment
No herbs were prescribed but only the patent remedy Er Ming Zuo Ci Wan *Tinnitus Pill that is Kind to the Left [Kidney]*.

This man is still under treatment and is gradually improving. Although tinnitus is difficult to treat, the prognosis in this case is relatively good due to his young age.

2. UPPER BURNER QI WEAK

CLINICAL MANIFESTATIONS

Intermittent tinnitus quite mild with a low sound and gradual onset, tiredness, slight breathlessness, pale complexion, slight spontaneous sweating.
Tongue: Pale, teeth-marks.
Pulse: Empty, especially in the right Front position.

This corresponds to deficiency of Lung-Qi with the deficient Lung-Qi unable to rise towards the head, thus causing tinnitus.

TREATMENT PRINCIPLE

Tonify Lung-Qi, promote the rising of clear Qi to the head.

ACUPUNCTURE

Ren-17 Shanzhong, BL-13 Feishu, LU-9 Taiyuan,

Ren-6 Qihai, Du-20 Baihui, T.B.-16 Tianyou, S.I.-19 Tinggong. Reinforcing method. Moxa may be used.

Explanation

- **Ren-17**, **BL-13** and **LU-9** tonify Lung-Qi.
- **Ren-6** tonifies Qi in general.
- **Du-20** and **T.B.-16** raise clear Qi to the head.
- **S.I.-19** is the main local point for this type of tinnitus.

HERBAL TREATMENT

Prescription

BU QI CONG MING TANG
Tonifying Qi Clear Hearing Decoction
Huang Qi *Radix Astragali membranacei* 12 g
Ren Shen *Radix Ginseng* 9 g
Sheng Ma *Rhizoma Cimicifugae* 3 g
Ge Gen *Radix Puerariae* 3 g
Man Jing Zi *Fructus Viticis* 3 g
Bai Shao *Radix Paeoniae albae* 6 g
Huang Bo *Cortex Phellodendri* 6 g
Zhi Gan Cao *Radix Glycyrrhizae uralensis prae-parata* 3 g

Explanation

- **Huang Qi** and **Ren Shen** tonify and raise Qi.
- **Sheng Ma**, **Ge Gen** and **Man Jing Zi** raise clear Qi and brighten the orifices.
- **Bai Shao** and **Huang Bo** make turbid Qi descend. Huang Bo makes turbid Qi descend via urination and Bai Shao directs Huang Bo to the Yin (turbid Qi) portion.
- **Gan Cao** harmonizes.

Variations

- If there are signs of Phlegm in the head add Bai Zhu *Rhizoma Atractylodis macrocephalae*, Tian Ma *Rhizoma Gastrodiae elatae* and Ban Xia *Rhizoma Pinelliae ternatae*.

Patent remedy

BU ZHONG YI QI WAN
Tonifying the Centre and Benefiting Qi Pill

Huang Qi *Radix Astragali membranacei*
Dang Shen *Radix Codonopsis pilosulae*
Zhi Gan Cao *Radix Glycyrrhizae uralensis prae-parata*
Bai Zhu *Rhizoma Atractylodis macrocephalae*
Dang Gui *Radix Angelicae sinensis*
Chen Pi *Pericarpium Citri reticulatae*
Sheng Ma *Rhizoma Cimicifugae*
Chai Hu *Radix Bupleuri*
Sheng Jiang *Rhizoma Zingiberis officinalis recens*
Da Zao *Fructus Ziziphi jujubae*

This remedy tonifies and raises Qi and may be used for tinnitus from deficient Lung-Qi not brightening the ears. Chai Hu benefits the ears.

3. HEART-BLOOD DEFICIENCY

CLINICAL MANIFESTATIONS

Intermittent tinnitus with low sound and gradual onset, dull-pale complexion, palpitations, insomnia, poor memory, slight anxiety.
Tongue: Pale and Thin.
Pulse: Weak or Choppy especially on the left Front position.

This tinnitus is due to deficient Heart-Blood not reaching the head.

TREATMENT PRINCIPLE

Tonify the Heart, nourish Blood.

ACUPUNCTURE

HE-5 Tongli, BL-15 Xinshu, Ren-14 Juque, Ren-17 Shanzhong, P-6 Neiguan, SP-6 Sanyinjiao, S.I.-19 Tinggong.

Explanation

- **HE-5** tonifies the Heart.
- **BL-15** and **Ren-14,** Back-Transporting and Front-Collecting point of the Heart respectively, tonify the Heart.
- **Ren-17** tonifies Heart-Qi.
- **P-6** tonifies Heart-Blood.

- **SP-6** nourishes Blood.
- **S.I.-19** is the main local point for this type of tinnitus.

HERBAL TREATMENT

Prescription

BU QI CONG MING TANG Variation
Tonifying Qi Clear Hearing Decoction
Huang Qi *Radix Astragali membranacei* 12 g
Ren Shen *Radix Ginseng* 9 g
Dang Gui *Radix Angelicae sinensis* 9 g
Shu Di Huang *Radix Rehmanniae glutinosae praeparata* 12 g
Long Yan Rou *Arillus Euphoriae longanae* 9 g
Sheng Ma *Rhizoma Cimicifugae* 3 g
Ge Gen *Radix Puerariae* 3 g
Man Jing Zi *Fructus Viticis* 3 g
Bai Shao *Radix Paeoniae albae* 6 g
Huang Bo *Cortex Phellodendri* 6 g
Zhi Gan Cao *Radix Glycyrrhizae uralensis praeparata* 3 g

Explanation

- **Dang Gui**, **Shu Di** and **Long Yan Rou** have been added to the original prescription to nourish Heart-Blood.

Patent remedy

REN SHEN LU RONG WAN
Ginseng-Cornu Cervi Pill
Ren Shen *Radix Ginseng*
Huang Qi *Radix Astragali membranacei*
Du Zhong *Cortex Eucommiae ulmoidis*
Ba Ji Tian *Radix Morindae officinalis*

Lu Rong *Cornu Cervi parvum*
Dang Gui *Radix Angelicae sinensis*
Niu Xi *Radix Achyranthis bidentatae seu Cyathulae*
Long Yan Rou *Arillus Longan*

This pill is suitable for tinnitus from deficiency of Heart-Blood.

The tongue presentation appropriate to this remedy is a Pale body.

Prognosis

Tinnitus is an extremely difficult condition to treat and results with acupuncture and/or herbs are not the best. However, it is always worth trying as Western medicine has absolutely nothing to offer for this condition. Obviously, the older the patient and the longer-lasting the condition, the more difficult it will be to treat.

Results are better for the Full than the Empty types. Of the Full types, the one from Liver-Fire is easier (or rather less difficult) to treat than the one from Phlegm-Fire. In any case, at least 10 treatments should be given before deciding whether it is working or not.

In tinnitus from Kidney deficiency it is essential that the patient takes adequate rest and restrains sexual activity. In tinnitus from Phlegm-Fire it is important for the patient to avoid eating dairy products and greasy-hot foods.

In tinnitus from Liver-Fire, the patient should be encouraged to relax and engage in moderate exercise. If Liver-Fire is caused by deep emotional problems, it may be necessary to recommend counselling.

Tiredness 12

虚
劳

Tiredness is one of the most common presenting symptoms in Western patients. Very often it is the main or only symptom of which a patient complains. Tiredness as a main presenting symptom is discussed in Chinese Medicine under the heading of "Exhaustion" (*Xu Lao*). The very term "Exhaustion" describes not only a symptom, i.e. tiredness, but also its underlying cause, i.e. a deficiency of the body's Qi. In fact, the term *Xu Lao*, derived from *xu* meaning "deficiency" and *lao* meaning "tiredness", means literally "tiredness from deficiency". However, tiredness is not necessarily always caused by a Deficiency; it can, sometimes, be caused by an Excess condition. A very simple example is the kind of tiredness which is experienced during a cold or influenza, i.e. an invasion of exterior Wind-Cold or Wind-Heat which are, by definition, Excess conditions. Of course, in many cases tiredness can be the result of an interaction of Deficiency and Excess. In this chapter, I will therefore also discuss some Excess causes of tiredness in addition to the Deficiency causes normally considered under "Exhaustion".

The "Classic of Difficulties" discusses the "five depletions" (*wu sun*) in chapter 14. It says:

In depletion of the skin [i.e. Lungs], the skin contracts and hair falls out; in depletion of the blood vessels [i.e. Heart], these become deficient and Blood cannot nourish the internal organs; in depletion of the muscles [i.e. Spleen], these become thin and food cannot nourish them; in depletion of the tendons [i.e. Liver], these weaken and cannot support the body and the hands cannot grasp; in depletion of the bones [i.e. Kidneys], these wither and the person cannot get up from bed . . . . In depletion of the Lungs tonify Qi; in depletion of the Heart harmonize Defensive Qi and Nutritive Qi; in depletion of the Spleen regulate the diet and protect the body from extremes of cold and heat; in depletion of the Liver soothe the Middle [with sweet herbs]; in depletion of the Kidneys nourish the Essence.[1]

The concept of "depletion" is similar to that of "exhaustion".

The "Prescriptions of the Golden Chest" by Zhang Zhong Jing introduces the term "Exhaustion" (*xu lao*) for the first time. It says in chapter 6: *"When the pulse is big but empty in male patients, it indicates extreme exhaustion from overexertion"*.[2]

The "Discussion on Causes and Symptoms of Diseases" (AD 610) by Chao Yuan Fang elaborates on the concept of Exhaustion by investigating its causes. Dr Chao considers Exhaustion to be due to the "6 Extremes" and the "7 Injuries". The "6 Extremes" are due to overexertion of the body leading to depletion of Qi, Blood, Tendons, Bones, Muscles and Essence. The "7 Injuries" refer to the damage inflicted on internal organs by various excesses which injure their energy. Thus:

– overeating injures the Spleen
– excessive and prolonged anger injures the Liver and makes Qi rise
– lifting excessive weights or sitting on damp ground injures the Kidneys
– exposure to cold and drinking cold liquids injure the Lungs
– excessive worrying and thinking injure the Heart
– wind, rain, cold and heat injure the body
– fear, anxiety and shock injure the Mind.[3]

The "Simple Questions" in chapter 23 lists five causes of Exhaustion:

Excessive use of the eyes injures Blood [i.e. the Heart]; excessive lying down injures Qi [i.e. the Lungs]; excessive sitting injures the muscles [i.e. the Spleen]; excessive standing injures the bones [i.e. the Kidneys]; excessive exercise injures the tendons [i.e. the Liver].[4]

Over the centuries various doctors discussed the treatment of Exhaustion according to their particular views and emphases. For example, Li Dong Yuan, author of the famous "Discussion on Stomach and Spleen" (1249), considered Stomach and Spleen deficiency to be the main cause of Exhaustion. Zhu Dan Xi, author of "Secrets of Dan Xi" (1347), placed the emphasis on Kidney- and Liver-Yin deficiency as a cause of Exhaustion and advocated nourishing Yin and clearing Heat. Zhang Jie Bin, author of the "Classic of Categories" (1624) and the "Complete Book of Jing Yue" (1624), advocated tonifying the Kidneys for the treatment of Exhaustion. Zhu Qi Shi (1463–1539) considered the Lungs, Spleen and Kidneys to be the three most important organs to treat in Exhaustion. He said in his book "Discussion on Exhaustion":

To treat Exhaustion there are three roots: Lungs, Spleen and Kidneys. Lungs are like the 'heaven'
of the internal organs, the Spleen is like the 'mother' of the body and the Kidneys are like the 'root' of life. Treat these three organs to treat Exhaustion.[5]

Dr Zhu indicated the Spleen and Lungs as the two main organs to treat in cases of chronic tiredness, the Spleen for Yang deficiency and the Lungs for Yin deficiency. Each of these can eventually lead to Kidney-Yang or Kidney-Yin deficiency and Yang-deficiency can lead to Yin-deficiency or vice versa. Dr Zhu says:

To treat Deficiency there are two interconnected systems: either the Lungs or the Spleen. Every [Deficiency] disease boils down to Yang or Yin deficiency. Yang deficiency can lead to Yin deficiency after a prolonged time . . . Yin deficiency can lead to Yang deficiency after a prolonged time . . . In Yang deficiency treat the Spleen, in Yin deficiency treat the Lungs.[6]

Aetiology

1. WEAK CONSTITUTION

A hereditary weakness of constitution is an obvious and frequent cause of chronic tiredness. A person's constitution is determined by several factors: the parents' constitution in general, the parents' health and age at the time of conception, the conditions of pregnancy and childhood development. Zhu Qi Shi considered the inherited constitution as one of the causes of chronic tiredness and he said: "*Inherited causes of tiredness are due to one of the parents being too old or to exhaustion or disease at the time of conception. [It can also be due] to the conditions of pregnancy . . .*"[7]

The causes and manifestations of poor hereditary constitution have already been discussed in the chapter on "Headaches" (ch. 1). It is important to point out, however, that a weak inherited constitution can manifest in any of the five main Yin organs, not only the Kidneys. Because the Kidneys store both the pre-natal and post-natal Essence some people identify an inherited weak constitution only with a Kidney weakness. This is not so; one can inherit a poor constitution in any of the five Yin organs. The signs of a poor hereditary constitution for each organ are as follows:

– *Heart*: nervousness and disturbed sleep in childhood, a bluish colour on the forehead, and a relatively deep midline crack on the tongue reaching the area just behind the tip.
– *Lungs*: a propensity to catching cold and chest diseases in childhood, a thin chest, a pale complexion and weak voice and a pulse in both Front positions which is felt more medial and running upwards towards the thumb (see Fig. 1.1 in chapter 1).
– *Spleen*: weak muscles and physical tiredness in childhood, a poor appetite and digestive disturbances in childhood and a sallow complexion.
– *Liver*: myopia and headaches in childhood, a greenish complexion, primary infertility or amenorrhoea in women.
– *Kidneys*: nocturnal enuresis and fears in childhood with a bluish colour on the chin, poor bone or brain development, primary infertility in women, sterility in men, premature ageing and greying of the hair.

2. OVERWORK

By "overwork" is meant here excessive work whether it be mental or physical, long hours of work without adequate rest and work under stressful conditions. A proper balance between rest and work is essential to health and many conditions of chronic tiredness are simply due to excessive work without adequate rest. Indeed, in many cases, rest is the only treatment required for chronic tiredness.

Overwork in the sense described above is one of the commonest causes of chronic tiredness, especially in modern industrial societies where the pace of life has become very fast indeed. Peer pressure, competitiveness, financial demands and a misguided "work ethic", all contribute to creating the conditions for overworking. In some societies, the very idea of rest seems to be old-fashioned and almost sinful.

When periods of work are alternated with proper rest, the body has a chance to recuperate and no ill effect will derive from work. Indeed, inactivity is also a cause of disease in Chinese medicine leading to stagnation of Qi and sometimes Lung-Qi deficiency. However, when a person overworks or works very long hours without adequate rest, the body has no time to recuperate. This leads the body to use reserves of energy, i.e. the Kidney-Essence. For this reason, a Kidney deficiency often results from overwork.

In Chinese medicine, overwork has been considered a cause of disease since early times and it would appear that working long hours under conditions of stress is not only a feature of our times but also of ancient China during certain historical periods. For example, conditions of life were difficult in China during the Yuan dynasty (1271–1368) and people had to work very hard under stress, which, as we know, depletes the Yin: some doctors think this was the reason why the School of Nourishing Yin (of which Zhu Dan Xi was the main advocate) developed during those times. Zhang Jie Bin wrote in his book "The Complete Book of Jing Yue" (1634): *"If one does not know one's limits of endurance and pushes oneself trying again and again, this will result in exhaustion"*.[8] This description fits admirably the behaviour of many people in our times.

"Overwork" is a general term which includes many different types of excessive work leading to disease. For example, work which involves standing for hours on end day after day without breaks to sit or lie down may injure the Kidneys. Excessive mental work and straining of the eyes at a computer monitor may weaken the Blood of both Heart and Liver. Mental work for long hours under conditions of great stress combined with irregular eating may weaken the Yin of both Stomach and Kidneys.

3. PHYSICAL OVEREXERTION

This includes both overexertion in the course of work and excessive exercising or sporting activities.

Excessive physical work without rest weakens the muscles and the Spleen. Excessive lifting injures the Kidneys.

Excessive jogging damages the tendons leading, after some years, to deficiency of Liver Blood or Liver-Yin and possible development of Liver-Wind. This would manifest with rigidity, numbness and spasms of the legs.

4. DIET

Improper diet is of course a very important cause of chronic tiredness. Irregular eating directly weakens the Stomach and Spleen and therefore very easily leads to chronic tiredness since the Stomach and Spleen are the origin of Qi and Blood.

First of all, slimming diets can lead to malnourishment of the body and obviously to tiredness by damaging the Spleen. In extreme cases they lead to anorexia which is, of course, a very severe case of chronic tiredness (apart from its obvious psychological implications).

Eating too much can also lead to chronic tiredness as it puts a strain on the Stomach and Spleen and causes retention of food.

Irregular eating habits are another very frequent cause of weakening of Stomach and Spleen: eating too late at night, eating in a hurry, discussing business while eating, reading while eating, having a "quick bite" standing up, going straight back to work after eating, eating too fast, eating in a state of emotional upset, etc. All these conditions weaken Stomach-Qi and, in the long run, Stomach-Yin.

Any imbalance in the type of food eaten can also weaken the Spleen and Stomach. Excessive consumption of cold-raw foods weakens Spleen-Yang, eating too much meat, spicy foods and alcohol leads to Stomach-Heat, eating too many sour foods (such as vinegar, yoghurt, sour apples, grapefruit, oranges, pickles) can stir up Liver-Yang, excessive consumption of dairy foods leads to Damp Phlegm, eating too much fried and greasy food leads to Damp-Heat. The first condition (Spleen-Yang deficiency) is a very frequent deficiency-cause of chronic tiredness. All the other conditions (Stomach-Heat, Liver-Yang rising, Damp-Phlegm and Damp-Heat) can be Excess-causes of chronic tiredness as will be explained shortly.

5. SEVERE ILLNESS

Any serious protracted illness can result in Spleen deficiency and therefore chronic tiredness. Examples of such illnesses are influenza, bronchitis, pneumonia, whooping cough, measles, meningitis, etc. In particular, Heat diseases can also lead to Yin deficiency as Heat has a tendency to "burn" body fluids.

An increasingly common cause of chronic tiredness is the deficiency of Qi and/or Yin that follows an invasion of exterior Wind-Heat, i.e. a bout of influenza, a common cold or an upper respiratory infection. This often results in myalgic encephalomyelitis (ME) which will be discussed separately (ch. 25).

6. EXCESSIVE SEXUAL ACTIVITY

Excessive sexual activity causes a deficiency of the Kidneys. As a cause of disease, it is more common in men than women. It is of course impossible to define a "normal" level of sexual activity as this depends on the person's constitution in general and his or her particular condition at the time. The stronger the constitution and the healthier the condition, the more a person can engage in sex without ill effects. On the other hand, a person of weak constitution or in poor health should curb his or her sexual activity. In any case, if someone experiences pronounced tiredness, lower back-ache and dizziness after sex, it certainly indicates that that level of sexual activity is excessive for him or her.

It is important for a practitioner of Chinese medicine to be aware of this particular cause of disease as most people do not know that excessive sexual activity could be detrimental or that they should abstain from sex during an acute illness.

7. CHILDBIRTH

Soon after childbirth a woman is obviously very tired because her Qi and Blood are depleted by the demands of pregnancy and delivery. Following childbirth a woman's body condition is very vulnerable and great care should be taken to eat well and rest. Unfortunately, the trend in modern industrial societies is for women to leave their beds shortly after childbirth and even to go back to work only a few days after. This definitely leads to deficiency of Liver-Blood and therefore to chronic tiredness. In some cases, it is also the cause of post-natal depression.

All the precautions that apply after childbirth also apply after a miscarriage. This is appreciated even less by women, most of whom just tend to carry on as usual immediately after a miscarriage. From the point of view of Qi and Blood, a miscarriage is as weakening as childbirth, often involving a substantial loss of blood. Indeed, there is a saying that declares: *"A miscarriage is more serious than childbirth".*[9]

8. "RECREATIONAL" DRUGS

Prolonged and continued use of drugs such as cannabis, LSD, cocaine or heroine is an important modern cause of chronic tiredness and lethargy. Researchers have called the state deriving from long-term use of cannabis "amotivational syndrome", consisting in a feeling of unease, a sense of not being fully effective, and gross lethargy.[10]

Pathology

Although the term Exhaustion (*xu lao*) by definition implies tiredness deriving from a deficiency, chronic tiredness can also result from an Excess condition as was remarked in the introduction to this chapter. There are basically three possibilities:

1. Deficiency
2. Combined condition of Deficiency and Excess (e.g. stagnation of Liver-Qi inducing a deficiency of Spleen-Qi and therefore tiredness)
3. Excess.

Whilst it is easy to understand how the first two conditions may result in tiredness, it may be more difficult to see how an Excess condition can cause tiredness. It basically does so by obstructing the proper movement, transformation and circulation of Qi and Blood. For example, stagnation of Liver-Qi is a frequent cause of tiredness. How does it cause tiredness even without a deficiency of Stomach and Spleen? The Liver ensures the smooth flow of Qi in all parts of the body and all organs and it regulates the entering/exiting and ascending/descending of Qi. It is easy to see therefore that if Liver-Qi is stagnant the proper direction of movement and circulation of Qi is impaired, necessarily resulting in tiredness. One can understand this concept by studying the herbal prescription Si Ni San *Four Rebellious Powder* (Chai Hu *Radix Bupleuri*, Bai Shao *Radix Paeoniae albae*, Zhi Shi *Fructus Citri aurantii immaturus* and Gan Cao *Radix Glycyrrhizae uralensis*), which resolves stagnation of Liver-Qi. One of the indications for the use of this prescription is cold hands: the hands are cold not from deficiency of Yang but because the stagnation of Liver-Qi obstructs a proper circulation of Qi. Exactly the same thinking can be applied to the symptom of tiredness: it can derive not only from a deficiency but also from the impairment in the movement and circulation of Qi caused by Liver-Qi stagnation.

The Excess conditions which are most likely to result in chronic tiredness are:

- Liver-Qi stagnation
- Liver-Yang rising
- Liver-Fire
- Liver-Wind
- Phlegm
- Dampness.

The first four conditions all pertain to the Liver and all hinge around the Liver function of ensuring the smooth flow of Qi. The last two conditions, Phlegm and Dampness, are very frequent Excess-causes of chronic tiredness. Although they both derive from a deficiency of Spleen-Qi which would cause tiredness in itself, Phlegm and Dampness also cause tiredness by themselves because they obstruct the movement and transformation of Qi.

Having differentiated whether tiredness is caused by a Deficiency or an Excess condition, in the case of Deficiency the next logical step is that of identifying the type, i.e. whether there is deficiency of Qi, Yang, Blood or Yin. Differentiating these four types of deficiency is extremely important to a successful treatment, particularly with herbs. Differentiating these four types of Deficiency is, however, closely linked to identifying the organ involved, which is the third step in diagnosing the cause of tiredness.

Of the Yin organs the one that is most frequently responsible for chronic tiredness is of course the Spleen. A Spleen deficiency is often accompanied by a Stomach deficiency and the two are the origin of Qi and Blood and therefore an extremely frequent Deficiency-cause of tiredness.

A Liver-Blood deficiency is also a frequent cause of chronic tiredness. The Liver regulates the volume of Blood according to physical activity, flowing to the muscles and tendons during exercise and flowing back to the Liver during rest. The flow of Blood back to the Liver during rest has a tonifying effect on the body and helps us to recuperate energy. For this reason a short period of rest lying down in the middle of the day helps the body to recuperate energy. This concept appeared first in chapter 9 of the "Simple Questions" where it says that *"The Liver has a regulating function [literally 'is the Root of stopping extremes'] . . .".*[11]

Most doctors agree that this means the Liver is responsible for endurance when Blood is abundant, and for tiredness when Blood is deficient.

The Liver is also responsible for chronic tiredness in Excess conditions such as Liver-Qi stagnation, Liver-Yang or Liver-Fire rising and Liver-Wind, as explained above.

The Lungs cause chronic tiredness in case of Lung-Qi or Lung-Yin deficiency. Either of these frequently follows a severe cold, influenza or upper respiratory infection.

Heart-Qi or Heart-Blood deficiency causing tiredness are often the result of long-standing emotional problems such as sadness or worry.

A Kidney deficiency is often the cause of chronic tiredness particularly in very long-standing conditions. In fact, a deficiency of any of the other Yin organs can lead to a Kidney deficiency after a long period of time. In particular,

Spleen deficiency often leads to Kidney-Yang deficiency, while a Liver-Blood deficiency often leads to Kidney-Yin deficiency.

To summarize, the three steps in identifying the cause of chronic tiredness are:

1. distinguish Deficiency and Excess
2. distinguish Qi, Yang, Blood or Yin Deficiency in case of Deficiency, distinguish which pathogenic factor is involved in case of Excess
3. identify the organ involved.

Differentiation and treatment

The patterns analyzed will be:

DEFICIENCY

Lung-Qi Deficiency
Spleen-Qi Deficiency
Heart-Qi Deficiency
Heart-Yang Deficiency
Spleen-Yang Deficiency
Kidney-Yang Deficiency
Heart-Blood Deficiency
Liver-Blood Deficiency
Spleen-Blood Deficiency
Lung-Yin Deficiency
Heart-Yin Deficiency
Stomach- and Spleen-Yin Deficiency
Liver-Yin Deficiency
Kidney-Yin Deficiency

EXCESS

Liver-Qi stagnation
Liver-Yang rising
Liver-Fire blazing
Liver-Wind
Phlegm
Dampness

Of course, these patterns do not occur in isolation but are very frequently combined. The following are examples of common combinations:

Lung-Qi and Spleen-Qi Deficiency

Spleen-Yang and Kidney-Yang Deficiency
Spleen-Blood and Liver-Blood Deficiency
Lung-Yin and Kidney-Yin Deficiency.

The combination of Deficiency with Excess patterns is also common. Examples are:

Spleen-Qi Deficiency with Phlegm or Dampness
Spleen-Qi Deficiency with Liver-Qi Stagnation
Liver-Blood Deficiency with Liver-Qi Stagnation
Liver-Blood Deficiency with Liver-Yang rising or Liver-Wind
Kidney-Yin Deficiency with Liver-Yang rising.

In all these cases, one needs to diagnose the primary aspect of the condition to choose the right prescription. This is especially important in combined conditions of Deficiency and Excess.

DEFICIENCY

QI DEFICIENCY

1. LUNG-QI DEFICIENCY

Clinical manifestations

Tiredness, slight breathlessness, low voice, pale-white complexion, slight spontaneous sweating, propensity to catching colds, timidity.
Pulse: Weak or Empty particularly on the left front position.
Tongue: slightly Pale.

This condition often results from an invasion of exterior Wind-Cold or Wind-Heat which goes to the chest. Prolonged coughing resulting from this situation may·induce Lung-Qi deficiency. This often occurs on a background of constitutional Lung deficiency and therefore a propensity to catching colds. The repeated bouts of colds and coughing further weaken the Lungs. A constitutional Lung deficiency (often a result of whooping cough in childhood) may be manifested on the tongue with two transversal cracks in the Lungs area (see Fig. 12.2, p. 333)

Treatment principle: tonify Lung-Qi.

Acupuncture

LU-9 Taiyuan, ST-36 Zusanli, Ren-6 Qihai all with reinforcing method. Moxa can be used.

Explanation

- **LU-9** tonifies Lung-Qi. As a Source point it is the best point to tonify a Yin organ.
- **ST-36** tonifies the Stomach and Qi in general. It is used according to the principle of "reinforcing Earth to tonify Metal" since Earth is the mother of Metal within the 5-element model.
- **Ren-6** tonifies Qi in general and the Lung channel deep pathway flows down to this point.

Herbal treatment

Prescription

BU FEI TANG
Tonifying the Lungs Decoction
Ren Shen *Radix Ginseng* 6 g
Huang Qi *Radix Astragali membranacei* 9 g
Wu Wei Zi *Fructus Schisandrae chinensis* 3 g
Shu Di Huang *Radix Rehmanniae glutinosae prae-parata* 12 g
Sang Bai Pi *Cortex Mori albae radicis* 3 g
Zi Wan *Radix Asteris tatarici* 3 g

Explanation

- **Ren Shen** and **Huang Qi** tonify Lung-Qi.
- **Wu Wei Zi** and **Shu Di Huang** tonify Lungs and Kidneys. The Kidneys are tonified according to the principle that they are the "root" of the Lungs.
- **Sang Bai Pi** and **Zi Wan** stimulate the descending of Lung-Qi and direct the prescription to the Lungs.

Variations

- In case of pronounced spontaneous sweating add: Mu Li *Concha Ostreae* and Ma Huang Gen *Radix Ephedrae*.
- In case of both Qi and Yin deficiency add: Bie Jia *Carapax Trionycis*, and Di Gu Pi *Cortex Lycii chinensis radicis*.

Patent remedy

BU ZHONG YI QI WAN
Tonifying the Centre and Benefiting Qi Pill

Huang Qi *Radix Astragali membranacei*
Dang Shen *Radix Codonopsis pilosulae*
Zhi Gan Cao *Radix Glycyrrhizae uralensis praeparata*
Bai Zhu *Rhizoma Atractylodis macrocephalae*
Dang Gui *Radix Angelicae sinensis*
Chen Pi *Pericarpium Citri reticulatae*
Sheng Ma *Rhizoma Cimicifugae*
Chai Hu *Radix Bupleuri*
Sheng Jiang *Rhizoma Zingiberis officinalis recens*
Da Zao *Fructus Ziziphi jujubae*

Explanation

This formula is suitable for both Lung-Qi and Spleen-Qi deficiency. It is excellent to relieve tiredness on both a physical and mental level.

2. SPLEEN-QI DEFICIENCY

Clinical manifestations

Poor appetite, tiredness, muscular weakness, slight uncomfortable feeling in the abdomen after eating, loose stools, sallow complexion.
Tongue: Pale with teeth marks.
Pulse: Empty, especially in the right Middle position.

If Stomach-Qi deficiency accompanies this pattern, in addition to the above manifestations there will be an uncomfortable sensation of the epigastrium after eating and a tongue coating without root.

This is by far the most common cause of chronic tiredness. The Spleen (with the Stomach) is the Root of Post-Heaven Qi and as such, it is the origin of Qi and Blood. All Qi and Blood made in the body originate from the Spleen and Stomach and if these two organs are weak, tiredness is one of the first and most common symptoms.

The tiredness would be more pronounced in the morning and it would also be characterized by a feeling of weakness of the muscles and lassitude.

Although this pattern is characterized by loss of appetite, it is not unusual in the different cultural milieu of Western societies for people with Spleen-Qi deficiency actually to eat more than normal, especially by constantly "picking". In any case, there are situations when Spleen-Qi is deficient and the Stomach has Heat which will cause people to feel hungry soon after eating.

Principle of treatment

Strengthen the Spleen, tonify Qi.

Acupuncture

ST-36 Zusanli, SP-3 Taibai, Ren-12 Zhongwan, BL-20 Pishu, BL-21 Weishu. All with reinforcing method. Moxa is applicable.

Explanation

– **ST-36** and **SP-3** tonify Stomach and Spleen Qi.
– **Ren-12** is the Front-Collecting point of the Stomach and it tonifies both Stomach and Spleen.
– **BL-20** and **BL-21** are the Back-Transporting points for Spleen and Stomach and they provide a very effective and strong stimulation in chronic deficiency of these two organs. They particularly have an effect in relieving tiredness.

Herbal treatment

Prescription

JIA WEI SI JUN ZI TANG
Four Gentlemen Decoction Variation
Ren Shen *Radix Ginseng* 9 g
Huang Qi *Radix Astragali membranacei* 9 g
Bai Zhu *Rhizoma Atractylodis macrocephalae* 6 g
Zhi Gan Cao *Radix Glycyrrhizae uralensis praeparata* 3 g
Fu Ling *Sclerotium Poriae cocos* 6 g
Bian Dou *Semen Dolichoris lablab* 6 g

Explanation

This is nothing but the *Four Gentlemen Decoction* with the addition of Huang Qi to tonify Qi and Bian Dou to tonify Spleen-Qi and stop loose stools.

(i) Patent remedy

LIU JUN ZI WAN
Six Gentlemen Pill
Dang Shen *Radix Codonopsis pilosulae*
Bai Zhu *Rhizoma Atractylodis macrocephalae*
Fu Ling *Sclerotium Poriae cocos*
Zhi Gan Cao *Radix Glycyrrhizae praeparata*
Chen Pi *Pericarpium Citri reticulatae*
Ban Xia *Rhizoma Pinelliae ternatae*

Explanation

This very famous pill tonifies Lung-Qi and Spleen-Qi and secondarily resolves Dampness and Phlegm. It is one of the most frequently used Spleen tonics.

The tongue presentation appropriate to this remedy is a Pale body.

(ii) Patent remedy

XIANG SHA LIU JUN ZI WAN
Saussurea-Amomum Six Gentlemen Pill
Dang Shen *Radix Codonopsis pilosulae*
Bai Zhu *Rhizoma Atractylodis macrocephalae*
Fu Ling *Sclerotium Poriae cocos*
Zhi Gan Cao *Radix Glycyrrhizae praeparata*
Chen Pi *Pericarpium Citri reticulatae*
Ban Xia *Rhizoma Pinelliae ternatae*
Mu Xiang *Radix Saussureae*
Sha Ren *Fructus seu Semen Amomi*

Explanation

This formula is used in preference to the previous one when there is also some stagnation of Qi giving rise to epigastric or abdominal distension and pain.

The tongue presentation appropriate to this remedy is a Pale body.

(iii) Patent remedy

SHEN LING BAI ZHU WAN
Ginseng-Poria-Atractylodes Pill
Ren Shen *Radix Ginseng* (or Dang Shen *Radix Codonopsis pilosulae*)
Fu Ling *Sclerotium Poriae cocos*

Bai Zhu *Rhizoma Atractylodis macrocephalae*
Jie Geng *Radix Platycodi grandiflori*
Shan Yao *Radix Dioscoreae oppositae*
Chen Pi *Pericarpium Citri reticulatae*
Sha Ren *Fructus seu Semen Amomi*
Lian Zi *Semen Nelumbinis*
Bian Dou *Semen Dolichoris lablab*
Yi Yi Ren *Semen Coicis lachryma jobi*
Zhi Gan Cao *Radix Glycyrrhizae uralensis praeparata*

Explanation

This remedy tonifies Stomach- and Spleen-Qi, resolves Dampness and stops diarrhoea. It is therefore particularly used if there is diarrhoea or loose stools. It is more wide-ranging in its effect than the Liu Jun Zi Wan *Six Gentlemen Pill* in so far as, besides tonifying Qi, it resolves Dampness and mildly tonifies Stomach-Yin.

The tongue presentation appropriate to this remedy is a Pale body with a sticky coating which is possibly rootless in the centre.

3. HEART-QI DEFICIENCY

Clinical manifestations

Tiredness, slight breathlessness on exercise, palpitations, slight spontaneous sweating, pale complexion, depression.
Tongue: Pale, midline crack reaching the tip.
Pulse: Empty, especially on the left Front position.

The tiredness in this pattern is slightly different from that in Spleen-Qi deficiency. In this case, the person feels not only physically tired and slightly breathless but also mentally tired.

Principle of treatment

Strengthen the Heart, tonify Qi.

Acupuncture treatment

HE-5 Tongli, P-6 Neiguan, BL-15 Xinshu, Ren-17 Shanzhong, Ren-6 Qihai. All with reinforcing method. Moxa is applicable.

Explanation

- **HE-5** and **P-6** tonify Heart-Qi.
- **BL-15** is the Back-Transporting point of the Heart and it tonifies Heart-Qi, especially with direct moxibustion.
- **Ren-17** is the Front-Collecting point of the Upper Burner and it tonifies both Lung and Heart Qi.
- **Ren-6** tonifies Qi in general.

Herbal treatment

Prescription

SI JUN ZI TANG Variation
Four Gentlemen Decoction Variation
Ren Shen *Radix Ginseng* 9 g
Bai Zhu *Rhizoma Atractylodis macrocephalae* 6 g
Fu Ling *Sclerotium Poriae cocos* 6 g
Zhi Gan Cao *Radix Glycyrrhizae uralensis praeparata* 3 g
Wu Wei Zi *Fructus Schisandrae chinensis* 4.5 g

Explanation

This simple variation of the *Four Gentlemen Decoction* only consists in the addition of Wu Wei Zi which enters the Heart.

Patent remedy

LING ZHI FENG WANG JIANG
Ganoderma-Royal Jelly Essence
Ling Zhi *Fructificatio Ganodermae lucidi*
Feng Wang Jiang *Royal jelly*
Dang Shen *Radix Codonopsis pilosulae*
Gou Qi Zi *Fructus Lycii chinensis*

Explanation

This formula (available in phials) tonifies both Heart-Qi and Heart-Blood and calms the Mind.

The tongue presentation appropriate to this remedy is a Pale and Thin body.

YANG DEFICIENCY

1. HEART-YANG DEFICIENCY

Clinical manifestations

Tiredness, weariness, shortness of breath on ex-ertion, slight sweating, feeling of cold, bright-pale face, cold limbs (especially hands), slight feeling of oppression or discomfort in the heart region.
Tongue: Pale, wet, Swollen.
Pulse: Weak-Deep. In severe cases it could be Knotted.

This pattern is similar to Heart-Qi deficiency and could be considered a progression of it. The tiredness and weariness are accentuated and are accompanied by a prominent feeling of cold, i.e. the more tired the person feels, the colder he or she feels. The feeling of tiredness is also accompanied by some breathlessness. The uncomfortable sensation in the chest is due to a slight stagnation of Blood in the chest following the deficiency of Yang Qi.

Principle of treatment

Tonify Qi, warm the Yang.

Acupuncture

HE-5 Tongli, P-6 Neiguan, BL-15 Xinshu, Ren-17 Shanzhong, Ren-6 Qihai and Du-14 Dazhui. All with reinforcing method. Moxa must be used.

Explanation

The points are the same as for Heart-Qi deficiency, with the addition of Du-14 which warms Heart-Yang when used with direct moxibustion.

Herbal treatment

Prescription

CHENG YANG LI LAO TANG
Assisting Yang and Regulating Tiredness Decoction
Ren Shen *Radix Ginseng* 9 g
Huang Qi *Radix Astragali membranacei* 9 g
Wu Wei Zi *Fructus Schisandrae chinensis* 4.5 g
Zhi Gan Cao *Radix Glycyrrhizae uralensis praeparata* 3 g
Gui Zhi *Ramulus Cinnamomi cassiae* 4.5 g
Sheng Jiang *Rhizoma Zingiberis offinalis recens* 3 slices
Bai Zhu *Rhizoma Atractylodis macrocephalae* 6 g

Chen Pi *Pericarpium Citri reticulatae* 3 g
Dang Gui *Radix Angelicae sinensis* 6 g
Da Zao *Fructus Ziziphi jujubae* 3 dates

Explanation

- **Ren Shen**, **Huang Qi**, **Wu Wei Zi** and **Zhi Gan Cao** in combination tonify Heart-Qi.
- **Gui Zhi** and **Sheng Jiang** warm Heart-Yang and warm the channels and blood vessels.
- **Bai Zhu**, **Chen Pi**, **Dang Gui** and **Da Zao** in combination strengthen the Spleen to make Blood. Even though this pattern involves Yang deficiency and not Blood deficiency, it is necessary to nourish Blood in order to strengthen the Heart as this governs Blood.

Variations

- In case of chest pain add: Yu Jin *Tuber Curcumae* and Chuan Xiong *Radix Ligustici wallichii*.
- In case of pronounced chilliness add: Fu Zi *Radix Aconiti carmichaeli praeparata*.

Patent remedy

REN SHEN LU RONG WAN
Ginseng-Cornu Cervi Pill
Ren Shen *Radix Ginseng*
Du Zhong *Cortex Eucommiae*
Ba Ji Tian *Radix Morindae officinalis*
Huang Qi *Radix Astragali membranacei*
Lu Rong *Cornu Cervi parvum*
Dang Gui *Radix Angelicae sinensis*
Niu Xi *Radix Achyranthis bidentatae seu Cyathulae*
Long Yan Rou *Arillus Euphoriae longanae*

Explanation

This formula can be used to tonify and warm Heart-Yang. It also tonifies Kidney-Yang.

The tongue presentation appropriate to this remedy is a Pale, Swollen and wet body.

2. SPLEEN-YANG DEFICIENCY

Clinical manifestations

Tiredness, muscular weakness, sallow complex-ion, poor appetite, feeling of cold, cold limbs, dislike of speaking, loose stools, slight abdominal pain.
Tongue: Pale, teeth marks, Swollen.
Pulse: Weak, especially in the right Middle position.

This pattern is basically the same as Spleen-Qi deficiency with the addition of cold symptoms, i.e. feeling of cold and cold limbs. The feeling of cold of the limbs usually extends to the upper arms and thighs and not just hands and feet.

The tiredness is characterized by a feeling of weakness of the muscles, a desire to lie down and sleepiness after meals, especially lunch. In Yang deficiency the tiredness is more likely to manifest with mental depression as well.

The slight abdominal pain is caused by deficiency-Cold in the abdomen.

Principle of treatment

Strengthen the Spleen and warm the Middle.

Acupuncture

ST-36 Zusanli, SP-3 Taibai, Ren-12 Zhongwan, BL-20 Pishu, BL-21 Weishu, Du-20 Baihui. All with reinforcing method. Moxa must be used.

Explanation

- **Du-20** with moxa tonifies and raises Yang. It can be used here to tonify Yang and lift the spirit. This point has a powerful uplifting effect on the mood of a person and relieves tiredness and depression. It would also be useful if there is chronic diarrhoea.

All the other points have been discussed under the Spleen-Qi deficiency pattern.

Herbal treatment

Prescription

LI ZHONG WAN
Regulating the Centre Decoction
Ren Shen *Radix Ginseng* 6 g or (**Dang Shen** *Radix Codonopsis pilosulae*) 12 g

Bai Zhu *Rhizoma Atractylodis macrocephalae* 9 g
Gan Jiang *Rhizoma Zingiberis officinalis* 5 g
Zhi Gan Cao *Radix Glycyrrhizae uralensis praeparata* 6 g

Explanation

This is the classical prescription from the "Discussion of Cold-induced Diseases" to tonify and warm Spleen-Yang.

– **Ren Shen** and **Bai Zhu** tonify Spleen-Qi.
– **Gan Jiang** warms the Middle and expels internal Cold.
– **Zhi Gan Cao** both tonifies Spleen-Qi and harmonizes.

Variations

– In case of pronounced internal Cold symptoms (such as a more severe abdominal pain and diarrhoea) add: Gao Liang Jiang *Rhizoma Alpiniae officinari* or Ding Xiang *Flos Caryophylli*.

Patent remedy

LI ZHONG WAN
Regulating the Centre Pill
Gan Jiang *Rhizoma Zingiberis officinalis*
Bai Zhu *Rhizoma Atractylodis macrocephalae*
Dang Shen *Radix Codonopsis pilosulae*
Gan Cao *Radix Glycyrrhizae uralensis*

Explanation

This remedy has the same ingredients and functions as the prescription of the same name.

The tongue presentation appropriate to this remedy is a Pale and wet body.

3. KIDNEY-YANG DEFICIENCY

Clinical manifestations

Extreme tiredness, exhaustion, listlessness, mental depression, lack of will-power, no desire to go out, soreness of the lower back, frequent-pale urination, bright-white complexion, feeling of cold, cold limbs especially legs, diarrhoea, weak knees, impotence in men, lack of sexual desire in both men and women. In severe cases there might be oedema of the ankles.
Tongue: Pale, Swollen.
Pulse: Deep-Slow-Weak.

This pattern, even more than that of Spleen-Yang deficiency, is characterized by mental depression together with extreme tiredness. The person feels weary, does not want to leave the house and lacks will power and initiative.

Bearing in mind that the Kidneys are the origin of the Yin and Yang energies for the whole body, it is quite possible and indeed frequent, for both the Yang and Yin of the Kidneys to be deficient simultaneously, albeit with the predominance of one over the other. Thus, for example, a person suffering from the above condition of Kidney-Yang deficiency, and manifesting many of the above symptoms, might well also suffer from night sweating which is a symptom of Kidney-Yin deficiency.

For this reason, when tonifying Kidney-Yang it is necessary to add herbs to tonify the Kidney-Essence as well (see below), and conversely, when tonifying Kidney-Yin it is necessary to add a few herbs to tonify Kidney-Yang.

Finally, chronic deficiency of Kidney-Yang deficiency nearly always "includes" deficiency of Spleen-Yang too. The Spleen and Kidneys are two organs which work in close coordination for the movement, transformation and excretion of body fluids. In disease, they affect each other and either a Spleen deficiency leads to Kidney deficiency, or a Kidney deficiency eventually affects the Spleen, especially in the case of Yang deficiency. Hence the need to tonify the Spleen as well as the Kidneys in a case of Kidney-Yang deficiency.

Principle of treatment

Warm and tonify Kidney-Yang, nourish Essence and Blood.

Acupuncture

KI-3 Taixi, KI-7 Fuliu, Ren-4 Guanyuan, SP-6 Sanyinjiao, BL-23 Shenshu, BL-20 Pishu. All with reinforcing method. Moxa must be used.

Explanation

- **KI-3** and **KI-7**, with moxa, tonify Kidney-Yang. KI-7 is particularly indicated if there is oedema of the ankles.
- **Ren-4** with moxa tonifies Kidney-Yang.
- **BL-23**, Back-transporting point of the Kidneys, with moxa, tonifies Kidney-Yang.
- **SP-6** and **BL-20** are used to tonify the Spleen, which is often necessary as explained above.

Herbal treatment

Prescription

YOU GUI WAN
Restoring the Right [Kidney] Pill
Fu Zi *Radix Aconiti carmichaeli praeparata* 3 g
Rou Gui *Cortex Cinnamomi cassiae* 3 g
Du Zhong *Cortex Eucommiae ulmoidis* 6 g
Shan Zhu Yu *Fructus Corni officinalis* 4.5 g
Tu Si Zi *Semen Cuscutae* 6 g
Lu Jiao Jiao *Colla Cornu Cervi* 6 g
Shu Di Huang *Radix Rehmanniae glutinosae praeparata* 12 g
Shan Yao *Radix Dioscoreae oppositae* 6 g
Gou Qi Zi *Fructus Lycii chinensis* 6 g
Dang Gui *Radix Angelicae sinensis* 4.5 g

Explanation

- **Shu Di Huang**, **Tu Si Zi**, **Shan Zhu Yu**, **Gou Qi Zi** and **Shan Yao** nourish Kidney, Liver and Spleen.
- **Du Zhong**, **Rou Gui**, **Fu Zi** and **Lu Jiao Jiao** tonify and warm Kidney-Yang and the Gate of Vitality.
- **Dang Gui** and **Lu Jiao Jiao** nourish Blood.

(i) Patent remedy

YOU GUI WAN
Restoring the Right [Kidney] Pill
Fu Zi *Radix Aconiti carmichaeli praeparata*
Rou Gui *Cortex Cinnamomi cassiae*
Du Zhong *Cortex Eucommiae ulmoidis*
Shan Zhu Yu *Fructus Corni officinalis*
Tu Si Zi *Semen Cuscutae*
Lu Jiao Jiao *Colla Cornu Cervi*
Shu Di Huang *Radix Rehmanniae glutinosae praeparata*
Shan Yao *Radix Dioscoreae oppositae*
Gou Qi Zi *Fructus Lycii chinensis*
Dang Gui *Radix Angelicae sinensis*

Explanation

This remedy has the same ingredients and functions as the above prescription of the same name. It is particularly indicated to tonify Kidney-Yang in women as it contains Lu Jiao Jiao, Shu Di Huang, Gou Qi Zi and Dang Gui which nourish Blood.

The tongue presentation appropriate to this remedy is a Pale and Swollen body.

(ii) Patent remedy

JIN GUI SHEN QI WAN
Golden Chest Kidney-Qi Pill
Gui Zhi *Ramulus Cinnamomi cassiae* (or Rou Gui *Cortex Cinnamomi cassiae*)
Fu Zi *Radix Aconiti carmichaeli praeparata*
Shu Di Huang *Radix Rehmanniae glutinosae praeparata*
Shan Yao *Radix Dioscoreae oppositae*
Shan Zhu Yu *Fructus Corni officinalis*
Ze Xie *Rhizoma Alismatis orientalis*
Fu Ling *Sclerotium Poriae cocos*
Mu Dan Pi *Cortex Moutan radicis*

Explanation

This very well-known remedy, sometimes marketed as "Sexoton", tonifies Kidney-Yang. It has the same ingredients and functions as the prescription of the same name. It is particularly indicated to reduce excessive urination, dribbling of urine, slight incontinence of urine or nocturia from Kidney-Yang deficiency.

The tongue presentation appropriate to this remedy is a Pale and wet body.

(iii) Patent remedy

GE JIE BU SHEN WAN
Gecko Tonifying the Kidneys Pill
Ge Jie *Gecko*
Lu Rong *Cornu Cervi parvum*
Ren Shen *Radix Ginseng*

Huang Qi *Radix Astragali membranacei*
Du Zhong *Cortex Eucommiae*
Gou Shen *Testis et Penis Canis*
Dong Chong Xia Cao *Sclerotium Cordicipitis chinensis*
Gou Qi Zi *Fructus Lycii chinensis*
Fu Ling *Sclerotium Poriae cocos*
Bai Zhu *Rhizoma Atractylodis macrocephalae*

Explanation

This pill, which also tonifies Kidney-Yang, is especially suitable to tonify the Kidney's grasping Qi. It can therefore be used if there is chronic asthma from Kidney-Yang deficiency.

The tongue presentation appropriate to this remedy is a Pale body.

(iv) Patent remedy

SHEN RONG HU GU WAN
Ginseng-Cornu Cervi-Os Tigris Pill
Ren Shen *Radix Ginseng*
Lu Rong *Cornu Cervi parvum*
Dang Gui *Radix Angelicae sinensis*
Hu Gu *Os Tigris*
Fang Ji *Radix Stephaniae tetrandae*
Fang Feng *Radix Ledebouriellae sesloidis*

Explanation

This pill tonifies Kidney-Yang, strengthens tendons and bones and expels Wind and Dampness. It is therefore suitable for rheumatic pains occurring against a background of Kidney-Yang deficiency.

The tongue presentation appropriate to this remedy is a Pale body.

(v) Patent remedy

QUAN LU WAN
Whole Deer Pill
Lu Rou *Caro Cervi*
Lu Rong *Cornu Cervi parvum*
Lu Wei *Penis et testis Cervi*
Lu Shen *Renes Cervi*
Lu Jiao Jiao *Colla Cornus Cervi*
Ren Shen *Radix Ginseng*

Bai Zhu *Rhizoma Atractylodis macrocephalae*
Fu Ling *Sclerotium Poriae cocos*
Gan Cao *Radix Glycyrrhizae uralensis*
Dang Gui *Radix Angelicae sinensis*
Chuan Xiong *Radix Ligustici wallichii*
Shu Di Huang *Radix Rehmanniae glutinosae praeparata*
Huang Qi *Radix Astragali membranacei*
Gou Qi Zi *Fructus Lycii chinensis*
Du Zhong *Cortex Eucommiae*
Niu Xi *Radix Achyranthis bidentatae seu Cyathulae*
Xu Duan *Radix Dipsaci*
Rou Cong Rong *Herba Cistanchis*
Suo Yang *Herba Cynomorii songarici*
Bai Ji Tian *Radix Morindae officinalis*
Tian Men Dong *Tuber Asparagi cochinchinensis*
Mai Men Dong *Tuber Ophiopogonis japonici*
Wu Wei Zi *Fructus Schisandrae chinensis*
Chen Xiang *Lignum Aquilariae*
Chen Pi *Pericarpium Citri reticulatae*

Explanation

This remedy strongly tonifies and warms Kidney-Yang and the Kidney-Essence. It is suitable for older people (over 40) and is useful also for allergic rhinitis.

The tongue presentation appropriate to this remedy is a Pale, Swollen and wet body.

Case history

A 61-year-old lady complained of lower back-ache since she was 13, following an attack of polio. The back-ache was better with rest, worse when standing. Her main complaint, however, was severe exhaustion. She also felt cold easily, had to pass water at night and her ankles were oedematous. Her urine had always previously been pale but recently it had occasionally been dark. She had also suffered from constipation for a long time. Her sleep was not good, and she frequently woke up at night with a dry mouth. Her memory was poor and she frequently felt dizzy and had a ringing in the ears. Finally, she also complained of mild palpitations and a slightly bitter taste.

She had given birth to three children. In the past she had had a myomectomy to remove some fibroids from the uterus, a bladder operation to correct a prolapse and finally a hysterectomy when she was 39.

Her pulse was very Deep, Weak and Slow (60). Both Rear positions (Kidneys) were especially Weak and Deep and both Front positions (Heart and Lungs) were relatively Overflowing.

Her tongue was Pale, Swollen and dry (Plate 12.1).

Diagnosis
This case is a good example of a simultaneous deficiency of both Kidney-Yang and Kidney-Yin, with a predominance of Kidney-Yang deficiency. The deficiency of Kidney-Yin led to the development of Heart Empty-Heat.

The manifestations of Kidney-Yang deficiency are: exhaustion, feeling of cold, constipation (stools not dry), nocturia with pale urine, oedema of the ankles, Deep, Weak and Slow pulse and a Pale tongue.

The manifestations of Kidney-Yin deficiency are: dizziness, tinnitus, dark urine (sometimes), poor memory, dry mouth, dry tongue.

The manifestations of Heart Empty-Heat are: insomnia, bitter taste, palpitations and the slightly Overflowing pulse in both Front positions.

This condition could be represented in a diagrammatic way as follows (Fig. 12.1).

Treatment principle
This patient was treated with both acupuncture and herbal medicine. The principle of treatment used was to tonify Kidney-Yang primarily and Kidney-Yin secondarily. It is not necessary to deal specifically with the Heart Empty-Heat since its manifestations are slight and will be cleared simply by treating the Kidney-Yin deficiency which is causing it.

Acupuncture
- **LU-7** Lieque on the right side and **KI-6** Zhaohai on the left, the opening points of the Directing Vessel were used each time to tonify the Kidneys.
- **ST-36** Zusanli, **SP-6** Sanyinjiao and **BL-20** Pishu were used to tonify the Spleen (it is always essential to tonify the Spleen in chronic deficiency of the Kidneys).
- **BL-23** Shenshu and **KI-7** Fuliu were used to tonify Kidney-Yang and resolve oedema.
- **Shiqizhuixia**, the extra point below the 5th lumbar vertebra, was used to relieve the back-ache.

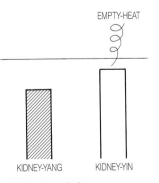

Fig. 12.1 Case-history's pathology

Herbal treatment
For the herbal treatment only patent remedies were used. Liu Wei Di Huang Wan *Six-Ingredient Rehmannia Pill* was given in the evening (8 pills) to nourish Kidney-Yin, and Quan Lu Wan *Whole-Deer Pill* was given in the morning (16 pills) to tonify Kidney-Yang.

She improved greatly even after only three acupuncture treatments.

BLOOD DEFICIENCY

1. HEART-BLOOD DEFICIENCY

Clinical manifestations

Tiredness which is worse at midday, palpitations, poor memory, insomnia or dream-disturbed sleep, dull-pale complexion, dizziness, pale lips.
Tongue: Pale and Thin. It may have a midline crack.
Pulse: Choppy or Fine.

This pattern arises from emotional problems such as sadness usually on a background of general deficiency of Qi and Blood. The tiredness is experienced more around midday which is the time of Heart activity (11 am to 1 pm). It is associated with palpitations and a slight anxiety.

This pattern is nearly always rooted in a deficiency of the Spleen, since it is Spleen-Qi that generates Blood.

Treatment principle

Nourish Blood, strengthen the Heart.

Acupuncture

HE-7 Shenmen, P-6 Neiguan, Ren-14 Juque, Ren-15 Jiuwei, Ren-4 Guanyuan, BL-17 Geshu (with moxa), BL-20 Pishu, ST-36 Zusanli, SP-6 Sanyinjiao. All with reinforcing method. Moxa can be used.

Explanation

- **HE-7** nourishes Heart-Blood and calms the Mind.
- **P-6** tonifies Heart-Qi and calms the Mind.

- **Ren-14** and **Ren-15** nourish Heart-Blood and calm the Mind.
- **Ren-4** nourishes Blood and calms the Mind.
- **BL-20** and **BL-17** (with moxa only) tonify Blood.
- **ST-36** and **SP-6** tonify Blood and Qi. SP-6 also calms the Mind.

Herbal treatment

Prescription

YANG XIN TANG
Nourishing the Heart Decoction
Ren Shen *Radix Ginseng* 6 g (or **Dang Shen** *Radix Codonopsis pilosulae* 12 g)
Huang Qi *Radix Astragali membranacei* 9 g
Fu Ling *Sclerotium Poriae cocos* 6 g
Zhi Gan Cao *Radix Glycyrrhizae uralensis prae-parata* 4.5 g
Dang Gui *Radix Angelicae sinensis* 6 g
Chuan Xiong *Radix Ligustici wallichii* 4.5 g
Wu Wei Zi *Fructus Schisandrae chinensis* 4.5 g
Bai Zi Ren *Semen Biotae orientalis* 6 g
Suan Zao Ren *Semen Ziziphi spinosae* 4.5 g
Yuan Zhi *Radix Polygalae tenuifoliae* 6 g
Rou Gui *Cortex Cinnamomi cassiae* 1.5 g
Ban Xia *Rhizoma Pinelliae ternatae* 4.5 g

Explanation

- **Ren Shen**, **Huang Qi**, **Fu Ling** and **Zhi Gan Cao** tonify Qi to generate Blood.
- **Dang Gui**, **Chuan Xiong**, **Wu Wei Zi**, **Bai Zi Ren**, **Suan Zao Ren** and **Yuan Zhi** nourish Blood and calm the Mind.
- **Rou Gui** and **Ban Xia** warm the Middle and tonify the Spleen to generate Blood.

Patent remedy

LING ZHI FENG WANG JIANG
Ganoderma-Royal Jelly Essence
Ling Zhi *Fructificatio Ganodermae lucidi*
Feng Wang Jiang *Royal jelly*
Dang Shen *Radix Codonopsis pilosulae*
Gou Qi Zi *Fructus Lycii chinensis*

Explanation

Although this remedy is not specific for the Heart, it tonifies Qi and nourishes Blood in general and may be used for this pattern.

The tongue presentation appropriate to this remedy is a Pale and Thin body.

2. LIVER-BLOOD DEFICIENCY

Clinical manifestations

Tiredness, feeling of weakness, cramps, blurred vision, propensity to being easily startled, numbness or tingling of limbs, scanty periods, brittle nails, dry skin and hair, dull-pale complexion, slight constipation.
Tongue: Pale and Thin, slightly dry.
Pulse: Choppy or Fine.

This is a very frequent cause of tiredness in women. It often derives from a deficiency of Spleen-Qi unable to make Blood.

In women, this pattern often causes scanty menstrual flow or no flow at all. It may also be manifested with dull vertical headaches occurring towards the end of the period.

Since Liver-Blood is the Yin part of the Liver which needs to "embrace" and root the Yang, a deficiency of Blood in the Liver often induces a slight stagnation of Liver-Qi, especially in women. In these cases, there may also be premenstrual tension and distension of the breasts, although all the other symptoms and signs (including the Pulse which is Choppy or Fine and not Wiry) point to Liver-Blood deficiency. The tiredness caused by Liver-Blood deficiency is very pronounced and is not easily alleviated by rest. It may result from chronic deficiency of Spleen-Qi, from excessive menstrual bleeding over a long period of time, from a diet deficient in blood-producing foods, or from childbirth.

Adequate rest, especially making a point of lying down for a short time in the afternoon, is essential to restore Liver-Blood. When lying down, the Blood flows back to the Liver and this regenerates both Blood and Qi.

Principle of treatment

Nourish Blood, tonify the Liver.

Acupuncture

BL-18 Ganshu, BL-20 Pishu, BL-17 Geshu, LIV-8 Ququan, ST-36 Zusanli, SP-6 Sanyinjiao and Ren-4 Guanyuan. All with reinforcing method. Moxa can be used.

Explanation

- **BL-18**, **BL-20** and **BL-17** nourish Liver-Blood.
- **LIV-8** nourishes Liver-Blood.
- **ST-36** and **SP-6** tonify the Spleen to produce Blood.
- **Ren-4** nourishes Blood and tonifies the uterus.

Herbal treatment

Prescription

BA ZHEN TANG
Eight Precious Decoction
Dang Gui *Radix Angelicae sinensis* 10 g
Chuan Xiong *Radix Ligustici wallichii* 5 g
Bai Shao *Radix Paeoniae albae* 8 g
Shu Di Huang *Radix Rehmanniae glutinosae prae-parata* 15 g
Ren Shen *Radix Ginseng* 3 g
Bai Zhu *Rhizoma Atractylodis macrocephalae* 10 g
Fu Ling *Sclerotium Poriae cocos* 8 g
Zhi Gan Cao *Radix Glycyrrhizae uralensis prae-parata* 5 g

Explanation

This prescription (already discussed in the chapter on Headaches, ch. 1) is the classical prescription to nourish Liver-Blood.

Variations

- In case of dry skin add: Shou Wu *Radix Polygoni multiflori*
- In case of blurred vision add: Gou Qi Zi *Fructus Lycii chinensis*.

Patent remedy

BA ZHEN WAN
Eight Precious Pill
Dang Gui *Radix Angelicae sinensis*
Chuan Xiong *Radix Ligustici wallichii*
Bai Shao *Radix Paeoniae albae*
Shu Di Huang *Radix Rehmanniae glutinosae prae-parata*
Ren Shen *Radix Ginseng*
Bai Zhu *Rhizoma Atractylodis macrocephalae*
Fu Ling *Sclerotium Poriae cocos*
Zhi Gan Cao *Radix Glycyrrhizae uralensis prae-parata*

Explanation

This very well-known pill tonifies Qi and Blood in general. In particular, it nourishes Liver-Blood and it is used in any gynaecological problem from Blood deficiency. In men, it can be used for chronic rheumatic pains occurring against a background of Blood deficiency.

The tongue presentation appropriate to this remedy is a Pale and Thin body.

3. SPLEEN-BLOOD DEFICIENCY

Clinical manifestations

Tiredness, loose stools, dull-pale complexion, poor appetite, pale lips, desire to lie down, slight palpitations.
Tongue: Pale, slightly Thin with teethmarks.
Pulse: Weak or Fine.

This situation is essentially the same as Spleen-Qi deficiency. However, since Spleen-Qi is also the origin of Blood, deficient Spleen-Qi can lead to Blood deficiency over a long period of time. Hence the slight palpitations and the Thin tongue, which are signs of Blood deficiency.

This pattern occurs very frequently in combination with either Heart-Blood or Liver-Blood deficiency and in some cases, with both. It is much more frequent in women than men. If accompanied by Heart-Blood deficiency, there would be more pronounced palpitations and insomnia. If accompanied by Liver-Blood deficiency there would be scanty periods, dizziness and blurred vision.

Principle of treatment

Tonify Qi and Blood, strengthen Spleen and Heart.

Acupuncture

ST-36 Zusanli, SP-3 Taibai, Ren-12 Zhongwan, BL-20 Pishu, BL-21 Weishu, BL-17 Geshu (with moxa only). All with reinforcing method. Moxa is applicable.

Explanation

- **ST-36** and **SP-3** tonify Stomach and Spleen Qi.
- **Ren-12** is the Front-Collecting point of the Stomach and it tonifies both Stomach and Spleen.
- **BL-20** and **BL-21** are the Back-Transporting points for Spleen and Stomach and they provide a very effective and strong stimulation in chronic deficiency of these two organs. They particularly have an effect in relieving tiredness.
- **BL-17** with direct moxa, nourishes Blood.

Herbal treatment

Prescription

GUI PI TANG
Tonifying the Spleen Decoction
Ren Shen *Radix Ginseng* 6 g (**Dang Shen** *Radix Codonopsis pilosulae* 12 g)
Huang Qi *Radix Astragali membranacei* 15 g
Bai Zhu *Rhizoma Atractylodis macrocephalae* 12 g
Dang Gui *Radix Angelicae sinensis* 3 g
Fu Shen *Sclerotium Poriae cocos pararadicis* 9 g
Suan Zao Ren *Semen Ziziphi spinosae* 9 g
Long Yan Rou *Arillus Euphoriae longanae* 12 g
Yuan Zhi *Radix Polygalae tenuifoliae* 9 g
Mu Xiang *Radix Saussureae* 6 g
Zhi Gan Cao *Radix Glycyrrhizae uralensis praeparata* 4 g
Sheng Jiang *Rhizoma Zingiberis officinalis recens* 3 slices
Hong Zao *Fructus Ziziphi jujubae* 5 dates

Explanation

- **Ren Shen, Huang Qi, Bai Zhu, Zhi Gan Cao, Sheng Jiang** and **Hong Zao** tonify Qi and strengthen the Spleen.
- **Dang Gui** nourishes the Liver and generates Blood.

- **Fu Shen**, **Suan Zao Ren** and **Long Yan Rou** nourish Blood and calm the Mind.
- **Yuan Zhi** calms the Heart and "firms Will Power".
- **Mu Xiang** regulates Qi and prevents the Qi and Blood tonics from giving rise to stagnation.

Patent remedy

GUI PI WAN
Tonifying the Spleen Pill
Ren Shen *Radix Ginseng* (Dang Shen *Radix Codonopsis pilosulae*)
Huang Qi *Radix Astragali membranacei*
Bai Zhu *Rhizoma Atractylodis macrocephalae*
Dang Gui *Radix Angelicae sinensis*
Fu Shen *Sclerotium Poriae cocos pararadicis*
Suan Zao Ren *Semen Ziziphi spinosae*
Long Yan Rou *Arillus Euphoriae longanae*
Yuan Zhi *Radix Polygalae tenuifoliae*
Mu Xiang *Radix Saussureae*
Zhi Gan Cao *Radix Glycyrrhizae uralensis praeparata*
Sheng Jiang *Rhizoma Zingiberis officinalis recens*
Hong Zao *Fructus Ziziphi jujubae*

Explanation

This very well-known remedy tonifies Spleen- and Heart-Blood and calms the Mind. It is excellent to tonify Spleen-Blood in chronic tiredness with insomnia from Blood deficiency. It is also used for bleeding from Qi deficiency.

The tongue presentation appropriate to this remedy is a Pale body.

YIN DEFICIENCY

1. LUNG-YIN DEFICIENCY

Clinical manifestations

Dry throat, dry cough, exhaustion, breathlessness, hoarse voice, feeling of heat in the afternoon, night sweating, 5-palm sweating, malar flush.
Tongue: Red without coating. It could be without coating only in the front part. There may be cracks in the Lung area (see Fig. 12.2).
Pulse: Fine and Rapid or Floating-Empty.

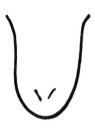

Fig. 12.2 Lung cracks

This pattern can occur in both young or old people. In young people it often follows a prolonged febrile disease which leads to exhaustion of the Yin and body fluids. In children, this can occur quite rapidly, in a matter of 2–3 weeks. In young adults it can happen after glandular fever, when the Yin is injured by prolonged Heat.

In old people, this pattern arises gradually as a result of a slow and progressive depletion of Yin. This does not mean, however, that every old person suffers from deficiency of Yin. In case of deficiency of Lung-Yin, it would occur only against a background of constitutional Lung weakness, which may also be in itself the consequence of a severe attack of whooping cough during childhood. People with constitutional Lung deficiency tend to be thin with a long and narrow rib cage.

Principle of treatment

Nourish Yin, generate fluids, strengthen the Lungs.

Acupuncture

LU-9 Taiyuan, Ren-17 Shanzhong, BL-43 Gaohuangshu, BL-13 Feishu, Du-12 Shenzhu, Ren-12 Zhongwan, ST-36 Zusanli, SP-6 Sanyinjiao. All with reinforcing method. No moxa.

Explanation

- **LU-9** and **Ren-17** tonify Lung-Qi and Lung-Yin (with acupuncture, tonification of Yin implies also tonification of Qi).
- **BL-43** nourishes Lung-Yin and is particularly indicated for chronic conditions.
- **BL-13** and **Du-12** tonify Lung-Qi.

- **Ren-12**, **ST-36** and **SP-6** tonify Stomach and Spleen and generate fluids. In particular, Ren-12 also tonifies the Lungs as the deep pathway of the Lung channel starts at this point.

Herbal treatment

Prescription

SHA SHEN MAI DONG TANG
Glehnia-Ophiopogon Decoction
Bei Sha Shen *Radix Glehniae littoralis* 9 g
Mai Men Dong *Tuber Ophiopogonis japonici* 9 g
Yu Zhu *Rhizoma Polygonati odorati* 6 g
Tian Hua Fen *Radix Trichosanthis* 4.5 g
Sang Ye *Folium Mori albae* 4.5 g
Bian Dou *Semen Dolichoris lablab* 4.5 g
Gan Cao *Radix Glycyrrhizae uralensis* 3 g

Explanation

- **Bei Sha Shen** moistens and nourishes Yin.
- **Mai Men Dong** nourishes Yin of Stomach and Lungs.
- **Yu Zhu** and **Tian Hua Fen** nourish Stomach and Lung Yin, generate fluids and clear Heat.
- **Sang Ye** clears Lung-Heat and stimulates the descending of Lung-Qi.
- **Bian Dou** tonifies Spleen Qi and Yin and is used according to the principle of "strengthening the Earth to promote Metal".
- **Gan Cao** harmonizes.

Variations

- In case of cough add Bai Bu *Radix Stemonae* or Kuan Dong Hua *Flos Tussilaginis farfarae*.
- In case of haemoptysis add Bai Mao Gen *Rhizoma Imperatae cylindricae*.
- In case of Empty-Heat add Di Gu Pi *Cortex Lycii chinensis radicis*.

Patent remedy

BA XIAN CHANG SHOU WAN
Eight Immortals Longevity Pill
Mai Men Dong *Tuber Ophiopogonis japonici*
Wu Wei Zi *Fructus Schisandrae chinensis*

Shu Di Huang *Radix Rehmanniae glutinosae praeparata*
Shan Yao *Radix Dioscoreae oppositae*
Shan Zhu Yu *Fructus Corni officinalis*
Ze Xie *Rhizoma Alismatis orientalis*
Fu Ling *Sclerotium Poriae cocos*
Mu Dan Pi *Cortex Moutan radicis*

Explanation

This remedy tonifies both Lung- and Kidney-Yin. These two are often deficient simultaneously.

The tongue presentation appropriate to this remedy is a Red body without coating in the front part.

2. HEART-YIN DEFICIENCY

Clinical manifestations

Exhaustion, mental restlessness, palpitations, insomnia, dream-disturbed sleep, propensity to be startled, poor memory, anxiety, "uneasiness", "fidgetiness", malar flush, feeling of heat in the afternoon or evening, "feeling hot and bothered", night sweating, dry mouth and throat, 5-palm heat.
Tongue: Red without coating, redder on the tip with a deep midline crack reaching the edge of the tip.
Pulse: Floating-Empty or Fine-Rapid.

This pattern is mostly seen in old people, though not exclusively. It is very often associated with (or caused by) a deficiency of Kidney-Yin. It is definitely caused by long-standing emotional problems which affect the Heart. These include sadness (as from the breaking off of relationships or bereavement), constant anxiety and worry and an excessively busy life (even if pleasurable) "always on the go".

This pattern is frequent in women during the menopause, when the decline of Kidney-Yin, associated with long-standing emotional problems as outlined above, gives rise to Heart-Yin deficiency.

Principle of treatment

Nourish Yin, strengthen the Heart, calm the Mind, if necessary, nourish Kidney-Yin.

Acupuncture

HE-7 Shenmen, HE-6 Yinxi, P-7 Daling, Ren-14 Juque, Ren-15 Jiuwei, Ren-4 Guanyuan, SP-6 Sanyinjiao, KI-6 Zhaohai, KI-3 Taixi. All with reinforcing method; no moxa.

Explanation

- **HE-7**, **P-7**, **Ren-14** and **Ren-15** calm the Mind and nourish the Heart.
- **HE-6** nourishes Heart-Yin and clears Heart Empty-Heat. In combination with KI-7 Fuliu, it stops sweating from Heart-Yin deficiency.
- **Ren-4**, **SP-6**, **KI-6** and **KI-3** can all nourish Kidney-Yin.

Herbal treatment

Prescription

TIAN WANG BU XIN DAN
Heavenly Emperor Tonifying the Heart Pill
Sheng Di Huang *Radix Rehmanniae glutinosae* 12 g
Xuan Shen *Radix Scrophulariae ningpoensis* 6 g
Mai Men Dong *Tuber Ophiopogonis japonici* 6 g
Tian Men Dong *Tuber Asparagi cochinchinensis* 6 g
Ren Shen *Radix Ginseng* 6 g
Fu Ling *Sclerotium Poriae cocos* 6 g
Wu Wei Zi *Fructus Schisandrae chinensis* 6 g
Dang Gui *Radix Angelicae sinensis* 6 g
Dan Shen *Radix Salviae miltiorrhizae* 6 g
Bai Zi Ren *Semen Biotae orientalis* 6 g
Suan Zao Ren *Semen Ziziphi spinosae* 6 g
Yuan Zhi *Radix Polygalae tenuifoliae* 6 g
Jie Geng *Radix Platycodi grandiflorae* 3 g

Explanation

- **Sheng Di Huang, Xuan Shen, Mai Dong** and **Tian Dong** nourish Yin of Kidneys and Heart.
- **Ren Shen** and **Fu Ling** tonify Qi.
- **Wu Wei Zi** nourishes Yin and calms the Mind.
- **Dang Gui** nourishes Blood.
- **Dan Shen, Bai Zi Ren, Suan Zao Ren** and **Yuan Zhi** calm the Mind.

– **Jie Geng** directs the herbs to the Upper Burner.

Patent remedy

TIAN WANG BU XIN DAN
Heavenly Emperor Tonifying the Heart Pill
Sheng Di Huang *Radix Rehmanniae glutinosae*
Xuan Shen *Radix Scrophulariae ningpoensis*
Mai Men Dong *Tuber Ophiopogonis japonicis*
Tian Men Dong *Tuber Asparagi cochinchinensis*
Ren Shen *Radix Ginseng*
Fu Ling *Sclerotium Poriae cocos*
Wu Wei Zi *Fructus Schisandrae chinensis*
Dang Gui *Radix Angelicae sinensis*
Dan Shen *Radix Salviae miltiorrhizae*
Bai Zi Ren *Semen Biotae orientalis*
Suan Zao Ren *Semen Ziziphi spinosae*
Yuan Zhi *Radix Polygalae tenuifoliae*
Jie Geng *Radix Platycodi grandiflori*

Explanation

This pill nourishes both Heart- and Kidney-Yin. It is particularly good to nourish the Yin of these two organs in chronic tiredness in women after menopause.

The tongue presentation appropriate to this remedy is a Red body without coating, with a Heart crack and possibly a redder and swollen tip.

3. STOMACH- AND SPLEEN-YIN DEFICIENCY

Clinical manifestations

Dry mouth and lips, no appetite, tiredness, dry stools, slight epigastric pain, malar flush, thirst with no desire to drink or with desire to drink in small sips only.
Tongue: normal body-colour, midline crack in the centre, rootless coating or no coating in the centre, transversal cracks on the sides indicating chronic Spleen-Qi and Spleen-Yin deficiency (see Fig. 12.3).
Pulse: Fine-Rapid, Floating-Empty on the right Middle position.

This pattern is a combination of Spleen-Qi deficiency and Stomach-Yin deficiency. Spleen-Yin deficiency manifests with dry lips and dry stools. This condition occurs in people over 50 after a lifelong history of overwork and irregular eating: for example, skipping meals, alternating days of eating very little with days of rich business lunches, eating late at night, eating in a hurry, eating standing up, discussing business while eating, etc.

Principle of treatment

Nourish Yin, strengthen Stomach and Spleen.

Acupuncture

ST-36 Zusanli, SP-6 Sanyinjiao, Ren-12 Zhongwan, ST-44 Neiting. All with reinforcing method. If the tongue-body is not Red, a little moxa can be used on ST-36.

Herbal treatment

Prescription

YI WEI TANG
Benefiting the Stomach Decoction
Bei Sha Shen *Radix Glehniae littoralis* 9 g
Mai Men Dong *Tuber Ophiopogonis japonici* 9 g
Sheng Di Huang *Radix Rehmanniae glutinosae* 12 g
Yu Zhu *Rhizoma Polygonati odorati* 6 g
Bing Tang *Brown sugar* 3 g

Explanation

– **Bei Sha Shen** and **Mai Men Dong** nourish Stomach-Yin.

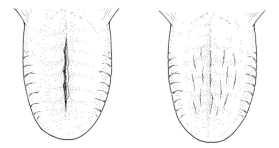

Fig. 12.3 Tongues in Stomach- and Spleen-Yin deficiency

- **Sheng Di Huang** nourishes Spleen- and Kidney-Yin.
- **Yu Zhu** nourishes Stomach-Yin and clears Heat.
- **Bing Tang** nourishes the Stomach and harmonizes the Middle.

Patent remedy

SHEN LING BAI ZHU WAN
Ginseng-Poria-Atractylodes Pill

Explanation

This remedy, which has already been mentioned under Spleen-Qi deficiency in this chapter, can also be used to nourish Stomach- and Spleen-Yin.

The tongue presentation appropriate to this remedy is a rootless coating and a body with a central Stomach crack and transversal Spleen cracks on the sides (Fig. 12.3).

Case history

A 37-year-old man had been suffering from extreme exhaustion for several years. His appetite was poor and he felt often nauseous. His mouth felt dry and he liked to sip liquids. He often developed a rash over his legs which was very itchy. He had a blood test which revealed him to be HIV-positive. His pulse was Floating-Empty and his tongue was completely peeled and had scattered Stomach cracks in the centre and transversal Spleen cracks on the sides (Plate 12.2).

Diagnosis
This is a very clear example of Stomach- and Spleen-Yin deficiency: the tongue could not show this condition more clearly.

Treatment principle
The treatment principle adopted was to nourish Stomach- and Spleen-Yin and clear Stomach Empty-Heat. He was treated with both acupuncture and herbs.

Acupuncture
The points, all needled with reinforcing method, were selected from the following:

- **Ren-12** Zhongwan, **ST-36** Zusanli and **SP-6** Sanyinjiao to nourish Stomach-Yin.
- **ST-44** Neiting to clear Stomach Empty-Heat and stop itching.
- **T.B.-6** Zhigou and **G.B.-31** Fengshi to expel Wind-Heat in order to eliminate the rash and itching.

Herbal treatment
The herbal treatment was based on a variation of Yi Wei Tang *Benefiting the Stomach Decoction*:

Bei Sha Shen *Radix Glehniae littoralis* 6 g
Mai Men Dong *Tuber Ophiopogonis japonici* 6 g
Sheng Di Huang *Radix Rehmanniae glutinosae* 9 g
Yu Zhu *Rhizoma Polygonati odorati* 6 g
Bing Tang *Brown sugar* 3 g
Shi Hu *Herba Dendrobii* 4 g
Tai Zi Shen *Radix Pseudostellariae heterophyllae* 6 g
Bian Dou *Semen Dolichoris lablab* 6 g

Explanation
- The first five herbs constitute the Yi Wei Tang to nourish Stomach-Yin.
- **Shi Hu** clears Stomach Empty-Heat.
- **Tai Zi Shen** and **Bian Dou** nourish Stomach- and Spleen-Yin.

This patient is making steady progress, reflected also in his T-cell count, and is still under treatment.

4. LIVER-YIN DEFICIENCY

Clinical manifestations

Headaches at the top of the head, tiredness which is worse in the afternoon, dizziness, tinnitus, blurred vision, dry eyes, irritability, numbness of the limbs, cramps, malar flush.
Tongue: Red, without coating, dry.
Pulse: Fine-Rapid or Floating-Empty.

Liver-Yin deficiency is a further stage of Liver-Blood deficiency. Its tiredness is characterized by being worse in the afternoon and is accompanied by a feeling of heat. Those who suffer from deficiency of Liver-Yin should definitely rest in the afternoon by lying down preferably between 1 and 3 pm, the opposite time to "Liver-hour" (1–3 am).

Principle of treatment

Nourish Yin, strengthen the Liver.

Acupuncture

Ren-4 Guanyuan, LIV-8 Ququan, SP-6 Sanyinjiao, ST-36 Zusanli. All with reinforcing method. If there are no signs of Empty-Heat and the tongue is not very Red, a little moxa can be used either on ST-36 or SP-6.

Explanation

- **Ren-4** nourishes Kidney- and Liver-Yin.
- **LIV-8** nourishes Liver-Yin.
- **SP-6** nourishes Liver-, Kidney- and Spleen-Yin.
- **ST-36** is added to tonify Blood to help to nourish Yin.

Herbal treatment

Prescription

BU GAN TANG
Tonifying the Liver Decoction
Dang Gui *Radix Angelicae sinensis* 9 g
Shu Di Huang *Radix Rehmanniae glutinosae praeparata* 9 g
Bai Shao *Radix Paeoniae albae* 9 g
Chuan Xiong *Radix Ligustici wallichii* 6 g
Mu Gua *Fructus Chaenomelis lagenariae* 6 g
Zhi Gan Cao *Radix Glycyrrhizae uralensis praeparata* 3 g
Mai Men Dong *Tuber Ophiopogonis japonici* 6 g
Suan Zao Ren *Semen Ziziphi spinosae* 3 g

Explanation

- The first four herbs constitute the Si Wu Tang *Four Substances Decoction* which nourishes Liver-Blood.
- **Mu Gua** and **Zhi Gan Cao**: one is sour (a taste which enters the Liver and astringes), the other sweet (a taste which is tonifying), in combination they nourish Yin.
- **Mai Men Dong** nourishes Yin.
- **Suan Zao Ren** is astringent, enters the Liver and calms the Mind (in case of irritability).

Patent remedy

LIU WEI DI HUANG WAN
Six-Ingredient Rehmannia Pill
Shu Di Huang *Radix Rehmanniae glutinosae praeparata*
Shan Yao *Radix Dioscoreae oppositae*
Shan Zhu Yu *Fructus Corni officinalis*
Ze Xie *Rhizoma Alismatis orientalis*
Fu Ling *Sclerotium Poriae cocos*
Mu Dan Pi *Cortex Moutan radicis*

Explanation

This remedy, more often used for Kidney-Yin deficiency, can also be used for Liver-Yin deficiency.

The tongue presentation appropriate to this remedy is a Red body which is peeled on the sides.

5. KIDNEY-YIN DEFICIENCY

Clinical manifestations

Soreness of the lower back, exhaustion, depression, lack of drive and will-power, weak legs and knees, dizziness, tinnitus, deafness, dry mouth and throat which are worse at night, night sweating, malar flush, disturbed sleep (waking up during the night), thin body.
Tongue: Red without coating.
Pulse: Floating-Empty or Rapid-Fine.

People suffering from Kidney-Yin deficiency feel completely exhausted. It is a type of exhaustion which is not eased by a short rest; it can be relieved only by regulating one's life and taking proper rest over a long period of time. Kidney-Yin deficiency is usually caused by overwork, irregular diet and excessive stress over a long period of time. In women, it can be caused by having too many children too close together. On a mental level, Kidney-Yin deficiency causes a person to feel depressed, lacking in drive and initiative as the Kidneys are the seat of Will-Power (*Zhi*).

Principle of treatment

Nourish Yin, strengthen the Kidneys, bolster the Will-Power.

Acupuncture

KI-3 Taixi, LU-7 Lieque and KI-6 Zhaohai, Ren-4 Guanyuan, SP-6 Sanyinjiao, BL-23 Shenshu, BL-52 Zhishi. All with reinforcing method; no moxa.

Explanation

- **KI-3** is the Source point and it nourishes Kidney-Yin.

- **LU-7** and **KI-6** in combination open the Directing Vessel (*Ren Mai*), nourish Kidney-Yin and moisten the throat.
- **Ren-4** and **SP-6** nourish Kidney-Yin and benefit fluids.
- **BL-23** and **BL-52** in combination, strengthen Will-Power and can improve one's drive and determination.

Herbal treatment

Prescription

ZUO GUI WAN
Restoring the Left [Kidney] Pill
Shu Di Huang *Radix Rehmanniae glutinosae praeparata* 12 g
Gou Qi Zi *Fructus Lycii chinensis* 6 g
Shan Yao *Radix Dioscoreae oppositae* 6 g
Gui Ban Jiao *Colla Plastri testudinis* 12 g
(Chuan) Niu Xi *Radix Cyathulae* 4 g
Shan Zhu Yu *Fructus Corni officinalis* 6 g
Tu Si Zi *Semen Cuscutae* 6 g
Lu Jiao Jiao *Colla Cornu Cervi* 6 g

Explanation

- **Shu Di Huang**, **Gou Qi Zi**, **Shan Yao** and **Gui Ban Jiao** nourish Kidney-Yin.
- **Shan Zhu Yu** is astringent and thus helps to nourish Yin and firms the Essence.
- **Tu Si Zi** and **Lu Jiao Jiao** tonify Kidney-Yang. They are added here according to the principle that because Kidney-Yin and Kidney-Yang share the same root, a long-term deficiency of one always implies also a slight deficiency of the other. A prescription made entirely of Yin-tonics would be too Yin and sticky: it needs a little Fire to set it in motion, i.e. some Kidney-Yang tonics. Lu Jiao Jiao is chosen here instead of Lu Rong as it tonifies both Kidney-Yang and Blood, and is thus more sticky and Yin than Lu Rong.
- **Niu Xi** directs the prescription to the Lower Burner, i.e. to the Kidneys.

(i) Patent remedy

ZUO GUI WAN
Restoring the Left [Kidney] Pill
Shu Di Huang *Radix Rehmanniae glutinosae praeparata*
Gou Qi Zi *Fructus Lycii chinensis*
Shan Yao *Radix Dioscoreae oppositae*
Gui Ban Jiao *Colla Plastri testudinis*
(Chuan) Niu Xi *Radix Cyathulae*
Shan Zhu Yu *Fructus Corni officinalis*
Tu Si Zi *Semen Cuscutae*
Lu Jiao Jiao *Colla Cornu Cervi*

Explanation

This pill nourishes Kidney-Yin and the Kidney-Essence. It is particularly indicated to treat complicated cases of a primary condition of Kidney-Yin deficiency with some symptoms of Kidney-Yang deficiency: this condition is more common in women. For example, a woman, typically over 40, may have all the symptoms and signs of Kidney-Yin deficiency such as hot flushes, night-sweating, malar flush, dizziness and dry throat, but may also suffer from cold feet and frequent-pale urination. For this reason, this remedy is particularly indicated for women.

The tongue presentation appropriate to this remedy is a Red and Thin body (but not too Red), with a rootless coating.

(ii) Patent remedy

LIU WEI DI HUANG WAN
Six-Ingredient Rehmannia Pill
Shu Di Huang *Radix Rehmanniae glutinosae praeparata*
Shan Yao *Radix Dioscoreae oppositae*
Shan Zhu Yu *Fructus Corni officinalis*
Ze Xie *Rhizoma Alismatis orientalis*
Fu Ling *Sclerotium Poriae cocos*
Mu Dan Pi *Cortex Moutan radicis*

Explanation

This is a very widely used remedy for any type of Kidney-Yin deficiency. It may be slightly difficult to digest and its dosage should be decreased if the patient experiences any digestive discomfort.

In complicated cases of a deficiency of both Yin and Yang of the Kidneys, this remedy, taken at night, can be used in conjunction with the Jin

Gui Shen Qi Wan *Golden Chest Kidney-Qi Pill* which should be taken in the morning. The dosage of these two pills should be adjusted according to whether the deficiency of Kidney-Yin or Kidney-Yang is primary.

The tongue presentation appropriate to this remedy is a Red body without coating.

(iii) Patent remedy

DA BU YIN WAN
Big Tonifying the Yin Pill
Shu Di Huang *Radix Rehmanniae glutinosae praeparata*
Gui Ban *Plastrum Testudinis*
Zhi Mu *Rhizoma Anemarrhenae asphodeloidis*
Huang Bo *Cortex Phellodendri*

Explanation

This remedy nourishes Kidney-Yin and clears Empty-Heat. It is particularly indicated when the symptoms of Empty-Heat are pronounced: these would include malar flush, a feeling of heat in the evening, hot flushes and a Red tongue without coating.

Case history

A 58-year-old woman complained of feeling very exhausted for the past 14 years. She had had a hysterectomy 15 years previously because her periods were very heavy and her uterus was prolapsed. Prior to that, she had had 4 miscarriages before having a child. After childbirth she suffered from post-natal depression manifesting with fits of crying and being deeply depressed. She felt emotionally worse after the hysterectomy. She also felt depressed, sweated at night, felt generally hot and suffered from dizziness and tinnitus. Her lower back ached most of the time. She had suffered from joint pain (hands, wrists and shoulders) for the past 16 years.

Her pulse was generally Weak and very Deep and Weak on both Rear positions (Kidneys). Her tongue was slightly Red while the sides were Pale. The coating had no root and the back of the tongue had no spirit.

Diagnosis
This case shows a deficiency of both Blood and Kidneys. In women, a deficiency of Blood very often overlaps with a deficiency of the Kidneys. This is due to the relationship between Blood and Uterus on the one hand and Kidney and Uterus on the other. In other words, the uterus is the common link in women between Blood and Kidney energy. A long-term deficiency of Blood weakens the Blood of the Uterus and eventually it weakens the Kidneys. In this case, she originally suffered from Blood deficiency (deriving from Spleen-Qi deficiency, as evidenced by the prolapsed uterus): this was still evident in the Pale sides of the tongue. The Blood deficiency is also a contributory factor to the chronic aches in the joints. The deficiency of Blood was aggravated after the four miscarriages and the childbirth, leading to the post-natal depression. The long-term deficiency of Blood eventually weakened the Kidneys (primarily Kidney-Yin) causing the depression, feeling of heat, night sweating, back-ache, dizziness and tinnitus. It is also evidenced by the Deep and Weak pulse in the Rear position, the slightly red colour of the tongue and the rootless coating.

Treatment principle
She was treated over a period of 12 months primarily with acupuncture. The main principle of treatment was to nourish Blood, nourish Kidney-Yin and remove obstructions from the channels.

Acupuncture
The main points used were **SP-6** Sanyinjiao, **KI-3** Taixi, **ST-36** Zusanli, **KI-7** Fuliu, **BL-23** Shenshu and **Ren-4** Guanyuan with reinforcing method to nourish Blood and Yin. Several other local and distal points were used in succession to remove obstructions from the channels and treat the Painful Obstruction Syndrome.

Herbal treatment
She was prescribed the Ba Zhen Wan *Eight Precious Pill* to nourish Blood and help to treat the chronic ache in the joints.

EXCESS

The main Excess patterns which can cause tiredness are:

- Liver-Qi stagnation
- Liver-Yang rising
- Liver-Fire
- Liver-Wind
- Phlegm
- Dampness.

There are other Excess conditions which cause chronic tiredness, notably those when some Heat (or Damp-Heat) remains in the body after an invasion of Wind-Heat. Called "residual pathogenic factor", this is one of the main causes of tiredness in many cases of myalgic encephalo-myelitis (ME) or post-viral syndrome, which is discussed in a separate chapter (ch. 25).

Another cause of tiredness is Latent Heat. This occurs when an exterior pathogenic factor (which may be Wind-Cold or Wind-Heat) enters the body in an insidious manner, causing no symptoms at the time of entry. The exterior pathogenic factor then lurks in the Interior and it changes into Heat, called Latent Heat. This Latent Heat then resurfaces after some months, typically (but not exclusively) in springtime, with symptoms of extreme tiredness, thirst and irritability. This is also discussed in a separate chapter (see ch. 25).

LIVER-QI STAGNATION

CLINICAL MANIFESTATIONS

Tiredness which is worse in the afternoon, depression, feeling of distension under the rib-cage or chest, sighing, nausea, poor appetite, belching, abdominal distension, "feeling wound-up", pre-menstrual tension and distension of the breasts in women.
Tongue: the body colour may be normal or, if severe, slightly Red on the sides.
Pulse: Wiry, especially on the left side. In women, the pulse may often feel Choppy or Fine. This reflects deficiency of Liver-Blood, which in women is often the underlying cause of Liver-Qi stagnation.

The tiredness deriving from stagnation of Liver-Qi is due to the impairment of the proper movement and direction of Qi. Liver-Qi aids the smooth flow of Qi and the ascending-descending of Qi. Tiredness is thus due not to a deficiency of Qi but to obstruction of Qi.

In men stagnation of Liver-Qi is usually a primary condition, i.e. it arises independently from emotional problems. It is often due to a state of tension over pressures at work or in the family. It may also be due to frustration over repression of the feminine side of a man on a psychological level.

In women, Liver-Qi stagnation is more often than not secondary to Liver-Blood deficiency. Liver-Blood and Liver-Qi represent the Yin and Yang aspects of the Liver and the two need to be harmonized. In particular, Liver-Blood needs to "anchor" or "embrace" Qi. If Liver-Blood is deficient and fails to embrace Qi, Liver-Qi becomes stagnant. Since this stagnation is secondary to Liver-Blood deficiency, the pulse may be Choppy or Fine even though the woman may display characteristic and prominent symptoms of Liver-Qi stagnation such as irritability, pre-menstrual tension and distension of the breasts.

The main characteristics of tiredness deriving from Liver-Qi stagnation are that it is worse in the afternoon especially between about 3 and 5 pm. It is *relieved* by slight exercise and it is associated with some mental depression or irritability.

In women suffering from deficiency of Liver-Blood, it is particularly beneficial to lie down around 1 to 3 pm in the afternoon. This has the effect of bringing the Blood back to the Liver and restoring energy.

The tiredness is relieved by mild exercise (such as a short walk in fresh air) because slight exercise temporarily eases stagnation of Liver-Qi. The Liver influences tendons and exercise of the tendons can therefore move Liver-Qi.

Finally, the most typical sign of stagnation of Liver-Qi is mental depression which can occur in various degrees, ranging from very mild to very severe. The person would also feel irritable and on a physical level this is reflected in a feeling of distension and discomfort under the rib-cage or chest. Frequent sighing is a sign of stagnation of Liver-Qi and an attempt by the body to relieve it.

PRINCIPLE OF TREATMENT

Soothe the Liver and regulate Qi.

ACUPUNCTURE

G.B.-34 Yanglingquan, LIV-3 Taichong, LIV-14 Qimen, LIV-13 Zhangmen, P-6 Neiguan, T.B.-6 Zhigou. All with reducing or even method.

Explanation

- **G.B.-34** moves Liver-Qi and influences the hypochondriac region.
- **LIV-3** is one of the main points to move Liver-Qi. In particular it affects the throat and is very calming.
- **LIV-14** relieves stagnation of Liver-Qi in the chest and rib-cage and it harmonizes Liver and Stomach.
- **LIV-13** relieves stagnation of Liver-Qi in the abdomen and harmonizes Liver and Spleen.
- **P-6** indirectly relieves stagnation of Liver-Qi and is particularly good in women. It also opens the chest, calms the Mind and stops irritability.
- **T.B.-6** regulates Liver-Qi and influences the sides of the body.

HERBAL TREATMENT

(a) Prescription

YUE JU WAN
Gardenia-Ligusticum Pill
Cang Zhu *Rhizoma Atractylodis lanceae* 6 g
Chuan Xiong *Radix Ligustici wallichii* 6 g
Xiang Fu *Rhizoma Cyperi rotundi* 6 g
Zhi Zi *Fructus Gardeniae jasminoidis* 6 g
Shen Qu *Massa Fermentata Medicinalis* 6 g

Explanation

This prescription uses five herbs for the "six stagnations", i.e. stagnation of Qi, Blood, Fire, Dampness, Phlegm and Food. Originally it was used for any of these six stagnations, while nowadays it is mostly used for Qi stagnation and mental depression.

- **Xiang Fu** is the emperor herb to move Qi and dispel stagnation (Qi stagnation).
- **Chuan Xiong** moves Blood and dispels stasis (Blood stagnation).
- **Zhi Zi** clears Heat and drains Fire (Fire stagnation).
- **Cang Zhu** dries Dampness (Dampness and Phlegm stagnation).
- **Shen Qu** promotes digestion and relieves retention of food (Food stagnation).

This prescription is very effective in relieving tiredness deriving mostly from stagnation of Liver-Qi, and also mental depression deriving from the same cause. Other symptoms and signs might include a feeling of tightness of the chest, epigastric and abdominal distension, nausea, a "heavy" feeling of the diaphragm, frequent sighing and a Wiry pulse.

The dosages of the individual herbs can be modified according to which of the six stagnations is predominant, thus increasing the relevant herb which becomes the emperor herb. For example, if stasis of Blood is predominant, the dose of Chuan Xiong is increased thus making this herb the emperor herb. Herbs can also be added according to which stagnation is predominant:

- For severe stagnation of Qi (and pain) add Mu Xiang *Radix Saussureae*.
- For severe Dampness add Fu Ling *Sclerotium Poriae cocos*, Ze Xie *Rhizoma Alismatis orientalis* and Hou Po *Cortex Magnoliae officinalis*.
- For severe stasis of Blood add Tao Ren *Semen Persicae* and Hong Hua *Flos Carthami tinctorii*.
- For severe Fire add Huang Lian *Rhizoma Coptidis*.
- For severe Phlegm add Ban Xia *Rhizoma Pinelliae ternatae*.
- For severe retention of food add Mai Ya *Fructus Hordei vulgaris germinatus* and Shan Zha *Fructus Crataegi*.

(b) Prescription

SI NI SAN
Four Rebellious Powder
Chai Hu *Radix Bupleuri* 6 g
Bai Shao *Radix Paeoniae albae* 9 g
Zhi Shi *Fructus Citri aurantii immaturus* 6 g
Zhi Gan Cao *Radix Glycyrrhizae uralensis praeparata* 6 g

Explanation

- **Chai Hu** moves Liver-Qi and ascends.
- **Zhi Shi** moves Liver-Qi and descends. These two herbs are therefore combined to harmonize and coordinate the ascending and

descending movement of Qi, thus dispelling stagnation of Qi.
- **Bai Shao** nourishes Blood and Yin and it pacifies Liver-Qi. It therefore regulates Liver-Qi by nourishing Liver-Blood.
- **Zhi Gan Cao** warms and harmonizes.

This formula is selected when there is some epigastric or abdominal pain and cold hands from Qi stagnation.

(c) Prescription

CHAI HU SU GAN TANG
Bupleurum Soothing the Liver Decoction
Chai Hu *Radix Bupleuri* 6 g
Bai Shao *Radix Paeoniae albae* 4.5 g
Zhi Ke *Fructus Citri aurantii* 4.5 g
Zhi Gan Cao *Radix Glycyrrhizae uralensis praeparata* 1.5 g
Chen Pi *Pericarpium Citri reticulatae* 6 g
Xiang Fu *Rhizoma Cyperi rotundi* 4.5 g
Chuan Xiong *Radix Ligustici wallichii* 4.5 g

Explanation

This is a variation of Si Ni San. The first four herbs are Si Ni San, except that Zhi Shi *Fructus Citri aurantii immaturus* is replaced with *Fructus Citri aurantii* and the dosage of Bai Shao *Radix Paeoniae albae* is reduced.

- **Chen Pi** and **Xiang Fu** move Qi.
- **Chuan Xiong** moves the Qi portion of Blood.

The impact of this prescription is therefore to move Liver-Qi, eliminate stagnation of Qi and stasis of Blood, and stop pain. This is one of the best prescriptions to move Liver-Qi both on a physical and psychological level.

(d) Prescription

XIAO YAO SAN
Free and Easy Wanderer Powder
Chai Hu *Radix Bupleuri* 6 g
Bo He *Herba Menthae* 4.5 g
Dang Gui *Radix Angelicae sinensis* 6 g
Bai Shao *Radix Paeoniae albae* 6 g
Bai Zhu *Rhizoma Atractylodis macrocephalae* 6 g
Fu Ling *Sclerotium Poriae cocos* 6 g

Zhi Gan Cao *Radix Glycyrrhizae uralensis praeparata* 3 g
Sheng Jiang *Rhizoma Zingiberis officinalis recens* 3 slices

Explanation

This is one of the most widely-used prescriptions to relieve stagnation of Qi and soothe the Liver. It has a very good psychological effect in relieving the typical irritability, moodiness or depression deriving from stagnation of Liver-Qi. In a case of tiredness deriving from stagnation of Liver-Qi, this prescription is particularly useful because, as well as moving Liver-Qi, it also tonifies Spleen-Qi and Liver-Blood.

This prescription is particularly effective and useful for women as, in women, stagnation of Liver-Qi is more likely to derive from Liver-Blood deficiency.

- **Chai Hu** and **Bo He** move Liver-Qi and relieve stagnation.
- **Bai Zhu** and **Fu Ling** tonify Spleen-Qi and drain Dampness.
- **Dang Gui** and **Bai Shao** nourish Liver-Blood. In addition, Bai Shao also pacifies the Liver.
- **Zhi Gan Cao** and **Sheng Jiang** harmonize.

(e) Prescription

WU GE KUAN ZHONG SAN
Five-Diaphragm Relaxing the Middle Powder
Bai Dou Kou *Fructus Amomi cardamomi* 1.5 g
Hou Po *Cortex Magnoliae officinalis* 9 g
Sha Ren *Fructus seu Semen Amomi* 4.5 g
Mu Xiang *Radic Saussureae* 3 g
Xiang Fu *Rhizoma Cyperi rotundi* 9 g
Qing Pi *Pericarpium Citri reticulatae viridae* 4.5 g
Chen Pi *Pericarpium Citri reticulatae* 4.5 g
Ding Xiang *Flos Caryophylli* 3 g
Zhi Gan Cao *Radix Glycyrrhizae uralensis praeparata* 6 g
Sheng Jiang *Rhizoma Zingiberis officinalis recens* 3 slices

Explanation

- **Bai Dou Kou**, **Hou Po** and **Sha Ren** fragrantly transform Dampness. Hou Po also opens the diaphragm and relaxes the chest.

- **Mu Xiang**, **Xiang Fu**, **Qing Pi** and **Chen Pi** move Qi and eliminate stagnation.
- **Ding Xiang** harmonizes the Middle and subdues rebellious Qi in the Middle Burner.
- **Zhi Gan Cao**, in a higher dose than when it is used only to harmonize, is here to soothe the Liver and eliminate stagnation. This is according to the principle that the sweet taste (pertaining to Earth) soothes the Liver (pertaining to Wood).
- **Sheng Jiang** harmonizes and regulates the Stomach.

This prescription regulates Qi, eliminates stagnation in the Middle Burner, resolves Dampness and opens the diaphragm.

It is used for the inclusive pattern called the "Five Diaphragms", which is composed of five separate patterns:

(i) *"Harassed diaphragm"*: knotted feeling in the chest, regurgitation of fluids, food does not descend, weight loss and breathlessness.

(ii) *"Sad diaphragm"*: feeling of fullness under the heart, hiccup, sour regurgitation, diarrhoea and difficult urination.

(iii) *"Qi diaphragm"*: fullness of chest and hypochondrium, choking feeling and vomiting of foul-smelling food.

(iv) *"Cold diaphragm"*: feeling of fullness and distension of abdomen and heart-region, cough, breathlessness, feeling of cold in the abdomen (literally "bitter and cold feeling in the abdomen"), borborygmi and umbilical pain.

(v) *"Heat diaphragm"*: 5-palm heat, dry mouth, mouth ulcers, hot limbs, dry lips, hot body, back ache, pain in the chest radiating to back and inability to eat much.

This prescription has a profound influence on the mental state and is very effective when tiredness is linked to mental depression and, on a physical level, with a feeling of tightness of the diaphragm as described above.

(i) Patent remedy

YUE JU WAN
Gardenia-Ligusticum Pill

Xiang Fu *Rhizoma Cyperi rotundi*
Cang Zhu *Rhizoma Atractylodis lanceae*
Shan Zhi Zi *Fructus Gardeniae jasminoidis*
Chuan Xiong *Radix Ligustici wallichii*
Shen Qu *Massa Fermentata Medicinalis*

Explanation

This is a magnificent remedy for chronic tiredness from Liver-Qi stagnation, especially in men. I have used this remedy for such cases over and over again, always with good results.

The tongue and pulse presentation appropriate to this remedy is a body with Red sides and a Wiry-Full pulse.

(ii) Patent remedy

XIAO YAO WAN
Free and Easy Wanderer Powder
Chai Hu *Radix Bupleuri*
Bo He *Herba Menthae*
Dang Gui *Radix Angelicae sinensis*
Bai Shao *Radix Paeoniae albae*
Bai Zhu *Rhizoma Atractylodis macrocephalae*
Fu Ling *Sclerotium Poriae cocos*
Zhi Gan Cao *Radix Glycyrrhizae uralensis praeparata*
Sheng Jiang *Rhizoma Zingiberis officinalis recens*

Explanation

This remedy is excellent for chronic tiredness from Liver-Qi stagnation, especially in women. This is because it contains Dang Gui and Bai Shao which nourish Liver-Blood as Liver-Blood deficiency is often, in women, the underlying cause of Liver-Qi stagnation.

The tongue and pulse presentation appropriate to this remedy is a Pale-Thin body and a pulse which is Weak and Choppy on the right and slightly Wiry on the left.

Case history

A young man of 28 complained of lack of vitality and fatigue for the past 2 years. He had also experienced a diminished sexual desire, nocturnal emissions (with dreams) once a week and he felt tired after sexual intercourse. He had a slight hypochondrial pain and a pronounced feeling of distension. His hands were usually cold. He was tall and thin. Although he made every effort to appear calm and relaxed, it was obvious that he was a very tense and somewhat rigid and demanding person. This conclusion was confirmed when his girl-friend sought treatment too! His tongue was very Red, the sides and tip were slightly redder and it had a thick yellow coating (Plate 12.3). His pulse was very Full and very Wiry.

Diagnosis
This is a good example of fatigue deriving from stagnation of Liver-Qi, as manifested by the Wiry pulse, Red tongue with redder sides, the hypochondrial pain and distension and the general tension and "uptight" feeling. His body shape was also a typical Wood type. There was also some Liver-Fire (red colour of the tongue, thick yellow coating) and Heart-Fire (red tip of the tongue). However, Liver-Fire and Heart-Fire here developed from stagnation of Liver-Qi, the prolonged stagnation imploding and giving rise to Heat.

This case is also a good example of a situation when symptoms and signs seem to point strongly to a certain pattern but the pulse and tongue contradict it. In such cases, on closer analysis, these symptoms and signs can usually be explained differently. In this case, this man's fatigue, lack of sexual desire, nocturnal emissions, tiredness after sex and cold hands, all seem to point to deficiency of Kidney-Yang. If this was the case, his pulse should have been Deep and Weak, possibly Slow, and his tongue should have been Pale. How to explain those symptoms and signs then? In this case, stagnation of Liver-Qi and its consequences can account for them. The decrease in sexual desire and the tiredness after sex are due to stagnant Liver-Qi obstructing the flow of Qi in the Lower Burner. The nocturnal emissions with dreams are due to Heart-Fire agitating the Mind. The presence of dreams indicates Fire. Had the nocturnal emissions been due to Kidney-Yang deficiency, they would have occurred without dreams. His cold hands are due not to deficiency of Yang, but to stagnant Liver-Qi obstructing the proper flow of Qi. If the feeling of cold had been due to deficiency of Yang, it would have affected the lower limbs too and would have been experienced throughout the limbs, rather than just at the extremities.

Treatment principle
The treatment principle applied was simply to soothe the Liver and relieve stagnation of Qi.

Acupuncture
As for acupuncture, the opening points of the Yang Heel Vessel (**BL-62** Shenmai on the left side and **S.I.-3** Houxi on the right) were used, and **HE-7** Shenmen was needled on the left side and **LIV-3** Taichong on the right side. Thus only four needles were used, two on one side and two on the other. This unilateral needling is particularly dynamic and powerful, while it also minimizes the number of needles. The Yang Heel Vessel is excellent to relieve stagnation of Qi in young men. HE-7 was used to calm the mind in combination with LIV-3, while this latter point also relieved stagnation of Liver-Qi and calmed the mind.

Herbal treatment
As for herbal treatment, the patent remedy Yue Ju Wan *Gardenia-Ligusticum Pill* was used to relieve stagnation of Qi and Fire. This pill (see above under "Stagnation of Liver-Qi") is excellent to clear Knotted Heat, i.e. Heat deriving from stagnation of Qi.

Only one acupuncture treament and two courses of the above patent remedy (for 2 months) were enough to restore this man's vitality and clear up the other symptoms.

Case history

A young man of 27 complained of feeling fatigued and very run-down for the past 5 years. He said he felt his whole body very tense. He also felt cold and his knees ached. His urination was frequent, his stools were loose and his sexual energy was weak. He was prone to colds and other respiratory infections.

His tongue was of a normal colour and slightly swollen on the whole of the right side. His pulse was Wiry on the left side and Weak on the right Front positions (Lung).

Diagnosis
This case is similar to the previous one. Here too, some symptoms and signs (frequent urination, loose stools, knee ache and weak sexual energy) seem to point to Kidney-Yang deficiency. However, the pulse and tongue contradict this. In this case too, most of the symptoms are due to stagnation of Liver-Qi, similar to the previous case. In addition, this young man shows a long-standing, underlying deficiency of Lung-Qi. This is evident from the Weak Lung pulse, his being prone to colds and the swelling on the whole right side of the tongue. In fact, on questioning, it emerged that he had had a long attack of glandular fever (mononucleosis) when he was 14, and that when he was 21 he had had a cough for 6 months and was suspected of having TB (which he did not). Thus, in this case the fatigue is primarily due to stagnant Liver-Qi impeding the proper flow of Qi. On trying to investigate the possible cause of Liver-Qi stagnation, it transpired that he felt "desperate" and "frustrated". His father had died when he was 14 and his mother when he was 22. Normally, bereavement tends to dissolve Qi and cause deficiency of Qi. However, people react emotionally to life's events in different

ways. In the case of this young man, the sadness from the bereavement had probably given way to anger about losing both parents in a few years.

Treatment principle
The treatment was aimed again primarily at soothing the Liver and relieving stagnation, and, secondarily at tonifying Lung-Qi. Only herbal medicine was used.

Herbal treatment
Initially he was prescribed a decoction of Yue Ju Wan *Gardenia-Ligusticum Pill* with the addition of only Zhi Gan Cao *Radix Glycyrrhizae uralensis praeparata* and Wu Wei Zi *Fructus Schisandrae chinensis* to tonify Lung-Qi. He reacted to this decoction with a dramatic improvement and after repeating another course, he was given the same prescription as a patent remedy for 3 months, producing a complete recovery.

Case history

A 74-year-old man complained of extreme tiredness and poor appetite. He did not have any other symptoms and had always been in good health. He was a keen gardener and had always been busy in the garden and the home. In the past year, however, he was always tired and mentally he could not "be bothered" to do anything.

His tongue was of a normal colour except for the sides which were slightly red. His pulse was Wiry and Full.

Diagnosis
The main problem in this case too is Liver-Qi stagnation impeding the proper flow of Qi and impairing the Stomach function (hence the poor appetite).

Treatment principle
The principle of treatment applied was to soothe the Liver and relieve stagnation.

Acupuncture
The acupuncture points used included: **L.I.-4** Hegu and **LIV-3** Taichong in combination to calm the Mind and soothe the Liver, **ST-36** Zusanli to tonify the Stomach, **Du-20** Baihui to lift the Mind, **BL-18** Ganshu (with even method) to pacify the Liver and **BL-21** Weishu (with reinforcing method) to tonify the Stomach. After a few treatments **BL-47** Hunmen was also needled with even method. This is the point on the outer Bladder line in correspondence with BL-18 Ganshu. The point BL-47 Hunmen acts on the mental aspect of the Liver, i.e. the Ethereal Soul, and it is very effective in relieving stagnation of Liver-Qi on a mental level in cases of depression.

Herbal treatment
As for herbal treatment, the patent remedy Yue Ju Wan *Gardenia-Ligusticum Pill* was also prescribed. The

treatment produced a complete cure in 6 sessions. He was in a much better frame of mind, his appetite returned and he started working in the house and garden again. His mental state and "drive" were so much improved that he later went on a trip to Australia to visit some relatives.

LIVER-YANG RISING

CLINICAL MANIFESTATIONS

Headaches of a throbbing character, dizziness, tinnitus, dry mouth and throat, short temper, insomnia and irritability.
Tongue: Red sides.
Pulse: Wiry, often only on the left side.

In women, Liver-Yang rising often arises from Liver-Blood deficiency, in which case the tongue may be Pale and the pulse Choppy.

Strictly speaking this is not an Excess pattern, but one which arises out of a combination of Deficiency and Excess. It is a deficiency of Liver-Blood or Liver-Yin or Kidney-Yin (or a combination of these) that gives rise to Liver-Yang rising.

Liver-Yang rising causes tiredness in much the same way as Liver-Qi stagnation, i.e. the derangement of Liver-Yang impairs the proper movement and direction of Qi which results in tiredness.

Additionally, the underlying deficiency of Liver and/or Kidneys also contributes to the feeling of tiredness. The tiredness deriving from Liver-Yang rising is also worse in the afternoon.

PRINCIPLE OF TREATMENT

Subdue Liver-Yang, nourish Liver and/or Kidneys.

ACUPUNCTURE

– **LIV-3** Taichong with reducing method to subdue Liver-Yang.
– **LIV-8** Ququan, **SP-6** Sanyinjiao, **KI-3** Taixi, **Ren-4** Guanyuan with reinforcing method to nourish Liver or Kidneys.
– **P-7** Daling (for women) or **HE-7** Shenmen (for men) with even method to calm the Mind.

HERBAL TREATMENT

(a) Prescription

TIAN MA GOU TENG YIN
Gastrodia-Uncaria Decoction
Tian Ma *Rhizoma Gastrodiae elatae* 9 g
Gou Teng *Ramulus Uncariae* 9 g
Shi Jue Ming *Concha Haliotidis* 6 g
Sang Ji Sheng *Ramulus Loranthi* 9 g
Du Zhong *Cortex Eucommiae ulmoidis* 9 g
Chuan Niu Xi *Radix Cyathulae* 9 g
Zhi Zi *Fructus Gardeniae jasminoidis* 6 g
Huang Qin *Radix Scutellariae baicalensis* 9 g
Yi Mu Cao *Herba Leonori heterophylli* 9 g
Ye Jiao Teng *Caulis Polygoni multiflori* 9 g
Fu Shen *Sclerotium Poriae cocos pararadicis* 6 g

Explanation

This prescription has already been explained in the chapter on Headaches (ch. 1).

(b) Prescription

ZHEN GAN XI FENG TANG
Pacifying the Liver and Subduing Wind Decoction
Huai Niu Xi *Radix Achyranthis bidentatae* 15 g
Dai Zhe Shi *Haematitum* 15 g
Long Gu *Os Draconis* 12 g
Mu Li *Concha Ostreae* 12 g
Gui Ban *Plastrum Testudinis* 12 g
Xuan Shen *Radix Scrophulariae ningpoensis* 12 g
Tian Men Dong *Tuber Asparagi cochinchinensis* 12 g
Bai Shao *Radix Paeoniae albae* 12 g
Yin Chen Hao *Herba Artemisiae capillaris* 6 g
Chuan Lian Zi *Fructus Meliae toosendan* 6 g
Mai Ya *Fructus Hordei vulgaris germinatus* 6 g
Gan Cao *Radix Glycyrrhizae uralensis* 6 g

Explanation

This prescription has already been explained in the chapter on Headaches (ch. 1).

The main difference between this prescription and the previous one is that the latter nourishes the Yin more and is therefore suitable when there is a pronounced deficiency of Liver and Kidney Yin. Note that Dai Zhe Shi is not suitable for long-term use and is contra-indicated in pregnancy. It could be eliminated from this prescription or replaced with Zhen Zhu *Margarita* which also sinks Liver-Yang.

(c) Prescription

LING JIAO GOU TENG TANG
Cornu Antelopis-Uncaria Decoction
Ling Yang Jiao *Cornu Antelopis* 4.5 g
Gou Teng *Ramulus Uncariae* 9 g
Sang Ye *Folia Mori albae* 6 g
Ju Hua *Flos Chrysanthemi morifolii* 9 g
Sheng Di Huang *Radix Rehmanniae glutinosae* 15 g
Bai Shao *Radix Paeoniae albae* 9 g
Chuan Bei Mu *Bulbus Fritillariae cirrhosae* 12 g
Zhu Ru *Caulis Bambusae in taeniis* 15 g
Fu Shen *Sclerotium Poriae cocos pararadicis* 9 g
Gan Cao *Radix Glycyrrhizae uralensis* 2.5 g

Explanation

This prescription has already been explained in the chapter on Headaches (ch. 1).

If Liver-Yang rising stems from Liver-Blood deficiency, the Si Wu Tang *Four Substances Decoction* could be added to any of the above prescriptions. If it stems from Liver-Yin deficiency, Yi Guan Jian *One Linking Decoction* could be added. If it stems from Kidney-Yin deficiency, Liu Wei Di Huang Wan *Six-Ingredient Rehmannia Pill* or Zuo Gui Wan *Restoring the Left [Kidney] Pill* could be added.

When the above prescriptions to subdue Liver-Yang are used to treat tiredness, then it will be necessary to use one of these tonifying prescriptions, or to increase the dosage of the tonifying herbs within the prescriptions. It would also be possible to reduce or eliminate the herbs which are more specific for headaches within those prescriptions, especially if they are minerals which are difficult to digest. For example, Shi Jue Ming *Concha Haliotidis* in Tian Ma Gou Teng Yin and Dai Zhe Shi *Haematitum* and Long Gu *Os Draconis* in Zhen Gan Xi Feng Tang.

(i) Patent remedy

QI JU DI HUANG WAN

Lycium-Chrysanthemum-Rehmannia Pill
Gou Qi Zi *Fructus Lycii chinensis*
Ju Hua *Flos Chrysanthemi morifolii*
Shu Di Huang *Radix Rehmanniae glutinosae praeparata*
Shan Yao *Radix Dioscoreae oppositae*
Shan Zhu Yu *Fructus Corni officinalis*
Ze Xie *Rhizoma Alismatis orientalis*
Fu Ling *Sclerotium Poriae cocos*
Mu Dan Pi *Cortex Moutan radicis*

Explanation

This pill is suitable only for Liver-Yang rising deriving from Liver- and Kidney-Yin deficiency.

The tongue presentation appropriate to this remedy is a Red body without coating.

(ii) Patent remedy

NAO LI QING
Brain Erecting and Clearing
Ci Shi *Magnetitum*
Dai Zhe Shi *Haematitum*
Ban Xia *Rhizoma Pinelliae ternatae*
Bing Pian *Borneol*
Zhen Zhu Mu *Concha margaritiferae*
Niu Xi *Radix Achyranthis bidentatae seu Cyathulae*
Bo He *Herba Menthae*

Explanation

This remedy treats only the Manifestation, i.e. Liver-Yang rising. In order to treat the Root simultaneously, it can be combined with the Ba Zhen Wan *Eight Precious Pill* if there is Liver-Blood deficiency, or Liu Wei Di Huang Wan *Six-Ingredient Rehmannia Pill* if there is Liver-Yin and/or Kidney-Yin deficiency.

LIVER-FIRE BLAZING

CLINICAL MANIFESTATIONS

Irritability, propensity to outbursts of anger, tiredness, tinnitus, deafness, temporal headache, dizziness, red face and eyes, thirst, bitter taste, dream-disturbed sleep, constipation with dry stools, dark-yellow urine, epistaxis, haematemesis, haemoptysis.
Tongue: Red body, redder on sides, yellow coating, dry.
Pulse: Full-Wiry-Rapid.

The appearance of a person suffering from this syndrome may belie the inner condition: he or she may complain of tiredness and look quite depressed and sad, and the face may be quite pale if the Spleen is also deficient. Judging by appearance and behaviour, one might deduce that the patient suffers from a Deficiency condition. However, careful observation of other manifestations, a Red tongue and a Full and Wiry pulse will clearly indicate the presence of Liver-Fire.

In this case tiredness is due to Liver-Fire blocking the circulation of Qi.

PRINCIPLE OF TREATMENT

Clear Fire, reduce the Liver.

ACUPUNCTURE

LIV-2 Xingjian. This is the main point to use, with reducing method. Other points to tonify Yin could be added, such as SP-6 Sanyinjiao and KI-3 Taixi, obviously with reinforcing method.

HERBAL TREATMENT

Prescription

LONG DAN XIE GAN TANG
Gentiana Draining the Liver Decoction
Long Dan Cao *Radix Gentianae scabrae* 6 g
Huang Qin *Radix Scutellariae baicalensis* 9 g
Shan Zhi Zi *Fructus Gardeniae jasminoidis* 9 g
Ze Xie *Rhizoma Alismatis orientalis* 9 g
Mu Tong *Caulis Akebiae* 9 g
Che Qian Zi *Semen Plantaginis* 9 g
Sheng Di Huang *Radix Rehmanniae glutinosae* 12 g
Dang Gui *Radix Angelicae sinensis* 9 g
Chai Hu *Radix Bupleuri* 9 g
Gan Cao *Radix Glycyrrhizae uralensis* 3 g

Explanation

- **Long Dan Cao** is the emperor herb in this prescription as it clears Liver-Fire.
- **Huang Qin** and **Shan Zhi Zi** clear Liver-Heat and are the minister herbs to help Long Dan Cao.
- **Ze Xie**, **Mu Tong** and **Che Qian Zi** are assistant herbs. They are cool and, as diuretics they expel Damp-Heat. They are included to clear Fire via urination.
- **Sheng Di** and **Dang Gui** nourish Yin, in order to prevent injury of Yin from Fire.
- **Chai Hu** is a messenger herb to direct the prescription to the Liver channel.
- **Gan Cao** harmonizes.

Patent remedy

LONG DAN XIE GAN WAN
Gentiana Draining the Liver Pill

Explanation

This pill has the same ingredients and indications as the prescription above.

The tongue presentation appropriate to this remedy is a Red body with redder sides and a dry-yellow coating.

LIVER-WIND

CLINICAL MANIFESTATIONS

Tremors, tic, numbness, tiredness, dizziness and paralysis.
Tongue: Red, Stiff, Deviated.
Pulse: Wiry, Firm.

There are three main types of Liver-Wind according to its aetiological factor, i.e. Heat (in the course of a febrile disease), Liver-Yang rising, or Liver-Blood deficiency. The type of Liver-Wind described here is mostly the one due to Liver-Yang rising and is frequently seen in old people, when it is often associated with Phlegm, in which case the tongue will have a sticky coating and the pulse will also be Slippery.

Tiredness is due to Liver-Wind obstructing the free circulation of Qi.

PRINCIPLE OF TREATMENT

Subdue Liver-Wind.

ACUPUNCTURE

LIV-3 Taichong, Du-16 Fengfu, G.B.-20 Fengchi, Du Mai (S.I.-3 Houxi and BL-62 Shenmai). All with reducing or even method.

HERBAL TREATMENT

TIAN MA GOU TENG YIN or ZHEN GAN XI FENG TANG
Both these prescriptions have been discussed under Liver-Yang rising.

Certain herbs that subdue Liver-Wind can be added:

- **Bai Ji Li** *Fructus Tribuli terrestris* extinguishes internal Wind.
- **Di Long** *Lumbricus* subdues internal Wind especially in old people. Di Long removes obstruction from the channels and is particularly indicated if there is numbness.
- **Jiang Can** *Bombyx batryticatus* extinguishes Wind and it also resolves Phlegm which often accompanies internal Wind in old people.

PHLEGM

CLINICAL MANIFESTATIONS

These vary according to the organ involved (which could be Lungs, Stomach, or Heart). General manifestations are: tiredness, lethargy, a slight feeling of dizziness, a feeling of heaviness of the body and cloudiness of the mind, numbness and chronic catarrh.
Tongue: Swollen, sticky coating.
Pulse: Slippery.

Tiredness is a very prominent symptom of Phlegm. It is due to Phlegm obstructing the circulation of Qi. Phlegm also impairs the transformation of Qi by the Spleen.

Tiredness is accompanied by a typical feeling of heaviness and "muzziness of the head". Thinking, memory and concentration are difficult.

PRINCIPLE OF TREATMENT

Resolve Phlegm, clear Lungs, Stomach, or Heart and tonify the Spleen.

ACUPUNCTURE

Ren-12 Zhongwan, ST-36 Zusanli, BL-20 Pishu, ST-8 Touwei, Du-20 Baihui, ST-40 Fenglong. Reinforcing method on all points except ST-40 which should be reduced.

- If the Phlegm is in the Lungs, reduce LU-5 Chize.

Explanation

- **Ren-12**, **ST-36** and **BL-20** tonify the Spleen to resolve Phlegm.
- **ST-8** resolves Phlegm from the head and relieves the feeling of muzziness of the head.
- **Du-20** promotes the rising of clear Yang to the head and the descending of turbid Qi from it.
- **LU-5** resolves Phlegm from the Lungs.

HERBAL TREATMENT

(a) Prescription

ER CHEN TANG
Two Old Decoction
Ban Xia *Rhizoma Pinelliae ternatae* 15 g
Chen Pi *Pericarpium Citri reticulatae* 12 g
Fu Ling *Sclerotium Poriae cocos* 9 g
Zhi Gan Cao *Radix Glycyrrhizae uralensis praeparata* 5 g
Sheng Jiang *Rhizoma Zingiberis officinalis recens* 3 g
Wu Mei *Fructus Pruni Mume* 1 plum

Explanation

- **Ban Xia** resolves Phlegm.
- **Chen Pi** and **Fu Ling** drain Dampness, which helps to resolve Phlegm.

This is the basic prescription to resolve Phlegm in any part of the body and any organ. It can be widely adapted to suit various conditions. Many other resolving-Phlegm prescriptions (e.g. Wen Dan Tang *Warming the Gall-Bladder Decoction* and Qing Qi Hua Tan Tang *Clearing Qi and Resolving Phlegm Decoction*) are variations of Er Chen Tang.

When used to treat tiredness, it should be adapted by adding one or two herbs to tonify the Spleen, such as Bai Zhu *Rhizoma Atractylodis macrocephalae*, Dang Shen *Radix Codonopsis pilosulae* or Huang Qi *Radix Astragali membranacei*.

(b) Prescription

WEN DAN TANG
Warming the Gall-Bladder Decoction
Ban Xia *Rhizoma Pinelliae ternatae* 6 g
Fu Ling *Sclerotium Poriae cocos* 5 g
Chen Pi *Pericarpium Citri reticulatae* 9 g
Zhu Ru *Caulis Bambusae in Taeniis* 6 g
Zhi Shi *Fructus Citri aurantii immaturus* 6 g
Zhi Gan Cao *Radix Glycyrrhizae uralensis praeparata* 3 g
Sheng Jiang *Rhizoma Zingiberis officinalis recens* 5 slices
Da Zao *Fructus Ziziphi jujubae* one date

Explanation

- **Ban Xia**, **Fu Ling** and **Chen Pi** form the Er Chen Tang *Two Old Decoction* which resolves Phlegm.
- **Zhu Ru** resolves Phlegm-Heat, calms the Mind and stops vomiting.
- **Zhi Shi** moves Qi and harmonizes the Stomach.

This is an excellent all-round prescription to resolve Phlegm-Heat from Lungs or Stomach. It is particularly indicated when the tongue has a sticky coating that is at the same time rough and dry-yellow. Very often this type of coating can

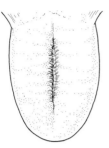

Fig. 12.4   Stomach crack with Stomach Phlegm-Heat

be observed inside a central midline crack (of the Stomach type, i.e. in the central portion only, not extending to the tip, see Fig. 12.4).

This prescription is excellent to relieve tiredness deriving from Phlegm-Heat. It also lifts the mood and relieves depression.

(c) Prescription

QING QI HUA TAN TANG
Clearing Qi and Resolving Phlegm Decoction
Dan Nan Xing *Rhizoma Arisaematis praeparata* 12 g
Gua Lou *Semen Trichosanthis* 9 g
Huang Qin *Radix Scutellariae baicalensis* 9 g
Zhi Shi *Fructus Citri aurantii immaturus* 9 g
Chen Pi *Pericarpium Citri reticulatae* 9 g
Fu Ling *Sclerotium Poriae cocos* 9 g
Xing Ren *Semen Pruni armeniacae* 9 g
Ban Xia *Rhizoma Pinelliae ternatae* 12 g

Explanation

- **Dan Nan Xing** is the emperor herb to resolve Phlegm.
- **Gua Lou** and **Huang Qin** are the minister herbs to clear Heat and resolve Phlegm.
- **Zhi Shi** and **Chen Pi** are added to move Qi, which helps to resolve Phlegm.
- **Fu Ling** and **Ban Xia** help to resolve Dampness and Phlegm.
- **Xing Ren** makes Lung-Qi descend, which, at the same time, treats cough and also helps to resolve Phlegm.

This prescription is indicated for Phlegm-Heat in the Lungs, with symptoms of cough with yellow sputum, breathlessness, tiredness, a Slippery pulse and a sticky yellow tongue coating.

In a case of chronic tiredness, it should be combined with one or two herbs to tonify the Spleen such as Bai Zhu *Rhizoma Atractylodis macrocephalae*, or with the prescription Si Jun Zi Tang *Four Gentlemen Decoction*.

This prescription is especially useful to treat the aftermath of an invasion of Wind-Heat which has penetrated in the Interior and generated Phlegm-Heat in the Lungs.

(d) Prescription

BEI MU GUA LOU SAN
Fritillaria-Trichosanthes Powder
Chuan Bei Mu *Bulbus Fritillariae cirrhosae* 5 g
Gua Lou *Semen Trichosanthis* 3 g
Tian Hua Fen *Radix Trichosanthis* 2.5 g
Fu Ling *Sclerotium Poriae cocos* 2.5 g
Chen Pi *Pericarpium Citri reticulatae* 2.5 g
Jie Geng *Radix Platycodi grandiflori* 2.5 g

Explanation

This prescription is for Phlegm and dryness of the Lungs. Although these two conditions might seem to be mutually exclusive, they are not. Phlegm is a *pathological* accumulation of fluids, whilst dryness is a lack of *physiological* fluids. In fact, in certain cases, chronic Phlegm can even lead to dryness, precisely because body fluids accumulate in a pathological way.

This prescription is therefore for very chronic cases of tiredness due to Phlegm and is more frequently used in old people. The main manifestations would include a cough with scanty sputum which is difficult to expectorate and a dry throat.

- **Chuan Bei Mu** is the emperor herb to resolve Phlegm from the Lungs, open the chest and stop cough.
- **Gua Lou** is the minister herb to clear Heat, resolve Phlegm, moisten dryness and open the diaphragm.
- **Tian Hua Fen** is the assistant herb to clear Heat, promote fluids and moisten dryness.
- **Fu Ling** and **Chen Pi** help the other herbs to resolve Phlegm by draining Dampness.
- **Jie Geng** makes Lung-Qi descend, resolves Phlegm and stops cough.

(e) Prescription

DAO TAN TANG
Conducting Phlegm Decoction
Ban Xia *Rhizoma Pinelliae ternatae* 6 g
Dan Nan Xing *Rhizoma Arisaematis praeparata* 3 g
Zhi Shi *Fructus Citri aurantii immaturus* 3 g
Fu Ling *Sclerotium Poriae cocos* 3 g
Chen Pi *Pericarpium Citri reticulatae* 3 g
Zhi Gan Cao *Radix Glycyrrhizae uralensis praeparata* 2 g
Sheng Jiang *Rhizoma Zingiberis officinalis recens* 3 g

Explanation

This prescription resolves Phlegm, moves Qi and resolves stagnation. It is particularly indicated when Phlegm and Qi are stagnating in the Middle Burner with symptoms of stuffiness and fullness of chest and epigastrium, nausea, poor appetite and cough.

– **Ban Xia** and **Nan Xing** resolve Phlegm.
– **Zhi Shi** moves Qi.
– **Fu Ling** and **Chen Pi** help to resolve Phlegm by draining Dampness.
– **Gan Cao** and **Sheng Jiang** harmonize.

(f) Prescription

DI TAN TANG
Washing away-Phlegm Decoction
Ban Xia *Rhizoma Pinelliae ternatae* 8 g
Dan Nan Xing *Rhizoma Arisaematis praeparata* 8 g
Zhu Ru *Caulis Bambusae in Taeniis* 2 g
Chen Pi *Pericarpium Citri reticulatae* 6 g
Fu Ling *Sclerotium Poriae cocos* 6 g
Zhi Shi *Fructus Citri aurantii immaturus* 6 g
Shi Chang Pu *Rhizoma Acori graminei* 3 g
Ren Shen *Radix Ginseng* (**Dang Shen** *Radix Codonopsis pilosulae*) 3 g
Zhi Gan Cao *Radix Glycyrrhizae uralensis praeparata* 2 g
Sheng Jiang *Rhizoma Zingiberis officinalis recens* 3 slices
Da Zao *Fructus Ziziphi jujubae* 3 dates

Explanation

– **Ban Xia**, **Zhu Ru** and **Nan Xing** resolve Phlegm. Nan Xing, in particular, resolves Wind-Phlegm.
– **Chen Pi** and **Fu Ling** help to resolve Phlegm by draining Dampness.
– **Zhi Shi** moves Qi and helps to resolve Phlegm.
– **Shi Chang Pu** opens the orifices.
– **Ren Shen** tonifies Qi.
– **Gan Cao**, **Sheng Jiang** and **Da Zao** harmonize.

This prescription is used for Wind-Phlegm, i.e. a combination of internal Wind and Phlegm. It is therefore used only in old people who are most likely to suffer from Wind-Phlegm, such as would occur after a stroke. Hence the addition of Shi Chang Pu which opens the orifices blocked by Phlegm. "Opening the orifices" in this case would address the symptom of slurred speech, for example.

Other manifestations would include numbness and paralysis of the limbs, tiredness, a tongue with a thick-sticky coating and a Slippery-Wiry pulse.

The above formulae to resolve Phlegm are compared and contrasted in Table 12.1.

(i) Patent remedy

ER CHEN WAN
Two Old Pill
Ban Xia *Rhizoma Pinelliae ternatae*
Chen Pi *Pericarpium Citri reticulatae*
Fu Ling *Sclerotium Poriae cocos*
Zhi Gan Cao *Radix Glycyrrhizae uralensis praeparata*
Sheng Jiang *Rhizoma Zingiberis officinalis recens*
Wu Mei *Fructus Pruni Mume*

Explanation

This is a general remedy which is suitable for a wide variety of types of Phlegm, especially if combined with acupuncture. It has the same ingredients and functions as the prescription of the same name.

The tongue presentation appropriate to this remedy is a Swollen body with a sticky coating.

(ii) Patent remedy

QING QI HUA TAN WAN
Clearing Qi and Resolving Phlegm Pill

Table 12.1   Comparison of Phlegm-resolving formulae

	Symptoms-signs	Tongue	Pulse	Pattern
Er Chen Tang	Expectoration of profuse, sticky-white sputum, feeling of oppression of the chest	Swollen, sticky-white coating	Slippery-Full	Cold Phlegm
Wen Dan Tang	Expectoration of scanty yellow sputum, a feeling of oppression and tightness of the chest, anxiety	Swollen, sticky-yellow coating, Stomach-crack with rough yellow coating in it	Slippery and Rapid	Hot Phlegm
Qing Qi Hua Tan Tang	Expectoration of profuse sticky-yellow coating, feeling of oppression of the chest	Swollen, sticky-yellow coating	Slippery and Rapid	Hot Phlegm
Bei Mu Gua Lou San	Expectoration of very scanty-dry sputum, dry mouth	Swollen, dry-sticky coating	Slightly Slippery and Empty	Dry Phlegm
Dao Tan Tang	Feeling of oppression of the epigastrium, distension	Swollen, Stomach crack	Slippery and Wiry	Phlegm and Qi stagnation
Di Tan Tang	Expectoration of scanty sputum, slurred speech	Swollen, no spirit	Slippery	Wind and Phlegm

Dan Nan Xing *Rhizoma Arisaematis praeparata*
Gua Lou *Semen Trichosanthis*
Huang Qin *Radix Scutellariae baicalensis*
Zhi Shi *Fructus Citri aurantii immaturus*
Chen Pi *Pericarpium Citri reticulatae*
Fu Ling *Sclerotium Poriae cocos*
Xing Ren *Semen Pruni armeniacae*
Ban Xia *Rhizoma Pinelliae ternatae*

Explanation

This remedy is suitable only for Phlegm-Heat affecting the Lungs. It has the same ingredients and functions as the prescription of the same name.

The tongue presentation appropriate to this remedy is a Swollen body with sticky-yellow coating.

DAMPNESS

CLINICAL MANIFESTATIONS

Tiredness and sleepiness, lethargy, feeling of heaviness of the body or head, no appetite, feeling of oppression of the chest or epigastrium, a sticky taste, urinary difficulty, turbid urine, excessive vaginal discharge, mucus in the stools, lack of concentration, a "muzzy" feeling of the head, dull headache, a sticky tongue coating and a Slippery pulse.

If Dampness combines with Heat there will be: thirst, dark urine, yellow vaginal discharge, mucus in the stools with a burning sensation of the anus on defecation, possibly blood in the stools, possibly night sweating and a sticky-yellow tongue coating.

If Dampness affects the Gall-Bladder and Liver there will be a bitter taste, hypochondrial pain and distension and possibly jaundice.

The tiredness deriving from Dampness has typical characteristics: it is associated with a feeling of heaviness of the body or head, and sleepiness and lethargy especially after lunch. It is not really relieved by rest because it does not derive from a deficiency. On the contrary, excessive rest may even aggravate it: for example, sleeping for a long time after lunch (more than half an hour) will tend to increase Dampness.

PRINCIPLE OF TREATMENT

Resolve Dampness, tonify the Spleen.

ACUPUNCTURE

SP-9 Yinlingquan, SP-6 Sanyinjiao, BL-22 Sanjiaoshu with reducing method. Ren-9 Shuifen, LU-7 Lieque and L.I.-4 Hegu with even method to resolve Dampness. BL-20 Pishu and Ren-12

Zhongwan with reinforcing method to tonify the Spleen. These are the general points to eliminate Dampness. Other points depend on the location of the Dampness.

- In the head: ST-8 Touwei, Du-20 Baihui and Du-23 Shangxing with even method.
- In the Stomach and Spleen: ST-21 Liangmen, Ren-10 Xiawan with even method.
- In the Intestines: ST-25 Tianshu, BL-25 Dachangshu, BL-27 Xiaochangshu, ST-27 Daju and ST-28 Shuidao, all with reducing or even method.
- In the Bladder: BL-28 Pangguangshu, Ren-3 Zhongji and BL-32 Ciliao with reducing or even method.
- In the Gall-Bladder: G.B.-34 Yanglingquan and G.B.-24 Riyue with reducing method.
- In the Liver: LIV-14 Qimen with reducing method.
- If Dampness combines with Heat: L.I.-11 Quchi with reducing method.

HERBAL TREATMENT

(a) Prescription

PING WEI SAN
Balancing the Stomach Powder
Cang Zhu *Rhizoma Atractylodis lanceae* 9 g
Chen Pi *Pericarpium Citri reticulatae* 6 g
Hou Po *Cortex Magnoliae officinalis* 6 g
Zhi Gan Cao *Radix Glycyrrhizae uralensis praeparata* 3 g
Sheng Jiang *Rhizoma Zingiberis officinalis recens* 3 g
Da Zao *Fructus Ziziphi jujubae* 3 dates

Explanation

- **Cang Zhu** is the emperor herb to dry Dampness.
- **Chen Pi** is the minister herb to assist Cang Zhu to dry Dampness.
- **Hou Po** is the assistant herb to fragrantly resolve Dampness and harmonize the Middle. It also moves Qi, which helps to resolve Dampness.
- **Zhi Gan Cao**, **Sheng Jiang** and **Da Zao** harmonize and regulate the Middle.

This is the main prescription to resolve Dampness in the Middle Burner.

(b) Prescription

HUO XIANG ZHENG QI SAN
Agastache Upright Qi Powder
Huo Xiang *Herba Agastachis* 9 g
Zi Su Ye *Folia Perillae frutescentis* 3 g
Bai Zhi *Radix Angelicae dahuricae* 3 g
Ban Xia *Rhizoma Pinelliae ternatae* 6 g
Chen Pi *Pericarpium Citri reticulatae* 6 g
Bai Zhu *Rhizoma Atractylodis macrocephalae* 6 g
Fu Ling *Sclerotium Poriae cocos* 3 g
Hou Po *Cortex Magnoliae officinalis* 6 g
Da Fu Pi *Pericarpium Arecae catechu* 3 g
Jie Geng *Radix Platycodi grandiflori* 6 g
Sheng Jiang *Rhizoma Zingiberis officinalis recens* 3 slices
Da Zao *Fructus Ziziphi jujubae* 3 dates
Zhi Gan Cao *Radix Glycyrrhizae uralensis praeparata* 3 g

Explanation

- **Huo Xiang** is the emperor herb to fragrantly resolve Dampness. It also harmonizes the Stomach.
- **Zi Su Ye** and **Bai Zhi** help Huo Xiang to resolve Dampness.
- **Ban Xia** and **Chen Pi** dry Dampness and harmonize the Stomach.
- **Bai Zhu** and **Fu Ling** strengthen the Spleen to resolve Dampness.
- **Hou Po** and **Da Fu Pi** move Qi and resolve Dampness. They also open the chest and relieve fullness.
- **Jie Geng** makes Lung-Qi descend and opens the diaphragm.
- **Sheng Jiang**, **Da Zao** and **Gan Cao** harmonize the prescription and regulate the Middle.

This prescription fragrantly resolves Dampness. It is especially suited to resolve Dampness from the head since it contains many aromatic herbs. It is more suited for Damp-Cold (white-sticky tongue coating) rather than Damp-Heat (yellow tongue coating).

(c) Prescription

LIAN PO YIN
Coptis-Magnolia Decoction
Huang Lian *Rhizoma Coptidis* 3 g
Hou Po *Cortex Magnoliae officianalis* 3 g
Shan Zhi Zi *Fructus Gardeniae jasminoidis* 9 g
Dan Dou Chi *Semen Sojae praeparatum* 9 g
Shi Chang Pu *Rhizoma Acori graminei* 3 g
Ban Xia *Rhizoma Pinelliae ternatae* 3 g
Lu Gen *Rhizoma Phragmitis communis* 15 g

Explanation

- **Huang Lian** clears Heat and dries Dampness.
- **Hou Po** fragrantly resolves Dampness and moves Qi (which in itself also helps to resolve Dampness).
- **Shan Zhi Zi** and **Dan Dou Chi** clear Heat. They specifically clear "hidden" Heat, i.e. any Heat remaining in the Interior after an invasion of Wind-Heat or Damp-Heat.
- **Shi Chang Pu** opens the orifices and helps to resolve Dampness. It is said to "awaken" the Spleen.
- **Ban Xia** resolves Phlegm, harmonizes the Stomach and stops vomiting.
- **Lu Gen** clears Heat and stops vomiting.

This prescription is excellent to clear Damp-Heat in Stomach and Spleen. It is especially suited to clear lingering Damp-Heat causing chronic tiredness. This frequently occurs after an invasion of either Wind-Heat or Damp-Heat. If the exterior pathogenic factor is not cleared properly, or if the person is in a state of weakness through overwork, it may linger in the Interior. In addition, Damp-Heat obstructs the Spleen: this in itself leads to the formation of Dampness and therefore a vicious circle is established. The main symptoms and signs indicating this prescription are a feeling of heaviness, thirst, a sticky taste, nausea, epigastric fullness, tiredness, lethargy, loose foul-smelling stools, a sticky-yellow tongue coating and a Slippery pulse.

(d) Prescription

HUO PO XIA LING TANG
Agastache-Magnolia-Pinellia-Poria Decoction

Huo Xiang *Herba Agastachis* 6 g
Bai Dou Kou *Fructus Amomi cardamomi* 2 g
Hou Po *Cortex Magnoliae officinalis* 3 g
Fu Ling *Sclerotium Poriae cocos* 9 g
Zhu Ling *Sclerotium Polypori umbellati* 4.5 g
Yi Yi Ren *Semen Coicis lachryma jobi* 12 g
Ze Xie *Rhizoma Alismatis orientalis* 4.5 g
Ban Xia *Rhizoma Pinelliae ternatae* 4.5 g
Dan Dou Chi *Semen Sojae praeparatum* 9 g
Xing Ren *Semen Pruni armeniacae* 9 g

Explanation

This prescription is more suited for the early stages of Dampness invading the body. The main manifestations would be a feeling of heaviness, epigastric fullness, tiredness, chilliness, a sticky-white tongue coating and a Slippery pulse.

- **Huo Xiang**, **Bai Dou Kou**, and **Hou Po** fragrantly resolve Dampness. Huo Xiang also releases the Exterior and, for this reason, this prescription is also suited in invasions of exterior Dampness.
- **Fu Ling**, **Zhu Ling**, **Yi Yi Ren** and **Ze Xie** drain Dampness.
- **Ban Xia** helps to drain Dampness by resolving Phlegm.
- **Dan Dou Chi** clears Heat and stops irritability.
- **Xing Ren** helps to drain Dampness by making Lung-Qi descend (and therefore move fluids downwards towards the Bladder and Kidneys).

(i) Patent remedy

PING WEI PIAN
Balancing the Stomach Tablet
Cang Zhu *Rhizoma Atractylodis lanceae*
Chen Pi *Pericarpium Citri reticulatae*
Hou Po *Cortex Magnoliae officinalis*
Zhi Gan Cao *Radix Glycyrrhizae uralensis praeparata*
Sheng Jiang *Rhizoma Zingiberis officinalis recens*
Da Zao *Fructus Ziziphi jujubae*

Explanation

This pill has the same ingredients and indications as the prescription above.

The tongue presentation appropriate to this remedy is a thick coating in the centre.

(ii) Patent remedy

HUO XIANG ZHENG QI WAN (PIAN)
Agastache Upright Qi Pill (Tablet)

Explanation

This remedy has the same ingredients and indications as the prescription of the same name above.

The tongue presentation appropriate to this remedy is a sticky-white coating.

(iii) Patent remedy

JIAN PI WAN
Strengthening the Spleen Pill
Dang Shen *Radix Codonopsis pilosulae*
Shan Zha *Fructus Crataegi*
Bai Zhu *Rhizoma Atractylodis macrocephalae*
Zhi Shi *Fructus Citri aurantii immaturus*
Chen Pi *Pericarpium Citri reticulatae*
Mai Ya *Fructus Hordei vulgaris germinatus*

Explanation

This pill resolves Dampness and mildly strengthens the Spleen.

The tongue presentation appropriate to this remedy is a Pale body with a thick coating in the centre.

Case history

A man of 34 complained of extreme tiredness, nausea, dizziness, headaches, thirst, loose stools, epigastric fullness and a feeling of heaviness. He also felt irritable and had been putting on weight. All these symptoms appeared after a prolonged stay in Sri Lanka.

His pulse was Rapid and Slippery and his tongue was slightly Red with red raised "pimples" and a sticky-yellow coating.

Diagnosis
All these manifestations clearly point to retention of Damp-Heat in the Interior, obviously contracted in Sri Lanka where the weather is hot and damp. The irritability derives from Heat and putting on weight

was due to Dampness. The red "pimples" on the tongue indicate Dampness.

Treatment principle
The principle adopted was to clear Heat and resolve Dampness from the Middle Burner.

Acupuncture
The acupuncture points chosen were simply aimed at tonifying the Spleen on the one hand (**Ren-12** Zhongwan, **ST-36** Zusanli and **BL-20** Pishu, reinforced) and at resolving Damp-Heat on the other hand (**SP-9** Yinlingquan, **SP-6** Sanyinjiao and **L.I.-11** Quchi, reduced).

Herbal treatment
The use of three courses of Lian Po Yin *Coptis-Magnolia Decoction* without any variations and four acupuncture treatments produced a complete recovery.

Case history

A 42-year-old woman complained of chronic fatigue for the previous 4 years. The symptoms had appeared after contracting influenza 4 years earlier; she still felt tired, her muscles ached and she had a feeling of heaviness. On interrogation, it emerged that she felt thirsty, irritable and had a feeling of heat in the evening. Her pulse was Rapid (92), slightly Slippery but Fine. Her tongue was Red, peeled in patches and with a thick coating elsewhere (Plate 12.4).

Diagnosis
These manifestations clearly point to retention of Damp-Heat mostly in the muscles, evidenced by the feeling of heaviness and ache. The pulse and tongue are also consistent with Damp-Heat. The Heat part of Damp-Heat obviously caused also a deficiency of Yin manifesting with thirst, irritability and feeling of heat. Her tongue clearly shows the two conditions of Damp-Heat with a sticky coating and Yin deficiency through a lack of coating in places.

Treatment principle
The treatment principle adopted was to resolve Damp-Heat primarily and nourish Yin secondarily.

Acupuncture
The acupuncture treatment was aimed at resolving Damp-Heat and tonifying the Spleen. The points used were:

- **ST-36** Zusanli, **SP-6** Sanyinjiao, **Ren-12** Zhongwan and **BL-20** Pishu (reinforced) to tonify the Spleen and nourish Stomach-Yin.
- **SP-9** Yinlingquan and **L.I.-11** Quchi (even method) to resolve Damp-Heat.

Herbal treatment
The herbal decoction Lian Po Yin *Coptis-Magnolia Decoction* was used with excellent results.

Western differential diagnosis

Chronic tiredness and debility can be due to many different causes, of which the seven most common ones will be discussed here.

1. CHRONIC NEPHRITIS

This can be pyelo- or glomerulonephritis. It consists in inflammation of the kidney pelvis or glomeruli or both. The main manifestations are severe tiredness, oedema, nausea, frequent urination and lower back-ache (see chapter 22).

2. GLANDULAR FEVER (MONONUCLEOSIS)

This is due to an infection from the Epstein-Barr virus. It manifests with debility, poor appetite, fever, swollen glands and, in prolonged cases, depression.

It usually occurs only in young adults and teenagers.

3. MYALGIC ENCEPHALOMYELITIS (ME)

This manifests with a general flu-like feeling, great tiredness, lethargy, muscle ache and poor memory (see chapter 25).

It is more common in young adults.

4. CARCINOMA

Carcinoma of any part of the body or in any organ can cause tiredness and debility. Tiredness is often the earliest presenting symptom. If it is accompanied by poor appetite, loss of weight and a sallow complexion in a middle-aged or elderly person, carcinoma should be suspected.

5. ADDISON'S DISEASE

This is due to hypofunction of the cortex of the adrenal glands. It is characterized by severe lassitude, poor appetite, nausea, vomiting, abdominal pain, giddiness, blurred vision, dyspnoea on exertion, palpitations, craving for salt, pigmentation of skin, weight loss and a low systolic blood pressure.

6. HYPOTHYROIDISM

This is due to insufficient secretion of thyroxine. It is more common in women. The main symptoms and signs are mental and physical debility, slow speech, somnolence, headache, feeling of cold, dyspnoea on exertion, obesity, sallow complexion, puffy eyes, coarse and dry skin, dry hair, scanty periods or amenorrhoea, oedema of legs, hypothermia and in severe cases, mental confusion.

Table 12.2   Causes of tiredness in Western medicine

Disease	Pathology	Symptoms	Signs
Nephritis	Inflammation of renal glomeruli	Tiredness, nausea	Polyuria, oedema
Glandular fever	Infection from Epstein-Barr virus	Tiredness, sweating	Swollen glands, fever
ME	Unknown	Tiredness, muscle ache, flu-like feeling	
Carcinoma	Malignancy	Tiredness	Loss of weight
Addison's disease	Adrenal hypofunction	Tiredness, lassitude, no appetite, nausea, giddiness, blurred vision, dyspnoea	Weight loss, pigmentation of skin, low systolic pressure (less than 110)
Hypothyroidism	Deficient secretion of thyroxine	Mental and physical debility, slow speech, somnolence, dyspnoea, feeling cold	Obesity, puffy face and eyes, coarse and dry skin, dry hair, oedema, hypothermia
Diabetes mellitus	Insulin deficiency	Thirst, hunger, tiredness	Loss of weight or obesity, polyuria, boils, dry tongue

7. DIABETES MELLITUS

This is due to insufficient secretion of insulin. At its onset, the main symptoms and signs are polyuria, thirst, hunger and loss of weight. The urine and blood contain glucose. During the chronic stage other manifestations include: obesity, pruritus vulvae, boils, peripheral neuritis, retinitis and a dry tongue.

The Western medical causes of tiredness are summarized in Table 12.2.

END NOTES

1. Nanjing College of Traditional Chinese Medicine 1979 A Revised Explanation of the Classic of Difficulties (*Nan Jing Jiao Shi* 难经校经), People's Health Publishing House, Beijing, pp. 28–29. The "Classic of Difficulties" itself was first published c. 100 BC.
2. Traditional Chinese Medicine Research Institute 1959 An Explanation of the Essential Prescriptions of the Golden Chest (*Jin Gui Yao Lue Yu Yi* 金匮要略语译), People's Health Publishing House, Beijing, p. 61. The "Essential Prescriptions of the Golden Chest" itself was written by Zhang Zhong Jing and first published c. AD 220.
3. Chao Yuan Fang AD 610 Discussion on Causes and Symptoms of Diseases (*Zhu Bing Yuan Hou Lun* 诸病源候论), cited in Zhang Bo Yu 1986 Chinese Internal Medicine (*Zhong Yi Nei Ke Xue* 中医内科学), Shanghai Science Publishing House, Shanghai, p. 281.
4. 1979 The Yellow Emperor's Classic of Internal Medicine — Simple Questions (*Huang Ti Nei Jing Su Wen* 黄帝内经素问), People's Health Publishing House, Beijing. First published c. 100 BC, p. 154.
5. Zhu Qi Shi 1988 Discussion on Exhaustion (*Li Xu Yuan Jian* 理虚元鉴), People's Health Publishing House, Beijing, p. 19. First published c. 1520.
6. Ibid., p. 21.
7. Ibid., p. 24.
8. Zhang Jie Bin The Complete Book of Jing Yue (*Jing Yue Quan Shu* 景岳全书). First published 1624; cited in: Zhang Bo Yu 1986 Chinese Internal Medicine, Shanghai Scientific Publishing House, Shanghai, p. 281.
9. Luo Yuan Qi 1986 Chinese Medicine Gynaecology (*Zhong Yi Fu Ke Xue* 中医妇科学), Shanghai Science Publishing House, Shanghai, p. 105.
10. D. R. Laurence 1973 Clinical Pharmacology, Churchill Livingstone, Edinburgh, p. 14.31.
11. Simple Questions, p. 68.

Chest Painful Obstruction Syndrome 13

胸
痹

The condition which goes under the name of "Chest Painful Obstruction" (Chest *Bi*) is characterized by a feeling of oppression and pain in the chest, extending to the shoulders. In severe cases the pain is greater than the sensation of oppression and in very severe cases there is a stabbing pain in the heart region on the left side of the chest extending to the left shoulder and down the left arm.

This type of condition is mentioned in the "Yellow Emperor's Classic of Internal Medicine". The "Simple Questions" in chapter 22 says: "*When the Heart is diseased there is pain in the centre of the chest, hypochondrial fullness and pain, pain between the scapulae and in both arms.*"[1] The "Spiritual Axis" in chapter 24 says: "*In true Heart pain the arms and legs are cyanotic and cold up to the elbows and knees and there is severe pain in the heart region . . .*".[2] This corresponds to a severe type of Chest Painful Obstruction.

During the Han dynasty, Zhang Zhong Jing in the "Essential Prescriptions from the Golden Chest" introduced the term "Chest Painful Obstruction" for the first time. In chapter 9 he says:

In Chest Painful Obstruction there is breathlessness, cough, pain in the chest and back, the Front-position pulse is Deep and Slow and in the Middle position it is Tight and Rapid. Use Trichosanthes-Allium-White Wine Decoction.[3]

Here "Slow" and "Rapid" do not refer to the actual rate of the pulse (which could not be Slow in one position and Rapid in another), but to the feeling of the pulse. In the same chapter he says: "*In Chest Painful Obstruction when the patient cannot lie down and heart pain extends to the back, use Trichosanthes-Allium-Pinellia Decoction.*"[4] The "Causes of Diseases and Treatment according to the Pulse" (1706) says:

Pain over the sternum indicates Chest Painful Obstruction . . . the internal causes of Chest Painful Obstruction are the 7 emotions and the 6 excessive desires. They stir Heart-Fire and affect the Lungs. They may also cause rebellious Qi to damage the Lung passages and Phlegm to accumulate and Qi to stagnate. Chest Painful Obstruction may also be caused by excessive consumption of hot-pungent foods which injure the Upper Burner and cause Blood to stagnate. This leads to a feeling of oppression and pain of the chest.[5]

Traditionally, there are three types of Chest Painful Obstruction:

(a) *Xin Tong* (Heart-pain): pain in the chest
(b) *Zhen Xin Tong* (True Heart-pain): pain in the chest with cyanosis of face, arms and feet
(c) *Jue Xin Tong* (Yang-Collapse Heart-pain): pain in the chest with cold limbs.

All these three types are the subject of this chapter.

From a Western medical perspective, Chest Painful Obstruction may correspond to several different diseases, pertaining to the heart or the lungs. If there is pain in the left side of the chest, palpitations and shortness of breath, it may correspond to heart diseases such as angina pectoris, myocardial infarction or coronary heart disease. If there is a cough, breathlessness and expectoration of phlegm, it may correspond to such lung diseases as chronic bronchitis, chronic tracheitis, pulmonary emphysema or cancer of the lungs. Examples of patterns corresponding to lung diseases may be "Turbid Phlegm stagnating in the chest" or "Spleen- and Heart-Yang deficiency". In some cases, Chest Painful Obstruction may correspond to chronic gastritis.

Aetiology and pathology

1. EXTERNAL PATHOGENIC FACTORS

External Cold can invade the chest and obstruct the circulation of Yang Qi in the chest. The obstruction of Yang Qi leads to Chest Painful Obstruction with the ensuing feeling of oppression and pain in the chest. External Cold is all the more likely to invade the body if there is a pre-existing deficiency of Yang. In particular, a deficiency of Yang of the Lungs or Heart will predispose the body to invasion of Cold in the chest.

The "Methods and Rules of Medicine" (1658) says: *"In Chest Painful Obstruction pain in the heart region is caused by Yang deficiency and invasion of Cold."*[6] The "Treatment Planning according to Syndrome Categories" (1839) says: *"In Chest Painful Obstruction Yang Qi of the chest does not move; after a long time Yin takes the place of Yang."*[7]

2. DIET

Irregular eating and excessive consumption of fats, sweets, dairy foods or cold-raw foods injure the Spleen and Stomach. As a result, these cannot transform food and transport food essences, and Phlegm is formed. Phlegm obstructs the blood vessels leading to stagnation of Qi and Blood. Stasis of Blood in the chest blocks the circulation of Yang Qi in the chest and this leads to Chest Painful Obstruction.

3. EMOTIONAL PROBLEMS

Worry, brooding and pensiveness injure the Spleen and Lungs. When Spleen- and Lung-Qi are weak, after some time, Qi may stagnate in the chest. Prolonged stagnation of Qi, on the other hand, may also lead to the formation of Phlegm in the chest. Both Qi stagnation and Phlegm contribute to Chest Painful Obstruction developing.

Anger, resentment, frustration and depression injure the Liver and prevent its Qi from flowing freely. Stagnant Liver-Qi may turn into Fire after a long period of time. Fire, on the other hand, burns body fluids and condenses them into Phlegm. Both stagnant Liver-Qi and Phlegm lead to stasis of Blood which obstructs the movement of Yang Qi. This causes Chest Painful Obstruction.

4. OLD AGE

Declining Kidney-Yang fails to warm the internal organs and may lead to Heart-Yang deficiency.

Declining Kidney-Yin fails to nourish the internal organs and may lead to Heart-Yin deficiency. If Heart-Yin is deficient, Heart-Yang cannot move and this leads to stagnation of Qi and Blood in the chest and Chest Painful Obstruction. In both these cases, the Root is the deficiency of Yin or Yang of Kidneys and Heart, and the Manifestation is the stagnation of Qi and Blood in the chest.

As for pathology, although from a Chinese viewpoint the Heart is central to the condition of Chest Painful Obstruction, other organs, notably the Lungs and Stomach, also play a prominent role. The Lungs govern Gathering Qi (*Zong Qi*) of the chest. This assists the Heart in pushing Blood through the blood vessels and if Gathering Qi is weak, the Heart lacks force in pumping and Blood may stagnate in the chest. The "Spiritual Axis" in chapter 75 says: "*If Gathering Qi does not descend, Blood will stagnate in the vessels.*"[8] Hence the importance of moving Qi in order to move Blood: the point Ren-17 Renzhong, where the Gathering Qi collects, is an important point to move Qi in the chest to relieve Blood stasis.

The Stomach also affects the Heart and Blood circulation: the Great Connecting channel of the Stomach gives the pulse the force to contract and dilate. This channel emerges from the Stomach and goes to the area below the left breast: the pulsation which can be felt here, called *Xu Li*, is the pulsation of the Great Connecting channel of the Stomach. Hence the importance of treating the Stomach to support the Heart and help to move Blood: the point ST-40 Fenglong, for example, is extremely important to open the chest and improve the circulation of Blood there. The point ST-36 Zusanli is very important to regulate the pulse and should always be needled when the pulse is irregular. Retention of food in the Stomach also affects the development of Chest Painful Obstruction: when food stagnates in the Middle Burner it may obstruct the circulation of Qi and Blood in the chest and prevents Heart-Qi and Lung-Qi from descending. This situation is actually very common in Western patients when it is often difficult to distinguish the chest from the epigastric symptoms. In treatment, it is therefore important to pay attention to the condition of the Middle Burner and, if there is retention of food (manifesting with sour regurgitation, belching, a feeling of fullness, lack of appetite, a thick-sticky tongue coating and a Slippery-Full pulse on the right Middle position), this should be treated with the addition of herbs such as Lai Fu Zi *Semen Raphani sativi*, Ji Nei Jin *Endothelium Corneum Gigeraiae Galli* or Mai Ya *Fructus Hordei vulgaris germinatus*.

Chest Painful Obstruction is always characterized by a combination of Deficiency and Excess. The Root of the disease is usually a deficiency of Spleen, Heart or Kidneys or a combination of these. The Manifestation is characterized mostly by stasis of Blood, Cold or Phlegm (Fig. 13.1).

The symptomatology of Chest Painful Obstruction is characterized by obstruction of blood vessels which leads to pain. Stasis of Blood is therefore nearly always present in this condition, either by itself or in combination with other factors. In long-standing conditions Phlegm is often present.

In chronic conditions there is an interaction between stasis of Blood and Phlegm, with one aggravating the other. The "Spiritual Axis" says in chapter 81: "*When body fluids are harmonized,*

ROOT

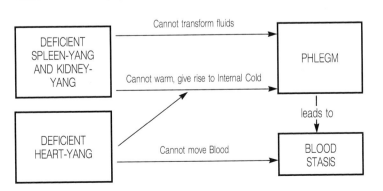

Fig. 13.1 Root and Manifestation of Chest Painful Obstruction

they are transformed into Blood."[9] Since body fluids provide the substance for the making of Blood, when they are pathologically transformed into Phlegm, Blood cannot be produced and moved properly and it stagnates. On the other hand, since there is a process of mutual exchange between Blood and body fluids, when Blood stagnates over a long period of time, it will interfere with the transformation of fluids and contribute to forming Phlegm. For this reason, in chronic conditions of Chest Painful Obstruction, especially in the elderly, stasis of Blood and Phlegm are both present.

If both Kidney and Heart Yang are deficient, body fluids accumulate and overflow towards the Heart and Lungs resulting in cough and oedema.

Differential diagnosis

It is important to differentiate Chest Painful Obstruction from other conditions with similar symptoms.

1. PHLEGM-FLUIDS IN CHEST-HYPOCHONDRIUM

In Chest Painful Obstruction there is a feeling of oppression and pain in the chest which may also extend to the shoulder or left breast. The pain is elicited by tiredness, exposure to cold, overeating or emotional stress. There is usually a history of breathlessness.

In the case of Phlegm-Fluids in chest and hypochondrium there is a feeling of distension and pain in the chest and hypochondrial region. The pain is continuous and is worse on breathing and turning one's body. There is also a feeling of fullness over the ribs and a cough with profuse white-watery sputum.

2. EPIGASTRIC PAIN

The pain of Chest Painful Obstruction may sometimes extend to the epigastrium and could be confused with epigastric pain, i.e. pain originating from a Stomach disharmony. However, with epigastric pain there is also belching, hiccups, sour regurgitation and other Stomach or Spleen symptoms which are absent in Chest Painful Obstruction.

3. TRUE HEART PAIN

True Heart pain is not so much a different condition as a further and serious development of Chest Painful Obstruction when there is severe stasis of Blood over a long period of time. True Heart pain is continuous and is accompanied by cold sweating, a pale-purplish face, cyanotic lips and limbs, a Minute or Knotted pulse and a Bluish-Purple tongue.

The pathogenic factor involved in Chest Painful Obstruction can be identified also according to the character of the pain.

A *distending* pain indicates stagnation of Qi; if accompanied by a *feeling of oppression or tightness* of the chest, it indicates Phlegm.

A *burning* pain denotes Heat (usually Phlegm-Heat), while a *very severe* pain indicates retention of Cold in the blood vessels.

A *stabbing* pain that is fixed and feels like a knife blade indicates stasis of Blood.

Deficiency of Yang should be differentiated from retention of (internal) Cold:

- *Retention of Cold*: exposure to cold aggravates it, the patient has no aversion to cold and the limbs feel cold to the touch
- *Yang deficiency*: the patient has aversion to cold, likes to curl up and cover up, feels cold, the face is pale and the limbs feel cold to the touch.

Treatment

The "Essential Prescriptions of the Golden Chest" by Zhang Zhong Jing (c. AD 220) advocates "penetrating Yang" as the main treatment for Chest Painful Obstruction. "Penetrating Yang" means moving Yang Qi and penetrating the blood vessels with warm and pungent herbs such as Gui Zhi *Ramulus Cinnamomi cassiae*.

The "Effective Formulae Tested by Physicians for Generations" (1349) by Wei Yi Lin introduced Su He Xiang Wan *Styrax Pill* with fragrant and warm herbs to move Yang Qi in the blood vessels.[10] This formula is widely used nowadays as a patent remedy for angina pectoris.

In later centuries many physicians resorted to moving Blood and eliminating stasis to treat Chest Painful Obstruction. For example, the "Standards of Diagnosis and Treatment" (1607) advocates using Hong Hua *Flos Carthami tinctorii*, Tao Ren *Semen Persicae*, Jiang Xiang *Lignum Dalbergiae odoriferae* and the formula Shi Xiao San *Breaking into a Smile Powder* for the treatment of Chest Painful Obstruction.[11]

The "Collection of Rhymes of Contemporary Formulae" (1801) recommends using Dan Shen Yin *Salvia Decoction* for Chest Painful Obstruction.[12] This formula is still widely used today, also as a patent remedy.

The "Correction of Errors in Medicine" (1830) by Wang Qing Ren introduced the formula Xue Fu Zhu Yu Tang *Blood-Mansion Eliminating Stasis Decoction* which is today one of the most important and widely-used prescriptions to move Blood and eliminate stasis especially in the chest.[13]

In Chest Painful Obstruction the Root is usually a Deficiency and the Manifestation is an Excess. It is always essential to differentiate clearly between the relative influence of Deficiency and Excess in the clinical manifestations of Chest Painful Obstruction. Once a Deficiency has been identified, one must further differentiate between deficiency of Qi, Yang, Blood or Yin. Once an Excess has been identified, one must further distinguish the pathogenic factor involved, e.g. Cold, Phlegm or Blood stasis.

Generally speaking, it is better to deal with the Manifestation first, i.e. eliminate the pathogenic factor. This would involve either expelling Cold or resolving Phlegm or moving Blood. Especially with herbal treatment, it is better to eliminate the obstruction of a pathogenic factor before tonifying the body's Qi. With acupuncture, it is possible to deal effectively with both the Root and Manifestation, i.e. tonify the body's Qi as well as eliminating the pathogenic factor.

In acute cases one must always concentrate on treating the Manifestation only (i.e. eliminate the pathogenic factor), whilst in the chronic phase in between acute attacks, one can turn one's attention to treating the Root (i.e. tonify the body's Qi).

Although the three main Excess conditions (Stasis of Blood, Phlegm and Cold) all derive from a deficiency (of Yang), they will be discussed separately because they correspond to acute stages during which one must treat the Manifestation rather than the Root.

The patterns discussed are:

EXCESS

Stagnation of Qi in the chest
Heart-Blood stasis
Turbid Phlegm stagnating in the chest
Stagnation of Cold in the chest

DEFICIENCY

Heart- and Kidney-Yin Deficiency
Qi and Yin Deficiency
Spleen- and Heart-Yang Deficiency

EXCESS CONDITIONS

1. STAGNATION OF QI IN THE CHEST

CLINICAL MANIFESTATIONS

Distending pain in the chest that moves from place to place and comes and goes, hypochondrial distension.
Tongue: not significant to diagnose this pattern.
Pulse: Wiry.

This is due to stagnation of Qi of the Liver and Heart. The feeling of distension, the moving of the pain from place to place and the fact that it comes and goes, are all typical of Qi stagnation.

TREATMENT PRINCIPLE

Move Qi, relax the chest, soothe the Liver and Heart, stop pain.

ACUPUNCTURE

Ren-17 Shanzhong, P-6 Neiguan, T.B.-6 Zhigou, G.B.-34 Yanglingquan, LIV-3 Taichong, BL-17 Geshu, BL-15 Xinshu, BL-18 Ganshu, BL-14 Jueyinshu. Reducing or even method.

Explanation

- **Ren-17** moves Qi in the chest. It is inserted horizontally usually downwards, but it can be slanted towards the direction of the area of pain.
- **P-6** moves Qi in the chest, relaxes and opens the chest, calms the Mind and settles the Ethereal Soul.
- **T.B.-6** and **G.B.-34** move Qi in the hypochondrial region.
- **LIV-3** moves Liver-Qi, relaxes the sinews, calms the Mind and settles the Ethereal Soul.
- **BL-17** relaxes the diaphragm and the chest.
- **BL-15** and **BL-18**, Back-Transporting points of the Heart and Liver respectively, move Heart- and Liver-Qi.
- **BL-14**, Back-Transporting point of the Pericardium, moves Qi in the chest.

HERBAL TREATMENT

Prescription

XUAN FU HUA TANG
Inula Decoction
Xuan Fu Hua *Flos Inulae* 9 g
Xiang Fu *Rhizoma Cyperi rotundi* 6 g
Su Geng *Radix Perillae frutescentis* 6 g
Yu Jin *Tuber Curcumae* 6 g
Zhi Ke *Fructus Citri aurantii* 6 g
Si Gua Luo *Fasciculus Luffae vascularis* 6 g

Explanation

- **Xuan Fu Hua** makes Qi descend in the chest.
- **Xiang Fu**, **Yu Jin** and **Zhi Ke** move Qi.
- **Su Geng** relaxes the chest.
- **Si Gua Luo** invigorates the channels in the chest.

Variations

- If there is stagnation of Heart-Qi from emotional problems and the patient is unhappy, taciturn and likes to be alone, add He Huan Pi *Cortex Albizziae julibrissin*.
- If there is stagnation of Qi on a background of Yin deficiency add Fu Shou *Fructus Citri sarcodactylis* which moves Qi without injuring Yin.
- If there is stagnation of Lung-Qi as well add Jie Geng *Radix Platycodi grandiflori*, Zi Wan *Radix Asteris tatarici* and Xing Ren *Semen Pruni armeniacae*.

2. HEART-BLOOD STASIS

CLINICAL MANIFESTATIONS

Pricking pain in the chest which is fixed and worse at night, palpitations.
Tongue: Purple, especially in the chest area or on the sides in correspondence with the chest area (Fig. 13.2).
Pulse: Deep and Choppy.

TREATMENT PRINCIPLE

Move Blood, eliminate stasis, invigorate the Connecting channels, stop pain.

ACUPUNCTURE

BL-13 Feishu, BL-14 Jueyinshu, BL-15 Xinshu, Ren-17 Shanzhong, Ren-14 Juque, P-4 Ximen, P-6 Neiguan, ST-40 Fenglong, SP-10 Xuehai, BL-17

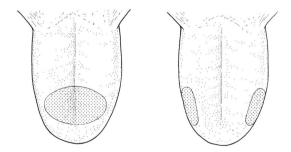

Fig. 13.2 Chest area on the tongue

Geshu, Du-12 Shenzhu, Du-11 Shendao, Du-10 Lingtai, S.I.-11 Tianzong. All needled with reducing or even method depending on the severity of the pain. The points on the Governing vessel (Du-12-11-10) can be alternated with those on the Directing vessel (Ren-17-14).

Explanation

- **BL-13** is used to stimulate the descending of Qi and to move Blood by moving Qi.
- **BL-14, Ren-17, BL-15** and **Ren-14** are the Back-Transporting and Front-Collecting points of Pericardium and Heart respectively. In acute cases they are used with reducing method. These are the main points. Ren-17 is needled horizontally downwards. If the chest pain extends towards the left side, this point can be needled horizontally towards the heart.
- **P-4** is the Accumulation point and as such stops pain and is specifically indicated in acute syndromes.
- **P-6** is the Connecting point and opening point of the Yin Linking vessel. It opens the chest, moves Qi and Blood and removes obstructions. It should be needled with reducing method.
- **ST-40** opens the chest (in combination with P-6) and it subdues rebellious Qi.
- **SP-10** moves Blood.
- **BL-17** moves Blood and relaxes the diaphragm.
- **Du-12-11-10** move Qi and Blood in the chest.
- **S.I.-11** moves Blood in the chest and it is chosen when the chest pain extends to the scapula.

HERBAL TREATMENT

(a) Prescription

XUE FU ZHU YU TANG
Blood Mansion Eliminating Stasis Decoction
Dang Gui *Radix Angelicae sinensis* 9 g
Sheng Di Huang *Radix Rehmanniae glutinosae* 9 g
Chi Shao *Radix Paeoniae rubrae* 6 g
Chuan Xiong *Radix Ligustici wallichii* 5 g
Tao Ren *Semen Persicae* 12 g

Hong Hua *Flos Carthami tinctorii* 9 g
Chai Hu *Radix Bupleuri* 3 g
Zhi Ke *Fructus Citri aurantii* 6 g
Niu Xi *Radix Cyathulae* 9 g
Jie Geng *Radix Platycodi grandiflori* 5 g
Gan Cao *Radix Glycyrrhizae uralensis* 3 g

Explanation

- **Dang Gui, Sheng Di, Chi Shao, Chuan Xiong, Tao Ren** and **Hong Hua** are a modified version of Tao Hong Si Wu Tang *Persica-Carthamus Four Substances Decoction* which moves Blood.
- **Chai Hu** and **Zhi Ke** move Qi in order to move Blood.
- **Niu Xi** directs the herbs downwards and **Jie Geng** directs them upwards. This movement in opposite directions makes the whole formula more dynamic in order to move Blood.
- **Gan Cao** harmonizes.

(b) Prescription

TAO HONG SI WU TANG Variation
Persica-Carthamus Four Substances Decoction Variation
Dang Gui *Radix Angelicae sinensis* 9 g
Shu Di Huang *Radix Rehmanniae glutinosae praeparata* 12 g
Bai Shao *Radix Paeoniae albae* 6 g
Chuan Xiong *Radix Ligustici wallichii* 6 g
Hong Hua *Flos Carthami tinctorii* 6 g
Tao Ren *Semen Persicae* 6 g
Huang Lian *Rhizoma Coptidis* 3 g
Dan Nan Xing *Rhizoma Arisaematis praeparata* 6 g
Zhu Ru *Caulis Bambusae in Taeniis* 6 g
San Qi *Radix Notoginseng* 3 g
Dan Shen *Radix Salviae miltiorrhizae* 9 g
Jiang Huang *Rhizoma Curcumae longae* 3 g

Explanation

This prescription is used when Phlegm and Heat accompany the stasis of Blood in the chest. The symptoms would be a feeling of oppression of the chest, a feeling of heat, thirst and a Red tongue.

- **Tao Hong Si Wu Tang** moves Blood.
- **Huang Lian**, **Dan Nan Xing** and **Zhu Ru** resolve Phlegm-Heat.
- **San Qi**, **Dan Shen** and **Jiang Huang** move Blood and eliminate stasis.

Variations

- If there are signs of Blood-Heat add Mu Dan Pi *Cortex Moutan radicis* and Chi Shao *Radix Paeoniae rubrae*.
- If there are signs of Cold add one or two of the following herbs: Chuan Xiong *Radix Ligustici wallichii*, Wu Ling Zhi *Excrementum Trogopteri*, Mo Yao *Myrrha* or Yan Hu Suo *Rhizoma Corydalis yanhusuo*.

(i) Patent remedy

GUAN XIN SU HE WAN
Styrax Coronary Pill
Su He Xiang *Styrax liquidis*
Bing Pian *Borneol*
Tan Xiang *Lignum Santali albi*
Ru Xiang *Gummi Olibanum*
Mu Hu Die *Semen Oroxyli indici*

Explanation

This pill is suitable for Chest Painful Obstruction from stasis of Blood or Cold. It is not to be taken for more than 2-3 months at a stretch.

The tongue presentation appropriate to this remedy is a Bluish-Purple tongue, especially in the chest area (see Fig. 13.2).

(ii) Patent remedy

FU FANG DAN SHEN PIAN
Compound-Formula Salvia Tablet
Dan Shen *Radix Salviae miltiorrhizae*
Bing Pian *Borneol*

Table 13.1 Formulae for Heart-Blood stasis

Formula	Differentiation
XUE FU ZHU YU TANG TAO HONG SI WU TANG	Heart-Blood stasis
Variation	Heart-Blood stasis with Phlegm-Heat

Explanation

This remedy is also suitable for Chest Painful Obstruction from stasis of Blood. It is milder than the previous patent remedy and can be taken for longer periods of time. It dilates the coronary arteries and increases the volume of blood in them.

The tongue presentation appropriate to this remedy is a slightly Purple tongue. As this remedy is for milder cases of stasis of Blood, it could also be prescribed when the stasis of Blood manifests with darkened veins under the tongue: this sign usually appears before the main body of the tongue becomes Purple.

(iii) Patent remedy

SU BING DI WAN
Styrax-Borneol Pill
Su He Xiang *Styrax liquidis*
Bing Pian *Borneol*

Explanation

This is suitable for Chest Painful Obstruction from stasis of Blood. In terms of strength, it is milder than Guan Xin Su He Wan but stronger than Fu Fang Dan Shen Pian.

The tongue presentation appropriate to this remedy is a Purple body in the chest area.

(iv) Patent remedy

DAN SHEN PIAN
Salvia Tablet
Dan Shen *Radix Salviae miltiorrhizae*

Explanation

This is suitable for Chest Painful Obstruction from stasis of Blood. It is the mildest of all the above remedies and can be used for a long time.

In this case, the tongue may be only slightly Purple, or not Purple at all and only show a slight darkening of the sub-lingual veins.

(v) Patent remedy

GUAN XIN GAO
Coronary Plaster
Su He Xiang *Styrax liquidis*

Explanation

This plaster for Chest Bi from stasis of Blood is applied to the umbilicus: this is based on the idea of treating the Pre-natal Qi to affect the Post-natal Qi. It is also intended to regulate Qi and Blood in the Governing, Directing and Penetrating Vessels, all of which originate from the area below the umbilicus. In particular the Penetrating Vessel subdues rebellious Qi in the chest and regulates Blood.

Case history

A 74-year-old man had been suffering from what had been diagnosed as angina pectoris for 1 year. The attacks were elicited by exercise, cold and eating. The pain in the chest was quite severe. He also complained of a feeling of heaviness in the legs. He looked generally quite strong and had no other symptoms. His voice and his spirit were strong. His tongue was Reddish-Purple with a yellow coating and his pulse was Wiry and Full.

Diagnosis

First of all, the condition is clearly one of Excess as evidenced by his strong voice and spirit, strong body, Full pulse and tongue with coating. As for the chest pain, this is due to stasis of Blood in the chest. Stasis of Blood is evident from the character of the pain, the purple colour of the tongue-body and the Wiry pulse. The feeling of heaviness in the legs is due to Dampness infusing downwards.

Treatment principle

The treatment principle used was to move Blood in the chest. This patient was treated with acupuncture only with good results.

Acupuncture

The main points used were aimed at moving Blood and eliminating stasis. These were:

– **P-6** Neiguan, **P-4** Ximen, **ST-40** Fenglong, **Ren-17** Shanzhong and **BL-14** Jueyinshu with even method. ST-40 was used not for its capacity of resolving Phlegm but because, in combination with P-6, it relaxes the chest and regulates the ascending and descending of Qi in the chest.

3. TURBID PHLEGM STAGNATING IN THE CHEST

CLINICAL MANIFESTATIONS

Pronounced feeling of oppression of the chest, pain in the chest extending to shoulder or upper back, breathlessness, feeling of heaviness, dizziness, expectoration of white sputum.
Tongue: Swollen body, sticky-white tongue coating.
Pulse: Slippery.

Phlegm obstructs the circulation of Qi in the chest and causes the typical feeling of oppression in the chest. Some patients may describe it as "heaviness" or "tightness". Phlegm causes some slight dizziness as it obstructs the rising of clear Yang to the chest.

In this condition, the feeling of oppression in the chest predominates over any pain.

This pattern very frequently occurs in combination with the first one, i.e. stasis of Blood in the chest. There is an interaction between Phlegm and stasis of Blood as they aggravate each other. The relative predominance of Phlegm or stasis of Blood can be easily evaluated according to pulse, tongue and symptoms (Table 13.2).

TREATMENT PRINCIPLE

Invigorate Yang, resolve Phlegm, open the orifices.

ACUPUNCTURE

P-6 Neiguan, BL-14 Jueyinshu, BL-15 Xinshu, Ren-17 Shanzhong, Ren-14 Juque, ST-40 Fenglong, Ren-12 Zhongwan, Ren-9 Shuifen, SP-6 Sanyinjiao, BL-13 Feishu, LU-7 Lieque, LU-9 Taiyuan. Reducing or even method, except for Ren-12 which should be reinforced. Moxa can be used.

Table 13.2 Comparison of Phlegm and stasis of Blood from symptoms, tongue and pulse

	Phlegm	Stasis of blood
Symptoms	Oppression of the chest	Pain in the chest
Tongue	Swollen body, sticky coating	Purple body
Pulse	Slippery	Choppy or Wiry

Explanation

- **P-6** opens the chest and invigorates Yang in the chest.
- **BL-14**, **BL-15**, **Ren-17** and **Ren-14** are respectively the Back-Transporting points and Front-Collecting points of Pericardium and Heart. They are the main points for Chest Painful Obstruction and, in this case, moxa can be used to invigorate Yang.
- **ST-40**, **Ren-12**, **Ren-9** and **SP-6** resolve Phlegm. ST-40 also opens the chest and subdues rebellious Qi in the chest.
- **BL-13** and **LU-7** open the Lung passages to facilitate the elimination of Phlegm.
- **LU-9** resolves Phlegm from the Lungs.

HERBAL TREATMENT

Prescription

GUA LOU XIE BAI BAN XIA TANG
Trichosanthes-Allium-Pinellia Decoction
Gua Lou *Fructus Trichosanthis* 12 g
Xie Bai *Bulbus Allii* 12 g
Ban Xia *Rhizoma Pinelliae ternatae* 12 g
Bai Jiu White rice wine 30 ml

Explanation

This is the classic prescription for Chest Painful Obstruction from Phlegm.

- **Gua Lou** resolves Phlegm and opens the chest.
- **Xie Bai** invigorates Yang in the chest.
- **Ban Xia** resolves Phlegm and subdues rebellious Qi.
- **White rice wine** invigorates Yang and dispels Cold Phlegm.

Variations

- In case of symptoms of Phlegm obstructing the head, such as pronounced dizziness, a feeling of muzziness of the head and blurred vision, add Shi Chang Pu *Rhizoma Acori graminei* and Yu Jin *Tuber Curcumae* to open the orifices.
- If there is a pronounced feeling of fullness and oppression of the chest add Hou Po *Cortex Magnoliae officinalis*.
- For copious expectoration of phlegm add Dan Nan Xing *Rhizoma Arisaematis praeparata*.
- For pronounced pain in the chest add Dan Shen *Radix Salviae miltiorrhizae*.
- If Phlegm is combined with some stasis of Blood one can use the following variation of the above prescription:

JIA WEI GUA LOU XIE BAI TANG
Trichosanthes-Allium Decoction Variation
GUA LOU *Fructus Trichosanthis* 15 g
XIE BAI *Bulbus Allii* 9 g
CHI SHAO *Radix Paeoniae rubrae* 6 g
HONG HUA *Flos Carthami tinctorii* 6 g
CHUAN XIONG *Radix Ligustici wallichii* 6 g
JIANG HUANG *Rhizoma Curcumae longae* 6 g

The last four herbs move Blood. Jiang Huang *Rhizoma Curcumae longae*, in particular, moves Qi and Blood in the shoulder area and is therefore used when the pain extends to this area.

- If Phlegm is combined with Heat with such manifestations as a feeling of heat, a bitter taste, a Red tongue with sticky-yellow coating and a Rapid pulse, use:
  HUANG LIAN WEN DAN TANG *Coptis Warming the Gall-Bladder Decoction* with XIAO XIAN XIONG TANG *Small Sinking [Qi of the] Chest Decoction*
  HUANG LIAN *Rhizoma Coptidis* 6 g
  FA BAN XIA *Rhizoma Pinelliae ternatae* 12 g
  GUA LOU *Fructus Trichosanthis* 30 g
  CHEN PI *Pericarpium Citri reticulatae* 6 g
  FU LING *Sclerotium Poriae cocos* 6 g
  ZHU RU *Caulis Bambusae in Taeniis* 6 g
  ZHI SHI *Fructus Citri aurantii immaturus* 6 g
  ZHI GAN CAO *Radix Glycyrrhizae uralensis praeparata* 3 g
  SHENG JIANG *Rhizoma Zingiberis officinalis recens* 5 slices
  DA ZAO *Fructus Ziziphi jujubae* one date

The above three prescriptions are compared in Table 13.3.

(a) Patent remedy

GUA LOU PIAN

Table 13.3 Comparison of formulae for Turbid Phlegm in chest

Formula	Differentiation
GUA LOU XIE BAI BAN XIA TANG	Phlegm
JIA WEI GUA LOU XIE BAI TANG	Phlegm and stasis of Blood
HUANG LIAN WEN DAN TANG and XIAO XIAN XIONG TANG	Phlegm-Heat

Trichosanthes Tablet
Gua Lou Ren *Fructus Trichosanthis*

Explanation

This remedy, composed of only one ingredient, is for chest pain from Phlegm.

The tongue presentation appropriate to this remedy is a Swollen tongue with a sticky-yellow coating.

(b) Patent remedy

SU HE XIANG WAN
Styrax Pill
Su He Xiang *Styrax liquidis*

Explanation

This pill, containing only one ingredient which opens the orifices, is suitable for Chest Painful Obstruction from Phlegm. It is stronger than the previous remedy.

The tongue presentation appropriate to this remedy is a Swollen tongue with a dirty-white-sticky coating.

Case history

A 59-year-old woman complained of a feeling of oppression and pain in the chest. She had experienced this since a heart attack 5 years previously. Her blood pressure was raised (180/100). She also suffered from pain and swelling of her knees, ankles and wrists.

She was quite overweight. Her tongue was very Pale and very Swollen (Plate 13.1). Her pulse was very Deep and Weak especially on both Rear positions.

Diagnosis
The pain and feeling of oppression in the chest are due to a combination of Phlegm and Cold stagnating in the chest, with predominance of Phlegm. This woman does not have many symptoms but the feeling of oppression in the chest, her being overweight and the very Swollen tongue are sufficient for a diagnosis of obstruction by Phlegm. This occurs on a background of severe deficiency of Yang of the Spleen and Kidneys. Again, she does not have many symptoms but the very Pale tongue and very Deep and Weak pulse on both Rear positions are definite signs of Kidney-Yang deficiency. We can also deduce Spleen-Yang deficiency from the presence of Phlegm. Both these conditions, i.e. Kidney deficiency and Phlegm, are contributory factors to the development of Painful Obstruction Syndrome from Cold and Dampness.

Treatment principle
This case (like most cases of Chest Painful Obstruction) is characterized by a combination of Deficiency (of Yang of Spleen and Kidneys) and Excess (itself a combination of Phlegm and Cold). The correct approach to treatment is to deal with the Excess condition during the acute or sub-acute stage and with the Deficiency afterwards. In this case, since this woman had quite a pronounced and distressing feeling of oppression and pain in the chest, attention was paid to treating the Excess condition, i.e. resolve Phlegm and dispel Cold. She was treated with acupuncture only and for the first 10 (weekly) sessions, the treatment was aimed at resolving Phlegm and removing obstruction from the chest.

Acupuncture
– **ST-40** Fenglong, **P-6** Neiguan, **P-4** Ximen, **Ren-17** Shanzhong, **BL-14** Jueyinshu, **Ren-9** Shuifen, **SP-6** Sanyinjiao, **Ren-12** Zhongwan and **BL-20** Pishu. All the points were needled with even method except the last two which were reinforced to tonify the Spleen to resolve Phlegm.

After these 10 sessions, attention was diverted to tonifying Spleen- and Kidney-Yang. The main signs to look for before changing the aim of treatment from resolving Phlegm to tonifying would be a reduction in the size of her swollen tongue and a marked decrease in the feeling of oppression and pain in the chest. The main points used to tonify Spleen- and Kidney-Yang were:
– **BL-20** Pishu, **BL-23** Shenshu, **Ren-12** Zhongwan, **ST-36** Zusanli, **KI-7** Fuliu, and **KI-3** Taixi. Reinforcing method and moxa were used. This lady was completely cured after another 10 sessions although she still comes for treatment every 3 months to prevent any recurrence.

Case history

A 66-year-old man complained of a feeling of oppression, tightness and mild ache in the chest. This had started over 20 years previously with recurring, sudden panic attacks characterized by breathlessness and an intense feeling of oppression in the chest like a "band around the chest". He also had the feeling he wanted to sigh but could not. Two years before the consultation he had also suffered a mild heart infarction. He felt occasionally dizzy and had recurrent bouts of a stabbing hypochondrial pain on the right side. His face was pale and his tongue was Bluish-Purple on the edges and Pale elsewhere. It was Swollen and had a very sticky tongue coating. His pulse was Slippery.

Diagnosis
This man's condition is characterized by Turbid Phlegm obstructing the chest (feeling of oppression and tightness of the chest, breathlessness, dizziness, Swollen tongue with sticky coating and Slippery pulse). Besides this central condition there is also some stagnation of Liver-Qi (feeling of needing to sigh) and Liver-Blood (stabbing hypochondrial pain and Bluish-Purple colour of the tongue's edges). Finally, the condition is characterized by Cold (Pale tongue and pale face).

Treatment principle
In spite of the very long duration of this problem, the condition was still primarily one of Excess as evidenced by the pulse. Attention was therefore paid to resolving Phlegm, moving Qi and Blood and expelling Cold. The herbal prescription chosen was aimed at resolving Phlegm as a primary objective, whilst with acupuncture some points were reinforced to tonify the body's Qi. Both acupuncture and herbs were used.

Acupuncture
With acupuncture some points were needled with even method:

- **P-6** Neiguan to move Qi and Blood in the chest and relieve the feeling of oppression and tightness.
- **ST-40** Fenglong to subdue rebellious Qi in the chest and resolve Phlegm.
- **GB-34** Yanglingquan to move Liver-Qi in the hypochondrium.
- **LIV-3** Taichong to move Liver-Qi, calm the Mind and settle the Ethereal Soul.
- **Ren-17** Shanzhong and **BL-14** Jueyinshu Front-Collecting point and Back-Transporting point of the Pericardium respectively, to move Qi in the chest and relieve the feeling of oppression and tightness.
- **LIV-14** Qimen to move Liver-Qi.
- **SP-6** Sanyinjiao to help to resolve Phlegm and calm the Mind.
- **SP-4** Gongsun on the left and P-6 Neiguan on the right to open the Penetrating vessel. This vessel is excellent to remove obstructions and subdue rebellious Qi in the chest.

Some points were needled with reinforcing method to tonify Qi:

- **ST-36** Zusanli and **Ren-12** Zhongwan to tonify Spleen-Qi to resolve Phlegm.

Herbal treatment
The formula used was a variation of two prescriptions: Gua Lou Xie Bai Ban Xia Tang *Trichosanthes-Allium-Pinellia Decoction* and Ban Xia Hou Po Tang *Pinellia-Magnolia Decoction.*

Gua Lou *Fructus Trichosanthis* 6 g
Xie Bai *Bulbus Allii* 4 g
Ban Xia *Rhizoma Pinelliae ternatae* 6 g
Hou Po *Cortex Magnoliae officinalis* 6 g
Su Ye *Folium Perillae frutescentis* 4 g
Fu Ling *Sclerotium Poriae cocos* 6 g
Gui Zhi *Ramulus Cinnamomi cassiae* 4 g
Zhi Shi *Fructus Citri aurantii immaturus* 4 g
Sheng Jiang *Rhizoma Zingiberis officinalis recens* 3 slices.

Gui Zhi was added to expel Cold and move Yang in the chest. Zhi Shi was added to move Liver-Qi and subdue rebellious Qi in the chest.

This patient showed a very marked improvement after a short time, with most of his symptoms disappearing or being greatly reduced in intensity.

Case history

A 56-year-old woman complained of palpitations with a dull ache in the chest extending upwards to the jaw and downwards to the left arm. She felt cold and sweaty during an attack. These attacks were becoming more frequent. She also complained of great tiredness, lack of appetite, a feeling of heaviness, dizziness and blurred vision. She also suffered from expectoration of profuse white phlegm.

Her pulse was Slippery and her tongue had a very sticky yellow coating.

Diagnosis
This is a clear example of chest pain due to Phlegm. The manifestations of Phlegm are dizziness, blurred vision, expectoration of phlegm, feeling of heaviness, Slippery pulse and a sticky tongue coating. The Phlegm is obviously caused by Spleen-Qi deficiency which accounts for the great tiredness and lack of appetite.

Treatment principle
This lady was treated with acupuncture only. The treatment was initially aimed at dealing with the Manifestation first, i.e. resolving Phlegm, and later with the Root, i.e. tonifying Spleen-Qi.

Acupuncture
The main points used to resolve Phlegm from the chest were:

– **ST-40** Fenglong, **LU-5** Chize, **SP-6** Sanyinjiao, **P-5** Jianshi, **P-4** Ximen, **Ren-17** Shanzhong, **Ren-9** Shuifen with even method.
– **Ren-12** Zhongwan with reinforcing method.

The main points used to tonify the Spleen were:

– **ST-36** Zusanli, **SP-3** Taibai, **BL-20** Pishu and **BL-21** Weishu with reinforcing method.

Case history

A 36-year-old woman had had an attack of viral pericarditis the previous year. At that time she had chest pain, felt very weak, was sweating and had a temperature. Since then, she had been feeling very tired, dizzy at times and her memory was poor. Her appetite was not very good and she had a constant desire to lie down. At times her mouth felt quite dry and she had a tendency to constipation. Her pulse was Rapid and Slippery and her tongue was Red with a sticky-yellow coating and a Stomach-type crack in the midline.

Diagnosis
This is a condition of combined Deficiency and Excess. There is some deficiency of Qi and Blood (tiredness, desire to lie down, poor appetite, poor memory) whilst the Excess is characterized by Phlegm (Slippery pulse and sticky tongue coating) and Heat (dry mouth, constipation, Red tongue with yellow tongue coating and Rapid pulse).

Treatment principle
Although the condition is one of both Deficiency and Excess, it is better to resolve Phlegm and clear Heat *before* tonifying Qi and Blood. Especially with herbal medicine, tonifying Qi and Blood in the presence of Phlegm and Heat may aggravate the condition. This is because most Qi and Blood tonics are "sticky" (therefore tending to aggravate Phlegm) and warm in nature (therefore tending to aggravate Heat). After a few weeks of treatment aimed at resolving Phlegm and clearing Heat, attention should be diverted to tonifying Qi and Blood.

Herbal treatment
In accordance with these principles the first prescription used was a variation of Gua Lou Xie Bai Ban Xia Tang *Trichosanthes-Allium-Pinellia Decoction*:

Gua Lou *Fructus Trichosanthis* 9 g
Xie Bai *Bulbus Allii* 4 g
Ban Xia *Rhizoma Pinelliae ternatae* 6 g
Bai Jiu Rice wine 15 ml
Huang Lian *Rhizoma Coptidis* 3 g
Dan Nan Xing *Rhizoma Arisaematis praeparata* 4 g
Zhu Ru *Caulis Bambusae in Taeniis* 6 g
Dan Shen *Radix Salviae miltiorrhizae* 4 g

Explanation
– Huang Lian was added to clear Stomach-Heat.
– Dan Nan Xing and Zhu Ru resolve Phlegm.
– Dan Shen moves Blood in the chest and stops pain.

After the patient had taken this formula for some weeks, attention was diverted to tonifying Qi and Blood. The main changes to look for to decide when to switch the aim of treatment to tonification are a lessening of the Red colour of the tongue body, a decrease in tongue coating, a less Rapid and less Slippery pulse and a disappearance of the thirst. The formula used was a variation of Liu Jun Zi Tang *Six Gentlemen Decoction*:

Bai Zhu *Rhizoma Atractylodis macrocephalae* 9 g
Dang Shen *Radix Codonopsis pilosulae* 6 g
Fu Ling *Sclerotium Poriae cocos* 6 g
Zhi Gan Cao *Radix Glycyrrhizae uralensis praeparata* 3 g
Ban Xia *Rhizoma Pinelliae ternatae* 9 g
Chen Pi *Pericarpium Citri reticulatae* 4 g
Huang Lian *Rhizoma Coptidis* 3 g
Gua Lou *Fructus Trichosanthis* 6 g

Gua Lou *Fructus Trichosanthis* and Huang Lian *Rhizoma Coptidis* were added to continue to resolve Phlegm and clear Heat.

4. STAGNATION OF COLD IN THE CHEST

CLINICAL MANIFESTATIONS

Severe cramping chest pain extending to the scapula, feeling of tightness of the chest, palpitations, breathlessness, difficulty in lying down, pale complexion, cold limbs. The chest pain is induced by exposure to cold and alleviated by warmth.

In very severe cases there would also be cyanosis of lips and nails, cold sweating, severe, continuous stabbing pain in the chest, the tongue would be Purple and the Pulse would be Knotted.

Tongue: Pale, Bluish-Purple.
Pulse: Deep-Weak-Tight.

This pattern is characterized by Cold obstructing the chest. Internal Cold derives from Yang deficiency with which this pattern would always be associated. However, it describes a relatively acute situation when the manifestations of Cold are predominant and the pain in the chest is severe. In such cases one should treat the Manifestation (i.e. the Cold) rather than the Root (i.e. Yang deficiency).

TREATMENT PRINCIPLE

Invigorate Yang (in herbal therapy with warm-pungent herbs), scatter Cold, remove obstruction.

ACUPUNCTURE

BL-14 Jueyinshu, BL-15 Xinshu, Ren-17 Shanzhong, Ren-14 Juque, P-6 Neiguan, Du-20 Baihui, Ren-6 Qihai, Ren-8 Shenque, ST-36 Zusanli. Even method, except on ST-36, Ren-6 and Ren-8 which should be reinforced. Moxa must be used.

Explanation

– **BL-14**, **BL-15**, **Ren-17**, **Ren-14** and **P-6**: the use of these points has already been explained above. They should be needled with reducing or even method depending on the severity of the chest pain.
– **Du-20** with direct moxa is used to raise the Yang.
– **Ren-6** and **Ren-8** with direct moxa are used to warm the Yang and expel Cold. Moxa cones are applied to Ren-8 after filling the umbilicus with salt.
– **ST-36** is used with moxa on needle and reinforced to tonify Yang and expel Cold.

HERBAL TREATMENT

(a) Prescription

GUA LOU XIE BAI BAI JIU TANG
Trichosanthes-Allium-White Wine Decoction
Gua Lou *Fructus Trichosanthis* 12 g
Xie Bai *Bulbus Allii* 12 g
Bai Jiu White rice wine 30 ml

Explanation

– **Gua Lou** opens the chest and resolves Phlegm.

– **Xie Bai** stops chest pain, invigorates Yang and dispels Cold.
– **Rice wine** invigorates Yang and dispels Cold. Its ascending movement will also act as a messenger to direct the other herbs to the chest.

(b) Prescription

ZHI SHI XIE BAI GUI ZHI TANG
Citrus-Allium-Cinnamomum Decoction
Zhi Shi *Fructus Citri aurantii immaturus* 12 g
Xie Bai *Bulbus Allii* 9 g
Gui Zhi *Ramulus Cinnamomi cassiae* 6 g
Gua Lou *Fructus Trichosanthis* 12 g
Hou Po *Cortex Magnoliae officinalis* 12 g

Explanation

– **Zhi Shi** makes Qi descend and therefore frees the chest relieving fullness and oppression.
– **Xie Bai** invigorates Yang, dispels Cold and stops chest pain.
– **Gui Zhi** invigorates Yang and dispels Cold from the blood vessels.
– **Gua Lou** frees the chest and resolves Phlegm.
– **Hou Po** opens the chest and relieves fullness. It also subdues rebellious Qi.

This prescription is more frequently used than the previous one as to that prescription's two main ingredients it adds Zhi Shi to move Qi and Gui Zhi to invigorate Yang in the blood vessels.

(c) Prescription

DANG GUI SI NI TANG
Angelica Four Rebellious Decoction
Dang Gui *Radix Angelicae sinensis* 12 g
Bai Shao *Radix Paeoniae albae* 9 g
Gui Zhi *Ramulus Cinnamomi cassiae* 9 g
Xi Xin *Herba Asari cum radice* 1.5 g
Zhi Gan Cao *Radix Glycyrrhizae uralensis praeparata* 5 g
Da Zao *Fructus Ziziphi jujubae* 8 pieces
Mu Tong *Caulis Akebiae* 3 g

Explanation

– **Dang Gui** and **Bai Shao** tonify Blood.

– **Gui Zhi** and **Xi Xin** are warm and pungent and warm the blood vessels. They also expel Cold from the blood vessels.
– **Zhi Gan Cao** and **Da Zao** on the one hand assist Dang Gui and Bai Shao to nourish Blood, and on the other hand help Gui Zhi and Xi Xin to warm the channels and blood vessels.
– **Mu Tong** penetrates the blood vessels and directs the other herbs to them.

This prescription would be particularly indicated if the hands are very cold.

(d) Prescription

LING GUI ZHU GAN TANG
Poria-Ramulus Cinnamomi-Atractylodes-Glycyrrhiza Decoction
Fu Ling *Sclerotium Poriae cocos* 12 g
Gui Zhi *Ramulus Cinnamomi cassiae* 9 g
Bai Zhu *Rhizoma Atractylodis macrocephalae* 6 g
Zhi Gan Cao *Radix Glycyrrhizae uralensis praeparata* 3 g

Explanation

This formula treats Phlegm-Fluids obstructing the epigastrium and chest with such manifestations as a feeling of fullness and oppression of the chest, a feeling of cold, coughing of white-watery-frothy sputum (characteristic of Phlegm-Fluids), shortness of breath and dizziness. The tongue would be Pale, Swollen, with teethmarks and a sticky-white coating.

Variations

These variations apply to all previous formulae.

– In case of very severe and stabbing pain in the chest, cold limbs, cold sweating, cyanosis of lips and Knotted pulse, use one of the two following prescriptions:

(i) Prescription

TONG MAI SI NI TANG and SU HE XIANG WAN
Penetrating the Blood Vessels Four-Rebellious Decoction and Styrax Pill

Tong Mai Si Ni Tang
FU ZI *Radix Aconiti carmichaeli praeparata* 15 g
GAN JIANG *Rhizoma Zingiberis officinalis* 9 g
ZHI GAN CAO *Radix Glycyrrhizae uralensis praeparata* 6 g

This prescription rescues the Yang and dispels Cold.

Su He Xiang Wan
SU HE XIANG *Styrax liquidis* 30 g
SHE XIANG *Secretio Moschus moschiferi* 60 g
BING PIAN *Borneol* 30 g
AN XI XIANG *Benzoinum* 60 g
MU XIANG *Radix Saussureae* 60 g
TAN XIANG *Lignum Santali albi* 60 g
CHEN XIANG *Lignum Aquilariae* 60 g
RU XIANG *Gummi Olibanum* 30 g
DING XIANG *Flos Caryophylli* 60 g
XIANG FU *Rhizoma Cyperi rotundi* 60 g
BI BA *Fructus Piperis longi* 60 g
SHUI NIU JIAO *Cornu Bufali* 60 g
ZHU SHA *Cinnabaris* 60 g
BAI ZHU *Rhizoma Atractylodis macrocephalae* 60 g
HE ZI *Fructus Terminaliae chebulae* 60 g

This formula treats pain in the chest from Cold. Note that the above dosages are for a pill, not a decoction. This formula is usually taken as a patent remedy. One particular way of using this formula is a plaster applied to the umbilicus. In the absence of a plaster the herbs of the above formula can be boiled and strained and the resulting liquid applied to the umbilicus as a hot compress. The umbilicus is on the Directing vessel and is also related to the Penetrating vessel and the Kidney's Original Qi. For these reasons, this method is applicable to treat Chest Painful Obstruction from Kidney deficiency.

(ii) Prescription

KUAN XIONG WAN
Opening the Chest Pill
GAO LIANG JIANG *Rhizoma Alpiniae officinari* 6 g
YAN HU SUO *Rhizoma Corydalis yanhusuo* 6 g
TAN XIANG *Lignum Santali albi* 6 g
BI BA *Fructus Piperis longi* 6 g
XI XIN *Herba Asari cum radice* 1.5 g
BING PIAN *Borneol* 3 g

Explanation. This formula eliminates Cold, opens the chest, moves Blood, resolves Phlegm and opens the orifices. It differs from the previous one in so far as it is hotter in nature and is therefore indicated for pronounced symptoms of Cold. This formula also exists as a patent remedy, the form in which it is normally used.

The previous six prescriptions are compared in Table 13.4.

Case history

A 70-year-old woman had been suffering from a feeling of oppression and pain in the chest for many years. The chest pain was elicited by exercise and exposure to cold. She was easily breathless and her complexion was pale.

Her tongue was Pale on the whole, Bluish-Purple on the sides in the chest area, and Swollen (Plate 13.2). Her pulse was Slippery, Deep and Weak.

Diagnosis
This is an example of stagnation of Cold in the chest occurring against a background of Yang deficiency. The tongue shows very clearly the location of Cold in the chest.

Treatment principle
The treatment principle followed was to expel Cold from the chest and tonify Yang.

Acupuncture
This patient was treated only with acupuncture and the points used were selected from the following:

– **P-6** Neiguan, **Ren-14** Juque and **BL-14** Jueyinshu to move Qi in the chest and stop pain. Even method.
– **Ren-17** Shanzhong with moxa to expel Cold from the chest.
– **Ren-6** Qihai with moxa to expel Cold in general.
– **ST-36** Zusanli and **BL-20** Pishu, with reinforcing method and moxa on needle, to tonify Yang.

Table 13.4 Comparison of formulae for Cold in the chest

Formula	Differentiation
GUA LOU XIE BAI BAI JIU TANG	Cold
ZHI SHI XIE BAI GUI ZHI TANG	Cold with stagnation of Qi
DANG GUI SI NI TANG	Cold, cold hands
LING GUI ZHU GAN TANG	Cold with Phlegm-Fluids
TONG MAI SI NI TANG and SU HE XIANG WAN	Severe Cold, collapse of Yang
KUAN XIONG WAN	Cold with some Phlegm obstructing the orifices

This patient made a gradual improvement over a period of 9 months until the feeling of oppression and pain in the chest subsided almost completely.

DEFICIENCY CONDITIONS

The Deficiency patterns always underlie the Excess ones. They are better discussed separately as they correspond to the chronic stage of the disease, in between attacks. In this stage, the treatment principle is to tonify the underlying deficiency.

The Deficiency patterns are:

1. Heart- and Kidney-Yin Deficiency
2. Qi and Yin Deficiency
3. Spleen- and Heart-Yang Deficiency.

1. HEART- AND KIDNEY-YIN DEFICIENCY

CLINICAL MANIFESTATIONS

A feeling of oppression and pain in the chest, palpitations, night sweating, insomnia, sore back and knees, tinnitus, dizziness, 5-palm heat.
Tongue: Red without coating with a Heart-crack.
Pulse: Fine-Rapid.

In this case, as in all cases of Deficiency, the pain in the chest is less severe than in the Excess conditions. In this pattern, besides the Yin deficiency, there is nearly always some Phlegm too which causes the feeling of oppression and pain in the chest.

All the other manifestations are typical of Yin deficiency.

TREATMENT PRINCIPLE

Nourish Yin, benefit the Kidneys, nourish the Heart, calm the Mind, stop pain.

ACUPUNCTURE

BL-14 Jueyinshu, BL-23 Shenshu, Ren-4 Guanyuan, KI-3 Taixi, P-6 Neiguan, Ren-17 Shanzhong, HE-6 Yinxi, KI-25 Shencang.

Explanation

- **BL-14**, **P-6** and **Ren-17** move Qi in the chest and stop pain.
- **BL-23**, **Ren-4** and **KI-3** tonify the Kidneys.
- **HE-6** nourishes Heart-Yin, calms the Mind, stops night sweating and relieves chest pain.
- **KI-25** is a local point for chest pain associated with a Kidney pattern.

HERBAL TREATMENT

(a) Prescription

ZUO GUI YIN
Restoring the Left [Kidney] Decoction
Shu Di Huang *Radix Rehmanniae glutinosae prae-parata* 12 g
Shan Zhu Yu *Fructus Corni officinalis* 6 g
Gou Qi Zi *Fructus Lycii chinensis* 6 g
Shan Yao *Radix Dioscoreae oppositae* 6 g
Fu Ling *Sclerotium Poriae cocos* 6 g
Zhi Gan Cao *Radix Glycyrrhizae uralensis prae-parata* 3 g

Explanation

This is a common formula to nourish Kidney-Yin.

(b) Prescription

TIAN WANG BU XIN DAN
Heavenly Emperor Tonifying the Heart Pill
Sheng Di Huang *Radix Rehmanniae glutinosae* 120 g
Xuan Shen *Radix Scrophulariae ningpoensis* 15 g
Tian Men Dong *Tuber Asparagi cochinchinensis* 60 g
Mai Men Dong *Tuber Ophiopogonis japonici* 60 g
Dan Shen *Radix Salviae miltiorrhizae* 15 g
Ren Shen *Radix Ginseng* 15 g
Fu Ling *Sclerotium Poriae cocos* 15 g
Suan Zao Ren *Semen Ziziphi spinosae* 60 g
Wu Wei Zi *Fructus Schisandrae chinensis* 15 g
Bai Zi Ren *Semen Biotae orientalis* 60 g
Yuan Zhi *Radix Polygalae tenuifoliae* 15 g
Jie Geng *Radix Platycodi grandiflori* 15 g
Zhu Sha *Cinnabaris* pill coating

Explanation

- **Sheng Di Huang** is the emperor herb to nourish Kidney-Yin.
- **Xuan Shen**, **Tian Men Dong** and **Mai Men Dong** assist Sheng Di to nourish Yin.
- **Dan Shen** enters the Heart and directs the formula to the Heart to calm the Mind.
- **Ren Shen** and **Fu Ling** tonify Qi.
- **Suan Zao Ren** and **Wu Wei Zi** absorb leakages (such as night sweating), nourish Yin and calm the Mind.
- **Bai Zi Ren**, **Yuan Zhi** and **Zhu Sha** calm the Mind.
- **Jie Geng** directs the formula to the Upper Burner, i.e. the Heart.

Variations

These variations apply to both above prescriptions.

- In case of Phlegm and a pronounced feeling of oppression in the chest add Gua Lou *Fructus Trichosanthis*.
- If there are symptoms and signs of Liver-Yang rising add Gou Teng *Ramulus Uncariae* and Shi Jue Ming *Concha Haliotidis*.
- In cases of pronounced chest pain add Dan Shen *Radix Salviae miltiorrhizae* (or increase it in Tian Wang Bu Xin Dan *Heavenly Emperor Tonifying the Heart Pill*).
- If there are signs of Blood deficiency as well as Yin deficiency add Shou Wu *Radix Polygoni multiflori*, Dang Gui *Radix Angelicae sinensis* and Dan Shen *Radix Salviae miltiorrhizae*.
- If there is mental restlessness and insomnia add (or increase the dosage if already in the prescription) Suan Zao Ren *Semen Ziziphi spinosae*, Wu Wei Zi *Fructus Schisandrae chinensis* and Long Chi *Dens Draconis*.
- In case of Empty-Heat signs add Gui Ban *Plastrum Testudinis* and Huang Bo *Cortex Phellodendri*.

The above two formulae are compared in Table 13.5.

Patent remedy

TIAN WANG BU XIN DAN
Heavenly Emperor Tonifying the Heart Pill

Table 13.5 Comparison of formulae for Heart- and Kidney-Yin deficiency

Formula	Differentiation
ZUO GUI YIN	Tonify Kidney-Yin
TIAN WANG BU XIN DAN	Tonify HE- and KI-Yin

Explanation

This remedy has the same ingredients and functions as the homonymous prescription above.

The tongue presentation appropriate to this remedy is a Red tongue without coating and possibly with cracks.

2. QI AND YIN DEFICIENCY

CLINICAL MANIFESTATIONS

A feeling of oppression and pain in the chest which comes and goes, palpitations, breathlessness, tiredness, dislike to speak, pale complexion, dizziness, blurred vision. All symptoms are aggravated by over-exertion.
Tongue: Red without coating.
Pulse: Fine or Weak.

This is deficiency of Qi and Yin of Heart, Lungs and Spleen. The Heart deficiency causes palpitations, while Lung deficiency causes breathlessness and pale complexion. When Yin is deficient the blood vessels lack nourishment, Blood cannot circulate properly and this causes the feeling of oppression and pain in the chest. This comes and goes and is much lighter than in Excess patterns.

TREATMENT PRINCIPLE

Tonify Qi, nourish Yin, move Blood, invigorate the Connecting channels.

ACUPUNCTURE

LU-9 Taiyuan, HE-5 Tongli, Ren-17 Shanzhong, BL-13 Feishu, BL-15 Xinshu, ST-36 Zusanli, P-6 Neiguan, SP-6 Sanyinjiao, Ren-4 Guanyuan. Reinforcing or even method as indicated below.

Explanation

- **LU-9**, **BL-13**, **HE-5** and **BL-15** tonify Lungs and Heart respectively. Reinforcing method.
- **Ren-17** and **P-6** move Qi and Blood in the chest. Even method.
- **ST-36**, **SP-6** and **Ren-4** tonify Qi and nourish Yin. Reinforcing method.

HERBAL TREATMENT

(a) Prescription

SHENG MAI SAN and REN SHEN YANG RONG TANG Variation
Generating the Pulse Powder and *Panax Nourishing and Flourishing Decoction*
Ren Shen *Radix Ginseng* 9 g
Wu Wei Zi *Fructus Schisandrae chinensis* 6 g
Mai Men Dong *Tuber Ophiopogonis japonici* 6 g
Bai Shao *Radix Paeoniae albae* 6 g
Dang Gui *Radix Angelicae sinensis* 6 g
Chen Pi *Pericarpium Citri reticulatae* 3 g
Huang Qi *Radix Astragali membranacei* 6 g
Bai Zhu *Rhizoma Atractylodis macrocephalae* 6 g
Zhi Gan Cao *Radix Glycyrrhizae uralensis praeparata* 3 g
Sheng Di Huang *Radix Rehmanniae glutinosae* 6 g
Fu Ling *Sclerotium Poriae cocos* 6 g
Yuan Zhi *Radix Polygalae tenuifoliae* 6 g
Sheng Jiang *Rhizoma Zingiberis officinalis recens* 3 slices
Da Zao *Fructus Ziziphi jujubae* 3 dates

Explanation

- **Ren Shen**, **Huang Qi**, **Bai Zhu**, **Fu Ling** and **Gan Cao** tonify Qi and benefit the Lungs.
- **Mai Dong**, **Sheng Di Huang**, **Dang Gui** and **Bai Shao** nourish Blood and Yin.
- **Yuan Zhi** and **Wu Wei Zi** tonify the Heart.
- **Chen Pi** counteracts the "stickiness" of the Blood and Yin tonics.
- **Sheng Jiang** and **Da Zao** harmonize.

Variations

- For pain in the chest add Dan Shen *Radix Salviae miltiorrhizae* and San Qi *Radix Notoginseng*.

(b) Prescription

ZHI GAN CAO TANG
Glycyrrhiza Decoction
Zhi Gan Cao *Radix Glycyrrhizae uralensis praeparata* 12 g
Ren Shen *Radix Ginseng* 6 g
Da Zao *Fructus Ziziphi jujubae* 10 dates
Sheng Di Huang *Radix Rehmanniae glutinosae* 30 g
Mai Men Dong *Tuber Ophiopogonis japonici* 10 g
E Jiao *Gelatinum Corii Asini* 6 g
Hei Zhi Ma (Hu Ma Ren) *Semen Sesami indici* 10 g
Sheng Jiang *Rhizoma Zingiberis officinalis recens* 9 g
Gui Zhi *Ramulus Cinnamomi cassiae* 9 g
Qing Jiu Rice wine 10 ml (added at the end)

Explanation

This formula tonifies Qi, Yang, Blood and Yin.

- **Zhi Gan Cao**, **Ren Shen** and **Da Zao** tonify Qi.
- **Sheng Di Huang** and **Mai Men Dong** nourish Yin.
- **E Jiao** and **Hu Ma Ren** nourish Blood.
- **Sheng Jiang**, **Gui Zhi** and **Rice wine** are warm and pungent and invigorate Yang in the blood vessels. They direct all the other tonics to the blood vessels to regulate the pulse. For this reason, this prescription is used for an irregular pulse or a pulse with the Knotted quality (slow and stopping at irregular intervals).

3. SPLEEN- AND HEART-YANG DEFICIENCY

CLINICAL MANIFESTATIONS

A feeling of oppression and dull pain in the chest, breathlessness, palpitations, sweating, feeling cold, cold limbs, bright-pale complexion, cyanosis of lips and nails, tiredness, poor appetite, insomnia.
Tongue: Pale or Bluish-Purple.
Pulse: Deep-Weak.

This is due to long-term deficiency of Spleen-Yang leading to deficiency of Heart-Yang. This manifests with a cold feeling, cold limbs, palpitations, insomnia, sweating, a bright-pale complexion and cyanosis of lips and nails. Deficient Heart-Yang fails to move Blood in the chest. Stasis of Blood causes pain and a feeling of oppression and a Purple tongue.

Long-term deficiency of Yang of the Spleen and Heart nearly always has its root in Kidney-Yang deficiency. This is especially so in old people. In this case, in addition to the above manifestations, there would also be sore back and knees, dizziness and frequent-pale urination.

TREATMENT PRINCIPLE

Tonify Qi, warm Yang, move Blood, invigorate the Connecting vessels.

ACUPUNCTURE

BL-15 Xinshu, Ren-14 Juque, HE-5 Tongli, BL-20 Pishu, Ren-12 Zhongwan, Ren-6 Qihai, ST-36 Zusanli, SP-6 Sanyinjiao, BL-23 Shenshu, Du-4 Mingmen, P-6 Neiguan, KI-25 Shencang, BL-13 Feishu. Moxa is applicable. All the points should be needled with reinforcing method except P-6 and KI-25 which should be needled with even method.

Explanation

- **BL-15**, **Ren-14** and **HE-5** with moxa, tonify Heart-Yang.
- **BL-20**, **Ren-12**, **Ren-6**, **ST-36** and **SP-6** tonify Spleen-Yang (with moxa).
- **BL-23** and **Du-4**, with moxa, warm Kidney-Yang.
- **P-6** opens the chest, stops pain and relieves a sensation of oppression.
- **KI-25** is a local point to move Qi and Blood in the chest when there is an underlying Kidney deficiency.
- **BL-13**, with moxa, tonifies Lung-Yang and strengthens the Gathering Qi which provides Qi to the Heart to move Blood.

HERBAL TREATMENT

Prescription

SHEN FU TANG and YOU GUI YIN
Panax-Aconitum Decoction and *Restoring the Right [Kidney] Decoction*
Ren Shen *Radix Ginseng* 9 g
Fu Zi *Radix Aconiti carmichaeli praeparata* 6 g
Shu Di Huang *Radix Rehmanniae glutinosae praeparata* 15 g
Shan Zhu Yu *Fructus Corni officinalis* 3 g
Shan Yao *Radix Dioscoreae oppositae* 6 g
Du Zhong *Cortex Eucommiae ulmoidis* 6 g
Rou Gui *Cortex Cinnamomi cassiae* 3 g
Gou Qi Zi *Fructus Lycii chinensis* 6 g
Zhi Gan Cao *Radix Glycyrrhizae uralensis praeparata* 3 g

Explanation

The formula Shen Fu Tang *Panax-Aconitum Decoction* strongly tonifies and warms the Yang. It is used for collapse of Yang. The formula You Gui Yin *Restoring the Right [Kidney] Decoction* tonifies and warms Kidney-Yang. This is necessary as chronic deficiency of Yang, especially in old people, nearly always derives from deficiency of Kidney-Yang.

Variations

– If both Yang and Yin are deficient add Mai Men Dong *Tuber Ophiopogonis japonici* and Wu Wei Zi *Fructus Schisandrae chinensis*.
– If, in addition to Heart and Spleen Yang deficiency, there are also pronounced signs of Kidney-Yang deficiency, add one or two of the following herbs: Rou Cong Rong *Herba Cistanchis*, Ba Ji Tian *Radix Morindae officinalis*, Du Zhong *Cortex Eucommiae ulmoidis*, Xu Duan *Radix Dipsaci* or Tu Si Zi *Semen Cuscutae*.
– If the deficiency of Heart-Yang is very severe with very cold hands, cold sweating on the forehead and cyanotic lips, face and nails, prevent collapse of Heart-Yang by increasing the dosage of Fu Zi *Radix Aconiti carmichaeli praeparata* and adding the following:

HONG SHEN *Radix Ginseng* (Red Ginseng) 30 g

LONG GU *Os Draconis* 30 g
MU LI *Concha Ostreae* 30 g

Alternatively, one can use the following three formulae together:

– SHEN FU TANG *Panax-Aconitum Decoction*
– SI NI TANG *Four Rebellious Decoction*
– SHENG MAI SAN *Generating the Pulse Powder*
– REN SHEN *Radix Ginseng* 30 g
– FU ZI *Radix Aconiti carmichaeli praeparata* 12 g
– GAN JIANG *Rhizoma Zingiberis officinalis* 6 g
– ZHI GAN CAO *Radix Glycyrrhizae uralensis praeparata* 6 g
– WU WEI ZI *Fructus Schisandrae chinensis* 9 g
– MAI MEN DONG *Tuber Ophiopogonis japonici* 12 g

The two combinations of formulae suggested above are compared in Table. 13.6.

Prognosis and prevention

Acupuncture and Chinese herbs are effective for Chest Painful Obstruction but the treatment will necessarily take several months if not longer. The most difficult types to treat are those from Phlegm and stasis of Blood. The tongue-body colour gives a good indication for prognosis: the more purple it is, the more difficult it will be to treat.

The prognosis necessarily depends also on the Western differentiation: ischaemic heart disease from an atheroma obstructing a coronary vessel and carcinoma of the lung are obviously the most difficult to treat.

As for prevention, it is essential that the patient takes regular exercise which is not too

Table 13.6 Comparison of formulae for Spleen- and Heart-Yang deficiency

Formula	Differentiation
SHEN FU TANG and YOU GUI YIN	Tonify Lung-, Spleen- and Kidney-Yang
SHEN FU TANG, SI NI TANG and SHENG MAI SAN	Collapse of Heart-Yang

strenuous. Chest Painful Obstruction is caused by stagnation of Qi-Blood-Cold or by Phlegm and all such conditions improve with moderate exercise. Brisk walking is an excellent exercise and, for those who have access to a teacher, *Tai Ji Chuan* or *Qi Gong* are ideal.

As for diet, it is extremely important not to eat dairy products or greasy-fried foods which lead to the production of Phlegm: this obstructs the chest and interacts with stasis of Blood.

If the patient is a smoker it is absolutely vital that he or she stops. Smoking is detrimental to Chest Painful Obstruction not only from a Western but also from a Chinese point of view. From a Western perspective nicotine contracts the blood vessels and would therefore aggravate stasis of Blood. From a Chinese viewpoint, tobacco is a toxic substance which is hot and drying: it dries up Blood in the vessels, which will contribute to the development of stasis of Blood.

Western differential diagnosis

From a Western medical point of view, the first broad differentiation to be made in a patient with chest pain is whether the pain originates from the lungs, heart or stomach/oesophagus.

The main causes are represented diagrammatically in Figure 13.3.

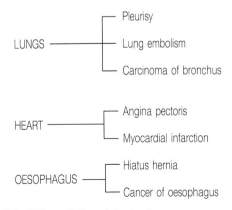

Fig. 13.3 Differentiation of chest pain

1. PLEURISY

This is an inflammation of the pleura. Its diagnosis should be fairly obvious as it occurs only during an acute febrile disease affecting the chest. The pain is worse below the nipple and is definitely worse on inhalation and coughing. The patient's breathing is rapid and shallow. There may be an unproductive cough. The temperature is raised.

The diagnosis of pleurisy can be confirmed with the help of a stethoscope. When this is placed over the chest (both front and back should be checked) a typical friction "rub" can be heard at the end of exhalation or inhalation. This is due to the rubbing together of the two pleural surfaces. This friction rub can be differentiated from other lung sounds as it does not disappear after coughing. It is therefore advisable, when an adventitious sound is heard, to ask the patient to cough: the pleural rub will not disappear whilst the sounds generated by mucus in the bronchi will.

2. LUNG EMBOLISM

This occurs when an embolus detaches from a thrombus and occludes (partially or totally) an artery in the lung. The main predisposing factors for this to happen are:

(a) slow circulation from dilatation and inefficiency of the veins such as that which occurs during pregnancy or in patients with varicose veins. It also affects people who have been confined to bed for a long time. It is particularly likely to occur within 10 days after surgery or childbirth
(b) pulmonary congestion deriving from mitral stenosis or congestive cardiac failure in the elderly
(c) trauma
(d) the contraceptive pill.

The manifestations of lung embolism vary in severity according to whether a lung artery is totally or partially occluded. If it is totally occluded there is a massive embolism and the patient is seized by an extremely severe chest pain and looks under shock. There is intense breathlessness, pallor, faintness, sweating and there may be collapse or even death. The blood pressure falls to very low levels and the jugular venous pressure is raised. From the point of view of Chinese medicine it corresponds to collapse of Yang and an acupuncturist would be extremely unlikely to ever encounter such a case as the patient would be hospitalized.

If the occlusion of the lung artery is only partial and temporary the manifestations are less dramatic. The patient feels a constriction in the chest and breathlessness. The pulse rate increases, there may be a temperature and there will be a dull area on the chest on percussion and auscultation. These symptoms and signs disappear after a while as the embolus moves on.

3. CARCINOMA OF BRONCHUS

This is more common in men over 40. It may manifest with a cough, a deep-seated chest pain, loss of appetite and loss of weight.

4. ISCHAEMIC HEART DISEASE

The term ischaemic heart disease indicates myocardial damage from an insufficient coronary blood supply. In most cases this is due to a narrowing of the coronary arteries from atherosclerosis, but in a few cases, it may also be due to aortic valve disease, severe anaemia or coronary embolism.

The most common cause of ischaemic heart disease is obstruction of a coronary artery by an atheroma, which is a plaque consisting of a core rich in cholesterol and other lipids, surrounded by fibrous tissue.

The clinical manifestations of this condition can be very varied as it can give rise to several consequences. For example, both cardiac infarction and angina pectoris (see below) may be a consequence of ischaemic heart disease. Other possible consequences of ischaemic heart disease are left ventricular failure and arrhythmia.

5. ANGINA PECTORIS

This is due to a recurrent spasm of a coronary artery. It is more common in men over 50. The chest pain is elicited by exercise, exposure to cold, a heavy meal, or excitement.

The main symptom is a recurrent chest pain which comes in bouts. It can vary in intensity from a slight prickling sensation to an intense stabbing pain. The pain may radiate to the shoulder or left arm. It is accompanied by a feeling of constriction in the chest, nausea or vomiting. The person becomes pale and motionless and the blood pressure is raised. The cardiac rhythm is not disturbed.

6. MYOCARDIAL INFARCTION

Myocardial infarction is usually due to coronary thrombosis or occlusion of a coronary artery by the release of an atheromatous plaque. This is another condition which an acupuncturist is unlikely to see in its acute stage, except by chance.

Myocardial infarction's main manifestation is a sudden and intense chest pain that may radiate to the left arm or to the neck, jaw or abdomen. The pain comes at rest. There is severe breathlessness, sweating, nausea and cyanosis of face, lips and nails. Twenty per cent of cases are fatal. The patient is restless, the pulse is fine and rapid and the blood pressure is decreased. The temperature may be raised.

From a Chinese point of view, it corresponds to collapse of Yang.

7. HIATUS HERNIA

This a common condition which acupuncturists are likely to see often in practice. It consists in the protrusion of the upper part of the stomach through the diaphragm into the thoracic cavity. This condition can cause chest pain. The pain is directly on the sternum and is elicited by swallowing or stooping. The pain may radiate to the region under the ribs or the space between the shoulder-blades. There is also nausea, belching and hiccups.

It is important in practice to differentiate a chest pain of this type from those caused by the heart or lungs.

Table 13.7 Causes of chest pain in Western medicine

Disease	Pathology	Symptoms	Signs
Pleurisy	Inflammation of pleura	Stabbing or lancinating pain below nipple, worse on inspiration, shallow breathing	Fever, friction rub on auscultation
Lung embolism	Embolus detached from thrombus occludes an artery in the lung	Feeling of constriction in chest, transient dyspnoea, haemoptysis	Friction rub on palpation, rapid pulse and breathing, oedema of legs
Carcinoma of bronchus	Malignancy	Dry cough, deep-seated chest pain, haemoptysis, poor appetite, tiredness	Loss of weight, wheeze, diminished breath sounds
Angina pectoris	Spasm of coronary arteries	Sudden bouts of severe chest pain radiating to left arm, feeling of constriction in the chest, nausea, vomiting	Pallor, patient motionless, raised blood pressure, cardiac rhythm not altered
Myocardial infarction	Thrombosis of atheromatous coronary arteries	Sudden, severe chest pain at rest which may radiate to left arm or shoulder, dyspnoea, nausea, vomiting, sweating	Pallor, patient restless, cyanosis of lips and nails, shock, feeble and rapid pulse, decreased blood pressure, raised temperature
Hiatus hernia	Protrusion of stomach-cardia through diaphragm into thoracic cavity	Nausea, vomiting, sternal pain, hiccup, regurgitation, dyspnoea	Heart may be displaced upwards away from affected side
Carcinoma of oesophagus	Malignancy	Retrosternal pain on swallowing, pain may radiate to costal margins or between scapulae, tiredness	Loss of weight, enlarged lymph nodes in neck

8. CARCINOMA OF OESOPHAGUS

This is more common in men over 40. It causes a pain on the sternum which is typically aggravated by swallowing. There is also excessive salivation, poor digestion, debility and loss of weight. The lymph nodes in the neck may be enlarged.

The causes of chest pain are summarized in Table 13.7.

END NOTES

1. 1979 The Yellow Emperor's Classic of Internal Medicine — Simple Questions (*Huang Ti Nei Jing Su Wen* 黄帝内经素问), People's Health Publishing House, Beijing. First published *c.* 100 BC, p. 146.
2. 1981 Spiritual Axis (*Ling Shu Jing* 灵枢经), People's Health Publishing House, Beijing. First published *c.* 100 BC, p. 62.
3. He Ren 1979 A Popular Guide to the Essential Prescriptions of the Golden Chest (*Jin Gui Yau Lue Tong Su Jiang Hua* 金匮要略通俗讲话), Shanghai Science Publishing House, p. 51. The "Essential Prescriptions of the Golden Chest" itself was written by Zhang Zhong Jing and first published *c.* AD 220.
4. Traditional Chinese Medicine Research Institute 1959 An Explanation of the Essential Prescriptions of the Golden Chest (*Jin Gui Yao Lue Yu Yi* 金匮要略语译), People's Health Publishing House, Beijing, p. 89. The "Essential Prescriptions of the Golden Chest" itself was written by Zhang Zhong Jing and first published *c.* AD 220.
5. Qin Jing Ming 1706 Causes of Diseases and Treatment according to the Pulse (*Zheng Yin Mai Zhi* 症因脉治), cited in Zhang Bo Yu 1986 Internal Medicine, Shanghai Science Publishing House, p. 108.
6. Shu Chang 1658 Methods and Rules of Medicine (*Yi Men Fa Lu* 医门法律), cited in Internal Medicine, p. 108.
7. Lin Shi Qin 1839 Treatment Planning according to Syndrome Categories (*Lei Zheng Zhi Cai* 类证治裁), cited in Internal Medicine, p. 108.
8. Spiritual Axis, p. 137.
9. Ibid., p. 153.
10. Wei Yi Lin 1349 Effective Formulae Tested by Physicians for Generations (*Shi Yi De Xiao Fang* 世医得效方), cited in Internal Medicine, p. 108.
11. Wang Ken Tang 1607 Standards of Diagnosis and Treatment (*Zheng Zhi Zhun Sheng* 证治准绳), cited in Internal Medicine, p. 108.
12. Chen Nian Zu 1801 Collection of Rhymes of Contemporary Formulae (*Shi Fang Ger Kuo* 时方歌括), cited in Internal Medicine, p. 108.
13. Wang Qing Ren 1830 Correction of Errors in Medicine (*Yi Lin Gai Cuo* 医林改错), cited in Internal Medicine, p. 108.

Epigastric pain 14

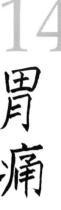

胃
痛

"Epigastric" indicates pain in the stomach area (Fig. 14.1). Although the pain may radiate towards the right or left costal margin, only if it *starts* in the epigastric area (i.e. roughly over the stomach) is it classified as epigastric pain.

Aetiology and pathology

1. EXTERNAL PATHOGENIC FACTORS

(a) COLD

External Cold can invade the Stomach directly, by-passing the skin and muscle energetic layers. As Cold contracts, it causes an acute and severe epigastric pain usually accompanied by vomiting. The tongue has a thick white coating and the pulse is Tight. This is an acute condition.

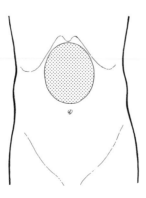

Fig. 14.1 Epigastric pain area

The "Simple Questions" in chapter 39 says: *"Cold invades the Stomach and Intestines . . . Blood cannot move, the Connecting channels are blocked and hence pain results."*[1]

(b) DAMPNESS

External Dampness can also invade the Stomach directly. This may be combined with either Cold or Heat according to season. During the summer months it is more likely to occur as Damp-Heat.

Dampness obstructs the descending of Stomach-Qi and causes a dull pain and nausea. It also causes a typical feeling of oppression and heaviness of the epigastrium. The tongue has a sticky coating (white or yellow according to whether Dampness combines with Cold or Heat) and the pulse is Slippery.

Dampness is a more frequent cause than Cold in acute stomach disorders, including food poisoning and many bacterial or viral infections affecting the stomach (manifesting with epigastric pain, fever, nausea and vomiting).

2. DIET

Diet is obviously the most important factor in Stomach disorders. The Stomach rots and ripens food: the Spleen transforms and transports the refined Food Essence up towards the Lungs, whilst the Stomach sends the waste down to the Intestines. The downward movement of Stomach-Qi is coordinated with the upward movement of Spleen-Qi, and the two together are absolutely crucial to ripen, transport and transform food essences and wastes in the Middle Burner.

The Stomach with its downward movement and the Spleen with its upward movement are like crucial crossroads in the Middle Burner. In disease, Qi easily flows in the wrong direction and, in the case of the Stomach, it may flow upwards leading to nausea, vomiting, hiccup or belching.

The nature of the food and the conditions in which it has been eaten very easily affect the Stomach. We will consider the quantity of food, the nature of food and the conditions of eating separately.

(a) QUANTITY OF FOOD

Problems with the quantity of food may lie in eating either too little or too much. In affluent industrialized countries it would seem strange that anyone could suffer from insufficient food intake, but even here there are pockets of extreme poverty and certain groups in the population may suffer nutritional deficiencies simply from not having enough food. Secondly, nutritional deficiencies can arise when people subject themselves to very strict slimming diets. In some cases these lead to severe anorexia. Thirdly, people may have a deficient diet not because they do not eat enough, but because they eat de-vitalized foods which are devoid of any nutritional value. Fourthly, although when properly applied vegetarian or vegan diets can be perfectly healthy and also ecologically and ethically sound, people who follow them may unwittingly deprive themselves of essential nutrients, seen from the point of view of Chinese dietary principles. For example, some vegetarians may tend to eat too much cheese (which produces Dampness) or salads (which produce Cold and injure Spleen-Yang). On the other hand, they will not eat warm Blood-producing foods such as meat, and there are few vegetarian foods with such a quality. A person who suffers from severe deficiency of Blood, for example, would benefit from a small amount of meat in the diet. Finally, old people who live alone often tend not to eat enough because they lack the stimulation of eating in company and "cannot be bothered" to cook for one person only.

Eating too little in the various ways described above causes a dull epigastric pain, tiredness and weak muscles.

Eating too much is of course a very frequent cause of stomach disorders! By this we mean eating too large meals, rather than constant nibbling which will be discussed below. Eating too much very simply leads to retention of food so that Stomach-Qi cannot descend. This causes sour regurgitation, epigastric pain and fullness, belching and foul breath.

Of course, there is no single fixed standard which lays down the ideal quantity of food eaten; much depends on a person's occupation and someone who is engaged in heavy physical work should obviously eat more than someone whose work is sedentary. As the amount of food eaten should be regulated according to one's physical activity, it follows that at week-ends, when most people are inactive, one should eat *less* than during the week; in most countries, the exact opposite happens when people tend to have large meals at week-ends.

(b) NATURE OF FOOD

The nature of food eaten is of paramount importance in Stomach disorders. Foods are classified according to their nature (hot, warm, cold, cool or neutral) and their taste (sour, bitter, sweet, pungent or salty). The subject of foods and their action in health and disease is a vast one and beyond the scope of this book. With regard to Stomach disorders, four broad categories of foods can be identified.

(i) *Cold foods:* these are raw vegetables, salads, fruit, cold drinks and ice-cream. An excessive consumption of these foods will tend to create Cold in the Spleen and Stomach and ensuing epigastric pain.

(ii) *Hot-spicy foods:* these include curries, spices, lamb, beef and alcohol. An excessive consumption of these foods produces Stomach-Heat which may manifest with a burning epigastric pain, thirst and a yellow tongue coating.

(iii) *Sugar and sweets:* an excessive consumption of these may tend to produce both Dampness and Heat in the Stomach.

(iv) *Greasy foods, fried foods and dairy foods:* an excessive consumption of these leads to the formation of Phlegm or Dampness in the Stomach.

Chinese dietary principles are very old and do not take into account the great changes that have occurred in the growing and production of food in the past few decades. Modern food is subject to considerable chemical manipulation and a great many of the food additives can obviously be a cause of stomach problems and indeed of many other disorders. For example, the correlation between artificial colourings and hyper-activity in children is well documented.

Modern food contains not only additives (such as flavourings, colourings, preservatives and emulsifiers) but also traces of drugs such as antibiotics and hormones found in milk and meat. Moreover, food and water are often contaminated with the residues of chemical pesticides and fertilizers. All these can obviously be causes of stomach disorders but a complete discussion of their role is beyond the scope of this book.

(c) CONDITIONS OF EATING

Chinese medicine and culture place as much emphasis on the conditions of eating as on the nature of the foods eaten. The Stomach is the main Yang organ and all Yang organs fill and empty in a rhythmical fashion. The "Simple Questions" in chapter 11 says: "... *the 6 Yang organs transform and digest and do not store . . . after food enters the mouth, the stomach is full and the intestines empty; when the food goes down, the intestines are full and the stomach empty.*"[2]

For this reason, Chinese medicine stresses the importance of eating according to a routine with regular meals taken at the same time every day and similar amounts for corresponding meals each day. It also stresses the importance of eating a good substantial breakfast and lunch and only a light evening meal.

Very many people, either because of habit or pressures of work, eat in very irregular conditions. The importance of having regular meals is very clear to diabetics who know that they must take the utmost care in this respect to keep a balance in their blood sugar. Similarly, normal people too should have regular meals to maintain a good balance of blood sugar throughout the day.

The main eating habits which cause stomach disorders are as follows:

(i) *Eating too fast or on the run:* this causes stagnation of Qi in the Stomach and retention of food. In a person who has eaten in this way for many years, the Stomach pulse on the right Middle position, just slightly distal to it (towards the thumb), feels quite Tight. This indicates stagnation of food in the oesophagus due to eating too fast or on the run. Eating on the run means eating a quick sandwich while working, or eating one's lunch in just a few minutes, or eating while driving.

(ii) *Eating late in the evening or night:* evening and night-time are times of Yin predominance. Eating at these times will therefore use up Stomach-Yin rather than Stomach-Qi: for this reason it causes Stomach-Yin deficiency. This may manifest on the tongue with a wide midline crack or scattered cracks (Fig. 12.3 in chapter 12). After many years of eating late the tongue may lose its coating completely and become Red.

On the pulse, Stomach-Yin deficiency may be felt with a Floating-Empty and soft quality on the right Middle position.

(iii) *Discussing work while eating:* this is a very common habit in modern industrialized societies where a lot of business is conducted during "business lunches". This also causes stagnation of Qi in the Stomach as the stress of business impairs the proper function of the Stomach and Spleen.

(iv) *Going straight back to work after eating:* this causes Stomach-Qi deficiency.

(v) *Eating when emotionally upset:* this causes stagnation of Qi in the Stomach and Liver and, in some cases, also Stomach-Heat. This is sadly an all too frequent occurrence in many families where meal times are an opportunity for family rows or stony silences. In children, this can affect their digestive system for life.

(vi) *Eating irregular amounts from day to day:* this happens, for example, when one eats a large and rich business lunch one day and skips lunch the next day. This causes Stomach-Qi deficiency.

(vii) *Not eating breakfast:* this is probably the most important meal of the day. The Stomach has its peak of activity between 7 and 9 a.m. and it is therefore natural to have a substantial meal in the morning. It also provides nourishment to sustain us throughout the day. Not eating breakfast causes Stomach-Qi deficiency and also Blood deficiency in women.

(viii) *Constant nibbling:* this causes stagnation of Qi in the Stomach and retention of food because, as explained above, the Stomach needs to be filled and emptied at regular intervals.

(ix) *Eating while reading or watching TV:* this causes stagnation of Qi in the Stomach and retention of food because reading diverts Qi away from the Stomach to the eyes. It is also often a cause of headaches on the forehead.

(x) *A sudden change in dietary habits:* this happens, for example, when a teenager moves from home to college, or when work circumstances change, forcing a change in dietary habits. These sudden changes are very frequent causes of stomach disorders and epigastric pain.

(xi) *Fasting:* fasting may be beneficial in those who have an Excess and Heat condition of the Stomach, manifested with a Full and Slippery pulse and a thick-yellow tongue coating. In most other cases, complete fasting on water or juices can weaken the Stomach and Spleen and lead to Stomach-Qi deficiency. In particular, those who already suffer from Stomach and Spleen Qi deficiency should not use fasting as a method of self-treatment.

(xii) *Eating too much at week-ends:* in most countries people tend to eat more at week-ends as they have more time to cook and relax. From the Chinese point of view this is not beneficial as it is actually appropriate to eat more during the week when one is active and needs the "fuel" provided by food, and less at week-ends when one is (usually) less active.

Case history

The following case history, although not related to epigastric pain, is a good example of irregular eating. A 42-year-old woman suffered from diabetes: when she came for her consultation it had just started and she was not on insulin. She was keen to avoid starting insulin. I made my diagnosis (of Stomach- and Spleen-Yin deficiency) and gave her Chinese herbs. Normally, if treatment is given straight away after the onset of diabetes and before insulin is started, this disease can be controlled completely. In this case, however, after 6 weeks of treatment, she was no better and had to resort to insulin. I re-checked my diagnosis, principle of treatment, and decoction used and could not understand why it had not worked at all.

I had discussed diet with her and told her what to eat: however, I had overlooked asking her about her eating habits. These turned out to be the worst possible: she was a sales representative and her job involved driving the whole day to visit various clients. She had no breakfast in the morning and left home in a rush; she did not have a proper lunch as she had no time for it, and this often consisted of a sandwich which she ate while driving and under great stress. She returned home at about 9 in the evening and was far too exhausted to cook, so that her evening meal consisted of a frozen "TV-dinner" cooked in the microwave and eaten while watching television. It should also be added that, in order to combat tiredness, she drank vast amounts of coffee every day. Her diet and eating habits provided the answer as to why the treatment had not worked. On reflection, it had been a mistake not to ask her about her eating habits before in order to advise her: this is very important to do especially in cases of Stomach- and Spleen-Yin deficiency.

3. EMOTIONAL PROBLEMS

Emotional problems have a profound influence on stomach disorders.

(a) ANGER

This term includes emotional states such as frustration and resentment. It causes either stagnation of Liver-Qi (if the anger is suppressed) or rising of Liver-Yang (if the anger is expressed). In both cases, it leads to the situation described in 5-Element terms as Wood overacting on Earth. If the predominant emotion is outright and expressed anger leading to Liver-Yang rising as well as Liver-Qi stagnation, it affects the Stomach more, preventing Stomach-Qi from descending. This causes epigastric pain, belching and nausea. If the predominant emotion is repressed frustration and resentment leading to Liver-Qi stagnation, it affects the Spleen more causing diarrhoea. The influence of Liver-Qi on the Stomach is an extremely frequent cause of Stomach patterns. In the case of epigastric pain, the pain stems from the centre but it extends towards the right or left hypochondrial region.

Both Liver-Yang rising and Liver-Qi stagnation usually stem from a deficiency of either Liver-Blood or Liver-Yin. Especially in women, they more frequently stem from Liver-Blood deficiency. It is important to differentiate whether the underlying condition is Liver-Blood or Liver-Yin deficiency as the herbal treatment is quite different in each case, nourishing Blood in the former case and nourishing Yin in the latter. In both cases it is also worth remembering that most moving-Qi herbs are pungent and warm and therefore tending to injure Blood and Yin: they should therefore be used with caution if there is deficiency of Blood or Yin. A few herbs such as Fu Shou *Fructus Citri sarcodactylis* and Lu Mei Hua *Flos Pruni mume Sieb. et zucc. var. viridicalyx Makino* move Qi without injuring Blood or Yin.

(b) PENSIVENESS AND WORRY

These affect the Spleen, Stomach and Lungs. In the case of the Stomach, they cause stagnation of Qi and retention of food.

4. OVER-EXERTION

Physical over-exertion weakens the Stomach and Spleen and may lead to a dull epigastric pain, tiredness and weak muscles. It usually causes Stomach-Qi deficiency.

5. OVERWORK

Mental overwork, working long hours and eating irregularly over several years cause deficiency of Stomach-Yin. This can manifest with cracks such as shown in Figure 12.3 in the chapter on "Tiredness" (ch. 12). After many years, the tongue will lose its coating entirely and become Red.

6. CONSTITUTIONAL WEAKNESS

An inherited constitutional weakness of the

Stomach is obviously a potential cause of stomach disorders. Such an inherited weakness manifests with digestive problems in early childhood such as poor appetite, vomiting or diarrhoea, and possibly also with weak and flabby muscles, low energy and a crack such as that shown in Figure 12.3 mentioned above.

7. WRONG TREATMENT

When used wrongly, Chinese herbs can injure the Stomach and Spleen. An excessive or wrong use of bitter-cold or moving-downward herbs can injure Stomach-Qi or Stomach-Yin and lead to epigastric pain.

Of course, the side-effects of very many Western drugs are also a frequent cause of epigastric pain. Anti-inflammatory agents used for rheumathoid arthritis are a particular case in point.

Diagnosis

Diagnostic symptoms and signs in epigastric pain include the nature, time and amelioration or aggravation of the pain.

(a) NATURE OF PAIN

- Severe: Excess condition
- Dull: Deficiency condition
- Stabbing: stasis of Blood
- Distending: stagnation of Qi
- Burning: Heat
- With a feeling of fullness: Dampness

(b) TIME OF PAIN

- In the morning: Deficiency
- In the afternoon: stagnation of Qi
- At night: stasis of Blood

(c) AMELIORATION/AGGRAVATION OF PAIN

- Better after eating: Deficiency

- Worse after eating: Excess
- Better with pressure: Deficiency
- Worse with pressure: Excess
- Better with application of heat or drinking hot fluids: Cold
- Better with rest: Deficiency
- Better with slight exercise: stagnation of Qi or Blood
- Better after vomiting: Excess condition
- Worse after vomiting: Deficiency condition

The manifestations of epigastric pain with regard to Deficiency/Excess and Heat/Cold can be summarized in tabular form (Table 14.1).

When diagnosing epigastric pain, questions about thirst, taste, belching, regurgitation, vomiting, fullness and distension are important.

(a) THIRST

- Intense thirst with desire to drink cold fluids: Full Heat
- Dry mouth with desire to sip fluids: Empty-Heat
- Absence of thirst: Cold
- Thirst without a desire to drink: Damp-Heat

(b) TASTE

- Sticky taste: Dampness
- Bitter taste: Heat
- Sweet taste: Damp-Heat
- Sour taste: retention of food
- Absence of taste: Spleen deficiency

Table 14.1 Character of epigastric pain according to Heat-Cold and Deficiency-Excess

	Deficiency	Excess
Heat	Dull pain, slight burning sensation, dry mouth, desire to sip fluids, tongue Red with wide midline crack, without coating	Intense burning pain, worse after eating, thirst with desire to drink cold fluids, tongue Red with dry yellow coating
Cold	Dull pain, preference for warm drinks and application of heat, no thirst, vomiting of thin fluids, Empty pulse	Severe spastic pain, no thirst, vomiting, thick-white tongue coating, Full-Tight pulse

(c) BELCHING

– Loud belching: Excess condition
– Quiet belching: Deficiency condition
– Better after belching: stagnation of Qi

(d) REGURGITATION

– Sour regurgitation: retention of food or stagnant Liver-Qi invading the Stomach.
– Regurgitation of thin fluids: Deficient-Cold condition or Phlegm-Fluids in Stomach

(e) NAUSEA/VOMITING

– Slight nausea: Deficiency
– Vomiting with loud sound: Excess
– Vomiting with low sound: Deficiency
– Vomiting soon after eating: Excess
– Vomiting some time after eating: Deficiency
– Vomiting of food: Excess
– Vomiting of thin fluids: Deficiency
– Sour vomiting: invasion of Stomach by Liver
– Vomiting of blood: Heat

(f) DISTENSION/OPPRESSION/ STUFFINESS/FULLNESS

These four sensations need to be differentiated clearly.

A feeling of *distension* (*zhang*) indicates stagnation of Qi. This type of sensation will be seldom referred to as "distension" by Western patients: more often than not patients will call it a feeling of "bursting", "being blown-up", "bloating", etc.

A feeling of *oppression* (*men*) denotes Dampness, Phlegm or also more severe stagnation of Qi. The translation of this term cannot adequately convey the image evoked by its Chinese character: this depicts a heart constrained by a door and, besides the physical sensation, it also implies a certain mental anguish associated with this feeling.

A feeling of *stuffiness* (*pi*) indicates Stomach-Qi deficiency or Stomach-Heat. Contrary to the previous two sensations which can be felt objectively on palpation (e.g. a distended or oppressed abdomen feels so on touch), the sensation of stuffiness is only subjective and the abdomen feels soft on touch.

A feeling of *fullness* (*man*) indicates retention of food or water and Dampness.

A feeling of an actual mass (on palpation) indicates stasis of Blood.

Differentiation and treatment

The patterns discussed will be the following:

EXCESS

Cold invading the Stomach
Retention of Food
Liver-Qi invading the Stomach
Stomach-Heat
Stomach-Fire
Stomach Phlegm-Fire
Stomach Damp-Heat
Stomach and Liver Heat
Stasis of Blood in the Stomach
Phlegm-Fluids in the Stomach

DEFICIENCY

Stomach and Spleen Deficient and Cold
Stomach-Yin Deficiency

EXCESS

1. COLD INVADING THE STOMACH

CLINICAL MANIFESTATIONS

Acute, severe epigastric pain with sudden onset, chilliness, desire for application of warmth on the stomach area, no thirst, desire for warm drinks, pain not alleviated by pressure, nausea, vomiting.
Tongue: thick-white coating.
Pulse: Full and Tight.

This is an acute condition which occurs when

external Cold invades the Stomach directly, without going through the skin and muscles first. Such direct invasion of Cold can only affect Stomach, Intestines or Uterus.

Cold contracts and this causes intense pain. It also prevents Stomach-Qi from descending, which causes nausea and vomiting.

The other symptoms (no thirst, desire for warm drinks and improvement with application of warmth) are obvious Cold symptoms.

TREATMENT PRINCIPLE

Scatter Cold, warm the Stomach, stop pain.

ACUPUNCTURE

ST-21 Liangmen, ST-34 Liangqiu, SP-4 Gongsun, Ren-13 Shangwan. Reducing method, moxa must be used. The application of the moxa box on the epigastrium while the needles on ST-21 are retained is particularly beneficial.

Explanation

- **ST-21** is used for Excess patterns of the Stomach.
- **ST-34** as Accumulation point stops pain.
- **SP-4** removes obstructions from the epigastrium and stops pain.
- **Ren-13** is used if there is nausea or vomiting.

HERBAL TREATMENT

In mild cases one can use:

(a) Prescription
SHENG JIANG HONG TANG TANG
Zingiber-brown sugar Decoction
This is simply a decoction of several slices of fresh ginger with the addition of one teaspoonful of Barbados sugar at the end. It scatters Cold and warms the Stomach.

In severe cases use:

(b) Prescription
LIANG FU WAN

Alpinia-Cyperus Pill
Gao Liang Jiang *Rhizoma Alpiniae officinari* 6 g
Xiang Fu *Rhizoma Cyperi rotundi* 10 g

Explanation

This is a simple formula to scatter Cold and warm the Stomach which is used in more severe cases.

- **Gao Liang Jiang** warms the Stomach and dispels Cold.
- **Xiang Fu** moves Qi and stops pain. Its moving-Qi action will help to expel Cold and also to relax the contraction caused by Cold.

Variations

- In case of very severe symptoms of Cold, such as intense pain and spitting of clear fluid, add Gan Jiang *Rhizoma Zingiberis officinalis* 3 g and Wu Zhu Yu *Fructus Evodiae rutaecarpae* 1.5 g. Both these herbs are very hot and pungent and should be used for short periods only. They should be stopped when thirst appears and spitting of thin fluid stops.
- If there are symptoms of stagnation of Qi, such as pronounced distension, add Chen Pi *Pericarpium Citri reticulatae* and Mu Xiang *Radix Saussureae*.
- If there are exterior symptoms such as a temperature and chilliness, add the formula Xiang Su San *Cyperus-Perilla Powder* which contains Xiang Fu *Rhizoma Cyperi rotundi*, Zi Su Ye *Folium Perillae frutescentis*, Chen Pi *Pericarpium Citri reticulatae* and Gan Cao *Radix Glycyrrhizae uralensis*.
- If there is a pronounced feeling of oppression of the epigastrium, no appetite, belching and vomiting add Zhi Shi *Fructus Citri aurantii immaturus*, Shen Qu *Massa Fermentata Medicinalis*, Ji Nei Jin *Endothelium Corneum Gigeraiae Galli*, Ban Xia *Rhizoma Pinelliae ternatae* and Sheng Jiang *Rhizoma Zingiberis officinalis recens*.

(i) Patent remedy

FU ZI LI ZHONG WAN
Aconitum Regulating the Centre Pill

Gan Jiang *Rhizoma Zingiberis officinalis*
Bai Zhu *Rhizoma Atractylodis macrocephalae*
Dang Shen *Radix Codonopsis pilosulae*
Gan Cao *Radix Glycyrrhizae uralensis*
Fu Zi *Radix Aconiti carmichaeli praeparata*

Explanation

This pill, which is very hot in energy, scatters Cold from the Middle Burner, stops pain and tonifies Stomach and Spleen. The pulse presentation in this case is Tight, Slow, Full and Deep.

The tongue presentation appropriate to this remedy is a Pale and wet body.

(ii) Patent remedy

HUO XIANG ZHENG QI WAN (PIAN)
Agastache Upright Qi Pill (Tablet)
Huo Xiang *Herba Agastachis*
Zi Su Ye *Folium Perillae frutescentis*
Bai Zhi *Radix Angelicae dahuricae*
Ban Xia *Rhizoma Pinelliae ternatae*
Chen Pi *Pericarpium Citri reticulatae*
Bai Zhu *Rhizoma Atractylodis macrocephalae*
Fu Ling *Sclerotium Poriae cocos*
Hou Po *Cortex Magnoliae officinalis*
Da Fu Pi *Pericarpium Arecae catechu*
Jie Geng *Radix Platycodi grandiflori*
Sheng Jiang *Rhizoma Zingiberis officinalis recens*
Da Zao *Fructus Ziziphi jujubae*
Zhi Gan Cao *Radix Glycyrrhizae uralensis praeparata*

Explanation

This pill is used in preference to the previous one when exterior Cold is combined with Dampness. This remedy releases the Exterior, expels Cold, resolves Dampness, stops pain and relieves nausea and vomiting.

The main symptoms of external Dampness invasion are a feeling of oppression of the epigastrium, nausea, vomiting, a feeling of heaviness, a sticky-white tongue coating and a Slippery pulse.

(iii) Patent remedy

KANG NING WAN

Health and Quiet Pill
Tian Ma *Rhizoma Gastrodiae elatae*
Bai Zhi *Radix Angelicae dahuricae*
Ju Hua *Flos Chrysanthemi morifolii*
Bo He *Herba Menthae*
Ge Gen *Radix Puerariae*
Tian Hua Fen *Radix Trichosanthis*
Cang Zhu *Rhizoma Atractylodis lanceae*
Yi Yi Ren *Semen Coicis lachryma jobi*
Fu Ling *Sclerotium Poriae cocos*
Mu Xiang *Radix Saussureae*
Hou Po *Cortex Magnoliae officinalis*
Chen Pi *Pericarpium Citri reticulatae*
Shen Qu *Massa Fermentata Medicinalis*
Huo Xiang *Herba Agastachis*
Gu Ya *Fructus Oryzae sativae germinatus*

Explanation

This well-known remedy is also for invasion of Cold and Dampness with such symptoms as a feeling of heaviness, pain, and oppression of the epigastrium, nausea, vomiting, headache and a sticky tongue coating which could be white or yellow. The pulse presentation for the use of this remedy is a pulse which is Slippery and slightly Wiry.

This remedy differs from the previous one in so far as it is more for epigastric pain than Dampness and it also treats a headache from exterior Cold-Dampness.

DIETARY ADVICE

In invasions of external Cold to the Stomach it is best to avoid cold foods such as salads and fruit and, most of all, iced drinks.

2. RETENTION OF FOOD

CLINICAL MANIFESTATIONS

Dull epigastric pain which is worse with pressure, feeling of distension and fullness, belching, sour regurgitation, foul breath, vomiting of undigested food, epigastric pain relieved after vomiting, loose stools or constipation.

Tongue: thick-sticky coating in the centre and root which could be white or yellow.
Pulse: Slippery.

This condition is very simply due to accumulation of undigested food in the stomach. This can result either from over-eating or from deficient Stomach-Qi being unable to make food descend.

The accumulation of undigested food in the Stomach causes the dull pain and characteristic feeling of distension and fullness. Undigested food obstructs the Stomach and prevents Stomach-Qi from descending: this causes belching, sour regurgitation, nausea and vomiting. The fact that vomiting relieves the pain indicates that the obstruction in the Stomach is of a substantial nature, i.e. accumulated undigested food. When the obstruction is of a non-substantial nature, such as stagnation of Qi, then the pain is not relieved by vomiting.

Whether there is constipation or loose stools depends on the relative strength of Spleen and Stomach. If the Spleen is deficient, the accumulated food in the Stomach prevents the Spleen from transforming food essences properly and this results in loose stools. If Spleen-Qi is relatively strong, then constipation may result from Stomach-Qi not descending and not moving the digestate downwards towards the Intestines.

The thick and sticky tongue coating in the centre and root reflects the accumulation of undigested food in the Stomach and Intestines. It will be white if there is Cold and yellow if there is Heat. The Slippery pulse reflects the accumulation of undigested food in the Stomach.

TREATMENT PRINCIPLE

Dissolve accumulation, eliminate stagnation and restore the descending of Stomach-Qi.

ACUPUNCTURE

Ren-13 Shangwan, Ren-10 Xiawan, ST-21 Liangmen, ST-20 Chengman, ST-44 Neiting, ST-45 Lidui, SP-4 Gongsun, P-6 Neiguan, ST-25 Tianshu. Reducing or even method.

Explanation

- **Ren-13** subdues rebellious Qi and relieves belching, sour regurgitation, nausea and vomiting.
- **Ren-10** stimulates the descending of Stomach-Qi.
- **ST-21** is suitable for Excess patterns of the Stomach and it stops pain.
- **ST-20** dissolves food accumulation and relieves fullness. Its name "Chengman" means "bearing fullness".
- **ST-44** and **ST-45** are distal points suitable for Excess patterns of the Stomach. They both stop epigastric pain. ST-44 clears Heat and ST-45 dissolves accumulation of food. In particular, ST-45 relieves insomnia caused by retention of food.
- **SP-4** and **P-6** in combination open the Penetrating Vessel. This is especially indicated in Excess patterns of the Stomach with obstructions in the epigastrium, rebellious Stomach-Qi and resulting feeling of distension and fullness.
- **ST-25**, Front-Collecting point of the Large Intestine, resolves retention of food by promoting the bowel movements.

HERBAL TREATMENT

Prescription

BAO HE WAN
Preserving and Harmonizing Pill
Shan Zha *Fructus Crataegi* 9 g
Shen Qu *Massa Fermentata medicinalis* 6 g
Lai Fu Zi *Semen Raphani sativi* 6 g
Ban Xia *Rhizoma Pinelliae ternatae* 6 g
Chen Pi *Pericarpium Citri reticulatae* 3 g
Fu Ling *Sclerotium Poriae cocos* 6 g
Lian Qiao *Fructus Forsythiae suspensae* 6 g

Explanation

- **Shan Zha** promotes digestion (especially of meat and fats) and dissolves food accumulation.
- **Shen Qu** promotes digestion (especially of alcohol, vinegar and rice) and dissolves food accumulation.

- **Lai Fu Zi** promotes digestion (especially of wheat and bread) and dissolves food accumulation.
- **Ban Xia**, **Chen Pi** and **Fu Ling** resolve Dampness, Phlegm and food accumulation.
- **Lian Qiao** clears Stomach-Heat which frequently results from retention of food. It can be eliminated if the tongue coating is not yellow.

Variations

- If there is a pronounced feeling of distension add Zhi Shi *Fructus Citri aurantii immaturus*, Sha Ren *Fructus seu Semen Amomi* and Bing Lang *Semen Arecae catechu*.
- If there is constipation add Da Huang *Rhizoma Rhei*, Hou Po *Cortex Magnoliae officinalis*, Zhi Shi *Fructus Citri aurantii immaturus* (these three herbs constitute the Xiao Cheng Qi Tang *Small Conducting Qi Decoction*), Mu Xiang *Radix Saussureae* and Xiang Fu *Rhizoma Cyperi rotundi*.
- If there is severe pain which is worse with pressure, constipation and a dry yellow tongue coating, add Da Cheng Qi Tang *Great Conducting Qi Decoction* (Da Huang *Radix Rhei*, Mang Xiao *Mirabilitum*, Hou Po *Cortex Magnoliae officinalis* and Zhi Shi *Fructus Citri aurantii immaturus*).
- If there is severe accumulation of food add Ji Nei Jin *Endothelium Corneum Gigeraiae Galli*, Mai Ya *Fructus Hordei vulgaris germinatus* and Gu Ya *Fructus Oryzae sativae germinatus*.

If the stagnation is not relieved promptly by the treatment the patient should be advised to fast for a few days. Even if the stagnation is relieved, the patient should eat less and eat easily-digestible foods.

(a) Patent remedy

BAO HE WAN
Preserving and Harmonizing Pill
Shan Zha *Fructus Crataegi*
Shen Qu *Massa Fermentata medicinalis*
Lai Fu Zi *Semen Raphani sativi*
Ban Xia *Rhizoma Pinelliae ternatae*
Chen Pi *Pericarpium Citri reticulatae*
Fu Ling *Sclerotium Poriae cocos*
Lian Qiao *Fructus Forsythiae suspensae*

Explanation

This pill has the same ingredients and functions as the homonymous prescription mentioned above. It is an excellent pill for general symptoms of retention of food. It is suitable for children who suffer from retention of food very easily.

The tongue presentation appropriate to this remedy is a thick coating which may be white or yellow.

(b) Patent remedy

QI XING CHA
Seven Stars Tea
Zhu Ye *Herba Lophatheri gracilis*
Gou Teng *Ramulus Uncariae*
Chan Tui *Periostracum Cicadae*
Shan Zha *Fructus Crataegi*
Gu Ya *Fructus Oryzae sativae germinatus*
Yi Yi Ren *Semen Coicis lachryma jobi*
Gan Cao *Radix Glycyrrhizae uralensis*

Explanation

This remedy resolves retention of food, drains Dampness, clears Heat and calms irritability. It is especially suitable for children with symptoms of retention of food and Heat such as poor digestion, epigastric and abdominal pain, restless sleep, irritability, a thick-yellow tongue coating and a Slippery and Rapid pulse.

(c) Patent remedy

MU XIANG SHUN QI WAN
Saussurea Subduing Qi Pill
Mu Xiang *Radix Saussureae*
Bai Dou Kou *Fructus Amomi cardamomi*
Cang Zhu *Rhizoma Atractylodis lanceae*
Sheng Jiang *Rhizoma Zingiberis officinalis recens*
Qing Pi *Pericarpium Citri reticulatae viridae*
Chen Pi *Pericarpium Citri reticulatae*
Fu Ling *Sclerotium Poriae cocos*

Chai Hu *Radix Bupleuri*
Hou Po *Cortex Magnoliae officinalis*
Bing Lang *Semen Arecae catechu*
Zhi Ke *Fructus Citri aurantii*
Wu Yao *Radix Linderae strychnifoliae*
Lai Fu Zi *Semen Raphani sativi*
Shan Zha *Fructus Crataegi*
Shen Qu *Massa Fermentata Medicinalis*
Mai Ya *Fructus Hordei vulgaris germinatus*
Gan Cao *Radix Glycyrrhizae uralensis*

Explanation

This remedy resolves retention of food and Dampness and moves Qi. It is indicated for retention of food accompanied by stagnation of Qi causing an epigastric pain which is more severe than that addressed by the previous two remedies.

DIETARY ADVICE

The patient should simply eat less and more slowly.

Case history

A 45-year-old woman had been suffering from epigastric pain for 2 years. The pain was dull, worse lying down, aggravated by pressing on the area, and accompanied by a slight nausea and acidity. When the pain was bad she also became constipated and her appetite decreased. She also had a slight feeling of fullness.

Besides this problem, she had also experienced some slight bleeding in between periods with light-fresh blood for 4 months.

Her pulse was Slippery on the whole and Weak on the right side. Her tongue was Pale with a slight Bluish-Purple tinge, teeth-marks and a sticky-white coating (Plate 14.1).

Diagnosis

This is a condition of mixed Deficiency and Excess. There is a deficiency of Spleen-Qi manifesting with poor appetite, dull epigastric pain, bleeding in between periods (Spleen-Qi not holding Blood), Weak pulse and Pale tongue with teeth-marks. The Excess condition, due to retention of food, manifests with constipation, nausea, pain which is worse for pressure and on lying down, the Slippery pulse and the sticky tongue coating. There is therefore a deficiency of Spleen- and Stomach-Qi, as well as retention of food. In addition, there is also the beginning of stasis of

Blood in the Stomach as evidenced by the slight Bluish-Purple tinge of the tongue body.

Treatment principle

The treatment principle adopted was to tonify Spleen-Qi and resolve retention of food. It was not necessary to deal with the stasis of Blood directly as this would be resolved by itself once Spleen-Qi is tonified and food retention is resolved.

She was treated with both acupuncture and Chinese herbs.

Acupuncture

The acupuncture points used were selected from the following:

- **Ren-12** Zhongwan, **ST-36** Zusanli, **SP-6** Sanyinjiao, **BL-20** Pishu and **BL-21** Weishu, with reinforcing method, to tonify Stomach- and Spleen-Qi;
- **Ren-11** Jianli, **ST-21** Liangmen and **ST-40** Fenglong, with even method, to promote the descending of Stomach-Qi to resolve retention of food;
- **P-6** Neiguan, with even method, to subdue rebellious Stomach-Qi (causing nausea and acidity).

Herbal treatment

The decoction used was a variation of Bao He Wan *Preserving and Harmonizing Pill*:

Shan Zha *Fructus Crataegi* 6 g
Shen Qu *Massa Fermentata medicinalis* 6 g
Lai Fu Zi *Semen Raphani sativi* 4 g
Ban Xia *Rhizoma Pinelliae ternatae* 6 g
Chen Pi *Pericarpium Citri reticulatae* 3 g
Fu Ling *Sclerotium Poriae cocos* 6 g
Mai Ya *Fructus Hordei vulgaris germinatus* 4 g
Zhi Shi *Fructus Citri aurantii immaturus* 4 g
Bai Shao *Radix Paeoniae albae* 9 g
Zhi Gan Cao *Radix Glycyrrhizae uralensis praeparata* 4 g
Bai Zhu *Rhizoma Atractylodis macrocephalae* 6 g

Explanation
- The first six herbs constitute the Bao He Wan which resolves retention of food. Lian Qiao was eliminated from it as, in this case, there were no signs of Heat.
- **Mai Ya** was added to resolve retention of food and move Qi in the epigastrium to relieve pain.
- **Zhi Shi** was added to promote the descending of Stomach-Qi to relieve food stagnation.
- **Bai Shao** and **Gan Cao** in combination, harmonize the Centre and stop pain.
- **Bai Zhu** tonifies Spleen-Qi.

This patient's epigastric pain was completely cured after three acupuncture sessions and three 5-packet courses of decoctions.

3. LIVER-QI INVADING THE STOMACH

CLINICAL MANIFESTATIONS

Epigastric distension and pain radiating towards

the right or left hypochondrium, belching, sighing, irritability, uncomfortable feeling of hunger. The pain comes in bouts clearly related to emotional tension.
Tongue: normal body colour or slightly Red sides.
Pulse: Wiry. It may be Wiry only on the left side.

This is an extremely common cause of epigastric pain. Stagnant Liver-Qi "invades" the Stomach horizontally and impairs the descending of Stomach-Qi. This results in stagnation of Qi in the Stomach and epigastric pain. From the 5-Element perspective it is called "Wood overacting on Earth". Liver-Qi stagnation is usually due to emotional problems such as anger, resentment or frustration.

TREATMENT PRINCIPLE

Soothe the Liver and regulate Qi.

ACUPUNCTURE

LIV-14 Qimen, P-6 Neiguan, ST-21 Liangmen, Ren-12 Zhongwan, ST-36 Zusanli, G.B.-34 Yanglingquan. Reducing or even method.

Explanation

– **LIV-14** is specific to harmonize Liver and Stomach.
– **P-6** regulates Liver-Qi, harmonizes the Stomach, subdues rebellious Stomach-Qi and calms the mind.
– **ST-21** stimulates the descending of Stomach-Qi, especially in Excess patterns.
– **Ren-12** and **ST-36** tonify Stomach-Qi. Strengthening Stomach-Qi prevents its being invaded by the Liver.
– **G.B.-34** soothes the Liver and eliminates stagnation. In combination with Ren-12, it eliminates stagnation in the epigastrium.

In cases of severe emotional tension other points can be added, especially the following combination:

– **P-7** Daling, **T.B.-3** Zhongzhu, **Du-24** Shenting and **G.B.-13** Benshen. P-7 and T.B.-3 could be used unilaterally, one on the left and the other on the right side.

This combination of points is very effective in eliminating stagnation of Liver-Qi and calming the Mind whenever there are severe emotional problems, especially if associated with relationship difficulties. It is particularly indicated for women. In men, it is better to replace P-7 with HE-7 Shenmen.

HERBAL TREATMENT
Prescription

CHAI HU SU GAN TANG
Bupleurum Soothing the Liver Decoction
Chai Hu *Radix Bupleuri* 6 g
Bai Shao *Radix Paeoniae albae* 4.5 g
Zhi Ke *Fructus Citri aurantii* 4.5 g
Zhi Gan Cao *Radix Glycyrrhizae uralensis praeparata* 1.5 g
Chen Pi *Pericarpium Citri reticulatae* 6 g
Xiang Fu *Rhizoma Cyperi rotundi* 4.5 g
Chuan Xiong *Radix Ligustici wallichii* 4.5 g

Explanation

– **Chai Hu**, **Bai Shao**, **Chuan Xiong** and **Xiang Fu** soothe the Liver and eliminate stagnation.
– **Chen Pi**, **Zhi Ke** and **Gan Cao** regulate Qi and harmonize the Stomach.

Variations

– If the pain is very severe add Yan Hu Suo *Rhizoma Corydalis yanhusuo* and Yu Jin *Tuber Curcumae*.
– In case of belching add Mei Gui Hua *Flos Rosae rugosae* and Fu Shou *Fructus Citri sarcodactylis*.
– If there are pronounced symptoms of rebellious Qi (such as belching, hiccup, nausea and vomiting) add Chen Xiang *Lignum Aquilariae* and Xuan Fu Hua *Flos Inulae*.
– If stagnant Liver-Qi leads to Liver-Fire, manifesting with a Red tongue with redder sides, a bitter taste and thirst, add Mu Dan Pi *Cortex Moutan radicis* and Shan Zhi Zi *Fructus Gardeniae jasminoidis*, remove Chai Hu *Radix Bupleuri* and increase the dosage of Bai Shao *Radix Paeoniae albae* and Gan Cao *Radix Glycyrrhizae uralensis*.

- If Liver-Fire begins to damage the Yin add Sheng Di Huang *Radix Rehmanniae glutinosae*, Mai Men Dong *Tuber Ophiopogonis japonici* and Chuan Lian Zi *Fructus Meliae toosendan*. In such a case it would be very important to avoid hot-spicy foods, alcohol and smoking.
- If there is sour regurgitation add Wa Leng Zi *Concha Arcae* and Wu Zei Gu *Os Sepiae*.
- If there are signs of Phlegm add a small dose of Bai Jie Zi *Semen Sinapis albae* (2 g) which resolves mucus from the gastric membrane.
- If there is epigastric distension soon after eating add Gu Ya *Fructus Oryzae sativae germinatus*, Mai Ya *Fructus Hordei vulgaris germinatus* and Lai Fu Zi *Semen Raphani sativi*.

In a condition such as this, clearly caused by emotional stress, it is important to explore with the patient the life situations and possibly emotional patterns which are at the root of the condition. If necessary, the help of a skilled counsellor or psychotherapist should be enlisted.

In cases of severe emotional tension the following herbs could be added:

- He Huan Pi *Cortex Albizziae julibrissin*, Suan Zao Ren *Semen Ziziphi spinosae* and Yu Jin *Tuber Curcumae*.

(a) Patent remedy

SHU GAN WAN
Pacifying the Liver Pill
Chuan Lian Zi *Fructus Meliae toosendan*
Jiang Huang *Rhizoma Curcumae longae*
Chen Xiang *Lignum Aquilariae*
Yan Hu Suo *Rhizoma Corydalis yanhusuo*
Mu Xiang *Radix Saussureae*
Bai Dou Kou *Fructus Amomi cardamomi*
Bai Shao *Radix Paeoniae albae*
Fu Ling *Sclerotium Poriae cocos*
Zhi Ke *Fructus Citri aurantii*
Chen Pi *Pericarpium Citri reticulatae*
Sha Ren *Fructus seu Semen Amomi*
Hou Po *Cortex Magnoliae officinalis*

Explanation

This pill primarily moves Liver-Qi. It is excellent for cases of stagnant Liver-Qi invading the Stomach causing epigastric pain and distension.

A pronounced feeling of epigastric distension and pain which is related to emotional stress and a Wiry pulse are the main manifestations indicating the use of this remedy.

(b) Patent remedy

MU XIANG SHUN QI WAN
Saussurea Subduing Qi Pill
This remedy, just mentioned above under "Retention of Food", is suitable also to treat stagnant Liver-Qi invading the Stomach. It is indicated if stagnation of Qi is accompanied by retention of food and Dampness in the Stomach.

Thus the main manifestations indicating the use of this pill are epigastric pain and fullness (rather than distension), a thick-sticky tongue coating and a Slippery-Wiry pulse.

Case history

A 38-year-old woman had been suffering from epigastric pain for 5 years. The pain radiated from the epigastrium to the right hypochondrium and was accompanied by a pronounced feeling of distension and belching. She also suffered from difficult bowel movements and the stools were often like small pebbles. She felt often depressed and irritable and found it difficult to establish permanent relationships with the opposite sex. Her periods were regular and normal in all ways, except that she suffered from premenstrual irritability and distension.

Her tongue was unremarkable, being only slightly Red on the sides. Her pulse was slightly Wiry on the left side.

Diagnosis
This is a clear condition of stagnation of Liver-Qi obviously deriving from emotional stress.

Treatment principle
The treatment principle adopted was to move Liver-Qi, eliminate stagnation, promote the descending of Stomach-Qi, calm the Mind and settle the Ethereal Soul. She was treated with acupuncture and herbs.

Acupuncture
The acupuncture points used were selected from the following:

- **P-6** Neiguan, with even method, to move Liver-Qi, subdue rebellious Stomach-Qi, calm the Mind and settle the Ethereal Soul. This is an excellent point, especially for women, for stagnation of Liver-Qi deriving from emotional stress, particularly that from relationship difficulties. At the same time, it

regulates the Upper and Middle Burner of the Stomach and stops epigastric pain.
- **ST-40** Fenglong, with even method, to harmonize the Stomach and subdue rebellious Stomach-Qi. It combines well with P-6, one on the right and the other on the left, to harmonize the Middle Burner.
- **Ren-12** Zhongwan and **ST-36** Zusanli, with reinforcing method, to strengthen the Stomach.
- **ST-21** Liangmen and **Ren-11**, with even method, to promote the descending of Stomach-Qi.
- **LIV-14** Qimen and **G.B.-34** Yanglingquan, with even method, to promote the free flow of Liver-Qi and move Qi. G.B.-34, in combination with Ren-12, moves Qi in the epigastrium.

Herbal treatment
The decoction used was a variation of Chai Hu Su Gan Tang *Bupleurum Soothing the Liver Decoction*:

Chai Hu *Radix Bupleuri* 4 g
Bai Shao *Radix Paeoniae albae* 9 g
Zhi Ke *Fructus Citri aurantii* 6 g
Zhi Gan Cao *Radix Glycyrrhizae uralensis praeparata* 4.5 g
Chen Pi *Pericarpium Citri reticulatae* 4 g
Xiang Fu *Rhizoma Cyperi rotundi* 4.5 g
Chuan Xiong *Radix Ligustici wallichii* 4.5 g
Mu Xiang *Radix Saussureae* 3 g
He Huan Pi *Cortex Albizziae julibrissin* 6 g
Dang Shen *Radix Codonopsis pilosulae* 6 g

Explanation
- The first seven herbs constitute the Chai Hu Su Gan Tang which moves Liver-Qi, eliminates stagnation and stops pain. The dosage of Bai Shao was increased to stop pain.
- **Mu Xiang** was added to move Qi in the epigastrium and stop pain.
- **He Huan Pi** was added to move Liver-Qi and relieve irritability and depression. This herb is particularly effective in treating depression from Liver-Qi stagnation.
- **Dang Shen** was added to tonify Spleen-Qi to prevent it being weakened by the stagnant Liver-Qi.

This patient was treated for 1 year with minor variations to the above treatment. With the help of some psychological counselling her epigastric pain disappeared and she became much happier in herself.

Case history

A 45-year-old man had been suffering from epigastric pain for 22 years. The pain radiated from the epigastrium to the right hypochondrial region. It was worse at night and better after eating. He belched a lot, his stools were slightly dry and he felt very tired.

His pulse was Fine, slightly Empty at the deep level in general, and Floating-Empty and very slightly Wiry on the right Middle position. His tongue was Red on the sides, Stiff and with a slightly rootless coating.

Diagnosis
This, like the previous one, is also a case of stagnant Liver-Qi invading the Stomach, but with a more complex condition. The stagnation of Liver-Qi is apparent from the radiation of the pain to the right hypochondrium, the belching, the Red sides of the tongue and the very slightly Wiry quality of the pulse. Because of the long duration of the condition, the stagnant Liver-Qi has weakened not only Stomach-Qi, but also Stomach-Yin. Stomach-Yin deficiency is apparent from the rootless coating on the tongue, the Stiff tongue body, the aggravation of the pain at night, the dry stools and the Floating-Empty quality on the right Middle position of the pulse. His tiredness is obviously caused by the long-standing deficiency of Stomach-Qi and Stomach-Yin.

Treatment principle
A two-stage treatment strategy was adopted: first move Liver-Qi, with caution so as not to injure Stomach-Yin further, and then tonify Stomach-Yin. It was decided to start by moving Liver-Qi first rather than tonifying Stomach-Yin to alleviate the epigastric pain.

He was treated with both acupuncture and herbs.

Acupuncture
The acupuncture points used were selected from the following:

- **Ren-12** Zhongwan, **ST-36** Zusanli and **SP-6** Sanyinjiao, with reinforcing method, to tonify Stomach-Qi and Stomach-Yin.
- **G.B.-34** Yanglingquan and **LIV-14**, with even method, to move Liver-Qi.
- **ST-21** Liangmen and **Ren-11** Jianli, with even method, to subdue rebellious Stomach-Qi and stop pain.

Herbal treatment
The decoction used first was a variation of Chai Hu Su Gan Tang *Bupleurum Soothing the Liver Decoction*:

Chai Hu *Radix Bupleuri* 4 g
Bai Shao *Radix Paeoniae albae* 9 g
Zhi Ke *Fructus Citri aurantii* 4 g
Zhi Gan Cao *Radix Glycyrrhizae uralensis praeparata* 4.5 g
Chen Pi *Pericarpium Citri reticulatae* 3 g
Xiang Fu *Rhizoma Cyperi rotundi* 4 g
Chuan Xiong *Radix Ligustici wallichii* 3 g
Mei Gui Hua *Flos Rosae rugosae* 4.5 g
Fu Shou *Fructus Citri sarcodactylis* 3 g
Tai Zi Shen *Radix Pseudostellariae* 6 g
Shan Yao *Radix Dioscoreae oppositae* 6 g
Mai Men Dong *Tuber Ophiopogonis japonici* 6 g
Yu Zhu *Rhizoma Polygonati odorati* 4 g

Explanation
- The first seven herbs constitute the Chai Hu Su Gan Tang to move Liver-Qi. The dosages of the moving-Qi herbs (which are warm and pungent) were all reduced in order not to injure Stomach-Yin.
- **Mei Gui Hua** and **Fu Shou** were added as they move Qi without injuring Yin.
- **Tai Zi Shen**, **Shan Yao** and **Mai Dong** were added to nourish Stomach-Yin.
- **Yu Zhu** was added to clear Stomach Empty-Heat.

After a few months during which the pain was greatly reduced, the decoction was changed and a variation of Huang Qi Jian Zhong Tang *Astragalus Strengthening the Centre Decoction* was used:

Huang Qi *Radix Astragali membranacei* 9 g
Bai Shao *Radix Paeoniae albae* 18 g
Gui Zhi *Ramulus Cinnamomi cassiae* 3 g
Zhi Gan Cao *Radix Glycyrrhizae uralensis praeparata* 6 g
Sheng Jiang *Rhizoma Zingiberis officinalis recens* 1 slice
Da Zao *Fructus Ziziphi jujubae* 5 dates
Yi Tang *Saccharum granorum* 30 g
Tai Zi Shen *Radix Pseudostellariae* 6 g
Mai Men Dong *Tuber Ophiopogonis japonici* 6 g
Yu Zhu *Rhizoma Polygonati odorati* 6 g
Mei Gui Hua *Flos Rosae rugosae* 4 g

Explanation
- The first seven herbs constitute the Huang Qi Jian Zhong Tang which tonifies Stomach-Qi and stops epigastric pain. The dosages of Sheng Jiang and Gui Zhi were reduced so as not to injure Stomach-Yin.
- **Tai Zi Shen**, **Mai Dong** and **Yu Zhu** were added to tonify Stomach-Yin.
- **Mei Gui Hua** was added to move Qi.

After a further 6 months of treatment with variations of this formula his pain went, his tongue-body colour became normal and his pulse lost the Floating-Empty quality.

DIETARY ADVICE

In stagnation of Liver-Qi affecting the Stomach it is important to advise the patient to eat slowly, avoid working or discussing business while eating and, most of all, avoid getting angry while eating.

4. STOMACH-HEAT

CLINICAL MANIFESTATIONS

Burning epigastric pain, thirst, irritability, sour regurgitation.

Tongue: dry, yellow tongue coating. The body colour may be Red if there is pronounced Heat, otherwise it could be normal.
Pulse: slightly Rapid, slightly Overflowing in the right Middle position.

This condition is usually due to excessive consumption of spicy foods such as curries, spices, lamb and alcohol.

TREATMENT PRINCIPLE

Clear Stomach-Heat, restore the descending of Stomach-Qi.

ACUPUNCTURE

ST-21 Liangmen, ST-44 Neiting. Reducing or even method.

Explanation

- **ST-21** is a local point for all Excess patterns of the Stomach.
- **ST-44** is the main distal point to clear Stomach-Heat.

HERBAL TREATMENT

Prescription

BAI HU TANG
White Tiger Decoction
Shi Gao *Gypsum fibrosum* 30 g
Zhi Mu *Radix Anemarrhenae asphodeloidis* 6 g
Geng Mi *Semen Oryzae sativae* 6 g
Gan Cao *Radix Glycyrrhizae uralensis* 3 g

Explanation

This is the famous formula to clear Stomach-Heat from the "Discussion of Cold-induced Diseases" by Zhang Zhong Jing (Han dynasty).

- **Shi Gao**, cold and pungent, is the main herb to clear Stomach-Heat.
- **Zhi Mu** clears Stomach-Heat and nourishes Yin fluids.

- **Geng Mi** is plain brown rice which nourishes Stomach fluids.
- **Gan Cao** harmonizes.

Variations

- For severe epigastric pain add Bai Shao *Radix Paeoniae albae* and increase Gan Cao *Radix Glycyrrhizae uralensis*.

Patent remedy

SAI MEI AN
Race [between] Rot and Peaceful [Health]
Ge Ke *Concha Cyclinae*
Han Shui Shi *Calcitum*
Wa Leng Zi *Concha Arcae*
Fu Long Gan *Terra Flava usta*
Bing Pian *Borneol*
Zhong Ju *Stalactitum*
Zhen Zhu *Margarita*

Explanation

This remedy can be used for several different stomach patterns as its main effect is to absorb stomach acids and reduce sour regurgitation. It is cold in nature and is therefore better indicated for Heat patterns of the Stomach.

As it contains many shells and minerals it may tend to weaken the Spleen if used continuously for a long time: it should not be used for more than a few weeks at a time.

DIETARY ADVICE

In Stomach-Heat one should avoid eating too much hot-energy food, such as game, lamb, beef and spices. Alcohol consumption should also be kept to a minimum.

5. STOMACH-FIRE

CLINICAL MANIFESTATIONS

Burning epigastric pain, thirst with desire to drink cold water, dry mouth, severe irritability, bleeding gums, vomiting of blood, red face, constipation.
Tongue: Red or Dark-Red body, yellow-dry coating.
Pulse: Rapid, Overflowing.

This pattern could be considered a further stage of Stomach-Heat. Heat and Fire are very similar in nature and share common manifestations. Fire, however, is a more substantial pathogenic factor than Heat and it differs from Heat in three respects:

(a) It dries up more (hence dry stools, dry mouth and dry tongue)
(b) It causes bleeding by agitating the Blood in the vessels (hence bleeding gums and vomiting of blood)
(c) It affects the Mind more (hence severe irritability).

When applying treatment with acupuncture the distinction between Heat and Fire is not crucial. In herbal treatment, however, this distinction is important as to clear Heat one uses pungent and cold herbs, while to clear Fire bitter and cold herbs are used.

TREATMENT PRINCIPLE

Clear Stomach-Fire, protect Stomach-Yin, restore the descending of Stomach-Fire.

ACUPUNCTURE

ST-44 Neiting, ST-45 Lidui, ST-21 Liangmen, SP-6 Sanyinjiao, Ren-13 Shangwan, BL-21 Weishu. Reducing or even method.

Explanation

- **ST-44** and **BL-21** clear Stomach-Fire.
- **ST-45** clears Stomach-Fire and calms the Mind. It is the main point to calm the Mind when it is disturbed by Stomach-Fire.
- **ST-21** is used in all Excess patterns of the Stomach.
- **SP-6** is used to protect Stomach-Yin, i.e. to prevent injury of Yin by Fire.

- **Ren-13** is used to subdue rebellious Stomach-Qi. In this case, Stomach-Qi rebels upwards due to the rising of Stomach-Fire, manifesting with bleeding gums and vomiting of blood.

HERBAL TREATMENT

(a) Prescription

XIE XIN TANG
Draining the Heart Decoction
Da Huang *Rhizoma Rhei* 6 g
Huang Lian *Rhizoma Coptidis* 3 g
Huang Qin *Radix Scutellariae baicalensis* 9 g

Explanation

In spite of its name, this formula can be used to clear Stomach-Fire as "Heart" in this case means the area below the heart, i.e. the epigastrium. It clears Fire by draining downwards via the bowel movements: this is the function of Da Huang *Rhizoma Rhei* in this formula. Huang Lian *Rhizoma Coptidis* and Huang Qin *Radix Scutellariae baicalensis* clear Stomach-Fire and assist Da Huang *Rhizoma Rhei* in clearing Fire.

(b) Prescription

QING WEI SAN
Clearing the Stomach Powder
Huang Lian *Rhizoma Coptidis* 5 g
Sheng Di Huang *Radix Rehmanniae glutinosae* 12 g
Mu Dan Pi *Cortex Moutan radicis* 9 g
Dang Gui *Radix Angelicae sinensis* 6 g
Sheng Ma *Rhizoma Cimicifugae* 6 g

Explanation

- **Huang Lian** and **Sheng Ma** clear Stomach-Heat or Stomach-Fire.
- **Sheng Di Huang** and **Mu Dan Pi** cool Blood and stop bleeding.
- **Dang Gui** is used here to direct the formula to the Blood portion in order to stop bleeding.

This formula is applicable to a further stage of Stomach-Fire. It addresses the situation when Stomach-Fire has entered Blood causing bleeding, and has begun to injure Yin. For these reasons, Mu Dan Pi *Cortex Moutan radicis* and Sheng Di Huang *Radix Rehmanniae glutinosae* are in this formula to cool Blood and stop bleeding, whilst the latter herb also nourishes Yin. Dang Gui *Radix Angelicae sinensis* is added to direct the other herbs to the Blood portion, thus helping the formula both to cool Blood and to stop bleeding.

The key manifestations of this pattern and formula are therefore bleeding gums or vomiting of Blood (indicating Stomach-Fire heating the Blood) and a Dark-Red tongue without coating in the centre but with a yellow-dry coating elsewhere (indicating Blood-Heat and injury of Stomach-Yin by Fire).

(c) Prescription

YU NU JIAN
Jade Woman Decoction
Shi Gao *Gypsum fibrosum* 30 g
Shu Di Huang *Radix Rehmanniae glutinosae praeparata* 18 g
Zhi Mu *Radix Anemarrhenae asphodeloidis* 4.5 g
Mai Men Dong *Tuber Ophiopogonis japonici* 6 g
Niu Xi *Radix Achyranthis bidentatae seu Cyathulae* 4.5 g

Explanation

This formula is similar to the previous one in so far as it is for Stomach-Fire injuring Yin. It differs from it in so far as it does not cool Blood. They both stop bleeding albeit in different ways. Yu Nu Jian stops bleeding simply by clearing Fire; Niu Xi *Radix Achyranthis bidentatae seu Cyathulae* is added to subdue rebellious Qi and, in the case of bleeding upwards such as in bleeding gums and vomiting of blood, to conduct Blood downwards. Qing Wei San stops bleeding by cooling Blood.

The differentiation between the three above formulae can be tabulated as shown in Table 14.2.

(a) Patent remedy

HUANG LIAN SU PIAN
Coptis Extract Tablet
Huang Lian *Rhizoma Coptidis*

Table 14.2   Comparison of Xie Xin Tang, Qing Wei San and Yu Nu Jian

	Xie Xin Tang	Qing Wei San	Yu Nu Jian
Bleeding Symptoms	Vomiting of blood, bleeding gums Severe irritability, feeling of heat, constipation, thirst with desire to drink cold water	Vomiting of blood, bleeding gums Irritability, thirst, toothache and headache, worse at night	Vomiting of blood, bleeding gums Irritability, toothache, headache
Signs	Red face and eyes, tongue ulcers	Malar flush	Malar flush
Tongue	Dry-yellow coating, Red body	Dark-Red body, no coating in the centre	Red body, no coating in the centre, dry-yellow elsewhere
Stomach pulse	Rapid and Overflowing	Rapid, Full in the middle level	Rapid, Floating-Empty in Stomach position

Explanation

This tablet, composed only of Huang Lian, drains Stomach-Fire and can treat epigastric pain which may be accompanied by either constipation or Damp-Heat diarrhoea. The tongue presentation appropriate to this remedy is a Red tongue body and a sticky-yellow coating.

(b) Patent remedy

JIA WEI XIANG LIAN PIAN
Supplemented Saussurea and Coptis Tablet
Mu Xiang *Radix Saussureae*
Bing Lang *Semen Arecae catechu*
Zhi Ke *Fructus Citri aurantii*
Hou Po *Cortex Magnoliae officinalis*
Wu Zhu Yu *Fructus Evodiae rutaecarpae*
Huang Lian *Rhizoma Coptidis*
Huang Bo *Cortex Phellodendri*
Huang Qin *Radix Scutellariae baicalensis*
Yan Hu Suo *Rhizoma Corydalis yanhusuo*
Bai Shao *Radix Paeoniae albae*
Dang Gui *Radix Angelicae sinensis*
Gan Cao *Radix Glycyrrhizae uralensis*

Explanation

This tablet specifically clears Stomach-Heat deriving from stagnation of Qi. Stagnant Qi over a long period of time easily turns into Heat: the correct treatment principle in this case is not to drain Fire, but to clear Heat with bitter herbs (such as Huang Lian, Huang Qin and Huang Bo here) and open and move Qi with pungent herbs (such as Wu Zhu Yu and Mu Xiang).

The main manifestation of such pattern would be a burning epigastric pain with distension, a tongue with Red sides and a yellow coating.

(c) Patent remedy

SAI MEI AN
Race [between] Rot and Peaceful [Health]

Explanation

This remedy, already explained above under "Stomach-Heat", is also suitable for epigastric pain from Stomach-Fire.

DIETARY ADVICE

Same as for Stomach-Heat.

6. STOMACH PHLEGM-FIRE

CLINICAL MANIFESTATIONS

Any of the symptoms and signs of Stomach-Fire can occur in Stomach Phlegm-Fire as well. In addition, there may be the following clinical manifestations: a feeling of oppression of the epigastrium, dry mouth but no desire to drink, mucus in the stools, nausea, vomiting, mental restlessness, in severe cases manic behaviour or manic-depression and insomnia.
Tongue: Red with a very sticky or slippery yellow coating. The tongue may have a wide Stomach-type crack in the centre with a rough, brush-like, dry yellow coating inside it (see Fig. 12.4 in ch. 12).
Pulse: Slippery, Rapid, Overflowing.

All the above symptoms and signs are due to Phlegm. A feeling of oppression in the chest is typical of Phlegm. The mouth feels dry because of the Fire, but there is no desire to drink because of the Phlegm. Since the Stomach is functionally related to the Large Intestine (Bright Yang), there may be mucus in the stools. Nausea or vomiting are due to Phlegm impairing the descending of Stomach-Qi. The tongue-crack illustrated above is typical of Stomach Phlegm-Fire and it almost invariably indicates that the Mind is affected by Phlegm-Fire resulting in manic-depression.

TREATMENT PRINCIPLE

Harmonize the Stomach, clear Fire, resolve Phlegm, calm the Mind.

ACUPUNCTURE

ST-21 Liangmen, Ren-12 Zhongwan, Ren-13 Shangwan, P-5 Jianshi, ST-40 Fenglong, P-7 Daling, Du-24 Shenting, G.B.-13 Benshen, ST-44 Neiting. All with reducing method, except for Ren-12 which should be reinforced.

Explanation

– **ST-21** is used for Stomach Excess patterns.
– **Ren-12** tonifies Stomach and Spleen to resolve Phlegm.
– **Ren-13** subdues rebellious Stomach-Qi and is used if there is nausea or vomiting.
– **P-5** resolves Phlegm from the Stomach and the Mind.
– **ST-40** resolves Phlegm.
– **P-7** resolves Phlegm and calms the Mind.
– **Du-24** and **G.B.-13** calm the Mind.
– **ST-44** clears Stomach-Fire.

HERBAL TREATMENT

Prescription

WEN DAN TANG
Warming the Gall-Bladder Decoction
Ban Xia *Rhizoma Pinelliae ternatae* 6 g
Fu Ling *Sclerotium Poriae cocos* 5 g

Chen Pi *Pericarpium Citri reticulatae* 9 g
Zhu Ru *Caulis Bambusae in Taeniis* 6 g
Zhi Shi *Fructus Citri aurantii immaturus* 6 g
Zhi Gan Cao *Radix Glycyrrhizae uralensis praeparata* 3 g
Sheng Jiang *Rhizoma Zingiberis officinalis recens* 5 slices
Da Zao *Fructus Ziziphi jujubae* one date

Explanation

– **Ban Xia**, emperor herb, resolves Phlegm, harmonizes the Stomach and stops nausea and vomiting.
– **Zhu Ru**, minister herb, clears Fire, resolves Phlegm, stops nausea and vomiting and calms the mind.
– **Zhi Shi**, assistant herb, moves Qi which helps to resolve Phlegm and makes Stomach-Qi descend.
– **Chen Pi** and **Fu Ling**, also assistant herbs, dry Dampness which helps to resolve Phlegm and harmonize the Stomach.
– **Sheng Jiang**, **Da Zao** and **Gan Cao**, messenger herbs, harmonize the Stomach and attune the decoction.

(a) Patent remedy

HUANG LIAN SU PIAN
Coptis Extract Tablet
Huang Lian *Rhizoma Coptidis*

Explanation

This tablet, already explained above, can be used for epigastric pain from Phlegm-Fire in the Stomach.

(b) Patent remedy

SAI MEI AN
Race [between] Rot and Peaceful [Health]

Explanation

This remedy, already explained under "Stomach-Heat", is also suitable to treat epigastric pain from Phlegm-Fire.

DIETARY ADVICE

The patient should avoid eating too many fried foods, and also avoid hot-energy foods as described for Stomach-Heat.

7. DAMP-HEAT IN THE STOMACH

CLINICAL MANIFESTATIONS

Feeling of oppression of the chest, dull epigastric pain, dry mouth, no desire to drink, a bitter taste, a sticky taste, nausea, vomiting. There may also be a frontal headache.
Tongue: Red with a sticky-yellow coating.
Pulse: Slippery, Rapid, slightly Weak-Floating in the right Middle position.

This is usually accompanied by Damp-Heat in the Spleen as well. It often derives from deficiency of Spleen-Qi being unable to transform fluids.

TREATMENT PRINCIPLE

Clear Heat, resolve Dampness, harmonize the Stomach.

ACUPUNCTURE

Ren-10 Xiawan, Ren-9 Shuifen, ST-21 Liangmen, SP-9 Yinlingquan, SP-6 Sanyinjiao, BL-20 Pishu, BL-21 Weishu, Ren-12 Zhongwan, ST-8 Touwei, L.I.-4 Hegu. All with reducing or even method except Ren-12 and BL-20 which should be reinforced.

Explanation

- **Ren-10**, **Ren-9** and **ST-21** promote the transformation of fluids and stimulate the descending of Stomach-Qi.
- **SP-9**, **SP-6** and **BL-21** clear Damp-Heat from the Stomach.
- **Ren-12** and **BL-20** tonify the Spleen to resolve Dampness.

- **ST-8** and **L.I.-4** resolve Dampness from the head and are used in case of frontal headaches.

HERBAL TREATMENT

Prescription

XIANG SHA PING WEI SAN
Saussurea-Amomum Regulating the Stomach Powder
Cang Zhu *Rhizoma Atractylodis lanceae* 12 g
Hou Po *Cortex Magnoliae officinalis* 9 g
Chen Pi *Pericarpium Citri reticulatae* 9 g
Zhi Gan Cao *Radix Glycyrrhizae uralensis praeparata* 3 g
Mu Xiang *Radix Saussureae* 6 g
Sha Ren *Fructus seu Semen Amomi* 6 g

Explanation

The first four herbs form the prescription Ping Wei San *Balancing the Stomach Powder* which moves Qi in the Middle, dries Dampness, stimulates the Spleen and harmonizes the Stomach. Mu Xiang *Radix Saussureae* and Sha Ren *Fructus seu Semen Amomi* further move Qi and dry Dampness.

Variations

- If there are pronounced signs of Heat (bitter taste, dry mouth and a dark-yellow tongue coating) add Huang Lian *Rhizoma Coptidis*.
- If there are pronounced signs of Dampness such as a very sticky tongue coating and a sticky taste add Huo Xiang *Herba Agastachis* and Pei Lan *Herba Eupatorii fortunei*.

(a) Patent remedy

SHEN QU CHA
Massa Fermentata Tea
Shen Qu *Massa Fermentata Medicinalis*
Fu Ling *Sclerotium Poriae cocos*
Huang Qin *Radix Scutellariae baicalensis*
Qiang Huo *Radix et Rhizoma Notopterygii*
Du Huo *Radix Angelicae pubescentis*
Mu Gua *Fructus Chaenomelis lagenariae*

Shan Yao *Radix Dioscoreae oppositae*
Jie Geng *Radix Platycodi grandiflori*
Qing Hao *Herba Artemisiae apiaceae*
Xiang Ru *Herba Elsholtziae splendentis*
Qing Pi *Pericarpium Citri reticulatae viridae*
Hu Po *Succinum*
Cao Guo *Fructus Amomi Tsaoko*
Gan Cao *Radix Glycyrrhizae uralensis*

Explanation

This tea resolves Dampness, clears Heat and moves Qi. It is therefore used for epigastric pain from Damp-Heat and some stagnation of Qi.

The main manifestations addressed by this tea would therefore be a feeling of heaviness and fullness of the epigastrium, nausea, a Slippery pulse and a sticky-yellow tongue coating.

(b) Patent remedy

KANG NING WAN
Health and Quiet Pill

Explanation

This pill, already explained above under "Cold invading the Stomach", is suitable also to treat Damp-Heat in the Stomach, although its main emphasis is on resolving Dampness rather than clearing Heat.

DIETARY ADVICE

The patient should avoid eating too many fried foods, bananas and peanuts.

8. STOMACH AND LIVER HEAT

CLINICAL MANIFESTATIONS

Burning epigastric pain, irritability, propensity to outbursts of anger, sour regurgitation, dry mouth, thirst, bitter taste.
Tongue: Red, redder on the sides, yellow coating.
Pulse: Wiry and Rapid.

This condition is due to stagnant Liver-Qi turning into Fire after a long time and Fire invading the Stomach. The manifestations that point to Liver-Heat are propensity to anger, bitter taste and Red sides of the tongue.

This pattern is due to long-standing emotional problems, of the same type that lead to stagnation of Liver-Qi.

TREATMENT PRINCIPLE

Soothe the Liver, clear Heat, harmonize the Stomach.

Acupuncture

LIV-14 Qimen, ST-21 Liangmen, G.B.-34 Yanglingquan, LIV-2 Xingjian, ST-44 Neiting, Du-24 Shenting, G.B.-13 Benshen. Reducing or even method.

Explanation

- **LIV-14** harmonizes Stomach and Liver and moves Liver-Qi.
- **ST-21** clears Stomach-Heat.
- **G.B.-34** moves Liver-Qi. It is necessary to do this as, in this case, Liver-Fire derives from long-term stagnation of Liver-Qi.
- **LIV-2** clears Liver-Fire.
- **ST-44** clears Stomach-Heat.
- **Du-24** and **G.B.-13** calm the Mind.

HERBAL TREATMENT

Prescription

HUA GAN JIAN and ZUO JIN WAN
Transforming the Liver Decoction (Variation) and *Left Metal Pill*
Chen Pi *Pericarpium Citri reticulatae* 6 g
Qing Pi *Pericarpium Citri reticulatae viridae* 4 g
Bai Shao *Radix Paeoniae albae* 9 g
Mu Dan Pi *Cortex Moutan radicis* 6 g
Shan Zhi Zi *Fructus Gardeniae jasminoidis* 6 g
Huang Lian *Rhizoma Coptidis* 6 g
Wu Zhu Yu *Fructus Evodiae rutaecarpae* 1.5 g

Explanation

- **Chen Pi** and **Qing Pi** move Qi and eliminate stagnation of Liver-Qi.
- **Bai Shao** soothes the Liver and stops pain.
- **Mu Dan Pi** and **Shan Zhi Zi** clear Liver-Fire.
- **Huang Lian**, bitter and cold, clears Stomach-Fire.
- **Wu Zhu Yu**, a pungent herb, eliminates stagnation and subdues rebellious Qi.

Variations

- If Heat is beginning to injure Yin add Fu Shou *Fructus Citri sarcodactylis* and Mei Gui Hua *Flos Rosae rugosae* which move Qi without injuring Yin, as most other moving-Qi herbs do.
- If the epigastric pain is very severe add Yan Hu Suo *Rhizoma Corydalis yanhusuo*.

DIETARY ADVICE

The patient should avoid eating too many fried foods as well as drinking too much alcohol, and in terms of eating conditions, avoid getting angry and worrying while eating.

It is also best to avoid eating too many sour foods, which include yoghurt, vinegar, cooking apples, pickles, oranges, grapefruit and gooseberries.

9. STASIS OF BLOOD IN THE STOMACH

CLINICAL MANIFESTATIONS

Stabbing epigastric pain which is worse with pressure and after eating, palpable masses in the epigastrium, vomiting of dark blood sometimes looking like coffee-grounds, dark complexion. The pain may be worse at night. There may be blood in the stools.
Tongue: Purple, possibly only in the centre.
Pulse: Choppy or Wiry or Firm.

This can only be a very chronic condition which takes a long time to develop. Stasis of Blood usually derives from stagnation of Qi over a long period of time. Stasis of Blood in the Stomach is often associated with stasis of Liver-Blood. It may also be the result of other Stomach patterns, principally Stomach-Fire or Retention of Food in the Stomach. A stabbing type of pain is typical of stasis of Blood and so is its possible aggravation at night. Because this is an Excess condition, the pain is worse with pressure and after eating. Because the Stomach is related to the Large Intestine (Bright Yang), the stasis of Blood may extend to the latter organ and cause blood in the stools. This blood would be dark, reflecting stasis of Blood. The purple colour of the tongue body indicates stasis of Blood; it may be Purple only in the centre.

Since this is a very chronic condition, it is inevitably accompanied by other patterns such as stasis of Liver-Blood, stagnation of Liver-Qi, retention of Cold (patterns of the Excess type) or deficiency of Qi or Yin (patterns of the Deficiency type).

Carcinoma of the stomach often manifests itself with this pattern.

TREATMENT PRINCIPLE

Move Blood, eliminate stasis, harmonize the Stomach, stop pain.

ACUPUNCTURE

Ren-10 Xiawan, ST-22 Guanmen, ST-34 Liangqiu, SP-10 Xuehai, BL-17 Geshu, SP-4 Gongsun, P-6 Neiguan, BL-18 Ganshu. Reducing or even method.

Explanation

- **Ren-10** stimulates the descending of Stomach-Qi.
- **ST-22** restores the descending of Stomach-Qi and dissolves accumulations in the epigastrium.
- **ST-34**, Accumulation point, stops pain and moves Qi and Blood.
- **SP-10** and **BL-17** move Blood and eliminate stasis.

– **SP-4** and **P-6** in combination open the Penetrating vessel and remove obstructions from the epigastrium. The Penetrating vessel is also called the "Sea of Blood" because it controls all the Blood Connecting channels. Its opening points can therefore also be used to move Blood and eliminate stasis.
– **BL-18** is used if there is stasis of Liver-Blood.

HERBAL TREATMENT

The formula used depends on whether the condition is primarily of the Excess or Deficiency type. Four prescriptions will be discussed, the first three for Excess conditions and the fourth for Deficiency ones.

(a) Prescription

SHI XIAO SAN
Breaking into a Smile Powder
Pu Huang *Pollen Typhae* 6 g
Wu Ling Zhi *Excrementum Trogopteri* 6 g

Explanation

This is a basic formula for stasis of Blood which can be adapted to reach any of the internal organs. It moves Blood, eliminates stasis and stops bleeding.

(b) Prescription

DAN SHEN YIN
Salvia Decoction
Dan Shen *Radix Salviae miltiorrhizae* 30 g
Tan Xiang *Lignum Santali albi* 5 g
Sha Ren *Fructus seu Semen Amomi* 5 g

Explanation

Although this formula is primarily for stasis of Blood in the chest, it can be adapted to treat stasis of Blood of the Stomach.

(c) Prescription

HUO LUO XIAO LING DAN

Miraculously Effective Invigorating the Connecting Channels Pill
Dang Gui *Radix Angelicae sinensis* 15 g
Dan Shen *Radix Salviae miltiorrhizae* 15 g
Ru Xiang *Gummi Olibanum* 15 g
Mo Yao *Myrrha* 15 g

Explanation

This is another general formula for stasis of Blood in various organs and also in the limbs (such as from sport injuries). Again, it would need to be adapted to Stomach conditions.

Variations

The following are variations which apply to all the above prescriptions.

– Some digestive herbs should be added to all the above prescriptions because some of the moving-Blood herbs (such as Mo Yao *Myrrha*, Ru Xiang *Gummi Olibanum* and Wu Ling Zhi *Excrementum Trogopteri*) are hard to digest. Digestive herbs include Mai Ya *Fructus Hordei vulgaris germinatus*, Gu Ya *Fructus Oryzae sativae germinatus*, Shan Zha *Fructus Crataegi* or Ji Nei Jin *Endothelium Corneum Gigeraiae Galli*. In particular, charred Shan Zha *Fructus Crataegi* is good to stop bleeding from the alimentary tract.
– In case of severe pain add Yan Hu Suo *Rhizoma Corydalis yanhusuo*.
– In case of stagnation of Qi add Zhi Ke *Fructus Citri aurantii*, Qing Pi *Pericarpium Citri reticulatae viridae* and Mu Xiang *Radix Saussureae*.
– If there is retention of Cold in the Stomach add Gui Zhi *Ramulus Cinnamomi cassiae* and either Gan Jiang *Rhizoma Zingiberis officinalis* or Gao Liang Jiang *Rhizoma Alpiniae officinari*.
– If there is bleeding from the alimentary tract (either vomiting of blood or blood in the stools) add San Qi *Radix Notoginseng*. In particular, if there is vomiting of blood add Niu Xi *Radix Achyranthis bidentatae seu Cyathulae* to attract Blood downwards.
– If there is vomiting of blood, acidity and sour regurgitation add Bai Ji *Rhizoma Bletillae*

striatae and Wu Zei Gu *Os Sepiae*. These two herbs reduce secretions of stomach-acids and protect the stomach mucosa in case of ulcers.

(d) Prescription

TIAO YING LIAN GAN YIN
Regulating Nutritive Qi and Restraining the Liver Decoction
Dang Gui *Radix Angelicae sinensis* 6 g
Chuan Xiong *Rhizoma Ligustici wallichii* 6 g
E Jiao *Gelatinum Asini* 6 g
Bai Shao *Radix Paeoniae albae* 9 g
Gou Qi Zi *Fructus Lycii chinensis* 6 g
Wu Wei Zi *Fructus Schisandrae chinensis* 3 g
Suan Zao Ren *Semen Ziziphi spinosae* 3 g
Fu Ling *Sclerotium Poriae cocos* 6 g
Chen Pi *Pericarpium Citri reticulatae* 4 g
Mu Xiang *Radix Saussureae* 3 g
Sheng Jiang *Rhizoma Zingiberis officinalis recens* 3 slices
Da Zao *Fructus Ziziphi jujubae* 3 dates

Explanation

- **Dang Gui**, **Chuan Xiong** and **E Jiao** nourish and move Blood.
- **Bai Shao**, **Gou Qi Zi**, **Wu Wei Zi** and **Suan Zao Ren** pacify the Liver and therefore regulate Liver-Blood. Bai Shao also stops pain.
- **Fu Ling** and **Chen Pi** counteract the "stickiness" of some of the above herbs.
- **Mu Xiang** moves Qi in order to move Blood.
- **Sheng Jiang** and **Da Zao** harmonize.

Variations

- If there is vomiting of blood or blood in the stools add Bai Ji *Rhizoma Bletillae striatae* and Xian He Cao *Herba Agrimoniae pilosae*.
- If the stasis of Blood derives from Cold on a background of Spleen-Yang deficiency (manifesting with cold limbs, a Pale tongue, tiredness and a Weak pulse) add the formula Li Zhong Wan *Regulating the Centre Decoction*.
- If the stasis of Blood occurs on a background of Yin deficiency, which is quite common in old people, add Sha Shen *Radix Glehniae*

littoralis, Sheng Di Huang *Radix Rehmanniae glutinosae*, Mai Men Dong *Tuber Ophiopogonis japonici*, Mu Dan Pi *Cortex Moutan radicis* and E Jiao *Gelatinum Asini* to nourish Yin, cool Blood and stop bleeding.
- If there has been loss of blood for a long time resulting in Heart-Blood deficiency manifesting with insomnia, palpitations, pale complexion and Pale tongue, add Gui Pi Tang *Tonifying the Spleen Decoction*.

(i) Patent remedy

YAN HU SUO ZHI TONG PIAN
Corydalis Stopping Pain Tablet
Yan Hu Suo *Rhizoma Corydalis yanhusuo*

Explanation

This tablet, composed of only Yan Hu Suo, moves Qi and Blood in the Stomach and stops pain.

(ii) Patent remedy

WU JIN WAN
Black Gold Pill
Yi Mu Cao *Herba Leonori heterophylli*
San Leng *Rhizoma Sparganii*
E Zhu *Rhizoma Curcumae zedoariae*
Xiang Fu *Rhizoma Cyperi rotundi*
Yan Hu Suo *Rhizoma Corydalis yanhusuo*
Wu Zhu Yu *Fructus Evodiae rutaecarpae*
Xiao Hui Xiang *Fructus Foeniculi vulgaris*
Mu Xiang *Radix Saussureae*
Bai Shao *Radix Paeoniae albae*
Chuan Xiong *Radix Ligustici wallichii*
Dang Gui *Radix Angelicae sinensis*
Shu Di Huang *Radix Rehmanniae glutinosae praeparata*
Bu Gu Zhi *Fructus Psoraleae corylifoliae*
Pu Huang *Pollen Typhae*
Ai Ye Tan *Folium Artemisiae carbonisatum*

Explanation

This moves Qi and Blood, stops pain and arrests bleeding. It is suitable to treat epigastric pain from Blood stasis with blood in the stools.

The tongue presentation appropriate to this remedy is a Reddish-Purple body.

Case history

A 45-year-old woman had been suffering from epigastric pain for 33 years. She had had a duodenal ulcer when she was 12. The pain was stabbing in character and radiated from the epigastrium to the right hypochondrial region. It was worse at night, was accompanied by nausea and was aggravated by emotional stress; she had had a lot of such stress recently, being in the process of a bitter divorce. Her periods were irregular, painful and the blood was very dark with clots. She often felt very tired. Her pulse was Wiry and Full and her tongue was Reddish-Purple, with a Spleen-type of swelling on the sides and a yellow coating.

Diagnosis
This is a clear condition of stasis of Blood affecting Liver and Stomach. This is apparent from the stabbing character of the pain, its aggravation at night, the painful periods with dark-clotted blood, the Wiry pulse and the Reddish-Purple tongue. Stasis of Liver-Blood implies stagnation of Liver-Qi: this was apparent from the nausea and the aggravation of the pain with emotional stress. Obviously, due to the very long duration of the problem, there was also some Spleen-Qi deficiency as evidenced by the swelling on the sides of the tongue and the tiredness.

Treatment principle
The treatment principle adopted was to move Liver-Qi and Liver-Blood, calm the Mind, settle the Ethereal Soul and tonify the Spleen. She was treated with acupuncture and herbs.

Acupuncture
The acupuncture points used were selected from the following:

– **Ren-12** Zhongwan, **ST-36** Zusanli and **SP-6** Sanyinjiao, with reinforcing method, to tonify Spleen-Qi. SP-6 also moves Blood and calms the Mind.
– **LIV-14** Qimen and **G.B.-34** Yanglingquan, with even method, to move Liver-Qi.
– **P-6** Neiguan, with even method, to move Liver-Qi, move Blood, subdue rebellious Stomach-Qi, harmonize the Upper and Middle Burners, calm the Mind and settle the Ethereal Soul.
– **SP-10** Xuehai and **BL-17** Geshu, with even method, to move Blood.

Herbal treatment
The decoction used was a variation of Tiao Ying Lian Gan Yin *Regulating Nutritive Qi and Restraining the Liver Decoction*:

Dang Gui *Radix Angelicae sinensis* 6 g
Chuan Xiong *Radix Ligustici wallichii* 4 g
Bai Shao *Radix Paeoniae albae* 9 g
Gou Qi Zi *Fructus Lycii chinensis* 6 g
Wu Wei Zi *Fructus Schisandrae chinensis* 3 g
Suan Zao Ren *Semen Ziziphi spinosae* 6 g
Fu Ling *Sclerotium Poriae cocos* 6 g
Chen Pi *Pericarpium Citri reticulatae* 4 g
Mu Xiang *Radix Saussureae* 3 g
Sheng Jiang *Rhizoma Zingiberis officinalis recens* 3 slices
Da Zao *Fructus Ziziphi jujubae* 3 dates
Dan Shen *Radix Salviae miltiorrhizae* 6 g
Yan Hu Suo *Rhizoma Corydalis yanhusuo* 6 g
He Huan Pi *Cortex Albizziae julibrissin* 6 g
Dang Shen *Radix Codonopsis pilosulae* 6 g

Explanation
– The first eleven herbs constitute the Tiao Ying Lian Gan Tang to harmonize the Liver and move Liver-Blood. E Jiao was removed as there was no deficiency of Blood.
– **Dan Shen** was added to help to move Blood and calm the Mind.
– **Yan Hu Suo** was added to move Blood in the Middle Burner and stop pain.
– **He Huan Pi** was added to move Liver-Qi, calm the Mind and settle the Ethereal Soul. It is very good for emotional problems related to Liver disharmonies.
– **Dang Shen** was added to tonify the Spleen.

This patient, also with the help of counselling, is gradually improving and is still being treated.

DIETARY ADVICE

The patient should be advised to avoid eating late at night and eating too fast.

10. PHLEGM-FLUIDS IN THE STOMACH

CLINICAL MANIFESTATIONS

Epigastric fullness and distension, nausea, vomiting of watery and frothy fluids, dry tongue and mouth without desire to drink, splashing sound in the stomach, feeling of fullness of the chest, loose stools, loss of weight, lethargy, dizziness, dull frontal headache.
Tongue: Swollen with a sticky coating.
Pulse: Deep-Slippery or Wiry-Fine.

Phlegm-Fluids are a form of Phlegm, seen only in very chronic conditions and usually in old people. They are characterized by expectoration (or vomiting as in this case) of white, watery and frothy fluids. The splashing sound in the epigastrium on movement is also characteristic of Phlegm-Fluids. All other symptoms and signs in this condition reflect Phlegm. The dry mouth is due to the accumulation of fluids into Phlegm-Fluids so that the normal fluids do not reach the mouth. The loss of weight, not normally associated with Phlegm conditions, is due to the chronic dysfunction of Stomach and Spleen.

TREATMENT PRINCIPLE

Resolve Phlegm, harmonize the Stomach, tonify the Spleen.

ACUPUNCTURE

Ren-10 Xiawan, Ren-12 Zhongwan, Ren-9 Shuifen, ST-36 Zusanli, ST-40 Fenglong, BL-20 Pishu, BL-21 Weishu. Even method, except for Ren-12, ST-36 and BL-20 which should be reinforced to tonify the Spleen.

Explanation

- **Ren-10** stimulates Stomach-Qi to descend.
- **Ren-9** promotes the transformation of fluids to resolve Phlegm.
- **Ren-12**, **ST-36** and **BL-20** tonify the Spleen.
- **ST-40** resolves Phlegm.
- **BL-21** regulates the Stomach.

HERBAL TREATMENT

Prescription

LING GUI ZHU GAN TANG
Poria-Ramulus Cinnamomi-Atractylodes-Glycyrrhiza Decoction
Fu Ling *Sclerotium Poriae cocos* 12 g
Gui Zhi *Ramulus Cinnamomi cassiae* 9 g
Bai Zhu *Rhizoma Atractylodis macrocephalae* 6 g
Zhi Gan Cao *Radix Glycyrrhizae uralensis praeparata* 3 g

Explanation

- **Fu Ling** resolves Phlegm by strengthening the Spleen and draining Dampness.
- **Gui Zhi** helps to transform fluids by warming the Yang.
- **Bai Zhu** strengthens the Spleen and drains Dampness.
- **Zhi Gan Cao** strengthens the Spleen and harmonizes.

This formula resolves Phlegm-Fluids in the epigastrium and should be opportunely modified to deal with epigastric pain.

Variations

- For fullness and pain of the epigastrium add Zhi Ke *Fructus Citri aurantii* and Hou Po *Cortex Magnoliae officinalis*.
- In case of vomiting add Ban Xia *Rhizoma Pinelliae ternatae*.

DIETARY ADVICE

The patient should avoid eating too much cold-energy foods and especially drinking iced drinks.

DEFICIENCY

1. STOMACH AND SPLEEN DEFICIENT AND COLD

CLINICAL MANIFESTATIONS

Dull epigastric pain which improves with pressure, after eating, and with the application of heat, vomiting of thin fluids, tiredness, poor appetite, chilliness, loose stools, pale complexion.
Tongue: Pale, white coating.
Pulse: Deep, Weak.

Some of the above manifestations reflect Spleen-Qi deficiency (tiredness, poor appetite and loose stools), whilst others indicate Stomach-Qi deficiency (dull epigastric pain). In this case, Yang-Qi is also deficient, resulting in feeling cold and cold limbs.

TREATMENT PRINCIPLE

Warm the Middle, strengthen the Spleen and Stomach.

ACUPUNCTURE

Ren-12 Zhongwan, P-6 Neiguan, ST-36 Zusanli, Ren-6 Qihai, BL-20 Pishu, BL-21 Weishu. All with reinforcing method, moxa is applicable.

Explanation

- **Ren-12**, **ST-36**, **BL-20** and **BL-21** tonify Spleen and Stomach. Moxa should be applied on the needle on ST-36. The moxa-box applied on the epigastrium is particularly effective to warm the Middle and stop epigastric pain.
- **P-6** stops nausea and pain.
- **Ren-6** with moxa warms the Yang and should be used if there are loose stools.

HERBAL TREATMENT

Prescription

HUANG QI JIAN ZHONG TANG
Astragalus Strengthening the Centre Decoction
Huang Qi *Radix Astragali membranacei* 9 g
Bai Shao *Radix Paeoniae albae* 18 g
Gui Zhi *Ramulus Cinnamomi cassiae* 9 g
Zhi Gan Cao *Radix Glycyrrhizae uralensis praeparata* 6 g
Sheng Jiang *Rhizoma Zingiberis officinalis recens* 10 g
Da Zao *Fructus Ziziphi jujubae* 12 dates
Yi Tang *Saccharum granorum* 30 g

Explanation

This formula is a variation of Xiao Jian Zhong Tang *Minor Strengthening the Centre Decoction*, in itself a variation of Gui Zhi Tang *Ramulus Cinnamomi Decoction*, with the addition of Yi Tang and the doubling of Bai Shao's dosage. Xiao Jian Zhong Tang *Minor Strengthening the Centre Decoction* warms the Middle, scatters Cold and stops pain. In it, Yi Tang *Saccharum*

granorum strengthens the Stomach and Spleen, Bai Shao *Radix Paeoniae albae* stops pain and Gui Zhi *Ramulus Cinnamomi cassiae* warms the Middle and scatters Cold. Sheng Jiang *Rhizoma Zingiberis officinalis recens* and Da Zao *Fructus Ziziphi jujubae* warm the Middle and pacify the Stomach. The addition of Huang Qi *Radix Astragali membranacei* reinforces this formula's action in strengthening the Spleen.

Variations

- If there is sour regurgitation add Wu Zhu Yu *Fructus Evodiae rutaecarpae* and Wu Zei Gu *Os Sepiae* and remove or reduce Yi Tang *Saccharum granorum*.
- In case of vomiting of thin fluids add Gan Jiang *Rhizoma Zingiberis officinalis*, Chen Pi *Pericarpium Citri reticulatae*, Ban Xia *Rhizoma Pinelliae ternatae* and Fu Ling *Sclerotium Poriae cocos* to warm the Stomach and resolve fluids.
- If there are pronounced symptoms of Cold such as vomiting of fluids, very cold limbs and very Pale tongue add the formula Da Jian Zhong Tang *Major Strengthening the Centre Decoction* which contains Chuan Jiao *Fructus Zanthoxyli bungeani*, Gan Jiang *Rhizoma Zingiberis officinalis*, Ren Shen *Radix Ginseng* and Yi Tang *Saccharum granorum*. This formula strongly warms the Middle, tonifies Stomach and Spleen, subdues rebellious Qi and stops pain. It is used for severe Stomach and Spleen Yang deficiency with accumulation of Cold and fluids in the stomach causing epigastric pain. Instead of this formula, either Li Zhong Wan *Regulating the Centre Pill* or Liang Fu Wan *Alpinia-Cyperus Pill* can be used.
- If there are confusing signs of both Cold and Heat, such as Cold in the Stomach (vomiting of thin fluids, white coating in the centre) and Heat in the Intestines (borborygmi and yellow coating on the root), use Gan Cao Xie Xin Tang *Glycyrrhiza Draining the Heart Decoction* which includes the following:

Ban Xia *Rhizoma Pinelliae ternatae* 9 g
Gan Jiang *Rhizoma Zingiberis officinalis* 6 g

Huang Qin *Radix Scutellariae baicalensis* 6 g
Huang Lian *Rhizoma Coptidis* 3 g
Zhi Gan Cao *Radix Glycyrrhizae uralensis praeparata* 12 g
Da Zao *Fructus Ziziphi jujubae* 4 dates

This formula benefits Qi, harmonizes the Stomach, relieves fullness and stops vomiting. Although it is called *"Draining the Heart Decoction"*, "Heart" here stands for the area under the heart, i.e. the epigastrium.

(a) Patent remedy

LIU JUN ZI PIAN
Six Gentlemen Tablet
Dang Shen *Radix Codonopsis pilosulae*
Bai Zhu *Rhizoma Atractylodis macrocephalae*
Fu Ling *Sclerotium Poriae cocos*
Zhi Gan Cao *Radix Glycyrrhizae uralensis praeparata*
Chen Pi *Pericarpium Citri reticulatae*
Ban Xia *Rhizoma Pinelliae ternatae*

Explanation

This very well-known tablet tonifies Stomach- and Spleen-Qi and resolves Dampness.

The tongue presentation appropriate to this remedy would be a slightly Pale tongue body and a thin, slightly sticky coating. The emphasis of this tablet is on tonifying Qi rather than resolving Dampness.

(b) Patent remedy

REN SHEN JIAN PI WAN
Ginseng Strengthening the Spleen Pill
Ren Shen *Radix Ginseng*
Bai Zhu *Rhizoma Atractylodis macrocephalae*
Zhi Shi *Fructus Citri aurantii immaturus*
Shan Zha *Fructus Crataegi*
Chen Pi *Pericarpium Citri reticulatae*
Mai Ya *Fructus Hordei vulgaris germinatus*

Explanation

This pill tonifies Spleen- and Stomach-Qi, moves Qi and resolves retention of food.

The tongue presentation appropriate to this remedy is a thick-sticky-white tongue coating and a Pale tongue body.

(c) Patent remedy

XIANG SHA LIU JUN ZI PIAN
Saussurea-Amomum Six Gentlemen Pill
Dang Shen *Radix Codonopsis pilosulae*
Bai Zhu *Rhizoma Atractylodis macrocephalae*
Fu Ling *Sclerotium Poriae cocos*
Zhi Gan Cao *Radix Glycyrrhizae uralensis praeparata*
Chen Pi *Pericarpium Citri reticulatae*
Ban Xia *Rhizoma Pinelliae ternatae*
Mu Xiang *Radix Saussureae*
Sha Ren *Fructus seu Semen Amomi*

Explanation

This pill tonifies Spleen- and Stomach-Qi, resolves Dampness and moves Qi. It is used when the epigastric pain is slightly more severe than in the patterns addressed by the previous two remedies.

(d) Patent remedy

XIANG SHA YANG WEI PIAN (I)
Saussurea-Amomum Nourishing the Stomach Tablet
Dang Shen *Radix Codonopsis pilosulae*
Bai Zhu *Rhizoma Atractylodis macrocephalae*
Zhi Gan Cao *Radix Glycyrrhizae uralensis praeparata*
Chen Pi *Pericarpium Citri reticulatae*
Mu Xiang *Radix Saussureae*
Sha Ren *Fructus seu Semen Amomi*
Mai Ya *Fructus Hordei vulgaris germinatus*
Shen Qu *Massa Fermentata Medicinalis*
Bai Dou Kou *Fructus Amomi cardamomi*

XIANG SHA YANG WEI PIAN (II)
Bai Zhu *Rhizoma Atractylodis macrocephalae*
Zhi Gan Cao *Radix Glycyrrhizae uralensis praeparata*
Chen Pi *Pericarpium Citri reticulatae*
Mu Xiang *Radix Saussureae*
Sha Ren *Fructus seu Semen Amomi*
Bai Dou Kou *Fructus Amomi cardamomi*
Fu Ling *Sclerotium Poriae cocos*

Ban Xia *Rhizoma Pinelliae ternatae*
Huo Xiang *Herba Agastachis*
Xiang Fu *Rhizoma Cyperi rotundi*
Hou Po *Cortex Magnoliae officinalis*
Zhi Ke *Fructus Citri aurantii*

Explanation

These two similar remedies with two different names both tonify Stomach- and Spleen-Qi, resolve Dampness and relieve retention of food.

They differ from the previous remedies in so far as they have a stronger action in resolving Dampness and retention of food. The tongue presentation would be a thick-sticky tongue coating and a Pale body.

(e) Patent remedy

SHEN LING BAI ZHU WAN (PIAN)
Ginseng-Poria-Atractylodes Pill (Tablet)
Ren Shen *Radix Ginseng* (or Dang Shen *Radix Codonopsis pilosulae*)
Fu Ling *Sclerotium Poriae cocos*
Bai Zhu *Rhizoma Atractylodis macrocephalae*
Jie Geng *Radix Platycodi grandiflori*
Shan Yao *Radix Dioscoreae oppositae*
Chen Pi *Pericarpium Citri reticulatae*
Sha Ren *Fructus seu Semen Amomi*
Lian Zi *Semen Nelumbinis nuciferae*
Bian Dou *Semen Dolichoris lablab*
Yi Yi Ren *Semen Coicis lachryma jobi*
Zhi Gan Cao *Radix Glycyrrhizae uralensis praeparata*

Explanation

This well-known remedy tonifies Stomach- and Spleen-Qi, resolves Dampness and stops diarrhoea.

The tongue presentation for this remedy is a Pale body with a Stomach crack in the middle and possibly rootless coating.

Case history

A 47-year-old woman had been suffering from epigastric pain for a few months. The pain was dull and improved with pressure and application of a hot-water bottle. Her appetite was poor and she felt easily tired. She easily felt cold. Her tongue was very Pale,

slightly Swollen and with transversal cracks on one side (Plate 14.2). Her pulse was Weak and Deep.

Diagnosis
This is a clear condition of Spleen and Stomach deficiency with internal Cold. The transversal cracks on the side of the tongue indicate very long-standing Spleen deficiency.

Treatment principle
The treatment principle adopted was to strengthen Stomach and Spleen and warm the Centre.

Herbal treatment
She was treated only with herbs and the decoction used was a variation of Huang Qi Jian Zhong Tang *Astragalus Strengthening the Centre Decoction*:

Huang Qi *Radix Astragali membranacei* 9 g
Bai Shao *Radix Paeoniae albae* 18 g
Gui Zhi *Ramulus Cinnamomi cassiae* 6 g
Zhi Gan Cao *Radix Glycyrrhizae uralensis praeparata* 6 g
Sheng Jiang *Rhizoma Zingiberis officinalis recens* 5 slices
Da Zao *Fructus Ziziphi jujubae* 5 dates
Yi Tang *Saccharum granorum* 30 g
Gan Jiang *Rhizoma Zingiberis officinalis* 3 g

Explanation
The original formula was left almost unchanged except for the addition of Gan Jiang to strengthen its action of warming the Middle Burner.

Due to the short duration of her problem, this condition was cleared up in a few weeks.

DIETARY ADVICE

The patient should avoid eating too much cold-energy foods such as salads and fruit, although a small amount of such food eaten in conjunction with cooked food is acceptable.

He or she should also make sure to eat enough in terms of quantity and not adhere too rigidly to various diets or food prohibitions on account of intolerances.

2. STOMACH-YIN DEFICIENCY

CLINICAL MANIFESTATIONS

Dull epigastric pain, dry mouth, desire to sip liquids, dry throat, dry stools, slight nausea.
Tongue: normal colour, dry, no coating, scattered cracks or a central wide Stomach-type crack (Fig. 12.3).

Pulse: Floating-Empty in the right Middle position.

If, in addition to Stomach-Yin deficiency, there is some Empty-Heat, there may be the following manifestations: feeling of heat, night sweating, malar flush, mental restlessness. The tongue would be Red (it may be Red only in the centre) and the pulse would be Rapid.

The Stomach's activity of "rotting and ripening" food produces a normal tongue coating. A lack of coating always reflects a deficiency of Stomach-Yin. Since the Stomach is the origin of body fluids, a Stomach-Yin deficiency implies a lack of body fluids. This causes a dry mouth and throat, dry tongue and dry stools. When Stomach-Yin is deficient Stomach-Qi fails to descend and this causes a slight nausea but not usually vomiting.

TREATMENT PRINCIPLE

Nourish Yin, benefit the Stomach, stop pain.

ACUPUNCTURE

Ren-12 Zhongwan, ST-36 Zusanli, SP-6 Sanyinjiao. Reinforcing method.

Explanation

– **Ren-12**, **ST-36** and **SP-6** nourish Stomach-Yin.

HERBAL TREATMENT

(a) Prescription

YI GUAN JIAN and BAI SHAO GAN CAO TANG
One Linking Decoction and *Paeonia-Glycyrrhiza Decoction*
Bei Sha Shen *Radix Glehniae littoralis* 9 g
Mai Men Dong *Tuber Ophiopogonis japonici* 9 g
Sheng Di Huang *Radix Rehmanniae glutinosae* 12 g
Gou Qi Zi *Fructus Lycii chinensis* 9 g
Dang Gui *Radix Angelicae sinensis* 6 g

Chuan Lian Zi *Fructus Meliae toosendan* 4.5 g
Bai Shao *Radix Paeoniae Albae* 9 g
Zhi Gan Cao *Radix Glycyrrhizae uralensis praeparata* 6 g

Explanation

Although the formula Yi Guan Jian *One Linking Decoction* is primarily for Liver-Yin deficiency, it can also be used for Stomach-Yin deficiency.

– **Bei Sha Shen** and **Mai Men Dong** nourish Stomach-Yin.
– **Sheng Di Huang** and **Gou Qi Zi** nourish the Liver and Kidneys and promote Stomach fluids.
– **Dang Gui** moves Liver-Blood and stops pain.
– **Chuan Lian Zi** moves Liver-Qi and stops pain.
– **Bai Shao** and **Gan Cao** harmonize Nutritive and Defensive Qi and stop pain.

(b) Prescription

YI WEI TANG
Benefiting the Stomach Decoction
Bei Sha Shen *Radix Glehniae littoralis* 9 g
Mai Men Dong *Tuber Ophiopogonis japonici* 9 g
Sheng Di Huang *Radix Rehmanniae glutinosae* 12 g
Yu Zhu *Rhizoma Polygonati odorati* 6 g
Bing Tang *Brown sugar* 3 g

Explanation

– **Bei Sha Shen, Yu Zhu** and **Mai Men Dong** nourish Stomach-Yin.
– **Sheng Di Huang** nourishes Yin.
– **Bing Tang** tonifies the Middle.

(c) Prescription

YANG WEI TANG
Nourishing the Stomach Decoction
Bei Sha Shen *Radix Glehniae littoralis* 9 g
Mai Men Dong *Tuber Ophiopogonis japonici* 6 g
Yu Zhu *Rhizoma Polygonati odorati* 6 g
Bian Dou *Semen Dolichoris lablab* 6 g
Sang Ye *Folium Mori albae* 4 g

Shi Hu *Herba Dendrobii* 6 g
Zhi Gan Cao *Radix Glycyrrhizae uralensis praeparata* 3 g

Explanation

This formula differs from the previous one in so far as it clears Empty-Heat besides nourishing Yin. Thus the main sign indicating the use of this formula is a Red tongue without coating, either all over or only in the centre.

- **Bei Sha Shen**, **Mai Men Dong** and **Yu Zhu** nourish Stomach-Yin.
- **Bian Dou** nourishes Spleen-Yin.
- **Shi Hu** clears Stomach Empty-Heat.
- **Sang Ye** assists Shi Hu in clearing Heat.
- **Zhi Gan Cao** tonifies the Middle and harmonizes.

Variations

- In case of pronounced acid regurgitation and some Liver-Heat, add Zuo Jin Wan *Left Metal Pill* which contains only Huang Lian *Rhizoma Coptidis* 15 g and Wu Zhu Yu *Fructus Evodiae rutaecarpae* 2 g. This formula clears Stomach-Heat and subdues rebellious Qi.
- In case of severe pain add Mei Gui Hua *Flos Rosae rugosae* and Fu Shou *Fructus Citri sarcodactylis* which move Qi without damaging Yin.
- If there is constipation with dry stools add Huo Ma Ren *Semen Cannabis sativae* and honey.

Patent remedy

SHEN LING BAI ZHU WAN (PIAN)
Ginseng-Poria-Atractylodes Pill (Tablet)

Explanation

This remedy, mentioned above under "Stomach and Spleen Deficient and Cold", may also be used for deficiency of Stomach-Yin. In this case, the tongue would be without coating in the centre and possibly with a Stomach crack.

DIETARY ADVICE

The patient should avoid eating drying foods, i.e. baked or broiled foods (including bread). It is beneficial to eat warm and moist foods such as soups, porridge, etc.

Case history

A 37-year-old man had been suffering from epigastric pain for many years. The pain was rather dull but persistent and was accompanied by slight nausea. The pain was better for pressure. His mouth felt always dry but he liked to sip liquids. His lips and stools were also often dry.

His tongue was slightly Red, without enough coating and with very clear Stomach and Spleen cracks (Plate 14.3): the Stomach crack runs vertically in the midline, while the Spleen cracks are transversal on the edges. His pulse was Floating-Empty on the right Middle position.

Diagnosis
This is a very clear example of Stomach- and Spleen-Yin deficiency. The latter often accompanies the former and its symptoms are dry lips and stools (apart from the transversal cracks on the edges of the tongue). Besides Yin deficiency, there is also some Stomach Empty-Heat as the tongue is Red.

Treatment principle
The treatment principle followed was to nourish Stomach- and Spleen-Yin and clear Empty-Heat. This patient was treated with acupuncture and herbs.

Acupuncture
The points were selected from the following (all with reinforcing method except for ST-44 Neiting):

- **ST-36** Zusanli, **Ren-12** Zhongwan and **SP-6** Sanyinjiao to nourish Stomach-Yin.
- **Ren-11** Jianli and **ST-44** Neiting to clear Stomach Empty-Heat.

Herbal treatment
The herbal formula used was a variation of Yang Wei Tang *Nourishing the Stomach Decoction*:

Bei Sha Shen *Radix Glehniae littoralis* 6 g
Mai Men Dong *Tuber Ophiopogonis japonici* 6 g
Yu Zhu *Rhizoma Polygonati odorati* 6 g
Bian Dou *Semen Dolichoris lablab* 6 g
Shi Hu *Herba Dendrobii* 4 g
Zhi Gan Cao *Radix Glycyrrhizae uralensis praeparata* 6 g
Tai Zi Shen *Radix Pseudostellariae heterophyllae* 6 g
Bai Shao *Radix Paeoniae albae* 6 g

Explanation
- The first six herbs constitute the Yang Wei Tang

which nourishes Stomach-Yin. Sang Ye *Folium Mori albae* was omitted as this patient did not have a dry throat.
- **Tai Zi Shen** was added to nourish Spleen-Yin.
- **Bai Shao** was added because, in combination with Gan Cao, it stops pain. For this reason, the dosage of Gan Cao was increased to 6 g.

Prognosis and prevention

Both acupuncture and Chinese herbs give excellent results in the treatment of epigastric pain. Of all the patterns discussed, the most difficult to treat are Stasis of Blood in the Stomach and Phlegm-Fluids in the Stomach. The easiest to treat, and probably the one that best reacts to acupuncture, is Liver-Qi invading the Stomach; this is also one of the most common patterns seen in epigastric pain.

Irrespective of the Western diagnosis, proper diagnosis and treatment as discussed in this chapter will yield results. For example, if a patient with epigastric pain is found to have a stomach ulcer, this should be treated according to the above identification of patterns and, if our diagnosis and treatment are correct, both acupuncture and Chinese herbs will promote the healing of such an ulcer.

Obviously, if a patient over 40 has been suffering from epigastric pain and poor digestion for some years, a Western diagnosis should always be sought to exclude the possibility of stomach cancer. This can also be treated with Chinese herbs (although not with acupuncture) but according to guidelines that differ from those given in this chapter.

As for prevention, this obviously follows on from the detailed aetiological factors mentioned in this chapter, particularly those regarding diet and eating habits.

Western differential diagnosis

From the perspective of a Western medical diagnosis the most important task is to differentiate between the organs from which the epigastric pain may stem. These can be:

- oesophagus (carcinoma of oesophagus)
- stomach (gastritis, gastric ulcer, perforated ulcer, carcinoma of stomach)
- duodenum (duodenal ulcer)
- pancreas (pancreatitis and carcinoma of pancreas)
- large intestine (appendicitis).

OESOPHAGUS

CARCINOMA OF OESOPHAGUS

This manifests with epigastric and sternal pain and dysphagia (difficulty in swallowing). In Western countries it occurs mostly in the elderly, whilst in China it is the commonest cancer of the alimentary canal.

STOMACH

1. GASTRITIS

This disease is confined to adults. It consists in inflammation of the stomach mucosa. It can be superficial (affecting only the superficial layers) or atrophic (with thinning of the mucosa).

The main manifestations are a diffuse and constant epigastric pain which occurs about 1 hour after eating, nausea, vomiting, sour regurgitation, belching and poor appetite. The tongue is coated and, in acute cases, there may be a slight temperature. In severe, acute cases there might be prostration and fainting as in shock with pallor and a rapid and feeble pulse.

2. GASTRIC ULCER

This is characterized by ulceration of the stomach's mucous membrane. Sympathetic stimuli inhibit the Brunner's glands which secrete a mucosa-protecting mucus. The stomach's lining thus becomes more vulnerable to acids.

Gastric ulcer causes epigastric pain which comes in bouts lasting for a few weeks at intervals of months. The pain occurs from 30 minutes to 2 hours after eating and it is not relieved by eating. There may also be nausea, regurgitation and distension.

If the ulcer perforates, this is a serious emergency and the patient should be hospitalized as soon as possible. It is characterized by a severe epigastric pain which soon spreads to the whole abdomen and is aggravated on coughing and deep breathing. The pain often radiates to the shoulder. The patient looks very distressed and under shock and, in contrast to the restlessness of a gall-bladder and renal colic, he or she is reluctant to move. The abdomen is rigid and does not move with breathing. The pain may deceptively subside about 6 hours after its onset. This may give the dangerous impression that improvement is taking place. This is followed, however, by a rise in the pulse rate and the patient's condition becomes more and more grave.

3. CARCINOMA OF THE STOMACH

This occurs only in middle age, usually after 40. The epigastric pain increases gradually over the years. There is also difficulty in swallowing, lack of appetite and vomiting. In advanced cases, the patient may vomit blood which looks like coffee-grounds. The patient looks increasingly cachectic and his or her complexion is sallow. There will be anaemia or melaena if there is chronic perforation. The liver may be enlarged with nodules.

DUODENUM
DUODENAL ULCER

This is characterized by ulceration of the duodenum associated with increased secretion of acid. The pain starts in the centre of the epigastrium and comes in bouts. It usually starts 2 to 3 hours after eating and it is relieved by eating little and frequently. Other symptoms are similar to those of gastric ulcer.

PANCREAS
1. PANCREATITIS

This is more common in men over 40. The epigastric pain has a sudden onset and is severe, gradually increasing. It may radiate to the back. There is also nausea, retching and vomiting which is relieved by sitting up and bending slightly forward.

The patient looks distressed and under shock and in 25% of cases there is jaundice from pressure of the head of the pancreas on the common bile duct.

2. CANCER OF THE PANCREAS

This is more common in men between 50 and 70. The epigastric pain starts as a dull ache which is worse lying down and at night. The patient is increasingly tired and there is vomiting, anorexia and loss of weight.

LARGE INTESTINE
APPENDICITIS

In a few cases, appendicitis may start with epigastric pain. However, it soon extends to the lower abdomen or umbilical area. For a description of the symptoms and signs see under "Abdominal pain" (ch. 16).

IRRITABLE BOWEL

More than a proper diagnosis, this term tends to be a catch-all for all cases of abdominal pain which do not have another explanation. It is important to remember, however, that in about 42% of cases, irritable bowel may present with epigastric pain (see also chapter 16 on "Abdominal pain"). However, it is equally important to bear in mind that, from the perspective of Chinese diagnosis, if the pain is in the epigastric region, it definitely indicates a Stomach pathology, and, in any case, the Stomach is closely related to the Large Intestine within the Bright Yang.

GALL-BLADDER
GALL STONES

Impaction of a gall stone sometimes presents with severe epigastric pain and vomiting. Sooner or later, however, the pain shifts to the right hypochondrial region.

END NOTES

1. 1979 The Yellow Emperor's Classic of Internal Medicine
— Simple Questions (*Huang Ti Nei Jing Su Wen*
黄帝内经素问), People's Health Publishing House,
Beijing. First published *c*. 100 BC, p. 219.
2. Ibid., p. 77.

Hypochondrial pain 15

胁
痛

Hypochondrial pain indicates pain under the rib-cage margin on both sides or one side only (Fig. 15.1).

Hypochondrial pain is always related to a Liver disharmony. The "Spiritual Axis" in chapter 20 says: *"When the disease is in the Liver there is hypochondrial pain on both sides."*[1] The "Simple Questions" in chapter 22 says: *"In Liver disease there is bilateral hypochondrial pain extending to the lower abdomen."*[2]

It is important to note that hypochondrial pain on either side is related to a Liver disharmony because of the bilateral pathway of the Liver channel.

Aetiology and pathology

1. EMOTIONAL STRAIN

Anger, resentment, frustration or hatred can all cause stagnation of Liver-Qi espe-

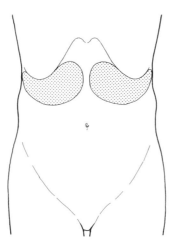

Fig. 15.1 Site of hypochondrial pain

419

cially when they are repressed and emotions are not shown. This is the most common cause of hypochondrial pain.

After a long time, stagnation of Liver-Qi may give rise to stasis of Liver-Blood.

2. EXTERNAL DAMP-HEAT

External Damp-Heat may invade the Liver channel and cause hypochondrial pain. This is very common in tropical countries, but it does occur in temperate countries in summertime.

3. DIET

Excessive consumption of dairy products and greasy-fried foods may lead to the formation of Damp-Heat in the Liver channel. Damp-Heat settles in the Liver channel rather than the Stomach and Spleen when the irregular diet is associated with emotional strain.

4. OVERWORK AND EXCESSIVE SEXUAL ACTIVITY

Both overwork and excessive sexual activity weaken Liver-Yin (as well as Kidney-Yin). Long-term deficiency of Liver-Yin may induce a secondary stagnation of Liver-Qi.

Secondary stagnation of Liver-Qi may also arise from a deficiency of Liver-Blood. This is very common in women suffering from Blood deficiency, which, in itself, may be caused by poor diet, childbirth or blood loss.

In terms of pathology, hypochondrial pain is always related to a Liver disharmony. A feeling of distension in this area indicates stagnation of Qi, while an intense, stabbing pain indicates Blood stasis. A feeling of fullness in this area indicates Damp-Heat.

The typical pulse of Liver-Qi stagnation is Wiry. There are many cases, however, when the symptoms all point very clearly to Liver-Qi stagnation and the pulse is not Wiry but Weak or Choppy. This indicates that, in such cases, Liver-Qi stagnation is secondary to either Liver-Blood or Liver-Yin deficiency. In such cases, although all symptoms point to Liver-Qi stagnation the pulse, being Weak or Choppy or Fine, reflects a deficiency of Liver-Blood or Liver-Yin.

Deficiency of Liver-Blood leading to stagnation of Liver-Qi is very common especially in women.

Differentiation and treatment

There are three Full patterns and one Empty pattern.

EXCESS

Stagnation of Liver-Qi
Stasis of Blood
Damp-Heat in the Liver and Gall-Bladder

DEFICIENCY

Deficiency of Liver-Blood
Deficiency of Liver-Yin

EXCESS CONDITIONS

1. STAGNATION OF LIVER-QI

CLINICAL MANIFESTATIONS

Hypochondrial pain and distension which is clearly related to the emotional state, a feeling of oppression in the chest, slight breathlessness, poor appetite, frequent sighing, belching.
Tongue: body-colour normal.
Pulse: Wiry. It may be Wiry only on the left side or only on the Left Middle position.

TREATMENT PRINCIPLE

Soothe the Liver and move Qi.

ACUPUNCTURE

G.B.-34 Yanglingquan, P-6 Neiguan, T.B.-6 Zhigou. Reducing or even method.

Explanation

- **G.B.-34** is the main point for hypochondrial pain and distension. It moves Liver-Qi and is specific for the hypochondrial area.
- **P-6** indirectly moves Liver-Qi due to the connection between Pericardium and Liver within the Terminal Yin, calms the Mind and settles the Ethereal Soul. It is excellent for hypochondrial pain deriving from emotional strain. In particular, it has the effect of encouraging the person to get in touch with repressed emotions.
- **T.B.-6** moves Liver-Qi in the hypochondrial region.

HERBAL TREATMENT

Prescription

CHAI HU SU GAN TANG
Bupleurum Soothing the Liver Decoction
Chai Hu *Radix Bupleuri* 6 g
Bai Shao *Radix Paeoniae albae* 4.5 g
Zhi Ke *Fructus Citri aurantii* 4.5 g
Zhi Gan Cao *Radix Glycyrrhizae uralensis praeparata* 1.5 g
Chen Pi *Pericarpium Citri reticulatae* 6 g
Xiang Fu *Rhizoma Cyperi rotundi* 4.5 g
Chuan Xiong *Radix Ligustici wallichii* 4.5 g

Explanation

This formula, which has already been explained in chapter 12, is *the* formula for distension and pain from Liver-Qi stagnation. It usually gives excellent results.

Variations

- If the pain is predominant add Qing Pi *Pericarpium Citri reticulatae viridae* and Yu Jin *Tuber Curcumae*.
- If Qi stagnation has given rise to Fire eliminate Chuan Xiong, reduce the dosage of Xiang Fu and add Mu Dan Pi *Cortex Moutan radicis*, Zhi Zi *Fructus Gardeniae jasminoidis* and Chuan Lian Zi *Fructus Meliae toosendan*.
- If Qi stagnation has given rise to Fire and this

has begun to injure Yin eliminate Chuan Xiong, reduce the dosage of Xiang Fu and add Dang Gui *Radix Angelicae sinensis*, Gou Qi Zi *Fructus Lycii chinensis*, Mu Dan Pi *Cortex Moutan radicis* and Mei Gui Hua *Flos Rosae rugosae*.
- If Liver-Qi stagnates horizontally and invades the Spleen causing diarrhoea add Bai Zhu *Rhizoma Atractylodis macrocephalae* and Fu Ling *Sclerotium Poriae cocos*.
- If Liver-Qi stagnates horizontally and invades the Stomach causing nausea add Ban Xia *Rhizoma Pinelliae ternatae*, Sha Ren *Fructus seu Semen Amomi* and Huo Xiang *Herba Agastachis*.

Patent remedy

SHU GAN WAN
Pacifying the Liver Pill
Chuan Lian Zi *Fructus Meliae toosendan*
Jiang Huang *Rhizoma Curcumae longae*
Chen Xiang *Lignum Aquilariae*
Yan Hu Suo *Rhizoma Corydalis yanhusuo*
Mu Xiang *Radix Saussureae*
Bai Dou Kou *Fructus Amomi cardamomi*
Bai Shao *Radix Paeoniae albae*
Fu Ling *Sclerotium Poriae cocos*
Zhi Ke *Fructus Citri aurantii*
Chen Pi *Pericarpium Citri reticulatae*
Sha Ren *Fructus seu Semen Amomi*
Hou Po *Cortex Magnoliae officinalis*

Explanation

This well-known pill moves Liver-Qi and may be used for hypochondrial pain from stagnation of Liver-Qi.

The pulse presentation appropriate to this remedy is a Wiry pulse, which may be so only on the left side.

2. STASIS OF LIVER-BLOOD

CLINICAL MANIFESTATIONS

Stabbing and fixed hypochondrial pain which is worse at night, feeling of a mass on palpation.

Tongue: Purple.
Pulse: Choppy.

TREATMENT PRINCIPLE

Soothe the Liver, move Qi and Blood and eliminate stasis.

ACUPUNCTURE

G.B.-34 Yanglingquan, P-6 Neiguan, T.B.-6 Zhigou, LIV-3 Taichong, SP-10 Xuehai, BL-17 Geshu, LIV-14 Qimen, BL-18 Ganshu. Reducing or even method.

Explanation

– **G.B.-34** is the main point for hypochondrial pain and distension. It moves Liver-Qi and is specific for the hypochondrial area. Moving Liver-Qi helps to move Liver-Blood.
– **P-6** indirectly moves Liver-Qi and Liver-Blood, calms the Mind and settles the Ethereal Soul. It is excellent for hypochondrial pain deriving from emotional strain.
– **T.B.-6** moves Liver-Qi in the hypochondrial region.
– **LIV-3** moves Liver-Blood, calms the Mind and settles the Ethereal Soul.
– **SP-10** and **BL-17** move Blood.
– **LIV-14** and **BL-18**, Front-Collecting and Back-Transporting point of the Liver respectively, regulate the Liver and move Qi and Blood.

HERBAL TREATMENT

Prescription

CHAI HU SU GAN TANG Variation
Bupleurum Soothing the Liver Decoction
Chai Hu *Radix Bupleuri* 6 g
Bai Shao *Radix Paeoniae albae* 4.5 g
Zhi Ke *Fructus Citri aurantii* 4.5 g
Zhi Gan Cao *Radix Glycyrrhizae uralensis praeparata* 1.5 g
Chen Pi *Pericarpium Citri reticulatae* 6 g

Xiang Fu *Rhizoma Cyperi rotundi* 4.5 g
Chuan Xiong *Radix Ligustici wallichii* 4.5 g
Yu Jin *Tuber Curcumae* 6 g
Yan Hu Suo *Rhizoma Corydalis yanhusuo* 6 g

Explanation

The first seven herbs constitute Chai Hu Su Gan Tang.

– **Yu Jin** and **Yan Hu Suo** strongly move Liver-Blood and stop pain. Yu Jin, in particular, is good for the emotional depression deriving from stagnation of Liver Qi and Blood.

Variations

– If there is constipation add Da Huang *Rhizoma Rhei*.
– If there are masses add San Leng *Rhizoma Sparganii*, E Zhu *Rhizoma Curcumae zedoariae* and Ze Lan *Herba Lycopi lucidi*.

3. DAMP-HEAT IN LIVER AND GALL-BLADDER

CLINICAL MANIFESTATIONS

Dull hypochondrial pain and fullness, a feeling of heaviness, a sticky taste, nausea, yellow sclera, dark urine.
Tongue: sticky-yellow tongue coating on one or both sides (Fig. 15.2).
Pulse: Slippery and slightly Rapid.

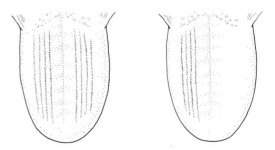

Fig. 15.2 Tongue coating in Gall-Bladder and Liver Damp-Heat

TREATMENT PRINCIPLE

Soothe the Liver, clear Heat and resolve Dampness.

ACUPUNCTURE

G.B.-34 Yanglingquan, BL-19 Danshu, G.B.-24 Riyue, L.I.-11 Quchi, SP-9 Yinlingquan, BL-20 Pishu and Ren-12 Zhongwan. Reducing or even method, except on the last two which should be reinforced.

Explanation

- **G.B.-34** moves Liver-Qi, soothes the hypochondrium and resolves Damp-Heat.
- **BL-19** and **G.B.-24**, Back-Transporting and Front-Collecting points of the Gall-Bladder respectively, clear Heat and resolve Dampness from the Gall-Bladder.
- **L.I.-11** and **SP-9** resolve Damp-Heat.
- **BL-20** and **Ren-12** tonify the Spleen to resolve Dampness.

HERBAL TREATMENT

Prescription

YIN CHEN HAO TANG
Artemisia capillaris Decoction
Yin Chen Hao *Herba Artemisiae capillaris* 30 g
Zhi Zi *Fructus Gardeniae jasminoidis* 15 g
Da Huang *Rhizoma Rhei* 9 g

Explanation

- **Yin Chen Hao** resolves Damp-Heat from the Liver and Gall-Bladder.
- **Zhi Zi** resolves Damp-Heat from the three Burners.

- **Da Huang** helps to clear Heat and resolve Dampness by moving downwards.

Variations

- If there is no constipation use vinegar-treated Da Huang and boil the decoction for longer than 30 minutes so that Da Huang clears Heat without moving downwards too strongly.
- If there is a Spleen deficiency add Bai Zhu *Rhizoma Atractylodis macrocephalae* and Fu Ling *Sclerotium Poriae cocos*.
- If there are gall stones add Jin Qian Cao *Herba Desmodii styracifolii*, Hai Jin Sha *Spora Lygodii japonici* and Yu Jin *Tuber Curcumae*.

Patent remedy

LI GAN PIAN
Benefiting the Liver Tablet
Jia Qian Cao *Herba Desmodii styracifolii*
Niu Dan *Fellis Bovis*

Explanation

This tablet drains Damp-Heat from the Liver and Gall-Bladder. The tongue presentation appropriate to this remedy is a Red body with a sticky, yellow coating on the sides.

DEFICIENCY CONDITIONS

1. LIVER-BLOOD DEFICIENCY

CLINICAL MANIFESTATIONS

Slight hypochondrial pain and distension, premenstrual tension, frequent sighing, depression, moodiness, dizziness, insomnia, tingling of limbs, blurred vision, scanty periods or amenorrhoea, tiredness.

Table 15.1 Differentiation between stagnation of Liver-Qi and Damp-Heat in Liver and Gall-Bladder

	Stagnation of Liver-Qi	Damp-Heat in Liver and Gall-Bladder
Emotions	Closely related to emotional state	Not so related to emotional state
Symptoms	No feeling of oppression of the chest	Feeling of oppression and fullness of chest and epigastrium
Fever	No fever	Fever, jaundice
Pulse	Wiry	Slippery
Tongue	Coating not sticky	Sticky coating

Tongue: Pale and Thin.
Pulse: Choppy or Fine. It may be very slightly Wiry on the left side or the left Middle position.

This is a very common condition especially in women, when stagnation of Liver-Qi is secondary to a deficiency of Liver-Blood.

TREATMENT PRINCIPLE

Nourish Blood, soothe the Liver and move Qi.

ACUPUNCTURE

ST-36 Zusanli, SP-6 Sanyinjiao, LIV-14 Qimen, Ren-4 Guanyuan, LIV-8 Ququan, G.B.-34 Yanglingquan, LIV-3 Taichong, P-6 Neiguan, T.B.-6 Zhigou, G.B.-41 Zulinqi. Reinforcing method on ST-36, SP-6, Ren-4 and LIV-8, even method on the others.

Explanation

– **ST-36**, **SP-6**, **Ren-4** and **LIV-8** nourish Liver-Blood.
– **LIV-14**, **G.B.-34**, **T.B.-6** and **LIV-3** move Liver-Qi.
– **P-6** moves Liver-Qi, calms the Mind and settles the Ethereal Soul.
– **G.B. -41** is used in women if there is also a feeling of distension of the breasts.

HERBAL TREATMENT

Prescription

XIAO YAO SAN
Free and Easy Wanderer Powder
Bo He *Herba Menthae* 3 g
Chai Hu *Radix Bupleuri* 9 g
Dang Gui *Radix Angelicae sinensis* 9 g
Bai Shao *Radix Paeoniae albae* 12 g
Bai Zhu *Rhizoma Atractylodis macrocephalae* 9 g
Fu Ling *Sclerotium Poriae cocos* 15 g
Gan Cao *Radix Glycyrrhizae uralensis* 6 g
Sheng Jiang *Rhizoma Zingiberis officinalis recens* 3 slices

Explanation

This formula, which has already been explained in chapter 1, moves Liver-Qi, nourishes Liver-Blood and tonifies Spleen-Qi.

Variations

– If the symptoms of Blood deficiency are pronounced increase the dosage of Dang Gui and add Shu Di Huang *Radix Rehmanniae glutinosae praeparata* and Shou Wu *Radix Polygoni multiflori*.
– If the symptoms of Qi stagnation are very pronounced add Xiang Fu *Rhizoma Cyperi rotundi* and Mu Xiang *Radix Saussureae*.
– If the Qi stagnation affects the breasts add Qing Pi *Pericarpium Citri reticulatae viridae*.
– If Qi stagnation is causing depression add He Huan Pi *Cortex Albizziae julibrissin*.

Patent remedy

XIAO YAO WAN
Free and Easy Wanderer Pill

Explanation

This pill has the same ingredients and functions as the homonymous formula explained above. It is ideal to treat stagnation of Liver-Qi, particularly in women, when it is secondary to Liver-Blood deficiency.

The tongue presentation appropriate to this remedy is a Pale and Thin body. The pulse presentation appropriate to this remedy is a pulse which is Weak and Choppy on the right and slightly Wiry on the left, or generally Fine and slightly Wiry on the left.

2. DEFICIENCY OF LIVER-YIN

CLINICAL MANIFESTATIONS

Slight hypochondrial pain, dryness of throat, eyes, skin and hair, tiredness, poor memory, insomnia, depression, scanty periods, dizziness.
Tongue: Red without coating.
Pulse: Floating-Empty.

TREATMENT PRINCIPLE

Soothe the Liver and nourish Liver-Yin.

ACUPUNCTURE

ST-36 Zusanli, SP-6 Sanyinjiao, Ren-4 Guanyuan, LIV-8 Ququan, KI-3 Taixi, G.B.-34 Yanglingquan, LIV-3 Taichong, P-6 Neiguan, T.B.-6 Zhigou, G.B.-41 Zulinqi. Reinforcing method on ST-36, SP-6, Ren-4, LIV-8 and KI-3 Taixi, even method on the others.

Explanation

These are the same points as for Liver-Blood deficiency with the addition of KI-3 Taixi to nourish Yin.

HERBAL TREATMENT

Prescription

YI GUAN JIAN
One Linking Decoction
Bei Sha Shen *Radix Glehniae littoralis* 10 g
Mai Men Dong *Tuber Ophiopogonis japonici* 10 g
Dang Gui *Radix Angelicae sinensis* 10 g
Sheng Di Huang *Radix Rehmanniae glutinosae* 30 g
Gou Qi Zi *Fructus Lycii chinensis* 12 g
Chuan Lian Zi *Fructus Meliae toosendan* 5 g

Explanation

This formula, which has already been explained in chapter 5, nourishes Liver-Yin.

Variations

− To enhance the Liver-Qi-moving effect of the formula add Mei Gui Hua *Flos Rosae rugosae* which moves Qi without injuring Yin.

Appendix

GALL-BLADDER STONES

Gall-Bladder stones are formed when there is an excess of cholesterol in relation to bile acids. Such changes in the relation between cholesterol and bile acids precede the formation of calculi and are dependent on the Liver. Thus, the free flow of Liver-Qi is the most important factor in maintaining normal bile acids and therefore stagnation of Liver-Qi is an important prerequisite for the formation of stones. When Liver-Qi stagnates, bile is not secreted properly or is secreted insufficiently. This leads to the accumulation of Damp-Heat in the Gall-Bladder. The steaming action of Heat on Dampness over a long time leads to the formation of stones.

There are three types of stones:

1. *Cholesterol stones* are composed almost entirely of cholesterol. They more often correspond to the pattern of Damp-Heat in the Liver and Gall-Bladder. They are usually single stones.
2. *Pigment stones*, which are always numerous, are composed of bile pigments. They are less common.
3. *Mixed stones* are the most common type. They consist of lamellated layers of cholesterol, calcium and bilirubin.

DIFFERENTIATION

Treatment must be differentiated according to the two main patterns appearing in gall stones, i.e. stagnation of Liver-Qi and Damp-Heat in Liver and Gall-Bladder. The two patterns may of course occur simultaneously and they often do.

1. STAGNATION OF LIVER-QI

Hypochondrial distension and pain, the former more marked than the latter, depression, moodiness, belching, frequent sighing and a Wiry pulse.

2. DAMP-HEAT IN LIVER AND GALL-BLADDER

Pain and fullness of the hypochondrium, bitter and sticky taste, poor appetite, feeling of fullness of the epigastrium, nausea, vomiting, yellow sclera, a sticky-yellow tongue coating and a Slippery pulse.

The differentiation between the pattern of stagnation of Liver-Qi and that of Damp-Heat in Liver and Gall-Bladder is illustrated in Table 15.1.

TREATMENT

1. STAGNATION OF LIVER-QI

Acupuncture

LIV-14 Qimen, LIV-3 Taichong, G.B.-34 Yanglingquan, Dannangxue. Reducing method.

Explanation

- **LIV-14** and **LIV-3,** Front-Collecting and Source points of the Liver, soothe the Liver, move Qi and stop pain.
- **G.B.-34** and **Dannangxue** regulate the Gall-Bladder and stop pain.

Herbal treatment

Prescription

CHAI HU SU GAN TANG Variation
Bupleurum Soothing the Liver Decoction
Chai Hu *Radix Bupleuri* 6 g
Bai Shao *Radix Paeoniae albae* 4.5 g
Zhi Ke *Fructus Citri aurantii* 4.5 g
Zhi Gan Cao *Radix Glycyrrhizae uralensis praeparata* 1.5 g
Chen Pi *Pericarpium Citri reticulatae* 6 g
Xiang Fu *Rhizoma Cyperi rotundi* 4.5 g
Chuan Xiong *Radix Ligustici wallichii* 4.5 g
Jin Qian Cao *Herba Desmodii styracifolii* 9 g
Hai Jin Sha *Spora Lygodii japonici* 9 g

Explanation

The first seven herbs constitute the Chai Hu Su Gan Tang which soothes the Liver and moves Qi.

- **Jin Qian Cao** and **Hai Jin Sha** dissolve stones.

Patent remedy

SHU GAN WAN
Pacifying the Liver Pill
Chuan Lian Zi *Fructus Meliae toosendan*
Jiang Huang *Rhizoma Curcumae longae*
Chen Xiang *Lignum Aquilariae*
Yan Hu Suo *Rhizoma Corydalis yanhusuo*
Mu Xiang *Radix Saussureae*
Bai Dou Kou *Fructus Amomi cardamomi*
Bai Shao *Radix Paeoniae albae*
Fu Ling *Sclerotium Poriae cocos*
Zhi Ke *Fructus Citri aurantii*
Chen Pi *Pericarpium Citri reticulatae*
Sha Ren *Fructus seu Semen Amomi*
Hou Po *Cortex Magnoliae officinalis*

Explanation

This pill moves Liver-Qi and is similar in action to the formula Chai Hu Su Gan Tang *Bupleurum Soothing the Liver Decoction* mentioned above.

2. DAMP-HEAT IN LIVER AND GALL-BLADDER

Acupuncture

G.B.-24 Riyue, ST-19 Burong, G.B.-34 Yanglingquan, Du-9 Zhiyang, SP-9 Yinlingquan. Reducing method.

Explanation

- **G.B.-24** and **G.B.-34** regulate the Gall-Bladder and resolve Damp-Heat.
- **ST-19** regulates the Gall-Bladder and stops pain.
- **Du-9** resolves Gall-Bladder Damp-Heat.
- **SP-9** resolves Damp-Heat.

Herbal treatment

(a) Prescription

DA CHAI HU TANG Variation
Big Bupleurum Decoction
Chai Hu *Radix Bupleuri* 15 g
Huang Qin *Radix Scutellariae baicalensis* 9 g
Ban Xia *Rhizoma Pinelliae ternatae* 9 g

Bai Shao *Radix Paeoniae albae* 9 g
Da Huang *Rhizoma Rhei* 6 g
Zhi Shi *Fructus Citri aurantii immaturus* 9 g
Sheng Jiang *Rhizoma Zingiberis officinalis recens* 15 g
Da Zao *Fructus Ziziphi jujubae* 5 dates
Jin Qian Cao *Herba Desmodii styracifolii* 9 g
Hai Jin Sha *Spora Lygodii japonici* 9 g

Explanation

- **Chai Hu** and **Huang Qin**, the two main ingredients of the Xiao Chai Hu Tang *Small Bupleurum Decoction*, regulate the Lesser Yang.
- **Ban Xia** resolves Phlegm.
- **Bai Shao** stops pain and moderates urgency.
- **Da Huang** clears Damp-Heat by moving downwards.
- **Zhi Shi** helps Da Huang to move downwards.
- **Sheng Jiang** and **Da Zao** harmonize.
- **Jin Qian Cao** and **Hai Jin Sha** dissolve stones.

(b) Prescription

Empirical formula
Jin Qian Cao *Herba Desmodii styracifolii* 30 g
Yin Chen Hao *Herba Artemisiae capillaris* 15 g
Yu Jin *Tuber Curcumae* 15 g
Zhi Ke *Fructus Citri aurantii* 9 g
Mu Xiang *Radix Saussureae* 9 g
Da Huang *Rhizoma Rhei* 9 g

Explanation

- **Jin Qian Cao** and **Yin Chen Hao** resolve Damp-Heat. Jin Qian Cao dissolves stones.
- **Yu Jin**, **Zhi Ke** and **Mu Xiang** move Liver-Qi.
- **Da Huang** resolves Damp-Heat by moving downwards.

(i) Patent remedy

LI GAN PIAN
Benefiting the Liver Tablet
Jia Qian Cao *Herba Desmodii styracifolii*
Niu Dan *Fellis Bovis*

Explanation

This tablet drains Damp-Heat from the Liver and Gall-Bladder and is used for acute or chronic hepatitis and chronic cholecystitis or cholelithiasis.

The tongue presentation appropriate to this remedy is a Red body and a sticky-yellow coating on the sides.

(ii) Patent remedy

LI DAN PIAN
Benefiting the Gall-Bladder Tablet
Huang Qin *Radix Scutellariae baicalensis*
Mu Xiang *Radix Saussureae*
Jin Qian Cao *Herba Desmodii styracifolii*
Jin Yin Hua *Flos Lonicerae japonicae*
Yin Chen Hao *Herba Artemisiae capillaris*
Chai Hu *Radix Bupleuri*
Da Qing Ye *Folium Isatidis seu Baphicacanthi*
Da Huang *Rhizoma Rhei*

Explanation

This tablet drains Damp-Heat from the Gall-Bladder and is used for acute or chronic cholecystitis and cholelithiasis. It can help to expel gall-bladder stones if they are under 1 cm in diameter.

It should be noted that this remedy contains Da Huang which moves downwards and should therefore not be used continuously for more than 2–3 months.

The tongue presentation appropriate to this remedy would be a very sticky-yellow coating which is thicker on the right side.

NOTES ON ACUPUNCTURE TREATMENT

Acupuncture can be used to facilitate the expulsion of gall stones and either set of points from the above two patterns may be used. It is important, however, to obtain the needling sensation and manipulate the needle with a reducing method very strongly. The needles should be retained for over 40 minutes and be manipulated at intervals. Treatment should be given every day for 10 days. Electricity can be used with high frequency and dense-sparse wave, connecting a local and a distal point, for example G.B.-24 and Dannangxue on the right side only. It is important to retain the needles for more than 40 minutes as cholecystography performed during acupuncture treatments has shown that acupuncture stimulates contractions of the gallbladder reaching a peak after 30 minutes. During the first 30 minutes large amounts of bile are accumulated in the gall-bladder. Then the contractions stop for about 10 minutes and suddenly, after 40 minutes, the gall-bladder orifice opens and the bile flows out.

If the stone is in the gall-bladder it can only be expelled if it is under 1 cm in diameter. If it is in the cystic duct, it can only be expelled if it is under 1.5 cm in diameter. Large, single stones are painful but relatively easy to excrete, whereas sand-like stones are less painful but more difficult to excrete. Successful expulsion with acupuncture occurs in 70% of cases.

Western differentiation

Whereas in Chinese medicine both sides of the hypochondrium are related to the Liver channel, in Western medicine obviously only the right side reflects a possible liver pathology. Thus an important distinction is that between right and left hypochondrial pain.

RIGHT HYPOCHONDRIAL PAIN

1. CHOLECYSTITIS OR CHOLELITHIASIS

Cholecystitis consists in inflammation of the gall-bladder with or without gall-stones. It is more frequent in women over 25. Cholesterol is maintained in solution in the bile by bile acids. Any factor which increases cholesterol (obesity, high fat diet) or decreases bile acids (bile stasis, liver disease) may lead to the formation of stones.

The hypochondrial pain may radiate to the right scapula and may be accompanied by nausea, vomiting and sweating. The right rectus muscle feels rigid on palpation and the patient is very restless during an acute attack.

2. CARCINOMA OF THE GALL-BLADDER

Carcinoma of the gall-bladder is more common in women over 50, but it is quite rare in general. The hypochondrial pain is similar to that of cholecystitis and there may be jaundice. In advanced cases the patient would be thin and exhausted. The gall-bladder is palpable and tender and its surface is felt to be irregular. The liver is also enlarged and the glands above the right clavicle may be enlarged.

3. HEPATITIS

Type A hepatitis may cause a right hypochondrial pain. The liver is enlarged and its surface feels smooth on palpation.

4. CARCINOMA OF THE LIVER

Carcinoma of the liver causes hypochondrial pain. The liver is enlarged and its surface feels irregular on palpation. There may be a single or multiple nodules.

LEFT HYPOCHONDRIAL PAIN

1. ACUTE PANCREATITIS

The onset of this disease is sudden with severe pain in the left hypochondrium extending to the epigastrium. The pain may also radiate to the left scapula. There may be nausea and vomiting and the patient looks very ill and pale as if suffering from shock.

2. CHRONIC PANCREATITIS

Chronic pancreatitis is more common in men over 50. The pain is in the left hypochondrium and may radiate to the epigastrium. Interestingly, the pain may also occur in the *right* hypochondrium (suggesting involvement of the Liver channel from a Chinese point of view). The pain is relieved by crouching forward or lying prone. This is a very typical sign of chronic pancreatitis.

END NOTES

1. 1981 Spiritual Axis (*Ling Shu Jing* 灵枢经), People's Health Publishing House, Beijing. First published *c.* 100 BC, p. 55.

2. 1979 The Yellow Emperor's Classic of Internal Medicine — Simple Questions (*Huang Ti Nei Jing Su Wen* 黄帝内经素问), People's Health Publishing House, Beijing. First published *c.* 100 BC, p. 146.

Abdominal pain 16

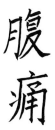

腹
痛

"Abdominal pain" indicates pain in any part of the abdomen below or just around the umbilicus (Fig. 16.1).

In this chapter I shall discuss abdominal pain which is intestinal in origin, not abdominal pain from gynaecological or other conditions. In women, it is not always easy to distinguish whether abdominal pain is of intestinal or gynaecological origin, also because the two conditions may well overlap.

Generally speaking, an abdominal pain which is clearly related to food intake or bowel movements and is associated with either constipation or diarrhoea, is purely of intestinal origin. An abdominal pain which is clearly related to the menstrual cycle, and is associated with irregular periods, dysmenorrhoea or mid-cycle pain, is of gynaecological origin.

However, as mentioned above, in women the two conditions may well overlap and it may be very difficult to distinguish between them. Indeed, from a purely Chinese medical perspective, it is not even that important to distinguish between the two conditions as some of their pathologies coincide: Cold in the Lower Burner, Damp-

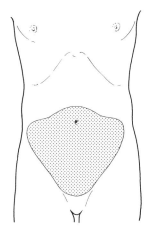

Fig. 16.1 Area of abdominal pain

Heat, stagnation of Qi or Blood. In other ways it is of course important to distinguish whether the pain is of intestinal or gynaecological origin, in order to advise the patient on life-style and diet and to have a better idea of prognosis.

The category of "abdominal pain" discussed here may also overlap with other conditions, particularly constipation, diarrhoea and abdominal masses. Generally speaking, the present chapter will discuss the condition when abdominal pain is the main presenting symptom, even though it may be accompanied by constipation or diarrhoea. Although these two conditions may also be accompanied by some abdominal pain, they are discussed under the categories of "Diarrhoea" (ch. 18) and "Constipation" (ch. 19) if the change in bowel habit is the main presenting manifestation. As for "abdominal masses", this condition may or may not present with pain. Again, if pain is the main presenting symptom the reader should use the differentiation and treatment given in this chapter. If an abdominal mass is the main sign, then one should use the differentiation and treatment given in the chapter on "Abdominal Masses" (ch. 17).

Finally, the area of abdominal pain illustrated in Figure 16.1 above includes the hypogastric region, i.e. the small, rounded area immediately above the pubic bone (Fig. 16.2).

Although abdominal pain of intestinal origin may be centred only in this region, a purely hypogastric pain is more often of urinary origin

and the reader should refer to the chapters on urinary diseases (chs 20–21).

Aetiology and pathology

1. EXTERNAL PATHOGENIC FACTORS

Cold and Dampness are the two pathogenic factors which most frequently cause abdominal pain.

External Cold may invade the Intestines directly without causing exterior symptoms first. This happens when a person is exposed to cold, especially when the body is wet after swimming. Invasion of the Intestines by Cold is also facilitated by excessive consumption of cold foods and especially cold drinks. For these two reasons (excessive consumption of cold drinks and exposure to cold after swimming), paradoxically, invasion of the Intestines by Cold is more common in summertime.

Women are more prone to invasions of the Intestines by Cold during and immediately after the periods and, even more so, after childbirth.

Cold contracts tissues and causes retardation of Qi and Blood, thus causing pain. Invasion of the Intestines by Cold is characterized by abdominal pain with a sudden onset and diarrhoea.

Dampness also invades the Intestines easily, entering the channels of the leg and flowing up towards the abdomen. Dampness obstructs the circulation of Qi in the abdomen and, besides the Intestines themselves, affects Spleen and Liver. This causes abdominal pain, a feeling of fullness and heaviness and possibly diarrhoea. The tongue coating will be thick and sticky and the pulse Slippery.

Dampness may combine with Cold or Heat. Invasion of external Damp-Heat is common in summertime even in northern countries such as Britain or the northern United States, but is, of course, even more common in southern European countries and the South of the USA.

2. EMOTIONAL STRESS

Emotional stress has a deep influence on the

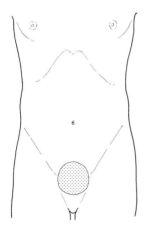

Fig. 16.2 Hypogastric area

circulation of Qi and Blood in the abdomen, particularly affecting the Liver and Spleen.

Anger (using this term in a broad sense which includes frustration and resentment) may cause stagnation of Liver-Qi in the Intestines and thus abdominal pain. This is a very frequent emotional cause of abdominal pain.

Pensiveness and *worry* affect the Spleen and Lungs. The Spleen is responsible for transforming and moving food essences in the Intestines, while Lung-Qi helps the Qi of the Intestines to descend. Pensiveness and worry impair the proper transformation of Spleen-Qi and the descent of Lung-Qi towards the Intestines. Both these conditions may cause abdominal pain.

3. IMPROPER DIET

Diet has of course a profound influence on the Intestines. Excessive consumption of cold and raw foods and ice-cold drinks weakens Spleen-Yang and leads to the formation of internal Cold. Cold contracts the Intestines and leads to stagnation of Qi and/or Blood which causes abdominal pain.

Excessive consumption of dairy foods and greasy foods leads to the formation of Dampness which obstructs the functions of the Spleen and Intestines: this causes abdominal pain. Excessive consumption of hot and spicy foods and alcohol may lead to Heat or Damp-Heat in the Intestines, which also causes abdominal pain.

Apart from the actual diet, eating habits also have a profound influence on the intestinal function. These have already been discussed in detail in the chapter on epigastric pain (ch. 14). First of all, simply eating too much leads to retention of food in the Stomach and Intestines and thus to abdominal pain. Eating irregularly, eating in a hurry, skipping meals, eating while discussing business, may all influence the function of the Intestines and lead to stagnation of Qi which causes abdominal pain.

In abdominal pain, a distinction is often made between substantial and non-substantial pain. Substantial abdominal pain (literally called "with form") is caused by stasis of Blood or retention of food. Any other type is non-substantial (literally called "without form"). A substantial abdominal pain improves after bowel movements, whilst a non-substantial one does not.

Diagnosis

There are some aspects of diagnosis which particularly apply to abdominal pain. These will be discussed under the following headings:

- nature of pain
- reaction to pressure
- reaction to food or drink
- reaction to bowel movement
- reaction to activity/rest
- reaction to heat
- tongue signs
- pulse signs.

NATURE OF PAIN

A dull pain is due to an Empty condition, whilst a severe pain is due to a Full condition.

A distending pain indicates stagnation of Qi. Patients often describe this as a "bloated" sensation.

A stabbing, fixed and intense pain indicates stasis of Blood, especially if it is associated with a fixed abdominal mass.

A feeling of fullness (which is more intense than "distension"), in Chinese called *man*, indicates retention of food or simply a more severe stagnation of Qi.

Both a feeling of distension (*zhang*) and of fullness (*man*) may be observed objectively as the abdomen will be distended or hard on pressure.

A feeling of stuffiness (*pi*) indicates an Empty condition together with some Dampness or Heat. Contrary to the feelings of fullness and distension, the feeling of stuffiness is entirely subjective as the patient's abdomen will feel soft on palpation.

REACTION TO PRESSURE

If an abdominal pain is eased by pressing the

area of pain this indicates an Empty condition. If it is aggravated by pressure this indicates a Full condition. The "Prescriptions of the Golden Chest" says: *"If an abdominal pain improves with pressure it indicates Deficiency, if it is aggravated by pressure it indicates Excess."*[1]

When diagnosing abdominal pain it is very important to check whether pressure alleviates or aggravates the pain as this test is very reliable. The following case history is a useful example.

Case history

A 35-year-old woman had been suffering from abdominal pain for 2 years. The pain was on the right side of the lower abdomen and was not related to the menstrual cycle. Although the pain was quite severe, she liked to press the area of pain and this afforded some relief. Her tongue was quite Purple and her pulse was very Fine, rather Deep and generally Weak.

As her tongue was definitely Purple and the pain was severe, indicating a Full condition, I adopted the treatment principle of moving Blood and eliminating stasis and used a variation of Shao Fu Zhu Yu Tang *Lower Abdomen Eliminating Stasis Decoction*, adding strong "breaking Blood" herbs such as Ze Lan *Herba Lycopi lucidi*. Although this provided some relief, it did not eliminate the pain completely and also made her feel rather tired. I therefore asked Professor Meng Jing Hua, one of my teachers from the Nanjing College of Traditional Chinese Medicine, to examine her on the occasion of his visit to Britain. He attached much more importance to the finding that her pain was alleviated by pressure or, at least, that she liked to press the area of pain. He also pointed out that her pulse was Fine and Weak. He therefore adopted the treatment principle of primarily tonifying and suggested a prescription that tonified Qi and Blood and only mildly moved Blood. This produced much better results in relieving the pain and she gained much more energy.

REACTION TO FOOD OR DRINK

Abdominal pain which improves with warm drinks, or is aggravated by ice-cold drinks, indicates a Cold condition. If it improves by drinking cold drinks, it is due to a Hot condition.

REACTION TO BOWEL MOVEMENT

If abdominal pain improves after bowel move-

ments it is said to be substantial in nature and usually due to either Blood stasis or retention of food. Both of these are Full types of abdominal pain.

Abdominal pain which is not influenced by bowel movements is also of the Full type but is non-substantial in nature and it may be due to Dampness, stagnation of Qi or Cold.

Abdominal pain which gets worse after bowel movements indicates an Empty condition.

REACTION TO ACTIVITY/REST

Abdominal pain which improves with slight exercise is due to Qi stagnation. If it improves with rest it is due to a Deficiency.

REACTION TO HEAT

If an abdominal pain improves with the application of heat, such as a hot-water bottle, this indicates that it is due to Cold in the Intestines. Unfortunately, this is not a completely reliable diagnostic sign because several other conditions are improved by the application of heat. Stagnation of Qi, stasis of Blood, and retention of food, for example, may all improve with the application of heat, as this has a moving effect on Qi and Blood.

TONGUE SIGNS

The condition of the Intestines is reflected in the root of the tongue and specifically in the coating of the root.

A thick coating indicates the presence of a pathogenic factor which may be Cold, Damp-Heat or retention of food. Obviously a white coating indicates Cold while a yellow or brown one indicates Heat. A grey or black coating indicates either Cold or Heat depending on whether it is wet or dry.

A sticky-yellow coating with red spots on the root indicates Damp-Heat and some stasis of Blood in the Intestines; the more red spots there are, the greater the Heat and stasis of Blood. If the colour of the coating on the root is not bright but dull and lifeless, it indicates that the condition is very long-standing.

The complete or, more usually, partial absence of coating in patches on the root of the tongue indicates deficiency of Qi and Yin of the Stomach and Intestines.

Stagnation of Qi in the Intestines does not show on the tongue, whilst stasis of Blood manifests with a purple colour on the sides of the tongue towards the root.

PULSE SIGNS

The Intestines are reflected in both Rear positions of the pulse. Although the left Rear position corresponds to the Small Intestine and the right one to the Large Intestine (some doctors reverse this), a pathology of the Intestines (whether Small or Large) is often reflected in both Rear positions having the same quality. If it is of gynaecological origin, one side or the other (more often the left) presents an abnormal quality. This may also be a useful sign to distinguish pain of intestinal origin from that of gynaecological origin in women.

Thus, if both Rear positions are Tight and the pulse is Slow, it indicates Cold in the Intestines.

If both Rear positions are Wiry, it indicates stagnation of Qi or stasis of Blood in the Intestines. If, besides being Wiry on these positions, the pulse is also Rapid and Slippery, it indicates Damp-Heat in the Intestines and possibly bleeding from the intestinal mucosa. This pulse finding is often seen in Crohn's disease or ulcerative colitis.

If both Rear positions are Wiry and Hollow it indicates prolonged bleeding from the gut. If the pulse is Rapid and both Rear positions are only slightly Hollow, it may indicate a forthcoming bleeding from the gut.

If both Rear positions are Slippery and Wiry, it indicates Damp-Heat and stagnation of Qi or Blood in the Intestines.

Differentiation and treatment

The *Excess* conditions are:

– Cold in the Intestines
– Damp-Heat in the Intestines
– Retention of Food
– Stagnation of Qi
– Stasis of Blood.

The *Deficiency* condition is:

– Deficiency of Qi and Empty-Cold in the Abdomen.

EXCESS CONDITIONS

1. COLD IN THE INTESTINES

CLINICAL MANIFESTATIONS

Intense abdominal pain which is aggravated by pressure and by consuming cold foods and drinks, and alleviated by application of warmth and drinking warm liquids, no thirst, pale urine, loose stools or constipation.
Tongue: white-sticky coating.
Pulse: Slippery-Full-Tight.

This is due to Full-Cold in the Intestines obstructing the circulation of Qi and Blood and therefore causing pain. Normally, the stools would be loose as Cold impairs Spleen-Yang, but in severe cases Cold may obstruct the descending of Qi of the Intestines causing constipation.

TREATMENT PRINCIPLE

Warm the Intestines and Spleen, scatter Cold and stop pain.

ACUPUNCTURE

ST-25 Tianshu, SP-15 Daheng, ST-27 Daju, Ren-10 Xiawan, SP-6 Sanyinjiao and ST-36 Zusanli. Reducing or even method. Moxa must be used.

Explanation

– **ST-25**, Front-Collecting point of the Large Intestine, with moxa, scatters Cold from the Intestines.

- **SP-15** with moxa, scatters Cold and promotes the descending of Qi in the Intestines.
- **ST-27** with moxa, expels Cold from the Intestines and stops pain.
- **Ren-10** promotes the descending of Stomach-Qi.
- **SP-6** stops abdominal pain.
- **ST-36** regulates the Intestines and promotes the descending of Qi.

HERBAL TREATMENT

Prescription

LIANG FU WAN and ZHENG QI TIAN XIANG SAN
Alpinia-Cyperus Pill and *Upright Qi Heavenly Fragrance Powder*
Gao Liang Jiang *Rhizoma Alpiniae officinari* 6 g
Xiang Fu *Rhizoma Cyperi rotundi* 6 g
Wu Yao *Radix Linderae strychnifoliae* 6 g
Gan Jiang *Rhizoma Zingiberis officinalis* 3 g
Zi Su Ye *Folium Perillae frutescentis* 6 g
Chen Pi *Pericarpium Citri reticulatae* 4.5 g

Explanation

- **Gao Liang Jiang**, **Gan Jiang** and **Su Ye** warm the Intestines and scatter Cold.
- **Wu Yao**, **Xiang Fu** and **Chen Pi** move Qi and stop pain.

Variations

- If the pain is very severe add Yan Hu Suo *Rhizoma Corydalis yanhusuo*.
- If, together with Cold, there is also Dampness add Fu Ling *Sclerotium Poriae cocos* and Yi Yi Ren *Semen Coicis lachryma jobi*.

2. DAMP-HEAT IN THE INTESTINES

CLINICAL MANIFESTATIONS

Abdominal pain which is worse with pressure and hot food, a feeling of heaviness and oppression of the chest, loose stools with foul smell, mucus and/or blood in the stools, a burning sensation of the anus, thirst, slight sweating, dark urine.
Tongue: Red body, thick-sticky-yellow coating.
Pulse: Slippery and Rapid.

TREATMENT PRINCIPLE

Clear Heat, resolve Dampness.

ACUPUNCTURE

ST-25 Tianshu, BL-25 Dachangshu, L.I.-11 Quchi, Ren-10 Xiawan, SP-9 Yinlingquan, SP-6 Sanyinjiao, T.B.-6 Zhigou and ST-37 Shangjuxu. Reducing or even method; no moxa.

Explanation

- **ST-25** and **BL-25**, Front-Collecting point and Back-Transporting point of the Large Intestine, resolve Damp-Heat.
- **L.I.-11** resolves Damp-Heat.
- **Ren-10** resolves Dampness and stimulates the descending of Qi in the Intestines.
- **SP-9** and **SP-6** resolve Damp-Heat. SP-6 is also specific for lower abdominal pain.
- **T.B.-6** clears Heat from the Intestines and promotes the bowel movements.
- **ST-37**, Lower Sea point of the Large Intestine, regulates the Large Intestine and stops diarrhoea.

HERBAL TREATMENT

(a) Prescription

DA CHENG QI TANG Variation
Great Conducting Qi Decoction Variation
Da Huang *Rhizoma Rhei* 12 g
Mang Xiao *Mirabilitum* 9 g
Hou Po *Cortex Magnoliae officinalis* 15 g
Zhi Shi *Fructus Citri aurantii immaturus* 12 g
Shan Zhi Zi *Fructus Gardeniae jasminoidis* 6 g

Explanation

This formula is suitable for an acute or sub-acute

case of abdominal pain from Damp-Heat. As it contains Da Huang, it should not be used for more than a few weeks at a time.

- The first four herbs constitute the Da Cheng Qi Tang which resolves Damp-Heat by moving downwards. It stops abdominal pain by removing obstruction of Damp-Heat from the Intestines.
- **Zhi Zi** resolves Damp-Heat.

(b) Prescription

SHAO YAO TANG
Paeonia Decoction
Bai Shao *Radix Paeoniae albae* 20 g
Dang Gui *Radix Angelicae sinensis* 9 g
Zhi Gan Cao *Radix Glycyrrhizae uralensis prae-parata* 5 g
Huang Lian *Rhizoma Coptidis* 5 g
Huang Qin *Radix Scutellariae baicalensis* 9 g
Da Huang *Rhizoma Rhei* 9 g
Mu Xiang *Radix Saussureae* 5 g
Bing Lang *Semen Arecae catechu* 5 g
Rou Gui *Cortex Cinnamomi cassiae* 2 g

Explanation

This formula is used for abdominal pain from Damp-Heat causing diarrhoea with mucus and blood in the stools.

- **Bai Shao** combined with **Dang Gui** regulates Blood, and combined with **Gan Cao** it stops pain. Bai Shao is used in a high dose to stop pain, absorb fluids and stop diarrhoea.
- **Huang Lian** and **Huang Qin** clear Heat and drain Dampness.
- **Da Huang** helps to drain Damp-Heat by moving downwards.
- **Mu Xiang** and **Bing Lang** move Qi, eliminate stagnation and stop pain. They are pungent and combine with the bitter herbs Huang Lian and Huang Qin so that the pungent taste of the former two herbs opens, and the bitter taste of the latter two makes Qi descend. This combination helps to drain Damp-Heat, move Qi and stop pain.
- **Rou Gui** is added partly to balance the coldness of the other herbs and partly

according to the principle of using Heat to conduct Heat downwards.

(c) Prescription

HUANG QIN TANG
Scutellaria Decoction
Huang Qin *Radix Scutellariae baicalensis* 9 g
Bai Shao *Radix Paeoniae albae* 9 g
Zhi Gan Cao *Radix Glycyrrhizae uralensis prae-parata* 3 g
Da Zao *Fructus Ziziphi jujubae* 4 dates

Explanation

This formula is similar to the previous one in action. It is simpler and suitable for a less severe case of abdominal pain.
- **Huang Qin** drains Damp-Heat.
- **Bai Shao** absorbs leakages and moderates urgency.
- **Gan Cao** and **Da Zao** harmonize.

(d) Prescription

BAI TOU WENG TANG
Pulsatilla Decoction
Bai Tou Weng *Radix Pulsatillae chinensis* 15 g
Huang Bo *Cortex Phellodendri* 12 g
Huang Lian *Rhizoma Coptidis* 4 g
Qin Pi *Cortex Fraxini* 12 g

Explanation

This prescription clears Heat, drains Dampness, resolves Fire-Poison and stops abdominal pain. It is suitable if there is diarrhoea with a lot of mucus and blood, the pulse is Rapid and Slippery on both Rear positions, and the tongue is Red with red points on the root and with a sticky-yellow coating.

- **Bai Tou Weng** and **Qin Pi** resolve Fire-Poison from the Intestines and stop abdominal pain.
- **Huang Bo** and **Huang Lian** clear Heat and drain Dampness.

Variations

These variations apply to all the above four prescriptions.

- If there is severe pain add Yan Hu Suo *Rhizoma Corydalis yanhusuo*.
- If the manifestations of Dampness are very pronounced add (or increase) Huang Qin *Radix Scutellariae baicalensis*, Huang Bo *Cortex Phellodendri* and Yi Yi Ren *Semen Coicis lachryma jobi*.
- If there is blood in the stools add Qian Cao Gen *Radix Rubiae cordifoliae*, Huai Hua *Flos Sophorae japonicae immaturus*, or Di Yu *Radix Sanguisorbae officinalis*. If the bleeding is profuse and occurs every day, integrate the treatment indicated in this chapter with the principles outlined in the chapter on bleeding (ch. 30).

3. RETENTION OF FOOD

CLINICAL MANIFESTATIONS

Abdominal pain which is worse on pressure and after eating, a feeling of fullness in the abdomen, belching, sour regurgitation, diarrhoea which relieves the abdominal pain, constipation.
Tongue: thick coating.
Pulse: Slippery.

This condition may manifest either with diarrhoea or constipation. If the Spleen is weak there will be a tendency to diarrhoea.

TREATMENT PRINCIPLE

Dissolve food accumulation, eliminate stagnation.

ACUPUNCTURE

Ren-10 Xiawan, Ren-6 Qihai, SP-15 Daheng, SP-16 Fuai, ST-27 Daju, T.B.-8 Sanyangluo, ST-36 Zusanli, BL-25 Dachangshu, BL-27 Xiaochangshu. Reducing or even method. Moxa may be used if symptoms of Cold accompany the food retention.

Explanation

- **Ren-10** promotes the descending of Qi from the Stomach.

- **Ren-6** moves Qi in the lower abdomen which helps to resolve food stagnation.
- **SP-15** and **SP-16** promote the transforming of the Spleen, move the bowels and relieve abdominal fullness.
- **ST-27** makes Qi descend and stops abdominal pain.
- **T.B.-8** regulates the Three Burners and promotes the bowel movement.
- **ST-36** tonifies the Stomach and promotes the descending of Stomach-Qi.
- **BL-25** and **BL-27**, Back-Transporting points of the Large and Small Intestine respectively, resolve food accumulation in the Intestines.

HERBAL TREATMENT

(a) Prescription

BAO HE WAN
Preserving and Harmonizing Pill
Shan Zha *Fructus Crataegi* 9 g
Shen Qu *Massa Fermentata Medicinalis* 6 g
Lai Fu Zi *Semen Raphani sativi* 6 g
Ban Xia *Rhizoma Pinelliae ternatae* 6 g
Chen Pi *Pericarpium Citri reticulatae* 3 g
Fu Ling *Sclerotium Poriae cocos* 6 g
Lian Qiao *Fructus Forsythiae suspensae* 6 g

Explanation

This formula is for a mild case of retention of food and has already been explained in the chapter on "Headaches" (ch. 1).

(b) Prescription

ZHI SHI DAO ZHI WAN
Citrus aurantius Eliminating Stagnation Pill
Da Huang *Rhizoma Rhei* 15 g
Zhi Shi *Fructus Citri aurantii immaturus* 12 g
Huang Lian *Rhizoma Coptidis* 6 g
Huang Qin *Radix Scutellariae baicalensis* 6 g
Fu Ling *Sclerotium Poriae cocos* 6 g
Ze Xie *Rhizoma Alismatis orientalis* 6 g
Bai Zhu *Rhizoma Atractylodis macrocephalae* 6 g
Shen Qu *Massa Fermentata Medicinalis* 12 g

Explanation

This formula is used for a more severe case of retention of food causing abdominal pain and constipation with a very pronounced feeling of fullness in the abdomen.

- **Da Huang** dissolves food accumulation by moving downwards.
- **Zhi Shi** makes Qi descend and helps Da Huang to move downwards. It also relieves abdominal fullness.
- **Huang Lian** and **Huang Qin** clear Heat and drain Dampness. They therefore help to resolve food retention when this has given rise to Heat and Dampness.
- **Fu Ling** and **Ze Xie** drain Dampness and help to resolve food accumulation.
- **Bai Zhu** tonifies the Spleen and resolves Dampness.
- **Shen Qu** is a digestive herb which resolves food retention.

(i) Patent remedy

BAO HE WAN
Preserving and Harmonizing Pill
Shan Zha *Fructus Crataegi*
Shen Qu *Massa Fermentata Medicinalis*
Lai Fu Zi *Semen Raphani sativi*
Ban Xia *Rhizoma Pinelliae ternatae*
Chen Pi *Pericarpium Citri reticulatae*
Fu Ling *Sclerotium Poriae cocos*
Lian Qiao *Fructus Forsythiae suspensae*

Explanation

This remedy has the same ingredients and functions as the homonymous prescription above. It is a general remedy for retention of food.

The tongue presentation appropriate to this remedy is a thick tongue coating which may be white or yellow.

(ii) Patent remedy

KANG NING WAN
Health and Quiet Pill
Tian Ma *Rhizoma Gastrodiae elatae*
Bai Zhi *Radix Angelicae dahuricae*

Ju Hua *Flos Chrysanthemi morifolii*
Bo He *Herba Menthae*
Ge Gen *Radix Puerariae*
Tian Hua Fen *Radix Trichosanthis*
Cang Zhu *Rhizoma Atractylodis lanceae*
Yi Yi Ren *Semen Coicis lachryma jobi*
Fu Ling *Sclerotium Poriae cocos*
Mu Xiang *Radix Saussureae*
Hou Po *Cortex Magnoliae officinalis*
Chen Pi *Pericarpium Citri reticulatae*
Shen Qu *Massa Fermentata Medicinalis*
Huo Xiang *Herba Agastachis*
Gu Ya *Fructus Oryzae sativae germinatus*

Explanation

This remedy has a more wide-ranging action than the previous one as it resolves food retention and Dampness, moves Qi, stops pain and arrests diarrhoea.

The tongue presentation appropriate to this remedy is a slightly Red body with a thick-yellow coating.

(iii) Patent remedy

ZI SHENG WAN
Life-Providing Pill
Dang Shen *Radix Codonopsis pilosulae*
Bai Zhu *Rhizoma Atractylodis macrocephalae*
Yi Yi Ren *Semen Coicis lachryma jobi*
Shen Qu *Massa Fermentata Medicinalis*
Chen Pi *Pericarpium Citri reticulatae*
Shan Zha *Fructus Crataegi*
Qian Shi *Semen Euryales ferocis*
Shan Yao *Radix Dioscoreae oppositae*
Bian Dou *Semen Dolichoris lablab*
Mai Ya *Fructus Hordei vulgaris germinatus*
Fu Ling *Sclerotium Poriae cocos*
Lian Zi *Semen Nelumbinis nuciferae*
Jie Geng *Radix Platycodi grandiflori*
Huo Xiang *Herba Agastachis*
Gan Cao *Radix Glycyrrhizae uralensis*
Bai Dou Kou *Fructus Amomi cardamomi*
Huang Lian *Rhizoma Coptidis*

Explanation

This pill simultaneously resolves food retention

and tonifies the Spleen. It is therefore suitable for chronic retention of food against a background of Spleen deficiency.

The tongue presentation appropriate to this remedy is a Pale body with a moderately thick-dirty coating.

4. STAGNATION OF QI

CLINICAL MANIFESTATIONS

Abdominal pain and distension which are clearly related to the emotional state, feeling bloated, constipation, irritability, moodiness, belching, borborygmi.
Tongue: there may be no change in the body colour, but in more severe cases it may be Red on the sides.

This is due to stagnation of Liver-Qi in the abdomen. If Liver-Qi invades the Spleen there will be tiredness and alternation of constipation with diarrhoea.

TREATMENT PRINCIPLE

Pacify the Liver and move Qi.

ACUPUNCTURE

Ren-6 Qihai, P-6 Neiguan, P-7 Daling, T.B.-6 Zhigou, G.B.-34 Yanglingquan, LIV-3 Taichong, BL-18 Ganshu, SP-6 Sanyinjiao. Reducing or even method.

Explanation

- **Ren-6** moves Qi in the abdomen, especially if combined with G.B.-34.
- **P-6** moves Liver-Qi indirectly (thanks to the Pericardium's relation with the Liver within the Terminal Yin channels), calms the Mind and settles the Ethereal Soul. It is a very important and effective point for this condition.
- **P-7** is used instead of P-6 if the emotional

stress is more severe, especially if due to the breaking up of relationships.
- **T.B.-6** moves Qi in the abdomen.
- **G.B.-34** moves Liver-Qi. In combination with Ren-6, it moves Liver-Qi in the lower abdomen.
- **LIV-3** and **BL-18** move Liver-Qi, stop pain, calm the Mind and settle the Ethereal Soul.
- **SP-6** soothes the Liver, stops abdominal pain and calms the Mind.

HERBAL TREATMENT

(a) Prescription

CHAI HU SU GAN TANG
Bupleurum Soothing the Liver Decoction
Chai Hu *Radix Bupleuri* 6 g
Bai Shao *Radix Paeoniae albae* 4.5 g
Zhi Ke *Fructus Citri aurantii* 4.5 g
Chen Pi *Pericarpium Citri reticulatae* 6 g
Xiang Fu *Rhizoma Cyperi rotundi* 4.5 g
Chuan Xiong *Radix Ligustici wallichii* 4.5 g
Zhi Gan Cao *Radix Glycyrrhizae uralensis praeparata* 1.5 g

Explanation

- **Chai Hu**, **Zhi Ke**, **Chen Pi** and **Xiang Fu** move Liver-Qi and promote the descending of Qi in the Intestines.
- **Bai Shao** pacifies the Liver, stops pain and calms the Mind.
- **Chuan Xiong** moves the Qi portion of Blood and stops pain.
- **Gan Cao** harmonizes and, in combination with Bai Shao, stops pain.

Variations

- If stagnant Liver-Qi invades the Spleen and there are pronounced symptoms of Spleen deficiency, especially diarrhoea, add Dang Shen *Radix Codonopsis pilosulae* and Huang Qi *Radix Astragali membranacei*.
- If stagnant Liver-Qi has turned into Fire add Zhi Zi *Fructus Gardeniae jasminoidis* and Mu Dan Pi *Cortex Moutan radicis*.
- If stagnant Liver-Qi has invaded the Spleen

and this, in turn, has led to the formation of Dampness add Fu Ling *Sclerotium Poriae cocos* and Cang Zhu *Rhizoma Atractylodis lanceae*.

- If pain is very severe add Yan Hu Suo *Rhizoma Corydalis yanhusuo*.
- If stagnation of Liver-Qi occurs against a background of Liver-Blood deficiency (common in women) add Dang Gui *Radix Angelicae sinensis* and increase the dosage of Bai Shao *Radix Paeoniae albae*.
- If stagnation of Liver-Qi occurs against a background of Liver-Yin deficiency (also common in women) add Dang Gui *Radix Angelicae sinensis* and Gou Qi Zi *Fructus Lycii chinensis*, and replace Xiang Fu with Chuan Lian Zi *Fructus Meliae toosendan*.

(b) Prescription

XIAO YAO SAN
Free and Easy Wanderer Powder
Bo He *Herba Menthae* 3 g
Chai Hu *Radix Bupleuri* 9 g
Dang Gui *Radix Angelicae sinensis* 9 g
Bai Shao *Radix Paeoniae albae* 12 g
Bai Zhu *Rhizoma Atractylodis macrocephalae* 9 g
Fu Ling *Sclerotium Poriae cocos* 15 g
Zhi Gan Cao *Radix Glycyrrhizae uralensis praeparata* 6 g
Sheng Jiang *Rhizoma Zingiberis officinalis recens* 3 slices

Explanation

This formula is used instead of the previous one when the stagnation of Liver-Qi occurs against a background of Liver-Blood deficiency, as frequently happens in women. It is also the main prescription to harmonize Liver and Spleen, when stagnant Liver-Qi invades the Spleen. Thus, the condition addressed by this formula is characterized by a combination of Excess (stagnation of Liver-Qi) and Deficiency (of Liver-Blood and Spleen-Qi). This is in contrast to the previous formula which addresses a purely Excess condition, i.e. just stagnation of Liver-Qi. Apart from other symptoms and signs, the pulse pictures appropriate to each of these two for-mulae can be clearly differentiated: the pulse picture appropriate to Chai Hu Su Gan Tang is a Wiry and Full pulse all over, whilst that appropriate to Xiao Yao San is a pulse which is slightly Weak on the right side (reflecting Spleen deficiency) and Fine and slightly Wiry on the left side (reflecting Liver-Blood deficiency and stagnation of Liver-Qi).

- **Bo He** and **Chai Hu** gently move Liver-Qi. Women are more sensitive to Chai Hu than men and this is another reason why this formula is so widely used in women's problems.
- **Dang Gui** and **Bai Shao** nourish Liver-Blood. Bai Shao also harmonizes the Liver and, together with Gan Cao, moderates urgency and stops pain.
- **Bai Zhu** and **Fu Ling** tonify the Spleen.
- **Zhi Gan Cao** tonifies the Spleen, stops pain and harmonizes.
- **Sheng Jiang** harmonizes.

Patent remedy

SHU GAN WAN
Pacifying the Liver Pill
Chuan Lian Zi *Fructus Meliae toosendan*
Jiang Huang *Rhizoma Curcumae longae*
Chen Xiang *Lignum Aquilariae*
Yan Hu Suo *Rhizoma Corydalis yanhusuo*
Mu Xiang *Radix Saussureae*
Bai Dou Kou *Fructus Amomi cardamomi*
Bai Shao *Radix Paeoniae albae*
Fu Ling *Sclerotium Poriae cocos*
Zhi Ke *Fructus Citri aurantii*
Chen Pi *Pericarpium Citri reticulatae*
Sha Ren *Fructus seu Semen Amomi*
Hou Po *Cortex Magnoliae officinalis*

Explanation

This remedy moves Liver-Qi and eliminates stagnation and is widely used for abdominal pain from Qi stagnation. It should be noted that it contains many warm and pungent herbs which, with prolonged use, may injure Yin. This remedy should therefore be used with caution if there is some Yin deficiency.

Case history

A 44-year-old man had been suffering from what had been diagnosed as irritable bowel syndrome. His bowel movements alternated between diarrhoea and constipation, the latter being more frequent. The stools were often small and round and he suffered abdominal pain on both lateral sides without much distending feeling. He also suffered from hiatus hernia which caused heartburn, belching and dry vomiting. His sleep was disturbed. His tongue was of a normal colour and only slightly Red on the sides; it had a very sticky coating all over. His pulse was Slippery and slightly Overflowing on the Stomach position.

Diagnosis
In this case there is stagnant Liver-Qi invading both Spleen and Stomach. The symptoms of stagnant Liver-Qi invading the Spleen are abdominal pain, diarrhoea and slightly Red sides of the tongue. The symptoms of stagnant Liver-Qi invading the Stomach are heartburn, belching, dry vomiting and a slightly Overflowing pulse on the Stomach position. The deficiency of Spleen-Qi has also given rise to Dampness causing the pulse to be Slippery and the tongue to have a sticky coating.

Treatment principle
The treatment principle adopted was to tonify the Spleen and move Liver-Qi. This patient was treated only with acupuncture.

Acupuncture
The points used were chosen from the following:

- **SP-4** Gongsun on the left with **P-6** Neiguan on the right, with even method, to open the Penetrating Vessel. This extraordinary vessel subdues rebellious Qi in the abdomen and chest and is therefore especially well indicated for stagnation of Liver-Qi in the abdomen and epigastrium.
- **Ren-13** Shangwan, with even method, to subdue rebellious Stomach-Qi.
- **ST-40** Fenglong, with reducing method, to resolve Dampness and Phlegm and subdue rebellious Stomach-Qi.
- **SP-6** Sanyinjiao, with even method, to resolve Dampness and stop abdominal pain.
- **SP-15** Daheng, with even method, to move the stools and eliminate stagnation in the Lower abdomen.
- **Ren-12** Zhongwan, with reinforcing method, to tonify Spleen-Qi.
- **G.B.-34** Yanglingquan, with even method, to move Liver-Qi and eliminate stagnation.
- **Ren-6** Qihai, with even method, to move Qi in the Lower abdomen.
- **ST-37** Shangjuxu, Lower Sea point of the Large Intestine, with even method, to regulate Qi of this organ.

- **ST-39** Xiajuxu, Lower Sea point of the Small Intestine, with even method, to stop abdominal pain.
- **BL-25** Dachangshu, Back-Transporting point of the Large Intestine, with even method, to regulate Qi of this organ and move the stools.
- **BL-20** Pishu, with reinforcing method, to tonify Spleen-Qi.
- **BL-18** Ganshu, with even method, to move Liver-Qi and eliminate stagnation.

After 10 treatments and advice on diet, this patient was completely cured. He is still seen every 3 months and his symptoms have not recurred.

Case history

A 45-year-old woman had been suffering from umbilical and abdominal pain for over 10 years. The abdominal pain, which was accompanied by distension, was worse after eating, after emotional upsets and when tired. The pain was relieved by pressure, by lying down and by the application of heat. The abdominal pain also extended to the hypogastric region and the pain in this area was aggravated when carrying heavy objects. The bowel movements were slightly constipated. Her voice was very weak and rather weepy in sound and her eyes lacked glitter and looked very sad. Her tongue was Red, redder on the sides and tip, with a yellow coating. It also had red points along the sides and on the tip. Her pulse was extremely Weak and Minute and very slightly Wiry on the left side.

Diagnosis
This is a complex condition characterized by a combination of Deficiency and Excess. First of all, there is stagnation of Liver-Qi and its symptoms are abdominal pain and distension which is aggravated by emotional stress and the slightly Wiry quality of the pulse on the left side. Stagnation of Liver-Qi has turned into Fire and this is shown by the Red colour of the tongue body and the fact that it is redder with red points on the sides. Liver-Fire has also affected the Heart giving rise to Heart-Fire as evidenced by the tongue's red tip with red points. The Red colour of the tongue and the redder colour with red points on the sides and tip clearly show the emotional origin of the problem. If there is Fire why does the abdominal pain improve with the application of heat? This is because heat improves not only abdominal pain which is caused by Cold, but also that caused by stagnation as heat moves Qi and Blood. The second question is: if there is stagnation of Liver-Qi and Liver-Fire, both Excess conditions, why is the pulse so Weak and Minute and only very slightly Wiry? The reason is that there is an underlying, very long-standing Deficiency condition of the Lungs and Spleen. In fact, the deficiency of the Lungs was, in my

opinion, at the root of the problem and caused by deep emotional problems such as sadness and grief. The look of her eyes and her voice confirmed this. Sadness affects Lungs and Heart and, after a long time, it gives rise to stagnation and Fire. It is even possible that the Lung deficiency was the origin of the stagnation of Liver-Qi: this happens when the deficient Lungs fail to control the Liver, or, in 5-Element terms, Metal fails to control Wood. The deficiency of Lungs and Spleen is evident from the Weak and Minute pulse, the aggravation of pain from tiredness and the weak voice. Finally, the hypogastric pain elicited by carrying weights is due to sinking of Spleen-Qi probably causing a slight prolapse of the bladder.

Treatment principle
The treatment principle adopted was to move Liver-Qi, tonify the Spleen, and strengthen the Lungs. It is not necessary to clear Liver-Fire, as when this derives from stagnation of Liver-Qi, it is sufficient to move Liver-Qi and eliminate stagnation. This patient was treated with acupuncture and patent remedies.

Acupuncture
The acupuncture points (with reducing or even method for those which eliminate stagnation or drain Fire and reinforcing for those which tonify Lungs and Spleen) were selected from the following:

- Ren-6 Qihai, to move Qi in the lower abdomen.
- LU-7 Lieque to tonify the Lungs and settle the Corporeal Soul. This point is particularly effective for sadness and grief affecting the Lungs.
- LIV-3 Taichong, **LIV-14** Qimen and **G.B.-34** Yanglingquan to move Liver-Qi.
- ST-36 Zusanli and **BL-20** to tonify the Spleen.
- ST-39 Xiajuxu to stop abdominal pain.
- SP-6 Sanyinjiao to regulate Liver and Spleen and stop abdominal pain.

Herbal treatment
The first patent remedy used was Yue Ju Wan *Gardenia-Ligusticum Pill* to move Liver-Qi and drain Fire. This pill is excellent for stagnation deriving from emotional stress. After a few weeks, attention was turned to treating the underlying deficiency of Spleen and Lungs as well with two remedies: Xiao Yao Wan *Free and Easy Wanderer Pill* to move Liver-Qi and tonify Spleen-Qi and Liu Jun Zi Wan *Six Gentlemen Pill* to tonify Lungs and Spleen.

This patient's reaction to treatment even surpassed my expectations as her abdominal pain went completely after only 2 acupuncture treatments. However, I continued to treat her for 3 months until there was an improvement in her pulse.

Case history

A 40-year-old man had been suffering from

abdominal pain and distension for "a long time". The distension was particularly pronounced and was aggravated by emotional strain. His bowel movements alternated between constipation and diarrhoea. He felt easily tired and was very tense. His tongue was slightly Red on the sides, Swollen, and had a yellow coating (Plate 16.1). His pulse was slightly Wiry and Rapid.

Diagnosis
This is a clear case of Liver-Qi stagnation. Stagnant Liver-Qi is just about to turn into Liver-Fire as evidenced by the slightly Red sides of the tongue.

Treatment principle
The principle of treatment used was to move Liver-Qi and eliminate stagnation. This patient was treated with herbs and acupuncture.

Acupuncture
The main acupuncture points, needled with reducing method to eliminate stagnation and reinforcing method to tonify the Spleen, were selected from the following:

- SP-4 Gongsun and **P-6** Neiguan to open the Penetrating Vessel and regulate Qi in the abdomen.
- HE-7 Shenmen to calm the Mind.
- LIV-3 Taichong and **G.B.-34** Yanglingquan to move Liver-Qi.
- Ren-6 Qihai to move Qi in the lower abdomen.
- BL-20 Pishu and **ST-36** Zusanli to tonify the Spleen.
- BL-18 Ganshu to move Liver-Qi.
- ST-39 Xiajuxu and **SP-6** Sanyinjiao to move Qi and stop abdominal pain.

Herbal treatment
The prescription used was a variation of Chai Hu Su Gan Tang *Bupleurum Soothing the Liver Decoction*:

Chai Hu *Radix Bupleuri*
Bai Shao *Radix Paeoniae albae*
Zhi Ke *Fructus Citri aurantii*
Gan Cao *Radix Glycyrrhizae uralensis*
Chen Pi *Pericarpium Citri reticulatae*
Xiang Fu *Rhizoma Cyperi rotundi*
Chuan Xiong *Radix Ligustici wallichii*
Zhi Zi *Fructus Gardeniae jasminoidis*
Mu Dan Pi *Cortex Moutan radicis*

Explanation
- The first seven herbs form the Chai Hu Su Gan Tang to move Liver-Qi, eliminate stagnation and stop pain. This formula is excellent to stop pain from stagnation.
- **Zhi Zi** and **Dan Pi** were added to clear Liver-Heat.

This patient showed 50% improvement after 5 acupuncture treatments and herbal decoctions and he is still being treated at the time of writing.

5. STASIS OF BLOOD

CLINICAL MANIFESTATIONS

Severe abdominal pain, masses in the abdomen, dark complexion.
Tongue: Purple.
Pulse: Deep and Choppy or Deep and Firm.

TREATMENT PRINCIPLE

Move Blood and eliminate stasis.

ACUPUNCTURE

Ren-6 Qihai, P-6 Neiguan, P-7 Daling, T.B.-6 Zhigou, G.B.-34 Yanglingquan, LIV-3 Taichong, BL-18 Ganshu, SP-6 Sanyinjiao, SP-10 Xuehai, BL-17 Geshu, KI-6 Zhaohai and LU-7 Lieque. Reducing or even method.

Explanation

- **Ren-6** moves Qi in the abdomen, especially if combined with G.B.-34. Moving Qi will help to move Blood.
- **P-6** indirectly moves Liver-Qi (because of the Pericardium's relation with the Liver within the Terminal Yin channels), calms the Mind, and settles the Ethereal Soul. It is a very important and effective point for this condition as it also moves Blood.
- **P-7** is used instead of P-6 if the emotional stress is stronger.
- **T.B.-6** moves Qi in the abdomen.
- **G.B.-34** moves Liver-Qi. In combination with Ren-6, it moves Liver-Qi in the lower abdomen.
- **LIV-3** and **BL-18**, in combination with BL-17 (see below), move Liver-Qi and Liver-Blood, stop pain, calm the Mind, and settle the Ethereal Soul.
- **SP-6** soothes the Liver, stops abdominal pain and calms the Mind.
- **SP-10** and **BL-17** regulate Blood and eliminate stasis.
- **KI-6** and **LU-7** in combination open the Yin Heel Vessel which removes obstructions and moves Qi and Blood in the Lower Burner.

HERBAL TREATMENT

Prescription

SHAO FU ZHU YU TANG
Lower Abdomen Eliminating Stasis Decoction
Xiao Hui Xiang *Fructus Foeniculi vulgaris* 6 g
Gan Jiang *Rhizoma Zingiberis officinalis* 2 g
Rou Gui *Cortex Cinnamomi cassiae* 1.5 g
Yan Hu Suo *Rhizoma Corydalis yanhusuo* 6 g
Mo Yao *Myrrha* 6 g
Pu Huang *Pollen Typhae* 6 g
Wu Ling Zhi *Excrementum Trogopteri* 4.5 g
Dang Gui *Radix Angelicae sinensis* 9 g
Chuan Xiong *Radix Ligustici wallichii* 4.5 g
Chi Shao Yao *Radix Paeoniae rubrae* 6 g

Explanation

- **Xiao Hui Xiang, Gan Jiang** and **Rou Gui** warm the Lower Burner and scatter Cold.
- **Yan Hu Suo, Mo Yao, Pu Huang** and **Wu Ling Zhi** move Blood and eliminate stasis. Yan Hu Suo is specific to stop pain from stasis of Blood.
- **Dang Gui, Chuan Xiong** and **Chi Shao** harmonize Blood.

Variations

This formula is warming and is therefore suitable for treating stasis of Blood with a background of Cold and Yang deficiency.

- If there are no prominent signs of Cold, eliminate Gan Jiang and Rou Gui or reduce their dosages.
- If there are signs of Heat, eliminate Gan Jiang and Rou Gui, increase the dosage of Chi Shao and add Mu Dan Pi *Cortex Moutan radicis*.
- If the abdominal pain follows abdominal surgery with resulting adhesions add Ze Lan *Herba Lycopi lucidi*, Hong Hua *Flos Carthami tinctorii*, and Tao Ren *Semen Persicae*.
- If there is bleeding from stasis of Blood increase the dosage of Pu Huang and add San Qi *Radix Notoginseng*.

DEFICIENCY CONDITIONS

DEFICIENCY OF QI AND EMPTY-COLD IN THE ABDOMEN

CLINICAL MANIFESTATIONS

Dull abdominal pain which comes in bouts and improves after rest, the application of warmth and pressure, tiredness, feeling cold, desire for warm drinks, loose stools, depression, slight breathlessness.
Tongue: Pale.
Pulse: Weak.

This is a condition of deficiency of Spleen-Yang with some internal Empty-Cold.

TREATMENT PRINCIPLE

Tonify Qi, warm Yang.

ACUPUNCTURE

ST-36 Zusanli, SP-6 Sanyinjiao, ST-37 Shangjuxu, ST-39 Xiajuxu, Ren-6 Qihai, Ren-12 Zhongwan, BL-20 Pishu, BL-21 Weishu, BL-25 Dachangshu. Reinforcing method. Moxa should be used.

Explanation

– **ST-36** and **SP-6** tonify Stomach and Spleen and promote the transformation and transportation of Qi in the abdomen. SP-6 also stops lower abdominal pain.
– **ST-37** and **ST-39** regulate the Large and Small Intestines. ST-39 is specific for abdominal pain.
– **Ren-6** moves Qi in the abdomen. With moxa, especially the moxa box, it is specific for abdominal pain from Empty-Cold.
– **Ren-12**, **BL-20** and **BL-21** regulate Stomach and Intestines.
– **BL-25**, Back-Transporting point of the Large Intestine, strengthens the descending movement of the Large Intestine.

HERBAL TREATMENT

Prescription

XIAO JIAN ZHONG TANG

Minor Strengthening the Centre Decoction
Yi Tang *Saccharum Granorum* 30 g
Bai Shao *Radix Paeoniae albae* 18 g
Gui Zhi *Ramulus Cinnamomi cassiae* 9 g
Sheng Jiang *Rhizoma Zingiberis officinalis recens* 10 g
Zhi Gan Cao *Radix Glycyrrhizae uralensis praeparata* 6 g
Da Zao *Fructus Ziziphi jujubae* 12 dates

Explanation

– **Yi Tang**, **Zhi Gan Cao** and **Da Zao** are sweet in taste: they tonify Qi and stop pain of an Empty nature.
– **Gui Zhi** and **Sheng Jiang** warm the channels and expel Cold.
– **Bai Shao**, in combination with Gan Cao, stops pain.

Variations

– If the condition is characterized by both a Deficiency and an Excess with pronounced Cold in the Intestines, add Gao Liang Jiang *Rhizoma Alpiniae officinari* and Gan Jiang *Rhizoma Zingiberis officinalis*.
– If the deficiency of Qi is pronounced add Huang Qi *Radix Astragali membranacei*: this addition transforms the above formula into Huang Qi Jian Zhong Tang *Astragalus Strengthening the Centre Decoction*.
– If there are pronounced symptoms of Dampness add Bai Zhu *Rhizoma Atractylodis macrocephalae*, Fu Ling *Sclerotium Poriae cocos* and Yi Yi Ren *Semen Coicis lachryma jobi*.
– If there are symptoms of retention of food add Shan Zha *Fructus Crataegi*, Lai Fu Zi *Semen Raphani sativi* and Shen Qu *Massa Fermentata Medicinalis*.

Patent remedy

LI ZHONG WAN
Regulating the Centre Pill
Gan Jiang *Rhizoma Zingiberis officinalis*
Bai Zhu *Rhizoma Atractylodis macrocephalae*
Dang Shen *Radix Codonopsis pilosulae*
Gan Cao *Radix Glycyrrhizae uralensis*

Explanation

This remedy tonifies Spleen-Yang and expels Cold from the abdomen. It is effective in abdominal pain from Deficient-Cold.

The tongue presentation appropriate to this remedy is a Pale and wet tongue.

Prognosis and prevention

Both acupuncture and Chinese herbs are very effective in abdominal pain. Acupuncture on its own can treat the patterns of stagnation of Qi, Cold in the Intestines and Qi deficiency with Empty-Cold very effectively. The other three patterns of Damp-Heat in the Intestines, retention of food and stasis of Blood also respond to acupuncture, but better results are obtained with herbal medicine or a combination of the two.

The easiest pattern to treat is that of stagnation of Qi, and the most difficult ones are those of Damp-Heat and stasis of Blood in the Intestines.

Other factors influencing the prognosis have to be based on the Western diagnosis. If the abdominal pain is caused by ulcerative colitis or Crohn's disease, the course of treatment will be very protracted indeed and it may take up to 2 years to effect a cure.

As for prevention, any patient who is prone to abdominal pain or has been cured of one, should follow certain precautions. In terms of diet, patients should avoid eating an excessive amount of cold-energy foods as these would aggravate not only Cold in the Intestines but also stagnation of Qi, Qi deficiency, stasis of Blood and retention of food. In particular, they should avoid drinking large amounts of cold drinks.

Moderate exercise is essential; this is especially important if the patient has been suffering from abdominal pain from Qi or Blood stagnation, but it will also alleviate Dampness and retention of food. The patient should also avoid sleeping for a long time (more than half an hour) after lunch as this tends to increase Dampness in the Intestines. However, a short nap (under half an hour) after lunch (a habit very rare in Anglo-Saxon countries, but quite common in Latin countries and in Asia) is beneficial to the Stom-ach. Patients should also avoid eating an excessive amount of sour foods: these have already been listed in the chapter on "Headaches" (ch. 1).

Finally, women who regularly practise meditation should not do so in a sitting position as this tends to increase (or cause) stagnation of Qi or Blood in the Lower Burner. However, meditation in a standing position is very beneficial for women.

Western differentiation

In abdominal pain *not* of gynaecological origin, the Western medical diagnosis must identify the organ involved. This may be:

– Kidney
– Appendix
– Large Intestine
– Small Intestine.

KIDNEY

PYELONEPHRITIS

Pyelonephritis is an inflammation of the kidney and its pelvis due to bacterial infection.

The pain normally starts in one loin but it may radiate to the lateral abdominal region.

RENAL CALCULUS

Renal stones are formed by precipitation in crystalline or granular form of acids in the urine. Stones may be made of uric acid, calcium oxalate or calcium phosphate.

The pain usually starts in one loin and radiates to the lateral abdominal region and then down to the groin. However, it may also start in the lateral abdominal region and radiate to the back. The pain, due to the violent contraction of kidney-pelvis and ureter, is sudden and very severe. It persists for 12–24 hours and is accompanied by frequency and difficulty of micturition, nausea, vomiting, sweating and sometimes shock.

From a Chinese perspective, this usually manifests with symptoms of Damp-Heat and, in chronic conditions, frequently occurs against a background of Kidney-Yin deficiency.

APPENDIX

APPENDICITIS

Appendicitis is one of the most difficult diagnoses to make in abdominal pain. The pain usually starts around the umbilicus and only settles in the right abdominal region when the inflammation spreads. It is accompanied by nausea and vomiting and the tongue coating is thick.

There is tenderness in the right lower quadrant on McBurney's point (Fig. 16.3).

From the acupuncture point of view, there is also deep tenderness on the extra point Lanweixue situated roughly half-way between ST-36 Zusanli and ST-37 Shangjuxu.

LARGE INTESTINE

DIVERTICULITIS

Diverticulitis consists in inflamed hernial protrusions in the colon. It is more common after 50. The pain is unilateral, more often on the left side, and is accompanied by alternation of constipation and diarrhoea.

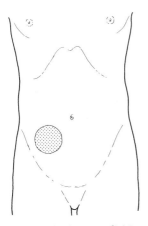

Fig. 16.3 McBurney's point in appendicitis

CARCINOMA OF COLON OR RECTUM

Carcinoma of the colon or rectum is more common over 50 years of age. Chronic ulcerative colitis is a predisposing factor.

There are three cardinal symptoms and signs for this condition:

– Lateral abdominal pain
– A change in bowel habit (towards either constipation or diarrhoea)
– Blood in the stools.

Thus, in an patient over 50 with the above symptoms and signs, a Western diagnosis is imperative.

The pain is usually lateral but it may also be umbilical. The stools may be thin and long. In advanced stages there is marked debility and loss of weight.

From a Chinese perspective, this usually manifests with symptoms of Damp-Heat and stasis of Blood.

IRRITABLE BOWEL SYNDROME

Irritable bowel syndrome consists in motor-secretory overactivity of the colon due to excessive parasympathetic stimulation.

The pain is lateral or diffuse in the whole lower abdominal region and it varies from a vague dragging ache to severe spastic pain. It is always accompanied by marked distension and usually alternation of constipation and loose stools. The stools are often small and round or small, thin and cigar-shaped. There is also fatigue and anxiety.

From the point of view of Chinese medicine, this usually manifests with symptoms of stagnant Liver-Qi invading the Spleen.

ULCERATIVE COLITIS

Ulcerative colitis consists in inflammation and ulceration of the intestinal mucosa. It is more common between the ages of 20 and 40.

The two main manifestations are abdominal pain and diarrhoea with mucus and blood.

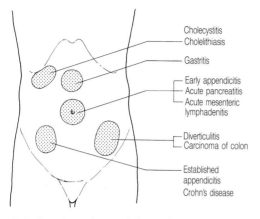

Fig. 16.4   Locations of acute abdominal pain

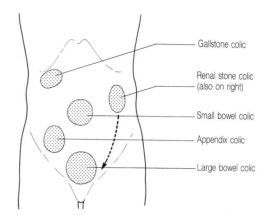

Fig. 16.5   Locations of abdominal colic

In Chinese medicine, this usually manifests with symptoms of Damp-Heat in the Intestines.

SMALL INTESTINE

CROHN'S DISEASE

Crohn's disease is characterized by localized areas of inflammation in the small intestine. In a few cases, it may also affect the large intestine.

The main clinical features are abdominal pain which occurs most frequently on the right side.

An abdominal mass may be palpable: this consists of inflamed loops of bowel bound together. Diarrhoea is usually present but, in contrast to ulcerative colitis, there is no mucus or blood, unless the large bowel is involved.

In chronic cases there may also be weight loss and low-grade fever.

Figure 16.4 summarizes the common locations of acute abdominal pain, while Figure 16.5 illustrates the locations of abdominal colic. By "colic" is meant a pain which is severe and paroxysmal in occurrence. It may be acute or chronic.

END NOTES

1. He Ren 1979 A Popular Guide to the Essential Prescriptions of the Golden Chest (*Jin Gui Yao Lue Tong Su Jiang Hua* 金匱要略通俗讲话), Shanghai Science Publishing House, Shanghai, p. 54. The "Essential Prescriptions of the Golden Chest" itself was written by Zhang Zhong Jing and first published *c.* AD 200.

Abdominal masses 17

积
聚

Abdominal masses are called *Ji Ju*. *Ji* indicates actual abdominal masses which are fixed and immovable; if there is an associated pain, its location is fixed. These masses are due to stasis of Blood. I shall call them "Blood masses". *Ju* indicates abdominal masses which come and go, do not have a fixed location and are movable. If there is an associated pain, it too comes and goes and changes location. Such masses are due to stagnation of Qi. I shall call them "Qi masses".

Actual abdominal lumps therefore pertain to the category of abdominal masses and specifically *Ji* masses, i.e. Blood masses.

Another name for abdominal masses was *Zheng Jia*, *Zheng* being equivalent to *Ji*, i.e. actual, fixed masses and *Jia* being equivalent to *Ju*, i.e. non-substantial masses from stagnation of Qi. The two terms *Zheng Jia* normally referred to abdominal masses occurring only in women; but although these masses are more frequent in women, they do occur in men as well.

The term *Ji Ju* appears in the "Classic of Difficulties" which clearly distinguishes the two types:

Ji masses pertain to Yin and Ju masses to Yang . . . When Qi accumulates it gives rise to Ji masses, when it gathers it gives rise to Ju masses. Ji masses arise from the Yin organs and Ju masses from the Fu organs. Ji masses have a fixed location and pain, and have boundaries above and below, and edges to the right and left [i.e. they have clearly defined borders]. Ju masses seem to start from nowhere, without a boundary above and below and with a moving pain.[1]

The "Prescriptions of the Golden Chest" by Zhang Zhong Jing says: *"Ji masses arise from the Yin organs and they cannot be moved; Ju masses arise from the Yang organs, they come and go, the pain has no fixed location, and they are easier to treat."[2]*

The "General Treatise on the Aetiology and Symptomatology of Diseases" (AD 610) says:

Abdominal masses are due to cold and heat not being regulated [i.e. exposure to extremes of weather], irregular diet and stagnation of the Qi of the Yin organs. If they do not move they are called Zheng; if they are movable they are called Jia. "Jia" implies the meaning of "false": this is because these masses can come and go and are not actual masses.[3]

Aetiology and pathology

1. EMOTIONAL STRAIN

Emotional strain is the most common cause of the formation of abdominal masses. Anger, especially when repressed, frustration, resentment, hatred can all lead to stagnation of Liver-Qi and, in the long run, to stasis of Liver-Blood. The Liver channel plays an important role in the movement of Qi in the lower abdomen and, in women, Liver-Blood plays a paramount role in the circulation of Blood in this area.

Anger and its related emotions are not the only ones leading to stagnation of Qi. Other emotions such as worry may also lead to stagnation of Qi and Blood but they affect more the Lungs and Heart and therefore the chest rather than the lower abdomen.

2. DIET

Diet is another important aetiological factor in the formation of abdominal masses. Irregular eating or the excessive consumption of cold and raw foods may lead to the formation of Cold in the lower abdomen. Cold contracts and naturally interferes with the circulation of Qi and Blood, especially Blood, and may lead to stasis of Blood.

Excessive consumption of greasy foods, on the other hand, impairs the Spleen and may lead to the formation of Dampness and Phlegm. If this settles in the lower abdomen, it leads to the formation of abdominal masses. There is also an interaction between Phlegm and stasis of Blood so that one may lead to or aggravate the other.

3. EXTERNAL PATHOGENIC FACTORS

External pathogenic factors are less important in the aetiology of abdominal masses. The most important pathogenic factor is external Cold which can invade the lower abdomen and impair the circulation of Blood, eventually leading to stasis of Blood. The "Spiritual Axis" in chapter 66 says: *"Ji masses are due to Cold."*[4]

External Dampness may invade the channels of the legs and then creep up the legs to settle in the lower abdomen where, in the long run, it transforms into Phlegm and may give rise to abdominal masses.

As for pathology, abdominal masses are always characterized by either stagnation of Qi or stasis of Blood, the former being non-substantial and the latter substantial masses. In addition to stagnation, there may also be Phlegm. However, in all cases of abdominal masses there is always an underlying deficiency of Qi. Deficient Qi fails to transport and transform and, leading to stagnation of Qi and Blood, it allows masses to form.

Masses from stagnation of Qi come and go, are movable on palpation and change location. If there is pain, the pain has no fixed location and is accompanied by a pronounced feeling of distension.

Masses from stasis of Blood are fixed in location, they are not movable on palpation and feel quite hard. If there is pain, the pain is fixed and stabbing in character.

Masses from Phlegm feel soft on palpation and have a fixed location. There is usually no pain.

Differentiation and treatment

The treatment of abdominal masses is always based on moving Qi and Blood. However, there are other factors to take into account depending on the stage of the disease. In the beginning stages of the condition the pathogenic factor (stagnation of Qi or stasis of Blood) is relatively weak and the body's Qi relatively strong. In the middle stage, the body's Qi is weakening and the pathogenic factor becoming more prominent. In the late stages, the pathogenic factor is very prominent and the masses very developed while the body's Qi is very weak. Thus, irrespective of the pathogenic factor involved, the principle of treatment must be guided by the stage of the condition:

- In the beginning stages primarily resolve the

pathogenic factor, i.e. move Qi and Blood and resolve Phlegm
- In the middle stages resolve the pathogenic factor and tonify the body's Qi simultaneously
- In the late stages primarily tonify the body's Qi and secondarily resolve the pathogenic factor.

Thus, the formulae given below are only a guideline. The approach adopted should be chosen according to the pattern of the disease, but the formulae must be modified in every case according to its stage.

Furthermore, all prescriptions indicated below should be modified with the addition of "softening" herbs, i.e. herbs which soften masses: this is particularly necessary for masses from stasis of Blood or Phlegm. Softening herbs are:

Yi Yi Ren *Semen Coicis lachryma jobi*
Zhe Bei Mu *Bulbus Fritillariae thunbergii*
Hai Zao *Herba Sargassii*
Kun Bu *Thallus Algae*
Chuan Shan Jia *Squama Manitis pentadactylae*
Xia Ku Cao *Spica Prunellae vulgaris*
Gui Ban *Plastrum Testudinis*
Mu Li *Concha Ostreae*
Jiang Can *Bombyx batryticatus*
Bie Jia *Carapax Trionycis*
Wa Leng Zi *Concha Arcae*
Hai Dai *Laminaria japonica*

As for the relative application of acupuncture and herbal medicine, especially for Blood masses, the herbal treatment is primary in relation to acupuncture.

The patterns discussed are:

QI MASSES

Liver-Qi stagnation
Retention of food and Phlegm

BLOOD MASSES

Stagnation of Qi and Blood
Stasis of Blood knotted in the Interior
Deficiency of Upright Qi and stasis of Blood

QI MASSES

1. LIVER-QI STAGNATION

CLINICAL MANIFESTATIONS

Movable abdominal masses which come and go, abdominal distension and pain which come and go with the masses, a feeling of discomfort in the hypochondrium, depression, moodiness, irritability, alternation of constipation and diarrhoea.
Tongue: the body colour may be normal or slightly Red on the sides. Thick coating on the root.
Pulse: Wiry.

TREATMENT PRINCIPLE

Soothe the Liver, eliminate stagnation, move Qi and dissolve masses.

ACUPUNCTURE

G.B.-34 Yanglingquan, Ren-6 Qihai, LIV-3 Taichong, T.B.-6 Zhigou, P-6 Neiguan, SP-6 Sanyinjiao, LU-7 Lieque and KI-6 Zhaohai. Reducing or even method.

Explanation

- **G.B.-34** and **Ren-6** in combination, move Liver-Qi in the lower abdomen.
- **LIV-3** moves Liver-Qi.
- **P-6** indirectly moves Liver-Qi and calms the Mind.
- **T.B.-6** moves Liver-Qi.
- **SP-6** moves Qi and soothes the Liver. Specifically, it treats the lower abdomen.
- **LU-7** and **KI-6** are used in women to open the Directing Vessel and move Qi in the lower abdomen. The Directing Vessel is specific for abdominal masses.

HERBAL TREATMENT

Prescription

XIAO YAO SAN
Free and Easy Wanderer Powder

Bo He *Herba Menthae* 3 g
Chai Hu *Radix Bupleuri* 9 g
Dang Gui *Radix Angelicae sinensis* 9 g
Bai Shao *Radix Paeoniae albae* 12 g
Bai Zhu *Rhizoma Atractylodis macrocephalae* 9 g
Fu Ling *Sclerotium Poriae cocos* 15 g
Gan Cao *Radix Glycyrrhizae uralensis* 6 g
Sheng Jiang *Rhizoma Zingiberis officinalis recens*
3 slices

Explanation

This formula, which has already been explained
in chapters 1 and 12, moves Liver-Qi in the
lower abdomen.

Variations

– In order to enhance the formula's moving-Qi
  effect add Xiang Fu *Rhizoma Cyperi rotundi*
  and Mu Xiang *Radix Saussureae*.
– If the stagnation and masses are very
  pronounced add Yan Hu Suo *Rhizoma
  Corydalis yanhusuo* and Yu Jin *Tuber Curcumae*.
– In an old person add Dang Shen *Radix
  Codonopsis pilosulae* or even better, Ren Shen
  Radix Ginseng.
– If, in addition to stagnation of Qi, there is
  some Dampness and Phlegm (a very common
  situation) increase the dosage of Fu Ling,
  reduce that of Dang Gui and add Sha Ren
  Fructus seu Semen Amomi, Cang Zhu *Rhizoma
  Atractylodis lanceae* and Huang Bo *Cortex
  Phellodendri*.

(i) Patent remedy

SHU GAN WAN
Pacifying the Liver Pill
Chuan Lian Zi *Fructus Meliae toosendan*
Jiang Huang *Rhizoma Curcumae longae*
Chen Xiang *Lignum Aquilariae*
Yan Hu Suo *Rhizoma Corydalis yanhusuo*
Mu Xiang *Radix Saussureae*
Bai Dou Kou *Fructus Amomi cardamomi*
Bai Shao *Radix Paeoniae albae*
Fu Ling *Sclerotium Poriae cocos*
Zhi Ke *Fructus Citri aurantii*

Chen Pi *Pericarpium Citri reticulatae*
Sha Ren *Fructus seu Semen Amomi*
Hou Po *Cortex Magnoliae officinalis*

Explanation

This remedy moves Liver-Qi and eliminates
stagnation. The pulse and tongue presentation
appropriate to this remedy is a Full and Wiry
pulse and a tongue body which is slightly Red
on the sides.

(ii) Patent remedy

XIAO YAO WAN
Free and Easy Wanderer Pill
Chai Hu *Radix Bupleuri*
Bo He *Herba Menthae*
Dang Gui *Radix Angelicae sinensis*
Bai Shao *Radix Paeoniae albae*
Bai Zhu *Rhizoma Atractylodis macrocephalae*
Fu Ling *Sclerotium Poriae cocos*
Zhi Gan Cao *Radix Glycyrrhizae uralensis prae-
parata*
Sheng Jiang *Rhizoma Zingiberis officinalis recens*

Explanation

This remedy moves Liver-Qi, tonifies Spleen-Qi
and nourishes Liver-Blood. The pulse presentation appropriate to this remedy is a pulse which
is Weak on the right side and Fine and slightly
Wiry on the left.

The tongue presentation appropriate to this
remedy is a Pale or normal-coloured body.

2. RETENTION OF FOOD AND PHLEGM

CLINICAL MANIFESTATIONS

Soft abdominal masses, which may be strip-like
in shape, abdominal distension, constipation or
diarrhoea, poor appetite, nausea and a feeling of
fullness.
Tongue: Swollen, with a sticky coating which is
thicker on the root.
Pulse: Slippery.

TREATMENT PRINCIPLE

Resolve food retention, regulate the bowels, move Qi and resolve Phlegm.

ACUPUNCTURE

Ren-12 Zhongwan, BL-20 Pishu, Ren-10 Xiawan, Ren-6 Qihai, L.I.-4 Hegu, ST-40 Fenglong, ST-36 Zusanli, BL-21 Weishu, ST-34 Lianqiu, SP-6 Sanyinjiao. Reducing or even method, except on Ren-12 and BL-20 which should be reinforced.

Explanation

- **Ren-12** and **BL-20** tonify the Spleen to resolve Phlegm and promote transformation of food.
- **Ren-10** promotes the descending of Stomach-Qi.
- **Ren-6** moves Qi in the lower abdomen.
- **L.I.-4** regulates the ascending and descending of Qi in the Stomach.
- **ST-40** resolves Phlegm and promotes the descending of Stomach-Qi.
- **ST-36** promotes the descending of Stomach-Qi and relieves constipation. If there is diarrhoea replace this with ST-37 Shangjuxu.
- **BL-21** and **ST-34**, Back-Transporting and Accumulation point respectively, promote the descending of Stomach-Qi.
- **SP-6** resolves Dampness and moves Qi in the lower abdomen.

HERBAL TREATMENT

Prescription

LIU MO TANG
Six Ground-Herbs Decoction
Mu Xiang *Radix Saussureae* 6 g
Wu Yao *Radix Linderae strychnifoliae* 6 g
Chen Xiang *Lignum Aquilariae* 4.5 g
Da Huang *Rhizoma Rhei* 6 g
Bing Lang *Semen Arecae catechu* 6 g
Zhi Shi *Fructus Citri aurantii immaturus* 6 g

Explanation

This formula moves Qi and resolves food reten-

tion in the lower abdomen. It is particularly used if there is constipation.

- **Mu Xiang**, **Wu Yao** and **Chen Xiang** regulate Qi, eliminate stagnation and make Qi descend.
- **Da Huang**, **Bing Lang** and **Zhi Shi** move downwards and make Qi descend.

Variations

- If there is diarrhoea, remove Da Huang and add Bai Zhu *Rhizoma Atractylodis macrocephalae* and Sha Ren *Fructus seu Semen Amomi*.
- To enhance the Phlegm-resolving effect of this formula add Ban Xia *Rhizoma Pinelliae ternatae*, Fu Ling *Sclerotium Poriae cocos*, Chen Pi *Pericarpium Citri reticulatae* and Zhe Bei Mu *Bulbus Fritillariae thunbergii*.
- If the retention of food is pronounced add Ping Wei San *Balancing the Stomach Powder* plus Shan Zha *Fructus Crataegi* and Shen Qu *Massa Fermentata Medicinalis*.
- If there is deficiency of Qi (which is always present in chronic conditions) use Xiang Sha Liu Jun Zi Tang *Saussurea-Amomum Six Gentlemen Decoction*, some herbs to move Qi in the lower abdomen, such as Xiang Fu *Rhizoma Cyperi rotundi*, and some to resolve Phlegm and lumps, such as Zhe Bei Mu *Bulbus Fritillariae thunbergii*.

BLOOD MASSES

1. STAGNATION OF QI AND BLOOD

CLINICAL MANIFESTATIONS

Hard and immovable abdominal masses, abdominal distension and pain.
Tongue: Purple.
Pulse: Wiry.

TREATMENT PRINCIPLE

Move Qi and Blood, remove obstructions from the Connecting channels and dissolve masses.

ACUPUNCTURE

G.B.-34 Yanglingquan, Ren-6 Qihai, LIV-3 Taichong, T.B.-6 Zhigou, P-6 Neiguan, SP-6 Sanyinjiao, LU-7 Lieque and KI-6 Zhaohai, SP-10 Xuehai, BL-17 Geshu. Reducing or even method.

Explanation

- **G.B.-34** and **Ren-6** in combination, move Liver-Qi in the lower abdomen.
- **LIV-3** moves Liver-Qi and Liver-Blood.
- **P-6** indirectly moves Liver-Qi and calms the Mind.
- **T.B.-6** moves Liver-Qi.
- **SP-6** moves Blood and soothes the Liver. Specifically, it treats the lower abdomen.
- **LU-7** and **KI-6** are used in women to open the Directing Vessel and move Qi in the lower abdomen. The Directing Vessel is specific for abdominal masses.
- **SP-10** and **BL-17** move Blood.

HERBAL TREATMENT

(a) Prescription

JIN LING ZI SAN and SHI XIAO SAN
Fructus Meliae toosendan Powder and *Breaking into a Smile Powder*
Jin Ling Zi (Chuan Lian Zi) *Fructus Meliae toosendan* 30 g
Yan Hu Suo *Rhizoma Corydalis yanhusuo* 30 g
Pu Huang *Pollen Typhae* 9 g
Wu Ling Zhi *Excrementum Trogopteri* 9 g

Explanation

The first formula (composed of the first two herbs) moves Liver-Qi and Liver-Blood and the second one moves Blood and stops pain in the lower abdomen.

(b) Prescription

DA QI QI TANG
Big Seven Qi Decoction
Qing Pi *Pericarpium Citri reticulatae viridae* 6 g
Chen Pi *Pericarpium Citri reticulatae* 4.5 g

Xiang Fu *Rhizoma Cyperi rotundi* 6 g
Jie Geng *Radix Platycodi grandiflori* 3 g
Huo Xiang *Herba Agastachis* 6 g
Rou Gui *Cortex Cinnamomi cassiae* 3 g
Yi Zhi Ren *Fructus Alpiniae oxyphyllae* 6 g
San Leng *Rhizoma Sparganii* 6 g
E Zhu *Rhizoma Curcumae zedoariae* 6 g
Zhi Gan Cao *Radix Glycyrrhizae uralensis praeparata* 3 g
Sheng Jiang *Rhizoma Zingiberis officinalis recens* 3 slices
Da Zao *Fructus Ziziphi jujubae* 3 dates

Explanation

This formula is selected if the stagnation of Qi and Blood in the lower abdomen derives from, or is associated with Cold in the abdomen.

- **Qing Pi**, **Chen Pi**, **Xiang Fu**, **Jie Geng** and **Huo Xiang** move Qi and harmonize the Stomach.
- **Rou Gui** and **Yi Zhi Ren** warm the Lower Burner and scatter Cold.
- **San Leng** and **E Zhu** "break" Blood and dissolve masses.
- **Gan Cao**, **Sheng Jiang** and **Da Zao** harmonize.

2. STASIS OF BLOOD KNOTTED IN THE INTERIOR

CLINICAL MANIFESTATIONS

Hard, immovable and painful masses in the abdomen, dark and withered complexion, feeling cold, amenorrhoea, painful periods.
Tongue: Purple.
Pulse: Choppy.

This is a condition of severe and chronic stasis of Blood with obvious masses. The dark and withered complexion reflects stasis of Blood and the cold feeling is due not to internal Cold, but to poor circulation of Blood.

TREATMENT PRINCIPLE

"Break" Blood, eliminate stasis, soften hardness, dissolve masses, regulate Spleen and Stomach.

ACUPUNCTURE

G.B.-34 Yanglingquan, Ren-6 Qihai, SP-4 Gongsun and P-6 Neiguan, SP-10 Xuehai, BL-17 Geshu, ST-29 Guilai, LIV-3 Taichong, SP-6 Sanyinjiao, LIV-8 Ququan, ST-36 Zusanli and BL-20 Pishu. Reducing or even method, except on LIV-8, ST-36 and BL-20 which should be reinforced.

Explanation

– **G.B.-34** and **Ren-6** move Qi and Blood in the abdomen.
– **SP-4** and **P-6** open the Penetrating Vessel and regulate Blood as this extraordinary vessel is the Sea of Blood and regulates all Blood-Connecting channels.
– **SP-10** and **BL-17** move Blood.
– **ST-29** moves Blood in the lower abdomen.
– **LIV-3** and **SP-6** move Liver-Blood.
– **LIV-8**, **ST-36** and **BL-20** nourish Blood.

HERBAL TREATMENT

(a) Prescription

GE XIA ZHU YU TANG
Eliminating Stasis below the Diaphragm Decoction
Dang Gui *Radix Angelicae sinensis* 9 g
Chuan Xiong *Radix Ligustici wallichii* 3 g
Chi Shao *Radix Paeoniae rubrae* 6 g
Hong Hua *Flos Carthami tinctorii* 9 g
Tao Ren *Semen Persicae* 9 g
Wu Ling Zhi *Excrementum Trogopteri* 9 g
Yan Hu Suo *Rhizoma Corydalis yanhusuo* 3 g
Xiang Fu *Rhizoma Cyperi rotundi* 3 g
Zhi Ke *Fructus Citri aurantii* 5 g
Wu Yao *Radix Linderae strychnifoliae* 6 g
Mu Dan Pi *Cortex Moutan radicis* 6 g
Gan Cao *Radix Glycyrrhizae uralensis* 9 g

Explanation

This formula is specific to move Blood, eliminate stasis, stop pain and dissolve masses in the lower abdomen.

– **Dang Gui**, **Chi Shao**, **Chuan Xiong**, **Hong Hua** and **Tao Ren**, a modified version of Tao Hong Si Wu Tang *Prunus-Carthamus Four Substances Decoction*, move Liver-Blood.
– **Wu Ling Zhi** and **Yan Hu Suo** "break" Blood, eliminate stasis, stop pain and dissolve masses.
– **Zhi Ke**, **Xiang Fu** and **Wu Yao** move Qi which helps to move Blood.
– **Dan Pi** clears any Liver-Heat which may derive from the hot herbs within the formula.
– **Gan Cao** harmonizes and stops pain.

(b) Prescription

GUI ZHI FU LING WAN
Ramulus Cinnamomi-Poria Pill
Gui Zhi *Ramulus Cinnamomi cassiae* 9 g
Fu Ling *Sclerotium Poriae cocos* 9 g
Chi Shao *Radix Paeoniae rubrae* 9 g
Mu Dan Pi *Cortex Moutan radicis* 9 g
Tao Ren *Semen Persicae* 9 g

Explanation

– **Gui Zhi** and **Fu Ling** in combination penetrate the channels and blood vessels of the Lower Burner so as to allow the Blood-moving herbs to reach that area.
– **Chi Shao**, **Dan Pi** and **Tao Ren** move Blood, eliminate stasis and dissolve masses.

Variations

The following variations apply to both above formulae.

– To enhance the mass-dissolving effect add San Leng *Rhizoma Sparganii*, E Zhu *Rhizoma Curcumae zedoariae* and Ze Lan *Herba Lycopi lucidi*, herbs which "break" Blood and dissolve masses.
– To soften hardness, a method of treatment which is necessary to dissolve masses, add one or two of the following herbs according to symptoms and signs: Zhe Bei Mu *Bulbus Fritillariae thunbergii*, Bie Jia *Carapax Trionycis*, Mu Li *Concha Ostreae*, Chuan Shan Jia *Squama Manitis pentadactylae*, Yi Yi Ren *Semen Coicis lachryma jobi*, Xia Ku Cao *Spica Prunellae vulgaris*, Hai Zao *Herba Sargassii* or Kun Bu *Thallus Algae*.

– If there is a deficiency of Blood, eliminate Yan Hu Suo, do not use Blood-"breaking" herbs, increase Dang Gui and add Shu Di Huang *Radix Rehmanniae glutinosae praeparata*.

(i) Patent remedy

JIN GU DIE SHANG WAN
Muscle and Bone Traumatic Injury Pill
San Qi *Radix Notoginseng*
Xue Jie *Sanguis Draconis*
Dang Gui *Radix Angelicae sinensis*
Ru Xiang *Gummi Olibanum*
Mo Yao *Myrrha*
Hong Hua *Flos Carthami tinctorii*

Explanation

This pill moves Blood and eliminates stasis. Although it is normally used for traumatic injuries of bones and ligaments, it can be used for masses from internal stasis of Blood.

The tongue presentation appropriate to this remedy is a Purple body.

(ii) Patent remedy

TONG JING WAN
Penetrating Menses Pill
E Zhu *Rhizoma Curcumae zedoariae*
San Leng *Rhizoma Sparganii*
Chi Shao *Radix Paeoniae rubrae*
Hong Hua *Flos Carthami tinctorii*
Chuan Xiong *Radix Ligustici wallichii*
Dang Gui *Radix Angelicae sinensis*
Dan Shen *Radix Salviae miltiorrhizae*

Explanation

This pill strongly "breaks" Blood and eliminates stasis. It is primarily used for menstrual irregularities deriving from stasis of Blood and it can therefore be used for Blood masses in the lower abdomen.

The tongue presentation appropriate to this remedy is a Purple body with purple spots on the sides.

Case history

A 45-year-old woman had been suffering from a myoma in the uterus which was about 2 cm in diameter. Her lower abdomen was generally distended and her periods were rather heavy, with dark-clotted blood. Apart from this, she was in good health. Her tongue was slightly Purple on the sides and her pulse was slightly Firm (i.e. Wiry at the deep level).

Diagnosis
This myoma was due to stasis of Blood of the Liver: this is confirmed by the Purple colour on the sides of her tongue and the dark colour of her menstrual blood.

Treatment principle
The treatment principle followed was to move Liver-Blood and eliminate stasis in the uterus. This patient was treated only with herbs.

Herbal treatment
The formula used was a variation of Ge Xia Zhu Yu Tang *Eliminating Stasis below the Diaphragm Decoction*:

Dang Gui *Radix Angelicae sinensis* 9 g
Chuan Xiong *Radix Ligustici wallichii* 3 g
Chi Shao *Radix Paeoniae rubrae* 6 g
Hong Hua *Flos Carthami tinctorii* 6 g
Tao Ren *Semen Persicae* 6 g
Wu Ling Zhi *Excrementum Trogopteri* 4 g
Yan Hu Suo *Rhizoma Corydalis yanhusuo* 6 g
Xiang Fu *Rhizoma Cyperi rotundi* 3 g
Zhi Ke *Fructus Citri aurantii* 6 g
Wu Yao *Radix Linderae strychnifoliae* 6 g
Mu Dan Pi *Cortex Moutan radicis* 6 g
Gan Cao *Radix Glycyrrhizae uralensis* 3 g
Yi Yi Ren *Semen Coicis lachryma jobi* 20 g
E Zhu *Rhizoma Curcumae zedoariae* 9 g

Explanation
– All the herbs but the last two form the Ge Xia Zhu Yu Tang with the dosages of some of the herbs reduced.
– **Yi Yi Ren** was added to soften the mass.
– **E Zhu** was added to "break" Blood.

This formula was given for 9 months, with slight variations, and produced a dispersal of the myoma.

Case history

A 27-year-old woman had been diagnosed as having a large cyst on one ovary (7.5 cm in diameter), a myoma between the uterus and the ovary, and endometriosis. This caused her some abdominal pain and discomfort. The abdomen felt hard on palpation. Her periods were painful, sometimes heavy and sometimes scanty, sometimes stopping and starting, and the menstrual blood was dark with clots. She had an excessive vaginal discharge, yellow in colour. Her tongue was Pale-Purple, Swollen and with a sticky coating all over which was yellow on the root. Her pulse was Slippery, slightly Firm (Wiry at the Deep level), Deep, and Weak on both Rear positions.

Diagnosis
The ovarian cyst and myoma were due to stasis of Blood, but there was also Damp-Heat in the Lower Burner contributing to the stagnation in that area. Underlying these two conditions, there was also a deficiency of the Kidneys.

Treatment principle
This patient's condition was very complex due to the presence of endometriosis, ovarian cyst and uterine myoma. The ovarian cyst was too large to be dissolved with herbal treatment but she did not want an operation. I therefore agreed to treat her in order first of all to tonify the general body condition, secondly to treat the endometriosis, and thirdly to attempt to shrink the cyst. The treatment principle was to move Liver-Blood, eliminate stasis in the uterus, resolve Damp-Heat and tonify the Kidneys.

She was treated only with herbs and the formula used was a variation of the two formulae Gui Zhi Fu Ling Wan *Ramulus Cinnamomi-Poria Pill* and Si Miao Tang *Four Wonderful Decoction*:

Gui Zhi *Ramulus Cinnamomi cassiae* 6 g
Fu Ling *Sclerotium Poriae cocos* 9 g
Chi Shao *Radix Paeoniae rubrae* 6 g
Mu Dan Pi *Cortex Moutan radicis* 6 g
Tao Ren *Semen Persicae* 6 g
Huang Bo *Cortex Phellodendri* 6 g
Cang Zhu *Rhizoma Atractylodis lanceae* 6 g
Yi Yi Ren *Semen Coicis lachryma jobi* 10 g
Niu Xi *Radix Achyranthis bidentatae seu Cyathulae* 6 g
Dang Gui *Radix Angelicae sinensis* 6 g
E Zhu *Rhizoma Curcumae zedoariae* 4 g
Tu Si Zi *Semen Cuscutae* 6 g
Lu Lu Tong *Fructus Liquidambaris taiwanianae* 4 g

Explanation
- The first 9 herbs constitute the two root formulae.
- **Dang Gui** was added to nourish and move Blood.
- **E Zhu** strongly moves Blood and dissolves masses.
- **Tu Si Zi** was added to tonify Kidney-Yang.
- **Lu Lu Tong** moves Qi and Blood, resolves Dampness and dissolves masses. It is specific for ovarian cysts.

This formula was used, with some variations, for about 9 months. After this time, her condition improved in so far as her periods were more regular, not painful and the blood was not clotted. The ovarian cyst also was reduced in size. Afterwards, the prescription was changed, introducing more tonifying herbs such as Bai Zhu *Rhizoma Atractylodis macrocephalae* and Dang Shen *Radix Codonopsis pilosulae*. This patient is still under treatment.

3. DEFICIENCY OF UPRIGHT QI AND STASIS OF BLOOD

CLINICAL MANIFESTATIONS

Hard and painful masses, sallow complexion, loss of weight, loss of appetite, exhaustion.
Tongue: Purple.
Pulse: Fine and Choppy.

This is a chronic condition of severe Blood stasis which has led to the formation of masses with an underlying deficiency of the body's Qi. From the point of view of Western medicine, it could correspond to carcinoma.

TREATMENT PRINCIPLE

Strongly tonify Qi and Blood, move Blood and eliminate stasis.

ACUPUNCTURE

Ren-4 Guanyuan, Ren-6 Qihai, Ren-8 Shenque, BL-23 Shenshu, BL-20 Pishu, ST-36 Zusanli, SP-6 Sanyinjiao, KI-3 Taixi, LU-7 Lieque and KI-6 Zhaohai, SP-10 Xuehai, BL-17 Geshu. Even method on the last two points and reinforcing method on all the others. Moxa should be used on Ren-4, Ren-6 or Ren-8.

Explanation

- **Ren-4** nourishes Blood and Yin and tonifies the Original Qi.
- **Ren-6** tonifies Qi.
- **Ren-8** tonifies the Original Qi and Essence.
- **BL-23**, **BL-20**, **ST-36**, **SP-6** and **KI-3** tonify Spleen and Kidneys.
- **LU-7** and **KI-6** open the Directing Vessel, move Qi in the abdomen and dissolve abdominal masses.
- **SP-10** and **BL-17** move Blood.

HERBAL TREATMENT

Prescription

BA ZHEN TANG and HUA JI WAN

Eight Precious Decoction and *Resolving Blood Masses Pill*

Dang Gui *Radix Angelicae sinensis* 10 g
Chuan Xiong *Radix Ligustici wallichii* 5 g
Bai Shao *Radix Paeoniae albae* 8 g
Shu Di Huang *Radix Rehmanniae glutinosae praeparata* 15 g
Ren Shen *Radix Ginseng* 3 g
Bai Zhu *Rhizoma Atractylodis macrocephalae* 10 g
Fu Ling *Sclerotium Poriae cocos* 8 g
Zhi Gan Cao *Radix Glycyrrhizae uralensis praeparata* 5 g
San Leng *Rhizoma Sparganii* 6 g
E Zhu *Rhizoma Curcumae zedoariae* 6 g
Wu Ling Zhi *Excrementum Trogopteri* 6 g
Su Mu *Lignum Sappan* 4.5 g
Xiang Fu *Rhizoma Cyperi rotundi* 6 g
Bing Lang *Semen Arecae catechu* 6 g
Xiong Huang *Realgar* 1.5 g
Wa Leng Zi *Concha Arcae* 15 g
A Wei *Herba Ferulae assafoetidae* 6 g
Hai Fu Shi *Pumice* 15 g

Explanation

The first eight herbs constitute the Eight Precious Decoction which tonifies Qi and Blood.

- **San Leng**, **E Zhu**, **Wu Ling Zhi** and **Su Mu** move Blood, eliminate stasis and dissolve masses. The first two herbs are stronger and they "break" Blood.
- **Xiang Fu** and **Bing Lang** move Qi to help to move Blood.
- **Xiong Huang** opens the orifices and helps to dissolve masses. This is a toxic substance and it can be omitted. It could be replaced with Shi Chang Pu *Rhizoma Acori graminei*.
- **Wa Leng Zi**, **A Wei** and **Hai Fu Shi** soften hardness and dissolve masses.

Variations

- If there is Yin deficiency add Sheng Di Huang *Radix Rehmanniae glutinosae* and Bei Sha Shen *Radix Glehniae littoralis*.

Patent remedy

BA ZHEN WAN and TONG JING WAN

Eight Precious Pill and *Penetrating the Menses Pill*
Dang Gui *Radix Angelicae sinensis*
Chuan Xiong *Radix Ligustici wallichii*
Bai Shao *Radix Paeoniae albae*
Shu Di Huang *Radix Rehmanniae glutinosae praeparata*
Ren Shen *Radix Ginseng*
Bai Zhu *Rhizoma Atractylodis macrocephalae*
Fu Ling *Sclerotium Poriae cocos*
Zhi Gan Cao *Radix Glycyrrhizae uralensis praeparata*
E Zhu *Rhizoma Curcumae zedoariae*
San Leng *Rhizoma Sparganii*
Chi Shao *Radix Paeoniae rubrae*
Hong Hua *Flos Carthami tinctorii*
Dan Shen *Radix Salviae miltiorrhizae*

Explanation

The first remedy tonifies Qi and Blood and the second "breaks" Blood and eliminates stasis in the lower abdomen.

The tongue presentation appropriate to this remedy is a Pale, Bluish-Purple body.

Prognosis and prevention

The subject of prognosis in abdominal masses cannot be separated from that of Western diagnosis. In the case of abdominal masses perhaps more than any other, a Western diagnosis is essential. Although Chinese medicine *is* effective in treating masses, we should never treat them blindly without first establishing what they really are.

As explained below, from a Western perspective, masses can be due to many different pathologies: enlarged organs, cysts, myomas ("fibroids"), spastic colon, masses of faeces and malignant tumours. The treatment and prognosis in each of these cases will obviously differ enormously. Furthermore, in addition to the above types of masses, one should add those that are non-substantial, i.e. due to Qi stagnation.

First of all, to make a prognosis from a Chinese perspective, we must differentiate between masses due to Qi and masses due to Blood accumulation: Qi masses are much easier to disperse than Blood masses. Acupuncture can be used to disperse Qi masses but Blood masses can be dispersed only with herbal medicine.

From a Western perspective, to mention the most common causes of masses, those due to a spasm in the colon or masses of faeces are the easiest to resolve. Ovarian cysts and uterine myomas can be dispersed only if they are very small (not more than 2 cm in diameter). There are three types of myomas: subserous (on the outside wall of the uterus), interstitial (within the wall of the uterus) and submucous (on the inside of the uterus). The interstitial myomas are the easiest (or better, the least difficult) to disperse.

Malignant tumours of the abdomen can also be treated with Chinese herbs and the prognosis varies according to the organ involved and the stage of the carcinoma: however, the differentiation and treatment outlined in this chapter do not apply to malignant tumours as their treatment needs a different approach. Of all malignant tumours, lymphomas respond best to treatment with Chinese herbs.

Finally, masses due to enlargement of organs can be dispersed by a combination of both acupuncture and herbs. In all the above cases, treatment will necessarily take a long time and patience is required from both the practitioner and the patient.

As for prevention, any patient who is prone to abdominal masses or has been cured of one should follow certain precautions. First of all, they should avoid the excessive consumption of cold-energy foods and especially cold drinks as these tend to lead to stasis in the lower abodmen. This is an important recommendation especially in countries such as the USA where people tend to consume large quantities of iced drinks. Women should pay particular care during the menstrual period and after childbirth: at these times, they should carefully avoid exposure to cold or dampness (for example, wearing a wet swimming suit on a windy beach, sitting on damp grass, etc.). Women who practise meditation concentrating the breath in the lower abdomen should do so in a standing rather than sitting position (see chapter 16 on "Abdominal pain"): this practice in a sitting position tends to increase or cause stagnation in the lower abdomen in women. Moderate exercise is vital to keep Qi moving in the lower abdomen. Even just brisk walking in the open air (although not in a city centre!) is an effective exercise. *Tai Ji Quan* is an excellent exercise to remove or prevent stagnation in the lower abdomen, and it is particularly suited to those over 40.

Finally, women should take care not to catch cold after sexual activity and also to avoid sex during the periods: both these activities lead to stasis of Blood in the lower abdomen.

Western differentiation

Masses which are sufficiently large or sufficiently close to the abdominal wall cause increased resistance to palpation. Obviously, only Blood masses may correspond to actual abdominal masses from the point of view of Western medicine. Qi masses, by their very nature, are not actual, physical masses.

From a Western diagnostic perspective, it is very important to establish whether a mass is in the abdominal wall or the abdominal cavity.

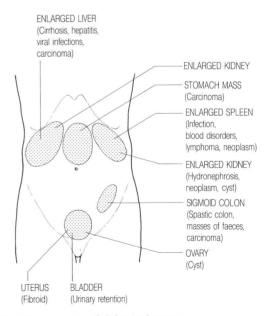

Fig. 17.1 Location of abdominal masses

This distinction can be easily made with a simple test. With the patient supine, ask him or her to raise the head in order to tense the abdominal muscles. If the mass is in the abdominal cavity, it will be shielded by the tensed muscles and will cease to be palpable. If the mass is in the abdominal wall it will still be felt through the tensed abdominal muscles.

The most common types of masses are summarized in Figure 17.1.

END NOTES

1. Nanjing College of Traditional Chinese Medicine 1979 A Revised Explanation of the Classic of Difficulties (Nan Jing Jiao Shi 难经校释), People's Health Publishing House, Beijing, p. 122. First published c. 100 BC.
2. He Ren 1979 A Popular Guide to the Essential Prescriptions of the Golden Chest (Jin Gui Yao Lue Tong Su Jiang Hua 金匮要略通俗讲话), Shanghai Science Publishing House, Shanghai, p. 83. The "Essential Prescriptions of the Golden Chest" itself was written by Zhang Zhong Jing and first published c. AD 220.
3. Chao Yuan Fang AD 610 General Treatise on the Aetiology and Symptomatology of Diseases (Zhu Bing Yuan Hou Zong Lun 诸病源候总论), cited in Internal Medicine, p. 187.
4. 1981 Spiritual Axis (Ling Shu Jing 灵枢经), People's Health Publishing House, Beijing. First published c. 100 BC, p. 122.

Diarrhoea 18

泄
泻

The term "diarrhoea" is defined as the passage of semi-formed or watery stools which are usually, but not always, passed more frequently than normal. In Chinese, the word "diarrhoea" (*Xie-xie*) is composed of two characters, both of which have the sound *xie*, one meaning "loose stools", the other "stools like water".

Acute seasonal diarrhoea is more frequent during summer and autumn.

Aetiology and pathology

1. INVASION OF EXTERNAL PATHOGENIC FACTORS

These can be Cold, Dampness and Summer-Heat.

Cold can invade the Intestines directly bypassing the body's Defensive-Qi portion. This happens when one is exposed to cold weather. Contrary to what one might expect, it happens more frequently in summertime when one is lightly dressed. If there is a spell of unseasonably cold weather, or if one stands in the wind after swimming with the body still wet, then Cold may invade the Intestines and cause diarrhoea and abdominal pain. The "Simple Questions" in chapter 39 says: "*When Cold invades the Small Intestine, this cannot transform [food] properly and diarrhoea and abdominal pain result.*"[1] The "Spiritual Axis" in chapter 29 says:

When Cold invades the Stomach there is abdominal pain and distension; when it invades the Intestines diarrhoea and borborygmi result. When the Stomach has Cold but the Intestines Heat, then distension and diarrhoea result.[2]

Summer-Heat also invades Intestines and Spleen and is a frequent cause of acute diarrhoea in summertime. In this case, the person will also have symptoms of invasion of the Defensive-Qi system by Summer-Heat, i.e. fever and aversion to cold. The "Simple Questions" in chapter 5 says: "*When Wind injures the body in Springtime, diarrhoea results in summertime*".[3]

Of the external pathogenic factors, Dampness is the one that most frequently causes diarrhoea. External Dampness penetrates the channels of the leg and flows up to the Spleen where it obstructs its function of transformation and transportation leading to diarrhoea.

2. IRREGULAR DIET

Diet is of course a frequent cause of acute or chronic diarrhoea. The most common cause of acute diarrhoea is eating spoiled food, too hot or too cold foods.

Chronic diarrhoea may be caused simply by over-eating or by the excessive consumption of cold, greasy or sweet foods. These impair the transforming and transporting of the Spleen, so that Spleen-Qi cannot ascend and diarrhoea results.

Zhang Jing Yue says in the "Complete Book of Jing Yue" (1634): "*Diarrhoea is either due to diet or invasion of a pathogenic factor ... when due to diet, there is Cold-Accumulation*".[4]

3. EMOTIONAL STRESS

Worry, pensiveness, brooding and excessive mental work weaken the Spleen and may cause chronic diarrhoea. Anger, which normally affects the Liver, may also affect the Spleen when one gets angry or frustrated after meals. This upsets the Spleen's transforming and transporting and leads to diarrhoea. Zhang Jing Yue says in the "Complete Book of Jing Yue": "*... if anger occurs during or after eating it injures Stomach and Spleen ... it affects both Liver and Spleen and Wood invades Earth ...*".[5]

4. OVERWORK, CHRONIC ILLNESS

Working long hours associated with irregular eating or physical overwork (including excessive exercise) weakens the Spleen and often leads to diarrhoea. Any chronic illness also inevitably weakens the Spleen and may lead to diarrhoea.

5. OVERWORK, EXCESSIVE SEXUAL ACTIVITY

Working long hours without adequate rest under conditions of stress may weaken the Kidneys. If a person has a tendency to Yang deficiency, it will lead to Kidney-Yang deficiency. When Kidney-Yang fails to nourish Spleen-Yang, the Spleen lacks the warmth necessary to transform and transport and this may result in diarrhoea.

Zhang Jing Yue in the "Complete Book of Jing Yue" says:

The Kidneys are the gate of the Stomach and they control the two [lower] orifices. Thus the opening and closing of the two [lower] orifices depends on the Kidneys. If Kidney-Yang is deficient and the Fire of the Gate of Vitality is declining ... Yin Qi is victorious and diarrhoea results.[6]

Thus diarrhoea is most of all related to the Spleen among the internal organs, and, of the pathogenic factors, it is most of all related to Dampness. Of the internal organs, the Liver and Kidneys also play a role. For this reason, Zhang Jing Yue says in the "Complete Book of Jing Yue": "*The root of diarrhoea cannot not be in the Spleen and Stomach*".[7] In any type of diarrhoea there is always an inversion in the movement of Spleen-Qi, i.e. Spleen-Qi descending instead of ascending. The Simple Questions in chapter 5 says: "*When clear Qi descends ... and turbid Qi ascends, there is diarrhoea*".[8]

Diagnosis

Acute diarrhoea with exterior symptoms such as fever and aversion to cold indicates invasion of Damp-Cold or Damp-Heat.

Foul-smelling diarrhoea accompanied by abdominal pain and borborygmi indicates retention of food.

Chronic diarrhoea with abdominal distension, belching, flatulence, fluctuating with the emotional state indicates that Liver-Qi is invading the Spleen.

Diarrhoea with frequent bowel movement and stools sometimes like water indicates long-term deficiency of Stomach and Spleen.

Early-morning diarrhoea with abdominal pain and borborygmi during the bowel movement with a feeling of cold indicates Kidney-Yang deficiency.

Pale-yellow stools indicate Liver and Gall-Bladder Damp-Heat.

Very dark stools indicate Heat. Very watery stools indicate Cold. Foul-smelling stools indicate Heat, whilst absence of a strong smell may indicate Cold (or of course, normality). A burning sensation in the anus during the bowel movement indicates Heat.

Abdominal pain which becomes worse after diarrhoea indicates a Deficiency condition, whilst if it lessens after diarrhoea it denotes an Excess condition.

Differentiation and treatment

According to the diagnostic guidelines given above, the most important differentiation to make is that between Excess and Deficiency and Cold and Heat.

As for the methods of treatment used to treat diarrhoea with herbal medicine the "Essential Readings of Medicine" (1637) by Li Zhong Zi lists nine methods:

- lightly draining Dampness for diarrhoea from invasion of external Dampness in the beginning stages: e.g. Fu Ling *Sclerotium Poriae cocos*
- raising Qi for diarrhoea from Spleen-Qi sinking: e.g. Huang Qi *Radix Astragali membranacei*
- expelling Cold for acute diarrhoea from Cold: e.g. Gan Jiang *Rhizoma Zingiberis officinalis* and Gao Liang Jiang *Rhizoma Alpiniae officinari*
- moving Qi for diarrhoea from Liver-Qi stagnation: e.g. Xiang Fu *Rhizoma Cyperi rotundi*
- moderate with sweet herbs for acute diarrhoea with increased frequency and abdominal pain: e.g. Gan Cao *Radix Glycyrrhizae uralensis* and Bai Shao *Radix Paeoniae albae*
- astringe with sour herbs for chronic diarrhoea with heavy loss of fluids: e.g. Qian Shi *Semen Euryales ferocis*

- dry the Spleen for chronic diarrhoea from internal Dampness and Spleen deficiency: e.g. Bai Zhu *Rhizoma Atractylodis macrocephalae* and Cang Zhu *Rhizoma Atractylodis lanceae*
- warm the Kidneys for chronic diarrhoea from Kidney- and Spleen-Yang deficiency: e.g. Rou Gui *Cortex Cinnamomi cassiae*
- fill-up Emptiness for chronic diarrhoea from severe deficiency of Spleen and Kidneys: e.g. Bai Zhu *Rhizoma Atractylodis macrocephalae* and Xu Duan *Radix Dipsaci*.

These methods of treatment are not mutually exclusive and may be combined. For example, one may simultaneously move Qi and dry the Spleen.

The patterns discussed are:

EXCESS

Retention of Cold-Dampness
Retention of Damp-Heat
Retention of Food
Liver-Qi stagnation

DEFICIENCY

Spleen and Stomach Deficiency
Kidney-Yang Deficiency

EXCESS CONDITIONS

1. RETENTION OF COLD-DAMPNESS

CLINICAL MANIFESTATIONS

Diarrhoea which, in severe cases, may be like water, abdominal pain, borborygmi, a feeling of oppression of the chest, no appetite, fever (not always present), aversion to cold, nasal obstruction, headache, feeling of heaviness.
Tongue: thick-sticky-white coating.
Pulse: Slippery-Slow.

This may be an external pattern when it is caused by exterior Dampness; the pattern may then become internal when Dampness is retained for a long time.

TREATMENT PRINCIPLE

Scatter Cold, fragrantly resolve Dampness.

ACUPUNCTURE

Ren-12 Zhongwan, BL-22 Sanjiaoshu, SP-9 Yinlingquan, SP-6 Sanyinjiao, Ren-6 Qihai with moxa on ginger, ST-25 Tianshu. Reducing or even method except on Ren-12 which should be reinforced.

Explanation

- **Ren-12** tonifies the Spleen to resolve Dampness.
- **BL-22**, **SP-9** and **SP-6** resolve Dampness in the Lower Burner.
- **Ren-6** with moxa on ginger expels Cold from the Intestines.
- **ST-25** stops diarrhoea.

HERBAL TREATMENT

Prescription

HUO XIANG ZHENG QI SAN
Agastache Upright Qi Powder
Huo Xiang *Herba Agastachis* 9 g
Hou Po *Cortex Magnoliae officinalis* 6 g
Da Fu Pi *Pericarpium Arecae catechu* 3 g
Zi Su Ye *Folium Perillae frutescentis* 3 g
Bai Zhi *Radix Angelicae dahuricae* 3 g
Ban Xia *Rhizoma Pinelliae ternatae* 6 g
Chen Pi *Pericarpium Citri reticulatae* 6 g
Bai Zhu *Rhizoma Atractylodis macrocephalae* 6 g
Fu Ling *Sclerotium Poriae cocos* 3 g
Jie Geng *Radix Platycodi grandiflori* 6 g
Sheng Jiang *Rhizoma Zingiberis officinalis recens* 3 slices
Da Zao *Fructus Ziziphi jujubae* 3 dates
Zhi Gan Cao *Radix Glycyrrhizae uralensis praeparata* 3 g

Explanation

- **Huo Xiang**, **Hou Po** and **Da Fu Pi** fragrantly resolve Dampness.

- **Zi Su Ye** harmonizes the Stomach.
- **Bai Zhi** expels Wind and releases the Exterior.
- **Ban Xia** and **Chen Pi** dry Dampness.
- **Bai Zhu** and **Fu Ling** dry and tonify the Spleen.
- **Jie Geng** helps to release the Exterior.
- **Sheng Jiang** and **Da Zao** help to harmonize the Stomach.
- **Gan Cao** harmonizes.

Variations

- If the exterior symptoms are pronounced add Jing Jie *Herba seu Flos Schizonepetae tenuifoliae* and Fang Feng *Radix Ledebouriellae sesloidis*.
- If symptoms of Dampness are predominant add *Rhizoma Atractylodis lanceae*, Zhu Ling *Sclerotium Polypori umbellati* and Yi Yi Ren *Semen Coicis lachryma jobi*.

Patent remedy

HUO XIANG ZHENG QI WAN
Agastache Upright Qi Pill

Explanation

This pill has the same ingredients and functions as the homonymous prescription above.

The tongue presentation appropriate to this remedy is a sticky-white coating.

2. RETENTION OF DAMP-HEAT

CLINICAL MANIFESTATIONS

Foul-smelling yellowish loose stools, abdominal pain, increased frequency of bowel movement, burning sensation in the anus, feeling of heat, thirst, scanty-dark urine.
Tongue: thick-sticky-yellow coating.
Pulse: Slippery-Rapid.

This may be an external pattern when it is caused by exterior Dampness; the pattern may then become internal when Dampness is retained for a long time.

TREATMENT PRINCIPLE

Clear Heat and resolve Dampness.

ACUPUNCTURE

Ren-12 Zhongwan, BL-22 Sanjiaoshu, SP-9 Yinlingquan, SP-6 Sanyinjiao, ST-25 Tianshu, BL-25 Dachangshu, L.I.-11 Quchi, reducing method no moxa.

Explanation

Most of these points have already been explained above for the Damp-Cold type. From the acupuncture perspective, the treatment of Damp-Cold and Damp-Heat differs only in the use of moxa.

- **L.I.-11** resolves Damp-Heat and stops diarrhoea from Heat. As a Sea point it treats the Yang organs and specifically diarrhoea (chapter 68 of the "Classic of Difficulties").

HERBAL TREATMENT

Prescription

GE GEN QIN LIAN TANG
Pueraria-Scutellaria-Coptis Decoction
Ge Gen *Radix Puerariae* 9 g
Huang Qin *Radix Scutellariae baicalensis* 9 g
Huang Lian *Rhizoma Coptidis* 4.5 g
Zhi Gan Cao *Radix Glycyrrhizae uralensis praeparata* 3 g

Explanation

- **Ge Gen** clears Heat and stops diarrhoea.
- **Huang Qin** and **Huang Lian** clear Heat and resolve Dampness.
- **Zhi Gan Cao** harmonizes.

Variations

- If there are pronounced symptoms of Dampness add Cang Zhu *Rhizoma Atractylodis lanceae* and Chen Pi *Pericarpium Citri reticulatae*.

- If the symptoms of Heat are pronounced add Jin Yin Hua *Flos Lonicerae japonicae*, Mu Tong *Caulis Akebiae* and Che Qian Zi *Semen Plantaginis*.
- If there is retention of food add Shen Qu *Massa Fermentata Medicinalis*, Mai Ya *Fructus Hordei vulgaris germinatus* and Shan Zha *Fructus Crataegi*.
- If the diarrhoea occurs in summertime and there are symptoms of Summer-Heat such as stools like water, sweating, irritability, thirst and dark urine add Huo Xiang *Herba Agastachis*, Xiang Ru *Herba Elsholtziae splendentis*, Bian Dou *Semen Dolichoris lablab* and He Ye *Folium Nelumbinis nuciferae*.

(i) Patent remedy

SHEN QU CHA
Massa Fermentata Tea
Qing Hao *Herba Artemisiae apiaceae*
Huang Qin *Radix Scutellariae baicalensis*
Xiang Ru *Herba Elsholtziae splendentis*
Qiang Huo *Radix et Rhizoma Notopterygii*
Du Huo *Radix Angelicae pubescentis*
Qing Pi *Pericarpium Citri reticulatae viridae*
Hu Po *Succinum*
Cao Guo *Fructus Amomi Tsaoko*
Mu Gua *Fructus Chaenomelis*
Jie Geng *Radix Platycodi grandiflori*
Shan Yao *Radix Dioscoreae oppositae*
Fu Ling *Sclerotium Poriae cocos*
Gan Cao *Radix Glycyrrhizae uralensis*
Shen Qu *Massa Fermentata Medicinalis*

Explanation

This remedy is suitable only for the beginning stages of an invasion of Damp-Heat in the Intestines causing nausea and diarrhoea.

The tongue presentation appropriate to this remedy is a sticky-yellow coating.

(ii) Patent remedy

BAO JI WAN
Protecting and Benefiting Pill
Chi Shi Zhi *Halloysitum rubrum*
Bai Zhi *Radix Angelicae dahuricae*

Ju Hua *Flos Chrysanthemi morifolii*
Bo He *Herba Menthae*
Ge Gen *Radix Puerariae*
Tian Hua Fen *Radix Trichosanthis*
Cang Zhu *Rhizoma Atractylodis lanceae*
Yi Yi Ren *Semen Coicis lachryma jobi*
Fu Ling *Sclerotium Poriae cocos*
Mu Xiang *Radix Saussureae*
Hou Po *Cortex Magnoliae officinalis*
Chen Pi *Pericarpium Citri reticulatae*
Shen Qu *Massa Fermentata Medicinalis*
Huo Xiang *Herba Agastachis*
Gu Ya *Fructus Oryzae sativae germinatus*

Explanation

This remedy, probably better known by its Cantonese name *"Po Chai Pill"*, resolves Damp-Heat and stops diarrhoea. It is used mostly for acute diarrhoea from Damp-Heat for which it is extremely effective.

The tongue presentation appropriate to this remedy is a sticky-yellow coating.

Case history

A 37-year-old man had been suffering from diarrhoea for 2 years. It started suddenly two years before in the autumn: at that time he had also a fever and nausea. He was prescribed antibiotics but these did not help at all. His bowel movements, of which he had 3–4 a day, were always very loose with some cramping pain during evacuation. He also suffered from a feeling of fullness and distension and his appetite was poor. His head felt muzzy, his thinking "foggy" and his body felt heavy. His tongue was Red with a thick, sticky-yellow coating (Plate 18.1). His pulse was Slippery.

Diagnosis
This is a very clear condition of Damp-Heat affecting the Intestines (diarrhoea with cramping pain, feeling of fullness, sticky-yellow tongue coating, Slippery pulse), the muscles (feeling of heaviness) and the head (muzzy head).

Treatment principle
The principle of treatment adopted was to resolve Dampness and clear Heat. He was treated with both acupuncture and herbs.

Acupuncture
The main acupuncture points used were:

- **ST-25** Tianshu to stop diarrhoea;
- **SP-9** Yinlingquan to resolve Damp-Heat;

- **ST-37** Shangjuxu for chronic diarrhoea;
- **BL-20** Pishu to tonify the Spleen to resolve Dampness;
- **BL-22** Sanjiaoshu to resolve Dampness from the Lower Burner;
- **BL-25** Dachangshu to clear Heat in the Intestines.

Herbal treatment
The herbal formula used was a variation of a combination of Ge Gen Qin Lian Tang *Pueraria-Scutellaria-Coptis Decoction* and Bai Tou Weng Tang *Pulsatilla Decoction*:

Ge Gen *Radix Puerariae* 9 g
Huang Qin *Radix Scutellariae baicalensis* 4 g
Huang Lian *Rhizoma Coptidis* 4.5 g
Zhi Gan Cao *Radix Glycyrrhizae uralensis praeparata* 3 g
Huang Bo *Cortex Phellodendri* 6 g
Bai Tou Weng *Radix Pulsatillae chinensis* 9 g
Qin Pi *Cortex Fraxini* 6 g
Zhi Ke *Fructus Citri aurantii* 4 g

Explanation
- The first four herbs form Ge Gen Qin Lian Tang which resolves Damp-Heat from the Intestines and stops diarrhoea.
- **Huang Bo**, **Qin Pi** and **Bai Tou Weng** clear Heat and stop diarrhoea.
- **Zhi Ke** was added to move Qi to help to resolve Dampness.

This patient started improving after three courses of five decoctions when his stools became normal at least some of the time. It took another 6 months to clear the condition completely.

Case history

A 55-year-old man had been suffering from diarrhoea for 3 years. His stools were always loose, often like water, and were mixed with mucus and blood. He had several movements a day, mostly in the morning, and these were also quite urgent. On interrogation, it transpired that he had actually had the very first symptoms at least 8 years before, when his bowel movements became more frequent, albeit without mucus or blood. In fact, his symptoms had started soon after a haemorrhoids operation when he started to suffer from frequency of bowel movements with bitty stools, flatulence and distension. I have in fact observed this connection between a haemorrhoids operation and bowel diseases in other cases.

His tongue was slightly Red, with a thin yellow coating and his pulse was slightly Slippery. He was a strongly-built man and he did not suffer from any other problem, neither had he had other problems in the past.

Diagnosis
As his tongue did not have a thick-sticky coating and

his pulse was only very slightly Slippery, I diagnosed that his diarrhoea was due mostly to Spleen deficiency and that the bleeding was due to deficient Spleen-Qi not holding Blood. I therefore treated him with prescriptions aimed at tonifying Spleen-Qi, first with Liu Jun Zi Tang *Six Gentlemen Decoction*, then with Bu Zhong Yi Qi Tang *Tonifying the Centre and Benefiting Qi Decoction*. After three months of treatment there was no improvement. It was at this time that I asked Prof. Shan Dao Wei, a teacher from Nanjing, to give his opinion. His diagnosis was different: he said that the main problem was Damp-Heat in the Intestines and that the bleeding was due to·Heat, not Qi deficiency. He pointed out that the presence of mucus in the stools indicates Dampness and also that the patient is a strong man with no previous history of any problem and his pulse is not Weak. He therefore concluded that the condition was purely one of Fullness, not Deficiency, and that, in Chinese medicine, it falls under the category of dysentery from Damp-Heat: this damages mucous membranes and capillaries leading to mucus and blood in the stools. He also said: *"In such a case, the more you tonify, the worse it will be"*. He therefore recommended a combination of three formulae: Bai Tou Weng Tang *Pulsatilla Decoction*, Xiang Lian Wan *Saussurea-Coptis Pill* and Ge Gen Qin Lian Tang *Pueraria-Scutellaria-Coptis Decoction*:

Bai Tou Weng *Radix Pulsatillae chinensis* 6 g
Qin Pi *Cortex Fraxini* 6 g
Huang Bo *Cortex Phellodendri* 6 g
Huang Lian *Rhizoma Coptidis* 3 g
Ge Gen *Radix Puerariae* 9 g
Huang Qin *Radix Scutellariae baicalensis* 4 g
Mu Xiang *Radix Saussureae* 6 g
Bai Shao *Radix Paeoniae albae* 9 g
Yi Yi Ren *Semen Coicis lachryma jobi* 12 g
Fu Ling *Sclerotium Poriae cocos* 9 g
Ma Chi Xian *Herba Portulacae oleraceae* 4 g
Chuan Xiong *Radix Ligustici wallichii* 3 g
Gan Cao *Radix Glycyrrhizae uralensis* 3 g

Explanation
- The first seven herbs constitute a combination of the above-mentioned formulae to drain Damp-Heat from the Intestines, move Qi and stop pain.
- **Bai Shao** was added as it is astringent and absorbing to help to stop diarrhoea. In combination with Gan Cao, it "moderates urgency" which means not only to stop pain, but also to calm any urgency, such as urgency of bowel movement in this case. Bai Shao also calms Blood in order to stop bleeding.
- **Yi Yi Ren** and **Fu Ling** were added to help to drain Dampness.
- **Ma Chi Xian** is specific to drain Damp-Heat from the Intestines.
- **Chuan Xiong** was added to direct the other herbs to the Blood portion in order to stop bleeding.

- **Gan Cao** harmonizes and, together with Bai Shao, it moderates urgency.

This formula proved to be right and this patient, who is still being treated, started improving straight away reporting a decrease in the number of bowel movements with normal stools some of the time. The bleeding from the bowel stopped after two months. This case history highlights the importance of a correct differentiation between Fullness and Emptiness with the consequent principle of treatment.

3. RETENTION OF FOOD

CLINICAL MANIFESTATIONS

Rotten-smelling loose stools, abdominal pain which is relieved by the bowel movement, borborygmi, bad digestion, feeling of fullness, belching, sour regurgitation, foul breath, no appetite.
Tongue: thick coating.
Pulse: Slippery.

TREATMENT PRINCIPLE

Dissolve food, eliminate stagnation.

ACUPUNCTURE

Ren-10 Xiawan, ST-21 Liangmen, ST-44 Neiting, ST-25 Tianshu, SP-4 Gongsun, Ren-12 Zhongwan. Reducing or even method on all points except Ren-12 which should be reinforced.

Explanation

- **Ren-10** stimulates the descending of Stomach-Qi.
- **ST-21** resolves retention of food.
- **ST-44** is used if retention of food is associated with Heat.
- **ST-25** stops diarrhoea.
- **SP-4** resolves retention of food.
- **Ren-12** tonifies the Spleen to resolve retention of food.

HERBAL TREATMENT

(a) Prescription

BAO HE WAN

Preserving and Harmonizing Pill
Shan Zha *Fructus Crataegi* 9 g
Shen Qu *Massa Fermentata Medicinalis* 6 g
Ban Xia *Rhizoma Pinelliae ternatae* 6 g
Chen Pi *Pericarpium Citri reticulatae* 3 g
Fu Ling *Sclerotium Poriae cocos* 6 g
Lian Qiao *Flos Forsythiae suspensae* 6 g
Lai Fu Zi *Semen Raphani* 6 g

Explanation

This formula has already been explained in the chapter on Headaches (ch. 1).

(b) Prescription

ZHI SHI DAO ZHI WAN
Citrus aurantius Eliminating Stagnation Pill
Da Huang *Radix Rhei* 15 g
Zhi Shi *Fructus Citri aurantii immaturus* 12 g
Huang Lian *Rhizoma Coptidis* 6 g
Huang Qin *Radix Scutellariae baicalensis* 6 g
Fu Ling *Sclerotium Poriae cocos* 6 g
Ze Xie *Rhizoma Alismatis orientalis* 6 g
Bai Zhu *Rhizoma Atractylodis macrocephalae* 6 g
Shen Qu *Massa Fermentata Medicinalis* 12 g

Explanation

This formula, already explained in chapter 16, is used for diarrhoea from retention of food if there is Heat as well. Note the use of Da Huang for diarrhoea rather than constipation.

– **Da Huang** and **Zhi Shi** move downward and eliminate Dampness by purging.
– **Huang Lian** and **Huang Qin** clear Damp-Heat.
– **Fu Ling** and **Ze Xie** drain Dampness.
– **Bai Zhu** and **Shen Qu** tonify the Spleen to resolve Dampness and resolve food accumulation.

Patent remedy

BAO HE WAN
Preserving and Harmonizing Pill
Shan Zha *Fructus Crataegi*

Shen Qu *Massa Fermentata Medicinalis*
Lai Fu Zi *Semen Raphani sativi*
Ban Xia *Rhizoma Pinelliae ternatae*
Chen Pi *Pericarpium Citri reticulatae*
Fu Ling *Sclerotium Poriae cocos*
Lian Qiao *Fructus Forsythiae suspensae*

Explanation

This remedy has the same ingredients and functions as the homonymous prescription above. It can be used for diarrhoea from retention of food and the tongue presentation is a very thick coating which could be either white or yellow.

4. LIVER-QI STAGNATION

CLINICAL MANIFESTATIONS

Diarrhoea often alternating with constipation, abdominal distension, belching, poor appetite, mental depression, moodiness, nervous tension, irritability.
Tongue: may not show much or the sides may be slightly Red.
Pulse: Wiry.

TREATMENT PRINCIPLE

Pacify the Liver, move Qi, strengthen the Spleen.

ACUPUNCTURE

Ren-12 Zhongwan, BL-20 Pishu, LIV-13 Zhangmen, G.B.-34 Yanglingquan, ST-36 Zusanli, SP-6 Sanyinjiao, ST-39 Xiajuxu.

Explanation

– **Ren-12**, **BL-20** and **ST-36** strengthen the Spleen; reinforcing method.
– **LIV-13** harmonizes Liver and Spleen; even method.
– **G.B.-34** moves Qi and pacifies the Liver; reducing method.
– **SP-6** tonifies the Spleen and relieves lower abdominal pain; even method.

– **ST-39** stops abdominal pain; reducing method.

HERBAL TREATMENT

Prescription

TONG XIE YAO FANG
Painful Diarrhoea Formula
Bai Zhu *Rhizoma Atractylodis macrocephalae* 9 g
Bai Shao *Radix Paeoniae albae* 6 g
Chen Pi *Pericarpium Citri reticulatae* 4.5 g
Fang Feng *Radix Ledebouriellae sesloidis* 6 g

Explanation

– **Bai Zhu** tonifies the Spleen.
– **Bai Shao** pacifies the Liver.
– **Chen Pi** moves Qi.
– **Fang Feng** harmonizes Liver and Spleen.

This formula is specific for painful diarrhoea from Liver-Qi stagnation and the condition it addresses is characterized by the fact that the abdominal pain is *not* relieved by the bowel movement.

Patent remedy

MU XIANG SHUN QI WAN and SHEN LING BAI ZHU WAN (PIAN)
Saussurea Subduing Qi Pill and *Ginseng-Poria-Atractylodes Pill (Tablet)*

Mu Xiang Shun Qi Wan

Mu Xiang *Radix Saussureae*
Bai Dou Kou *Fructus Amomi cardamomi*
Cang Zhu *Rhizoma Atractylodis lanceae*
Sheng Jiang *Rhizoma Zingiberis officinalis recens*
Qing Pi *Pericarpium Citri reticulatae viridae*
Chen Pi *Pericarpium Citri reticulatae*
Fu Ling *Sclerotium Poriae cocos*
Chai Hu *Radix Bupleuri*
Hou Po *Cortex Magnoliae officinalis*
Bing Lang *Semen Arecae catechu*
Zhi Ke *Fructus Citri aurantii*
Wu Yao *Radix Lynderae strychnifoliae*
Lai Fu Zi *Semen Raphani sativi*
Shan Zha *Fructus Crataegi*

Shen Qu *Massa Fermentata Medicinalis*
Mai Ya *Fructus Hordei vulgaris germinatus*
Gan Cao *Radix Glycyrrhizae uralensis*

Shen Ling Bai Zhu Wan (Pian)

Ren Shen *Radix Ginseng* (or Dang Shen *Radix Codonopsis pilosulae*)
Fu Ling *Sclerotium Poriae cocos*
Bai Zhu *Rhizoma Atractylodis macrocephalae*
Jie Geng *Radix Platycodi grandiflori*
Shan Yao *Radix Dioscoreae oppositae*
Chen Pi *Pericarpium Citri reticulatae*
Sha Ren *Fructus seu Semen Amomi*
Lian Zi *Semen Nelumbinis nuciferae*
Bian Dou *Semen Dolichoris lablab*
Yi Yi Ren *Semen Coicis lachryma jobi*
Zhi Gan Cao *Radix Glycyrrhizae uralensis praeparata*

Explanation

The first remedy moves Liver-Qi and resolves retention of food, while the second one tonifies Spleen-Qi and stops diarrhoea. In the case of diarrhoea, it is better to combine a Qi-moving remedy with one to tonify the Spleen and stop diarrhoea as stagnant Liver-Qi often invades the Spleen and interferes with its transforming and transporting.

DEFICIENCY CONDITIONS

1. SPLEEN AND STOMACH DEFICIENCY

CLINICAL MANIFESTATIONS

Loose stools, sometimes like water, thin stools, sometimes with mucus, increased frequency of bowel movement, poor appetite, slight abdominal distension, a feeling of oppression of the chest, a sallow complexion, tiredness.
Tongue: Pale, teeth marks.
Pulse: Weak

TREATMENT PRINCIPLE

Strengthen the Spleen and benefit the Stomach.

ACUPUNCTURE

Ren-12 Zhongwan, BL-20 Pishu, BL-21 Weishu, ST-36 Zusanli, SP-6 Sanyinjiao, Ren-6 Qihai moxa on ginger, ST-25 Tianshu, ST-37 Shangjuxu, Du-20 Baihui; reinforcing method.

Explanation

- **Ren-12**, **BL-20**, **BL-21**, **ST-36** and **SP-6** tonify Stomach and Spleen.
- **Ren-6** tonifies Qi. Moxa on ginger on this point is the best method for intestinal problems from a deficient and cold Spleen.
- **ST-25** and **ST-37** stop diarrhoea.
- **BL-20** raises Spleen-Qi and helps to stop diarrhoea.

HERBAL TREATMENT

Prescription

SHEN LING BAI ZHU SAN
Ginseng-Poria-Atractylodes Powder
Ren Shen *Radix Ginseng* 6 g (or **Dang Shen** *Radix Codonopsis pilosulae* 12 g)
Bai Zhu *Rhizoma Atractylodis macrocephalae* 9 g
Fu Ling *Sclerotium Poriae cocos* 12 g
Zhi Gan Cao *Radix Glycyrrhizae uralensis praeparata* 6 g
Bian Dou *Semen Dolichoris lablab* 12 g
Shan Yao *Radix Dioscoreae oppositae* 12 g
Lian Zi *Semen Nelumbinis nuciferae* 12 g
Sha Ren *Fructus seu Semen Amomi* 4.5 g
Yi Yi Ren *Semen Coicis lachryma jobi* 10 g
Jie Geng *Radix Platycodi grandiflori* 6 g

Explanation

This is the main formula to tonify Spleen-Qi and stop diarrhoea from Spleen and Stomach deficiency.

- **Ren Shen**, **Bai Zhu**, **Fu Ling** and **Gan Cao** form the Si Jun Zi Tang *Four Gentlemen Decoction* which tonifies Stomach- and Spleen-Qi.
- **Bian Dou**, **Shan Yao** and **Lian Zi** tonify the Spleen and Stomach. Bian Dou and Shan Yao also tonify Spleen-Yin; Lian Zi is also astringent and stops diarrhoea.

- **Sha Ren** and **Yi Yi Ren** resolve Dampness, the former via sweating, the latter via urination.
- **Jie Geng** is added to carry the formula to the Upper Burner and the Lungs, so that it also tonifies Lung-Qi. Jie Geng is sometimes described as having the same function as that of an oar of a boat.

Patent remedy

SHEN LING BAI ZHU WAN (PIAN)
Ginseng-Poria-Atractylodes Pill (Tablet)

Explanation

This remedy has the same ingredients and indications as the homonymous formula above.

The tongue presentation appropriate to this remedy is a Pale body with a rootless coating in the centre, and possibly a Stomach crack.

Case history

A 37-year-old man had been suffering from diarrhoea for 5 years. His stools were always loose and occasionally like water. He was often very tired and his head felt muzzy.

His pulse was very Weak on the right side and his tongue was Pale and Swollen.

Diagnosis
This is a clear case of Spleen-Qi deficiency with some Dampness and Phlegm. It is Dampness and Phlegm in the head that cause it to feel muzzy.

Treatment principle
The treatment principle used was to tonify Spleen-Qi and resolve Dampness. This patient was treated with acupuncture and a patent remedy.

Acupuncture
The main acupuncture points used (with reinforcing method) were:

- **ST-36** Zusanli, **SP-6** Sanyinjiao, **BL-20** Pishu, **BL-21** Weishu and **Ren-12** Zhongwan to tonify Stomach and Spleen.
- **ST-25** Tianshu and **Ren-6** Qihai with moxa on ginger to tonify Qi and stop diarrhoea.
- **ST-37** Shangjuxu, Lower Sea point of the Large Intestine, is specific to stop chronic diarrhoea.

Herbal treatment
The remedy used was Shen Ling Bai Zhu Wan *Ginseng-Poria-Atractylodis Pill* which is specific to tonify Spleen-Qi and stop chronic diarrhoea.

This patient's condition was cured after 9 months of treatment.

2. KIDNEY-YANG DEFICIENCY

CLINICAL MANIFESTATIONS

Early-morning diarrhoea, abdominal pain, borborygmi which stop after the bowel movement, weak back and knees.
Tongue: Pale, teeth marks.
Pulse: Weak and Deep.

TREATMENT PRINCIPLE

Warm the Kidneys, strengthen the Spleen, stop diarrhoea and fill-up Emptiness.

ACUPUNCTURE

Ren-12 Zhongwan, BL-20 Pishu, ST-36 Zusanli, SP-6 Sanyinjiao, BL-23 Shenshu, BL-25 Dachangshu, ST-25 Tianshu, Ren-6 Qihai, Du-20 Baihui. Reinforcing method and moxa.

Explanation

- **Ren-12**, **BL-20**, **ST-36** and **SP-6** tonify the Spleen.
- **BL-23** tonifies Kidney-Yang.
- **BL-25** and **ST-25** Back-Transporting and Front-Collecting points of the Large Intestine treat chronic diarrhoea.
- **ST-37** Lower Sea point of the Large Intestine stops chronic diarrhoea.
- **Ren-6** with moxa, tonifies Qi and stops diarrhoea. Indirect moxibustion on ginger is a very effective method of treating this type of diarrhoea.
- **Du-20** raises sinking Qi.

HERBAL TREATMENT

Prescription

SI SHEN WAN
Four Spirits Pill

Bai Dou Kou *Fructus Cardamomi rotundi* 6 g
Bu Gu Zhi *Fructus Psoraleae corylifoliae* 12 g
Wu Wei Zi *Fructus Schisandrae chinensis* 6 g
Wu Zhu Yu *Fructus Evodiae rutaecarpae* 3 g
Sheng Jiang *Rhizoma Zingiberis officinalis recens* 3 slices
Hong Zao *Fructus Ziziphi jujubae* 3 dates

Explanation

- **Bai Dou Kou** and **Wu Zhu Yu** warm Spleen and Kidneys.
- **Bu Gu Zhi** strengthens Kidney-Yang and stops leakage.
- **Wu Wei Zi** is astringent and stops leakage.

Variations

- If there are pronounced cold symptoms add Fu Zi *Radix Aconiti carmichaeli praeparata* and Gan Jiang *Rhizoma Zingiberis officinalis*.
- In an old person with very long-standing diarrhoea and symptoms of sinking Qi add Huang Qi *Radix Astragali membranacei*, Dang Shen *Radix Codonopsis pilosulae* and Bai Zhu *Rhizoma Atractylodis macrocephalae*.

Patent remedy

FU ZI LI ZHONG WAN
Aconitum Regulating the Centre Pill
Gan Jiang *Rhizoma Zingiberis officinalis*
Bai Zhu *Rhizoma Atractylodis macrocephalae*
Dang Shen *Radix Codonopsis pilosulae*
Gan Cao *Radix Glycyrrhizae uralensis*
Fu Zi *Radix Aconiti carmichaeli praeparata*

Explanation

This remedy tonifies Spleen- and Kidney-Yang and expels internal Cold. It can be used for chronic diarrhoea from Spleen- and Kidney-Yang deficiency and the tongue presentation is a very Pale, Swollen and wet tongue body.

Case history

A 38-year-old man had been suffering from diarrhoea since he was 16. His stools were always loose and occasionally like water, and he had up to 8 bowel movements a day, all in the morning. His sleep was poor as he woke up frequently during the night, feeling his throat dry. He also suffered from tinnitus and impotence. His pulse was Fine and Deep and his tongue was slightly Red and Swollen, with the coating slightly peeled in patches.

Diagnosis
This is a complicated condition of deficiency of both Kidney-Yang and Kidney-Yin. The symptoms of Kidney-Yang deficiency are: impotence, diarrhoea in the mornings and Swollen tongue. The symptoms of Kidney-Yin deficiency are: Red tongue, peeled coating, tinnitus, insomnia and dry throat.

Treatment principle
As the diarrhoea was his main concern because the frequency of bowel movements in the morning severely interfered with his work, attention was directed at treating this first. In order to treat the diarrhoea, Kidney-Yang should be tonified and warmed. However, he suffered from a deficiency of both Kidney-Yin and Kidney-Yang, and tonifying and warming the latter with a Kidney-Yang herbal formula, would definitely aggravate the former. In such complex cases of deficiency of both Yin and Yang, acupuncture is often preferable to herbal medicine as, with acupuncture, the Kidneys can be strengthened in general, without any special emphasis on Yin or Yang.

Acupuncture
The main points used (with reinforcing method) were chosen from the following:

- **ST-37** Shangjuxu and **BL-25** Dachangshu to stop chronic diarrhoea.
- **BL-23** Shenshu, **KI-7** Fuliu, **Ren-4** Guanyuan and **Ren-6** Qihai to tonify the Kidneys.
- **HE-7** Shenmen and **KI-6** Zhaohai to calm the Mind and promote sleep.

This patient needed treatment for over a year in order to achieve a cure as his condition was very long-standing.

Prognosis

Diarrhoea responds very well to treatment with acupuncture and herbs. Acute diarrhoea responds practically immediately and acupuncture and herbs (or patent remedies) are probably the medicine of choice in this condition. For example, for acute diarrhoea from Damp-Heat, the patent remedy Po Chai Pill is extremely effective.

As for chronic diarrhoea, this naturally takes longer to treat and occasionally, it may be very stubborn. If it is due to Kidney-Yang deficiency, male patients should reduce the level of their sexual activity.

Western differentiation

In Western medicine, diarrhoea is first of all differentiated between acute or chronic. Acute diarrhoea is further differentiated between infective and non-infective. Infective diarrhoea ("food poisoning") may be due to infection of various organisms such as salmonella, *Escherichia coli*, staphylococcus or clostridium. Non-infective causes include mostly poisonous plants (such as mushrooms) but most of all, medicinal drugs. Drugs which most commonly cause diarrhoea as a side-effect are antibiotics, antimitotic (against cancer) drugs and digitalis.

Chronic diarrhoea is classified as inflammatory or non-inflammatory. The two most common causes of inflammatory chronic diarrhoea are Crohn's disease and ulcerative colitis. In more recent years, AIDS may also be a cause.

Non-inflammatory causes include irritable bowel and neoplasm.

INFLAMMATORY CAUSES OF CHRONIC DIARRHOEA

CROHN'S DISEASE

This is characterized by a chronically inflamed and greatly thickened small intestine with narrowing of its lumen and ulceration of the mucosa.

Its main manifestations are diarrhoea and abdominal pain with stools which may rarely contain mucus and blood.

From the point of view of Chinese medicine, this condition often corresponds to Damp-Heat in the Intestines.

ULCERATIVE COLITIS

This is characterized by ulceration of the large

intestine. It is often accompanied by iritis, arthritis and erythema nodosum.

The main clinical manifestations include diarrhoea with blood and mucus in the stools and abdominal pain.

From the Chinese point of view, this condition often corresponds to Damp-Heat and stasis of Blood in the Intestines.

AIDS

Diarrhoea is common in this disease and it is caused by a secondary infection of the bowel by a wide variety of pathogenic organisms.

NON-INFLAMMATORY CAUSES OF CHRONIC DIARRHOEA

IRRITABLE BOWEL

This term is usually used in Western medicine in all cases of abdominal pain and alternation of diarrhoea and constipation for which no abnormality may be found on sigmoidoscopy, colonoscopy or barium enema. Rather than a

Table 18.1 Causes of diarrhoea in Western medicine

ACUTE		CHRONIC	
Infectious	Non-infectious	Inflammatory	Non-inflammatory
Salmonella Escherichia Staphylococcus Clostridium	Poisonous plants Drugs	Crohn's disease Ulcerative colitis AIDS	Irritable bowel Neoplasm

specific "disease", it is a diagnostic refuge whenever a specific cause cannot be found.

The clinical manifestations include abdominal pain and distension and diarrhoea which often alternates with constipation.

From a Chinese perspective, this condition often corresponds to stagnant Liver-Qi invading the Spleen.

NEOPLASM

A malignant cancer of the large intestine may cause diarrhoea. This would be accompanied by abdominal pain.

The causes of diarrhoea are summarized in Table 18.1.

END NOTES

1. 1979 The Yellow Emperor's Classic of Internal Medicine — Simple Questions (*Huang Ti Nei Jing Su Wen* 黄帝内经素问), People's Health Publishing House, Beijing. First published *c.* 100 BC, p. 220.
2. 1981 Spiritual Axis (*Ling Shu Jing* 灵枢经), People's Health Publishing House, Beijing. First published *c.* 100 BC, p. 69.
3. Simple Questions, p. 35.
4. Zhang Jing Yue 1986 Complete Book of Jing Yue (*Jing Yue Quan Shu* 景岳全书), Shanghai Scientific Publishing House, Shanghai, p. 415. First published in 1624.
5. Ibid., p. 415.
6. Ibid., p. 415.
7. Ibid., p. 415.
8. Simple Questions, p. 32.

Constipation 19

便
秘

The term constipation is used to describe the slow movement of unduly firm contents through the large bowel leading to infrequent passing of small hard stools. Thus "constipation" may indicate several different signs among which are:

– bowel movements which do not occur daily
– dry stools
– difficult defaecation
– abnormal shape of stools.

Views on what constitutes constipation vary widely. It is not infrequent to hear doctors saying, quite wrongly, that it does not matter if one has a bowel movement only twice a week. On the other hand, some naturopaths believe that it is normal and desirable to have up to four bowel movements a day.

The quantity of stools passed varies from culture to culture. In rural Africa about 400–500 g of stools are passed by an adult. In contrast, in Western countries an adult passes about 80–120 g of stools a day.[1] Similarly, the transit time of the stools in the bowel averages 1.5 days in rural Africa and 3 days in Western countries. Interestingly, constipation has affected Western societies for a long time. Jonathan Swift (the author of "Gulliver's Travels") wrote a book entitled "Human Ordure" describing various types of stools he had observed in Dublin in 1733. He said: *"The fifth type [of stools] are those voided in small, firm, round Balls, Buttons or Bullets . . . I have observed these [types] to flourish mostly about Colleges, Schools and most places of publik Education."*[2] His description fits perfectly the type of stools passed by those who suffer from constipation today.

Normally, the bowels should open every day and the stools should be light-brown in colour, roughly cylindrical in shape and a few inches long.

Aetiology

The main aetiological factors are as follows:

1. DIET

Diet is of course an important cause of constipation. Excessive consumption of hot foods dries up the fluids of Stomach and Intestines and may cause constipation by drying up the stools so that they cannot be moved properly.

Conversely, excessive consumption of cold foods may block the Spleen function of transportation so that stools cannot be moved downwards.

Apart from the nature of foods eaten, lack of fibre in food is of course a major cause of constipation in Western industrialized countries. Lack of fibre in the diet is a modern cause of disease not contemplated in the old classics of Chinese medicine as it would not have been a problem in the times at which they were written. The importance of this factor has, however, lessened considerably over the past 10 years or so as awareness about the importance of fibre in the diet has increased tremendously.

2. EMOTIONAL STRESS

Emotional stress affects the bowel movements mostly through the Liver and Spleen. Emotional problems such as anger, resentment or frustration over a long period of time may cause stagnation of Liver-Qi. Stagnant Liver-Qi obstructs the smooth flow of Qi in the Lower Burner and leads to constipation and abdominal distension and pain. This is constipation of an Excess nature.

Excessive mental work, too much thinking and worrying, brooding, all affect the Spleen and slow down its transportation of food in the Intestines, leading to constipation. This is constipation of a Deficient nature and is *not* accompanied by distension and pain.

3. LACK OF EXERCISE

Lack of exercise is another very important cause of constipation in Western industrialized societies. Exercise stimulates the peristalsis of the Large Intestine and, from a Chinese perspective, lack of exercise weakens Spleen-Qi and may also cause stagnation of Liver-Qi. Deficient Spleen-Qi over a long period of time fails to provide Qi to move the stools and therefore may result in constipation, while stagnant Liver-Qi may cause it by failing to move Qi in the Intestines.

4. OVERWORK AND CHILDBIRTH

Excessive physical work weakens the Spleen and injures muscles. Deficient Spleen-Qi fails to move the stools in the Large Intestine and may cause constipation. The same situation may follow childbirth in women who have a pre-existing condition of Spleen deficiency.

Overwork in the sense of working long hours without adequate rest for many years weakens the Kidneys. If it weakens Kidney-Yin it may cause constipation from dryness. If it weakens Kidney-Yang, it may cause constipation by leading to internal Cold.

5. FEBRILE DISEASE

If external Wind-Heat is not expelled, it easily progresses to the Interior and turns into interior Heat, usually affecting the Lungs and/or the Stomach. At this stage, corresponding to the Bright-Yang stage of the 6 Stages or Qi Level of the 4 Levels, there is a high fever and pronounced symptoms of Heat such as intense thirst, profuse sweating, a Red tongue and a Rapid pulse. This type of Heat during a febrile disease tends to injure fluids very quickly and cause dryness. This affects Lungs, Stomach and Intestines where it dries up the stools and causes constipation.

Heat that causes dryness and constipation during a febrile disease is called Fire. Constipation with abdominal pain and pronounced dryness are the main symptoms which distinguish Fire from Heat. It is for this reason that at this stage of a febrile disease with constipation (or merely with dry stools), the treatment principle is to drain Fire by moving downwards. In herbal medicine, the practitioner uses one of the three moving-downwards formulae, i.e. Da Cheng Qi Tang *Great Conducting Qi Decoction*, Xiao Cheng

Qi Tang *Small Conducting Qi Decoction* or Tiao Wei Cheng Qi Tang *Regulating the Stomach Conducting Qi Decoction*. With acupuncture, one can use the combination of T.B.-6 Zhigou with SP-15 Daheng.

Pathology

As for the pathology, the organs mostly involved in constipation are the Stomach, the Large Intestine, the Spleen, the Liver and the Kidneys; the key factors for a healthy bowel function are a good supply of fluids in Stomach and Intestines and a strong Qi to move the stools along the digestive system.

STOMACH

The Stomach is the origin of fluids and is very closely linked to the Intestines. If the Stomach is affected by Heat or if it suffers from Yin deficiency, the fluids are deficient in the Stomach and Large Intestine and the stools dry up so that they cannot be moved properly.

In acute febrile diseases at the Qi Level (of the 4 Levels) there is often Fire drying up the fluids in the Stomach and Large Intestine and therefore the stools. This causes constipation. In this case the stools are very dry.

LARGE INTESTINE

The Large Intestine is functionally related to the Stomach (within the Bright-Yang channels) and is affected by Stomach-Heat or Stomach-Yin deficiency as described above. This causes constipation from Heat or Yin deficiency.

The Large Intestine receives water from the Small Intestine, reabsorbs some fluids and excretes stools. Cold is obstructing and it may affect the Large Intestine by blocking its excretion of stools. This causes constipation of the Cold type. In this case the stools are not dry.

SPLEEN

Although Spleen-Qi normally ascends and its pathology usually involves diarrhoea, deficient Spleen-Qi may also cause constipation. It may do so because the movement of wastes and stools in the Large Intestine relies on Spleen-Qi. Thus, if Spleen-Qi is deficient and it does not provide enough Qi to move the stools in the bowel, constipation may ensue. In this case the stools may be thin and long.

LIVER

Liver-Qi ensures the smooth flow of Qi in every organ. In the Lower Burner, it ensures a smooth movement of stools in the Large Intestine. If Liver-Qi stagnates, it causes stagnation of Qi in the Lower Burner and the Large Intestine so that the stools are knotted and cannot move downwards. In this case the stools are small and round like pebbles.

KIDNEYS

The Kidneys control the two lower orifices — urethra and anus — and they therefore influence defaecation. Kidney-Yin deficiency involves deficiency of fluids: this affects the Large Intestine as there are not enough fluids to moisten the stools which therefore cannot move smoothly downwards. Wu Ju Tong (1758–1836) in his book "Differentiation of Warm Diseases" says: *"When fluids are deficient there is not enough water to make the boat move."*[3] "Boat" here stands for stools. In this case the stools are dry.

Although Kidney-Yang deficiency will normally cause diarrhoea, it may also cause constipation. This happens when Yang Qi in the Lower Burner is so deficient that it cannot move the stools. On the other hand, Kidney-Yang deficiency over a long period of time will lead to Cold in the Lower Burner which further obstructs the movement of the stools. In this case the stools are not dry and defaecation is very difficult, succeeding only with great strain.

Thus, to summarize, constipation may be caused by:

– Heat
– Stagnation of Qi

– Deficiency (of Qi, Yang, Blood or Yin)
– Interior Cold.

Since stagnation of Qi is a Full pattern, constipation is therefore simply due to Heat, Cold, Fullness, or Emptiness.

Diagnosis

When diagnosing the causes and type of constipation, it is important to take into account the following factors:

– Stools shape
– Moisture of stools
– Pain
– Effort of defaecation
– Colour.

STOOLS SHAPE

Stools which are round and small like pebbles indicate Heat if they are very dry or Liver-Qi stagnation if they are not dry.

Long and thin stools like pencils indicate Spleen-Qi deficiency. It should be kept in mind that they may indicate carcinoma of the bowel. Figure 19.1 shows normal stools, stools in Liver-Qi stagnation, and in Spleen deficiency.

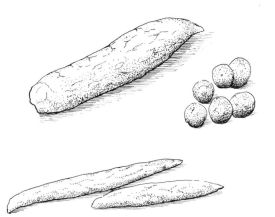

Fig. 19.1   Normal stools, stools in Liver-Qi stagnation, and stools in Spleen deficiency

MOISTURE OF STOOLS

Dry stools indicate Heat or deficiency of Yin. Apart from other symptoms and signs, thirst and dryness of the mouth are an important differentiating symptom. With Heat, there is intense thirst with desire to drink large amounts of cold water. With Yin deficiency there is only a dryness of the mouth with desire to sip water.

Loose stools which are hesitant and difficult to come out indicate Spleen-Qi deficiency with stagnation of Liver-Qi.

Watery, explosive stools splashing in all directions indicates either Damp-Heat (in which case the stools are yellow and frothy) or Damp-Cold.

PAIN

Constipation with abdominal pain points to stagnation of Liver-Qi or Cold. Pain from stagnation of Liver-Qi is not too severe and is accompanied by pronounced distension. Pain from Cold is severe and spastic.

EFFORT OF DEFAECATION

Difficult defaecation with great effort indicates deficiency of Qi or Yang. This is also confirmed by a feeling of exhaustion after the bowel movement.

Cramps after defaecation indicate Cold or stagnation of Qi.

COLOUR

– Pale stools indicate Dampness, usually Damp-Heat in the Gall-Bladder
– Dark stools indicate Heat
– Green stools in children indicate Cold.

Differentiation and treatment

The main patterns appearing with constipation are:

Heat

1. Chronic Interior Heat
2. Acute heat in febrile disease

Qi

Stagnation of Liver-Qi

Deficiency

1. Qi Deficiency
2. Blood Deficiency
3. Yang Deficiency
4. Yin Deficiency

Cold

HEAT

1. CHRONIC INTERIOR HEAT

HEAT IN THE STOMACH AND LARGE INTESTINE

Clinical manifestations

Dry stools, infrequent bowel movements, thirst, scanty-dark urine, red face, feeling of heat, abdominal pain, dry mouth, foul breath.
Tongue: Red with yellow coating and red points around the centre and on the root.
Pulse: Rapid and Slippery.

HEAT IN THE LIVER

Clinical manifestations

Dry stools, infrequent bowel movements, thirst, bitter taste, dark urine, headache, irritability, red face, blood-shot eyes.
Tongue: Red, redder on the sides, dry-yellow coating.
Pulse: Wiry and Rapid.

Treatment principle

Clear Heat, drain Fire (of Large Intestine or Liver), moisten the Intestines.

Acupuncture

L.I.-4 Hegu, L.I.-11 Quchi, T.B.-6 Zhigou, SP-14 Fuji, SP-15 Daheng, ST-44 Neiting, ST-28 Shuidao, Waishuidao, ST-29 Guilai, Waiguilai, LIV-2 Xingjian. Reducing method.

Explanation

– **L.I.-4** clears Heat in the Large Intestine and moves the stools.
– **L.I.-11** clears Heat in the Large Intestine.
– **T.B.-6** clears Heat, opens the Triple Burner and promotes the bowel movement.
– **SP-14** and **SP-15** move downwards.
– **ST-44** clears Stomach-Heat.
– **ST-28** and **ST-29** clear Heat and promote the bowel movement. When used for constipation, they only need be needled on the left side to affect the descending colon.
– **Waishuidao** and **Waiguilai**, extra points which are located one *cun* lateral to ST-28 and ST-29 respectively, have similar actions to these two points and promote the bowel movements. They also only need be needled on the left side.
– **LIV-2** is used if there is Liver-Fire.

Herbal treatment

Stomach and Large Intestine Heat

Prescription

MA ZI REN WAN
Cannabis Pill
Huo Ma Ren *Semen Cannabis sativae* 9 g
Da Huang *Rhizoma Rhei* 6 g
Xing Ren *Semen Pruni armeniacae* 4.5 g
Zhi Shi *Fructus Citri aurantii immaturus* 6 g
Hou Po *Cortex Magnoliae officinalis* 4.5 g
Bai Shao *Radix Paeoniae albae* 4.5 g

Explanation.
– **Huo Ma Ren** moistens the Intestines and moves downwards.
– **Da Huang** clears Heat and moves downwards.
– **Xing Ren** and **Zhi Shi** help the first two herbs to move downwards.
– **Hou Po** regulates Qi and relieves fullness.
– **Bai Shao** is sour and absorbing and it is used to prevent injury of fluids from Heat.

Liver-Fire

Prescription

DANG GUI LONG HUI WAN
Angelica-Gentiana-Aloe Pill
Dang Gui *Radix Angelicae sinensis* 30 g
Long Dan Cao *Radix Gentianae scabrae* 15 g
Lu Hui *Herba Aloes* 15 g
Shan Zhi Zi *Fructus Gardeniae jasminoidis* 6 g
Huang Lian *Rhizoma Coptidis* 4 g
Huang Bo *Cortex Phellodendri* 6 g
Huang Qin *Radix Scutellariae baicalensis* 6 g
Da Huang *Rhizoma Rhei* 9 g
Mu Xiang *Radix Saussureae* 5 g
She Xiang *Secretio Moschus moschiferi* 1.5 g
Qing Dai *Indigo Naturalis* 6 g

Explanation.
- **Dang Gui** enters the Liver and moves the stools.
- **Long Dan Cao** drains Liver-Fire.
- **Lu Hui** drains Liver-Fire and moves the stools.
- **Zhi Zi**, **Huang Lian**, **Huang Bo** and **Huang Qin** drain Fire in the Intestines.
- **Da Huang** drains Fire and moves downward.
- **Mu Xiang** moves Qi: it is added to help the downwards movement of stools.
- **She Xiang** opens the orifices: it is added to help Da Huang to move downwards. As this is not a substance in common use (and it is also extremely expensive) it can be replaced by Shi Chang Pu *Rhizoma Acori graminei* (6 g).
- **Qing Dai** enters the Liver and resolves Fire-Poison.

This prescription is a very strong one with many bitter and cold herbs. It should be used only for severe cases of Liver-Fire and only for a relatively short time. If the symptoms of Liver-Fire are not very severe, the previous formula (Ma Zi Ren Wan) can be used simply with the addition of Long Dan Cao to drain Liver-Fire.

Variations.
- If fluids have been injured add Sheng Di Huang *Radix Rehmanniae glutinosae*, Xuan Shen *Radix Scrophulariae ningpoensis* and Mai Men Dong *Tuber Ophiopogonis japonici*.

(i) Patent remedy

LONG DAN XIE GAN WAN
Gentiana Draining the Liver Pill
Long Dan Cao *Radix Gentianae scabrae*
Huang Qin *Radix Scutellariae baicalensis*
Shan Zhi Zi *Fructus Gardeniae jasminoidis*
Ze Xie *Rhizoma Alismatis orientalis*
Mu Tong *Caulis Akebiae*
Che Qian Zi *Semen Plantaginis*
Sheng Di Huang *Radix Rehmanniae glutinosae*
Dang Gui *Radix Angelicae sinensis*
Chai Hu *Radix Bupleuri*
Gan Cao *Radix Glycyrrhizae uralensis*

Explanation. This remedy can be used for constipation from Liver-Fire. The tongue presentation appropriate to this remedy is a Red body with redder sides and a dry-yellow coating.

(ii) Patent remedy

CAI FENG ZHEN ZHU AN CHUANG WAN
Colourful Phoenix Pearl Hiding Boils Pill
Zhen Zhu *Margarita*
Sheng Di Huang *Radix Rehmanniae glutinosae*
Nan Sha Shen *Radix Adenophorae*
Xuan Shen *Radix Scrophulariae ningpoensis*
Jin Yin Hua *Flos Lonicerae japonicae*
Huang Bo *Cortex Phellodendri*
Da Huang *Rhizoma Rhei*
Ling Yang Jiao *Cornu Antelopis*

Explanation. This pill nourishes Yin, promotes fluids, drains Fire and moves the stools. It is suitable for constipation caused by Fire in the Large Intestines, when Fire has begun to injure Yin and particularly if accompanied by acne.

The tongue presentation appropriate to this remedy is a Red body without coating in the centre but with a dry yellow coating elsewhere.

(iii) Patent remedy

MING MU SHANG QING PIAN
Brightening the Eyes Clearing Upward Tablet
Shan Zhi Zi *Fructus Gardeniae jasminoidis*
Dang Gui *Radix Angelicae sinensis*
Huang Lian *Rhizoma Coptidis*
Ju Hua *Flos Chrysanthemi morifolii*

Da Huang *Rhizoma Rhei*
Huang Qin *Radix Scutellariae baicalensis*
Lian Qiao *Fructus Forsythiae suspensae*
Bai Ji Li *Fructus Tribuli terrestris*
Chan Tui *Periostracum Cicadae*
Mai Dong *Tuber Ophiopogonis japonici*
Shi Gao *Gypsum fibrosum*

Explanation.   Although this is a remedy which is usually used for eye problems deriving from Liver-Fire, it can be used for constipation from the same cause as it contains Da Huang and Dang Gui which move the stools.

The tongue presentation appropriate to this remedy is a Red body with redder sides and a dry-yellow coating.

(iv) Patent remedy

RUN CHANG WAN
Moistening the Intestines Pill
Huo Ma Ren *Semen Cannabis sativae*
Tao Ren *Semen Persicae*
Qiang Huo *Radix et Rhizoma Notopterygii*
Dang Gui *Radix Angelicae sinensis*
Da Huang *Rhizoma Rhei*

Explanation.   This remedy clears Intestine-Heat and moves downwards. It is suitable for constipation from Heat in the Stomach and Intestines. The tongue presentation appropriate to this remedy is a Red body with a dry-yellow coating.

Please note that some books describe this remedy as being suitable for chronic constipation in the elderly or in women after childbirth: but it cannot be appropriate in such cases as it contains Da Huang which should not be used for months on end, especially in old people or people in a weak condition (such as women after childbirth).

Case history

A 34-year-old woman had been suffering from constipation for 10 years. She had only 2–3 bowel movements a week and the stools were dry and small. Her breath had a bad smell. Apart from this, she had no other symptoms. Her tongue-body colour was normal but it had a dry-yellow coating which was thicker on the root. Her pulse was unremarkable.

Diagnosis
This is a case of Heat in the Intestines. Dry and small stools indicate Heat and this is confirmed by the yellow tongue coating and the breath smell which indicates that there is Heat also in the Stomach.

Treatment principle
The treatment principle adopted was to clear Heat in the Intestines and benefit fluids. This patient was treated with both acupuncture and herbs.

Acupuncture
The main acupuncture points used were:

- **SP-15** Daheng to clear Heat in the Intestines and move the stools.
- **ST-25** Tianshu and **L.I.-11** Quchi to clear Intestine-Heat.
- **ST-44** Neiting to clear Stomach-Heat.
- **Ren-10** Xiawan to promote the descending of Stomach-Qi.
- **ST-36** Zusanli to promote the bowel movements.

The points were all needled with even method, except for ST-36 which was reinforced.

Herbal treatment
The herbal formula used was a variation of Ma Zi Ren Wan *Cannabis Pill*:

Huo Ma Ren *Semen Cannabis sativae* 9 g
Da Huang *Rhizoma Rhei* 6 g
Xing Ren *Semen Pruni armeniacae* 4.5 g
Zhi Shi *Fructus Citri aurantii immaturus* 6 g
Hou Po *Cortex Magnoliae officinalis* 4.5 g
Bai Shao *Radix Paeoniae albae* 4.5 g
Huang Lian *Rhizoma Coptidis* 3 g
Ku Shen *Radix Sophorae flavescentis* 4.5 g

Explanation
- The first six herbs constitute the original formula.
- **Huang Lian** was added to clear Stomach-Heat.
- **Ku Shen** was added to clear Intestine-Heat.

After a few weeks, Da Huang was removed and replaced with Dang Gui. This patient improved slowly and gradually over the course of one year.

Case history

A 62-year-old woman sought treatment for what had been diagnosed 4 years previously as Parkinson's disease. She had a very slight tremor of her arm, dragged her foot slightly and her handwriting had been getting progressively smaller (a typical symptom of this disease). Apart from this, she had also been suffering from constipation more or less "for her whole life". She resorted to taking up to 10 Senokot (an anthraquinone-based laxative) a day. Because she took laxatives every day it was difficult to find out how her stools would have been without them. She also suffered from back-ache, dizziness, tinnitus, night-sweating, poor sleep (waking up during the night) and a dry throat at night with a desire to sip water. She often felt hot. Her tongue was Red, redder on the sides, with a very dry, yellow-black coating (Plate 19.1). Her pulse was Full, Wiry, Slippery and slightly Rapid.

Diagnosis
This is a rather complex condition. There is obviously Liver-Wind, manifested by the tremor of the arm. This most probably arose from Liver-Fire as evidenced by the Rapid and Full pulse, the Red tongue with yellow coating, the constipation and the feeling of heat. There was also some Phlegm as shown by the Slippery pulse. Thus, in this case Wind, Fire and Phlegm are all contributing to her condition. Her other symptoms of back-ache, dizziness, tinnitus, poor sleep and dry throat at night, point to a deficiency of Kidney-Yin. Rather than being the cause of the rising of Liver-Wind, the Kidney-Yin deficiency is probably the result of Liver-Fire injuring the Yin. We can come to this conclusion from observation of the tongue and pulse: the tongue shows the presence of Fire rather than Empty-Heat as it is Red with a yellow coating (rather than without coating), and her pulse is Full, Slippery and Wiry (rather than Fine or Floating-Empty).

Treatment principle
The treatment principle is to drain Liver-Fire, extinguish Liver-Wind, resolve Phlegm and nourish Kidney-Yin.

As for the constipation, although she did not consider this to be her main problem as she consulted me for her Parkinson's disease, it is related to the underlying condition of Liver-Fire and it is necessary to drain it by moving downwards.

This patient was treated only with herbs (as she was receiving acupuncture from a colleague who referred her to me for herbal treatment).

Herbal treatment
I used a variation of Ban Xia Bai Zhu Tian Ma Tang *Pinellia-Atractylodes-Gastrodia Decoction*, which is a formula to extinguish Wind and resolve Phlegm:

Ban Xia *Rhizoma Pinelliae ternatae* 9 g
Bai Zhu *Rhizoma Atractylodis macrocephalae* 6 g
Tian Ma *Rhizoma Gastrodiae elatae* 9 g
Chen Pi *Pericarpium Citri reticulatae* 4 g
Fu Ling *Sclerotium Poriae cocos* 6 g
Zhi Gan Cao *Radix Glycyrrhizae uralensis praeparata* 3 g
Sheng Jiang *Rhizoma Zingiberis officinalis recens* 3 slices
Da Zao *Fructus Ziziphi jujubae* 3 dates
Da Huang *Rhizoma Rhei* 6 g
Mang Xiao *Mirabilitum* 6 g
Di Long *Pheretima aspergillum* 6 g
Sheng Di Huang *Radix Rehmanniae glutinosae* 9 g

Explanation
- The first eight herbs constitute the original formula which extinguishes Wind-Phlegm.

- **Da Huang** and **Mang Xiao** were added to drain Fire by moving downwards.
- **Di Long** was added to extinguish Wind and stop tremors.
- **Sheng Di Huang** was added to nourish Yin.

This formula was administered for about 3 months with slight variations. After 3 months, her bowel movements became normal and regular without the use of laxatives and her tongue was less dry. At this point, the formula was changed to the following variation of the same prescription:

Ban Xia *Rhizoma Pinelliae ternatae* 9 g
Bai Zhu *Rhizoma Atractylodis macrocephalae* 6 g
Tian Ma *Rhizoma Gastrodiae elatae* 9 g
Chen Pi *Pericarpium Citri reticulatae* 4 g
Fu Ling *Sclerotium Poriae cocos* 6 g
Zhi Gan Cao *Radix Glycyrrhizae uralensis praeparata* 3 g
Sheng Jiang *Rhizoma Zingiberis officinalis recens* 3 slices
Da Zao *Fructus Ziziphi jujubae* 3 dates
Sheng Di Huang *Radix Rehmanniae glutinosae* 9 g
Di Long *Pheretima aspergillum* 6 g
Gou Teng *Ramulus Uncariae* 6 g
Ju Hua *Flos Chrysanthemi morifolii* 4 g

Explanation
- The first eight herbs constitute the same original formula Ban Xia Bai Zhu Tian Ma Tang to extinguish Wind-Phlegm.
- **Sheng Di** was added to nourish Yin.
- **Di Long**, **Gou Teng** and **Ju Hua** were added to extinguish Liver-Wind.

This patient is making very good progress also with the Parkinson's symptoms and she is still being treated.

2. ACUTE HEAT IN FEBRILE DISEASE

Constipation, dry stools, abdominal pain and fullness, red face, thirst, dry mouth, profuse sweating, feeling of heat, high fever.
Tongue: Red with dry yellow coating.
Pulse: Overflowing and Rapid.

TREATMENT PRINCIPLE

Drain Fire and move downwards.

ACUPUNCTURE

T.B.-6 Zhigou, SP-15 Daheng, L.I.-11 Quchi,

ST-44 Neiting, L.I.-4 Hegu, ST-28 Shuidao and ST-29 Guilai. Reducing method.

Explanation

- **T.B.-6** drains Fire from the Three Burners and, in combination with SP-15, moves downwards.
- **SP-15** moves downwards.
- **L.I.-11** clears Heat in the Intestines.
- **ST-44** clears Stomach Heat.
- **L.I.-4** clears Heat in the Intestines and moves downwards.
- **ST-28** and **ST-29** clear Heat and promote the bowel movements.

HERBAL TREATMENT

Prescription

DA CHENG QI TANG
Great Conducting Qi Decoction
Da Huang *Rhizoma Rhei* 12 g
Mang Xiao *Mirabilitum* 9 g
Hou Po *Cortex Magnoliae officinalis* 15 g
Zhi Shi *Fructus Citri aurantii immaturus* 12 g

Explanation

- **Da Huang** drains Fire by moving downwards. It is the main herb for Fire in the Stomach corresponding to either the Organ pattern of the Bright-Yang pattern (within the 6 Stages) or the Intestines-Dry-Heat pattern at Qi level (within the 4 Levels).
- **Mang Xiao** helps Da Huang to move downwards.
- **Hou Po** relieves fullness and regulates Qi.
- **Zhi Shi** makes Qi descend and therefore helps the first two herbs to move downwards. It also relieves abdominal distension and pain.

Patent remedy

QING FEI YI HUO PIAN
Clearing the Lungs and Eliminating Fire Tablet
Huang Qin *Radix Scutellariae baicalensis*
Da Huang *Rhizoma Rhei*
Shan Zhi Zi *Fructus Gardeniae jasminoidis*

Tian Hua Fen *Radix Trichosanthis*
Jie Geng *Radix Platycodi grandiflori*
Zhi Mu *Radix Anemarrhenae asphodeloidis*
Qian Hu *Radix Peucedani*
Ku Shen *Radix Sophorae flavescentis*

Explanation

This remedy clears Lung-Fire by moving downwards. It is suitable for acute constipation from Fire in the Lungs and Intestines during a febrile disease, corresponding to either the Bright-Yang-Organ pattern within the 6 Stages, or the Intestine-Dry-Heat pattern within the 4 Levels.

The tongue presentation appropriate to this remedy is a Red tongue with a very dry yellow or even black coating.

QI

STAGNATION OF LIVER-QI

CLINICAL MANIFESTATIONS

Constipation with stools shaped like pebbles but not dry, desire to open the bowels but difficulty in doing so, belching, abdominal distension, irritability.
Tongue: may be of a normal colour or slightly Red on the sides.
Pulse: Wiry. It may be Wiry only on the left side.

TREATMENT PRINCIPLE

Pacify the Liver, regulate Qi, make Qi descend, eliminate stagnation.

ACUPUNCTURE

Ren-10 Xiawan, G.B.-34 Yanglingquan, Ren-6 Qihai, LIV-3 Taichong, SP-15 Daheng.

Explanation

- **Ren-10** stimulates the descending of Qi.
- **G.B.-34** and **Ren-6**, in combination, move Liver-Qi in the lower abdomen.
- **LIV-3** moves Qi and pacifies the Liver.
- **SP-15** moves downwards.

HERBAL TREATMENT

Prescription

LIU MO TANG
Six Ground-Herbs Decoction
Mu Xiang *Radix Saussureae* 6 g
Wu Yao *Radix Linderae strychnifoliae* 6 g
Chen Xiang *Lignum Aquilariae* 4.5 g
Da Huang *Rhizoma Rhei* 6 g
Bing Lang *Semen Arecae catechu* 6 g
Zhi Shi *Fructus Citri aurantii immaturus* 6 g

Explanation

– **Mu Xiang**, **Wu Yao** and **Chen Xiang** regulate Qi, eliminate stagnation and make Qi descend.
– **Da Huang**, **Bing Lang** and **Zhi Shi** move downwards and make Qi descend.

Variations

– If there are Heat signs add Huang Qin *Radix Scutellariae baicalensis* and Zhi Zi *Fructus Gardeniae jasminoidis*.

(i) Patent remedy

XIAO YAO WAN
Free and Easy Wanderer Pill
Chai Hu *Radix Bupleuri*
Bo He *Herba Menthae*
Dang Gui *Radix Angelicae sinensis*
Bai Shao *Radix Paeoniae albae*
Bai Zhu *Rhizoma Atractylodis macrocephalae*
Fu Ling *Sclerotium Poriae cocos*
Zhi Gan Cao *Radix Glycyrrhizae uralensis praeparata*
Sheng Jiang *Rhizoma Zingiberis officinalis recens*

Explanation

This famous remedy moves Liver-Qi, tonifies Spleen-Qi and nourishes Liver-Blood. It is suitable for chronic constipation from Liver-Qi stagnation especially in women, and especially if there is also an underlying Liver-Blood deficiency.

The pulse presentation appropriate to this remedy is pulse which is Weak and Choppy on the right and slightly Wiry on the left, or Fine in general and slightly Wiry on the left.

(ii) Patent remedy

MU XIANG SHUN QI WAN
Saussurea Subduing Qi Pill
Mu Xiang *Radix Saussureae*
Bai Dou Kou *Fructus Amomi cardamomi*
Cang Zhu *Rhizoma Atractylodis lanceae*
Sheng Jiang *Rhizoma Zingiberis officinalis recens*
Qing Pi *Pericarpium Citri reticulatae viridae*
Chen Pi *Pericarpium Citri reticulatae*
Fu Ling *Sclerotium Poriae cocos*
Chai Hu *Radix Bupleuri*
Hou Po *Cortex Magnoliae officinalis*
Bing Lang *Semen Arecae catechu*
Zhi Ke *Fructus Citri aurantii*
Wu Yao *Radix Linderae strychnifoliae*
Lai Fu Zi *Semen Raphani sativi*
Shan Zha *Fructus Crataegi*
Shen Qu *Massa Fermentata Medicinalis*
Mai Ya *Fructus Hordei vulgaris germinatus*
Gan Cao *Radix Glycyrrhizae uralensis*

Explanation

This remedy moves Liver-Qi and subdues rebellious Qi. It is suitable for constipation from stagnation of Liver-Qi which is more severe than that addressed by the previous remedy.

The pulse presentation appropriate to this remedy is pulse which is Wiry in its overall quality.

DEFICIENCY

1. QI DEFICIENCY

Desire to open the bowels but difficulty in doing so, great effort to open bowels, feeling of exhaustion afterwards, thin and long stools which are not dry, pale complexion, tiredness.
Tongue: Pale
Pulse: Empty.

This pattern is due to either Spleen- or Lung-Qi deficiency or both. If there is Spleen deficiency there will also be muscular weakness and poor appetite. If there is Lung deficiency there will be slight breathlessness on exertion and a weak voice.

The constipation here is due to deficient Spleen-Qi not moving the stools in the intestines or to deficient Lung-Qi not providing enough Qi to the Large Intestine for the effort of defaecation. This pattern is common in old people, women after childbirth or anyone after a long, severe illness.

TREATMENT PRINCIPLE

Tonify Qi and moisten the Intestines.

ACUPUNCTURE

BL-21 Weishu, BL-25 Dachangshu, SP-15 Daheng, ST-36 Zusanli, Ren-6 Qihai, SP-6 Sanyinjiao. Reinforcing method.

Explanation

- **BL-21** tonifies Stomach-Qi and is chosen also because, due to the descending movement of Stomach-Qi, it will stimulate the bowel movement.
- **BL-25**, Back-Transporting point of the Large Intestine stimulates the bowel movement.
- **SP-15** stimulates the bowel movement.
- **ST-36** and **SP-6** tonify Qi and promote the bowel movement.
- **Ren-6** tonifies Qi in the Lower Burner.

HERBAL TREATMENT

Prescription

HUANG QI TANG
Astragalus Decoction
Huang Qi *Radix Astragali membranacei* 9 g
Chen Pi *Pericarpium Citri reticulatae* 4.5 g
Huo Ma Ren *Semen Cannabis sativae* 6 g
Feng Mi *Mel* 1 teaspoonful

Explanation

- **Huang Qi** tonifies Spleen- and Lung-Qi.

- **Chen Pi** is combined with Huang Qi to prevent the formation of Dampness when tonifying.
- **Huo Ma Ren** moves downwards by moistening the Intestines.
- **Honey** mildly tonifies Qi and moistens the Intestines to move downwards.

Variations

- If there is very pronounced Qi deficiency add Dang Shen *Radix Codonopsis pilosulae* and Shan Yao *Radix Dioscoreae oppositae*.
- If there are symptoms of sinking Qi and prolapse of the anus, use Bu Zhong Yi Qi Tang *Tonifying the Centre and Benefiting Qi Decoction* instead, with the dosage of Bai Zhu *Rhizoma Atractylodis macrocephalae* increased to 30 g.

2. BLOOD DEFICIENCY

CLINICAL MANIFESTATIONS

Dry stools, difficulty of defaecation, dull-pale complexion, dizziness, numbness of the limbs, blurred vision.
Tongue: Pale or normal.
Pulse: Empty.

TREATMENT PRINCIPLE

Nourish Blood, moisten the Intestines.

ACUPUNCTURE

ST-36 Zusanli, SP-6 Sanyinjiao, Ren-4 Guanyuan, SP-15 Daheng, BL-23 Shenshu, BL-20 Pishu, BL-25 Dachangshu. Reinforcing method.

Explanation

- **ST-36** and **SP-6** nourish Blood. ST-36 also promotes the bowel movement.
- **Ren-4** nourishes Blood.
- **SP-15** promotes the bowel movement.
- **BL-23** and **BL-20** nourish Blood.

- **BL-25**, Back-transporting point of the Large Intestine, promotes the bowel movement in chronic constipation.

HERBAL TREATMENT

Prescription

RUN CHANG WAN Variation
Moistening the Intestines Pill
Dang Gui *Radix Angelicae sinensis* 9 g
Sheng Di Huang *Radix Rehmanniae glutinosae* 12 g
Huo Ma Ren *Semen Cannabis sativae* 6 g
Tao Ren *Semen Persicae* 4.5 g
Zhi Ke *Fructus Citri aurantii* 6 g

Explanation

- **Dang Gui** and **Sheng Di Huang** nourish Blood and Yin and moisten the Intestines.
- **Huo Ma Ren** moves the bowels by moistening and it mildly nourishes Blood.
- **Tao Ren** moisten the Intestines.
- **Zhi Ke** moves Qi in the Intestines and prevents griping.

Da Huang *Rhizoma Rhei* was removed from the original formula, making it more suitable for chronic constipation.

Variations

- If the stools are very dry add Wu Ren Wan *Five Seeds Pill* (Tao Ren *Semen Persicae*, Xing Ren *Semen Pruni armeniacae*, Bai Zi Ren *Semen Biotae orientalis*, Song Zi Ren *Semen Pini tabulaeformis*, Yu Li Ren *Semen Pruni*, Chen Pi *Pericarpium Citri reticulatae*).

Patent remedy

BA ZHEN WAN
Eight Precious Decoction
Dang Gui *Radix Angelicae sinensis*
Chuan Xiong *Radix Ligustici wallichii*
Bai Shao *Radix Paeoniae albae*
Shu Di Huang *Radix Rehmanniae glutinosae praeparata*

Ren Shen *Radix Ginseng*
Bai Zhu *Rhizoma Atractylodis macrocephalae*
Fu Ling *Sclerotium Poriae cocos*
Zhi Gan Cao *Radix Glycyrrhizae uralensis praeparata*

Explanation

Although of the constituents of this formula only Dang Gui actually moves the stools, the remedy nourishes Blood and may be helpful, in conjunction with acupuncture, in the treatment of chronic constipation from Blood deficiency.

The tongue presentation appropriate to this remedy is a Pale and Thin tongue.

Case history

A 39-year-old woman had been suffering from constipation for 20 years. She had only two bowel movements a week but her stools were not particularly dry or small. Her periods were rather scanty and she suffered from pre-menstrual tension. Her memory was poor. Her tongue was Pale and partially peeled (Plate 19.2), and her pulse was generally Choppy.

Diagnosis
This is a clear example of constipation from Blood deficiency: this is apparent from the Pale tongue, the Choppy pulse, the poor memory and the scanty periods. A Pale and peeled tongue (often referred to as "chicken-flesh tongue", i.e. looking like uncooked chicken) indicates severe Blood deficiency. There is also some stagnation of Liver-Qi originating from deficiency of Liver-Blood.

Treatment principle
The treatment principle followed was to nourish Liver-Blood and moisten the Intestines. This patient was treated with herbs.

Herbal treatment
The formula used was a variation of Run Chang Wan *Moistening the Intestines Pill*:

Dang Gui *Radix Angelicae sinensis* 9 g
Shu Di Huang *Radix Rehmanniae glutinosae praeparata* 12 g
Huo Ma Ren *Semen Cannabis sativae* 6 g
Tao Ren *Semen Persicae* 4.5 g
Zhi Ke *Fructus Citri aurantii* 6 g
Shou Wu *Radix Polygoni multiflori* 9 g
Chai Hu *Radix Bupleuri* 4.5 g
Yu Li Ren *Semen Pruni* 6 g
Zhi Gan Cao *Radix Glycyrrhizae uralensis praeparata* 3 g
Hong Zao *Fructus Ziziphi jujubae* 3 dates

Explanation
- **Dang Gui**, **Shu Di**, **Huo Ma Ren** and **Shou Wu** nourish Blood. Dang Gui, Huo Ma Ren and Shou Wu also move the stools.
- **Tao Ren** moistens the Intestines and moves the stools.
- **Zhi Ke** moves Qi to help to move the stools.
- **Chai Hu** moves Liver-Qi.
- **Yu Li Ren** moistens the Intestines and moves the stools.
- **Zhi Gan Cao** and **Hong Zao** harmonize. Hong Zao also mildly nourishes Blood.

Due to the long duration of this patient's problem, it took over a year to restore normal bowel movements.

3. YANG DEFICIENCY

CLINICAL MANIFESTATIONS

Difficulty in defaecation, exhaustion and sweating after defaecation, stools *not* dry, sore back and knees, feeling cold, frequent-pale urination.
Tongue: Pale and wet.
Pulse: Deep and Weak.

This is a pattern of mostly Kidney-Yang deficiency. Normally, when Kidney-Yang is deficient the stools are loose. However, it may also have the opposite effect when the deficient Kidney-Yang fails to move Qi in the Intestines and the bowels do not move. In addition, when Kidney-Yang is deficient, internal Cold results and this contracts the muscles in the Lower Burner, again impairing the normal bowel peristalsis.

TREATMENT PRINCIPLE

Tonify the Kidneys, warm the Lower Burner and moisten the Intestines.

ACUPUNCTURE

ST-36 Zusanli, SP-6 Sanyinjiao, BL-23 Shenshu, BL-25 Dachangshu, Ren-4 Guanyuan, KI-7 Fuliu. Reinforcing method. Moxa should be used.

Explanation

- **ST-36** and **SP-6**, with moxa on the needle, tonify Yang. ST-36 promotes the bowel movement.
- **BL-23** and **KI-7** tonify Kidney-Yang. Direct moxa may be used on BL-23.
- **BL-25** stimulates the Intestines and promotes the bowel movement.
- **Ren-4**, with direct moxa, tonifies Kidney-Yang and the Original Qi.

HERBAL TREATMENT

Prescription

JI CHUAN JIAN
Benefit the River Decoction
Dang Gui *Radix Angelicae sinensis* 9 g
Niu Xi *Radix Achyranthis bidentatae seu Cyathulae* 6 g
Rou Cong Rong *Herba Cistanchis* 6 g
Ze Xie *Rhizoma Alismatis orientalis* 4.5 g
Zhi Ke *Fructus Citri aurantii* 3 g
Sheng Ma *Rhizoma Cimicifugae* 1.5 g

Explanation

- **Dang Gui** moistens the Intestines and promotes the bowel movement.
- **Niu Xi** has a descending movement and therefore promotes the bowel movement.
- **Rou Cong Rong** tonifies Kidney-Yang and promotes the bowel movement. It is one of the very few Kidney-Yang tonics which promote the bowel movement.
- **Ze Xie** drains Dampness via urination: it therefore has a downwards movement and helps Rou Cong Rong to move downwards. Because it also clears Empty-Heat, it prevents excessive heating from Rou Cong Rong.
- **Zhi Ke** moves Qi in the lower abdomen and helps the other herbs to stimulate the bowels.
- **Sheng Ma** has an ascending movement and it raises clear Yang to the top. Raising the clear Yang towards the upper part of the body makes it easier for the impure Qi to flow downwards, and this therefore stimulates the bowel movement.

Case history

A 61-year-old woman had been suffering from

persistent constipation for many years. She had only about two bowel movements a week but her stools were not dry. She often felt exhausted after the bowel movement. Her other symptoms included great weariness and exhaustion, feeling cold, a lack of will-power and spirit of initiative, back-ache, dizziness, and tinnitus. Her tongue was Pale and Swollen and her pulse was Deep and Weak.

Diagnosis
This patient suffered from Kidney-Yang deficiency, which was also the cause of the constipation. The symptoms of Kidney-Yang deficiency are back-ache, dizziness, tinnitus, a cold feeling, exhaustion and Pale-Swollen tongue. Her lack of will-power and initiative was also due to the deficiency of Kidney-Yang and its mental aspect, the Will-Power (*Zhi*).

Treatment principle
The treatment principle adopted was to tonify and warm Kidney-Yang and moisten the Intestines. She was treated with both acupuncture and herbs.

Acupuncture
The main acupuncture points used (with reinforcing method) included:

– **ST-36** Zusanli, with moxa, to tonify Qi and Yang and move the stools.
– **Ren-4** Guanyuan and **BL-23** Shenshu to tonify Kidney-Yang.
– **SP-15** Daheng to move the stools.
– **SP-6** Sanyinjiao and **KI-3** Taixi to tonify the Kidneys and move the stools.

Herbal treatment
The herbal prescription used was a variation of Ji Chuan Jian *Benefit the River Decoction*:

Dang Gui *Radix Angelicae sinensis* 9 g
Huai Niu Xi *Radix Achyranthis bidentatae* 6 g
Rou Cong Rong *Herba Cistanchis* 6 g
Ze Xie *Rhizoma Alismatis orientalis* 4.5 g
Zhi Ke *Fructus Citri aurantii* 3 g
Sheng Ma *Rhizoma Cimicifugae* 1.5 g
Shu Di Huang *Radix Rehmanniae glutinosae praeparata* 9 g
Huo Ma Ren *Semen Cannabis sativae* 6 g
Hu Tao Rou *Semen Juglandis regiae* 6 g
Zhi Gan Cao *Radix Glycyrrhizae uralensis praeparata* 3 g

Explanation
– The first six herbs constitute the original formula which tonifies Kidney-Yang and moves the stools.
– **Shu Di Huang** tonifies the Kidneys and strengthens Will-Power.
– **Huo Ma Ren** moves the stools.
– **Hu Tao Rou** tonifies Kidney-Yang.
– **Zhi Gan Cao** harmonizes.

After 18 months of treatment the patient had much more energy and her bowels became regular.

4. YIN DEFICIENCY

CLINICAL MANIFESTATIONS

Dry stools, thirst with desire to sip water, dry mouth and throat especially in the evening, sore back and knees, dizziness, tinnitus, night-sweating.
Tongue: Red without coating, cracks.
Pulse: Floating-Empty.

This condition is very frequent in elderly people with Kidney-Yin deficiency. The tongue will be Red: in quite advanced cases it will completely lack coating; in less serious cases it may only partially lack coating or have a rootless coating; and in still milder cases it may have a normal colour with a dry rootless coating.

TREATMENT PRINCIPLE

Nourish Yin, tonify the Kidneys and moisten the Intestines.

ACUPUNCTURE

ST-36 Zusanli, SP-6 Sanyinjiao, Ren-4 Guanyuan, KI-3 Taixi, KI-6 Zhaohai, BL-23 Shenshu, BL-25 Dachangshu, SP-15 Daheng. Reinforcing method, no moxa.

Explanation

– **ST-36** and **SP-6** nourish Stomach-Yin. ST-36 also promotes the bowel movement.
– **Ren-4**, **KI-3** and **KI-6** nourish Kidney-Yin. KI-6 also promotes the bowel movement.
– **BL-23** tonifies the Kidneys.
– **BL-25** and **SP-15** promote the bowel movement.

HERBAL TREATMENT

(a) Prescription

ZENG YE TANG
Increasing Fluids Decoction
Xuan Shen *Radix Scrophulariae ningpoensis* 18 g

Mai Men Dong *Tuber Ophiopogonis japonici* 12 g
Sheng Di Huang *Radix Rehmanniae glutinosae* 12 g

Explanation

All these three herbs nourish Stomach- and Kidney-Yin. This formula originally was for dryness in the Intestines after a Bright Yang-Organ pattern condition in the course of a febrile disease. Such a pattern is characterized by Fire which dries up the body fluids and causes severe dryness in the Intestines and therefore constipation. Apart from its original use, this formula may be used simply to nourish Yin and moisten the Intestines in chronic constipation from Yin deficiency.

Variations

– In order to enhance the effect of this formula on bowel movement add Huo Ma Ren *Semen Cannabis sativae* and Yu Li Ren *Semen Pruni*.

(b) Prescription

TONG YOU TANG
Penetrating the Deep Decoction
Sheng Di Huang *Radix Rehmanniae glutinosae* 12 g
Shu Di Huang *Radix Rehmanniae glutinosae praeparata* 12 g
Dang Gui *Radix Angelicae sinensis* 12 g
Tao Ren *Semen Persicae* 4.5 g
Hong Hua *Flos Carthami tinctorii* 4.5 g
Sheng Ma *Rhizoma Cimicifugae* 3 g
Zhi Gan Cao *Radix glycyrrhizae uralensis praeparata* 3 g

Explanation

– **Sheng Di Huang** and **Shu Di Huang** nourish Yin and Blood.
– **Dang Gui** nourishes Blood and moistens the Intestines.
– **Tao Ren** and **Hong Hua** move Blood. Tao Ren also moistens the Intestines.
– **Sheng Ma** raises the clear Yang and, by so doing, helps the impure Qi to descend. This helps to stimulate the bowel movement.
– **Zhi Gan Cao** harmonizes.

This formula is suitable if there is also some stasis of Blood and the tongue is slightly Purple.

COLD

Internal Cold in the Intestines can derive either from an invasion of external Cold or from Yang deficiency, particularly of the Spleen and/or Kidneys. Cold contracts the muscles and prevents the proper movement and transformation of Qi in the Intestines. It can therefore cause constipation. If it derives from Yang deficiency, then constipation results not only from the contracting action of Cold, but also from the deficient Yang-Qi being unable to push the stools through the Intestines. In such cases, the condition is characterized by a combination of Deficiency and Excess.

Constipation from Cold is nearly always accompanied by quite severe abdominal pain.

CLINICAL MANIFESTATIONS

Difficult defaecation, stools *not* dry, no bowel movement for several days, spastic abdominal pain, pale urine, pale face, cold limbs, feeling cold.
Tongue: Pale and wet. Thick-white coating on the root.
Pulse: Deep-Slow-Full-Tight. If Cold derives from Yang deficiency the pulse will be Deep-Slow-Fine, with a slightly Tight quality on both Rear positions only.

TREATMENT PRINCIPLE

Warm the Yang, scatter Cold, promote bowel movement.

ACUPUNCTURE

Ren-6 Qihai, Ren-8 Shenque, KI-18 Shiguan, BL-23 Shenshu, BL-25 Dachangshu, BL-26 Guanyuanshu. Reducing method in case of Full condition with internal Cold or reinforcing method if there is deficiency of Yang. Moxa is applicable in either case.

Explanation

- **Ren-6** with moxa, moves Qi and expels Cold from the Lower Burner.
- **Ren-8**, with indirect moxa cones on salt, scatters Cold from the Intestines.
- **KI-18** expels Cold from the abdomen and promotes the bowel movement.
- **BL-23** with moxa tonifies Kidney-Yang.
- **BL-25**, Back-transporting point of the Large Intestine, with moxa, expels Cold from the Intestines and promotes the bowel movement.
- **BL-26** with moxa expels Cold from the Intestines and promotes the bowel movement.

HERBAL TREATMENT

(1) PRESCRIPTION

DA HUANG FU ZI TANG
Rheum-Aconitum Decoction
Da Huang *Rhizoma Rhei* 9 g
Fu Zi *Radix Aconiti carmichaeli praeparata* 9 g
Xi Xin *Herba Asari cum radice* 3 g

Explanation

This formula is for Full-Cold in the Intestines and should not be used if there is any deficiency.

- **Da Huang** moves downwards. Although it is cold, it is used in this formula, combined with the other two herbs which are very hot, to move downwards.
- **Fu Zi** warms the Lower Burner and scatters Cold.
- **Xi Xin** scatters Cold.

(2) PRESCRIPTION

WEN PI TANG
Warming the Spleen Decoction
Da Huang *Rhizoma Rhei* 9 g

Fu Zi *Radix Aconiti carmichaeli praeparata* 6 g
Gan Jiang *Rhizoma Zingiberis officinalis* 4.5 g
Ren Shen *Radix Ginseng* 9 g
Zhi Gan Cao *Radix Glycyrrhizae uralensis praeparata* 3 g

Explanation

- **Da Huang** moves downwards.
- **Fu Zi** and **Gan Jiang** scatter Cold.
- **Ren Shen** and **Zhi Gan Cao** tonify Qi.

This prescription is used when there is internal Cold in the Intestines on a background of Spleen-Yang deficiency.

(3) PRESCRIPTION

JI CHUAN JIAN Variation
Benefit the River Decoction Variation
Dang Gui *Radix Angelicae sinensis* 9 g
Niu Xi *Radix Achyranthis bidentatae seu Cyathulae* 6 g
Rou Cong Rong *Herba Cistanchis* 6 g
Ze Xie *Rhizoma Alismatis orientalis* 4.5 g
Zhi Ke *Fructus Citri aurantii* 3 g
Sheng Ma *Rhizoma Cimicifugae* 1.5 g
Rou Gui *Cortex Cinnamomi cassiae* 3 g

Explanation

The original formula Ji Chuan Jian tonifies Kidney-Yang and promotes the bowel movement. With the addition of Rou Gui, it tonifies Kidney-Yang, promotes the bowel movement and expels internal Cold from the Intestines. This formula is therefore suitable for a combination of Cold obstructing the Intestines with a background of Kidney-Yang deficiency.

Prognosis

Both acupuncture and Chinese herbs are very effective in the treatment of constipation. However, chronic constipation may take a long time to be cured. The more long-standing it is, and the more the patient has resorted to laxatives, the longer it will take to cure. Thus, one should not be surprised if a case of chronic constipation of over 10 years' duration takes more than 1 year to be cured.

Western differentiation

There is no Western medical differentiation of constipation as such, as it is considered a symptom rather than a "disease". In our practice, the main possibilities to keep in mind are acute appendicitis and intestinal obstruction in acute constipation, and bowel carcinoma in chronic constipation.

ACUTE APPENDICITIS (see also "Abdominal pain", ch. 16)

This usually presents with an umbilical pain which gradually moves and settles on the McBurney's point on the right iliac fossa. There is also vomiting, foul breath and constipation. However, it must be emphasized that constipation is not an absolutely distinguishing sign of acute appendicitis as this may also present with diarrhoea.

INTESTINAL OBSTRUCTION

At all ages adhesions and hernias are common causes of obstruction. In children, intussusception is a frequent cause. This consists in the prolapse of one part of the intestine into the lumen of an immediately adjacent part. In the elderly a volvulus (the torsion of a loop of intestine) or tumour are the most likely causes.

Bowel cancer is the second most frequent cancer in men over 50 after lung cancer. It may present with either constipation or diarrhoea. In any case, it is characterized by a fairly sudden change of bowel habit, blood in the stools, and abdominal pain (see also "Abdominal pain", ch. 16).

As for medication, many patients suffering from chronic constipation take laxatives, most of them based on Senna fruits (*Cassia angustifolia*). These contain anthraquinones which stimulate the bowel peristalsis. From a Chinese perspective, these purgatives are somewhat similar to Da Huang *Rhizoma Rhei* (which also contains anthraquinones) and are really indicated only in Full conditions. They are therefore not suitable for long-term use as a laxative for chronic constipation. Their long-term use will tend to weaken the Spleen. Thus, if a patient has been resorting to such laxatives for many years, their use should be given up gradually as the herbal decoction based on differentiation of patterns takes effect.

END NOTES

1. Burkitt D 1980 Don't Forget Fibre in your Diet, Martin Dunitz, London, p. 47.
2. Ibid., p. 49.

3. Wu Ju Tong 1978 Differentiation of Warm Diseases (Wen Bing Tiao Bian 温病条辨), People's Health Publishing House, Beijing. First published 1798, p. 68.

Painful-Urination 20
Syndrome 淋証

Painful-Urination Syndrome, called *Lin* in Chinese, refers to a condition of urinary dysfunction characterized by frequency, scanty urine, pain, urgency and difficulty. Some doctors aptly describe this condition as: "The patient wants to urinate but the urine does not flow freely and he or she has distension and pain; when the patient does not want to urinate, there is some dribbling." The term *Lin* has been used in Chinese medicine since the time of the "Yellow Emperor's Classic of Internal Medicine" (*c*. 100 BC). It first appears in the "Simple Questions", chapter 71:

Diseases [of a particular time of year] will be characterized by a hot sensation, oedema of the face and eyes, sleepiness, nasal discharge, epistaxis, sneezing, yawning, vomiting, dark or bloody urine and painful-urination syndrome.[1]

The "Prescriptions of the Golden Chest" in chapter 11 calls this condition *Lin Bi*, i.e. obstructive urinary dysfunction: "*. . . Heat in the Lower Burner causes blood in the urine and obstructive urinary dysfunction . . .*"[2]

Over the centuries, Painful-Urination Syndrome has been classified in various ways. The "Classic of the Secret Transmission" by Hua Tuo (Han dynasty) in chapter 44 distinguishes eight types of Painful-Urination Syndrome: Cold, Hot, Qi, Fatigue, Sticky, Sand, Deficient and Excess types.[3]

The "General Treatise on the Aetiology and Symptomatology of Diseases" by Chao Yuan Fang (AD 610) distinguishes seven types of Painful-Urination Syndrome: Stone, Fatigue, Qi, Blood, Sticky, Cold and Hot.[4] The "Medical Secrets of an Official" (AD 752) by Wang Tao differentiates five types of Painful-Urination Syndrome, i.e. Stone, Qi, Sticky, Fatigue and Hot.[5]

Pathology

Although there are several types of Painful-Urination Syndrome, Heat is frequently present in most of them. As cited above, the "Prescriptions of the Golden Chest" (chapter 11) relates Painful-Urination Syndrome to Heat in the Lower Burner. The "Essential Methods of Dan Xi" (1481) by Zhu Dan Xi says: "*There are five types of Painful-Urination Syndrome but all have Heat.*"[6]

The "General Treatise on the Aetiology and Symptomatology of Diseases" quoted above says: *"Painful-Urination Syndrome is due to Kidney deficiency and Bladder Heat."*[7]

The "Complete Book of Jing Yue" (1624) says:

In the beginning stages, Painful-Urination Syndrome cannot not be due to Heat and there is no need to differentiate . . . in chronic Painful-Urination Syndrome there is less pain and difficulty but Dampness persists, the urine is turbid, Central Qi is weak and the Fire of the Gate of Vitality feeble.[8]

Most doctors in modern China emphasize the importance of Heat or Damp-Heat in Painful-Urination Syndrome especially in the acute stage. Although Damp-Heat is certainly the most common pathological condition in Painful-Urination Syndrome, it is by no means the only one and, in modern China, it tends perhaps to be over-emphasized.

The main pathological conditions seen in Painful-Urination Syndrome are:

- Dampness and Damp-Heat
- Stagnation of Qi
- Qi deficiency
- Kidney deficiency.

DAMPNESS

Dampness is the most important and common pathological factor in Painful-Urination Syndrome. It may be of external origin developing from exterior Dampness or internally generated from Spleen deficiency. Dampness settles in the Lower Burner and obstructs the urinary passages causing difficulty in urination and, in extreme cases, retention of urine. Dampness may also make the urine cloudy or turbid.

Dampness more often combines with Heat but it may also combine with Cold. Besides causing urinary difficulty, Damp-Heat causes burning during urination.

Dampness at the acute stage is a purely Full condition, whereas in chronic states it always occurs on a background of Spleen and/or Kidney deficiency.

STAGNATION OF QI

Stagnation of Qi in the Lower Burner affects mostly Liver and Triple Burner channels. Stagnation of Qi in the Liver channel, which flows through the genitalia, interferes with the Bladder function of Qi transformation and the Triple Burner function of keeping the Water passages open and free. This causes urinary dysfunction, hypogastric distension and pain. If there is pain, this typically occurs before urination.

QI DEFICIENCY

Deficiency of Spleen-Qi involves deficiency of Central Qi, i.e. the Qi which pulls up the internal organs in the midline of the body. Sinking Spleen-Qi causes frequency and dribbling of urine.

Qi deficiency affects the urinary function also via the Lungs. Lung-Qi descends to communicate not only with the Kidneys but also the Bladder as it provides strength to the Bladder for urination. Thus, deficient Lung-Qi, especially in old people, may sometimes cause urinary retention or Painful-Urination Syndrome.

KIDNEY DEFICIENCY

Kidney deficiency is a common background to Painful-Urination Syndrome. The balance between Kidney-Yang and Kidney-Yin regulates the amount of urine excreted. When Kidney-Yang is deficient there is excessive urination, when Kidney-Yin is deficient, urination is scanty.

In Painful-Urination Syndrome, Kidney-Yang deficiency causes dribbling, while Kidney-Yin deficiency causes the urine to be scanty. Besides this, when deficient Kidney-Yang fails to transform fluids it may lead to the formation of Dampness. Thus Dampness in the Lower Burner is often found against a background of Kidney-Yang deficiency. In chronic conditions, however, it may also be found against a background of Kidney-Yin deficiency, either because Kidney-Yang deficiency has changed into Kidney-Yin deficiency or because the Empty-Heat arising from Kidney-Yin deficiency has condensed the body fluids and caused Dampness to form.

On the other hand, Dampness itself may induce a deficiency of the Kidneys. Damp-Cold may weaken Kidney-Yang while Damp-Heat may injure Kidney-Yin.

The organs which are most involved in Painful-Urination Syndrome are the Spleen, Kidneys, Lungs, Bladder, Liver, Triple Burner and Small Intestine.

SPLEEN

The Spleen transforms and transports fluids and its deficiency leads to the formation of Dampness which may settle in the urinary system.

KIDNEYS

The influence of the Kidneys on the urinary function has just been described above.

LUNGS

The relationship between Lungs and Bladder has also been described above.

BLADDER

The Bladder not only stores and excretes urine but also transforms it by the power of Qi. This is the very last stage in the transformation of fluids in the urinary function. However, this Bladder function is subordinate to Kidney-Yang which provides the Qi for the Bladder's function of transformation.

LIVER

The Liver spreads Qi smoothly in every part of the body and therefore also in the Lower Burner. Specifically, its channel flows to the genitalia and urethra. Stagnation of Liver-Qi affects the Bladder so that it cannot transform urine properly. This leads to hypogastric distension and Painful-Urination Syndrome.

Long-term stagnation of Liver-Qi often leads to Liver-Fire. Although Liver-Fire normally rises, it may also infuse downwards to the Bladder and cause Painful-Urination Syndrome with intense burning pain. When would Liver-Fire infuse downwards rather than flare upwards as it is in its nature to do? If someone stands for long periods of time or lifts heavy weights every day, Qi stagnates in the Lower Burner and the emotional stress which would normally make Liver-Fire flare up, will instead make it infuse downwards.

TRIPLE BURNER

The Triple Burner is responsible for keeping Qi and Water passages open at all stages of the process of Qi and fluids metabolism. In the Lower Burner, it ensures the smooth and free opening and patency of the Water passages. "Excretion" and "free passage" are the key words used in the "Simple Questions" to describe the function of the Triple Burner with regard to fluids. The Lower Burner is compared to a "ditch" through which fluids are excreted: *"The Triple Burner is the official in charge of irrigation and it controls the Water passages."*[9]

Qi stagnation or Dampness affect the Lower Burner and cause urinary dysfunction and Painful-Urination Syndrome.

SMALL INTESTINE

The Small Intestine separates clear fluids from turbid ones and sends the latter to the Bladder. Thus, there is a direct connection between the Small Intestine and the Bladder, also confirmed by their channels' connection within the Greater-Yang channels.

In disease, Small Intestine Fire may affect the Bladder causing Heat Painful-Urination Syndrome. Small Intestine Fire, in turn, may derive from Heart-Fire. It is because of this connection between the Heart and Small Intestine that

Heart-Fire may cause some types of Heat Painful-Urination Syndrome.

There are six types of Painful-Urination Syndrome which will be discussed in detail below. All types are manifested with difficulty and pain on urination (which may radiate to the hypogastrium), dribbling of urine, sacral ache and frequency of micturition.

The six types of Painful-Urination Syndrome are:

Heat Painful-Urination Syndrome
Stone Painful-Urination Syndrome
Qi Painful-Urination Syndrome
Blood Painful-Urination Syndrome
Cloudy Painful-Urination Syndrome
Fatigue Painful-Urination Syndrome

HEAT PAINFUL-URINATION SYNDROME

Heat usually manifests as Damp-Heat which originates either externally or internally from a Spleen deficiency. When Dampness persists over a long period of time it tends to turn into Damp-Heat, especially in someone who eats excessive amounts of spicy foods.

Dampness obstructs the Water passages and causes urinary difficulty while Heat causes burning on micturition.

STONE PAINFUL-URINATION SYNDROME

When Damp-Heat is retained for a long time, Heat evaporates fluids, condenses Dampness and precipitates it to form stones or sand.

QI PAINFUL-URINATION SYNDROME

There are two types of Qi Painful-Urination Syndrome, one from stagnation of Liver-Qi and the other from deficiency and sinking of Spleen-Qi. The former is characterized by a pronounced feeling of distension and pain in the hypogastrium, the latter by a dragging and bearing down sensation in the area.

Liver-Qi stagnation usually derives from emotional stress and affects the Lower Burner and Bladder when the person either stands for long periods of time or has a very sedentary occupation with no exercise.

BLOOD PAINFUL-URINATION SYNDROME

This is due to either Heat or Empty-Heat pushing the Blood out of the vessels. Blood-Heat is usually related to Liver-Fire, while Empty-Heat affecting the Blood derives from Kidney-Yin deficiency. In either case, there is blood in the urine and burning on micturition.

CLOUDY PAINFUL-URINATION SYNDROME

This is characterized by Dampness preventing the proper transformation of fluids and separation of clear from turbid in the Lower Burner. Its main manifestation is difficulty in urination and cloudy urine.

This condition can also develop from a deficiency of the Kidneys and Original Qi being unable to provide Qi to separate clear from turbid in the urinary system.

FATIGUE PAINFUL-URINATION SYNDROME

This is a chronic condition which can develop from any of the other types of Painful-Urination Syndrome. It is due to deficiency of the Kidneys and its main manifestations are difficulty and frequency of micturition without much pain, and a feeling of exhaustion. The attacks typically come in bouts when the person is overtired.

Thus, the six types of Painful-Urination Syndrome could be described in a nutshell as follows:

- Heat Painful-Urination Syndrome: burning on urination
- Stone Painful-Urination Syndrome: urinary stones or sand
- Qi Painful-Urination Syndrome:

Full type: hypogastric distension
Empty type: frequency of urination with
bearing down feeling
- Blood Painful-Urination Syndrome: blood in
  urine
- Cloudy Painful-Urination Syndrome: cloudy
  urine
- Fatigue Painful-Urination Syndrome:
  frequent urination and exhaustion.

From a Western medical perspective Painful-Urination Syndrome may correspond to several different conditions such as cystitis, urethritis, urinary retention, prostatitis, urinary calculi or TB of the kidney.

The condition which an acupuncturist or herbalist is most commonly usually called upon to treat is cystitis. Both acupuncture and herbal medicine, on their own or in combination, give excellent results in cystitis and there is usually no need to resort to antibiotics.

Any of the types of Painful-Urination Syndrome may be seen in cystitis, but of these, Heat and Blood Painful-Urination Syndrome are the most typical manifestations. These two types could be said to correspond to a true cystitis, i.e. a bacterial infection of the bladder. In such cases, there is intense burning on micturition, frequency and the tongue is Red with a yellow coating and red spots on the root. However, very many patients complain only of frequency, difficulty and hypogastric distension with little or no pain, the tongue is not Red and there is no thick yellow coating and red spots on its root. Moreover, from a Western point of view, no bacteria can be cultured from the urine, though the patient is still diagnosed as having "cystitis" and antibiotics are prescribed. The term "urethral syndrome" has been applied to this category of patients who are predominantly women. These cases usually correspond to other types of Painful-Urination Syndrome, especially the Qi or Fatigue types.

The use of antibiotics is not generally called for in treating Painful-Urination Syndrome and in the cases just outlined above, it is even less justified as there is no true infection of the bladder. In other words, Chinese diagnosis can give guidelines not only for the use of Chinese herbs and acupuncture but, in certain conditions, even for the use of Western drugs. Thus, if there are signs of Heat, Damp-Heat or Blood-Heat in the Bladder with intense burning and a Red tongue with a yellow coating and red spots on the root, then antibiotics may be more justified, they will usually work and cause fewer side-effects. If, on the contrary, the "cystitis" manifests with symptoms and signs of Qi or Fatigue Painful-Urination Syndrome, to administer antibiotics is even more futile: they will usually not work at all or work only temporarily, and will cause more side-effects such as a Candida infection.

Some doctors correlate different types of Painful-Urination Syndrome to different Western diseases as follows:

- Heat Painful-Urination Syndrome: acute
  infection of urinary tract, acute nephritis,
  cystitis
- Blood Painful-Urination Syndrome: TB of
  kidney, carcinoma of bladder or kidney
- Stone Painful-Urination Syndrome: urinary
  calculi
- Cloudy Painful-Urination Syndrome:
  urethritis
- Fatigue Painful-Urination Syndrome: chronic
  prostatitis.[10]

Except for Stone Painful-Urination Syndrome, which by definition corresponds to urinary calculi, the above correlations are given only as a guideline as there is never an exact correspondence between Chinese symptoms and Western diseases.

Aetiology

1. EXTERNAL DAMPNESS

External Dampness is a very common aetiological factor in urinary diseases. It penetrates the channels in the legs and then flows upwards to settle in the Bladder, uterus or Intestines.

External Dampness is contracted by sitting on damp grass, living in a damp environment or damp house, wading in water, keeping a wet swimming suit on after swimming, being exposed to early-morning dampness while jogging and sweating, etc. Women are particularly prone to invasion of Dampness during their period or after childbirth.

2. DIET

Excessive consumption of sweets, sugar, dairy foods and greasy foods leads to the formation of Dampness which, if it settles in the urinary system, causes Painful-Urination Syndrome.

Excessive consumption of spicy foods and alcohol may generate Heat which combines with Dampness and causes Damp-Heat in the Lower Burner. This is an extremely important factor in Painful-Urination Syndrome, particularly Heat or Cloudy Painful-Urination Syndrome.

Long-standing Dampness may condense under the action of Heat to form urinary stones or "sand". This is called Stone Painful-Urination Syndrome.

The Heat part of Damp-Heat may injure the blood vessels in the urinary tract and cause blood in the urine. This is called Blood Painful-Urination Syndrome.

Finally, long-standing retention of Dampness may weaken Spleen-Qi and lead to Qi Painful-Urination Syndrome.

Thus, Damp-Heat may be the origin of different types of Painful-Urination Syndrome, i.e. Heat, Sticky, Stone, Blood and Qi Painful-Urination Syndrome.

3. EXCESSIVE SEXUAL ACTIVITY

Excessive sexual activity weakens the Kidneys and leads to either Cloudy or Fatigue Painful-Urination Syndrome, depending on whether Dampness or Deficiency is the predominant resulting factor.

Deficient Kidney-Yang fails to provide Qi to the Bladder and this causes dribbling of urine and Fatigue Painful-Urination Syndrome.

4. OLD AGE AND CHRONIC ILLNESS

Old age and chronic illness weaken Qi in general and may lead to sinking of Spleen-Qi which causes dribbling of urine or difficulty in urination and Qi or Fatigue Painful-Urination Syndrome.

Sinking Spleen-Qi causes Qi Painful-Urination Syndrome while Kidney deficiency causes Fatigue Painful-Urination Syndrome.

5. EMOTIONAL STRESS

Emotional stress influences urinary dysfunction but always with the concomitant action of other aetiological factors.

Emotional factors which cause Liver-Qi stagnation (such as anger, frustration and resentment) may cause Qi Painful-Urination Syndrome. Intense rage leading to Liver-Fire may cause Heat Painful-Urination Syndrome when Liver-Fire infuses downwards.

Long-standing grief, sadness and anxiety may all lead to Heart-Fire. This, in turn, may be transmitted to the Small Intestine to which the Heart is interiorly-exteriorly related. Because of the connection between the Small Intestine and Bladder channels (within the Greater-Yang channels), Fire is transmitted to the Bladder causing Heat Painful-Urination Syndrome.

6. EXCESSIVE LIFTING OR STANDING

Excessive lifting of heavy objects or standing may cause stagnation of Qi in the Lower Burner. This prevents the Triple Burner from ensuring that the Water passages are open and it therefore causes stagnation of fluids in the urinary tract. Eventually, it will lead to Dampness which obstructs the urinary tract and causes Cloudy Painful-Urination Syndrome.

A particular case of stagnation of Qi in the Lower Burner is the one caused by a hysterectomy. Very often, when the uterus is surgically removed, the stagnation of Qi and Blood affecting it is transmitted to its nearest organ, i.e. the Bladder. It is for this reason that many women suffer from recurrent "cystitis" after a hysterectomy.

Diagnosis

In diagnosing Painful-Urination Syndrome one must take into account the following aspects:

- Frequency of urination
- Ease or difficulty of urination
- Colour of urine
- Pain
- Hypogastric sensations.

FREQUENCY OF URINATION

Frequent urination indicates either deficiency of Kidney-Yang or sinking of Spleen-Qi if the urine is pale. If the urine is dark and micturition painful, frequency is due to Damp-Heat.

Scanty urination with dark urine indicates deficiency of Kidney-Yin.

EASE OR DIFFICULTY OF URINATION

Difficulty in micturition so that the flow of urine is hesitant or fitful indicates Dampness obstructing the Water passages.

Weak-stream micturition is due either to Dampness obstructing the Water passages or to deficient Kidney-Yang unable to push the urine along.

COLOUR OF URINE

Pale urine indicates deficiency of Kidney-Yang, while dark urine indicates either deficiency of Kidney-Yin or Heat in the Bladder.

Cloudy urine indicates Dampness while rusty-coloured urine may indicate the presence of blood.

Blood in the urine is due either to Blood-Heat (which may be Full- or Empty-Heat) or to Qi deficiency. If the colour of the blood is dark and there are small clots, it indicates Blood stasis. The "Essential Methods of Dan Xi" says: "In Blood Painful-Urination Syndrome . . . if the colour of the blood is fresh it indicates Heart and Small Intestine Full-Heat; if it is dark, it indicates Empty-Cold in the Kidneys and Bladder."[11]

PAIN

Burning pain in the urethra during urination is due to Heat or Damp-Heat. Pain before urination indicates stagnation of Qi, while pain after urination indicates deficiency of Qi.

Pain over the hypogastrium indicates stagnation of Liver-Qi or Liver-Fire.

Pain over the sacrum is due to a Kidney deficiency.

HYPOGASTRIC SENSATIONS

A feeling of distension in the hypogastric area indicates stagnation of Liver-Qi. Intense pain is due either to stasis of Liver-Blood or to Liver-Fire.

A feeling of fullness over the hypogastrium indicates Dampness, while a dragging, bearing-down feeling indicates sinking of Spleen-Qi.

This area should be palpated and its tone and texture assessed. If it feels hard and distended it indicates stagnation of Qi or Dampness. If it is soft and flaccid, it indicates a deficiency of the Kidneys and the Original Qi.

TONGUE

The root of the tongue reflects problems of the Bladder, Intestines or Kidneys. Problems of the Bladder or of the Intestines will be reflected in the coating. This, however, presents similar signs for both types of problem and the two cannot be distinguished from the tongue only. Thus, a thick yellow and sticky coating with red spots on the root indicates Damp-Heat, which may be either in the Bladder or in the Intestines.

A sticky and dull-dirty coating on the root indicates long-standing retention of Dampness and usually Cloudy Painful-Urination Syndrome.

No coating on the root or coating that is partially peeled may indicate a deficiency of Kidney-Yin and Fatigue Painful-Urination Syndrome, but may also, however, be due to a pathology of the Intestines.

Thus observation of the root of the tongue in urinary problems must always be closely checked against the pulse findings. If both Rear positions of the pulse present the same abnormal quality, then the problem is most probably in the Intestines. If only the left Rear position of the pulse presents an abnormal quality, then the problem is most probably in the Bladder.

PULSE

On the pulse, the Bladder is reflected on the left Rear position. If this is Wiry it indicates either stagnation of Liver-Qi affecting the Bladder if it is Slow, or Bladder Heat if it is Rapid.

A Slippery quality on the left Rear position indicates Dampness, Damp-Heat if it is Rapid and Damp-Cold if it is Slow.

A Weak-Floating quality on the same position indicates long-standing retention of Dampness and Qi deficiency.

By rolling the finger proximally on the left Rear position, one can feel the prostate position. If this feels Full and Slippery it may indicate prostatic hypertrophy. This is often the cause of Painful-Urination Syndrome, especially Qi Painful-Urination Syndrome or Fatigue Painful-Urination Syndrome.

Differentiation and treatment

I shall discuss six types of Painful-Urination Syndrome:

Heat
Stone
Qi
Blood
Sticky
Fatigue.

All types are manifested with difficulty and pain on urination (which may radiate to the hypogastrium), dribbling of urine, sacral ache and frequency of micturition.

As always in Chinese medicine, it is essential to distinguish between Full and Empty conditions. Generally speaking, the beginning stages of Painful-Urination Syndrome are characterized

by Fullness, e.g. Dampness, Heat, stones and Qi stagnation. The chronic stage is characterized by Emptiness, e.g. Qi deficiency, Spleen-Qi sinking, Lung-Qi deficiency and Kidney deficiency.

Three of the six types of Painful-Urination Syndrome are always Full or always Empty in character.

These are:

Heat Painful-Urination Syndrome — Full type
Stone Painful-Urination Syndrome — Full type
Fatigue Painful-Urination Syndrome — Empty type.

Each of the other three categories of Painful-Urination Syndrome can be either of the Full or Empty type. These may be summarized in tabular form (Table 20.1).

In the beginning stages when Fullness is evident the main principle of treatment is to clear Heat, resolve Dampness, drain Water and open the Water passages. In the late stages when Deficiency is predominant the main principle of treatment is to tonify Qi, drain Dampness and open the Water passages.

HEAT PAINFUL-URINATION SYNDROME

CLINICAL MANIFESTATIONS

Frequent, scanty and difficult urination, burning pain on urination, dark urine with a strong smell, hypogastric pain, a bitter taste, nausea, pain on the sacrum, constipation, thirst.
Tongue: yellow-sticky coating on the root with red spots.
Pulse: Slippery on the left Rear position and slightly Rapid.

– If it occurs with an invasion of exterior Wind: aversion to cold, shivers, fever, headache, aches in the body and a Floating pulse.

Table 20.1 Types if Qi, Blood and Cloudy Painful-Urination Syndrome

Painful urination syndrome	Full type	Empty type
Qi	Stagnation of Qi	Sinking Qi
Blood	Blood Heat	Blood Empty-Heat
Sticky	Dampness	Dampness with Qi deficiency

Although this is called Heat Painful-Urination Syndrome, the condition is one of Damp-Heat in the Bladder, with Heat predominant. There are two other possible conditions when Bladder-Heat is transmitted from Liver-Fire or from Heart-Fire. In these cases, in addition to the above manifestations, there would be the following symptoms and signs:

LIVER-FIRE

Irritability, headache, dizziness, tinnitus, a Red tongue with redder sides and a Wiry-Rapid pulse.

HEART-FIRE

Insomnia, tongue ulcers, mental restlessness, a Red tongue with a redder tip and a Rapid pulse which is Overflowing on the left Front position.

TREATMENT PRINCIPLE

Clear Heat, drain Dampness, open the Water passages.

- For Liver-Fire: soothe the Liver and drain Fire.
- For Heart-Fire: drain Heart-Fire and calm the Mind.
- If with an exterior invasion: release the Exterior, expel Wind and open the Water passages.

ACUPUNCTURE

Ren-3 Zhongji, BL-28 Pangguangshu, BL-22 Sanjiaoshu, SP-9 Yinlingquan, BL-66 Tonggu, BL-63 Jinmen, L.I.-11 Quchi. Reducing method, no moxa.

- For Liver-Fire: LIV-2 Xingjian and SP-6 Sanyinjiao, with reducing method.
- For Heart-Fire: HE-8 Shaofu, S.I.-2 Qiangu, with reducing method.
- If with an exterior invasion: L.I.-4 Hegu, LU-7 Lieque and T.B.-5 Waiguan, reducing method.

EXPLANATION

- **Ren-3** and **BL-28**, respectively Front-Collecting and Back-Transporting point of the Bladder, clear Heat and drain Dampness from the Bladder.
- **BL-22**, Back-Transporting point of the Triple Burner, drains Dampness from the Lower Burner.
- **SP-9** drains Damp-Heat from the Lower Burner.
- **BL-66** clears Bladder-Heat.
- **BL-63**, Accumulation point, stops pain in the Bladder channel.
- **L.I.-11** is used if symptoms of Heat (such as fever) are very pronounced.
- **LIV-2** drains Liver-Fire.
- **SP-6** clears Heat and cools Blood, drains Dampness from the Lower Burner and calms the Mind.
- **HE-8** drains Heart-Fire and calms the Mind.
- **S.I.-2** clears Small Intestine Heat. This is used because Fire is transmitted from the Heart to the Bladder via the Small Intestine.
- **L.I.-4** and **T.B.-5** release the Exterior and expel Wind.
- **LU-7** releases the Exterior, expels Wind and opens the Water passages.

HERBAL TREATMENT

(1) PRESCRIPTION

BA ZHENG TANG
Eight Corrections Powder
Bian Xu *Herba Polygoni avicularis* 6 g
Che Qian Zi *Semen Plantaginis* 9 g
Qu Mai *Herba Dianthi* 6 g
Mu Tong *Caulis Akebiae* 6 g
Hua Shi *Talcum* 9 g
Da Huang *Rhizoma Rhei* 6 g
Zhi Zi *Fructus Gardeniae jasminoidis* 6 g
Zhi Gan Cao *Radix Glycyrrhizae uralensis praeparata* 6 g

Explanation

- **Bian Xu, Che Qian Zi, Qu Mai, Mu Tong**

and **Hua Shi** all drain Damp-Heat from the Bladder and open the Water passages.
- **Da Huang** clears Heat by moving downwards. This method is sometimes combined with that of clearing Heat via urination, as all the previous herbs do.
- **Zhi Zi** drains Damp-Heat from the Three Burners.
- **Zhi Gan Cao** harmonizes and stops pain.

This is the main prescription to drain Damp-Heat from the Bladder.

Variations

- If symptoms of Dampness are very pronounced add Fu Ling *Sclerotium Poriae cocos* and Zhu Ling *Sclerotium Polypori umbellati*.
- If constipation is pronounced increase Da Huang *Rhizoma Rhei* and add Zhi Shi *Fructus Citri aurantii immaturus*.
- If there are symptoms of exterior invasion with alternation of hot and cold sensations and a bitter taste, add the formula Xiao Chai Hu Tang *Small Bupleurum Decoction*.
- If Heat has begun to injure Yin add Sheng Di Huang *Radix Rehmanniae glutinosae*, Zhi Mu *Radix Anemarrhenae asphodeloidis* and Bai Mao Gen *Rhizoma Imperatae cylindricae* (to prevent bleeding from Empty-Heat).

(2) PRESCRIPTION

LONG DAN XIE GAN TANG
Gentiana Draining the Liver Decoction
Long Dan Cao *Radix Gentianae scabrae* 6 g
Huang Qin *Radix Scutellariae baicalensis* 9 g
Shan Zhi Zi *Fructus Gardeniae jasminoidis* 9 g
Ze Xie *Rhizoma Alismatis orientalis* 9 g
Mu Tong *Caulis Akebiae* 9 g
Che Qian Zi *Semen Plantaginis* 9 g
Sheng Di Huang *Radix Rehmanniae glutinosae* 12 g
Dang Gui *Radix Angelicae sinensis* 9 g
Chai Hu *Radix Bupleuri* 9 g
Gan Cao *Radix Glycyrrhizae uralensis* 3 g

Explanation

This formula, which has already been explained in chapters 1 and 10, is used if Damp-Heat in the Bladder is transmitted from Liver-Fire. The formula needs little modification as it drains Damp-Heat both in the head (such as in otitis media) and in the Lower Burner (such as in Painful-Urination Syndrome). In fact, Ze Xie, Mu Tong and Che Qian Zi within the prescription will drain Damp-Heat from the Bladder, and Zhi Zi drains Damp-Heat from the Three Burners.

(3) PRESCRIPTION

DAO CHI SAN
Eliminating Redness Powder
Sheng Di Huang *Radix Rehmanniae glutinosae* 15 g
Mu Tong *Caulis Akebiae* 3 g
Gan Cao *Radix Glycyrrhizae uralensis* 6 g
Zhu Ye *Herba Lophatheri gracilis* 6 g

Explanation

This formula is used if Damp-Heat in the Bladder derives from Heart-Fire (via Small Intestine Fire).

- **Sheng Di Huang** clears Heat and cools Blood.
- **Mu Tong** clears the Heart and drains Damp-Heat from the Bladder.
- **Zhu Ye** clears the Heart and clears Heat from the Bladder.
- **Gan Cao** harmonizes, smooths out roughness and stops pain.

(a) PATENT REMEDY

TE XIAO PAI SHI WAN
Especially-Effective Discharging Stones Pill
Jin Qian Cao *Herba Desmodii styracifolii*
Hai Jin Sha *Spora Lygodii japonici*
Bai Zhi *Radix Angelicae dahuricae*
Chuan Xin Lian *Herba Andrographis paniculatae*
Chuan Niu Xi *Radix Cyathulae*
Wu Hua Guo Gen *Radix Fici*
Huang Lian *Rhizoma Coptidis*
Da Huang *Rhizoma Rhei*
Niu Da Li *Radix Millettiae speciosae*
San Qi *Radix Notoginseng*
Hu Po *Succinum*

Explanation

This remedy drains Damp-Heat from the Bladder and expels urinary stones. It can be used in Heat Painful-Urination Syndrome to drain Damp-Heat even if there are no stones.

The tongue presentation appropriate to this remedy is a sticky-yellow coating and red spots on the root.

(b) PATENT REMEDY

LONG DAN XIE GAN WAN
Gentiana Draining the Liver Pill
Long Dan Cao *Radix Gentianae scabrae*
Huang Qin *Radix Scutellariae baicalensis*
Shan Zhi Zi *Fructus Gardeniae jasminoidis*
Ze Xie *Rhizoma Alismatis orientalis*
Mu Tong *Caulis Akebiae*
Che Qian Zi *Semen Plantaginis*
Sheng Di Huang *Radix Rehmanniae glutinosae*
Dang Gui *Radix Angelicae sinensis*
Chai Hu *Radix Bupleuri*
Gan Cao *Radix Glycyrrhizae uralensis*

Explanation

This pill drains Liver-Fire in the Upper and Lower Burners. It is suitable to treat Heat Painful-Urination Syndrome deriving from Liver-Fire.

The tongue presentation appropriate to this remedy is a Red body, with redder sides and a sticky-yellow coating and red spots on the root.

Case history

A 30-year-old woman had been suffering from what had been diagnosed as recurring cystitis. During the attacks her micturition was very frequent and scanty, with a burning pain during urination. The urine was darker than normal. She had been prescribed antibiotics which helped for a while but then the attacks returned. She had lost her father the year before and felt very sad. Her tongue was slightly Red, with a markedly redder tip with red points, and the root had a yellow coating with red spots (Plate 20.1). Her pulse was slightly Rapid, slightly Wiry on the left-Rear position and slightly Overflowing in the left-Front position.

Diagnosis

This is a case of Heat Painful-Urination Syndrome from Heart-Fire affecting the Small Intestine and, from this organ, infusing down to the Bladder. Heart-Fire is evident from the red tip of the tongue with red points and the Overflowing pulse on the Heart position. The condition of Heart-Fire obviously developed from the sadness and grief following her father's death as although these two emotions dissolve Qi, they can also lead to stagnation of Qi in the chest and, in the long run, stagnant Qi can implode to cause Heart-Fire. The Heat in the Bladder is very evident from the burning on urination, the dark urine and the red spots and yellow coating on the root of the tongue.

Treatment principle

The treatment principle adopted was to clear Heart-Fire, calm the Mind, clear Bladder Heat, resolve Dampness, moderate urgency and stop pain. She was treated only with acupuncture.

Acupuncture

The main points used, with reducing method, were selected from the following:

– **HE-8** Shaofu and **S.I.-2** Qiangu to clear Heart-Fire and Small-Intestine Heat. HE-8 also calms the Mind.
– **SP-9** Yinlingquan to drain Damp-Heat and open the water passages.
– **Ren-3** Zhongji, Front-Collecting point of the Bladder, to clear Bladder-Heat and open the water passages.
– **BL-63** Jinmen, Accumulation point of the Bladder, to clear Bladder-Heat, moderate urgency and stop pain.

This patient's problem was cleared after 6 treatments, but she continued to receive treatment, at longer intervals, for a further 6 months to deal with her sadness and grief following the death of her father.

Case history

A 51-year-old man had been suffering from painful micturition for 18 months. His urination was frequent and there was intense burning during micturition; the urine was dark and there were traces of blood. Just a few days before he came for the consultation, a carcinoma of the bladder had been diagnosed. Apart from the above symptoms, he also experienced a pronounced feeling of heat and thirst and he was often constipated. His tongue was Reddish-Purple with a thick-yellow and sticky coating all over, but thicker on the root. His pulse was very Full, Slippery and Wiry.

Diagnosis

This is a clear example of Heat Painful-Urination

Syndrome with Damp-Heat in the Bladder and Fire in general. There was also some stasis of Blood as shown by the Purple colour of the tongue: the carcinoma of the bladder evidently is of Blood-stasis type.

Treatment principle
My treatment was combined and coordinated with the treatment he was receiving from the hospital. This consisted in administration of the BCG vaccine which provokes a shedding of the bladder's mucosa. At the time of consultation he had not yet started this treatment and my treatment principle was therefore to drain Fire, resolve Damp-Heat, move Blood and soften hardness.

Herbal treatment
The formula used was a variation of Ba Zheng Tang *Eight Corrections Decoction*:

Che Qian Zi *Semen Plantaginis* 9 g
Bian Xu *Herba Polygoni avicularis* 6 g
Da Huang *Rhizoma Rhei* 6 g
Mu Tong *Caulis Akebiae* 3 g
Qu Mai *Herba Dianthi* 6 g
Zhi Zi *Fructus Gardeniae jasminoidis* 6 g
Gan Cao *Radix Glycyrrhizae uralensis* 6 g
Huang Bo *Cortex Phellodendri* 6 g
Yi Yi Ren *Semen Coicis lachryma jobi* 20 g
Deng Xin Cao *Medulla Junci effusi* 4 g
Tian Kui Zi *Rhizoma Semiaquiligiae adoxoides* 9 g
Shi Shang Bai *Herba Selaginellae doederleinii* 9 g
Chi Shao *Radix Paeoniae rubrae* 6 g
Qian Cao Gen *Radix Rubiae cordifoliae* 6 g
Bai Shao *Radix Paeoniae albae* 9 g

Explanation
- The first eight herbs form the Ba Zheng San, with Huang Bo replacing Hua Shi as the former is stronger in resolving Damp-Heat.
- **Yi Yi Ren** and **Deng Xin Cao** resolve Damp-Heat from the Bladder.
- **Tian Kui Zi** and **Shi Shang Bai** resolve Damp-Heat from the Bladder and have an anti-cancer effect.
- **Chi Shao** and **Qian Cao Gen** move Blood and stop bleeding.
- **Bai Shao**, in combination with Gan Cao, stops pain and moderates urgency.

The patient took this prescription for about 1 month, until he started the hospital treatment. Once this was started, the treatment principle was changed: this was necessary because the drug was attacking the carcinoma directly and had debilitating side-effects. Attention was therefore directed at tonifying Qi with a variation of Bu Zhong Yi Qi Tang *Tonifying the Centre and Benefiting Qi Decoction*:

Huang Qi *Radix Astragali membranacei* 15 g
Bai Zhu *Rhizoma Atractylodis macrocephalae* 6 g
Dang Shen *Radix Codonopsis pilosulae* 12 g
Dang Gui *Radix Angelicae sinensis* 6 g
Chen Pi *Pericarpium Citri reticulatae* 3 g

Sheng Ma *Rhizoma Cimicifugae* 3 g
Chai Hu *Radix Bupleuri* 3 g
Fu Ling *Sclerotium Poriae cocos* 6 g
Xiao Ji *Herba Cephalanoplos segeti* 6 g

Explanation
- The first seven herbs constitute the Bu Zhong Yi Qi Tang.
- **Fu Ling** was added to resolve Dampness.
- **Xiao Ji** was added to stop bleeding from the bladder as the drug treatment causes profuse bleeding.

While he was having the drug treatment, the Chinese herbs helped him to boost his energy and minimize the side-effects. After 3 months of drug treatment, the tongue coating had reduced considerably, but the tongue body was still Reddish-Purple and his pulse was still Full, Slippery and Wiry. In addition, the tongue had also lost its "spirit" on the root indicating a Kidney deficiency. The carcinoma in the bladder had gone. Thus, although from the point of view of Western medicine he was "cured", the tongue and pulse showed that this was not the case. In particular, the very Full, Slippery and Wiry pulse showed that the pathogenic factors (i.e. the stasis of Blood and Damp-Heat causing the carcinoma) were still present and, furthermore, the lack of spirit on the root of the tongue showed a Kidney deficiency. Thus the principle of treatment was changed again to nourish Kidney-Yin, resolve Damp-Heat and move Blood. The formula used was a variation of Zhi Bo Di Huang Wan *Anemarrhena-Phellodendron-Rehmannia Pill*:

Zhi Mu *Radix Anemarrhenae asphodeloidis* 6 g
Huang Bo *Cortex Phellodendri* 6 g
Sheng Di Huang *Radix Rehmanniae glutinosae* 9 g
Shan Yao *Radix Dioscoreae oppositae* 6 g
Shan Zhu Yu *Fructus Corni officinalis* 4 g
Ze Xie *Rhizoma Alismatis orientalis* 6 g
Fu Ling *Sclerotium Poriae cocos* 6 g
Mu Dan Pi *Cortex Moutan radicis* 6 g
Yi Yi Ren *Semen Coicis lachryma jobi* 15 g
Tian Kui Zi *Rhizoma Semiaquilegiae adoxoides* 9 g
Shi Shang Bai *Herba Selaginellae doederleinii* 9 g
Bai Hua She She Cao *Herba Oldenlandiae diffusae* 6 g
Huang Qi *Radix Astragali membranacei* 12 g
E Zhu *Rhizoma Curcumae zedoariae* 6 g

Explanation
- The first eight herbs constitute the root formula.
- **Yi Yi Ren** was added to drain Damp-Heat and soften hardness.
- **Tian Kui Zi**, **Shi Shang Bai** and **Bai Hua She She Cao** resolve Damp-Heat and have an anti-cancer effect.
- **Huang Qi** tonifies Qi, and raises immunity to combat and prevent cancer.
- **E Zhu** breaks Blood and has an anti-cancer effect.

This patient continued to take variations of the above prescription for 6 months, after which his general energy improved and he had no recurrence of the cancer. His tongue lost its Purple colour and regained its spirit on the root, and the pulse became much less Full, Slippery and Wiry. He is still under treatment and he will probably need to be for some time, until his pulse loses its Full, Slippery and Wiry quality completely. From a Chinese perspective, this would indicate that the cancer has definitely gone.

Case history

A 47-year-old man had been diagnosed as having carcinoma of the bladder 4 years before. This had been operated on at the time and he had no symptoms for the following 3 years. After that, he developed papillomas in the bladder. His symptoms included: burning on urination, occasional blood in the urine, frequency and difficulty of urination, dark urine, back-ache, slight dizziness and chilliness. He had been suffering from frequent urination for many years before he developed cancer. On closer interrogation, in fact it transpired that he had two types of frequency of urination: sometimes his urination was frequent, profuse and pale, and at other times he had a frequent *desire* to urinate but his urine was scanty and dark.

His tongue was of a normal colour, slightly Pale on the sides, and had a dirty-sticky coating on the root. His pulse was slightly Slippery, slightly Weak and particularly Weak on the left Rear position.

Diagnosis
The burning on urination, the dark urine with occasional blood and the frequency and difficulty of urination, all pointed to Heat Painful-Urination Syndrome. This occurred, however, against a background of Kidney-Yang deficiency (slightly Pale tongue, chilliness, Weak Kidney pulse and frequency of urination since childhood).

Treatment principle
The treatment principle adopted was to resolve Damp-Heat in the Bladder first, and then tonify Kidney-Yang. This patient was treated only with herbs.

Herbal treatment
The formula used initially was a variation of Ba Zheng Tang *Eight Corrections Powder* and Xiao Ji Yin Zi *Cephalanoplos Decoction*. As there is some overlap between the ingredients of these two decoctions, they can be used in combination without an excessive number of herbs:

Bian Xu *Herba Polygoni avicularis* 6 g
Che Qian Zi *Semen Plantaginis* 6 g
Qu Mai *Herba Dianthi* 6 g
Mu Tong *Caulis Akebiae* 6 g

Hua Shi *Talcum* 9 g
Zhi Zi *Fructus Gardeniae jasminoidis* 6 g
Zhi Gan Cao *Radix Glycyrrhizae uralensis praeparata* 6 g
Xiao Ji *Herba Cephalanoplos segeti* 6 g
Ou Jie *Nodus Nelumbinis nuciferae rhizomatis* 6 g
Zhu Ye *Herba Lophatheri gracilis* 4 g
Shu Di Huang *Radix Rehmanniae glutinosae praeparata* 9 g
Dang Gui *Radix Angelicae sinensis* 4 g
Tian Kui Zi *Rhizoma Semiaquilegiae adoxoides* 6 g
Shi Shang Bai *Herba Selaginellae doederleinii* 6 g

Explanation
- The first seven herbs constitute the Ba Zheng Tang which clears Heat and resolves Dampness from the Bladder. Da Huang was eliminated because his tongue did not have a thick or dry tongue coating.
- The next five herbs are part of the Xiao Ji Yin Zi which clears Heat and cools Blood in the Bladder and stops hematuria. Pu Huang was eliminated as the urinary bleeding was not very pronounced; other herbs were eliminated as already contained in the first formula. Sheng Di Huang was replaced with Shu Di Huang as he had deficiency of Kidney-Yang.
- **Tian Kui Zi** and **Shi Shang Bai** were added as they are specific anti-carcinogenic herbs which enter the Bladder.

After taking this formula, which treats only the Manifestation (i.e. Damp-Heat in the Bladder), for 2 months, the treatment principle was changed diverting attention to treating the Root and the Manifestation simultaneoulsy, i.e. tonifying the Kidneys and resolving Damp-Heat from the Bladder. The formula used was a variation of Zhi Bo Di Huang Wan *Anemarrhena-Phellodendron-Rehmannia Pill*:

Shu Di Huang *Radix Rehmanniae glutinosae praeparata* 24 g
Shan Zhu Yu *Fructus Corni officinalis* 12 g
Shan Yao *Radix Dioscoreae oppositae* 12 g
Ze Xie *Rhizoma Alismatis orientalis* 9 g
Fu Ling *Sclerotium Poriae cocos* 9 g
Mu Dan Pi *Cortex Moutan radicis* 9 g
Zhi Mu *Radix Anemarrhenae asphodeloidis* 9 g
Huang Bo *Cortex Phellodendri* 9 g
Fu Pen Zi *Fructus Rubi* 4 g
Tu Si Zi *Semen Cuscutae* 6 g
Tian Kui Zi *Rhizoma Semiaquilegiae adoxoides* 6 g
Shi Shang Bai *Herba Selaginellae doederleinii* 6 g

Explanation
- The first 8 herbs constitute the Zhi Bo Di Huang Wan which tonifies the Kidneys and resolves Damp-Heat from the Bladder.
- **Fu Pen Zi** and **Tu Si Zi** were added to tonify Kidney-Yang.
- **Tian Kui Zi** and **Shi Shang Bai** were added as they are herbs which have an anti-carcinogenic effect and enter the Bladder.

Two months after taking this decoction he had a further cystoscopy which showed that his papillomas had completely gone. In the meantime, his symptoms also had all gone.

STONE PAINFUL-URINATION SYNDROME

CLINICAL MANIFESTATIONS

Stones or sand in the urine, difficult urination which may stop suddenly, hypogastric pain, sacral pain, blood in urine.
Tongue: Red, with a thick-sticky coating on the root.
Pulse: Wiry on the left Rear position and Rapid.

TREATMENT PRINCIPLE

Clear Heat, drain Dampness, open the Water passages, expel the stones.

ACUPUNCTURE

BL-22 Sanjiaoshu, ST-28 Shuidao, SP-9 Yinlingquan, Ren-6 Qihai, Ren-3 Zhongji, BL-28 Pangguangshu, BL-63 Jinmen, BL-39 Weiyang, KI-2 Rangu. Reducing method, no moxa.

EXPLANATION

– **BL-22** drains Dampness from the Lower Burner.
– **ST-28** promotes the transformation of fluids in the Lower Burner.
– **SP-9** drains Damp-Heat from the Lower Burner.
– **Ren-6** moves Qi in the Lower Burner. Moving Qi helps to transform fluids and drain Dampness.
– **Ren-3** and **BL-28**, Front-Collecting and Back-Transporting points of the Bladder respectively, drain Dampness from the Bladder.
– **BL-63** removes obstructions from the Bladder channel.
– **BL-39**, Lower Sea point of the Triple Burner

(specifically the Lower Burner), in combination with **KI-2**, removes obstructions from the Bladder and frees the Water passages.

HERBAL TREATMENT

(1) PRESCRIPTION

SHI WEI SAN
Pyrrosia Powder
Shi Wei *Folium Pyrrosiae* 9 g
Dong Kui Zi *Semen Abutiloni seu Malvae* 6 g
Qu Mai *Herba Dianthi* 6 g
Che Qian Zi *Semen Plantaginis* 6 g
Hua Shi *Talcum* 6 g

Explanation

All these herbs drain Damp-Heat, open the Water passages and relieve urinary dysfunction.

Variations

– To enhance the stone-dissolving effect of this formula add Jin Qian Cao *Herba Desmodii styracifolii*, Hai Jin Sha *Spora Lygodii japonici* and Ji Nei Jin *Endothelium Corneum Gigeraiae Galli*.
– If there is sacral pain add Bai Shao *Radix Paeoniae albae* and Gan Cao *Radix Glycyrrhizae uralensis*.
– If there is blood in the urine add Xiao Ji *Herba Cephalanoplos segeti*, Sheng Di Huang *Radix Rehmanniae glutinosae*, and Ou Jie *Nodus Nelumbinis nuciferae rhizomatis*.
– If there is fever add Pu Gong Ying *Herba Taraxaci mongolici cum Radice*, Huang Bo *Cortex Phellodendri*, and Da Huang *Rhizoma Rhei*.
– In a chronic condition of urinary calculi with Dampness in the Lower Burner and deficiency of Qi and Blood, instead of the above formula, use the formulae Er Shen San *Two Spirits Powder* (which contains Hai Jin Sha *Spora Lygodii japonici* and Hua Shi *Talcum*) and Ba Zhen Tang *Eight Precious Decoction*.
– In a chronic condition with Damp-Heat in the

Lower Burner and Yin deficiency, use Zhi Bo Di Huang Wan (also called Zhi Bo Ba Wei Wan) *Anemarrhena-Phellodendron-Rehmannia Pill* in combination with Shi Wei San *Pyrrosia Powder*.

(2) PRESCRIPTION

SAN JIN TANG
Three-Gold Decoction
Jin Qian Cao *Herba Desmodii styracifolii* 15 g
Hai Jin Sha *Spora Lygodii japonici* 9 g
Ji Nei Jin *Endothelium Corneum Gigeraiae Galli* 6 g
Dong Kui Zi *Semen Abutiloni seu Malvae* 6 g
Shi Wei *Folium Pyrrosiae* 6 g
Qu Mai *Herba Dianthi* 6 g

Explanation

– **Jin Qian Cao**, **Hai Jin Sha** and **Ji Nei Jin** dissolve urinary stones.
– **Dong Kui Zi**, **Shi Wei** and **Qu Mai** drain Damp-Heat.

For a fuller discussion of the acupuncture treatment of urinary calculi see the appendix to this chapter.

PATENT REMEDY

TE XIAO PAI SHI WAN
Especially-Effective Discharging Stones Pill

Explanation

This remedy already mentioned above is specific to drain Damp-Heat from the Bladder and expel or dissolve urinary stones.

QI PAINFUL-URINATION SYNDROME

CLINICAL MANIFESTATIONS

Full type: difficult and painful urination, hypogastric pain and distension, irritability, Wiry and Deep pulse.
Empty type: difficult urination, weak stream, slight hypogastric distension, tiredness, Pale tongue, Weak pulse.

TREATMENT PRINCIPLE

Full type: move Qi, eliminate stagnation, open the Water passages.
Empty type: tonify and raise Qi, open the Water passages.

ACUPUNCTURE

Ren-3 Zhongji, Ren-5 Shimen, BL-28 Pang-guangshu, LIV-3 Taichong, LIV-5 Ligou, LIV-8 Ququan, BL-64 Jinggu, SP-6 Sanyinjiao, ST-36 Zusanli, Ren-6 Qihai, Du-20 Baihui, LU-7 Lieque, KI-6 Zhaohai, S.I.-3 Houxi and BL-62 Shenmai. Reducing or even method for the Full type and reinforcing method and moxa for the Empty type.
Ancient prescription: KI-1 Yongquan, G.B.-34 Yanglingquan and Ren-5 Shimen ("Gatherings from Eminent Acupuncturists" 1529).[12]

EXPLANATION

– **Ren-3** and **BL-28**, respectively Front-Collecting and Back-Transporting point of the Bladder, regulate Qi in the Bladder.
– **Ren-5**, Front-Collecting point of the Triple Burner, eliminates stagnation in the Lower Burner.
– **LIV-3** moves Liver-Qi and eliminates stagnation.
– **LIV-5** moves Liver-Qi in the Liver Connecting channel which flows to the urethra and genitalia.
– **LIV-8** moves Liver-Qi in the Liver channel in the hypogastric region.
– **BL-64**, Source point, can be used in the Empty type to strengthen the Bladder function.
– **SP-6** regulates Qi, soothes the Liver, opens the Water passages and stops pain.
– **ST-36** tonifies Qi and is used mostly for the Empty type.
– **Ren-6** moves Qi in the Lower Burner.

- **Du-20** raises Qi and relieves stagnation of Qi in the hypogastrium.
- **LU-7** and **KI-6** in combination open the Directing Vessel. This can be used in women to regulate Qi in the hypogastrium, with Ren-6 in Full conditions and Du-20 in empty ones.
- **S.I.-3** and **BL-62** in combination open the governing Vessel. This can be used in men to regulate Qi in the hypogastrium, with Ren-6 in Full conditions and Du-20 in Empty ones.

HERBAL TREATMENT

(1) PRESCRIPTION

CHEN XIANG SAN
Aquilaria Powder
Chen Xiang *Lignum Aquilariae* 9 g
Shi Wei *Folium Pyrrosiae* 6 g
Hua Shi *Talcum* 6 g
Dong Kui Zi *Semen Abutiloni seu Malvae* 6 g
Dang Gui *Radix Angelicae sinensis* 6 g
Wang Bu Liu Xing *Semen Vaccariae segetalis* 6 g
Bai Shao *Radix Paeoniae albae* 6 g
Chen Pi *Pericarpium Citri reticulatae* 4.5 g
Gan Cao *Radix Glycyrrhizae uralensis* 3 g

Explanation

This formula is specific for Painful-Urination Syndrome from Qi stagnation.

- **Chen Xiang** regulates Qi.
- **Shi Wei**, **Hua Shi** and **Dong Kui Zi** drain Dampness from the Bladder and open the Water passages.
- **Dang Gui**, **Wang Bu Liu Xing** and **Bai Shao** regulate Blood.
- **Chen Pi** drains Dampness and moves Qi.
- **Gan Cao** harmonizes and, in combination with Bai Shao, it smooths roughness and stops pain.

Variations

- To enhance this formula's moving Qi action add Xiang Fu *Rhizoma Cyperi rotundi*, Wu Yao *Radix Linderae strychnifoliae* and Xiao Hui Xiang *Fructus Foeniculi vulgaris*.

- If there is Blood stasis add Hong Hua *Flos Carthami tinctorii*, Tao Ren *Semen Persicae* and Niu Xi *Radix Achyranthis bidentatae seu Cyathulae*.

(2) PRESCRIPTION

BU ZHONG YI QI TANG
Tonifying the Centre and Benefiting Qi Decoction
Huang Qi *Radix Astragali membranacei* 12 g
Ren Shen *Radix Ginseng* 9 g
Bai Zhu *Rhizoma Atractylodis macrocephalae* 9 g
Dang Gui *Radix Angelicae sinensis* 6 g
Chen Pi *Pericarpium Citri reticulatae* 6 g
Sheng Ma *Rhizoma Cimicifugae* 3 g
Chai Hu *Radix Bupleuri* 3 g

Explanation

This formula, which has already been explained in chapter 1, is for Painful-Urination Syndrome from deficiency and sinking of Qi. It raises clear Qi and makes turbid Qi descend and, by so doing, it separates clear and turbid in the urinary system and relieves Painful-Urination Syndrome.

(a) PATENT REMEDY

QIAN LIE XIAN WAN
Prostate Gland Pill
Wang Bu Liu Xing *Semen Vaccariae segetalis*
Mu Dan Pi *Cortex Moutan radicis*
Chi Shao *Radix Paeoniae rubrae*
Huang Qi *Radix Astragali membranacei*
Bai Jiang *Herba Patriniae seu Thlaspi*
Qian Hu *Radix Peucedani*
Gan Cao *Radix Glycyrrhizae uralensis*
Mu Xiang *Radix Saussureae*
Mu Tong *Caulis Akebiae*

Explanation

This remedy tonifies Qi, moves Qi and Blood, promotes the separation of the clear from the turbid and drains Damp-Heat. It can be used for Qi Painful-Urination Syndrome of the Full type, i.e. from Qi stagnation.

The tongue presentation appropriate to this remedy in connection with this condition is a tongue body with slightly Red sides.

(b) PATENT REMEDY

BU ZHONG YI QI WAN
Tonifying the Centre and Benefiting Qi Pill

Explanation

This pill has the same ingredients and functions as the homonymous prescription mentioned above. It is suitable to treat Qi Painful-Urination Syndrome of the Empty type, i.e. from deficiency and sinking of Qi.

The tongue presentation appropriate to this remedy is a Pale body.

(c) PATENT REMEDY

JIE JIE WAN
Dispel Swelling Pill
Sheng Di Huang *Radix Rehmanniae glutinosae*
Huang Qi *Radix Astragali membranacei*
Dang Shen *Radix Codonopsis pilosulae*
Nu Zhen Zi *Fructus Ligustri lucidi*
Che Qian Zi *Semen Plantaginis*
Huai Niu Xi *Radix Achyranthis bidentatae*
Dan Shen *Radix Salviae miltiorrhizae*
Ze Xie *Rhizoma Alismatis orientalis*
Tu Si Zi *Semen Cuscutae*
Sang Piao Xiao *Ootheca Mantidis*

Explanation

This remedy tonifies Qi, nourishes Kidney-Yin, resolves Dampness and moves Blood. It is normally used for prostatic hypertrophy occurring against a background of Qi and Kidney-Yin deficiency. In this case, it can be used for Qi Painful-Urination Syndrome of the Empty type, i.e. from deficiency of Qi and Yin.

The tongue presentation appropriate to this remedy is a Red body with rootless coating on the whole, but also sticky on the root and with red spots.

Case history

A 30-year-old woman had been suffering for 6 months from what had been diagnosed as "cystitis". Her urination was frequent and there was pain and distension in the hypogastrium, but no burning during micturition. Urine tests showed no infection. Apart from this, she frequently experienced abdominal distension and she suffered from premenstrual tension with irritability and breast distension. In the past, she had suffered from depression. She also had some lower back-ache, dizziness and slight tinnitus. Her tongue was of a normal colour except for Red sides. Her pulse was Weak on both Rear positions and slightly Wiry on the left side.

Diagnosis

This is Qi Painful-Urination Syndrome of the Excess-type, i.e. from stagnation of Liver-Qi. The symptoms of this are pain and distension of the hypogastrium: there are also other general symptoms of Liver-Qi stagnation such as abdominal distension, premenstrual tension, the depression in the past, and a Wiry pulse. Apart from this, this patient also had some deficiency of the Kidneys as shown by the backache, dizziness and tinnitus, at this moment in time, without pronounced symptoms of either Yin or Yang deficiency.

Treatment principle

The treatment principle adopted was to pacify the Liver, eliminate stagnation and tonify the Kidneys. She was treated only with acupuncture.

Acupuncture

The main points used (with reinforcing method to tonify the Kidneys and even method to pacify the Liver) were selected from the following:

- **LU-7** Lieque and **KI-6** Zhaohai to open the Directing Vessel and move Qi in the urinary system.
- **Ren-3** Zhongji to move Qi in the Bladder and hypogastric region.
- **LIV-5** Ligou and **LIV-3** Taichong to move Liver-Qi in the hypogastrium.
- **SP-6** Sanyinjiao to pacify the Liver.
- **KI-3** Taixi and **BL-23** Shenshu to tonify the Kidneys.

This patient's condition was cleared in 8 treatments as this type of Painful-Urination Syndrome usually responds very quickly to treatment. She continued to receive occasional treatment after that to treat the underlying Kidney deficiency.

Case history

A 70-year-old woman had been suffering from

painful urination for 2 years. She experienced pain before or during urination and also had pain and distension over the hypogastrium. The micturition was sometimes "reluctant" and the urine was rather dark. All urine and blood tests had proven negative. One year before her consultation she had had an acute episode of urinary retention and had to go to hospital for catheterization. She also suffered from lower back-ache, and a sore and "tired throat" which was also dry at night. Her tongue was Dark-Red, dry with some cracks and the root had red spots and yellow coating. Her pulse was Deep and Wiry, particularly so on the left-Rear position.

Diagnosis
This is a combination of two types of Painful-Urination Syndrome: Qi (of the Excess variety) and Heat Painful-Urination Syndrome against a background of Kidney-Yin deficiency. The symptoms of Qi Painful-Urination Syndrome are pain before urination, pain and distension of the hypogastrium and a Wiry pulse. The symptoms of Heat Painful-Urination Syndrome, in this case Damp-Heat, are pain during micturition, slight retention of urine (from Dampness obstructing the Water passages) and a yellow coating and red spots on the root of the tongue. The symptoms of Kidney-Yin deficiency are a dry throat at night, back-ache and a Red, dry and cracked tongue.

Treatment principle
This patient was treated only with acupuncture. The principle of treatment adopted was to clear Bladder-Heat, resolve Dampness, move Qi, eliminate stagnation and nourish Kidney-Yin.

Acupuncture
The main points used, using reinforcing method to nourish Kidney-Yin and even method to clear Damp-Heat and move Qi, were chosen from the following:

- **SP-9** Yinlingquan and **SP-6** Sanyinjiao to resolve Damp-Heat from the urinary passages.
- **LIV-5** Ligou and **LIV-3** Taichong to move Qi and eliminate stagnation from the urinary passages.
- **L.I.-11** Quchi and **KI-2** Rangu to clear Heat and cool Blood.
- **KI-6** Zhaohai and **Ren-4** Guanyuan to nourish Kidney-Yin and soothe the throat.
- **LU-7** Lieque and **KI-6** Zhaohai in combination to open the Directing vessel which will move Qi in the Lower Burner, nourish Kidney-Yin and soothe the throat.
- **BL-63** Jinmen and **LIV-6** Zhongdu, both Accumulation points, to stop pain and remove obstructions from the channels.

This patient was treated for 3 months at fortnightly intervals. There was a very marked improvement in her condition after 6 treatments and she continued to receive treatment every 3 months to maintain the improvement and continue nourishing Kidney-Yin.

Case history

A 35-year-old man had been suffering from painful urination for 1 year. Before and during micturition he had a stinging pain which extended to the tip of the penis. He also had a feeling of distension in the hypogastrium and a tingling in the left big toe. A week before his urinary problem started, he had sciatica with pain at the back of the left leg. Two years before the consultation he had suffered from depression for which he took antidepressants. His tongue was slightly Red on the sides and had a yellow coating on the root. His pulse was slightly Rapid, Wiry on the left side, more so on the left-Rear position which was also Tight.

Diagnosis
This is a combination of Qi and Heat Painful-Urination Syndromes with predominance of the former. The symptoms of the former are the pain before micturition extending to the penis, the feeling of distension of the hypogastrium, the tingling of the left big toe (Liver channel) and the Wiry pulse. Symptoms of Heat Painful-Urination Syndrome are the pain during micturition, the yellow coating on the root of the tongue, and the Wiry-Tight pulse on the left-Rear position indicating Heat in the Bladder. Normally the Tight pulse quality indicates Cold, but when it is combined with a Wiry quality and the pulse is Rapid, it can indicate Heat in an organ.

Treatment principle
The principle of treatment adopted was to pacify the Liver, eliminate stagnation and clear Bladder-Heat. This patient was treated only with acupuncture.

Acupuncture
The points used (with even method) were selected from the following:

- **BL-62** Shenmai on the left and **S.I.-3** Houxi on the right, to open the Yang Heel Vessel and move Qi in the hypogastrium. The use of this vessel is indicated by the Wiry and Tight quality on the left-Rear position. This vessel is used to absorb "excess Yang" and stagnation of Qi is a form of excess Yang.
- **Ren-3** Zhongji to clear Bladder-Heat.
- **LIV-5** Ligou and **LIV-3** Taichong to pacify the Liver and eliminate stagnation from the hypogastrium, urethra and penis. LIV-5 is the Connecting point and the Connecting channel flows from this point to the external genitalia and penis in men.
- **SP-6** Sanyinjiao to pacify the Liver and moderate urgency.

This patient's condition was cleared in 10

treatments, after which, in order to maintain the improvement, he was prescribed a course of the pills Shu Gan Wan *Pacifying the Liver Pill* to pacify the Liver and eliminate stagnation. This patent remedy could not have been used before, in conjunction with acupuncture, as all its ingredients are warm, which would have aggravated the condition of Bladder-Heat.

Case history

A 47-year-old woman had been suffering from frequency of urination and hypogastric pain for 4 years. The pain was slight and confined to the hypogastric region and there was no burning on micturition. She also had an ache in the sacral region. The urine was pale and she often had to pass water at night. These symptoms started 3 months after a hysterectomy. Her pulse was generally Weak, more so on both Rear positions. Her tongue was very Pale, with a white and yellow sticky coating, and the root had no spirit (Plate 20.2).

Diagnosis
This is a condition of Qi Painful-Urination Syndrome of the Deficiency type. There is deficiency and sinking of Spleen- and Kidney-Qi: this latter is obvious from the frequent urination, pale urine, nocturia, Pale tongue and Weak pulse on both Kidney positions. This condition started after the hysterectomy (which was done due to the presence of myomas); as so often happens after this operation, the stagnation present in the uterus is transferred to the closest organ, i.e. the bladder. Thus, there was also an element of stagnation within the deficiency of Qi, and this was apparent from the slight hypogastric pain.

Treatment principle
The treatment principle adopted was to tonify and raise Spleen-Qi and tonify and warm Kidney-Yang. This patient was treated with acupuncture and two patent remedies.

Acupuncture
The acupuncture points used (with reinforcing method) were selected from the following:

- **LU-7** Lieque and **KI-6** Zhaohai to open the Directing Vessel, tonify the Kidneys and, at the same time, move Qi in the lower abdomen.
- **Du-20** Baihui was used to raise Qi.
- **KI-3** Taixi, with moxa on the needle, to tonify and warm Kidney-Yang.
- **BL-23** Shenshu to tonify Kidney-Yang.
- **Ren-4** Guanyuan, with direct moxa cones, to warm the Uterus (or rather the area where the uterus should have been) and tonify Kidney-Yang. This point combines well with Du-20 to raise Qi and tonify the Kidneys.

Herbal treatment
The patent remedies used were Bu Zhong Yi Qi Wan *Tonifying the Centre and Benefiting Qi Pill* to tonify and raise Spleen-Qi and Jin Suo Gu Jing Wan *Golden Lock Consolidating the Essence Pill* to tonify the Kidneys and stop frequency.

With these two remedies, it took only two treatments to clear this patient's condition completely. In fact, even after only one treatment her urine was darker and there was no frequency or pain.

BLOOD PAINFUL-URINATION SYNDROME

CLINICAL MANIFESTATIONS

Full type (Blood Heat): difficult urination, burning pain on urination, blood in the urine which could take the form of small clots, fullness and pain in the hypogastrium, mental restlessness, Red tongue and Rapid pulse which feels Full at the middle level.

Empty type (Blood Empty-Heat from Yin deficiency): pale blood in urine, slight discomfort on urination, not much pain, sore back, depression, feeling of heat in the evening, Red and peeled tongue, Rapid and Floating-Empty pulse.

TREATMENT PRINCIPLE

Full type: clear Heat, cool Blood, stop bleeding, open the Water passages.
Empty type: clear Empty-Heat, cool Blood, nourish Yin, stop bleeding, open the Water passages.

ACUPUNCTURE

LIV-3 Taichong, KI-2 Rangu, Ren-3 Zhongji, BL-28 Pangguangshu, BL-63 Jinmen, SP-10 Xuehai, BL-17 Geshu, SP-6 Sanyinjiao, Ren-4 Guanyuan, KI-6 Zhaohai. Reducing method for the Full type and reinforcing method for the Empty type. No moxa should be used.

Ancient prescription: KI-1 Yongquan, KI-6 Zhaohai, KI-10 Yingu and SP-6 Sanyinjiao ("Compendium of Acupuncture" 1601).[13]

- **LIV-3** and **KI-2** cool the Blood and open the Water passages.
- **Ren-3** and **BL-28** clear Bladder-Heat.

- **BL-63** stops bleeding.
- **SP-10** and **BL-17** cool the Blood.
- **SP-6** cools the Blood, drains Dampness from the Lower Burner and opens the Water passages.
- **Ren-4** and **KI-6**, with reinforcing method, nourish Yin. These two points are used for the Empty type.

HERBAL TREATMENT

(1) PRESCRIPTION

XIAO JI YIN ZI
Cephalanoplos Decoction
Xiao Ji *Herba Cephalanoplos segeti* 30 g
Ou Jie *Nodus Nelumbinis nuciferae rhizomatis* 6 g
Pu Huang *Pollen Typhae* 9 g
Hua Shi *Talcum* 15 g
Mu Tong *Caulis Akebiae* 9 g
Zhu Ye *Herba Lophatheri gracilis* 9 g
Zhi Zi *Fructus Gardeniae jasminoidis* 9 g
Sheng Di Huang *Radix Rehmanniae glutinosae* 30 g
Dang Gui *Radix Angelicae sinensis* 6 g
Gan Cao *Radix Glycyrrhizae uralensis* 6 g

Explanation

This prescription is specific for Blood Painful-Urination Syndrome from Blood-Heat.

- **Xiao Ji** cools Blood, stops bleeding and opens the Water passages. It should be used in a large dose.
- **Ou Jie** and **Pu Huang** help Xiao Ji to stop bleeding. Pu Huang stops bleeding without congealing Blood as it also moves Blood.
- **Hua Shi**, **Mu Tong** and **Zhu Ye** clear Heat, drain Dampness and open the Water passages.
- **Zhi Zi** drains Damp-Heat from the Three Burners.
- **Sheng Di** cools Blood and nourishes Yin.
- **Dang Gui** helps to nourish Yin by nourishing Blood. It also helps the other herbs to stop bleeding by entering Blood.
- **Gan Cao** harmonizes.

(2) PRESCRIPTION

ZHI BO DI HUANG WAN (also called ZHI BO BA WEI WAN)
Anemarrhena-Phellodendron-Rehmannia Pill (Anemarrhena-Phellodendron Eight-Ingredient Pill)
Shu Di Huang *Radix Rehmanniae glutinosae praeparata* 24 g
Shan Zhu Yu *Fructus Corni officinalis* 12 g
Shan Yao *Radix Dioscoreae oppositae* 12 g
Ze Xie *Rhizoma Alismatis orientalis* 9 g
Fu Ling *Sclerotium Poriae cocos* 9 g
Mu Dan Pi *Cortex Moutan radicis* 9 g
Zhi Mu *Radix Anemarrhenae asphodeloidis* 9 g
Huang Bo *Cortex Phellodendri* 9 g

Explanation

This formula is used for Blood Painful-Urination Syndrome, i.e. Blood Empty-Heat from Yin deficiency.

Variations

These variations apply to both above formulae.

- If bleeding is profuse add Qian Cao Gen *Radix Rubiae cordifoliae*.
- If there are signs of Blood stasis add Hong Hua *Flos Carthami tinctorii* and Tao Ren *Semen Persicae*.

(a) PATENT REMEDY

QIAN LIE XIAN WAN
Prostate Gland Pill

Explanation

This pill, already mentioned above, drains Damp-Heat and moves Blood. Because of this latter function, it can be used to treat Blood Painful-Urination Syndrome of the Full type, i.e. from Blood-Heat with stasis of Blood.

The tongue presentation appropriate to this remedy, in connection with this condition, is a Reddish-Purple body with a yellow coating and red spots on the root.

(b) PATENT REMEDY

YUNNAN TE CHAN TIAN QI PIAN
Yunnan Specially-Prepared Notoginseng Tablet
San Qi *Radix Notoginseng*

Explanation

This remedy, which moves Blood and stops bleeding, can be used, in conjunction with others, to treat the Manifestation of Blood Painful-Urination Syndrome, i.e. blood in the urine.

(c) PATENT REMEDY

ZHI BO BA WEI WAN
Anemarrhena-Phellodendron Eight-Ingredient Pill
Shu Di Huang *Radix Rehmanniae glutinosae praeparata*
Shan Zhu Yu *Fructus Corni officinalis*
Shan Yao *Radix Dioscoreae oppositae*
Ze Xie *Rhizoma Alismatis orientalis*
Fu Ling *Sclerotium Poriae cocos*
Mu Dan Pi *Cortex Moutan radicis*
Zhi Mu *Radix Anemarrhenae asphodeloidis*
Huang Bo *Cortex Phellodendri*

Explanation

This remedy nourishes Kidney-Yin and drains Damp-Heat from the Bladder. It can be used to treat chronic Blood Painful-Urination Syndrome deriving from deficiency of Kidney-Yin with Empty-Heat in the Blood.

The tongue presentation appropriate to this remedy is a Red and peeled body but with a sticky-yellow, rootless coating and red spots on the root.

NOTE

Blood in the urine may be due in Western medicine to many different conditions. It should also always be kept in mind that the most common cause of haematuria in men over 50 is carcinoma of the bladder. For these reasons, persistent haematuria should *never* be treated without a proper Western diagnosis.

CLOUDY PAINFUL-URINATION SYNDROME

CLINICAL MANIFESTATIONS

Full type (Dampness): turbid or cloudy urine like rice soup (it may look as if it had patches of oil floating on it); possibly with blood or a sediment looking like cotton wool after some time; difficult urination, a sticky tongue coating and a Full-Slippery pulse.
Empty type (Qi deficiency with some Dampness): cloudy or turbid urine, slight difficulty in urination, tiredness, dizziness, lower back-ache, a Pale tongue with sticky coating and a Weak-Floating pulse.

TREATMENT PRINCIPLE

Full type: drain Dampness, clear Heat, separate the clear from the turbid, open the Water passages.
Empty type: tonify Qi, strengthen the Kidneys, separate the clear from the turbid, drain Dampness and open the Water passages.

ACUPUNCTURE

Ren-3 Zhongji, BL-22 Sanjiaoshu, BL-28 Pangguangshu, BL-23 Shenshu, KI-7 Fuliu, Ren-6 Qihai, Ren-9 Shuifen, ST-28 Shuidao, SP-9 Yinlingquan, SP-6 Sanyinjiao. Reducing or even method in the Full type and reinforcing method in the Empty one.
Ancient prescription for the Empty-type: direct moxa on SP-6 Sanyinjiao, 7 cones ("Compendium of Acupuncture" 1601).[14]

EXPLANATION

– **Ren-3** and **BL-28** drain Dampness from the Bladder.
– **BL-22** promotes the transformation of fluids and the separation of clear from turbid in the Lower Burner.
– **BL-23** and **KI-7** should be reinforced in the Empty type to strengthen the Kidneys and the Bladder function of Qi transformation.

- **Ren-6** moves Qi in the Lower Burner and helps the transformation of fluids there.
- **Ren-9** and **ST-28** promote the transformation of fluids and the separation of clear from turbid.
- **SP-9** and **SP-6** drain Dampness from the Lower Burner.

HERBAL TREATMENT

(1) PRESCRIPTION

CHENG SHI BI XIE YIN
Dioscorea Decoction of the Cheng Clan
Bi Xie *Rhizoma Dioscoreae hypoglaucae* 9 g
Shi Chang Pu *Rhizoma Acori graminei* 6 g
Che Qian Zi *Semen Plantaginis* 6 g
Huang Bo *Cortex Phellodendri* 6 g
Fu Ling *Sclerotium Poriae cocos* 9 g
Bai Zhu *Rhizoma Atractylodis macrocephalae* 6 g
Lian Zi *Semen Nelumbinis nuciferae* 6 g
Dan Shen *Radix Salviae miltiorrhizae* 4.5 g

Explanation

This prescription is for the Full type of Cloudy Painful-Urination Syndrome with symptoms of Damp-Heat and a yellow-sticky tongue coating.

- **Bi Xie** and **Chang Pu** separate the clear from the turbid in the urinary tract and drain Dampness.
- **Che Qian Zi** and **Huang Bo** drain Damp-Heat.
- **Fu Ling** and **Bai Zhu** tonify the Spleen and drain Dampness.
- **Lian Zi** and **Dan Shen** clear the Heart, move Blood, open the Water passages and separate the clear from the turbid.

Variations

- If there is distension of the hypogastrium add Wu Yao *Radix Linderae strychnifoliae* and Xiang Fu *Rhizoma Cyperi rotundi*.
- If there is blood in the urine add Xiao Ji *Herba Cephalanoplos segeti*, Ou Jie *Nodus Nelumbinis nuciferae rhizomatis* and Bai Mao Gen *Rhizoma Imperatae cylindricae*.

(2) PRESCRIPTION

BI XIE FEN QING YIN
Dioscorea Separating the Clear Decoction
Bi Xie *Rhizoma Dioscoreae hypoglaucae* 12 g
Yi Zhi Ren *Fructus Alpiniae oxyphyllae* 9 g
Wu Yao *Radix Linderae strychnifoliae* 9 g
Shi Chang Pu *Rhizoma Acori graminei* 9 g

Explanation

This formula is used for Cloudy Painful-Urination Syndrome from Damp-Cold.

- **Bi Xie** separates the clear from the turbid in the urinary system and is specific for cloudy urine.
- **Yi Zhi Ren** warms the Lower Burner and expels Cold.
- **Wu Yao** warms the Kidneys, moves Qi and opens the Water passages in the Lower Burner.
- **Shi Chang Pu** opens the orifices and helps Bi Xie to separate the clear from the turbid.

(3) PRESCRIPTION

GAO LIN TANG
Cloudy Painful-Urination Syndrome Decoction
Shan Yao *Radix Dioscoreae oppositae* 12 g
Qian Shi *Semen Euryales ferocis* 6 g
Sheng Di Huang *Radix Rehmanniae glutinosae* 9 g
Long Gu *Os Draconis* 12 g
Mu Li *Concha Ostreae* 12 g
Bai Shao *Radix Paeoniae albae* 6 g
Dang Shen *Radix Codonopsis pilosulae* 6 g

Explanation

This formula is for the Empty type of Painful-Urination Syndrome, i.e. a chronic case characterized by deficiency of Qi and some Dampness.

- **Shan Yao** tonifies Qi and relieves urinary dysfunction.
- **Qian Shi** and **Sheng Di** nourish Yin.
- **Long Gu**, **Mu Li** and **Bai Shao** absorb and reduce urination.
- **Dang Shen** tonifies Qi.

Variations

– If there is Spleen and Kidney deficiency use Bu Zhong Yi Qi Tang *Tonifying the Centre and Benefiting Qi Decoction* together with Qi Wei Du Qi Tang *Seven-Ingredient Capital Qi Decoction* (which is the Liu Wei Di Huang Wan *Six-Ingredient Rehmannia Pill* plus Wu Wei Zi *Fructus Schisandrae chinensis*).

PATENT REMEDY

QIAN JIN ZHI DAI WAN

Thousand Gold Pieces Stopping Leukorrhoea Pill
Da Qing Ye *Folium Isatidis seu Baphicacanthi*
Dang Shen *Radix Codonopsis pilosulae*
Mu Li *Concha Ostreae*
Mu Xiang *Radix Saussureae*
Dang Gui *Radix Angelicae sinensis*
Yan Hu Suo *Rhizoma Corydalis yanhusuo*
Xu Duan *Radix Dipsaci*
Bai Zhu *Rhizoma Atractylodis macrocephalae*
Xiao Hui Xiang *Fructus Foeniculi vulgaris*

Explanation

This remedy tonifies and moves Qi and absorbs discharges. Although it is primarily for chronic vaginal discharge, it is suitable to treat chronic Cloudy Painful-Urination Syndrome against a background of Qi deficiency.

The tongue presentation appropriate to this remedy is a Pale body with a dirty-dull-white coating on the root.

Case history

A 65-year-old man had been suffering from slight retention of urine for 2 years. Although his urination was very frequent, also at night, the urine was scanty and hesitant in coming out. It was also cloudy. His GP had prescribed antibiotics, treating his problem as "cystitis": the antibiotics did not help his condition at all. His tongue had a sticky-yellow coating on the root and his pulse was generally Slippery, Full and Rapid. On the position proximal to the left Rear one, felt rolling the finger proximally, the pulse was very Full, Tight and Slippery. This is the position where the prostate may be felt.

Diagnosis
This is a condition of Cloudy Painful-Urination Syndrome of the Full-type with Damp-Heat in the Bladder. Most of his symptoms (retention of urine, frequency, cloudy urine, sticky coating and Slippery pulse) are due to Dampness. The Full, Tight and Slippery quality on the prostate pulse position almost certainly indicates either prostatic hypertrophy or carcinoma of the prostate. Judging by his age and the very Full, Slippery and Rapid quality of his pulse I suspected he might have carcinoma of the prostate. I advised him to insist that his GP refer him to a consultant for a proper diagnosis. In the meanwhile, I started treating him, giving him a variation of the formula Cheng Shi Bi Xie Yin *Dioscorea Decoction of the Cheng Clan*:

Bi Xie *Rhizoma Dioscoreae hypoglaucae* 9 g
Shi Chang Pu *Rhizoma Acori graminei* 6 g
Che Qian Zi *Semen Plantaginis* 6 g
Huang Bo *Cortex Phellodendri* 6 g
Fu Ling *Sclerotium Poriae cocos* 9 g
Bai Zhu *Rhizoma Atractylodis macrocephalae* 6 g
Lian Zi *Semen Nelumbinis nuciferae* 6 g
Dan Shen *Radix Salviae miltiorrhizae* 4.5 g
Yi Yi Ren *Semen Coicis lachryma jobi* 15 g
Tian Kui Zi *Rhizoma Semiaquilegiae adoxoides* 9 g

Explanation
– The first eight herbs constitute the root formula.
– **Yi Yi Ren** was added to drain Dampness and soften hardness (i.e. for the prostatic hypertrophy or carcinoma).
– **Tian Kui Zi** was added to drain Damp-Heat, dissolve swelling and combat cancer.

By using this decoction he seemed to improve for 2 or 3 weeks, only to deteriorate each time. After 3 months he went to see a consultant and had tests and the diagnosis of carcinoma of the prostate was confirmed.

FATIGUE PAINFUL-URINATION SYNDROME

CLINICAL MANIFESTATIONS

Difficult urination coming in bouts, no burning, frequency, dribbling after micturition, dragging feeling in the hypogastrium, exhaustion, sore back, depression, feeling cold.
Tongue: Pale.
Pulse: Weak.

This is a chronic condition with deficiency of Kidney-Yang.

TREATMENT PRINCIPLE

Tonify and raise Qi, strengthen the Kidneys, open the Water passages.

ACUPUNCTURE

BL-23 Shenshu, Ren-4 Guanyuan, BL-28 Pang-guangshu, Du-20 Baihui, ST-36 Zusanli, SP-6 Sanyinjiao, SP-9 Yinlingquan, Ren-6 Qihai, KI-3 Taixi, Du-4 Mingmen. Reinforcing method. Moxa should be used.

EXPLANATION

- **BL-23** and **Ren-4** tonify the Kidneys. Direct moxa can be used on Ren-4 to tonify Kidney-Yang.
- **BL-28** strengthens the Bladder's function and opens the Water passages.
- **Du-20** raises clear Qi and separates the clear from the turbid.
- **ST-36** and **SP-6** tonify Qi. SP-6 also opens the Water passages and drains Dampness from the Lower Burner.
- **SP-9** drains Dampness from the Lower Burner.
- **Ren-6** tonifies Qi in the Lower Burner. It combines well in this condition with Du-20 (with moxa) to strengthen Qi in the Lower Burner, raise Qi and harmonize Governing and Directing Vessels.
- **KI-3** tonifies the Kidneys.
- **Du-4**, with moxa, tonifies Kidney-Yang and strengthens the Fire of the Gate of Vitality.

HERBAL TREATMENT

(1) PRESCRIPTION

WU BI SHAN YAO WAN
Incomparable Dioscorea Pill
Shan Yao *Radix Dioscoreae oppositae* 15 g
Rou Cong Rong *Herba Cistanchis* 9 g
Tu Si Zi *Semen Cuscutae* 9 g
Ba Ji Tian *Radix Morindae officinalis* 6 g
Du Zhong *Cortex Eucommiae ulmoidis* 6 g
Shu Di Huang *Radix Rehmanniae glutinosae prae-parata* 9 g
Shan Zhu Yu *Fructus Corni officinalis* 6 g
Niu Xi *Radix Achyranthis bidentatae seu Cyathulae* 6 g
Wu Wei Zi *Fructus Schisandrae chinensis* 4.5 g

Chi Shi Zhi *Halloysitum rubrum* 6 g
Ze Xie *Rhizoma Alismatis orientalis* 6 g
Fu Shen *Sclerotium Poriae cocos pararadicis* 6 g

Explanation

This formula is for Dampness in the Bladder against a background of Kidney-Yang deficiency.

- **Shan Yao** tonifies Spleen and Kidneys and relieves urinary dysfunction.
- **Rou Cong Rong**, **Tu Si Zi**, **Ba Ji Tian** and **Du Zhong** tonify Kidney-Yang.
- **Shu Di**, **Shan Zhu Yu** and **Niu Xi** tonify the Kidneys and Liver.
- **Wu Wei Zi** and **Chi Shi Zhi** are astringent and they help to nourish the Kidneys.
- **Ze Xie** drains Dampness and prevents excessive heating from the other herbs.
- **Fu Shen** drains Dampness and calms the Mind.

(2) PRESCRIPTION

BU ZHONG YI QI TANG
Tonifying the Centre and Benefiting Qi Decoction
Huang Qi *Radix Astragali membranacei* 12 g
Ren Shen *Radix Ginseng* 9 g
Bai Zhu *Rhizoma Atractylodis macrocephalae* 9 g
Dang Gui *Radix Angelicae sinensis* 6 g
Chen Pi *Pericarpium Citri reticulatae* 6 g
Sheng Ma *Rhizoma Cimicifugae* 3 g
Chai Hu *Radix Bupleuri* 3 g

Explanation

This formula, which has already been explained in chapter 1, is used if there is deficiency and sinking of Spleen-Qi causing frequency of urination and a dragging feeling in the hypogastrium.

(3) PRESCRIPTION

ZHI BO DI HUANG WAN
Anemarrhena-Phellodendron-Rehmannia Pill
Shu Di Huang *Radix Rehmanniae glutinosae prae-parata* 24 g
Shan Zhu Yu *Fructus Corni officinalis* 12 g

Shan Yao *Radix Dioscoreae oppositae* 12 g
Ze Xie *Rhizoma Alismatis orientalis* 9 g
Fu Ling *Sclerotium Poriae cocos* 9 g
Mu Dan Pi *Cortex Moutan radicis* 9 g
Zhi Mu *Radix Anemarrhenae asphodeloidis* 9 g
Huang Bo *Cortex Phellodendri* 9 g

Explanation

This prescription is chosen if there is deficiency of Kidney-Yin and Empty-Heat with such symptoms as scanty-dark urine with slight burning. It is suitable to treat chronic, recurrent cystitis occurring against a background of Kidney-Yin deficiency and Bladder Damp-Heat.

The tongue presentation is a Red and peeled tongue with red spots and a sticky-yellow coating on the root.

(4) PRESCRIPTION

YOU GUI WAN
Restoring the Right (Kidney) Pill
Fu Zi *Radix Aconiti carmichaeli praeparata* 3 g
Rou Gui *Cortex Cinnamomi cassiae* 3 g
Du Zhong *Cortex Eucommiae ulmoidis* 6 g
Shan Zhu Yu *Fructus Corni officinalis* 4.5 g
Tu Si Zi *Semen Cuscutae* 6 g
Lu Jiao Jiao *Colla Cornu Cervi* 6 g
Shu Di Huang *Radix Rehmanniae glutinosae praeparata* 12 g
Shan Yao *Radix Dioscoreae oppositae* 6 g
Gou Qi Zi *Fructus Lycii chinensis* 6 g
Dang Gui *Radix Angelicae sinensis* 4.5 g

Explanation

This formula, which has already been explained in chapter 1, is used if there is a pronounced deficiency of Kidney-Yang.

(a) PATENT REMEDY

BU ZHONG YI QI WAN
Tonifying the Centre and Benefiting Qi Pill

Explanation

This remedy, which has already been explained in chapter 1, is suitable to treat Fatigue Painful-Urination Syndrome deriving from Spleen-Qi deficiency.

The tongue presentation appropriate to this remedy is a Pale body.

(b) PATENT REMEDY

ZHI BO BA WEI WAN
Anemarrhena-Phellodendron Eight-Ingredient Pill

Explanation

This remedy is suitable to treat Fatigue Painful-Urination Syndrome deriving from deficiency of Kidney-Yin.

The tongue presentation appropriate to this remedy is a Red and peeled body with a sticky-yellow coating and red spots on the root.

(c) PATENT REMEDY

JIE JIE WAN
Dispel Swelling Pill

Explanation

This remedy, already explained above, is suitable for Fatigue Painful-Urination Syndrome deriving from Qi deficiency and Dampness.

The tongue presentation appropriate to this remedy is a Pale body with a sticky coating on the root.

Case history

A 45-year-old woman had been suffering from difficult urination and frequency for 3 years. There was some dribbling after micturition and a dragging feeling with a slight pain in the hypogastrium, together with general exhaustion, a sore back, depression, and a cold feeling. All these symptoms were always immediately aggravated from overwork. Her urinary symptoms started 2 months after a hysterectomy operation which had been done due to very heavy bleeding. Her tongue was Pale and her pulse very Weak and Fine, especially so on both Rear positions.

Diagnosis
This is a condition of Fatigue Painful-Urination

Syndrome against a background of Kidney-Yang deficiency. As for a previous patient whose case history was presented in the section on Qi Painful-Urination Syndrome, the urinary symptoms started after a hysterectomy: this was due to the transferral of a condition of stagnation from the uterus to the nearest organ, i.e. the bladder. The heavy menstrual bleeding which prompted her to have the hysterectomy itself, was obviously due to the deficiency and sinking of Spleen- and Kidney-Qi, the same causes of the subsequent Painful-Urination Syndrome.

Treatment principle
The principle of treatment adopted was to tonify Spleen-Qi and Kidney-Yang. This patient was treated only with acupuncture.

Acupuncture
The points used (with reinforcing method) were the following:

- **LU-7** Lieque on the right and **KI-6** Zhaohai on the left to open the Directing vessel, tonify the Kidneys and move Qi in the lower abdomen.
- **Ren-4** Guanyuan with direct moxa cones to tonify and warm Kidney-Yang.
- **Du-20** Baihui to raise Qi: this point combines well with Ren-4 Guanyuan.
- **KI-3** Taixi with moxa on needle to tonify and warm Kidney-Yang.
- **BL-20** Pishu and **BL-23** Shenshu to tonify Spleen- and Kidney-Yang.

This patient was treated for over 9 months as her energy was very low and this produced an improvement of about 70% in her symptoms.

Appendix

Urinary calculi

The "Classic of the Secret Transmission" (*c.* AD 200) by Hua Tuo mentions urinary stones in chapter 44:

A dull abdominal pain, difficulty and pain on micturition and emaciation indicate urinary stones . . . Stones are caused by Qi deficiency and Heat . . . [their formation] is similar to the evaporation of sea water by fire to produce salt.[15]

Thus urinary stones or sand derive from Dampness which is precipitated (like a crystal formation) into solid stones under the condensing action of Heat.

From a Western medical perspective, urinary calculi are formed by the precipitation in crystalline (stones) or granular (sand) form of acids present in the urine. These acids are uric acid, oxalate or phosphates. Thus, different kinds of stones may be formed from different acids. The main components may be calcium (as found in cheese and milk), oxalate (spinach and rhubarb), uric acid (liver, kidney, fish-roe, and sardines) or phosphate (very widespread in many foodstuffs).

AETIOLOGY

1. EXCESSIVE SEXUAL ACTIVITY

Excessive sexual activity may weaken Kidney-Yin and lead to a concentration of urine which, after years, may give rise to stones.

2. DIET

The excessive consumption of cheese, milk, spinach, rhubarb, liver, kidney, fish-roe and sardines may all contribute to the formation of urinary stones.

3. LACK OF EXERCISE

Lack of exercise leads to stagnation in the Lower Burner which may contribute to the formation of stones.

4. LOSS OF FLUIDS

Persistent and long-standing loss of fluids from sweating in certain occupations can be a factor in the formation of stones.

PATHOLOGY

This is characterized by two conditions: a deficiency of Spleen and Kidneys, and Heat.

The deficient Spleen and Kidneys fail to transform fluids in the Lower Burner resulting in the accumulation of Dampness. Heat, on the other hand, evaporates fluids and condenses Dampness into stones or sand.

CLINICAL MANIFESTATIONS
ACUTE STAGE

Clinical manifestations depend on the location of the stones in the urinary tract. The main symptom is pain. This is located in one loin, the lateral abdominal region, the groin or the urethra depending on the location of the stone in the kidney, kidney-pelvis, ureter or urethra (Fig. 20.1).

The pain is of a colicky nature and is very intense, coming in waves. The patient is restless, sweats and may look under shock.

Other manifestations include burning pain on micturition, interrupted flow of micturition, frequency, urgency and blood in urine. The urine will be dark.

Other general symptoms and signs may include shivering, fever, thirst, lumbago and lassitude. The tongue will have a thick-yellow coating with red spots on the root. The pulse will be Rapid and Wiry on the left Rear position.

CHRONIC STAGE

At the chronic stage, the stone is not moving in the urinary tract and therefore there is no colicky pain. There are three conditions:

DAMP-HEAT

This is characterized by burning on urination, difficulty in micturition, dark urine, yellow-sticky tongue coating on the root and a Rapid and Slippery pulse.

KIDNEY-YIN DEFICIENCY

Repeated attacks of urinary-stones pain, dull ache in the back, dark urine, prickly pain in the urethra on micturition, insomnia, dry mouth, night-sweating, Red tongue without coating and a Floating-Empty pulse.

KIDNEY-YANG DEFICIENCY

In long-standing cases Kidney-Yin deficiency may turn into Kidney-Yang deficiency. In this case there would be a long history of repeated colicky attacks, a sore back, chilliness, depression, exhaustion and a Weak-Deep pulse. If Kidney-Yang deficiency develops from Kidney-Yin deficiency the tongue would *not* change from Red to Pale but stay Pale.

TREATMENT
ACUTE STAGE

The treatment in the acute colicky stage is aimed at expelling the stones and stopping pain.

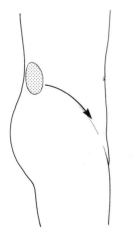 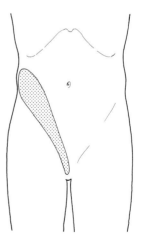

Fig. 20.1 Area of pain in renal colic

ACUPUNCTURE

Main prescription

BL-23 Shenshu, ST-25 Tianshu, Ren-6 Qihai, SP-9 Yinlingquan, LIV-3 Taichong and KI-3 Taixi. Reducing method. In the acute stage, moxa may be used to tonify Yang and facilitate the movement of the stone, even if there is Kidney-Yin deficiency.

Insert the needles deeply. Obtain the needling sensation to radiate horizontally for ST-25 and Ren-6 and vertically (upwards) for SP-9, LIV-3 and KI-3. Ideally, the needling sensation from these last three points should radiate all the way to the abdomen. If possible, two practitioners can manipulate the points in the back and front at the same time. Retain the needles for 1 hour or even longer and manipulate them every time the pain returns.

Use the points unilaterally. If the stones have not moved after 5 treatments, use distal points bilaterally and apply electrical stimulation with high frequency.

Other points according to location of pain

Other points are chosen according to the location of pain which follows the movement of the stones along the urinary tract.

- Stones in the kidney (lumbar-loin pain): BL-23 Shenshu, BL-22 Sanjiaoshu, G.B.-25 Jingmen and BL-52 Zhishi.
- Stones in upper ureter (loin and upper-abdomen pain): ST-25 Tianshu, SP-15 Daheng, BL-23 Shenshu and BL-24 Qihaishu.
- Stones in middle-lower ureter (pain lower abdomen): ST-27 Daju, ST-28 Shuidao, ST-29 Guilai and BL-26 Guanyuanshu.
- Stones in the bladder (hypogastric pain): Ren-3 Zhongji, Ren-2 Qugu, BL-32 Ciliao and BL-28 Pangguangshu.

Other points according to channel

- Liver channel: LIV-3 Taichong and LIV-8 Ququan.
- Stomach channel: ST-36 Zusanli.
- Kidney channel: KI-10 Yingu, SP-9 Yinlingquan and BL-39 Weiyang.

HERBAL TREATMENT

Prescription

SHI WEI SAN
Pyrrosia Powder
Shi Wei *Folium Pyrrosiae* 9 g
Dong Kui Zi *Semen Abutiloni seu Malvae* 6 g
Qu Mai *Herba Dianthi* 6 g
Che Qian Zi *Semen Plantaginis* 6 g
Hua Shi *Talcum* 6 g

Explanation

All these herbs in this formula, already explained in this chapter, drain Damp-Heat, open the Water passages and relieve urinary dysfunction.

Variations

- The above formula can be taken as a decoction together with Hu Po *Succinum* and Chen Xiang *Lignum Aquilariae* (3 g of each) ground into a powder.
- To strengthen the stone-expelling power add Jin Qian Cao *Herba Desmodii styracifolii* and Hai Jin Sha *Spora Lygodii japonici*. Jin Qian Cao can be drunk as an infusion every day also to prevent the formation of new stones after some have been expelled.
- If there is stagnation of Qi add Xiang Fu *Rhizoma Cyperi rotundi*, Wu Yao *Radix Linderae strychnifoliae* and Yan Hu Suo *Rhizoma Corydalis yanhusuo*.
- If there is stasis of Blood with a stabbing pain add Tao Ren *Semen Persicae* and Yan Hu Suo *Rhizoma Corydalis yanhusuo*.
- If there is hematuria add Da Ji *Herba Cirsii japonici*, Xiao Ji *Herba Cephalanoplos segeti* and Qian Cao Gen *Radix Rubiae cordifoliae*.
- If there are signs of Yin deficiency add Bie Jia *Carapax Trionycis* and Sheng Di Huang *Radix Rehmanniae glutinosae*.
- If there is Qi deficiency add Huang Qi *Radix Astragali membranacei*.
- If there is Kidney-Yang deficiency add Hu Tao Rou *Semen Juglandis regiae* and Gou Ji *Rhizoma Cibotii barometz*. Hu Tao Rou (walnut) is good to dissolve urinary calculi, also eaten as a nut.

– If there are signs of Fire and constipation add Da Huang *Rhizoma Rhei*.

CHRONIC STAGE

For the treatment at the chronic stage one must distinguish the pattern.

ACUPUNCTURE

Damp-Heat

BL-22 Sanjiaoshu, ST-28 Shuidao, SP-9 Yinlingquan, ST-36 Zusanli, Ren-6 Qihai. Even method.

Kidney deficiency

BL-23 Shenshu, Ren-6 Qihai, Ren-4 Guanyuan, SP-6 Sanyinjiao and KI-3 Taixi. Reinforcing method. Moxa for Kidney-Yang deficiency, no moxa for Kidney-Yin deficiency.

HERBAL TREATMENT

(a) Prescription

ZHI BO BA WEI WAN
Anemarrhena-Phellodendron Eight-Ingredient Pill

Explanation

This formula, already explained in this chapter, is suitable to treat both patterns as it simultaneously nourishes Kidney-Yin and resolves Damp-Heat.

(b) Prescription

JIN GUI SHEN QI WAN and WU LING SAN
Golden Chest Kidney-Qi Pill and *Five "Ling" Powder*

Explanation

These two formulae, already explained in this chapter, tonify and warm Kidney-Yang and resolve Dampness.

Patent remedy

TE XIAO PAI SHI WAN
Especially-Effective Discharging Stones Pill

Explanation

This pill, already mentioned above, is specific to drain Damp-Heat and either expel or dissolve urinary stones.

The tongue presentation appropriate to this remedy is a sticky-yellow coating and red spots on the root.

PROGNOSIS

The successful expulsion of stones depends on the location, shape and size of the stone, the timing of treatment and the body condition.

LOCATION

Generally, the higher the stone the more difficult it is to expel. If the stone is in the upper ureter and there is hydronephrosis (swelling of the kidney), it will be difficult to expel. If it is in the middle-lower ureter or bladder it will be easier to expel.

SHAPE AND SIZE

If the stone is rounded it will be easier to expel even if it is big, but not if it is larger than 1 cm. If the stone is irregularly shaped it will be difficult to expel even if it is small.

If the stone moves downwards, which can be gauged by the movement of the pain, and then impacts in the ureter blocking it, there will be severe pain. In this case add KI-7 Fuliu and KI-3 Taixi manipulated with vigorous reducing method to change the position of the stone.

TIME OF TREATMENT

Best results are obtained if treatment is given at the time of pain. If there is pain after needling it indicates that the expulsion of the stone is imminent.

BODY CONDITION

The weaker the body condition of the patient, the more difficult it will be to expel the stone. If the Kidneys are very deficient, it will be even more difficult.

The treatment is effective in about 70% of cases. Advise the patient to drink more and to take exercise.

Prognosis and prevention

Chinese medicine, with acupuncture and herbs, is extremely effective in treating both acute and chronic Painful-Urination Syndrome. Indeed, in acute cases, either acupuncture or herbs, or a combination of the two, can give almost immediate relief. In chronic cases too, acupuncture and/or herbs provide the necessary tonification to eliminate the cause of recurrent urinary problems.

The most difficult Painful-Urination Syndrome to treat is the Stone type.

As for prevention, any patient who is prone to recurrent episodes of Painful-Urination Syndrome should observe certain precautions. Men should moderate their sexual activity as this depletes Kidney-Qi, a deficiency of which is at the basis of most kinds of chronic Painful-Urination Syndrome. Men should also avoid sexual activity soon after a period of heavy physical work, especially that which involves lifting or carrying weights, as this habit could lead to Blood Painful-Urination Syndrome.

Women should also moderate their sexual activity, but for different reasons. In women, sexual activity may induce some Heat or stagnation of Qi in the Lower Burner: it could therefore aggravate particularly the Heat or Qi types of Painful-Urination Syndrome.

Both men and women should definitely avoid the excessive consumption of spicy and very hot foods (including alcohol) which would aggravate not only the Heat type, but also other types of Painful-Urination Syndrome. The excessive consumption of greasy foods and dairy products would aggravate the Cloudy Painful-Urination Syndrome.

Patients who are prone to the Fatigue type of Painful-Urination Syndrome should definitely avoid lifting heavy weights (including heavy suitcases or shopping bags) as this will weaken Kidney-Qi and may even induce sinking of Spleen-Qi: these two factors may lead to Qi or Fatigue Painful-Urination Syndrome.

Having sex while the bladder is full and there is an urge to urinate may lead to Qi Painful-Urination Syndrome (of the Excess type, i.e. from stagnation of Qi).

Finally, standing for long hours may both weaken Kidney-Qi and cause stagnation of Qi in the Lower Burner causing Qi Painful-Urination Syndrome.

Western differentiation

From a Western medical perspective Painful-Urination Syndrome may correspond to cystitis, urethritis, prostatitis, urinary calculi or TB of the kidney.

CYSTITIS

Cystitis is probably the most common condition of the Painful-Urination Syndromes to be seen by acupuncturists and herbalists. It consists of a bacterial infection of the bladder.

The main manifestations are frequency, dysuria, burning pain on micturition and tenderness in the hypogastrium. The urine is darker than normal and has a strong odour. There may be blood and, on microscopic examination, organisms.

Cystitis is more frequent in women, often induced by sexual intercourse, and infection is usually due to *Escherichia coli*, although in a high number of patients no organism can be cultured from the urine.

From a Chinese perspective, it often corresponds to Heat Painful-Urination Syndrome.

URETHRITIS

Urethritis consists in inflammation of the urethra. This condition is also more common in women. Its main manifestations are a burning pain on urination and possibly cloudy urine.

From the point of view of Chinese medicine, it may manifest with symptoms corresponding to Heat or Cloudy Painful-Urination Syndrome.

PROSTATITIS AND PROSTATIC HYPERTROPHY

Prostatitis is an inflammation of the prostate, while prostatic hypertrophy consists in enlargement of the prostate gland. However, there are similarities between these two conditions as the inflamed prostate is also swollen.

The main manifestations are difficulty in urination, weak-stream, hypogastric distension and pain on urination.

In Chinese medicine this condition may correspond to Qi, Cloudy or Fatigue Painful-Urination Syndrome.

URINARY CALCULI

The pathology and symptomatology of urinary calculi have already been described in the appendix above and also in the chapter on "Abdominal Pain" (ch. 16).

In Chinese medicine this corresponds, by definition, to Stone Painful-Urination Syndrome.

TB OF THE KIDNEYS

Tuberculosis of the kidney is always secondary to tuberculosis elsewhere. It develops in the kidney first and may then affect the bladder and prostate. It is more frequent in young people.

The main manifestations are haematuria and dysuria due to secondary involvement of the bladder. Blood Painful-Urination Syndrome would be a typical manifestation of TB of the kidney.

END NOTES

1. 1979 The Yellow Emperor's Classic of Internal Medicine — Simple Questions (*Huang Ti Nei Jing Su Wen* 黄帝内经素问), People's Health Publishing House, Beijing. First published *c*. 100 BC, p. 464.
2. He Ren 1981 A New Explanation of the Essential Prescriptions of the Golden Chest (*Jin Gui Yao Lue Xin Jie* 金匮要略新解), Zhejiang Science Publishing House, p. 82. The "Essential Prescriptions of the Golden Chest" itself was written by Zhang Zhong Jing and first published *c*. AD 200.
3. Hua Tuo (?-AD 208) The Classic of the Secret Transmission (*Zhong Zang Jing* 中藏经), Jiangsu Science Publishing House, 1985, p. 51.
4. Chao Yuan Fang AD 610 General Treatise on the Aetiology and Symptomatology of Diseases (*Zhu Bing Yuan Hou Lun* 诸病源候总论), cited in Zhang Bo Yu 1986 Internal Medicine (*Zhong Yi Nei Ke Xue* 中医内科学), Shanghai Science Publishing House, Shanghai, p. 233.
5. Wang Tao AD 752 Medical Secrets of an Official (*Wai Tai Mi Yao* 外台秘要), cited in Internal Medicine, p. 233.
6. Zhu Dan Xi 1481 Essential Methods of Dan Xi (*Dan Xi Xin Fa* 丹溪心法), cited in Internal Medicine, p. 233.
7. General Treatise on the Aetiology and Symptomatology of Diseases, cited in Internal Medicine, p. 233.
8. Zhang Jing Yue 1624 Complete Book of Jing Yue (*Jing Yue Quan Shu* 景岳全书), Shanghai Science Publishing House, Shanghai, p. 505.
9. Simple Questions, p. 59.
10. Dr Sheng Can Ruo 1982 Advanced International Acupuncture Course at the Nanjing College of Traditional Chinese Medicine.
11. Essential Methods of Dan Xi, cited in Internal Medicine, p. 238.
12. Gao Wu 1529 Gatherings from Eminent Acupuncturists (*Zhen Jiu Ju Ying* 针灸聚英), cited in Yang Jia San 1989 Acupuncture, People's Hygiene Publishing House, Beijing, p. 665.
13. Yang Ji Zhou 1601 Compendium of Acupuncture (*Zhen Jiu Da Cheng* 黄帝内经素问), cited in Yang Jia San 1989 Acupuncture (*Zhen Jiu Xue* 针灸学), People's Health Publishing House, Beijing, p. 665.
14. Ibid., p. 1180.
15. The Classic of the Secret Transmission, p. 51.

Enuresis and incontinence (retention of urine — blood in the urine)

21 遺
尿

This chapter discusses different symptoms involving a loss of control of urination.

Enuresis indicates an involuntary discharge of urine, i.e. the person passes urine without realizing it. This usually happens to children in nocturnal enuresis.

Incontinence means inability to control the voiding of urine. The urine is passed involuntarily; the person involved knows he or she is doing it, but cannot hold it back. This happens to old people or to those suffering from certain neurological diseases such as multiple sclerosis.

In less severe cases, there may only be urgency of urination (i.e. the person has to go quickly once the urge comes or will be incontinent) or difficulty in holding urine. In yet other cases, a person may be only slightly incontinent and pass urine only on coughing or jumping. All these less severe conditions share the same aetiology, pathology and treatment as true enuresis and incontinence.

Aetiology and pathology

1. WEAK CONSTITUTION

Weak constitution is a cause of nocturnal enuresis in children. Constitutionally-deficient Kidneys are unable to control fluids and fail to provide Qi to the Bladder: this results in nocturnal enuresis.

2. SHOCK

Prenatal or perinatal shock in children can be a cause of nocturnal enuresis. This can be observed in a bluish colour on the child's chin.

3. OLD AGE

The natural decline of Qi occurring with ageing may cause incontinence in old people. This is due to a decline not only of Kidney-Qi, but also of Lung- and Spleen-Qi.

4. EXCESSIVE SEXUAL ACTIVITY

Excessive sexual activity weakens Kidney-Yang and may lead to inability of the Kidneys to control fluids and therefore to slight incontinence.

5. CHRONIC COUGH

The persistent strain caused by a chronic cough may lead to incontinence in a mechanical way from the strain on the bladder and, in an energetic way, from deficient Lung-Qi not controlling the Bladder.

6. CHILDBIRTH

The weakening of the Kidney energy occurring in some women after childbirth may cause a slight incontinence.

The pathology of enuresis and incontinence is always characterized by Deficiency. This may be a deficiency of the Lungs, Spleen or Kidneys. Lung-Qi communicates downwards with the Bladder and the Lungs, which govern Qi in general, also provide Qi to the Bladder to control urine. Thus deficient Lung-Qi is unable to control the Bladder and urine leaks out.

Spleen-Qi raises Qi in general and a sinking Spleen-Qi may be unable to control urine which leaks out. The Kidneys obviously control urination directly as the balance of Kidney-Yang and Kidney-Yin influences urination and also because Kidney-Yang provides Qi to the Bladder to control and transform urine.

There is, however, a Full type of enuresis. This occurs to some children in whom nocturnal enuresis is due, not to a deficiency, but to Liver-Fire infusing downwards to the Bladder. These tend to be tense and highly-strung children.

Differentiation and treatment

The patterns discussed are:

DEFICIENCY

Lung-Qi Deficiency

Spleen-Qi Deficiency
Kidney-Yang Deficiency
Kidney-Yin Deficiency

EXCESS

Liver-Fire infusing downwards

DEFICIENCY

1. LUNG-QI DEFICIENCY

CLINICAL MANIFESTATIONS

Frequent urge to urinate with inability to contain it, slight incontinence often on coughing or sneezing, dribbling, weak voice, tiredness, slight sweating, shortness of breath.
Tongue: Pale.
Pulse: Weak.

TREATMENT PRINCIPLE

Warm and tonify Lung-Qi.

ACUPUNCTURE

BL-13 Feishu, Du-12 Shenzhu, Du-20 Baihui, LU-7 Lieque, Ren-6 Qihai, BL-23 Shenshu, BL-28 Pangguangshu, BL-53 Baohuang. Reinforcing method; moxa is applicable.

Explanation

- **BL-13** and **Du-12** tonify Lung-Qi. Direct moxa on these points is particularly effective to tonify Qi and Yang. It is especially useful in this condition to use Fire (moxa) to contain Water.
- **Du-20** is used, with moxa, to raise Qi and therefore contain urine.
- **LU-7** is the best point on the Lung channel to affect the Water passages.
- **Ren-6** tonifies Qi in general and specifically, Qi in the lower abdomen.
- **BL-23**, with moxa, tonifies Kidney-Yang and reduces urination.

- **BL-28** and **BL-53** strengthen the Bladder function.

HERBAL TREATMENT

Prescription

BU ZHONG YI QI TANG
Tonifying the Centre and Benefiting Qi Decoction
Huang Qi *Radix Astragali membranacei* 12 g
Ren Shen *Radix Ginseng* 9 g
Bai Zhu *Rhizoma Atractylodis macrocephalae* 9 g
Dang Gui *Radix Angelicae sinensis* 6 g
Chen Pi *Pericarpium Citri reticulatae* 6 g
Sheng Ma *Rhizoma Cimicifugae* 3 g
Chai Hu *Radix Bupleuri* 3 g

Explanation

This formula, which has already been explained in chapter 1, tonifies and raises Qi. By tonifying Lung-Qi and raising Qi it restrains the leaking of urine.

Patent remedy

BU ZHONG YI QI WAN
Tonifying the Centre and Benefiting Qi Pill

Explanation

This remedy has the same ingredients and functions as the homonymous prescription. It is excellent to tonify and raise Qi to stop incontinence from Qi deficiency.

The tongue presentation appropriate to this remedy is a Pale tongue.

2. SPLEEN-QI DEFICIENCY

CLINICAL MANIFESTATIONS

Slight incontinence, urgency, frequent desire to go and inability to contain it, loose stools, tiredness, poor appetite.
Tongue: Pale.
Pulse: Weak.

TREATMENT PRINCIPLE

Tonify and raise Spleen-Qi.

ACUPUNCTURE

BL-20 Pishu, ST-36 Zusanli, Ren-12 Zhongwan, Du-20 Baihui, Ren-6 Qihai, BL-23 Shenshu, BL-28 Pangguangshu, BL-53 Baohuang. Reinforcing method; moxa is applicable.

Explanation

- **BL-20**, **ST-36** and **Ren-12** tonify Spleen-Qi.
- All the other points have been explained above.

HERBAL TREATMENT

Prescription

BU ZHONG YI QI TANG
Tonifying the Centre and Benefiting Qi Decoction

Explanation

See above.

Patent remedy

BU ZHONG YI QI WAN
Tonifying the Centre and Benefiting Qi Decoction

Explanation

See above.

3. KIDNEY-YANG DEFICIENCY

CLINICAL MANIFESTATIONS

Frequent urination, nocturia (waking up to urinate at night), slight dribbling, nocturnal enuresis in children, incontinence in old people, pale urine, exhaustion, dizziness, tinnitus, weak and sore back and knees, feeling of cold.
Tongue: Pale and wet.
Pulse: Weak and Deep.

It is important to remember that children, apart from the enuresis, will not have any of the above symptoms of Kidney deficiency.

TREATMENT PRINCIPLE

Tonify and warm the Kidneys.

ACUPUNCTURE

BL-23 Shenshu, Du-4 Mingmen, KI-7 Fuliu, Ren-6 Qihai, Ren-4 Guanyuan, Du-20 Baihui, BL-28 Pangguangshu, BL-53 Baohuang, BL-32 Ciliao, SP-6 Sanyinjiao, HE-7 Shenmen and Yintang. Reinforcing method and moxa on all points except HE-7 and Yintang which should be needled with even method.

Explanation

– **BL-23**, **Du-4**, **KI-7** and **Ren-4** (with moxa) strengthen Kidney-Yang.
– **Ren-6** tonifies Qi in general.
– **Du-20** raises Qi.
– **BL-28** and **BL-53** tonify the Bladder.
– **BL-32** strengthens the Bladder function and also has some general tonic properties.
– **SP-6** tonifies the Kidneys.
– **HE-7** and **Yintang** are used for enuresis in children to calm the Mind. This is necessary as children with enuresis nearly always suffer from an underlying fear and insecurity.

Modern prescription

Some doctors alternate the following two combination of points (both with needle and moxa stick):

(i) SP-6 Sanyinjiao, Ren-4 Guanyuan and BL-23 Shenshu
(ii) Ren-4 Guanyuan, Ren-3 Zhongji, BL-23 Shenshu, BL-28 Pangguangshu and KI-3 Taixi.

Ancient prescription

HE-7 Shenmen and BL-40 Weizhong ("The ABC of Acupuncture" AD 282).[1] This is an interesting combination of points which harmonizes Heart and Kidneys, regulates the Lower Burner and calms the Mind. It is particularly suited to nervous or slightly hyperactive children with nocturnal enuresis.

HERBAL TREATMENT

Prescription

SUO QUAN WAN and JIN GUI SHEN QI WAN
Contracting the Spring Pill and *Golden Chest Kidney-Qi Pill*
Yi Zhi Ren *Fructus Alpiniae oxyphyllae* 9 g
Wu Yao *Radix Linderae strychnifoliae* 6 g
Shan Yao *Radix Dioscoreae oppositae* 9 g
Fu Zi *Radix Aconiti carmichaeli praeparata* 3 g
Gui Zhi *Ramulus Cinnamomi cassiae* 3 g
Shu Di Huang *Radix Rehmanniae glutinosae praeparata* 24 g
Shan Zhu Yu *Fructus Corni officinalis* 12 g
Ze Xie *Rhizoma Alismatis orientalis* 9 g
Mu Dan Pi *Cortex Moutan radicis* 9 g
Fu Ling *Sclerotium Poriae cocos* 9 g

Explanation

– The first three herbs constitute the Suo Quan Wan which stops enuresis or incontinence from deficiency of Kidney-Yang.
– The other herbs constitute the Jin Gui Shen Qi Wan (obviously without Shan Yao as it is already included in the first formula) which tonifies Kidney-Yang.

(i) Patent remedy

JIN SUO GU JING WAN
Golden Lock Consolidating the Essence Pill
Qian Shi *Semen Euryales ferocis*
Lian Xu *Stamen Nelumbinis nuciferae*
Long Gu *Os Draconis* (calcined)
Mu Li *Concha Ostreae* (calcined)
Lian Zi *Semen Nelumbinis nuciferae*
Sha Yuan Ji Li *Semen Astragali membranacei*

Explanation

This pill tonifies the Kidneys and absorbs leakages. It is quite neutral and not very Yang in nature: it can therefore be combined with other remedies to treat nocturnal enuresis or incontinence.

(ii) Patent remedy

NAN XING BU SHEN WAN

Male Gender Tonifying the Kidneys Pill
Shu Di Huang *Radix Rehmanniae glutinosae prae-*
parata
Shan Yao *Radix Dioscoreae oppositae*
Shan Zhu Yu *Fructus Corni officinalis*
Ze Xie *Rhizoma Alismatis orientalis*
Fu Ling *Sclerotium Poriae cocos*
Mu Dan Pi *Cortex Moutan radicis*
Rou Gui *Cortex Cinnamomi cassiae*
Fu Zi *Radix Aconiti carmichaeli praeparata*
Wu Wei Zi *Fructus Schisandrae chinensis*
Che Qian Zi *Semen Plantaginis*

Explanation

This remedy, a variation of Jin Gui Shen Qi Wan *Golden Chest Kidney-Qi Pill*, tonifies Kidney-Yang and Kidney-Essence and absorbs leakages. It is suitable to treat incontinence in old people with an underlying deficiency of Kidney-Yang.

The tongue presentation appropriate to this remedy is a Pale body.

(iii) Patent remedy

ZHUANG YAO JIAN SHEN PIAN
Invigorating the Back and Strengthening the Kidneys Tablet
Gou Ji *Rhizoma Cibotii barometz*
Huai Niu Xi *Radix Achyranthis bidentatae*
Du Zhong *Cortex Eucommiae ulmoidis*
Jin Ying Zi *Fructus Rosae laevigatae*
Sang Ji Sheng *Ramus Loranthi*
Dong Chong Xia Cao *Sclerotium Cordicipitis chinensis*
Fu Ling *Sclerotium Poriae cocos*
Fu Pen Zi *Fructus Rubi*

Explanation

This remedy tonifies and warms Kidney-Yang and Kidney-Essence and absorbs leakages. It is stronger than the previous two and is suitable to treat incontinence in middle-aged or old people with deficiency of Kidney-Yang and Kidney-Essence.

The tongue presentation appropriate to this remedy is a Pale and wet tongue body.

Case history

A 47-year-old woman had been suffering from frequency of urination for over 10 years. Her urination was very frequent in daytime and she got up twice a night to pass water. She was also slightly incontinent when jumping or coughing. She felt always very tired and was easily cold. Even in summertime, when she came for treatment she had to wear small dance socks to keep her feet warm as she lay on the couch to receive acupuncture. Her lower back ached and she often felt dizzy. Her memory was poor and sometimes she had tinnitus. Her tongue was Pale and her pulse was Weak and Deep.

Diagnosis
This is a clear example of Kidney-Yang deficiency and Kidney-Qi not Firm.

Treatment principle
The treatment principle adopted was to tonify and raise Qi, consolidate Bladder-Qi and tonify and warm Kidney-Yang. She was treated initially with acupuncture and patent remedies.

Acupuncture
The acupuncture points used (with reinforcing method) were selected from the following:

- **LU-7** Lieque and **KI-6** Zhaohai to open the Directing Vessel and tonify the Kidneys.
- **Du-20** Baihui to raise Qi to stop incontinence.
- **Ren-12** Zhongwan to tonify Qi in general and Spleen-Qi in particular.
- **Ren-6** Qihai to tonify and raise Qi in the lower abdomen. It combines well with Du-20 to tonify and raise Qi to treat enuresis, incontinence and prolapses.
- **ST-36** Zusanli and **SP-6** Sanyinjiao to tonify Stomach and Spleen.
- **KI-3** Taixi with moxa on needle to tonify and warm the Kidneys.
- **Ren-4** Guanyuan with moxa box to tonify and warm the Kidneys.
- **BL-23** Shenshu and **BL-20** Pishu to tonify Kidney-Yang and Spleen-Yang respectively.

Herbal treatment
The patent remedies used were three: Jin Gui Shen Qi Wan *Golden Chest Kidney-Qi Pill* (10 pills in the morning) to tonify Kidney-Yang, Bu Zhong Yi Qi Wan *Tonifying the Centre and Benefiting Qi Pill* (10 pills at lunchtime) to tonify and raise Qi, and Jin Suo Gu Jing Wan *Golden Lock Consolidating the Essence Pill* (10 pills in the evening) to absorb leakages. The combination of acupuncture and these remedies produced an improvement of about 70% in her urinary symptoms and she also felt much better in general. She later had a consultation with Prof. Zhou Zhong Ying on the occasion of his visit to England

and he prescribed a variation of Suo Quan Wan *Contracting the Spring Pill* as a decoction:

Shan Yao *Radix Dioscoreae oppositae* 10 g
Yi Zhi Ren *Fructus Alpiniae oxyphyllae* 10 g
Wu Yao *Radix Linderae strychnifoliae* 10 g
Tu Si Zi *Semen Cuscutae* 10 g
Yin Yang Huo *Herba Epimedii* 5 g
Shu Di Huang *Radix Rehmanniae glutinosae praeparata* 10 g
Huang Qi *Radix Astragali membranacei* 12 g
Chuan Jiao Zi *Semen Zanthoxyli bungeani* 3 g
Fu Pen Zi *Fructus Rubi* 10 g
Zhi Gan Cao *Radix Glycyrrhizae uralensis praeparata* 3 g

Explanation
- The first three herbs constitute the Suo Quan Wan to warm the Kidneys and stop incontinence.
- **Tu Si Zi** and **Yin Yang Huo** tonify and warm Kidney-Yang.
- **Shu Di Huang** tonifies the Kidneys.
- **Huang Qi** tonifies and raises Qi.
- **Chuan Jiao** warms the Kidneys.
- **Fu Pen Zi** warms the Kidneys and reduces urination.
- **Gan Cao** harmonizes.

She stopped the patent remedies and took this decoction for 2 months: this produced a further improvement in her urinary symptoms which disappeared almost completely. She also felt a lot more energy. After 3 months of taking this decoction, she asked to change to taking it as a powder. We did this, but, interestingly, the powders did not work as well as the decoction, and she herself decided to go back to the decoction for a further 2 months, after which she did not need to take it any longer.

4. KIDNEY-YIN DEFICIENCY

CLINICAL MANIFESTATIONS

Incontinence of urine but in scanty amounts, dribbling after urination, dark urine, dry throat, dizziness, tinnitus, night-sweating, 5-palm heat, insomnia.
Tongue: Red without coating.
Pulse: Floating-Empty.

TREATMENT PRINCIPLE

Tonify the Kidneys and nourish Yin.

ACUPUNCTURE

Ren-4 Guanyuan, KI-3 Taixi, SP-6 Sanyinjiao, BL-23 Taixi, BL-28 Pangguangshu. Reinforcing method, no moxa.

Explanation

- **Ren-4**, **KI-3** and **SP-6** nourish Kidney-Yin.
- **BL-23** and **BL-28** tonify Kidney-Qi and strengthen the Bladder function. Points in the back are used as, although there is a deficiency of Yin, it is still necessary to tonify the Yang within the Yin to control fluids.

HERBAL TREATMENT

Prescription

SANG PIAO XIAO SAN
Ootheca Mantidis Powder
Sang Piao Xiao *Ootheca Mantidis* 9 g
Long Gu *Os Draconis* 15 g
Gui Ban *Plastrum Testudinis* 15 g
Dang Gui *Radix Angelicae sinensis* 9 g
Ren Shen *Radix Ginseng* 9 g
Fu Shen *Sclerotium Poriae cocos pararadicis* 6 g
Yuan Zhi *Radix Polygalae tenuifoliae* 6 g
Shi Chang Pu *Rhizoma Acori graminei* 6 g

Explanation

- **Sang Piao Xiao** is astringent and stops leaking of urine and enuresis.
- **Long Gu** and **Gui Ban** are absorbing and help to restrain urine. They nourish Kidney-Yin and Long Gu also calms the Mind.
- **Dang Gui** helps the previous two to nourish Yin by nourishing Blood.
- **Ren Shen** and **Fu Shen** tonify Qi in order to control urine. Fu Shen also calms the Mind.
- **Yuan Zhi** and **Chang Pu** open the Heart orifices and calm the Mind.

Calming the Mind is necessary in enuresis or incontinence from Kidney-Yin deficiency as Empty-Heat affecting the Pericardium and Triple Burner (Minister Fire) may affect the Bladder function.

Variations

- If the symptoms and signs of Yin deficiency

and Empty-Heat are very pronounced add the formula Zhi Bo Di Huang Wan *Anemarrhena-Phellodendron-Rehmannia Pill.*

Patent remedy

JIN SUO GU JING WAN
Golden Lock Consolidating the Essence Pill

Explanation

This pill, already explained above, is quite neutral in character and can therefore be used for enuresis or incontinence from an underlying deficiency of Kidney-Yin. It may be combined with other remedies which nourish Kidney-Yin such as Liu Wei Di Huang Wan *Six-Ingredient Rehmannia Pill.*

EXCESS

LIVER-FIRE INFUSING DOWNWARDS

CLINICAL MANIFESTATIONS

Nocturnal enuresis in children, grinding teeth at night, restless sleep, nightmares, waking up crying, thirst, bitter taste, hypochondrial pain.
Tongue: Red with redder sides, yellow coating.
Pulse: Wiry and Rapid.

Enuresis in children can be classified in two broad categories: on the one hand quiet and shy children, on the other rather hyperactive and nervous children. The pattern of Kidney deficiency pertains to the former group, while that of Liver-Fire pertains to the latter group.

TREATMENT PRINCIPLE

Soothe the Liver, drain Fire, calm the Mind and settle the Ethereal Soul.

ACUPUNCTURE

LIV-2 Xingjian, HE-7 Shenmen, SP-6 Sanyinjiao, Yintang, BL-28 Pangguangshu. Reducing method on all points except BL-28 which should be reinforced.

Explanation

- **LIV-2** drains Liver-Fire.
- **HE-7** and **Yintang** calm the Mind.
- **SP-6** regulates the Water passages and calms the Mind.
- **BL-28** strengthens the Bladder function.

HERBAL TREATMENT

Prescription

LONG DAN XIE GAN TANG
Gentiana Draining the Liver Decoction
Long Dan Cao *Radix Gentianae scabrae* 6 g
Huang Qin *Radix Scutellariae baicalensis* 9 g
Shan Zhi Zi *Fructus Gardeniae jasminoidis* 9 g
Ze Xie *Rhizoma Alismatis orientalis* 9 g
Mu Tong *Caulis Akebiae* 9 g
Che Qian Zi *Semen Plantaginis* 9 g
Sheng Di Huang *Radix Rehmanniae glutinosae* 12 g
Dang Gui *Radix Angelicae sinensis* 9 g
Chai Hu *Radix Bupleuri* 9 g
Gan Cao *Radix Glycyrrhizae uralensis* 3 g

Explanation

This formula, which has already been explained in chapters 1 and 10, drains Liver-Fire.

Variations

- To enhance the Bladder function and stop enuresis add Sang Piao Xiao *Ootheca Mantidis* and Ji Nei Jin *Endothelium Corneum Gigeraiae Galli.*

Patent remedy

LONG DAN XIE GAN WAN and JIN SUO GU JING WAN
Gentiana Draining the Liver Pill and *Golden Lock Consolidating the Essence Pill*

Explanation

The first remedy, the ingredients of which are the same as the prescription above, drains Liver-Fire; the second one, the ingredients of which have already been listed in this chapter (p. 528), absorbs leakages. The two together can be used to treat enuresis or incontinence from Liver-Fire. This combination is particularly useful to treat enuresis in nervous children.

Case history

An 11-year-old boy had been suffering from nocturnal enuresis from birth. He never had a dry night. He appeared to be a very tense child with a nervous tic of his eyes. His tongue was Red, with redder sides and tip and red points on the sides and tip, and a yellow coating. His pulse was Full and Wiry.

Diagnosis
This boy's condition is very clearly Liver-Fire. This is very often seen in tense and nervous children.

Treatment principle
The principle of treatment adopted was to drain Liver-Fire, absorb leakages, calm the Mind and settle the Ethereal Soul. He was treated with acupuncture and two patent remedies.

Acupuncture
The acupuncture points used (with reducing method) were selected from the following:
- **LIV-2** Xingjian to drain Liver-Fire and settle the Ethereal Soul.
- **HE-7** Shenmen to calm the Mind.
- **SP-6** Sanyinjiao to pacify the Liver.

Herbal treatment
The patent remedies used were Long Dan Xie Gan Wan *Gentiana Draining the Liver Pill* and Jin Suo Gu Jing Wan *Golden Lock Consolidating the Essence Pill* to drain Liver-Fire and absorb leakages.

This boy was treated every week for 10 weeks after which he managed to stay dry 5 nights out of 7. He is still under treatment to achieve a complete cure.

Case history

A 10-year-old girl had been suffering from nocturnal enuresis since birth. She did not wet the bed every day, like the boy in the previous case history, but about twice a week. When she was 5 she had had a bout of cystitis with burning on urination. She was a shy and quiet child with a pale complexion and a bluish tinge on her chin. Her tongue was Pale but with red points along the left side and on the root. Her pulse was very slightly Wiry on the left side and otherwise normal.

Diagnosis
This child manifests symptoms from both Full and Empty types of patterns causing enuresis. There is a Kidney deficiency manifesting with a Pale tongue: this deficiency was probably due to fright (which may even have occurred *in utero*) as the bluish tinge on her chin shows. Besides this, there is some Liver-Fire and Damp-Heat in the Bladder, manifesting with the red points along the left side and on the root and the Wiry pulse on the left. The cystitis episode she had when she was 5 would seem to confirm this.

Treatment principle
The treatment principle adopted was to tonify the Kidneys, absorb leakages, calm the Mind, settle the Ethereal Soul and pacify the Liver. She was treated with acupuncture and patent remedies.

Acupuncture
The acupuncture points used (with even method to pacify the Liver and reinforcing method to tonify the Kidneys) were selected from the following:

- **HE-7** Shenmen to calm the Mind.
- **LIV-2** Xingjian to clear Liver-Fire and settle the Ethereal Soul.
- **SP-6** Sanyinjiao, **KI-3** Taixi, **Ren-4** Guanyuan and **BL-23** Shenshu to tonify the Kidneys.

Herbal treatment
The patent remedies used were Zhen Zhu San *Pearl Powder* to calm the Mind and settle the Ethereal Soul and Jin Suo Gu Jing Wan *Golden Lock Consolidating the Essence Pill* to absorb leakages.

This girl was treated for 3 months (once a week) and this produced an improvement of 80%. She also became calmer and, at the same time, more confident.

Prognosis

Acupuncture and herbs can give good results in the treatment of enuresis and incontinence.

As for enuresis in children, if the child is under 10, a brief course of acupuncture may sometimes suffice to produce a cure; if the child is over 10, enuresis is more difficult to treat. Of the two types of enuresis, the Deficiency type is easier to treat than the Excess one from Liver-Fire.

As for incontinence, it usually responds to treatment with acupuncture and herbs in a few months, unless it is due to a neurological disease such as multiple sclerosis, in which case it may not respond to treatment at all or may respond only very slowly.

Appendix

The conditions of retention of urine and blood in the urine will be dealt with only in tabular form.

Retention of urine ranges from scanty and difficult urination (without pain) to total absence of urination. If there is scanty and difficult urination with pain, then it falls under the heading of Painful-Urination Syndrome.

From a Western medical perspective, urinary retention may be due to episiotomy after childbirth, bladder stones, prostatic hypertrophy and carcinoma of the prostate. Although acupuncture and herbal medicine are effective for this condition, in advanced cases when the prostate is grossly enlarged the possibility of combining Chinese medicine with Western medicine should be discussed with the patient. In particular, in the case of benign prostatic hypertrophy, Western medicine can help with a relatively simple

procedure consisting of enlarging the urethra with a catheter.

Blood in the urine is characterized by the presence of frank or occult blood in the urine without pain. If it is accompanied by pain it falls under the category of Painful-Urination Syndrome.

If there are large amounts of blood in the urine, the urine will be smoky-coloured, bright-red or reddish-brown. Haematuria may be caused by nephritis, endocarditis, polyarteritis, systemic lupus erythematosus (if it affects the kidney), TB of the kidney, polycystic disease, haemorrhagic disease, tumour of the kidney, infection of the lower urinary tract and carcinoma of the prostate or bladder. When blood is present in the urine a *cause* should always be sought and found in Western medicine. It is therefore essential to get a good Western diagnosis from a specialist.

It is convenient to classify haematuria into

Table 21.1   Patterns in retention of urine

Burner	Pattern	Manifestations		Treatment principle	Acupuncture	Herbs
		Urinary	General			
Upper	Lung-Heat	Dysuria, dribbling	Dry throat, thirst, cough	Clear Heat, promote descending of Lung-Qi	LU-7,LU-5 L.I.-11, Ren-3 reducing m.	Huang Qin Qing Fei Yin
	Heart-Heat	Blood in urine	Insomnia, red tongue, red tip	Clear Heart, clear Heat	HE-8,S.I.-2 Ren-3,BL-28, KI-2 reducing m.	Dao Chi San
Middle	Damp-Heat	Turbid urine	Oppression epigastrium, feeling of heaviness, sticky tongue coating	Resolve Dampness, tonify Qi	Ren-12, BL-20,SP-6, SP-9,Ren-3 reducing m.	Jia Wei Wu Ling San
	Central Qi deficient	Pale urine	Tiredness, shortness of breath	Tonify Qi, raise Yang	Du-20,Ren-12 Ren-6,BL-20, SP-6, Ren-3 BL-28 reinforcing m.	Bu Zhong Yi Qi Tang
Lower	Damp-Heat in Bladder	Burning on urination, dribbling, distension hypogastrium	Sticky-yellow tongue coating	Resolve Dampness, clear Heat	Ren-3,BL-28 SP-9,BL-22, BL-40,BL-32 reducing m.	Tong Guan Wan
	Stagnation of Essence	Dribbling	Distension of hypogastrium Purple tongue	Move Blood	SP-10,BL-17, SP-6,LIV-5, Ren-6,ST-29 reducing m.	Dai Di Dang Wan
	Kidney-Yang deficiency	Dribbling, pale urine, weak-stream	Lower abdomen cold, sore back, loose stools	Warm and tonify Kidney-Yang	BL-28,BL-23, Du-4,Ren-4, moxa	Jin Gui Shen Qi Wan

Table 21.2 Patterns of blood in the urine

Type	Pattern	Manifestations	Treatment principle	Acupuncture	Herbs
Full	Liver-Fire Blazing	Burning pain, pain in hypogastrium, bitter taste, dizziness, Wiry pulse, Red tongue	Drain Liver-Fire	LIV-2, SP-6, SP-10, Ren-3, reducing m.	Jia Wei Xiao Yao San or Long Dan Xie Gan Tang
	Small Intestine Fire	Burning on urination, insomnia, dry mouth, red tip of tongue	Clear Heart, cool Blood	HE-8, S.I.-2, Ren-3, L.I.-11, KI-2, reducing m.	Dao Chi San plus Zhi Zi, Qu Mai, Hu Po Xiao Ji Yin Zi
	Heat in Lower Burner	Burning on urination, difficulty, yellow coating, Wiry pulse	Clear Heat, cool Blood, resolve Dampness	SP-6, SP-9, SP-10, L.I.-11, T.B.-6, Ren-5, Ren-3, KI-2, LIV-3, reducing m.	
Empty	Kidney deficiency	No pain, exhaustion, hesitancy, sore back, weak-stream	Tonify Kidneys	KI-3, BL-23, Ren-4, Ren-5, BL-28, KI-6	Yin deficiency: Liu Wei Di Huang Wan Yang deficiency: Lu Jia Jiao Tang
	Lung and Kidney deficiency	No pain, dry mouth, hesitancy, sore back, weak voice	Tonify Lungs and Kidneys	LU-7, LU-9, KI-6, KI-3, BL-23, Ren-3, BL-28	Liu Wei Di Huang Wan and Sheng Mai San
	Spleen deficient not controlling blood	No pain, tiredness, poor appetite, bearing-down sensation	Tonify and raise Qi	Ren-12, ST-36, SP-6, Du-20, BL-20, Ren-3, BL-28	Gui Pi Tang

Table 21.3 Causes of haematuria

Type	Disease	Symptoms	Signs
Pre-renal	Endocarditis Drugs: Warfarin, sulphonamides	Malaise, rigours, weakness	Sweating, petechiae, fever at night
Renal	Glomerulo-nephritis	Malaise, poor appetite, ache in loins, headache	Pallor, oedema face and legs, scanty dark urine, hypertension, fever
	Pyelo-nephritis	Malaise, frequency, dysuria, ache loins	Fever
	Cancer of kidney (rare)	Ache loins	Palpable tumour
Post-Renal	Cystitis	Frequency, dysuria, pain in urethra and hypogastrium	Haematuria
	Cancer of bladder	Hypogastric distension	Haematuria
	Prostatic hypertrophy	Urinary retention and difficulty	Profuse haematuria
	Cancer of prostate	Frequency, nocturia, hesitancy, debility, back-ache	Weak-stream, nocturia
Stones	Stones	*Bladder*: pain on micturition *Ureter*: pain in lateral abdomen *Kidney*: pain in loin	Haematuria

pre-renal, renal and post-renal depending on whether the cause resides in organs above the kidney, in the kidney itself or in organs below the kidney, i.e. bladder or prostate. Table 21.3 lists the most common of these conditions.

When blood appears only at the beginning of micturition, the source of bleeding is *below* the bladder. When blood is uniformly mixed with urine, it may come from anywhere *above* the urethra.

The patterns causing retention of urine in Chinese medicine are summarized in Table 21.1.

The patterns of blood in the urine are summarized in Table 21.2.

END NOTES

1. Huang Fu Mi AD 282 The ABC of Acupuncture (*Zhen Jiu Jia Yi Jing* 针灸甲乙经), cited in Chen You Bang 1990 Chinese Acupuncture Therapy (*Zhong Guo Zhen Jiu Zhi Liao Xue* 中国针灸治疗学), China Scientific Publishing House, p. 458.

Oedema 22
(nephritis) 水
肿

Oedema consists in retention of fluids under the skin which may occur around the eyes, face, limbs and abdomen. In the "Yellow Emperor's Classic of Internal Medicine" it is called "Water". This should not be interpreted as Water in a 5-Element sense, but as a pathological overflowing of body fluids into the space under the skin. Chapter 61 of the "Simple Questions" discusses oedema and relates it to the Kidneys and the Lungs saying that " . . . *the Kidneys are the root and the Lungs the end [of this disease].*"[1] In chapter 74 it says: "*A feeling of fullness and swelling from Dampness is due to the Spleen.*"[2] Thus, the "Simple Questions" identifies the Lungs, Spleen and Kidneys as the three organs primarily responsible for oedema. The "General Treatise on the Aetiology and Symptomatology of Diseases" (AD 610) also relates oedema to the Spleen and Stomach. It says:

The Kidneys govern Water and Stomach and Spleen govern Earth. Earth overacts on Water, Stomach and Spleen are exteriorly-interiorly related and the Stomach is the Sea of Food. When the Stomach is deficient it cannot transform Water [i.e. fluids], Water overflows out of the channels . . . and is retained under the skin causing oedema.[3]

Dr Zhu Dan Xi in "Essential Methods of Dan Xi" (1481) distinguishes Yang oedema from Yin oedema:

Yang oedema is characterized by swelling, mental restlessness, dark urine and constipation. Yin oedema is characterized by swelling without mental restlessness or dark urine but with loose stools.[4]

The differentiation between Yang oedema and Yin oedema is widely followed today albeit with a different interpretation.

Aetiology

1. EXTERNAL WIND

Exterior Wind-Cold or Wind-Heat invades the Defensive-Qi portion where Defensive-Qi and fluids circulate. Wind impairs the circulation of Lung-Qi in the Defensive-Qi portion so that Lung-Qi cannot disperse fluids: these accumulate under the skin causing oedema, usually of the face and hands. This is a Full type of oedema with acute onset. This type of exterior Wind, which may present with the character of Heat or Cold, is called "Wind-Water".

Acute nephritis usually starts with symptoms of an exterior invasion of Wind-Water with oedema of the face.

2. EXTERIOR DAMPNESS

Exterior Damp-Heat may invade the Stomach and Spleen and impair their function of transforming and transporting fluids. Fluids stagnate and are retained under the skin causing oedema. This is not a common cause of oedema in temperate climates.

Exterior Cold-Dampness may invade the body and if it is retained for a long time it interferes with the transformation of fluids and may lead to oedema.

3. DIET

Irregular eating and eating too many dairy products and greasy foods impairs the Spleen's function of transforming and transporting fluids, leading to oedema.

4. OVERWORK AND EXCESSIVE SEXUAL ACTIVITY

Overwork and excessive sexual activity weaken the Kidneys and impair their function of transforming fluids, possibly leading to oedema.

5. FIRE-POISON FROM SORES OR CARBUNCLES

Fire-Poison deriving from carbuncles, furuncles or sores may impede the clearing and excreting of turbidity from the space between skin and muscles therefore leading to retention of fluids there and oedema.

Pathology

The most important distinction with oedema, as with all other diseases, is that between Full type and Empty type. Oedema of the Full type, also called Yang oedema, derives from external Wind-Water, external Dampness or Fire-Poison. Oedema of the Empty type, also called Yin oedema, arises from a deficiency of the Spleen and/or Kidneys.

The three Yin organs most involved in oedema are the Lungs, Spleen and Kidneys as these are the three organs responsible for dispersing, transforming, transporting and excreting fluids. Of the other organs, the Triple Burner plays an important role in the metabolism of fluids. The Upper Burner diffuses fluids, like a fine spray, to the space between skin and muscles, the Middle Burner transforms fluids and sends turbid fluids downward and the Lower Burner further transforms and excretes fluids.

Yang oedema may develop into Yin oedema and vice versa. For example, after a long period Yang oedema may be transformed into Yin oedema because the retained fluids impair the Spleen and Kidneys. On the other hand, after repeated invasions of external Dampness Yin oedema may turn into Yang oedema.

In any case, whether it is Yang or Yin oedema, it is important to remember that oedema in itself is a Full condition, or the Full aspect of a condition. For example, although Yin oedema derives from a deficiency of the Spleen and/or Kidneys, the fluids retained in the form of oedema are the Full aspect of the condition. Thus, in this example, the Root of the condition is characterized by Emptiness of Spleen and/or Kidneys, while the Manifestation is characterized by Fullness in the form of oedema. This has important implications in treatment as oedema, as a Manifestation, calls for draining with herbs which resolve oedema, or by reducing acupuncture points which resolve oedema.

From a diagnostic point of view, Yin oedema is characterized by marked pitting on pressure, with the skin being very slow to bounce back to normal. In Yang oedema there is little or no pitting on pressure.

Differentiation and treatment

As a general principle, oedema of the upper part of the body is treated by diaphoresis, while oedema of the lower part is treated by diuresis.

Thus to treat oedema of the upper part of the body one uses some herbs which expel Wind, such as Ma Huang *Herba Ephedrae*, Fang Feng *Radix Ledebouriellae sesloidis*, Fu Ping *Herba Lemnae seu Spirodelae* and Bai Zhi *Radix Angelicae dahuricae*, and some herbs which fragrantly resolve Dampness, such as Cang Zhu *Rhizoma Atractylodis lanceae*, Da Fu Pi *Pericarpium Arecae catechu* and Hou Po *Cortex Magnoliae officinalis*.

To treat oedema of the lower part of the body use herbs which promote diuresis, such as Fu Ling *Sclerotium Poriae cocos*, Zhu Ling *Sclerotium Polypori umbellati*, Ze Xie *Rhizoma Alismatis orientalis* and Yi Yi Ren *Semen Coicis lachryma jobi*.

In Yin oedema from Spleen and Kidney Yang deficiency, one uses herbs which tonify Yang and move fluids, such as Fu Zi *Radix Aconiti carmichaeli praeparata*, Rou Gui *Cortex Cinnamomi cassiae* or Gui Zhi *Ramulus Cinnamomi cassiae*.

The patterns discussed are:

YANG OEDEMA

Wind-Water invading the Defensive-Qi portion
Fire-Poison
Dampness
Damp-Heat

YIN OEDEMA

Spleen-Yang Deficiency
Kidney-Yang Deficiency

YANG OEDEMA

1. WIND-WATER INVADING THE DEFENSIVE-QI PORTION

CLINICAL MANIFESTATIONS

Oedema of eyes and face with sudden onset, aversion to cold, fever, aches in muscles, retention of urine.
Tongue: no change in the body colour.
Pulse: Floating-Slow.

TREATMENT PRINCIPLE

Release the Exterior, expel Wind, open the Water passages, stimulate the Lung's dispersing of fluids.

ACUPUNCTURE

L.I.-4 Hegu, T.B.-5 Waiguan, LU-7 Lieque, BL-12 Fengmen, BL-13 Feishu, L.I.-6 Pianli, L.I.-10 Shousanli, Du-26 Renzhong, Ren-17 Shanzhong, ST-36 Zusanli. Reducing method; cupping may be applied to BL-12 and BL-13.

Explanation

- **L.I.-4**, **T.B.-5**, **LU-7**, **BL-12** and **BL-13** release the Exterior, expel Wind and restore the Lung's dispersing and descending function.
- **L.I.-6** opens the Water passages and resolves acute oedema of the upper limbs and face.
- **L.I.-10** is an important local point for the arms, used here to resolve oedema.
- **Du-26** is used as a local point for facial oedema. The old name of this point was *Shuigou* which means "water ditch".
- **Ren-17** stimulates the descending of Lung-Qi.
- **ST-36** harmonizes Nutritive and Defensive Qi and removes fluids from the space between skin and muscles.

Ancient prescriptions

- Oedema of face and limbs with fever: KI-6 Zhaohai, Du-26 Renzhong, L.I.-4 Hegu, ST-36 Zusanli, G.B.-41 Zulinqi, L.I.-11 Quchi and ST-36 Zusanli ("Great Compendium of Acupuncture" 1601).
- Oedema of upper body: Du-26 Renzhong with reducing method and Ren-9 Shuifen with direct moxa cones ("Great Compendium of Acupuncture" 1601).

HERBAL TREATMENT

Prescription

YUE BI JIA ZHU TANG
Overstepping Maidservant Decoction plus Atrac-tylodes
Ma Huang *Herba Ephedrae* 9 g
Shi Gao *Gypsum fibrosum* 18 g
Sheng Jiang *Rhizoma Zingiberis officinalis recens*
9 g
Gan Cao *Radix Glycyrrhizae uralensis* 5 g
Da Zao *Fructus Ziziphi jujubae* 5 dates
Bai Zhu *Rhizoma Atractylodis macrocephalae* 9 g

Explanation

This is a variation of the formula Yue Bi Tang which, in itself is a variation of Ma Xing Shi Gan Tang *Ephedra-Prunus-Gypsum-Glycyrrhiza Decoction* without Xing Ren.

The formula Yue Bi Tang is specific to release the Exterior, expel Wind-Water and resolve oedema. The addition of Bai Zhu gives it a stronger effect in resolving oedema.

- **Ma Huang** releases the Exterior, expels Wind, restores the Lung's dispersing function, regulates the Water passages and resolves oedema.
- **Shi Gao** clears Heat. This formula can therefore be used for the intermediate stage between the Greater Yang and Yang Ming patterns.
- **Sheng Jiang** helps Ma Huang to expel Wind-Cold and also to resolve oedema.
- **Da Zao**, in combination with Sheng Jiang, regulates Defensive and Nutritive Qi and therefore helps to resolve oedema from the space between skin and muscles.
- **Gan Cao** harmonizes.
- **Bai Zhu** tonifies Qi, dries Dampness and resolves oedema.

The "overstepping maidservant" in the curious name of this decoction could signify the fluids overflowing into the space between skin and muscles. Other books translate this as *Maidservant from Yue Decoction*, "Yue" being southern China.

Variations

- To enhance the oedema-resolving effect, add

Fu Ping *Herba Lemnae seu Spirodelae*, Ze Xie *Rhizoma Alismatis orientalis* and Fu Ling *Sclerotium Poriae cocos*.
- If there are pronounced symptoms of Wind-Cold eliminate Shi Gao and add Fang Feng *Radix Ledebouriellae sesloidis* and Gui Zhi *Ramulus Cinnamomi cassiae*.

2. FIRE-POISON

CLINICAL MANIFESTATIONS

Oedema of any part of the body, sores, carbuncles or furuncles.
Tongue: Red with a sticky-yellow coating.
Pulse: Slippery and Rapid.

TREATMENT PRINCIPLE

Tonify Lungs and Spleen, drain Dampness, clear Heat and resolve Fire-Poison.

ACUPUNCTURE

Ren-12 Zhongwan, BL-20 Pishu, Ren-9 Shuifen, ST-28 Shuidao, BL-22 Sanjiaoshu, SP-9 Yinlinquan, LU-7 Lieque, BL-13 Feishu, L.I.-11 Quchi. Reducing method except on Ren-12, BL-20 and BL-13 which should be reinforced. No moxa.

Explanation

- **Ren-12** and **BL-20** tonify the Spleen to resolve Dampness and oedema.
- **Ren-9**, **ST-28** and **BL-22** promote the transformation of fluids and resolve oedema.
- **SP-9** resolves Dampness.
- **LU-7** stimulates the Lung's dispersing of fluids.
- **BL-13** tonifies Lung-Qi.
- **L.I.-11** resolves Fire-Poison.

HERBAL TREATMENT

Prescription

MA HUANG LIAN QIAO CHI XIAO DOU TANG and WU WEI XIAO DU YIN

Ephedra-Forsythia-Phaseolus Decoction and *Five-Ingredient Resolving Poison Decoction*

Ma Huang *Herba Ephedrae* 9 g
Xing Ren *Semen Pruni armeniacae* 6 g
Sang Bai Pi *Cortex Mori albae radicis* 6 g
Lian Qiao *Fructus Forsythiae suspensae* 6 g
Chi Xiao Dou *Semen Phaseoli calcarati* 9 g
Zhi Gan Cao *Radix Glycyrrhizae uralensis praeparata* 3 g
Sheng Jiang *Rhizoma Zingiberis officinalis recens* 3 slices
Da Zao *Fructus Ziziphi jujubae* 3 dates
Jin Yin Hua *Flos Lonicerae japonicae* 9 g
Pu Gong Ying *Herba Taraxaci mongolici cum Radice* 3.5 g
Zi Hua Di Ding *Herba Violae cum radice* 3.5 g
Ju Hua *Flos Chrysanthemi morifolii* 3.5 g
Zi Bei Tian Kui *Herba Begoniae fimbristipulatae* 3.5 g

Explanation

The first eight herbs constitute the Ma Huang Lian Qiao Chi Xia Dou prescription which clears Heat, resolves Dampness and stimulates the dispersing and descending of Lung-Qi. It specifically drains Dampness from the skin. The last five herbs constitute the Wu Wei Xiao Du Yin which resolves Fire-Poison and is specific to treat boils, carbuncles and sores from Fire-Poison.

3. DAMPNESS

CLINICAL MANIFESTATIONS

Oedema of whole body or legs, scanty urination, a feeling of heaviness, a feeling of oppression of the chest.
Tongue: Swollen, sticky coating.
Pulse: Slippery.

TREATMENT PRINCIPLE

Strengthen the Spleen, resolve Dampness, benefit Yang and resolve oedema.

ACUPUNCTURE

Ren-12 Zhongwan, BL-20 Pishu, BL-21 Weishu, ST-36 Zusanli, Ren-9 Shuifen, ST-28 Shuidao, Ren-6 Qihai, SP-9 Yinlingquan, SP-6 Sanyinjiao, BL-22 Sanjiaoshu. Reinforcing method on Ren-12, BL-20, BL-21 and ST-36, even method on the others. Moxa is applicable.

Explanation

– **Ren-12**, **BL-20**, **BL-21** and **ST-36** tonify Stomach and Spleen.
– **Ren-9** and **ST-28** resolve oedema.
– **Ren-6**, with moxa, tonifies and moves Yang-Qi which will help to move and transform fluids and resolve oedema.
– **SP-9** and **SP-6** resolve Dampness.
– **BL-22** stimulates the transformation and excretion of fluids in the Lower Burner.

HERBAL TREATMENT

Prescription

WU PI SAN and WEI LING TANG
Five Peels Powder and *Stomach Poria Decoction*
Sheng Jiang Pi *Cortex Rhizomae Zingiberis officinalis recens* 9 g
Sang Bai Pi *Cortex Mori albae radicis* 9 g
Chen Pi *Pericarpium Citri reticulatae* 9 g
Da Fu Pi *Pericarpium Arecae catechu* 9 g
Fu Ling Pi *Cortex Poriae cocos* 9 g
Cang Zhu *Rhizoma Atractylodis lanceae* 6 g
Hou Po *Cortex Magnoliae officinalis* 6 g
Chen Pi *Pericarpium Citri reticulatae* 4 g
Gan Cao *Radix Glycyrrhizae uralensis* 3 g
Bai Zhu *Rhizoma Atractylodis macrocephalae* 6 g
Fu Ling *Sclerotium Poriae cocos* 6 g
Zhu Ling *Sclerotium Polypori umbellati* 6 g
Ze Xie *Rhizoma Alismatis orientalis* 6 g
Gui Zhi *Ramulus Cinnamomi cassiae* 3 g

Explanation

The first five herbs constitute the Wu Pi San which is specific to resolve oedema from Lung and Spleen deficiency.

The rest of the herbs constitute the Wei Ling Tang (in itself composed of Ping Wei San *Balancing the Stomach Powder* and Wu Ling San *Five*

"Ling" Powder) which resolves Dampness, harmonizes the Stomach, promotes diuresis and resolves oedema.

Patent remedy

WU LING SAN
Five "Ling" Powder
Bai Zhu *Rhizoma Atractylodis macrocephalae*
Fu Ling *Sclerotium Poriae cocos*
Zhu Ling *Sclerotium Polypori umbellati*
Ze Xie *Rhizoma Alismatis orientalis*
Gui Zhi *Ramulus Cinnamomi cassiae*

Explanation

This remedy, which has the same ingredients and functions as the homonymous prescription, is specific to resolve oedema.

4. DAMP-HEAT

CLINICAL MANIFESTATIONS

Oedema of legs or abdomen, thin and shiny skin, a feeling of oppression of the chest, thirst without desire to drink, scanty-dark urine.
Tongue: sticky-yellow tongue coating.
Pulse: Slippery-Rapid.

TREATMENT PRINCIPLE

Clear Heat and resolve Dampness.

ACUPUNCTURE

L.I.-11 Quchi, SP-9 Yinlingquan, SP-6 Sanyinjiao, Ren-9 Shuifen, ST-28 Shuidao, BL-22 Sanjiaoshu. Reducing method.

Explanation

- **L.I.-11** resolves Damp-Heat and clears Heat.
- **SP-9** and **SP-6** resolve Damp-Heat from the Lower Burner.
- **Ren-9** promotes the transformation of fluids

and the separation of clear from turbid. It resolves oedema.
- **ST-28** promotes the transformation of fluids in the Lower Burner and resolves oedema.
- **BL-22**, Back-Transporting point of the Lower Burner, promotes the transformation and excretion of fluids in the Lower Burner.

HERBAL TREATMENT

Prescription

SHU ZAO YIN ZI
Dredging and Digging Decoction
Qiang Huo *Radix et Rhizoma Notopterygii* 6 g
Qin Jiao *Radix Gentianae macrophyllae* 6 g
Da Fu Pi *Pericarpium Arecae catechu* 6 g
Fu Ling Pi *Cortex Poriae cocos* 6 g
Sheng Jiang Pi *Cortex Rhizomae Zingiberis officinalis recens* 6 g
Ze Xie *Rhizoma Alismatis orientalis* 6 g
Mu Tong *Caulis Akebiae* 3 g
Jiao Mu *Fructus Zanthoxyli schinifolii* 1.5 g
Chi Xiao Dou *Semen Phaseoli calcarati* 6 g
Shang Lu *Radix Phytolaccae acinosae* 6 g
Bing Lang *Semen Arecae catechu* 6 g

Explanation

This formula is specific to drain Damp-Heat and resolve oedema by promoting both urination and bowel evacuation.

- **Qiang Huo** and **Qin Jiao** expel Wind-Dampness and release the Exterior. Their function is to help to resolve oedema by sweating.
- **Da Fu Pi**, **Fu Ling Pi** and **Sheng Jiang Pi** resolve oedema.
- **Ze Xie**, **Mu Tong**, **Jiao Mu**, **Chi Xiao Dou**, **Shang Lu** and **Bing Lang** drain Damp-Heat and promote urination and defecation.

Variations

- If oedema is severe and there is breathlessness and scanty urination with symptoms of fluids in the lungs add both Wu Ling San *Five "Ling" Powder* and Wu Pi San *Five Peels Powder*.

– If the Heat part of Damp-Heat has injured the Yin fluids and there is a complex picture of both retention of fluids in the form of oedema and deficiency of fluids from Yin deficiency, the treatment method of draining fluids to resolve oedema may injure Yin further. In this case use Zhu Ling Tang *Polyporus Decoction*:

Zhu Ling *Sclerotium Polypori umbellati* 9 g
Fu Ling *Sclerotium Poriae cocos* 9 g
Ze Xie *Rhizoma Alismatis orientalis* 9 g
Hua Shi *Talcum* 9 g
E Jiao *Gelatinum Corii Asini* 9 g

– If Damp-Heat has affected the Bladder and there is blood in the urine add Xiao Ji *Herba Cephalanoplos segeti* and Bai Mao Gen *Rhizoma Imperatae cylindricae*.

YIN OEDEMA

1. SPLEEN-YANG DEFICIENCY

CLINICAL MANIFESTATIONS

Oedema of the abdomen and/or legs, pitting on pressure, feeling of oppression of the chest and abdomen, loose stools, pale face, tiredness, scanty urine.
Tongue: Pale, Swollen, teeth-marks.
Pulse: Weak and Fine.

TREATMENT PRINCIPLE

Tonify and warm the Spleen and resolve oedema.

ACUPUNCTURE

Ren-12 Zhongwan, ST-36 Zusanli, BL-20 Pishu, BL-21 Weishu, SP-6 Sanyinjiao, Ren-6 Qihai, Ren-9 Shuifen, ST-28 Shuidao, BL-22 Sanjiaoshu. Reducing or even method on Ren-9, ST-28 and BL-22, reinforcing method on the others. Moxa should be used.

Explanation

– **Ren-12**, **ST-36**, **BL-20**, **BL-21** and **SP-6** tonify Stomach and Spleen.

– **Ren-6** tonifies Qi in general and helps to resolve oedema, especially in the abdomen. Direct moxa on ginger is particularly effective.
– **Ren-9**, **ST-28** and **BL-22** promote the transformation of fluids and resolve oedema.

HERBAL TREATMENT

Prescription

SHI PI YIN
Strengthening the Spleen Decoction
Fu Zi *Radix Aconiti carmichaeli praeparata* 6 g
Gan Jiang *Rhizoma Zingiberis officinalis* 6 g
Fu Ling *Sclerotium Poriae cocos* 6 g
Mu Gua *Fructus Chaenomelis lagenariae* 6 g
Bai Zhu *Rhizoma Atractylodis macrocephalae* 6 g
Hou Po *Cortex Magnoliae officinalis* 6 g
Mu Xiang *Radix Saussureae* 6 g
Da Fu Pi *Pericarpium Arecae catechu* 6 g
Cao Guo *Fructus Amomi Tsaoko* 6 g
Zhi Gan Cao *Radix Glycyrrhizae uralensis praeparata* 3 g

Explanation

This formula tonifies and warms the Spleen and resolves Dampness and oedema.

– **Fu Zi** and **Gan Jiang** warm the Spleen and Kidneys and expel Cold.
– **Fu Ling** resolves Dampness.
– **Mu Gua** resolves Wind-Dampness and transforms turbidity from the Middle Burner.
– **Bai Zhu** tonifies Spleen-Qi.
– **Hou Po**, **Da Fu Pi** and **Cao Guo** fragrantly resolve Dampness.
– **Mu Xiang** moves Qi, which helps to resolve Dampness.
– **Gan Cao** harmonizes.

Variations

– If Qi deficiency is pronounced add Dang Shen *Radix Codonopsis pilosulae* and Huang Qi *Radix Astragali membranacei*.
– If urine is scanty add Gui Zhi *Ramulus Cinnamomi cassiae* and Ze Xie *Rhizoma Alismatis orientalis*.

Patent remedy

LI ZHONG WAN
Regulating the Centre Pill
Gan Jiang *Rhizoma Zingiberis officinalis*
Bai Zhu *Rhizoma Atractylodis macrocephalae*
Dang Shen *Radix Codonopsis pilosulae*
Gan Cao *Radix Glycyrrhizae uralensis*

Explanation

This remedy tonifies Spleen-Yang and expels internal Cold. Although it does not treat the Manifestation directly, it can be used for oedema to treat the Root (Spleen-Yang deficiency).

2. KIDNEY-YANG DEFICIENCY

CLINICAL MANIFESTATIONS

Oedema of the whole body or legs, pitting on pressure, sore back and knees, feeling cold especially in the back and legs, urination scanty or profuse but very pale, tiredness, depression, bright-white complexion.
Tongue: Pale, Swollen.
Pulse: Deep-Weak.

TREATMENT PRINCIPLE

Tonify and warm the Kidneys and resolve oedema.

ACUPUNCTURE

Ren-4 Guanyuan, BL-23 Shenshu, BL-20 Pishu, ST-36 Zusanli, KI-7 Fuliu, BL-22 Sanjiaoshu, ST-28 Shuidao. Reinforcing method on all points except the last two. Moxa should be used.

Explanation

- **Ren-4**, with moxa, tonifies Kidney-Yang.
- **BL-23** and **KI-7** tonify Kidney-Yang.
- **BL-20** and **ST-36** tonify the Spleen. In oedema from Kidney-Yang deficiency it is essential to tonify the Spleen as well.
- **BL-22** and **ST-28** resolve oedema.

HERBAL TREATMENT

Prescription

JI SHENG SHEN QI WAN and ZHEN WU TANG
Kidney-Qi Pill from "Ji Sheng Fang" and *True Warrior Decoction*
Fu Zi *Radix Aconiti carmichaeli praeparata* 3 g
Gui Zhi *Ramulus Cinnamomi cassiae* 3 g
Shu Di Huang *Radix Rehmanniae glutinosae praeparata* 24 g
Shan Zhu Yu *Fructus Corni officinalis* 12 g
Shan Yao *Radix Dioscoreae oppositae* 12 g
Ze Xie *Rhizoma Alismatis orientalis* 9 g
Mu Dan Pi *Cortex Moutan radicis* 9 g
Fu Ling *Sclerotium Poriae cocos* 9 g
Niu Xi *Radix Achyranthis bidentatae seu Cyathulae* 6 g
Che Qian Zi *Semen Plantaginis* 6 g
Bai Zhu *Rhizoma Atractylodis macrocephalae* 12 g
Bai Shao *Radix Paeoniae albae* 6 g
Sheng Jiang *Rhizoma Zingiberis officinalis recens* 3 slices

Explanation

The first eight herbs constitute the Jin Gui Shen Qi Wan *Golden Chest Kidney-Qi Pill*. Niu Xi and Che Qian Zi are added to drain Dampness from the Lower Burner.

The Zhen Wu Tang, already explained in chapter 3, tonifies and warms the Spleen and resolves oedema.

Variations

- If urination is very copious and the urine very pale, omit Ze Xie and Che Qian Zi and add Tu Si Zi *Semen Cuscutae* and Bu Gu Zhi *Fructus Psoraleae corylifoliae*.

Patent remedy

JIN GUI SHEN QI WAN
Golden Chest Kidney-Qi Pill
Gui Zhi *Ramulus Cinnamomi cassiae* (or Rou Gui *Cortex Cinnamomi cassiae*)
Fu Zi *Radix Aconiti carmichaeli praeparata*
Shu Di Huang *Radix Rehmanniae glutinosae praeparata*

Shan Yao *Radix Dioscoreae oppositae*
Shan Zhu Yu *Fructus Corni officinalis*
Ze Xie *Rhizoma Alismatis orientalis*
Fu Ling *Sclerotium Poriae cocos*
Mu Dan Pi *Cortex Moutan radicis*

Explanation

This remedy, with the same ingredients and functions as the homonymous prescription, tonifies Kidney-Yang and can be used to treat the Root in oedema.

The tongue presentation appropriate to this remedy is a Pale, Swollen and wet body.

Case history

A 52-year-old woman had been suffering from oedema of the ankles for 2 years. She also suffered from early-morning diarrhoea and she felt always cold. Her tongue was Pale and wet and her pulse was Deep and Weak.

Diagnosis
This is oedema from Kidney-Yang deficiency which is also confirmed by the early-morning diarrhoea and the cold feeling.

Treatment principle
The treatment principle adopted was to tonify Spleen- and Kidney-Yang and resolve oedema. She was treated only with acupuncture.

Acupuncture
The points used (with reinforcing method to tonify Spleen and Kidneys and even method to resolve oedema) were selected from the following:

- **ST-36** Zusanli, **SP-6** Sanyinjiao, **BL-20** Pishu and **BL-21** Weishu to tonify Spleen and Stomach. According to chapter 35 of the "Spiritual Axis" ST-36 should always be used in oedema as it encourages the return of fluids from the space between skin and muscles into the channels.[5]
- **BL-23** Shenshu and **KI-7** Fuliu to tonify Kidney-Yang.
- **BL-22** Sanjiaoshu, **Ren-9** Shuifen, **SP-9** Yinlingquan and **SP-6** Sanyinjiao to drain Dampness and resolve oedema.

This patient was treated weekly for the first 3 months and fortnightly thereafter; it took 12 months to resolve the oedema completely.

Case history

A 48-year-old woman had been suffering from oedema of the lower legs from the age of 15. She had been taking Moduretic (a diuretic) for 12 years. She felt cold in general but often had a burning feeling in her feet. Her urine was sometimes dark. She also suffered from lower back-ache and loose stools. Her tongue was slightly Red and Stiff. Her pulse was very Fine and extremely Weak on both Rear positions.

Diagnosis
This case is interesting as there are some signs of Kidney-Yin deficiency and yet her main problem is chronic oedema which is, in theory, always due to Kidney-Yang deficiency. There certainly is a Kidney-Yang deficiency as shown by the general cold feeling, the oedema itself, the back-ache, the loose stools and the very Weak pulse. However, there are also a few signs of Kidney-Yin deficiency: the slightly Red and Stiff tongue (which, apart from Wind, may indicate Yin deficiency), the burning sensation of her feet and the dark urine. Obviously the primary condition is Kidney-Yang deficiency but, as often happens in women, this can overlap with Kidney-Yin deficiency. Since she has been suffering from Kidney-Yang deficiency for a very long time, her condition is just at the point of transition from Yang to Yin deficiency. Without treatment, her tongue would become redder and redder and she would develop more Yin-deficiency symptoms such as a feeling of heat, hot flushes and night-sweating. There is also another possible interpretation of the presence of Kidney-Yin deficiency symptoms: it could be that the long-term use of diuretics has depleted Kidney-Yin. By removing Water (a Yin substance) from the body, diuretics may quite possibly lead to a deficiency of Kidney-Yin.

Treatment principle
The treatment principle adopted was to tonify Kidney-Yang and resolve oedema. As there is also a deficiency of Kidney-Yin, the action of the warm herbs which tonify Kidney-Yang was moderated by the addition of some cool herbs to nourish Yin.

She was treated with both acupuncture and herbs.

Acupuncture
The main points used (with reinforcing method to tonify the Kidneys and even method to resolve oedema) were selected from the following:

- **ST-36** Zusanli, **SP-6** Sanyinjiao, **BL-20** Pishu and **BL-21** Weishu to tonify Spleen and Stomach.
- **BL-23** Shenshu and **KI-7** Fuliu to tonify Kidney-Yang.
- **BL-22** Sanjiaoshu, **Ren-9** Shuifen, **SP-9** Yinlingquan and **SP-6** Sanyinjiao to drain Dampness and resolve oedema.
- **KI-3** Taixi and **Ren-4** Guanyuan, without moxa, to nourish Kidney-Yin.

Herbal treatment
The prescription used was a variation of Zhen Wu

Tang *True Warrior Decoction* and Wu Ling San *Five "Ling" Powder*:

Fu Zi *Radix Aconiti carmichaeli praeparata* 4 g
Bai Zhu *Rhizoma Atractylodis macrocephalae* 9 g
Fu Ling *Sclerotium Poriae cocos* 15 g
Bai Shao *Radix Paeoniae albae* 6 g
Sheng Jiang *Rhizoma Zingiberis officinalis recens* 3 slices
Zhu Ling *Sclerotium Polypori umbellati* 6 g
Ze Xie *Rhizoma Alismatis orientalis* 6 g
Gui Zhi *Ramulus Cinnamomi cassiae* 6 g
Gou Ji *Rhizoma Cibotii barometz* 6 g
Chi Xiao Dou *Semen Phaseoli calcarati* 9 g
Tian Men Dong *Tuber Asparagi cochinchinensis* 6 g

Explanation
- The first five herbs constitute the Zhen Wu Tang which tonifies Spleen- and Kidney-Yang and resolves oedema.
- The next three herbs constitute Wu Ling San (minus Fu Ling and Bai Zhu which are already in the first formula) which resolves oedema.
- **Gou Ji** tonifies Kidney-Yang.
- **Chi Xiao Dou** drains Dampness.
- **Tian Men Dong** nourishes Kidney-Yin and is added to temper the hot energy of the Yang tonics. Ze Xie (contained in Wu Ling San) would also perform this function.

As this patient had been suffering from oedema for 33 years and had resorted to the use of diuretics for 12, the treatment necessarily took a long time (2 years) and, although she improved by about 70%, the oedema was never resolved completely.

Prognosis

Acute oedema can be resolved fairly easily using acupuncture and/or herbs but chronic oedema usually requires a lengthy treatment of at least several months. The oedema from Kidney-Yang deficiency is more difficult to treat than the one from Spleen-Yang deficiency.

Western medicine differentiation

Oedema consists in the excessive accumulation of interstitial fluid, and it may be either localized or generalized.

From a Western medical viewpoint there are very many causes of oedema and the main ones are summarized in Table 22.1.

Appendix

Acute nephritis

Acute nephritis is an inflammation of the kidney glomeruli. It starts with an acute onset and its two main manifestations are oedema of the face and eyes and blood in the urine. Other manifestations include symptoms of exterior invasion such as aversion to cold, fever, headache and a sore throat. Still other manifestations include nausea and vomiting.

AETIOLOGY AND PATHOLOGY

1. INVASION OF EXTERNAL WIND

External Wind invades the Lung Defensive-Qi portion and may interfere with the Lung's dispersing of Qi in the Water passages of the Upper Burner. This causes fluids to overflow in the space between skin and muscles. This type of Wind is called Wind-Water.

2. INFECTION

Nephritis may develop from a transmission of

Table 22.1 Main causes of oedema in Western medicine

Oedema				
Localized		Bilateral		
Inflammatory	Venous	Above diaphragm	Below diaphragm	
– Boils	– Phlebitis	– Acute nephritis	Cardiovascular	Kidney
– Carbuncles	– Varicosities			
– Cellulitis			Congestive cardiac	Chronic nephritis
– Abscesses			failure	

infection from other sites in the body. It may develop from laryngitis, pharyngitis, tonsillitis, scarlet fever and skin infections from boils, carbuncles or eczema.

3. EXTERNAL DAMPNESS

Invasion of external Dampness can impair the function of the Spleen and lead to accumulation of body fluids and oedema in acute nephritis.

Acute nephritis falls under the category of Yang oedema and it is characterized mainly by Fullness in the form of Wind-Water, Dampness or Fire-Poison. The main principle of treatment is therefore to expel pathogenic factors.

DIFFERENTIATION AND TREATMENT

The main principle of treatment is to expel the predominant pathogenic factor, i.e.:

- Wind-Water: expel Wind-Water by releasing the Exterior and promoting sweat
- Dampness: resolve Dampness, invigorate Yang and promote diuresis
- Fire-Poison: drain Fire, resolve Poison and promote diuresis. Occasionally it is necessary to drain Fire-Poison by purgation. The principle of draining Fire-Poison was not used in the past for nephritis. It has been developed in modern times with good results in the treatment of nephritis.

The patterns discussed are:

ACUTE NEPHRITIS

Invasion of External Wind-Water
Dampness
Fire-Poison

1. INVASION OF EXTERNAL WIND-WATER
CLINICAL MANIFESTATIONS

Oedema of face and eyes of sudden onset gradually spreading to limbs, shiny skin, pitting resolves quickly, aversion to cold, fever, sore throat, body aches, cough, coarse breathing.
Tongue: thin-white coating if Wind-Cold, slightly Red on the sides and/or front if Wind-Heat.
Pulse: Floating-Tight if Wind-Cold, Floating-Rapid if Wind-Heat.

TREATMENT PRINCIPLE

Expel Wind-Water, release the Exterior, promote sweating. Although the herbs used promote sweating, many of them also open the Water passages and therefore also promote diuresis. Thus the patient may not necessarily be obviously sweating after taking the decoction.

ACUPUNCTURE

See under Yang oedema from Wind-Water.

HERBAL TREATMENT

(a) Prescription

LING GUI FU PING TANG
Poria-Cinnamomum-Spirodela Decoction
Fu Ling *Sclerotium Poriae cocos* 9 g
Gui Zhi *Ramulus Cinnamomi cassiae* 6 g
Fu Ping *Herba Lemnae seu Spirodelae* 9 g
Xing Ren *Semen Pruni armeniacae* 9 g
Ze Xie *Rhizoma Alismatis orientalis* 9 g
Ban Xia *Rhizoma Pinelliae ternatae* 9 g
Zhi Gan Cao *Radix Glycyrrhizae uralensis praeparata* 3 g

Explanation

This formula is used if there is a prevalence of Wind-Cold.

- **Fu Ling** and **Gui Zhi** in combination invigorate Yang and transform Water. Gui Zhi also releases the Exterior and expels Wind-Cold.
- **Fu Ping** drains Dampness and is specific to resolve oedema.

- **Xing Ren** helps to release the Exterior and regulate Water by stimulating the descending of Lung-Qi.
- **Ze Xie** transforms Water and resolves oedema by promoting diuresis.
- **Ban Xia** helps to resolve Water by resolving Phlegm.
- **Gan Cao** harmonizes.

(b) Prescription

YUE BI JIA ZHU TANG
Overstepping Maidservant Decoction plus Atractylodes
Ma Huang *Herba Ephedrae* 9 g
Shi Gao *Gypsum fibrosum* 18 g
Sheng Jiang *Rhizoma Zingiberis officinalis recens* 9 g
Gan Cao *Radix Glycyrrhizae uralensis* 5 g
Da Zao *Fructus Ziziphi jujubae* 5 dates
Bai Zhu *Rhizoma Atractylodis macrocephalae* 9 g

Explanation

This formula, already explained above, is used if there is a predominance of Wind-Heat.

(c) Prescription

EMPIRICAL PRESCRIPTION BY PROF. ZHOU ZHONG YING
Fu Ping *Herba Lemnae seu Spirodelae* 9 g
Fang Feng *Radix Ledebouriellae sesloidis* 9 g
Zi Su Ye *Folium Perillae frutescentis* 6 g
Ma Huang *Herba Ephedrae* 9 g
Xing Ren *Semen Pruni armeniacae* 6 g
Sheng Jiang Pi *Cortex Rhizomae Zingiberis officinalis recens* 6 g

Explanation

- **Fu Ping** releases the Exterior, expels Wind-Water and resolves oedema.
- **Fang Feng**, **Su Ye** and **Ma Huang** expel Wind-Cold, release the Exterior and regulate the Water passages of the Upper Burner.
- **Xing Ren** helps the previous herbs to release the Exterior by promoting the descending of Lung-Qi.
- **Sheng Jiang Pi** resolves oedema.

Variations

These variations apply to all three previous formulae.

- If urination is scanty add Ze Xie *Rhizoma Alismatis orientalis* (or increase it if it is already in the prescription) and Chi Xiao Dou *Semen Phaseoli calcarati*.
- If symptoms of Heat are pronounced add Lian Qiao *Fructus Forsythiae suspensae* and Chai Hu *Radix Bupleuri*.
- If there is blood in the urine add Xiao Ji *Herba Cephalanoplos segeti* and Bai Mao Gen *Rhizoma Imperatae cylindricae*.
- If the throat is sore and swollen add She Gan *Rhizoma Belamcandae chinensis* and Da Qing Ye *Folium Isatidis seu Baphicacanthi*.
- If there is an underlying deficiency of Qi add Huang Qi *Radix Astragali membranacei* and Fang Ji *Radix Aristolochiae seu Cocculi*.

2. DAMPNESS

CLINICAL MANIFESTATIONS

Oedema of the legs, a feeling of oppression of the chest, abdominal distension, nausea, a feeling of heaviness, scanty urination.
Tongue: sticky coating.
Pulse: Slippery.

TREATMENT PRINCIPLE

Resolve Dampness, invigorate Yang and promote diuresis.

ACUPUNCTURE

See under Yang oedema, Dampness type.

HERBAL TREATMENT

Prescription

WU LING SAN Variation
Five "Ling" Powder Variation
Fu Ling *Sclerotium Poriae cocos* 6 g

Zhu Ling *Sclerotium Polypori umbellati* 6 g
Bai Zhu *Rhizoma Atractylodis macrocephalae* 6 g
Ze Xie *Rhizoma Alismatis orientalis* 6 g
Gui Zhi *Ramulus Cinnamomi cassiae* 6 g
Dang Shen *Radix Codonopsis pilosulae* 6 g
Huang Qi *Radix Astragali membranacei* 9 g
Chuan Xiong *Radix Ligustici wallichii* 4.5 g
Yi Mu Cao *Herba Leonori heterophylli* 4.5 g

Explanation

- The formula Wu Ling San resolves oedema from the Lower Burner.
- **Dang Shen** and **Huang Qi** tonify the Spleen to resolve Dampness and transform fluids.
- **Chuan Xiong** and **Yi Mu Cao** move Blood. Because of the relationship of interchange between fluids and Blood, moving Blood helps to transform fluids and resolve oedema.

Variations

- If there is breathlessness add Ma Huang *Herba Ephedrae* and Xing Ren *Semen Pruni armeniacae*.
- If there is pronounced chilliness add Fu Zi *Radix Aconiti carmichaeli praeparata* and Gui Zhi *Ramulus Cinnamomi cassiae*.
- If there are also exterior symptoms and sweating add Huang Qi *Radix Astragali membranacei*, Fang Feng *Radix Ledebouriellae sesloidis* and Fang Ji *Radix Stephaniae tetrandae*. Huang Qi and Fang Ji in combination promote diuresis.

Patent remedy

WU LING SAN
Five "Ling" Powder

Explanation

This remedy has already been explained above under "Yang oedema".

3. FIRE-POISON

CLINICAL MANIFESTATIONS

Dark or cloudy and scanty urine, mild oedema, blood in the urine, burning sensation on micturition, fever, sore throat, cough.
Tongue: Red with a sticky-yellow coating.
Pulse: Slippery-Rapid.

This corresponds to acute nephritis from an infection with haematuria as its main manifestation.

TREATMENT PRINCIPLE

Clear Heat, resolve Poison, cool Blood and promote diuresis.

ACUPUNCTURE

See under Yang oedema, Fire-Poison.

HERBAL TREATMENT

(a) Prescription

SI MIAO SAN
Four Wonderful Powder
Cang Zhu *Rhizoma Atractylodis lanceae* 6 g
Huang Bo *Cortex Phellodendri* 9 g
Niu Xi *Radix Achyranthis bidentatae seu Cyathulae* 6 g
Yi Yi Ren *Semen Coicis lachryma jobi* 9 g

Explanation

This formula resolves Damp-Heat and Fire-Poison from the Lower Burner.

- **Cang Zhu** and **Huang Bo** form the Er Miao San *Two Wonderful Powder* which resolves Damp-Heat from the Lower Burner.
- **Niu Xi**, added to the previous two herbs, forms the San Miao San *Three Wonderful Powder*. Niu Xi directs the formula to the Lower Burner, lower back and legs.
- **Yi Yi Ren**, added to the previous three herbs, forms the Si Miao San. The addition of Yi Yi Ren allows the formula to treat Fire-Poison as well as Damp-Heat. Yi Yi Ren also resolves oedema and treats swollen feet.

(b) Prescription

EMPIRICAL PRESCRIPTION FROM PROF. ZHOU ZHONG YING

Ma Huang *Herba Ephedrae* 3 g
Lian Qiao *Fructus Forsythiae suspensae* 9 g
Huang Bo *Cortex Phellodendri* 9 g
Jin Yin Hua *Flos Lonicerae japonicae* 9 g
Zi Hua Di Ding *Herba Violae cum radice* 9 g
Pu Gong Ying *Herba Taraxaci mongolici cum Radice* 9 g
Yi Yi Ren *Semen Coicis lachryma jobi* 15 g
Chi Xiao Dou *Semen Phaseoli calcarati* 9 g

Explanation

- **Ma Huang** opens the Water passages and resolves oedema by sweating.
- **Lian Qiao**, **Huang Bo**, **Jin Yin Hua**, **Zi Hua Di Ding** and **Pu Gong Ying** resolve Fire-Poison.
- **Yi Yi Ren** and **Chi Xiao Dou** resolve Dampness and Fire-Poison and promote diuresis.

(c) Prescription

XIAO JI YIN ZI Variation
Cephalanoplos Decoction Variation
Xiao Ji *Herba Cephalanoplos segeti* 30 g
Ou Jie *Nodus Nelumbinis nuciferae rhizomatis* 6 g
Pu Huang *Pollen Typhae* 9 g
Hua Shi *Talcum* 15 g
Mu Tong *Caulis Akebiae* 9 g
Zhu Ye *Herba Lophatheri gracilis* 9 g
Gan Cao *Radix Glycyrrhizae uralensis* 6 g
Huang Bo *Cortex Phellodendri* 6 g
Lian Qiao *Fructus Forsythiae suspensae* 6 g
Chi Xiao Dou *Semen Phaseoli calcarati* 9 g
Bai Mao Gen *Rhizoma Imperatae cylindricae* 9 g

Explanation

This variation omits Zhi Zi, Sheng Di Huang and Dang Gui and adds Huang Bo, Lian Qiao, Chi Xiao Dou and Bai Mao Gen to drain Damp-Heat, clear Heat, promote diuresis and stop bleeding.

Variations

These variations apply to all three previous prescriptions.

- If oedema is very pronounced add Fang Feng *Radix Ledebouriellae sesloidis* and Fu Ping *Herba Lemnae seu Spirodelae*.
- If there is tonsillitis add She Gan *Rhizoma Belamcandae chinensis*, Niu Bang Zi *Fructus Arctii lappae* and Xuan Shen *Radix Scrophulariae ningpoensis*.
- If the urine is very dark and there is intense burning on micturition add Che Qian Cao *Herba Plantaginis*.
- If there is blood in the urine add Xiao Ji *Herba Cephalanoplos segeti* (or increase it if is already present), Zhi Zi *Fructus Gardeniae jasminoidis* and Yi Mu Cao *Herba Leonori heterophylli* to move Blood, cool Blood, stop bleeding and promote diuresis.

Chronic nephritis

"Chronic nephritis" is a Western medical term identifying a disease characterized by inflammation of the kidney glomeruli. In Chinese medicine, its complex of symptoms and signs may fall under different categories, such as "Oedema" or "Exhaustion". Its main signs are oedema of the ankles, albuminuria and hypertension.

Chronic nephritis may develop from acute nephritis. In many cases, however, it develops insidiously without apparent symptoms. Acute nephritis broadly corresponds to "Yang Water" or "Yang oedema" in Chinese medicine, whilst chronic nephritis broadly corresponds to "Yin Water", "True Water" or "Stone Water". As explained above, "Water" here refers *not* to Water in a 5-Element sense, but to Water as a pathogenic factor, i.e. the accumulation of body fluids in oedema.

The three cardinal signs of chronic nephritis are oedema, proteinuria and hypertension.

OEDEMA

Oedema is due to dysfunction of Lungs, Spleen and Kidneys as explained above under "Oedema".

Zhang Jing Yue (1563-1640) said: *"Oedema is due to the transformation of Essence and Blood into Water and is mostly deficient in nature."*[6]

Although chronic nephritis by its very nature is always due to a deficiency of the Lungs, Spleen and Kidneys, nearly always there is also some Dampness or Damp-Heat. For this reason, adopting the treatment principle of simply warming and tonifying Spleen and Kidneys may not be enough. Attention should be paid to draining Dampness as well with such herbs as Huang Bo *Cortex Phellodendri*, Hua Shi *Talcum* or Che Qian Zi *Semen Plantaginis*. With acupuncture, one needs to use points such as SP-9 Yinlingquan, SP-6 Sanyinjiao, Ren-9 Shuifen, BL-22 Sanjiaoshu, and ST-28 Shuidao, with even method.

It is possible to differentiate between conditions of Deficient character and conditions of Excess character according to the severity of the oedema. If oedema is severe, it indicates a predominance of Dampness, therefore an Excess pattern. This is treated by warming Yang and resolving Dampness. If oedema is slight or even absent, it denotes a deficiency of Spleen- and Kidney-Yang, i.e. a Deficient pattern. This is treated by tonifying Spleen and Kidneys.

There are, however, other factors that also play a part in the pathogenesis of oedema. Stasis of Blood can also be a causative factor of oedema. This is due to the interaction and interchange between Blood and Body Fluids. The "Discussion of Prescriptions of the Golden Chest" (*c.* AD 220) by Zhang Zhong Jing says: *"When Blood is not harmonized it gives rise to Water."*[7] The "Discussion on Blood Syndromes" (1884) by Tang Zong Hai says: *"Pouring [and overflowing] stagnant Blood gives rise to oedema and swelling, Blood turning into Water . . . "*[8]

PROTEINURIA

Proteinuria is due to leakage of Essence from the Kidneys. The Kidneys store the Essence and if they are deficient, Essence may leak out. The seepage of protein in the urine is viewed as a sign of such leakage in Chinese medicine. This is due to the sinking of Spleen- and Kidney-Qi.

To treat proteinuria, besides strengthening the Spleen and Kidneys and using astringent herbs which also nourish the Essence (such as Wu Wei Zi *Fructus Schisandrae chinensis*) to stop leakage, some doctors advocate moving Blood too. They base this view on the fact that when the Original Qi of the Kidneys is severely deficient, it cannot reach the blood vessels and this leads to stasis of Blood.[9] With acupuncture, one needs to strengthen the Essence with points such as Ren-4 Guanyuan, BL-23 Shenshu, BL-52 Zhishi, G.B.-39 Xuanzhong, and Jinggong extra points (0.5 *cun* lateral to BL-52), with reinforcing method and moxa.

HYPERTENSION

Hypertension can be due to either Kidney-Yang or Kidney-Yin deficiency. If Kidney-Yang is deficient Yin (Water) accumulates, Yang does not move, the blood vessels cannot relax, Blood cannot flow properly and this causes hypertension.

If Kidney-Yin is deficient it fails to nourish Liver-Yin which leads to hyperactivity of Liver-Yang. The rising of Liver-Yang and Liver-Wind causes high blood pressure and its typical symptoms of headache, dizziness and tinnitus. With acupuncture, one needs to tonify the Kidneys with BL-23 Shenshu and KI-3 Taixi and subdue Liver-Yang with LIV-3 Taichong and G.B.-20 Fengchi.

Anaemia is often present and this is due to deficiency of the Spleen in failing to make Blood and of the Kidneys in failing to nourish Marrow.

Haematuria is often present in chronic nephritis. Its pathology is usually very complicated. Three main factors may be responsible and these often occur simultaneously. They are as follows:

(a) A deficient Spleen-Qi is unable to hold Blood in the vessels
(b) In very chronic cases deficiency of Yang can lead to deficiency of Yin with Empty-Heat. Empty-Heat pushes blood out of the vessels
(c) Stasis of Blood in the vessels may also cause bleeding.

The colour of the urine will vary according to the predominant condition. It will be bright red if Spleen-Qi deficiency predominates, dark red if there is Empty-Heat and dark with clots or brown if there is stasis of Blood.

Bearing in mind the above three factors, the principle of treatment in cases of haematuria is to tonify Qi, nourish Yin, cool Blood and eliminate stasis. To tonify Kidney-Qi and Kidney-Yin one can use Shan Zhu Yu *Fructus Corni officinalis*, Du Zhong *Cortex Eucommiae ulmoidis*, Shu Di Huang *Radix Rehmanniae glutinosae praeparata*, Gou Qi Zi *Fructus Lycii chinensis*, Nu Zhen Zi *Fructus Ligustri lucidi*, or Xu Duan *Radix Dipsaci*. If there is a pronounced deficiency of Spleen-Qi Huang Qi *Radix Astragali membranacei* can be used. In cases of deficiency of Yin with Empty-Heat affecting the Blood one can select Sheng Di Huang *Radix Rehmanniae glutinosae*, Mu Dan Pi *Cortex Moutan radicis*, Bai Mao Gen *Rhizoma Imperatae cylindricae*, Qian Cao Gen *Radix Rubiae cordifoliae* or Han Lian Cao *Herba Ecliptae prostratae*. If Heat signs are pronounced add Huang Bo *Cortex Phellodendri* and Zhi Mu *Radix Anemarrhenae asphodeloidis*. In cases of stasis of Blood add Yi Mu Cao *Herba Leonori heterophylli*, San Qi *Radix Notoginseng* or Tao Ren *Semen Persicae*.

TREATMENT

The treatment of the Manifestation is based on three main methods: sweating, promoting urination and purging. The treatment of the Root is based on tonifying.

Sweating is used for only one type of "Yang oedema", i.e. acute nephritis characterized by invasion of the Lungs by Wind-Water. In such a case, sweating is used because it releases the Exterior and expels Wind, of which Wind-Water is a type.

Promoting urination is used for chronic nephritis with oedema and Dampness. Within this method of treatment it is important to distinguish Excess from Deficiency and Cold from Heat.

1. Excess pattern of Dampness:
   (a) Cold Dampness: warm Yang and promote urination
   (b) Hot Dampness: clear Heat and promote urination
2. Deficiency pattern: warm and tonify Spleen and Kidneys.

The purging method is used only in very severe cases of oedema when the above methods of treatment are unsuccessful. For light purging, one can use large doses of Bing Lang *Semen Arecae catechu* (30 g) and Yu Li Ren *Semen Pruni* (24 g). The purging method should not be used if the patient's body condition is very weak. In these cases, one should tonify first and then purge. If after purging the patient feels better, is in better spirits and has more appetite, one can continue using purging herbs combined with tonic ones. One should never use purging in patients with heart disease (in a Western medical sense) or who are suffering from bleeding from the alimentary canal. After purging and improvement of the symptoms, one can tonify the Spleen and Kidneys, still combining the tonic herbs with herbs which gently resolve Dampness.

Finally, if Dampness turns into Phlegm and combines with Heat, it may manifest with nausea, vomiting and mental confusion. In this case three different methods of treatment are available depending on the case:

1. warm Yang and subdue rebellious Qi (causing the nausea and vomiting)
2. clear Heat and open the orifices
3. use purging.

It will be noted that each of the treatment methods mentioned corresponds to a certain category of herbs and prescriptions in herbal medicine. The definition of the treatment method therefore gives an immediate indication of the category of herbs and prescriptions to use. In acupuncture, the connection is not so direct and other considerations guide the choice of points (such as the channel involved, the balance of points, etc.).

The patterns of chronic nephritis discussed are:

1. Spleen- and Kidney-Yang deficiency
2. Spleen- and Kidney-Yang deficiency, Water overflowing
3. Spleen-Kidney Yang deficiency, Yin rebelling upwards
4. Spleen and Kidney deficiency, Essence leaking
5. Kidney- and Heart-Yang deficiency Qi-Blood stagnant.

1. SPLEEN- AND KIDNEY-YANG DEFICIENCY

In a chronic disease such as nephritis, both Spleen and Kidneys are involved. These organs work in very close coordination to transform, transport and excrete Body Fluids and, in a chronic disease, deficiency of one often causes deficiency of the other.

Clinical manifestations

Sallow complexion, dizziness, tinnitus, listlessness, mental depression, poor appetite, soreness and weakness of the lower back, slight oedema. The tongue would be Pale and Swollen and the pulse Deep and Weak. All these manifestations reflect Spleen- and Kidney-Yang deficiency.

Principle of treatment

Tonify the Spleen, strengthen the Kidneys, warm Yang.

Acupuncture

- ST-36 Zusanli, KI-7 Fuliu, Ren-12 Zhongwan, BL-20 Pishu and BL-23 Shenshu with reinforcing method to tonify Spleen- and Kidney-Yang. Moxa is applicable.
- SP-6 Sanyinjiao, SP-9 Yinlingquan, BL-22 Sanjiaoshu and Ren-9 Shuifen with even method to eliminate Dampness and oedema.

Herbal treatment

(a) Prescription

BU ZHONG YI QI TANG Variation
Tonifying the Centre and Benefiting Qi Decoction
Huang Qi *Radix Astragali membranacei* 15 g
Dang Shen *Radix Codonopsis pilosulae* 15 g
Bai Zhu *Rhizoma Atractylodis macrocephalae* 15 g
Fu Ling *Sclerotium Poriae cocos* 10 g
Shan Yao *Radix Dioscoreae oppositae* 15 g
Chai Hu *Radix Bupleuri* 6 g
Zhi Gan Cao *Radix Glycyrrhizae uralensis praeparata* 3 g
Lu Jiao *Cornu Cervi* 10 g

Explanation

All the herbs, except Lu Jiao and Shan Yao, belong to the prescription Bu Zhong Yi Qi Tang *Tonifying the Centre and Benefiting Qi Decoction* which tonifies Spleen-Qi and promotes the raising of clear Qi and the descending of turbid Qi. Lu Jiao is added to tonify Kidney-Yang and Shan Yao to tonify both Spleen and Kidneys.

If albuminuria is pronounced together with severe symptoms of Qi deficiency, increase the dose of Huang Qi *Radix Astragali membranacei* and Dang Shen *Radix Codonopsis pilosulae*.

(b) Prescription

WEI LING TANG
Stomach "Ling" Decoction
Cang Zhu *Rhizoma Atractylodis lanceae* 6 g
Hou Po *Cortex Magnoliae officinalis* 6 g
Chen Pi *Pericarpium Citri reticulatae* 4 g
Gan Cao *Radix Glycyrrhizae uralensis* 3 g
Bai Zhu *Rhizoma Atractylodis macrocephalae* 6 g
Fu Ling *Sclerotium Poriae cocos* 6 g
Zhu Ling *Sclerotium Polypori umbellati* 6 g
Ze Xie *Rhizoma Alismatis orientalis* 6 g
Gui Zhi *Ramulus Cinnamomi cassiae* 3 g

Explanation

This prescription is a combination of Ping Wei San (the first four herbs) and Wu Ling San (the last five herbs). The two together dry Dampness (with fragrant herbs such as Cang Zhu and Hou Po) and drain Dampness via urination (with such herbs as Fu Ling, Zhu Ling and Ze Xie).

The prescription as it stands does not tonify the Spleen and Kidneys and should therefore be modified by increasing the dosage of Bai Zhu *Rhizoma Atractylodis macrocephalae* and adding Xu Duan *Radix Dipsaci*.

(c) Prescription

SHEN LING BAI ZHU SAN
Ginseng-Poria-Atractylodes Powder
Ren Shen *Radix Ginseng* 6 g (or **Dang Shen** *Radix Codonopsis pilosulae* 12 g)
Bai Zhu *Rhizoma Atractylodis macrocephalae* 9 g

Fu Ling *Sclerotium Poriae cocos* 12 g
Zhi Gan Cao *Radix Glycyrrhizae uralensis praeparata* 6 g
Bian Dou *Semen Dolichoris lablab* 12 g
Shan Yao *Radix Dioscoreae oppositae* 12 g
Lian Zi *Semen Nelumbinis nuciferae* 12 g
Sha Ren *Fructus seu Semen Amomi* 4.5 g
Yi Yi Ren *Semen Coicis lachryma jobi* 10 g
Jie Geng *Radix Platycodi grandiflori* 6 g

Explanation

This prescription tonifies Spleen and Stomach and is particularly used if there is diarrhoea. In this case, other herbs should be added to tonify Kidney-Yang: Xu Duan *Radix Dipsaci* for instance, or Du Zhong *Cortex Eucommiae ulmoidis*.

(d) Prescription

PI SHEN SHUANG BU TANG
Decoction tonifying both Spleen and Kidneys
Dang Shen *Radix Codonopsis pilosulae* 12 g
Bai Zhu *Rhizoma Atractylodis macrocephalae* 12 g
Fu Ling *Sclerotium Poriae cocos* 15 g
Zhi Gan Cao *Radix Glycyrrhizae uralensis praeparata* 6 g
Du Zhong *Cortex Eucommiae ulmoidis* 9 g
Tu Si Zi *Semen Cuscutae* 12 g
Shan Zhu Yu *Fructus Corni officinalis* 6 g
Shu Di Huang *Radix Rehmanniae glutinosae praeparata* 12 g

Explanation

The first four herbs are the Si Jun Zi Tang *Four Gentlemen Decoction* which tonifies Spleen-Qi.

- **Du Zhong** and **Tu Si Zi** tonify Kidney-Yang.
- **Shan Zhu Yu** and **Shu Di Huang** tonify the Kidneys.

One should add to this prescription some herbs to resolve Dampness such as Yi Yi Ren *Semen Coicis lachryma jobi* and Zhu Ling *Sclerotium Polypori umbellati*.

(e) Prescription

SHI PI YIN Variation
Strengthening the Spleen Decoction Variation

Huang Qi *Radix Astragali membranacei* 15 g
Dang Shen *Radix Codonopsis pilosulae* 9 g
Bai Zhu *Rhizoma Atractylodis macrocephalae* 9 g
Fu Ling *Sclerotium Poriae cocos* 12 g
Gan Jiang *Rhizoma Zingiberis officinalis* 6 g
Fu Zi *Radix Aconiti carmichaeli praeparata* 6 g
Hou Po *Cortex Magnoliae officinalis* 9 g
Da Fu Pi *Pericarpium Arecae catechu* 9 g
Che Qian Zi *Semen Plantaginis* 9 g
Mu Xiang *Radix Saussureae* 6 g

Explanation

- **Huang Qi**, **Dang Shen**, **Bai Zhu** and **Fu Ling** tonify the Spleen and drain Dampness.
- **Gan Jiang** and **Fu Zi** warm the Spleen and Kidneys and thus help to resolve Dampness and oedema.
- **Hou Po**, **Da Fu Pi** and **Che Qian Zi** transform and drain Dampness. Da Fu Pi resolves oedema.
- **Mu Xiang** moves Qi. Because the moving-Qi action helps to eliminate Dampness, one or two moving-Qi herbs are often added to such a prescription.

(i) Patent remedy

BU ZHONG YI QI WAN
Tonifying the Centre and Benefiting Qi Pill
Huang Qi *Radix Astragali membranacei*
Dang Shen *Radix Codonopsis pilosulae*
Zhi Gan Cao *Radix Glycyrrhizae uralensis praeparata*
Bai Zhu *Rhizoma Atractylodis macrocephalae*
Dang Gui *Radix Angelicae sinensis*
Chen Pi *Pericarpium Citri reticulatae*
Sheng Ma *Rhizoma Cimicifugae*
Chai Hu *Radix Bupleuri*
Sheng Jiang *Rhizoma Zingiberis officinalis recens*
Da Zao *Fructus Ziziphi jujubae*

Explanation

This remedy tonifies and raises Qi. The tongue presentation appropriate to this remedy is a Pale tongue.

(ii) Patent remedy

SHEN LING BAI ZHU WAN (PIAN)
Ginseng-Poria-Atractylodes Pill (Tablet)
Ren Shen *Radix Ginseng* (or Dang Shen *Radix Codonopsis pilosulae*)
Fu Ling *Sclerotium Poriae cocos*
Bai Zhu *Rhizoma Atractylodis macrocephalae*
Jie Geng *Radix Platycodi grandiflori*
Shan Yao *Radix Dioscoreae oppositae*
Chen Pi *Pericarpium Citri reticulatae*
Sha Ren *Fructus seu Semen Amomi*
Lian Zi *Semen Nelumbinis nuciferae*
Bian Dou *Semen Dolichoris lablab*
Yi Yi Ren *Semen Coicis lachryma jobi*
Zhi Gan Cao *Radix Glycyrrhizae uralensis praeparata*

Explanation

This remedy tonifies Lung-, Stomach- and Spleen-Qi and resolves Dampness.

The tongue presentation appropriate to this remedy is a Pale tongue with a rootless coating in the centre.

(iii) Patent remedy

FU ZI LI ZHONG WAN
Aconitum Regulating the Centre Pill
Gan Jiang *Rhizoma Zingiberis officinalis*
Bai Zhu *Rhizoma Atractylodis macrocephalae*
Dang Shen *Radix Codonopsis pilosulae*
Gan Cao *Radix Glycyrrhizae uralensis*
Fu Zi *Radix Aconiti carmichaeli praeparata*

Explanation

This remedy tonifies Spleen- and Kidney-Yang. The tongue presentation appropriate to this remedy is a Pale and wet body.

2. SPLEEN- AND KIDNEY-YANG DEFICIENCY, WATER OVERFLOWING

This pattern is almost the same as the previous one, characterized by deficiency of Yang of the Spleen and Kidneys. The main difference is that there is pronounced oedema (called "Water overflowing"). When Spleen- and Kidney-Yang are deficient they fail to transform, transport and excrete fluids, so that these accumulate and give rise to oedema. Severe deficiency of Kidney-Yang also involves failing of the Fire of the Gate of Vitality. When this Fire is deficient it fails to warm the organs which rely on heat for their physiological functions: thus the Bladder is unable to transform urine and becomes cold, the Lower Burner fails to transform and excrete fluids and the Small Intestine cannot separate fluids.

Clinical manifestations

A sallow complexion, anaemia, oedema of the whole body, ache in the lower back, abdominal fullness, chilliness, mental depression, loose stools, cold limbs, scanty or profuse urine, pronounced albuminuria, a Pale and Swollen tongue and a Deep and Weak pulse.

All these are clear symptoms and signs of severe Spleen- and Kidney-Yang deficiency. When the Yang of these two organs is deficient the urine is usually abundant and clear. However, in severe cases, Kidney-Yang can be so deficient that it does not transport fluids to the Bladder at all and the urination becomes scanty. This condition may be clearly differentiated from scanty urination due to Kidney-Yin deficiency, from the absence of thirst.

Principle of treatment

Warm the Kidneys, strengthen Yang, stoke the Fire of the Gate of Vitality, strengthen the Spleen, eliminate Water.

Acupuncture

The acupuncture treatment for this pattern would be almost exactly the same as for the previous one, with only two differences. First of all, more moxa would be needed and the point Du-4 Mingmen should be added (with moxa) to strongly tonify and warm the Fire of the Gate of Vitality. Secondly, the points used to eliminate oedema should be needled with reducing method because the pathogenic factor (in this case "Water overflowing") is strong and predominant.

Herbal treatment

(a) Prescription

ZHEN WU TANG Variation
True Warrior Decoction Variation
Fu Zi *Radix Aconiti carmichaeli praeparata* 10 g
Bai Zhu *Rhizoma Atractylodis macrocephalae* 12 g
Fu Ling *Sclerotium Poriae cocos* 15 g
Bai Shao *Radix Paeoniae albae* 6 g
Sheng Jiang *Rhizoma Zingiberis officinalis recens* 3 slices
Ze Xie *Rhizoma Alismatis orientalis* 12 g
Dong Gua Pi *Cortex Fructi Benincasae hispidae* 12 g
Yu Mi Xu *Stylus Zeae mays* 30 g

Explanation

The first five herbs form the *True Warrior Decoction* which is specific for oedema from Spleen- and Kidney-Yang deficiency.

– **Ze Xie**, **Dong Gua Pi** and **Yu Mi Xu** all drain Dampness and resolve oedema.

(b) Prescription

ZHEN WU TANG and WU LING SAN
True Warrior Decoction and *Five "Ling" Powder*
Fu Zi *Radix Aconiti carmichaeli praeparata* 9 g
Bai Zhu *Rhizoma Atractylodis macrocephalae* 15 g
Fu Ling *Sclerotium Poriae cocos* 12 g
Bai Shao *Radix Paeoniae albae* 12 g
Sheng Jiang *Rhizoma Zingiberis officinalis recens* 9 g
Zhu Ling *Sclerotium Polypori umbellati* 9 g
Ze Xie *Rhizoma Alismatis orientalis* 6 g
Gui Zhi *Ramulus Cinnamomi cassiae* 6 g

Explanation

The first five herbs make up the prescription Zhen Wu Tang which tonifies Kidney-Yang and resolves oedema. The last three herbs are part of the prescription Wu Ling San which drains Dampness and promotes diuresis; its other two ingredients, Bai Zhu *Rhizoma Atractylodis macrocephalae* and Fu Ling *Sclerotium Poriae cocos*, are already included as they form part of Zhen Wu Tang.

(c) Prescription

BU QI YI SHEN TANG
Tonify Qi and Benefit the Kidneys Decoction
Dang Shen *Radix Codonopsis pilosulae* 30 g
Huang Qi *Radix Astragali membranacei* 15 g
Fu Zi *Radix Aconiti carmichaeli praeparata* 10 g
Yin Yang Huo *Herba Epimedii* 9 g
Chai Hu *Radix Bupleuri* 6 g
Chi Shao *Radix Paeoniae rubrae* 12 g
Chuan Xiong *Radix Ligustici wallichii* 6 g
Yi Mu Cao *Herba Leonori heterophylli* 9 g
Da Huang *Rhizoma Rhei* 3 g
San Qi *Radix Notoginseng* 3 g

Explanation

– **Dang Shen** and **Huang Qi** tonify Spleen Qi. Huang Qi also resolves oedema.
– **Fu Zi** and **Yin Yang Huo** tonify and warm Kidney-Yang.
– **Chai Hu** moves Qi. It is added here to move Qi in order to move Blood.
– **Chi Shao**, **Chuan Xiong**, **Yi Mu Cao**, **Da Huang** and **San Qi** all move Blood. Moving-Blood herbs are used here because stasis of Blood can contribute to the formation of oedema (see above).

(d) Prescription

GUI FU LI ZHONG TANG and JIN GUI SHEN QI WAN Variation
Cinnamomum-Aconitum Regulating the Centre Decoction and *Golden Chest Kidney-Qi Pill* Variation
Fu Zi *Radix Aconiti carmichaeli praeparata* 6 g
Rou Gui *Cortex Cinnamomi cassiae* 6 g
Bai Zhu *Rhizoma Atractylodis macrocephalae* 9 g
Gan Jiang *Rhizoma Zingiberis officinalis* 3 g
Shu Di Huang *Radix Rehmanniae glutinosae praeparata* 12 g
Shan Zhu Yu *Fructus Corni officinalis* 6 g

Shan Yao *Radix Dioscoreae oppositae* 12 g
Fu Ling *Sclerotium Poriae cocos* 12 g
Ze Xie *Rhizoma Alismatis orientalis* 9 g

Explanation

The prescription Li Zhong Tang tonifies Spleen-Yang and expels Cold. Its variation Gui Fu Li Zhong Tang tonifies both Spleen and Kidney Yang. The prescription Jin Gui Shen Qi Wan (from which Mu Dan Pi *Cortex Moutan radicis* has been eliminated) tonifies Kidney-Yang.

Patent remedy

JIN GUI SHEN QI WAN
Golden Chest Kidney-Qi Pill

Explanation

This pill, already mentioned above under Yin Oedema, tonifies and warms Kidney-Yang.

The tongue presentation appropriate to this remedy is a Pale and wet body.

3. SPLEEN-KIDNEY YANG DEFICIENCY, YIN REBELLING UPWARDS

Clinical manifestations

This pattern is basically the same as the previous one, the only difference being that it is character-ized by uprising of Yin (or "Water") in the chest causing nausea and vomiting. These two symp-toms distinguish this pattern from the previous one.

Other clinical manifestations include a greyish complexion, a feeling of oppression of the chest, abdominal distension, constipation and scanty urination in addition to other common symp-toms and signs of Spleen- and Kidney-Yang deficiency (see previous pattern). The tongue would be Pale and Swollen with a sticky-white coating and the pulse would be Deep and Slow.

Principle of treatment

Warm the Yang, subdue rebellious Yin.

Acupuncture

BL-20 Pishu, BL-23 Shenshu, SP-4 Gongsun and P-6 Neiguan, Ren-13 Shangwan, Ren-17 Shanzhong, Ren-9 Shuifen, LU-5 Chize, Du-4 Mingmen, KI-7 Fuliu. Moxa should be used.

Explanation

- **BL-20**, **BL-23**, **Du-4** and **KI-7** tonify and warm Spleen and Kidneys.
- **SP-4** and **P-6** are the opening points of the Penetrating vessel and, as such, they open the chest and relieve stagnation in the upper part of the body.
- **Ren-13** subdues rebellious Stomach-Qi and stops vomiting.
- **Ren-17** opens the chest and stimulates the descending of Lung-Qi.
- **Ren-9** promotes the transformation of fluids and resolves oedema.
- **LU-5** resolves Phlegm from the Lungs and stimulates the descending of Lung-Qi.

Herbal treatment

Prescription

Empirical prescription
Fu Zi *Radix Aconiti carmichaeli praeparata* 9 g
Dang Shen *Radix Codonopsis pilosulae* 15 g
Fu Ling *Sclerotium Poriae cocos* 15 g
Chen Pi *Pericarpium Citri reticulatae* 6 g
Hou Po *Cortex Magnoliae officinalis* 3 g
Ban Xia *Rhizoma Pinelliae ternatae* 9 g
Da Huang *Rhizoma Rhei* 9 g
Sheng Jiang *Rhizoma Zingiberis officinalis recens* 9 g

Explanation

- **Fu Zi** tonifies Kidney-Yang.
- **Dang Shen** tonifies Spleen-Yang.
- **Fu Ling**, **Chen Pi** and **Hou Po** drain and transform Dampness.
- **Ban Xia** subdues rebellious Qi and stops nausea and vomiting.
- **Da Huang** promotes the bowel movements and thus helps to resolve oedema by purging.
- **Sheng Jiang** warms the Yang and helps to stop nausea and vomiting.

4. SPLEEN AND KIDNEY DEFICIENCY, ESSENCE LEAKING

Clinical manifestations

This pattern is characterized by severe and chronic deficiency of Spleen and Kidneys and pronounced albuminuria. As explained above, the presence of protein in the urine is seen in Chinese medicine as a leakage of Kidney-Essence.

Other clinical manifestations include a withered and sallow complexion, mental depression, soreness of the lower back, weakness of the knees, a Pale tongue and a Weak Pulse.

Principle of treatment

Strengthen the Spleen, tonify Kidney-Yang, nourish Yin and Essence.

Acupuncture

The same as for the previous pattern.

Herbal treatment

Prescription

JIN GUI SHEN QI WAN and WU ZI YAN ZONG WAN Variation
Golden Chest Kidney-Qi Pill and *Five-Seed Developing Ancestors Pill* Variation
Sheng Di Huang *Radix Rehmanniae glutinosae* 12 g
Shu Di Huang *Radix Rehmanniae glutinosae praeparata* 12 g
Shan Zhu Yu *Fructus Corni officinalis* 6 g
Shan Yao *Radix Dioscoreae oppositae* 12 g
Rou Gui *Cortex Cinnamomi cassiae* 3 g
Huang Qi *Radix Astragali membranacei* 12 g
Dang Shen *Radix Codonopsis pilosulae* 15 g
Bai Zhu *Rhizoma Atractylodis macrocephalae* 9 g
Fu Ling *Sclerotium Poriae cocos* 15 g
Gou Qi Zi *Fructus Lycii chinensis* 12 g
Tu Si Zi *Semen Cuscutae* 15 g
Jin Ying Zi *Fructus Rosae laevigatae* 9 g
Lu Jiao Shuang *Cornu Cervi deglutinatum* 15 g

Explanation

- **Sheng Di**, **Shu Di**, **Shan Zhu Yu** and **Shan Yao** nourish Liver- and Kidney-Yin.

- **Rou Gui** warms Kidney-Yang.
- **Huang Qi**, **Dang Shen**, **Bai Zhu** and **Fu Ling** tonify the Spleen and drain Dampness.
- **Gou Qi Zi**, **Tu Si Zi**, **Jin Ying Zi** and **Lu Jiao Shuang** consolidate the Kidneys and nourish Essence.

5. KIDNEY- AND HEART-YANG DEFICIENCY QI-BLOOD STAGNANT

Clinical manifestations

This pattern is seen only in old people with severe deficiency of Kidney- and Heart-Yang causing Phlegm-Fluids to overflow upwards towards the Heart.

There are some symptoms and signs of Kidney-Yang deficiency such as a lower back-ache, difficulty in walking, chilliness, tinnitus, dizziness, blurred vision, profuse urination at night, a Pale tongue and a Deep and Weak pulse. The symptoms and signs of Heart-Yang deficiency with Phlegm-Fluids overflowing are palpitations, breathlessness and a dull headache. The headache is due to failure of Heart Qi and Blood to reach the head.

When Yang is deficient over a long period of time, it often gives rise to stasis of Blood. The main manifestations of this would be pain in the limbs and a Bluish-Purple tongue. Due to the interchange between Blood and Body Fluids, the stasis of Blood contributes to the derangement of Body Fluids and oedema.

Principle of treatment

Tonify Kidney and Heart, warm the Yang.

Acupuncture

- Reinforce ST-36 Zusanli, KI-7 Fuliu, Pishu BL-20 and Shenshu BL-23 to tonify Spleen- and Kidney-Yang. Moxa must be used.
- Reinforce BL-15 Xinshu to tonify Heart-Yang (with moxa).
- Reduce (or even method) SP-6 Sanyinjiao, SP-9 Yinlingquan, BL-22 Sanjiaoshu, ST-28 Shuidao and Ren-9 Shuifen to eliminate Dampness and oedema.

Herbal treatment

Prescription

YI SHEN TONG MAI TANG
Benefit the Kidneys-Penetrate the Blood Vessels Decoction
Hong Shen *Radix Ginseng (Red Ginseng)* 6 g
Gou Qi Zi *Fructus Lycii chinensis* 10 g
Shan Zhu Yu *Fructus Corni officinalis* 6 g
Fu Ling *Sclerotium Poriae cocos* 15 g
Dang Gui *Radix Angelicae sinensis* 12 g
Chi Shao *Radix Paeoniae rubrae* 6 g
Hong Hua *Flos Carthami tinctorii* 6 g
Ze Lan *Herba Lycopi lucidi* 6 g
Wang Bu Liu Xing *Semen Vaccariae segetalis* 15 g
Chuan Xiong *Radix Ligustici wallichii* 12 g
Dan Shen *Radix Salviae miltiorrhizae* 12 g
Gui Zhi *Ramulus Cinnamomi cassiae* 4.5 g

Explanation

- **Hong Shen** tonifies Spleen- and Kidney-Yang.
- **Gou Qi Zi** and **Shan Zhu Yu** tonify Liver and Kidneys.
- **Fu Ling** expels Dampness.
- **Dang Gui**, **Chi Shao**, **Hong Hua**, **Ze Lan**, **Wang Bu Liu Xing**, **Chuan Xiong** and **Dan Shen** move Blood.
- **Gui Zhi** moves Yang, which is necessary to move fluids.

Patent remedy

DU ZHONG BU TIAN SU
Eucommia Benefiting Heaven Pill
Du Zhong *Cortex Eucommiae ulmoidis*
Gou Qi Zi *Fructus Lycii chinensis*
Huang Qi *Radix Astragali membranacei*
Dang Shen *Radix Codonopsis pilosulae*
Dang Gui *Radix Angelicae sinensis*
Sheng Di Huang *Radix Rehmanniae glutinosae*
Ba Ji Tian *Radix Morindae officinalis*
Shan Zhu Yu *Fructus Corni officinalis*
Rou Cong Rong *Herba Cistanchis*
Lian Zi *Semen Nelumbinis nuciferae*
Bai Zi Ren *Semen Biotae orientalis*

Explanation

This remedy tonifies Kidney-Yang, strengthens the Essence, and nourishes Heart-Blood.

The tongue presentation appropriate to this remedy is a Pale and Thin body.

Prevention

DIET

The most important dietary precaution to take is to avoid excessive consumption of salt and drinking too much. A small amount of salt is essential to health and, from the Chinese dietary point of view, it tonifies the Kidneys. In excess, however, salt harms both the Kidneys and the Heart and it dries Blood. This drying effect can lead to further derangement of Body Fluids and therefore aggravate oedema.

Excessive drinking also weakens the Kidneys. Many people erroneously believe that drinking large amounts of fluid "flushes" the Kidneys. All that it does is to put an extra strain on the Kidneys; eventually this weakens them. Drinking in excess, especially drinking cold fluids, will weaken the Kidneys and may aggravate oedema. Of course, the opposite is also true. Some people following certain diets advocate drastically cutting down the amount of fluids ingested. This is also mistaken and can be dangerous.

REST

No method of treatment is more obvious and yet more ignored than simple rest. This means short periods of resting, preferably lying down, alternated with periods of work. In the particular case of the Kidneys, lying down increases the flow of blood through the glomeruli and therefore helps the kidney function. From a Chinese viewpoint, resting is essential to restore the Kidney and Liver energy. If a person with a Kidney deficiency leads a very hectic life and overworks, no therapy will ever be completely successful without adequate rest. For a complete discussion of this question see the chapter on "Tiredness" (ch. 12).

END NOTES

1. 1979 The Yellow Emperor's Classic of Internal Medicine — Simple Questions (*Huang Ti Nei Jing Su Wen* 黄帝内经素问), People's Health Publishing House, Beijing. First published *c.* 100 BC, p. 326.
2. Ibid., p. 538.
3. Chao Yuan Fang AD 610 General Treatise on the Aetiology and Symptomatology of Diseases (*Zhu Bing Yuan Hou Lun* 诸病源候论), cited in Internal Medicine, p. 221.
4. Zhu Dan Xi 1481 Essential Methods of Dan Xi (*Dan Xi Xin Fa* 丹溪心法), cited in Internal Medicine, p. 221.
5. 1981 Spiritual Axis (*Ling Shu Jing* 灵枢经), People's Health Publishing House, Beijing. First published *c.* 100 BC, p. 75.
6. Yao Jiu Jiang 1989 in Journal of Chinese Medicine (*Zhong Yi Za Zhi* 中医杂志), Vol. 30, no. 8, p. 16.
7. Discussion of the Essential Prescriptions of the Golden Chest (*Jin Gui Yao Lue Fang Lun* 金匮要略方论) *c.* AD 220 cited in Li Tao Hua 1979 Patterns and Treatment of Kidney Diseases (*Shen Yu Shen Bing de Zheng Zhi* 肾与肾病的证治) Hebei People's Publishing House, Hebei, p. 87.
8. Tang Zong Hai 1884 "Discussion on Blood" (*Xue Zheng Lun* 血证论) in "Patterns and Treatment of Kidney Diseases", p. 87.
9. Yao Jiu Jiang 1989 in Journal of Chinese Medicine, op. cit., p. 16.

Painful Obstruction Syndrome 23 痹症

"Painful Obstruction Syndrome" indicates pain, soreness or numbness of muscles, tendons and joints from invasion of external Wind, Cold or Dampness. It is probably the most universal of all diseases affecting practically everyone at some time or another of one's life in all parts of the globe. Due to exposure to climatic factors, it is probably also one of the oldest afflictions of mankind. Painful Obstruction Syndrome is called *"Bi"*, which evokes the idea of "obstruction". In Chinese medicine it means pain, soreness or numbness due to obstruction in the circulation of Qi and Blood in the channels caused by invasion of exterior Wind, Cold or Dampness. The "Origin of Complicated Diseases" (1773) says:

Bi means obstruction. The three evils [Wind, Cold and Dampness] invade the body, obstruct the channels, Qi and Blood cannot circulate . . . [so that] after some time Painful Obstruction Syndrome develops.[1]

The invasion of external climatic factors is due to a pre-existing and temporary deficiency of the body's Qi and Blood which allows the Wind, Cold and Dampness to penetrate. The "Discussion on the Origin of All Illnesses" (AD 610) says:

Painful Obstruction Syndrome is due to the combined invasion of Wind, Cold and Dampness, causing swelling and pain. It is due to a weak body condition and the space between skin and muscles being open, which allows the Wind to penetrate.[2]

In another chapter it says: *Painful Obstruction Syndrome is due to deficiency of Qi and Blood which allows Wind to penetrate.*

The "Treatment Strategies for Assorted Syndromes" (1839) says:

Painful Obstruction Syndrome . . . is due to deficiency of Nutritive and Defensive Qi and to the space between skin and muscles being open, thus allowing Wind-Cold-Dampness to ride the deficiency. Qi becomes obstructed by the pathogenic factors, it cannot circulate, it stagnates, Qi and Blood congeal, and in time Painful Obstruction Syndrome develops.[3]

Thus, the relative strength of the climatic pathogenic factors and the body's Qi at any given time is crucial to the development of Painful Obstruction Syndrome. This explains why we can be exposed to climatic factors every day for long periods without developing Painful Obstruction Syndrome. It is only when the climatic factors are *temporarily* and *relatively* stronger than our body's Qi, that they become pathogenic and cause Painful Obstruction Syndrome.

It is important to stress however, that the deficiency of body's Qi necessary for the development of Painful Obstruction Syndrome is only *relative*, i.e. in relation to the strength of climatic pathogenic factors. It is not an absolute deficiency, otherwise that would mean that anyone who develops Painful Obstruction Syndrome suffers from deficiency of Qi or Blood, which is not the case. Thus, Painful Obstruction Syndrome is an affliction of the *channels alone*, not the internal organs.

However, in chronic Painful Obstruction Syndrome and in the elderly, internal factors (deficiency of Qi and Blood) are important contributory factors to the development of the disease as will be explained shortly.

Painful Obstruction Syndrome is by definition an affliction of the channels rather than the internal organs. The pain and soreness are caused by obstruction in the circulation of Qi and Blood in the channels by exterior Wind, Cold or Dampness. It may be useful here to revise the structure of main and secondary channels and the energetic role of the Five Transporting points on the limbs as this will be relevant when we discuss the treatment of Painful Obstruction Syndrome.

To each main channel corresponds a network of secondary channels formed by Connecting channels, Muscle channels and Cutaneous Regions.

The *Connecting channels* (*Luo* channels) connect the Yin and Yang paired channels at the level of the limbs. For example, the Lung and Large Intestine channels are connected in the forearm via their respective Connecting points, LU-7 Lieque and L.I.-6 Pianli respectively. More important than this, in the context of Painful Obstruction Syndrome, the Connecting channels represent a network which distributes Qi to more superficial parts of the body, not covered by the main channels. For this reason the Connecting channels are called *Luo Mai* as opposed to *Jing Mai* which are the main channels. *Luo* conveys the idea of "net", whilst *Jing* conveys the idea of longitudinal line. Thus the main channels are longitudinal lines, whilst the Connecting channels are a network of channels irrigating the more superficial regions of the body. In particular, the Connecting channels branch out into a smaller network of tiny channels of which there are three types, the Minute, Superficial and Blood channels.

Any external manifestation on the skin is a reflection of an imbalance in these smaller channels. For example a discolouration on the skin reflects the presence of a pathogenic factor in the Superficial channels, bluish or greenish indicating Cold, and red indicating Heat. Small venules appearing on the skin reflect the state of the Blood channels, red indicating Heat in the Blood and purple indicating stasis of Blood.

The *Muscle channels* basically integrate muscles and sinews within the channel system. They are also more superficial than the main channels and run alongside muscles. They are involved in any muscular pathology such as muscular weakness or stiffness that may appear in Painful Obstruction Syndrome.

The *Cutaneous regions* represent twelve areas of the skin under the influence of the twelve channels. They are the most superficial areas of the channels and the zones through which pathogenic factors penetrate the body to cause Painful Obstruction Syndrome. They are, of course, also the areas through which therapy is effected by inserting the acupuncture needles.

Of the Transporting points along the channels below elbows and knees, three are particularly important in the pathogenesis and treatment of Painful Obstruction Syndrome.

The *Stream* (*Shu*) point is the point at which external pathogenic factors such as Cold, Dampness and Wind penetrate the channel. It is also the point of concentration of Defensive Qi.

The *River* (*Jing*) point is the point from which pathogenic factors are deviated to joints and sinews where they settle. This is why pathogenic factors can settle in a joint for a long time without penetrating deeper and affecting the internal organs.

The *Connecting* (*Luo*) point is the starting point of the Connecting channel. Since these channels flow in the surface affecting muscles and sinews, the Connecting point has an important application in the treatment of Painful Obstruction Syndrome.

Within the flow of Qi dynamics, joints are important areas of convergence of Qi and Blood. Through joints, Yin- and Yang-Qi meet, Exterior and Interior converge and Qi and Blood enter and exit. Joints are also the places where pathogenic factors converge after penetrating the channels, causing obstruction to the flow of Qi and hence local stagnation of Qi and Blood. This stagnation accounts for the pain caused by external pathogenic factors in Painful Obstruction Syndrome. Invasion of pathogenic factors is made easier if the body condition is weak leading to malnourishment of the joints. It is also made easier if the joints are weakened by over-use through work or certain sports. In these cases, the external pathogenic factors penetrate the body and settle in the joints more easily due to the pre-existing condition of deficiency of Qi and Blood.

Finally, the anatomical entity *Cou Li* described in ancient texts should be mentioned. The term *Cou Li* indicates on the one hand the striae of skin, muscles and internal organs, and on the other hand, the "space between the skin and muscles". It is with this last meaning that the term is used in the context of Painful Obstruction Syndrome. The "space between skin and muscles" is the space where body fluids circulate (giving rise to sweat) and where Defensive Qi moves, protecting the body from external pathogenic factors. When the Defensive Qi is deficient and the body condition is weak, the space between skin and muscles is said to be "open" and thus prone to invasion of Wind, Cold and Dampness.

Aetiology

This is by definition invasion of external pathogenic factors such as Wind, Cold or Dampness.

Wind is the most pernicious of all pathogenic factors and one that is almost always combined with the others. Exposure to wind is an extremely important cause of Painful Obstruction Syndrome. Even though in modern industrial societies housing is generally good and our life is relatively more sheltered from climatic pathogenic factors, dictates of fashion or simply ignorance lead many people to be exposed to disease-inducing weather conditions. For example, people living in cold and rainy countries may tend to be over-enthusiastic at the slightest spell of sunny weather and wear very little clothing even though temperatures may still be low. It is also not infrequent to see joggers running in extremely cold and damp weather with very little on: they also sweat profusely which opens the pores and facilitates the invasion of external Wind, Cold and Dampness.

Some doctors think that "Wind" as an aetiological factor in Chinese Medicine indicates a sudden change of weather and the consequent inability of the body to adapt to it, rather than actual wind. The body is more prone to invasion of Wind during spells of unseasonable weather: this applies not only when it is unseasonably cold, but also when it is unseasonably warm.

Apart from being exposed to adverse weather conditions, Painful Obstruction Syndrome can of course develop also from exposure to other conditions, such as sitting on damp surfaces, wading in water, living in a damp environment, etc.

Although the only aetiological factor in Painful Obstruction Syndrome is weather, there are other predisposing factors. First of all, excessive sport or work activities may predispose one to develop Painful Obstruction Syndrome. For example, excessive aerobic exercise or jogging may put a strain on the spine and lead to backache. The constant repetition of a certain movement in one's work is an obvious predisposing factor too, as this causes stagnation of Qi and Blood in an area which becomes more prone to invasion of exterior pathogenic factors. For example, the wrists in car mechanics become prone to stagnation of Qi and Blood through repeated use of wrenches, spanners and screw-drivers.

Another very important predisposing factor is an underlying deficiency of Blood or Yin which leads to malnourishment of the channels so that they become prone to invasion of external pathogenic factors. Particularly in chronic Painful Obstruction Syndrome or in the elderly, an underlying deficiency of Blood or Yin is nearly always a factor. In treatment, it is important not only to expel Wind, Cold or Damp, but also to nourish Blood or Yin.

Accidents also predispose one to Painful Obstruction Syndrome. An accident causes either stagnation of Qi (if light) or Blood (if serious) in an area. Even though one may seemingly recover perfectly well after an accident, some stagnation of Blood may remain in the area. Years later, exposure to external pathogenic factors leads to the development of Painful Obstruction Syndrome in that particular area. This often explains the unilateral development of Painful Obstruction Syndrome as the climatic factors of Wind, Cold or Dampness settle in the area where there is a pre-existing condition of stagnation of Blood caused by the accident.

Finally, emotional problems are also contributing factors in the origin of Painful Obstruction Syndrome either by causing stagnation of Qi (such as from anger or resentment) which affects the channels, or by causing depletion of Qi and Blood (such as from sadness, grief and shock) which leads to malnourishment of the channels.

Differentiation

Since very ancient times Painful Obstruction Syndrome has been classified according to the predominant pathogenic factor, i.e. Wind, Cold or Dampness. For example the "Simple Questions" in chapter 43 says: *"The three pathogenic factors of Wind, Cold and Dampness give rise to Painful Obstruction Syndrome".*[4] Zhang Jie Bin (1563–1640) says:

Painful Obstruction Syndrome means obstruction . . . Wind-Cold-Dampness obstruct the channels, Qi and Blood cannot circulate properly. Wind moves and changes rapidly and causes Wandering Painful Obstruction Syndrome. Cold (a Yin pathogenic factor) invades the muscles, tendons and bones, it gathers and knots and is difficult to disperse; this obstructs the movement of Yang-Qi which causes severe pain and hence Painful Obstruction Syndrome. Fixed Painful Obstruction Syndrome [is characterized by] heaviness, obstruction to circulation and pain caused by Dampness in the muscles.[5]

There are therefore three main types according to causative factor:

1. WIND PAINFUL OBSTRUCTION SYNDROME (OR WANDERING PAINFUL OBSTRUCTION SYNDROME)

This is caused by Wind and is characterized by soreness and pain of muscles and joints, limitation of movement, with the pain moving from joint to joint. In acute cases the pulse would be Floating and slightly Rapid.

2. DAMP PAINFUL OBSTRUCTION SYNDROME (OR FIXED PAINFUL OBSTRUCTION SYNDROME)

This is caused by Dampness and is characterized by pain, soreness and swelling in muscles and joints with a feeling of heaviness and numbness of the limbs, the pain being fixed in one place and aggravated by damp weather. In acute cases the pulse would be Slow and slightly Slippery.

3. COLD PAINFUL OBSTRUCTION SYNDROME (OR ACHING PAINFUL OBSTRUCTION SYNDROME)

This is caused by Cold and is characterized by a severe pain in a joint or muscle with limitation of movement, usually unilateral. In acute cases the pulse is Tight.

4. HEAT PAINFUL OBSTRUCTION SYNDROME

This originates from any of the previous three types when the exterior pathogenic factor turns into Heat in the Interior and gives rise to Heat Painful Obstruction Syndrome. This happens especially with an underlying deficiency of Yin.

It is characterized by pain and heat in the joints which feel hot to the touch, redness and swelling of joints, limitation of movement and severe pain. In acute cases there would be thirst, a fever which does not abate after sweating and a Slippery and Rapid pulse.

In this case, sweating does not bring the temperature down or reduce the pain because it is due to Damp-Heat. Thus, this syndrome is characterized not just by Heat, but Damp-Heat. In fact, Dampness is the primary aspect of this syndrome and Heat the secondary one.

5. BONE PAINFUL OBSTRUCTION SYNDROME

This only occurs in chronic cases and develops from any of the previous four types. Persistent obstruction of the joints by pathogenic factors leads to retention of body fluids which turn into Phlegm which further obstructs the joints and channels. This leads to muscular atrophy and swelling and deformity of the bones in the joints, which is an extreme form of Phlegm. At this stage, Painful Obstruction Syndrome becomes an interior syndrome affecting not only muscles, joints and channels, but also the internal organs.

In prolonged cases of Bone Painful Obstruction Syndrome other pathological conditions may play a part in the development of the disease. First of all, the obstruction in the circulation of Qi, Blood and Body Fluids caused by Phlegm may lead to stasis of Blood. The stasis of Blood in the channels further obstructs proper circulation and therefore is another cause of pain. In many cases of chronic Painful Obstruction Syndrome, stasis of Blood is a factor. For example, Cold and Dampness are frequent causes of Painful Obstruction Syndrome of the lower back. After repeated episodes of invasion of the lower back by Cold and Dampness, the prolonged retention of pathogenic factors may lead to chronic stasis of Blood in the area. The ache then becomes more or less constant and more severe. Stasis of Blood also causes pronounced stiffness due to stagnant Blood not nourishing and moistening sinews.

Finally, another important factor in chronic Painful Obstruction Syndrome is deficiency of the Liver and Kidneys. It is this deficiency that allows the retention of Phlegm and stasis of Blood. Liver-Blood nourishes the sinews and

when the Liver is deficient the sinews and tendons are not nourished, which leads to ache and stiffness of joints. The Kidneys nourish bones and when they are deficient the bones are deprived of nourishment and this allows Phlegm to build up in the joints in the form of swellings.

To sum up, the factors which may be present in chronic Painful Obstruction Syndrome are as follows (see also Fig. 23.1, p. 571):

(i) a general deficiency of Qi and Blood which predisposes the body to invasions of external pathogenic factors
(ii) the formation of Phlegm in the joints in the form of swellings due to improper transformation of Body Fluids
(iii) stasis of Blood due to the long-standing obstruction in the circulation of Blood caused both by the external pathogenic factors and by Phlegm
(iv) deficiency of Liver and Kidneys which leads to malnourishment of sinews and bones, the former causing ache and stiffness, the latter contributing to the settling of Phlegm in the joints.

To summarize the five types of Painful Obstruction Syndrome in a nutshell, we can say:

1. *Wind Painful Obstruction Syndrome*: pain moving from joint to joint
2. *Damp Painful Obstruction Syndrome*: fixed pain with soreness, heaviness, numbness and swelling of the joints
3. *Cold Painful Obstruction Syndrome*: severe pain in one joint
4. *Heat Painful Obstruction Syndrome*: very severe pain, hot-red-swollen joints
5. *Bony Painful Obstruction Syndrome*: painful joints with swelling and bone deformities.

However, having differentiated Painful Obstruction Syndrome according to the causative pathogenic factor, most doctors agree that all three factors (Wind, Cold and Dampness) are present in *every* case, and each case can only be differentiated according to the predominance of one factor over the others. This consideration is important in treatment, especially in treatment with herbs. In fact, although herbal prescriptions for Painful Obstruction Syndrome put the emphasis on expelling one of the pathogenic factors, many of them include herbs to expel the other two.

A different classification of Painful Obstruction Syndrome appears in the "Yellow Emperor's Classic of Internal Medicine — Simple Questions". The "Simple Questions" in chapter 43 classifies Painful Obstruction Syndrome according to the tissue and organ affected. It says:

The 5 Yin organs are related to the five tissues where a chronic disease can lodge itself. In Bone Painful Obstruction Syndrome the pathogenic factor reaches the Kidneys; in Sinew Painful Obstruction Syndrome it reaches the Liver; in Blood Vessel Painful Obstruction Syndrome it reaches the Heart; in Muscle Painful Obstruction Syndrome it reaches the Spleen and in Skin Painful Obstruction Syndrome it reaches the Lungs.[6]

It then says:

Painful Obstruction Syndrome in the bones is serious, in the blood vessels it leads to Blood stasis, in the sinews it causes stiffness, in the muscles it leads to weakness and in the skin it causes Cold.[7]

The "Simple Questions" thus classifies Painful Obstruction Syndrome according to the tissue affected and it deduces which tissue is affected by the main manifestation, i.e. bone deformities in Bone Painful Obstruction Syndrome, Blood stasis in Blood Vessel Painful Obstruction Syndrome, stiffness in Sinew Painful Obstruction Syndrome, weakness in Muscle Painful Obstruction Syndrome and feeling of cold in Skin Painful Obstruction Syndrome. It also determines a difference in severity among the different types. In the same chapter it says:

When Painful Obstruction Syndrome affects the organs it causes death, when it is situated in the bones or sinews it becomes chronic, when it is situated in the muscles or skin it easily goes.[8]

Treatment

The aim of the treatment is simply to expel the pathogenic factors which have invaded the channels, and eliminate the resulting local stagnation of Qi and Blood in the channels.

The treatment of Painful Obstruction Syndrome is a channel treatment by definition and it only involves treating the internal organs as a secondary aim. The most obvious and notable exception to this, however, is chronic Painful Obstruction Syndrome which does require treatment of the internal organs too.

As a general principle, since the three pathogenic factors of Wind, Cold and Dampness are usually all present in Painful Obstruction Syndrome (although with the predominance of one or two), the treatment is aimed at expelling Wind, scattering Cold and resolving Dampness. The "Essential Readings from Medical Masters" (1637) says:

To treat Wind Painful Obstruction Syndrome principally expel Wind, but secondarily also scatter Cold and resolve Dampness and also nourish Blood. To extinguish Wind, treat Blood; if Blood is harmonized, Wind is automatically expelled. To treat Cold Painful Obstruction Syndrome primarily scatter Cold, but secondarily also expel Wind and dry Dampness, and also tonify Fire. If Heat moves, Cold goes, proper circulation removes pain. To treat Damp Painful Obstruction Syndrome primarily dry Dampness, but secondarily also expel Wind and scatter Cold, and also tonify the Spleen. If the Earth is strong, Dampness goes, if Qi is strong there is no numbness [a symptom of Dampness].[9]

This passage highlights two important principles in the treatment of Painful Obstruction Syndrome: first, that it is usually necessary to expel all three pathogenic factors, and secondly, that it is also necessary to treat the internal organs. This means treating Blood (i.e. the Liver) in the case of Wind, tonifying Fire (i.e. Kidney-Yang) in the case of Cold and strengthening the Spleen in the case of Dampness.

The "Enlightenment of Medical Theory" (1732) confirms all of the above in almost the same words and adds: *"To treat exterior problems first of all expel the pathogenic factors, then also treat the internal organs and Upright Qi".[10]*

The treatment of chronic Painful Obstruction Syndrome, in particular, requires a more comprehensive approach. Besides expelling pathogenic factors, it is necessary to nourish Blood, nourish Liver and Kidneys, resolve Phlegm or move Blood, depending on the predominant underlying condition.

Prof. Qiu Mao Liang advocates benefiting the Kidneys and strengthening the Governing Vessel to treat chronic Painful Obstruction Syndrome.[11] The main reason for this approach is that the penetration of external pathogenic factors which cause Painful Obstruction Syndrome is closely dependent on the strength of the Kidneys and the Governing Vessel. The Defensive Qi which protects the body from invasion of pathogenic factors is Yang in nature and has its root in Kidney-Yang and the Governing Vessel.

When pathogenic factors invade the body to cause Painful Obstruction Syndrome, they will go through the skin, the space between skin and muscles, the channels, the sinews and the bones. The Liver nourishes the sinews and the Kidneys the bones: thus the strength of sinews and bones depends on the nourishment, not only of Blood and Essence of the Liver and Kidneys, but also on the evaporation of fluids by Kidney-Yang which leads to the formation of synovial fluid. When Liver and Kidneys are weak, Blood and Essence are depleted, Kidney-Yang cannot evaporate fluids, the Defensive Qi is feeble and external pathogenic factors invade the body causing Painful Obstruction Syndrome. Thus, "benefiting the Kidneys" involves both nourishing Liver-Blood and Kidney-Essence and strengthening Kidney-Yang and the Governing Vessel. Strengthening the Governing Vessel is necessary as this extraordinary vessel is Yang in nature, arises from the Kidneys and spreads Defensive Qi all over the back along the Greater-Yang channels: these form the first line of defense from invasion of external pathogenic factors also because, as will be remembered, the Greater-Yang channels "open towards the Exterior".

Strengthening the Governing Vessel with acupuncture simply means reinforcing (also with moxa) points along this vessel, especially Du-4 Mingmen, Du-12 Shenzhu and Du-14 Dazhui, and opening the vessel with the points S.I.-3 Houxi and BL-62 Shenmai. A particular combination to warm Yang and strengthen the Governing Vessel is direct moxa on Ren-4 Guanyuan and Du-14 Dazhui.

With herbal medicine, strengthening the Governing Vessel is achieved by using some of the following substances:

Lu Rong *Cornu Cervi parvum* (the most important one)
Lu Jiao *Cornu Cervi*
Lu Jiao Jiao *Colla Cornu Cervi*
Lu Jiao Shuang *Cornu Cervi deglutinatum*
Fu Zi *Radix Aconiti carmichaeli praeparata*
Rou Gui *Cortex Cinnamomi cassiae*

Finally, another reason for adopting the treatment principle of benefiting the Kidneys and strengthening the Governing Vessel is to be able to reduce the dosage of herbs. In fact, many formulae for Painful Obstruction Syndrome contain pungent and scattering herbs which are not suitable for long-term use. By benefiting the Kidneys and strengthening the Governing Vessel the body resistance is raised, the efficacy of the herbs is increased and therefore their dosages can be correspondingly reduced.

ACUPUNCTURE TREATMENT

GENERAL PRINCIPLES

In general, the treatment is based on the choice of points from four possible groups:

1. distal points
2. local points (including *Ah Shi* points)
3. adjacent points
4. points according to pattern
5. general points.

1. DISTAL POINTS

These are the points below elbows and knees which can treat problems further up along the channel. One or more of these points must always be used to treat Painful Obstruction Syndrome. Distal points "open" the channel, eliminate stagnation of Qi and help to expel pathogenic factors. They are used with reducing method in acute cases and even method in chronic cases.

Distal points are chosen according to the channel and area involved. As a general principle, the more distal along a channel a point is, the further up along the channel it extends its influence. For example, the point G.B.-34 Yanglingquan affects the shoulder joint, while the point G.B.-39 Xuanzhong affects the neck. Of course, this is not an absolute rule as it has many exceptions. For example, the point G.B.-41 Zulinqi (which is below the point G.B.-39 Xuanzhong and should therefore affect an area above the neck), can affect the hip and breast. Since the distal points are by definition those below elbows and knees, it follows that in the case of wrists, fingers, ankles and toes, there are no distal points, with few exceptions. Or, to put it differently, in these cases the distal and local points coincide.

Distal points do not always need to be chosen from the affected channel as distal points on one channel can affect another. This particularly applies to channels of the same polarity on upper and lower limb, and especially the Yang ones, e.g. Greater Yang (Small Intestine and Bladder), Lesser Yang (Triple Burner and Gall Bladder) and Bright Yang (Large Intestine and Stomach) which connect in the face area directly. As was explained in the chapter on "Headaches" (ch. 1), for the purpose of treatment, one could almost look upon the Yang channels of arm and leg as one channel. This connection opens up possibilities in terms of treatment as distal points can be chosen not only on the affected channel but also on its related channel of the same polarity and opposite potential (e.g. Large Intestine and Stomach within the Bright-Yang system).

Distal points of related Yang channels can also be chosen according to the correspondence of joints in the upper and lower limbs:

Shoulder = Hip
Elbow = Knee
Wrist = Ankle

For example, if tenderness and swelling appears in the wrist along the Triple Burner channel, one can use a distal point on the channel of the same polarity and opposite potential, i.e. the Gall Bladder channel. Because of the correspondence between wrist and ankle, the point

will be G.B.-40 Qiuxu. This principle of choice of points will be expanded upon and extended to Yin channels in Appendix 1 (see Appendix 1 and Table I.3). In the meanwhile, the correspondence among Yang-channel points according to joint is illustrated in Table 23.1 (p. 596).

The main distal points for Painful Obstruction Syndrome according to channels are:

Lungs: LU-7 Lieque
Large Intestine: L.I.-4 Hegu
Stomach: ST-40 Fenglong
Spleen: SP-5 Shangqiu
Heart: HE-5 Tongli
Small Intestine: S.I.-3 Houxi
Bladder: BL-60 Kunlun
Kidneys: KI-4 Dazhong
Pericardium: P-6 Neiguan
Triple Burner: T.B.-5 Waiguan
Gall-Bladder: G.B.-41 Zulinqi
Liver: LIV-5 Ligou

The choice of distal points must also be made on the basis of the area involved. The main distal points according to areas are:

Neck: G.B.-39 Xuanzhong, S.I.-3 Houxi, T.B.-5 Waiguan, T.B.-8 Sanyangluo, Bl-60 Kunlun. Secondary points: ST-40 Fenglong and KI-4 Dazhong.
Shoulder: T.B.-5 Waiguan, L.I.-4 Hegu, LU-7 Lieque, T.B.-1 Guanchong, L.I.-1 Shangyang, ST-38 Tiaokou, BL-58 Feiyang.
Elbow: L.I.-4 Hegu, T.B.-5 Waiguan, L.I.-1 Shangyang.
Wrist: ST-36 Zusanli, SP-5 Shangqiu, G.B.-40 Qiuxu.
Fingers: no distal points (see above).
Lower back: BL-40 Weizhong, BL-60 Kunlun, BL-59 Fuyang, BL-62 Shenmai.
Sacrum: BL-40 Weizhong, BL-58 Feiyang.
Hip: G.B.-41 Zulinqi, BL-62 Shenmai.
Knee: SP-5 Shangqiu, S.I.-5 Yanggu.
Ankle: no distal points.
Toes: L.I.-4 Hegu.

2. LOCAL POINTS

The main local points according to area are:

Neck: BL-10 Tianzhu, G.B.-20 Fengchi.
Shoulder: L.I.-15 Jianyu, T.B.-14 Jianliao, Jian-neiling (extra-point).
Elbow: L.I.-11 Quchi, T.B.-10 Tianjing, S.I.-8 Xiaohai.
Wrist: T.B.-4 Yangchi, L.I.-5 Yangxi, S.I.-5 Yanggu, S.I.-4 Wangu, P-7 Daling.
Fingers: T.B.-3 Zhongzhu, L.I.-3 Sanjian, Baxie (extra points).
Lower back: BL-23 Shenshu, BL-26 Guanyuanshu, BL-25 Dachangshu, BL-24 Qihaishu, Shiqizhui-xia (extra point), Du-3 Yaoyangguan.
Sacrum: BL-32 Ciliao, Shiqizhuixia, BL-27 Xiao-changshu, BL-28 Pangguangshu.
Hip: G.B.-30 Huantiao, G.B.-29 Juliao.
Knee: Xiyan (extra points), ST-36 Zusanli, SP-9 Yinlingquan, LIV-7 Xiguan, LIV-8 Ququan, KI-10 Yingu, G.B.-34 Yanglingquan, BL-40 Weizhong, SP-10 Xuehai.
Ankle: SP-5 Shangqiu, G.B.-40 Qiuxu, ST-41 Jiexi, BL-60 Kunlun.
Toes: Bafeng (extra points), SP-3 Taibai.

Ah Shi points (points which are tender on pressure) are also local points and form an important part of the acupuncture treatment of Painful Obstruction Syndrome. In most cases, these will coincide with normal channel points, but if other points are tender on pressure, they can be needled in addition to normal points.

3. ADJACENT POINTS

The main adjacent points according to areas are:

Neck: G.B.-21 Jianjing, Du-14 Dazhui, BL-11 Dashu.
Shoulder: S.I.-9 Jianzhen, S.I.-10 Naoshu, S.I.-11 Tianzong, S.I.-12 Bingfeng, S.I.-13 Quyuan, S.I.-14 Jianwaishu, S.I.-15 Jianzhongshu, T.B.-15 Tianliao, G.B.-21 Jianjing, L.I.-14 Binao, T.B.-13 Naohui.
Elbow: L.I.-13 Wuli, L.I.-10 Shousanli, L.I.-14 Binao.
Wrist: T.B.-5 Waiguan, LU-7 Lieque.
Fingers: T.B.-5 Waiguan.
Lower back: no adjacent points.
Sacrum: BL-23 Shenshu.
Hip: G.B.-31 Fengshi.
Knee: SP-10 Xuehai, ST-34 Liangqiu.

Ankle: KI-7 Fuliu, G.B.-34 Yanglingquan, ST-36 Zusanli.
Toes: SP-4 Gongsun, ST-41 Jiexi, G.B.-34 Yanglingquan, SP-9 Yinlingquan.

4. POINTS ACCORDING TO PATTERN

The main points to use according to pattern are:

(a) Wind Painful Obstruction Syndrome

BL-12 Fengmen, G.B.-31 Fengshi, G.B.-39 Xuanzhong, Du-14 Dazhui, T.B.-6 Zhigou, BL-17 Geshu, BL-18 Ganshu. All these points expel Wind, apart from the last two which nourish Blood and are chosen according to the principle of "nourishing Blood in order to extinguish Wind".

In acute cases, one uses the reducing method and in chronic cases the even method. In case of Wind Painful Obstruction Syndrome, it is particularly important to try and obtain the propagation of the needling sensation along the channel. The use of points according to syndrome is especially important for Wind Painful Obstruction Syndrome as, in this case, the pain moves from joint to joint.

The "Compendium of Acupuncture" (1601) suggests the use of LU-5 Chize and G.B.-38 Yangfu for Wind Painful Obstruction Syndrome.[12]

(b) Cold Painful Obstruction Syndrome

ST-36 Zusanli, Ren-6 Qihai, S.I.-5 Yanggu, Bl-10 Tianzhu, Du-14 Dazhui, Du-3 Yaoyangguan, BL-23 Shenshu, Ren-4 Guanyuan. In this case, one uses the reinforcing method and moxa. Moxa on the needle is the best form of moxibustion for Cold Painful Obstruction Syndrome. It combines the benefit of needling with that of the heat penetrating the muscle and joint via the needle.

The "Compendium of Acupuncture" suggests the following points for Cold Painful Obstruction Syndrome: L.I.-11 Quchi, LU-7 Lieque, G.B.-30 Huantiao, G.B.-31 Fengshi, BL-40 Weizhong, SP-5 Shangqiu, LIV-4 Zhongfeng, G.B.-41 Zulinqi.

(c) Damp Painful Obstruction Syndrome

SP-9 Yinlingquan, SP-6 Sanyinjiao, G.B.-34

Yanglingquan, ST-36 Zusanli, BL-20 Pishu. Use the reducing method in acute cases and even method in chronic ones. BL-20 should be reinforced in either case. Moxa is also applicable. If the joints are swollen (as they usually are in Damp Painful Obstruction Syndrome), one can lightly tap the affected joint with the plum-blossom needle until very tiny droplets of blood appear and then direct the smoke of burning moxa onto it.

The "Compendium of Acupuncture" suggests using BL-17 Geshu for Damp Painful Obstruction Syndrome.

(d) Heat Painful Obstruction Syndrome

ST-43 Xiangu, L.I.-4 Hegu, L.I.-11 Quchi, Du-14 Dazhui. Use the reducing method in acute cases and even method in chronic ones. Positively no moxa. Note the use of Dazhui for both Cold Painful Obstruction Syndrome and Heat Painful Obstruction Syndrome (as well as Wind Painful Obstruction Syndrome). When used with moxa, this point tonifies Yang, whilst when used with needle only (with reducing method) it clears Heat.

(e) Bone Painful Obstruction Syndrome

BL-11 Dashu and G.B.-39 Xuanzhong, with even method.

(f) Chronic Painful Obstruction Syndrome

(i) Qi-Blood Deficiency

Reinforce ST-36 Zusanli, SP-6 Sanyinjiao, Ren-4 Guanyuan, LIV-8 Ququan, BL-20 Pishu and BL-23 Shenshu.

(ii) Phlegm in joints

ST-40 Fenglong, SP-9 Yinlingquan, SP-6 Sanyinjiao, Ren-12 Zhongwan, Ren-9 Shuifen, BL-20 Pishu. Ren-12 and BL-20 should be reinforced, while all the others should be reduced or needled with even method.

(iii) Stasis of Blood

SP-10 Xuehai, BL-17 Geshu, P-6 Neiguan, SP-6 Sanyinjiao, L.I.-11 Quchi, all with reducing or even method.

(iv) Deficiency of Liver and Kidneys

Reinforce LIV-8 Ququan, KI-3 Taixi, SP-6 Sanyinjiao, G.B.-39 Xuanzhong, BL-18 Ganshu, BL-23 Shenshu, Ren-4 Guanyuan, BL-11 Dashu, G.B.-34 Yanglingquan, ST-36 Zusanli.

5. GENERAL POINTS

Some of the points mentioned above are general points which treat the condition underlying each pattern. These are:

Wind: nourish Blood with BL-17 Geshu.
Cold: tonify Yang with Du-14 Dazhui (direct moxa) and BL-23 Shenshu.
Dampness: tonify the Spleen with BL-20 Pishu.

The principles of selection of points are summarized in Figure 23.1.

Case history

A 42-year-old woman complained of severe pain in the joints of the fingers, shoulder and knees. The joints were also swollen and felt hot to the touch. This had started 4 months previously in February after planting 100 trees in her garden. It started with pain in one finger only, then spreading to all fingers which also became swollen. At that time she also felt cold, lost her voice, had a sore throat, a temperature and felt generally achy. Since then she had a recurrent sore throat every 10 days accompanied by ache in all joints. All her muscles generally ached and felt heavy, she felt lethargic most of the time and she put on weight.

Her tongue was Red, with a thick-sticky-yellow coating. The coating was thicker in the Lung area (i.e. just behind the tip). Her pulse was Rapid and Slippery.

Diagnosis
This is a clear case of Heat Painful Obstruction Syndrome. Originally when her symptoms started in February, she suffered from invasion of Wind-Cold-Damp in the joints: Wind, because the pain started in one finger and moved to other joints, Cold, because she felt cold, and Damp, because the joints were swollen. She also had symptoms of invasion of Wind-Cold in the Lung Defensive Qi portion: aversion to cold, temperature, sore throat and ache in muscles. After some time, Cold turned into Heat, Dampness settled in the body and the condition turned into Heat

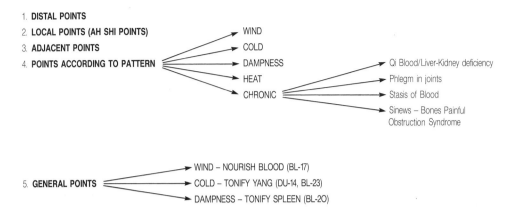

1. **DISTAL POINTS**
2. **LOCAL POINTS (AH SHI POINTS)**
3. **ADJACENT POINTS**
4. **POINTS ACCORDING TO PATTERN** → WIND
   → COLD
   → DAMPNESS
   → HEAT
   → CHRONIC → Qi Blood/Liver-Kidney deficiency
   → Phlegm in joints
   → Stasis of Blood
   → Sinews – Bones Painful Obstruction Syndrome

5. **GENERAL POINTS** → WIND – NOURISH BLOOD (BL-17)
   → COLD – TONIFY YANG (DU-14, BL-23)
   → DAMPNESS – TONIFY SPLEEN (BL-20)

Fig. 23.1   Principles of selection of points

Painful Obstruction Syndrome characterized by Dampness (swelling of joints) and Heat (hot joints). In addition, she also had general symptoms and signs of Damp-Heat such as achy muscles, feeling of heaviness, lethargy, weight-gain, a sticky-yellow tongue coating and a Slippery-Rapid pulse. She also had signs of a residual pathogenic factor (in the form of Wind-Damp-Heat) as evidenced by the recurrent sore throats and the thick yellow coating in the Lung area on the tongue. This latter sign usually indicates the presence of a residual pathogenic factor after an exterior invasion which has not been cleared properly.

Treatment principle
She was treated with acupuncture and the treatment was aimed at clearing Heat, resolving Damp, and removing obstructions from the channels.

Acupuncture
The main points used were:

– **L.I.-11** Quchi, **ST-43** Xiangu and **Du-14** Dazhui to clear Heat;
– **SP-9** Yinlingquan to resolve Dampness;
– **L.I.-15** Jianyu and **Baxie** points as local points.

All the points were needled with reducing method since the condition was still fairly acute and the pattern still Full on the whole. She made a complete recovery after 21 weekly treatments.

Case history

A 35-year-old woman had been suffering from rheumathoid arthritis for the past 4 years. When it first started all her small joints were painful, swollen and hot. After a few months, some of her joints developed bone deformities. Her tongue was Red with a sticky-yellow coating and her pulse was Slippery and Rapid.

Diagnosis
This is a clear example of Heat Painful Obstruction Syndrome complicated by Phlegm in the joints as evidenced by the swelling and bone deformities.

Treatment principle
The treatment principle adopted was to clear Heat, resolve Dampness, and remove obstructions from the channels.

Acupuncture
The main points used were a selection of the following:

– **L.I.-11** Quchi to clear Damp-Heat;
– **T.B.-5** Waiguan, **T.B.-6** Zhigou and **ST-43** Xiangu to expel Wind-Heat and clear obstructions from the joints;
– **ST-40** Fenglong and **SP-9** Yinlingquan to resolve Phlegm;
– **BL-11** Dashu, Gathering point for bones, to prevent further deterioration of the bones;
– **Du-14** Dazhui to clear Heat.

Case history

A 39-year-old woman had been suffering from what was diagnosed as rheumathoid arthritis for the previous two years. Her wrists and feet were painful and swollen. The pain was aggravated by damp and rainy weather and improved with heat. This was her presenting problem. On interrogation, it transpired that she also suffered from lower back-ache, she felt easily cold, she had to pass water at night twice and she felt often exhausted. She also occasionally had dull headaches affecting the whole head and sometimes she sweated at night.

Her tongue was slightly Pale, Stiff and slightly Deviated. Her pulse was Deep and Weak.

Diagnosis
The pain and swelling of wrists and feet were clearly

due to invasion of Wind, Cold and Dampness, predominantly Dampness and Cold. Dampness is indicated by the swelling and Cold by the fact that it is aggravated by rainy weather and improved by warm weather.

This occurred against a background of Liver and Kidney deficiency, especially Kidney as clearly shown by the back-ache, the cold feeling, nocturia and exhaustion. The Deep and Weak pulse also shows deficiency of Kidney-Yang. Her tongue, being Stiff and Deviated, shows also the very beginning of Liver-Wind. Liver-Wind can develop from long-standing deficiency of Liver and Kidney Yin deficiency. How could it develop in this case from Kidney-Yang deficiency? The reason is that Kidney-Yin and Kidney-Yang have a common root and that they are often both deficient especially in women, albeit in different degrees. In this case, Kidney-Yang is predominantly deficient (cold feeling, nocturia) but there is also a slight and lesser Kidney-Yin deficiency (night sweating, Red and Stiff tongue). The slight Kidney-Yin deficiency gave rise to slight Liver-Wind, the only evidence of which is the Stiff and Deviated tongue. A Stiff tongue can indicate both Liver-Wind and Yin deficiency.

Treatment principle
The treatment was aimed at removing Dampness and Cold from the joints while simultaneously nourishing Liver and Kidneys. Only acupuncture was used.

Acupuncture
The main points used were:

– **L.I.-10** Shousanli (warm needle), **ST-36** Zusanli (warm needle) to expel Damp and Cold from the channels;
– **G.B.-40** Qiuxu and **SP-5** Shangqiu (both warm needle) as local points to expel Cold and Damp from the feet channels;
– **KI-3** Taixi, **KI-7** Fuliu, **BL-23** Shenshu and **BL-18** Ganshu were tonified to nourish Liver and Kidneys.

She started to improve after the first treatment and steadily progressed until most of the pain and swelling disappeared after eight treatments. She also noticed a great improvement in her energy and the nocturia decreased.

HERBAL TREATMENT

The patterns discussed are:

Wind Painful Obstruction Syndrome
Cold Painful Obstruction Syndrome
Damp Painful Obstruction Syndrome
Heat Painful Obstruction Syndrome

Chronic Painful Obstruction Syndrome
 Qi-Blood Deficiency and Liver-Kidney Deficiency
 Phlegm stagnating in joints
 Stasis of Blood in joints
 Sinews-Bones Painful Obstruction Syndrome

In the way of review, the main expelling Wind-Dampness herbs classified as warm or cold are:

WARM

Du Huo *Radix Angelicae pubescentis*
Wu Shao She *Zaocys Dhumnades*
Hai Feng Teng *Caulis Piperis*
Wu Jia Pi *Cortex Acanthopanacis radicis*
Can Sha *Excrementum Bombycis mori*
Mu Gua *Fructus Chaenomelis lagenariae*
Song Jie *Lignum Pini Nodi*
Tian Xian Teng *Caulis Aristolochiae debilis*
Wei Ling Xian *Radix Clematidis chinensis*

COLD

Xi Xian Cao *Herba Siegesbeckiae orientalis*
Fang Ji *Radix Stephaniae tetrandae*
Qin Jiao *Radix Gentianae macrophyllae*
Sang Zhi *Ramulus Mori albae*
Hai Tong Pi *Cortex Erythrinae variegatae*
Si Gua Luo *Fasciculus Luffae vascularis*
Kuan Jin Teng *Ramus Tinosporae sinensis*
Luo Shi Teng *Caulis Trachelospermi jasminoidis*
Ren Dong Teng (or Yin Hua Teng) *Caulis Lonicerae japonicae*

Most of these herbs expel Wind-Dampness and treat Painful Obstruction Syndrome as their main function. Some of them also have other important functions which may need to be taken into account when prescribing, notably:

Xi Xian Cao — calms the Mind
Fang Ji — resolves oedema
Qin Jiao — clears Empty-Heat
Mu Gua — benefits fluids (is astringent)
Si Gua Luo — moves Blood.

There are other herbs, not in the expelling-

Wind Dampness category which are very frequently used for Painful Obstruction Syndrome:

Ji Xue Teng *Caulis Millettiae seu Caulis Spatholobi*: nourishes Blood and is used for chronic Painful Obstruction Syndrome with an underlying deficiency of Blood.

Fang Feng *Radix Ledebouriellae sesloidis*: resolves Dampness and is used for Damp Painful Obstruction Syndrome.

Du Zhong *Cortex Eucommiae ulmoidis*: tonifies Yang and is used for Cold Painful Obstruction Syndrome especially of the lower part of the body.

Gui Zhi *Ramulus Cinnamomi cassiae*: tonifies and moves Yang and is used for Cold Painful Obstruction Syndrome especially of the upper part of the body.

Qiang Huo *Radix et Rhizoma Notopterygii*: expels Wind and is used for Wind Painful Obstruction Syndrome especially of the neck.

Niu Xi *Radix Achyranthis bidentatae seu Cyathulae*: moves Blood and is used for chronic Painful Obstruction Syndrome of the lower back and knees.

Dang Gui *Radix Angelicae sinensis*: nourishes Blood and is used for chronic Painful Obstruction Syndrome with an underlying Blood deficiency.

Sang Ji Sheng *Ramus Loranthi*: nourishes Liver-Blood and is used for chronic Painful Obstruction Syndrome with an underlying Blood deficiency.

Bai Zhu *Rhizoma Atractylodis macrocephalae*: tonifies Qi and dries Dampness and is used for Damp Painful Obstruction Syndrome.

Cang Zhu *Rhizoma Atractylodis lanceae*: dries Dampness and is used for Damp Painful Obstruction Syndrome.

Ru Xiang *Gummi Olibanum*: moves Blood and is used for chronic Painful Obstruction Syndrome with an underlying stasis of Blood and very painful and stiff joints.

Yi Yi Ren *Semen Coicis lachryma jobi*: drains Dampness and is used for Damp Painful Obstruction Syndrome with swollen joints.

Mu Tong *Caulis Akebiae*: invigorates the Connecting channels and is used for Heat Painful Obstruction Syndrome with numbness of the limbs.

Lu Jiao *Cornu Cervi*: tonifies Kidney-Yang and strengthens the Governing Vessel and is used for chronic Painful Obstruction Syndrome with underlying Yang deficiency and internal Cold.

Some herbs specifically affect the limbs and are therefore used for Painful Obstruction Syndrome of elbows, knees, wrists, ankles, fingers and toes:

Sang Zhi *Ramulus Mori albae*
Gui Zhi *Ramulus Cinnamomi cassiae* (upper limbs)
Ji Xue Teng *Caulis Millettiae seu Spatholobi* (lower limbs)
Luo Shi Teng *Caulis Trachelospermi jasminoidis*
Tian Xian Teng *Caulis Aristolochiae debilis*
Kuan Jin Teng *Ramus Tinosporae sinensis*
Hai Feng Teng *Caulis Piperis*
Ren Dong Teng (or Yin Hua Teng) *Caulis Lonicerae japonicae*

Most of the vines (recognizable by the term *teng* in their Chinese name) affect the limbs.

Finally, insects or animal substances have an important role to play in the treatment of chronic Painful Obstruction Syndrome. This may be characterized by Blood stasis, Phlegm in joints and long-term obstruction of the channels. Certain insects or animal substances remove turbidity and Phlegm, move Blood, eliminate stasis and open the channels. They are therefore particularly indicated for chronic Painful Obstruction Syndrome in old people. The various insects and animal substances can be differentiated as follows:

Cold-Dampness: Wu Shao She *Zaocys Dhumnades* and Can Sha *Excrementum Bombycis mori*, combined with Fu Zi *Radix Aconiti carmichaeli praeparata* and Cang Zhu *Rhizoma Atractylodis lanceae*.
Heat: Di Long *Pheretima aspergillum*, combined with Shi Gao *Gypsum fibrosum*.
Phlegm: Jiang Can *Bombyx batryticatus*, combined with Dan Nan Xing *Rhizoma Arisaematis praeparata* and Ban Xia *Rhizoma Pinelliae ternatae*.
Stasis of Blood: Di Bie Chong *Eupolyphaga seu Opisthoplatia*, combined with Hong Hua *Flos Carthami tinctorii* and Tao Ren *Semen Persicae*.
Severe pain: Quan Xie *Buthus Martensi* and Wu Gong *Scolopendra subspinipes*, combined with Yan Hu Suo *Rhizoma Corydalis yanhusuo*.

Swelling of joints: Feng Fang *Polistes mandarinus* and Jiang Can *Bombyx batryticatus*, combined with Yi Yi Ren *Semen Coicis lachryma jobi.*
Lower back-ache: Wu Shao She *Zaocys Dhumnades*, Feng Fang *Polistes mandarinus* and Di Bie Chong *Eupolyphaga seu Opisthoplatia.*

There are three other animal products used in Painful Obstruction Syndrome:

Zi He Che *Placenta hominis* to nourish Essence and Marrow in chronic Painful Obstruction Syndrome with an underlying Kidney deficiency.
Lu Jiao *Cornu Cervi* and **Lu Rong** *Cornu Cervi parvum* to strengthen the Governing Vessel as mentioned above.
Chuan Shan Jia *Squama Manitis pentadactylae* to move Blood in chronic Painful Obstruction Syndrome with an underlying stasis of Blood.

It should be remembered that most insects are drying and, especially in old people, they should be combined with Yin-nourishing herbs such as Sheng Di Huang *Radix Rehmanniae glutinosae*, Mai Men Dong *Tuber Ophiopogonis japonici* or Shi Hu *Herba Dendrobii.*

1. WIND PAINFUL OBSTRUCTION SYNDROME

TREATMENT PRINCIPLE

Expel Wind, remove obstructions from the channels.

(a) Prescription

FANG FENG TANG
Ledebouriella Decoction
Fang Feng *Radix Ledebouriellae sesloidis* 6 g
Ma Huang *Herba Ephedrae* 3 g
Qin Jiao *Radix Gentianae macrophyllae* 3 g
Xing Ren *Semen Pruni armeniacae* 2 g
Ge Gen *Radix Puerariae* 3 g
Rou Gui *Cortex Cinnamomi cassiae* 1.5 g
Fu Ling *Sclerotium Poriae cocos* 3 g
Dang Gui *Radix Angelicae sinensis* 3 g
Huang Qin *Radix Scutellariae baicalensis* 2 g
Gan Cao *Radix Glycyrrhizae uralensis* 2 g

Sheng Jiang *Rhizoma Zingiberis officinalis recens* 3 slices
Da Zao *Fructus Ziziphi jujubae* 3 dates

Explanation

- **Fang Feng** and **Ma Huang** expel Wind.
- **Qin Jiao** helps the first two to expel Wind.
- **Xing Ren** helps to expel Wind by stimulating the descending of Lung-Qi.
- **Ge Gen** relaxes the sinews and expels Wind.
- **Fu Ling** expels Dampness.
- **Dang Gui** nourishes Blood and is added according to the principle of "nourishing Blood in order to extinguish Wind".
- **Rou Gui** is very warm and is added to expel Cold, as Wind is often combined with Cold.
- **Huang Qin** is cold and is added to balance all the other ingredients most of which are warm or hot.
- **Sheng Jiang** helps to expel Wind and Cold.
- **Gan Cao** and **Da Zao** harmonize the Middle.

(b) Prescription

Empirical prescription from Dr Jiao Shu De
Gui Zhi *Ramulus Cinnamomi cassiae* 9 g
Fu Zi *Radix Aconiti carmichaeli praeparata* 6 g
Bai Zhu *Rhizoma Atractylodis macrocephalae* 9 g
Qiang Huo *Radix et Rhizoma Notopterygii* 9 g
Du Huo *Radix Angelicae pubescentis* 9 g
Wei Ling Xian *Radix Clematidis chinensis* 10 g
Fang Ji *Radix Stephaniae tetrandae* 9 g
Dang Gui *Radix Angelicae sinensis* 9 g
Gan Cao *Radix Glycyrrhizae uralensis* 5 g

Explanation

This formula differs from the previous one in so far as it is warmer in energy and is more specific for the spine.

- **Gui Zhi** expels Wind and scatters Cold.
- **Fu Zi** scatters Cold.
- **Bai Zhu** drains Dampness. Thus, the first three herbs eliminate Wind, Cold and Dampness, the three pathogenic factors causing Painful Obstruction Syndrome.
- **Qiang Huo**, **Du Huo**, **Wei Ling Xian** and

Fang Ji expel Wind and Dampness and remove obstructions from the channels.

- **Dang Gui** nourishes Blood and is added according to the principle of nourishing Blood in order to extinguish Wind.
- **Gan Cao** harmonizes.

Variations

The following variations apply to both prescriptions.

- If the pain is in the upper part of the body consider adding (or increasing the dosage of) one of the following: Qiang Huo *Radix et Rhizoma Notopterygii*, Bai Zhi *Radix Angelicae dahuricae*, Wei Ling Xian *Radix Clematidis chinensis*, Jiang Huang *Radix Curcumae longae* or Chuan Xiong *Radix Ligustici wallichii*.
- If the pain is in the lower part of the body choose from: Du Huo *Radix Angelicae pubescentis*, Niu Xi *Radix Achyrantis bidentatae* or Bi Xie *Radix Dioscoreae hypoglaucae*.
- For pain in the lower back add one or more of the following herbs: Du Zhong *Radix Eucommiae ulmoidis*, Sang Ji Sheng *Ramulus Loranthi*, Yin Yang Huo *Herba Epimedii*, Ba Ji Tian *Radix Morindae* or Xu Duan *Radix Dipsaci*.

(i) Patent remedy

FENG SHI PIAN
Wind-Dampness Tablet
Ma Huang *Herba Ephedrae*
Gui Zhi *Ramulus Cinnamomi cassiae*
Fang Feng *Radix Ledebouriellae sesloidis*
Du Huo *Radix Angelicae pubescentis*
Quan Xie *Buthus Martensi*
Ma Qian Zi *Semen Strychnotis*
Du Zhong *Cortex Eucommiae ulmoidis*
Niu Xi *Radix Achyranthis bidentatae seu Cyathulae*
Gan Cao *Radix Glycyrrhizae uralensis*

Explanation

This tablet expels Wind and scatters Cold. It can be used for the acute stage of Painful Obstruction Syndrome from Wind-Cold.

It is important to note that this tablet contains Ma Qian Zi which is a toxic herb: the remedy should therefore only be used for a short time (two-three weeks). It is contraindicated in pregnancy and in hypertensive patients.

(ii) Patent remedy

ZHUI FENG HUO XUE PIAN
Expelling Wind and Moving Blood Tablet
Gui Zhi *Ramulus Cinnamomi cassiae*
Du Huo *Radix Angelicae pubescentis*
Ma Huang *Herba Ephedrae*
Fang Feng *Radix Ledebouriellae sesloidis*
Di Feng *Cortex Illici*
Qiang Huo *Radix et Rhizoma Notopterygii*
Ru Xiang *Gummi Olibanum*
Zi Ran Tong *Pyritum*
Mo Yao *Myrrha*
Du Zhong *Cortex Eucommiae ulmoidis*
Qian Nian Jian *Rhizoma Homalomenae occultae*
Mu Gua *Fructus Chaenomelis lagenariae*
Niu Xi *Radix Achyranthis bidentatae seu Cyathulae*
Gan Cao *Radix Glycyrrhizae uralensis*
Feng Mi *Mel*

Explanation

This tablet expels Wind-Cold and moves Blood. It is suitable for acute or sub-acute Cold Painful Obstruction Syndrome, especially of the upper part of the body, with some stasis of Blood.

It is contraindicated in pregnancy.

(iii) Patent remedy

TIAN MA HU GU WAN
Gastrodia-Tiger Bone Pill
Tian Ma *Rhizoma Gastrodiae elatae*
Gao Ben *Rhizoma et Radix Ligustici sinensis*
Hu Gu *Os Tigris*
Chuan Xiong *Radix Ligustici wallichii*
Du Zhong *Cortex Eucommiae ulmoidis*
Dang Gui *Radix Angelicae sinensis*
Ren Shen *Radix Ginseng*

Explanation

This pill expels Wind and is used to treat sub-acute Wind Painful Obstruction Syndrome. It is particularly indicated to treat elderly people.

2. COLD PAINFUL OBSTRUCTION SYNDROME

TREATMENT PRINCIPLE

Warm the channels, scatter Cold, expel Wind, eliminate Dampness.

(a) Prescription

WU TOU TANG
Radix Aconiti Decoction
Wu Tou *Radix Aconiti carmichaeli* 3 g
Ma Huang *Herba Ephedrae* 3 g
Bai Shao *Radix Paeoniae alba* 3 g
Gan Cao *Radix Glycyrrhizae uralensis* 3 g
Huang Qi *Radix Astragali membranacei* 3 g

Explanation

- **Wu Tou** and **Ma Huang** warm the channels, scatter Cold, resolve Dampness and stop pain.
- **Bai Shao** and **Gan Cao** in combination, stop pain.
- **Huang Qi** consolidates the Exterior and stops pain.

(b) Prescription

WU FU MA XIN GUI JIANG TANG
Aconitum-Ephedra-Asarum-Cinnamomum-Zingiber Decoction
Wu Tou *Radix Aconiti carmichaeli* 3 g
Fu Zi *Radix Aconiti carmichaeli praeparata* 1.5 g
Ma Huang *Herba Ephedrae* 3 g
Xi Xin *Herba Asari cum radice* 1.5 g
Gui Zhi *Ramulus Cinnamomi cassiae* 3 g
Gan Jiang *Rhizoma Zingiberis officinalis* 1.5 g
Gan Cao *Radix Glycyrrhizae uralensis* 2 g

Explanation

- **Wu Tou**, **Fu Zi** and **Gan Jiang** warm the channels, scatter Cold and stop pain.
- **Ma Huang**, **Xi Xin** and **Gui Zhi** scatter Cold, expel Wind and resolve Dampness.
- **Gan Cao** harmonizes.

(c) Prescription

GUI ZHI FU ZI TANG
Cinnamomum-Aconitum Decoction
Fu Zi *Radix Aconiti carmichaeli* 3 g
Gui Zhi *Ramulus Cinnamomi cassiae* 6 g
Gan Cao *Radix Glycyrrhizae uralensis* 3 g
Sheng Jiang *Rhizoma Zingiberis officinalis recens* 3 slices
Da Zao *Fructus Ziziphi jujubae* 3 dates

Explanation

- **Fu Zi** and **Gui Zhi** warm the channels and scatter Cold.
- **Gan Cao**, **Sheng Jiang** and **Da Zao** benefit the Middle and harmonize.

Variations

- If the pain is in shoulders or elbows add Qiang Huo *Rhizoma et Radix Notopterygii* or Jiang Huang *Rhizoma Curcumae longae*.
- If the pain is in the knees add Huai Niu Xi *Radix Achyranthis bidentatae*.
- If the pain is in the spine choose from Du Zhong *Radix Eucommiae ulmoidis*, Sang Ji Sheng *Ramulus Loranthi* or Xu Duan *Radix Dipsaci*.

(i) Patent remedy

FENG SHI LING PIAN
Wind-Dampness Efficacious Tablet
Chuan Wu *Radix Aconiti carmichaeli*
San Qi *Radix Notoginseng*
Ren Shen *Radix Ginseng*
Duan Jie Shen *Radix Cynanchi wallichii*

Explanation

This tablet tonifies Qi and Yang and scatters Cold. It is used for Cold Painful Obstruction Syndrome.

(ii) Patent remedy

XIAO HUO LUO DAN
Small Invigorating the Connecting Vessels Pill
Chuan Wu *Radix Aconiti carmichaeli*

Cao Wu *Radix Aconiti kusnezoffii*
Dan Nan Xing *Rhizoma Arisaemae praeparata*
Ru Xiang *Gummi Olibanum*
Mo Yao *Myrrha*
Di Long *Pheretima aspergillum*

Explanation

This remedy strongly scatters Cold, expels Wind-Dampness and moves Blood. It is used for acute or sub-acute Painful Obstruction Syndrome from Cold.

It should be noted that this remedy is extremely hot in energy and one should therefore be absolutely certain not only that there is pronounced internal Cold, but also that there is no Heat anywhere in the body. In doubt, it is better not to use this pill. It is also contraindicated in pregnancy.

3. DAMP PAINFUL OBSTRUCTION SYNDROME

TREATMENT PRINCIPLE

Drain Dampness, remove obstruction from the channels, expel Wind, scatter Cold.

(a) Prescription

YI YI REN TANG
Coix Decoction
Yi Yi Ren *Semen Coicis lachryma jobi* 6 g
Cang Zhu *Rhizoma Atractylodis lanceae* 6 g
Qiang Huo *Radix et Rhizoma Notopterygii* 3 g
Du Huo *Radix Angelicae pubescentis* 6 g
Fang Feng *Radix Ledebouriellae sesloidis* 6 g
Wu Tou *Radix Aconiti carmichaeli* 1.5 g
Ma Huang *Herba Ephedrae* 3 g
Gui Zhi *Ramulus Cinnamomi cassiae* 3 g
Dang Gui *Radix Angelicae sinensis* 6 g
Chuan Xiong *Rhizoma Ligustici wallichii* 3 g
Sheng Jiang *Rhizoma Zingiberis officinalis recens* 3 slices
Gan Cao *Radix Glycyrrhizae uralensis* 3 g

Explanation

– **Yi Yi Ren** and **Cang Zhu** drain Dampness.

– **Qiang Huo**, **Du Huo** and **Fang Feng** expel Wind and Dampness.
– **Wu Tou**, **Ma Huang** and **Gui Zhi** warm the channels and scatter Cold.
– **Dang Gui** and **Chuan Xiong** nourish and move Blood.
– **Sheng Jiang** and **Gan Cao** harmonize.

Variations

– If there is pronounced swelling of the joints, one may add one of the following herbs: Bi Xie *Rhizoma Dioscoreae hypoglaucae*, Mu Tong *Caulis Akebiae* or Jiang Huang *Rhizoma Curcumae longae*.
– If there is pronounced numbness, add Hai Tong Pi *Cortex Erythrinae variegatae* or Xi Xian Cao *Herba Siegesbeckiae orientalis*.

(b) Prescription

CHUAN BI TANG
Eliminating Painful Obstruction Syndrome Decoction
Qiang Huo *Radix et Rhizoma Notopterygii* 6 g
Du Huo *Radix Angelicae pubescentis* 6 g
Qin Jiao *Radix Gentianae macrophyllae* 6 g
Hai Feng Teng *Caulis Piperis* 3 g
Gui Zhi *Ramulus Cinnamomi cassiae* 3 g
Dang Gui *Radix Angelicae sinensis* 6 g
Chuan Xiong *Rhizoma Ligustici wallichii* 3 g
Ru Xiang *Resina Olibani* 3 g
Mu Xiang *Radix Saussureae* 3 g
Sang Zhi *Ramus Mori albae* 6 g
Gan Cao *Radix Glycyrrhizae uralensis* 3 g

Explanation

This formula is used if the distinction between Wind, Cold and Dampness is not clear.

– **Qiang Huo**, **Du Huo**, **Qin Jiao**, **Hai Feng Teng** and **Gui Zhi** expel Wind, drain Dampness and scatter Cold.
– **Dang Gui**, **Chuan Xiong**, **Ru Xiang**, **Mu Xiang**, **Sang Zhi** and **Gan Cao** move Blood, remove obstructions from the channels and stop pain.

(c) Prescription

MA HUANG LIAN QIAO CHI XIAO DOU TANG Variation
Ephedra-Forsythia-Phaseolus Decoction
Ma Huang *Herba Ephedrae* 5 g
Lian Qiao *Fructus Forsythiae suspensae* 15 g
Chi Xiao Dou *Semen Phaseoli calcarati* 30 g
Fang Feng *Radix Ledebouriellae sesloidis* 10 g
Gui Zhi *Ramulus Cinnamomi cassiae* 5 g
Chi Shao *Radix Paeoniae rubrae* 10 g
Gan Cao *Radix Glycyrrhizae uralensis* 3 g
Hai Feng Teng *Caulis Piperis* 6 g
Qiang Huo *Radix et Rhizoma Notopterygii* 15 g
Sheng Jiang *Rhizoma Zingiberis officinalis recens* 3 slices

Explanation

This formula is used if Dampness combines with Heat and is not too severe, causing red-swollen-hot joints, fever, thirst and a Floating-Rapid pulse, at the acute stage.

- **Ma Huang** expels Wind.
- **Lian Qiao** expels Wind-Heat.
- **Chi Xiao Dou** drains Dampness and clears Heat.
- **Fang Feng** and **Qiang Huo** expel Wind and Dampness.
- **Gui Zhi** penetrates the channels.
- **Chi Shao** clears Heat and penetrates the blood vessels.
- **Gan Cao** harmonizes.
- **Hai Feng Teng** expels Wind and Dampness from the channels.
- **Sheng Jiang** harmonizes.

(d) Prescription

GUI SHAO XI CAO TANG
Angelica-Paeonia-Siegesbeckia Decoction
Dang Gui *Radix Angelicae sinensis* 15 g
Chi Shao *Radix Paeoniae rubrae* 15 g
Bai Shao *Radix Paeoniae albae* 15 g
Xi Xian Cao *Herba Siegesbeckiae orientalis* 30 g
Qin Jiao *Radix Gentianae macrophyllae* 10 g
Wei Ling Xian *Radix Clematidis chinensis* 15 g
Di Long *Lumbricus* 10 g
Fang Feng *Radix Ledebouriellae sesloidis* 10 g
Sheng Di *Radix Rehmanniae glutinosae* 30 g
Ru Xiang *Resina Olibani* 6 g
Mo Yao *Resina Myrrhae* 6 g
Sang Zhi *Ramulus Mori albae* 15 g

Explanation

This prescription is used if the joints are still swollen after an acute attack and all the acute symptoms and signs have gone.

- **Dang Gui**, **Chi Shao**, **Sheng Di** and **Bai Shao** harmonize Blood.
- **Xi Xian Cao**, **Qin Jiao**, **Sang Zhi** and **Wei Ling Xian** expel Wind-Damp and remove obstructions from the channels.
- **Di Long** expels Wind and removes obstructions from the channels, particularly in chronic cases.
- **Fang Feng** expels Wind and Dampness.
- **Ru Xiang** and **Mo Yao** move Blood, eliminate stasis and stop pain.

(e) Prescription

SAN MIAO SAN
Three Wonderful Powder
Cang Zhu *Rhizoma Atractylodis lanceae* 15 g
Huang Bo *Cortex Phellodendri* 12 g
Niu Xi *Radix Cyathulae* 6 g

Explanation

This is for Damp-Heat affecting the legs (or one leg) and causing the knee joint to be hot, red, painful and swollen.

- **Cang Zhu** and **Huang Bo** form the Er Miao San *Two Wonderful Powder* which drains Damp-Heat from the Lower Burner and legs. With the addition of **Niu Xi**, it is used for pain, numbness and swelling of the leg and knee joint.

Patent remedy

GUAN JIE YAN WAN
Arthritis Pill
Xi Xian Cao *Herba Siegesbeckiae orientalis*
Cang Zhu *Rhizoma Atractylodis lanceae*

Yi Yi Ren *Semen Coicis lachryma jobi*
Fang Ji *Radix Stephaniae tetrandae*
Huai Niu Xi *Radix Achyranthis bidentatae*
Qin Jiao *Radix Gentianae macrophyllae*
Rou Gui *Cortex Cinnamomi cassiae*
Sheng Jiang *Rhizoma Zingiberis officinalis recens*
Ma Huang *Herba Ephedrae*
Du Huo *Radix Angelicae pubescentis*

Explanation

This pill drains Dampness and expels Wind. It is used to treat acute or sub-acute Damp Painful Obstruction Syndrome with swollen and painful joints.

The tongue presentation appropriate to this remedy is a Swollen body with a sticky coating. It is contraindicated in pregnancy.

4. HEAT PAINFUL OBSTRUCTION SYNDROME

TREATMENT PRINCIPLE

Clear Heat, remove obstructions from the channels, expel Wind and drain Dampness.

(a) Prescription

BAI HU JIA GUI ZHI TANG
White Tiger Ramulus Cinnamomi Decoction
Shi Gao *Gypsum fibrosum* 30 g
Zhi Mu *Rhizoma Anemarrhenae asphodeloidis* 9 g
Gan Cao *Radix Glycyrrhizae uralensis* 3 g
Geng Mi *Semen Oryzae sativae* 6 g
Gui Zhi *Ramulus Cinnamomi cassiae* 5 g

Explanation

This formula is suitable only for the acute stage of Heat Painful Obstruction Syndrome.

- The **White Tiger Decoction** clears Heat and promotes Stomach fluids.
- **Gui Zhi** expels Wind and removes obstructions from the channels.

(b) Prescription

XUAN BI TANG

Clearing Painful Obstruction Syndrome Decoction
Fang Ji *Radix Stephaniae tetrandae* 6 g
Can Sha *Excrementum Bombycis mori* 6 g
Xing Ren *Semen Pruni armeniacae* 3 g
Hua Shi *Talcum* 12 g
Lian Qiao *Fructus Forsythiae suspensae* 6 g
Shan Zhi Zi *Fructus Gardeniae jasminoidis* 6 g
Yi Yi Ren *Semen Coicis lachryma jobi* 6 g
Chi Xiao Dou *Semen Phaseoli calcarati* 6 g
Ban Xia *Rhizoma Pinelliae ternatae* 6 g

Explanation

This prescription is suitable for a sub-acute stage of Heat Painful Obstruction Syndrome.

- **Fang Ji** and **Can Sha** expel Wind and Dampness.
- **Xing Ren** stimulates the descending of Lung-Qi and thus helps to eliminate Wind.
- **Hua Shi**, **Lian Qiao** and **Shan Zhi Zi** clear Heat.
- **Yi Yi Ren** and **Chi Xiao Dou** drain Dampness.
- **Ban Xia** resolves Phlegm and thus helps to drain Dampness.

(c) Prescription

XI JIAO SAN
Cornu Bisontis Decoction
Sheng Di Huang *Radix Rehmanniae glutinosae* 9 g
Xi Jiao *Cornu bisontis* 12 g
Xuan Shen *Radix Scrophulariae ningpoensis* 6 g
Mai Men Dong *Tuber Ophiopogonis japonici* 6 g
Fang Ji *Radix Stephaniae tetrandae* 6 g
Jiang Huang *Rhizoma Curcumae longae* 6 g
Qin Jiao *Radix Gentianae macrophyllae* 6 g
Hai Tong Pi *Cortex Erythrinae variegatae* 3 g

Explanation

This formula is used if Heat Painful Obstruction Syndrome turns into Fire which damages body fluids and causes red-swollen and very painful joints which are worse at night together with irritability, thirst, a Red tongue without coating and a Rapid pulse.

- **Sheng Di**, **Xi Jiao**, **Xuan Shen**, and **Mai Dong** nourish Yin and cool Blood. Since the rhino is a protected species and its horn cannot be used, Xi Jiao is always replaced by Shui Niu Jiao, the water-buffalo horn, in a higher dose.

– **Fang Ji**, **Jiang Huang**, **Qin Jiao**, and **Hai Tong Pi** clear Heat, drain Dampness, remove obstructions from the channels and stop pain.

(d) Prescription

Empirical prescription by Dr Jiao Shu De
Dang Gui *Radix Angelicae sinensis* 9 g
Yi Yi Ren *Semen Coicis lachryma jobi* 12 g
Ku Shen *Radix Sophorae flavescentis* 6 g
Hua Shi *Talcum* 12 g
Ban Xia *Rhizoma Pinelliae ternatae* 9 g
Huang Qin *Radix Scutellariae baicalensis* 9 g
Lian Qiao *Fructus Forsythiae suspensae* 6 g
Fang Feng *Radix Ledebouriellae sesloidis* 9 g
Qin Jiao *Radix Gentianae macrophyllae* 6 g
Hai Tong Pi *Cortex Erythrinae variegatae* 9 g
Gan Cao *Radix Glycyrrhizae uralensis* 6 g

Explanation

This formula is suitable for chronic Heat Painful Obstruction Syndrome occurring against a background of Blood deficiency. This is a very common occurrence in the type of patients we see with chronic rheumathoid arthritis with swollen and painful joints flaring up occasionally.

– **Dang Gui** nourishes Blood to extinguish Wind.
– **Yi Yi Ren**, **Ku Shen**, **Hua Shi**, and **Ban Xia** drain Dampness and resolve Phlegm.
– **Huang Qin** and **Lian Qiao** clear Heat.
– **Fang Feng**, **Qin Jiao** and **Hai Tong Pi** expel Wind-Dampness.
– **Gan Cao** harmonizes.

(e) Prescription

Empirical prescription by Dr Jiao Shu De
Dang Gui *Radix Angelicae sinensis* 9 g
Sheng Di Huang *Radix Rehmanniae glutinosae* 12 g
Zhi Mu *Rhizoma Anemarrhenae asphodeloidis* 6 g
Huang Qin *Radix Scutellariae baicalensis* 6 g

Lian Qiao *Fructus Forsythiae suspensae* 6 g
Yi Yi Ren *Semen Coicis lachryma jobi* 12 g
Ku Shen *Radix Sophorae flavescentis* 6 g
Hua Shi *Talcum* 9 g
Ban Xia *Rhizoma Pinelliae ternatae* 9 g
Fang Ji *Radix Aristolochiae seu Cocculi* 6 g
Fang Feng *Radix Ledebouriellae sesloidis* 6 g
Hai Tong Pi *Cortex Erythrinae variegatae* 6 g
Gan Cao *Radix Glycyrrhizae uralensis* 6 g

Explanation

This formula is suitable for chronic Heat Painful Obstruction Syndrome with swollen, hot and painful joints flaring up occasionally, occurring against a background of Yin deficiency.

– **Dang Gui** nourishes Blood to extinguish Wind.
– **Sheng Di** and **Zhi Mu** nourish Yin.
– **Huang Qin** and **Lian Qiao** clear Heat.
– **Yi Yi Ren**, **Ku Shen**, **Hua Shi** and **Ban Xia** drain Dampness and resolve Phlegm.
– **Fang Ji**, **Fang Feng** and **Hai Tong Pi** expel Wind-Dampness and remove obstructions from the channels.
– **Gan Cao** harmonizes.

Variations

The following variations are applicable to all the previous formulae.

– Other herbs that may be added are: Huang Bo *Cortex Phellodendri* to clear Heat, and Hai Tong Pi *Cortex Erythrinae variegatae*, Wei Ling Xian *Radix Clematidis chinensis* or Sang Zhi *Ramulus Mori albae* to expel Wind and Dampness.
– If there are red maculae, add Mu Dan Pi *Cortex Moutan radicis*, Sheng Di *Radix Rehmanniae glutinosae*, Chi Shao Yao *Radix Paeoniae rubrae* and Di Fu Zi *Fructus Kochiae*.

Some doctors apply the theory of the 4 Levels, based on Heat patterns at the Defensive-Qi, Qi, Nutritive-Qi and Blood Level, to the treatment of Heat Painful Obstruction Syndrome. Briefly, the symptoms and formulae for each Level would be as follows.

Defensive-Qi Level

Pain, redness and swelling of the joints with acute onset, the skin feeling hot to the touch, fever, sore throat, shivering. This corresponds to the acute, beginning stage of Heat Painful Obstruction Syndrome.

Use Yin Qiao San *Lonicera-Forsythia Powder* plus Luo Shi Teng *Caulis Trachelospermi jasminoidis* and Si Gua Luo *Fasciculus Luffae vascularis*. If the upper limbs are affected add Sang Zhi *Ramulus Mori albae* and Bo He *Herba Menthae*. If the lower limbs are affected add Niu Xi *Radix Achyranthis bidentatae seu Cyathulae*.

Qi Level

Painful, red, hot, swollen joints, worse with movement, feeling of heat, thirst, constipation, dark urine, Rapid pulse and Red tongue with yellow coating. If there is Dampness the joints would be very swollen and there would be a feeling of heaviness.

This could correspond to acute attacks of chronic Heat Painful Obstruction Syndrome.

The formula to use for Heat is Bai Hu Tang *White Tiger Decoction* plus Huang Qin *Radix Scutellariae baicalensis*, Zhi Zi *Fructus Gardeniae jasminoidis*, Lian Qiao *Fructus Forsythiae suspensae*, Qin Jiao *Radix Gentianae macrophyllae*, Si Gua Luo *Fasciculus Luffae vascularis* and Ren Dong Teng *Caulis Lonicerae japonicae*.

For Damp-Heat use Lian Po Yin *Coptis-Magnolia Decoction* plus Huang Qin *Radix Scutellariae baicalensis*, Huang Bo *Cortex Phellodendri*, Yi Yi Ren *Semen Coicis lachryma jobi*, Fu Ling *Sclerotium Poriae cocos*, Zhu Ling *Sclerotium Polypori umbellati*, Xi Xian Cao *Herba Siegesbeckiae orientalis* and Ren Dong Teng *Caulis Lonicerae japonicae*. If the upper limbs are affected add, Huo Xiang *Herba Agastachis* and Pei Lan *Herba Eupatorei fortunei*. If the lower limbs are affected add Cang Zhu *Rhizoma Atractylodis lanceae*, Niu Xi *Radix Achyranthis bidentatae seu Cyathulae* and Fang Ji *Radix Stephaniae tetrandae*.

Nutritive-Qi Level

Maculae on the legs, low-grade fever or a feeling of heat, irritability, Rapid and Fine pulse and Red tongue without coating.

Use Qing Ying Tang *Clearing Nutritive Qi Decoction* plus Dang Gui *Radix Angelicae sinensis*, Sang Zhi *Ramulus Mori albae*, Ji Xue Teng *Caulis Millettiae seu Caulis Spatholobi*, Xi Xian Cao *Herba Siegesbeckiae orientalis* and Dan Shen *Radix Salviae miltiorrhizae*.

Blood Level

Painful and swollen joints in bouts, joints cannot be extended fully, low-grade fever or a feeling of heat, palpitations, dizziness, Fine pulse, Reddish-Purple tongue without coating.

Use the following prescription: Dang Gui *Radix Angelicae sinensis*, Chi Shao *Radix Paeoniae rubrae*, Dan Shen *Radix Salviae miltiorrhizae*, Di Gu Pi *Cortex Lycii chinensis radicis*, Qing Hao *Herba Artemisiae apiaceae*, Chai Hu *Radix Bupleuri*, Dang Shen *Radix Codonopsis pilosulae*, Bai Zhu *Rhizoma Atractylodis macrocephalae*, Huang Qi *Radix Astragali membranacei*, Sang Zhi *Ramulus Mori albae*, Qin Jiao *Radix Gentianae macrophyllae*, Bie Jia *Carapax Trionycis* and Wu Shao She *Zaocys dhumnades*.

If there is stasis of Blood add Hong Hua *Flos Carthami tinctorii* and Tao Ren *Semen Persicae*.

Case history

A 2½-year-old girl had been suffering from juvenile arthritis for 2 months before the consultation. The attack started with a swelling of the knees which became hot and painful; the pain then went to the neck. Since then, she had bouts of pain and swelling moving from the knee to the neck. She had no other problem and her appetite and bowel movements were normal. Her tongue was slightly Red.

Diagnosis
This is acute Heat Painful Obstruction Syndrome characterized by Heat, Dampness and Wind. The Heat shows in the hot joints, the Dampness in the swelling of the joints and the Wind in the movement of the pain from one joint to the other.

Treatment principle
The treatment principle adopted was to clear Heat, resolve Dampness, expel Wind, and remove obstructions from the channels.

Herbal treatment
This little girl was treated only with herbs in the form of decoctions. The prescription used was a variation

of Bai Hu Jia Gui Zhi Tang *White Tiger Ramulus Cinnamomi Decoction*:

Shi Gao *Gypsum fibrosum* 15 g
Zhi Mu *Rhizoma Anemarrhenae asphodeloidis* 6 g
Gan Cao *Radix Glycyrrhizae uralensis* 3 g
Geng Mi *Semen Oryzae sativae* 6 g
Gui Zhi *Ramulus Cinnamomi cassiae* 5 g
Cang Zhu *Rhizoma Atractylodis lanceae* 4 g
Yi Yi Ren *Semen Coicis lachryma jobi* 6 g
Fang Feng *Radix Ledebouriellae sesloidis* 4 g

Explanation
– The first five herbs constitute the Bai Hu Jia Gui Zhi Tang which clears Heat and expels Wind.
– **Cang Zhu** and **Yi Yi Ren** were added to drain Dampness. Yi Yi Ren also has the function of clearing Heat via urination.
– **Fang Feng** was added to expel Wind and resolve Dampness.

These herbs were given as a decoction diluted in water in small doses throughout the day. After two months of taking this decoction with slight variations, all her pain and swelling went.

5. CHRONIC PAINFUL OBSTRUCTION SYNDROME

The above prescriptions are for the acute or semi-acute cases of Painful Obstruction Syndrome. The majority of cases we see in practice are chronic and therefore both channels and internal organs are involved. Several internal conditions may either derive from or accompany invasion of the channels by Wind-Cold-Dampness. The factors contributing to chronic Painful Obstruction Syndrome are summarized in Figure 23.2.

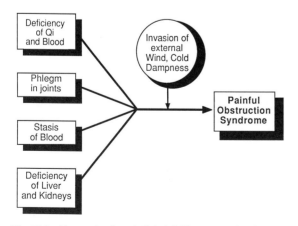

Fig. 23.2 Factors in chronic Painful Obstruction Syndrome

(a) QI-BLOOD DEFICIENCY AND LIVER-KIDNEY DEFICIENCY

Treatment principle

Expel pathogenic factors, tonify Qi and Blood, nourish Liver and Kidneys.

(i) Prescription

DU HUO JI SHENG TANG
Angelica pubescens-Loranthus Decoction
Du Huo *Radix Angelicae pubescentis* 9 g
Xi Xin *Herba Asari cum radice* 3 g
Fang Feng *Radix Ledebouriellae sesloidis* 6 g
Qin Jiao *Radix Gentianae macrophyllae* 6 g
Sang Ji Sheng *Ramus Loranthi* 6 g
Du Zhong *Radix Eucommiae ulmoidis* 6 g
Huai Niu Xi *Radix Achyranthis bidentatae* 6 g
Dang Gui *Radix Angelicae sinensis* 6 g
Chuan Xiong *Radix Ligustici wallichii* 6 g
Sheng Di Huang *Radix Rehmanniae glutinosae* 6 g
Bai Shao *Radix Paeoniae albae* 6 g
Ren Shen *Radix Ginseng* 6 g
Fu Ling *Sclerotium Poriae cocos* 6 g
Rou Gui *Cortex Cinnamomi cassiae* 6 g
Gan Cao *Radix Glycyrrhizae uralensis* 6 g

Explanation

– **Du Huo** is the emperor herb and is used to simultaneously expel Wind-Dampness and benefit the tendons. It acts primarily on the lower part of the body, i.e. lower back and knees.
– **Xi Xin** scatters Cold from the channels.
– **Fang Feng** and **Qin Jiao** expel Wind and drain Dampness.
– **Sang Ji Sheng**, **Du Zhong** and **Niu Xi** nourish Liver and Kidneys and benefit tendons and bones.
– **Dang Gui**, **Chuan Xiong**, **Sheng Di Huang** and **Bai Shao** (the Si Wu Tang *Four Substances Decoction*) nourish and harmonize Blood. This helps to expel Wind according to the principle that in order to expel Wind, it is necessary to harmonize Blood.
– **Ren Shen** and **Fu Ling** tonify Qi and strengthen the Spleen.
– **Rou Gui** scatters Cold and enters the Blood

vessels. This last property helps to expel Cold and Wind in accordance to the principle mentioned above.

- **Gan Cao** helps to tonify Qi and harmonizes.

Note: this prescription treats mostly the lower part of the body. It has an overall hot energy and should therefore be modified in case of deficiency of Kidney-Yin or in case of some Heat signs. For example, Xi Xin and Rou Gui should be decreased in dose or eliminated. In case of Kidney-Yin deficiency the dosage of Du Zhong could be reduced.

(ii) Prescription

QIN JIAO SI WU TANG
Gentiana macrophylla Four Substances Decoction
Dang Gui *Radix Angelicae sinensis* 6 g
Sheng Di Huang *Radix Rehmanniae glutinosae* 6 g
Bai Shao *Radix Paeoniae albae* 6 g
Chuan Xiong *Radix Ligustici wallichii* 6 g
Qin Jiao *Radix Gentianae macrophyllae* 6 g
Yi Yi Ren *Semen Coicis lachryma jobi* 6 g
Can Sha *Excrementum Bombycis mori* 6 g
Gan Cao *Radix Glycyrrhizae uralensis* 3 g

Explanation

This prescription is specific for Wind Painful Obstruction Syndrome occurring against a background of Blood deficiency.

- **Dang Gui**, **Sheng Di**, **Bai Shao** and **Chuan Xiong** form the Si Wu Tang *Four Substances Decoction* and nourish and harmonize Blood.
- **Qin Jiao** and **Can Sha** expel Wind and Dampness.
- **Yi Yi Ren** expels Dampness.
- **Gan Cao** harmonizes.

(iii) Prescription

Empirical prescription by Dr Jiao Shu De
Xu Duan *Radix Dipsaci* 6 g
Bu Gu Zhi *Fructus Psoraleae corylifoliae* 6 g
Gu Sui Bu *Rhizoma Gusuibu* 6 g
Yin Yang Huo *Herba Epimedii* 6 g
Gui Zhi *Ramulus Cinnamomi cassiae* 4 g
Fang Feng *Radix Ledebouriellae sesloidis* 6 g

Ma Huang *Herba Ephedrae* 3 g
Du Huo *Radix Angelicae pubescentis* 6 g
Wei Ling Xian *Radix Clematidis chinensis* 9 g
Kuan Jin Teng *Ramus Tinosporae sinensis* 9 g
Song Jie *Lignum Pini Nodi* 6 g
Zhi Mu *Rhizoma Anemarrhenae asphodeloidis* 6 g
Cang Zhu *Rhizoma Atractylodis lanceae* 6 g
Niu Xi *Radix Achyranthis bidentatae seu Cyathulae* 6 g
Shan Jia *Squama Manitis pentadactylae* 6 g
Chi Shao *Radix Paeoniae rubrae* 6 g
Bai Shao *Radix Paeoniae albae* 9 g

Explanation

- **Xu Duan**, **Bu Gu Zhi**, **Gu Sui Bu** and **Yin Yang Huo** tonify Kidney-Yang and benefit the bones.
- **Gui Zhi**, **Fang Feng** and **Ma Huang** expel Wind.
- **Du Huo**, **Wei Ling Xian**, **Kuan Jin Teng** and **Song Jie** expel Wind and Dampness and remove obstructions from the channels.
- **Zhi Mu** clears any Heat that might derive from the many hot herbs in the prescription.
- **Cang Zhu** dries Dampness.
- **Niu Xi**, **Shan Jia**, **Chi Shao** and **Bai Shao** move Blood. Niu Xi also nourishes sinews and bones.

This formula tonifies Kidney-Yang, benefits bones, expels Wind-Dampness, dries Dampness and moves Blood. It is suitable only for conditions characterized by a definite Yang deficiency and internal Cold.

(iv) Prescription

Prescription by Zhu Dan Xi (1281–1358)
Cang Zhu *Rhizoma Atractylodis lanceae* 6 g
Huang Bo *Cortex Phellodendri* 6 g
Fang Ji *Radix Stephaniae tetrandae* 6 g
Qiang Huo *Radix et Rhizoma Notopterygii* 6 g
Wei Ling Xian *Radix Clematidis chinensis* 9 g
Gui Zhi *Ramulus Cinnamomi cassiae* 4 g
Bai Zhi *Radix Angelicae dahuricae* 6 g
Chuan Xiong *Radix Ligustici wallichii* 6 g
Tao Ren *Semen Persicae* 6 g
Hong Hua *Flos Carthami tinctorii* 6 g

Dan Nan Xing *Rhizoma Arisaematis praeparata* 6 g
Long Dan Cao *Radix Gentianae scabrae* 6 g
Shen Qu *Massa Fermentata Medicinalis* 9 g

Explanation

This formula expels Wind from the Upper Burner, clears Heat and drains Dampness from the Lower Burner, and moves Blood and resolves Phlegm in the Middle Burner. It therefore treats Painful Obstruction Syndrome stemming from all three Burners.

- **Cang Zhu** and **Huang Bo** drain Dampness from the Lower Burner and treat the legs and knees.
- **Fang Ji** resolves Dampness and moves Water.
- **Qiang Huo** and **Wei Ling Xian** expel Wind-Dampness and remove obstructions from the channels.
- **Gui Zhi** scatters Cold, warms the channels, penetrates the Connecting channels, expels Wind and removes obstructions from the channels of hands and shoulders.
- **Bai Zhi** expels Wind from the head.
- **Chuan Xiong** moves Blood in the centre.
- **Tao Ren** and **Hong Hua** move Blood and eliminate stasis.
- **Dan Nan Xing** resolves Phlegm from the joints.
- **Long Dan Cao** drains Liver-Fire.
- **Shen Qu** regulates the Middle Burner.

Patent remedy

DU HUO JI SHENG WAN
Angelica pubescens-Loranthus Pill

Explanation

This well-known remedy has the same ingredients and indications as the homonymous prescription above. It is for chronic Painful Obstruction Syndrome, especially of the back and legs, against a background of Blood deficiency and Kidney-Yang deficiency.

The tongue presentation appropriate to this remedy is a Pale and Swollen body.

Patent remedy

JI XUE TENG QIN GAO PIAN
Millettia Liquid Extract Tablet
Ji Xue Teng *Caulis Millettiae seu Caulis Spatholobi*

Explanation

This tablet, composed of only Ji Xue Teng, expels Wind-Dampness, nourishes Blood and strengthens sinews.

It is for Painful Obstruction Syndrome, especially of the back and legs, against a background of Blood deficiency.

The tongue presentation appropriate to this remedy is a Pale and Thin body.

Patent remedy

DU ZHONG HU GU WAN
Eucommia-Tiger Bone Pill
Ren Shen *Radix Ginseng*
Bai Zhu *Rhizoma Atractylodis macrocephalae*
Dang Gui *Radix Angelicae sinensis*
Chuan Xiong *Radix Ligustici wallichii*
Ji Xue Teng *Caulis Millettiae seu Caulis Spatholobi*
San Qi *Radix Notoginseng*
Du Zhong *Cortex Eucommiae ulmoidis*
Hu Gu *Os Tigris*
Mu Gua *Fructus Chaenomelis lagenariae*
Yin Yang Huo *Herba Epimedii*
Wu Shao She *Zaocys dhumnades*
Lu Lu Tong *Fructus Liquidambaris taiwanianae*
Cang Zhu *Rhizoma Atractylodis lanceae*
Xun Gu Feng *Rhizoma seu Herba Aristolochiae*
Wei Ling Xian *Radix Clematidis chinensis*
Shi Nan Teng *Ramus Photiniae*
Sang Zhi *Ramulus Mori albae*

Explanation

This pill expels Wind-Dampness, tonifies Kidney-Yang and strengthens sinews and bones. It is used to treat chronic Painful Obstruction Syndrome, especially of the back and legs, against a background of Kidney-Yang deficiency.

The tongue presentation appropriate to this remedy is a Pale, Swollen and wet body. It is contraindicated in pregnancy.

Patent remedy

JIAN BU HU QIAN WAN
Vigorous Walk [like] Stealthy Tiger Pill
Mu Gua *Fructus Chaenomelis lagenariae*
Huai Niu Xi *Radix Achyranthis bidentatae*
Hu Gu *Os Tigris*
Qin Jiao *Radix Gentianae macrophyllae*
Dang Gui *Radix Angelicae sinensis*
Ren Shen *Radix Ginseng*
Feng Mi *Mel*

Explanation

This pill expels Wind-Dampness, nourishes Liver-Yin and strengthens the sinews. It is used for Chronic Painful Obstruction Syndrome, especially of the back and legs, against a background of Liver-Blood or Liver-Yin deficiency.

The tongue presentation appropriate to this remedy is a Pale-Thin or Red-Thin and Peeled body.

(b) PHLEGM STAGNATING IN JOINTS

Treatment principle

Resolve Phlegm, eliminate stasis, expel Wind, remove obstructions from the channels.

Prescription

TAO HONG YIN Variation
Persica-Carthamus Decoction Variation
Tao Ren *Semen Persicae* 6 g
Hong Hua *Flos Carthami tinctorii* 6 g
Chuan Xiong *Radix Ligustici wallichii* 6 g
Dang Gui (Wei) *Radix Angelicae sinensis* ("tail" only) 6 g
Wei Ling Xian *Radix Clematidis chinensis* 6 g
Ban Xia *Rhizoma Pinelliae ternatae* 6 g
Dan Nan Xing *Rhizoma Arisaematis praeparata* 6 g

Explanation

- **Tao Ren**, **Hong Hua**, **Chuan Xiong**, and **Dang Gui (Wei)**, move Blood, eliminate stasis and penetrate the blood vessels.
- **Wei Ling Xian** expels Wind-Damp and removes obstructions from the channels.
- **Ban Xia** and **Dan Nan Xing** resolve Phlegm.

(c) STASIS OF BLOOD IN JOINTS

Treatment principle

Move Blood, eliminate stasis, expel Wind-Dampness.

Prescription

HUO LUO XIAO LING DAN
Miraculously Effective Invigorating the Connecting Channels Pill
Dang Gui *Radix Angelicae sinensis* 15 g
Dan Shen *Radix Salviae miltiorrhizae* 15 g
Ru Xiang *Gummi Olibanum* 15 g
Mo Yao *Myrrha* 15 g

Explanation

This formula is used for chronic Painful Obstruction Syndrome with stasis of Blood in the joints.

- **Dang Gui** nourishes and moves Blood.
- **Dan Shen**, **Ru Xiang** and **Mo Yao** move Blood and eliminate stasis. Ru Xiang, in particular, moves Blood in the channels.

(d) SINEWS-BONES PAINFUL OBSTRUCTION SYNDROME

This deserves to be discussed separately as it is one of the most common types of Painful Obstruction Syndrome seen in a Western practice. Sinews-Bones Painful Obstruction Syndrome is a type of Damp Painful Obstruction Syndrome characterized by swelling of the joints. From a Western point of view it broadly corresponds to chronic rheumathoid arthritis.

The symptoms can be differentiated into 3 groups according to the stage:

Beginning stage: swelling of the joints, numbness and a feeling of heaviness.
Middle stage: swelling and pain of joints, contraction of tendons, limitation of joint movement.
Late stage: pain from buttocks to heels and from lower back to occiput.

The treatment principle also varies according to the stage:

Beginning stage: resolve Dampness, remove obstructions from the channels and penetrate the Connecting channels.
Middle stage: resolve Dampness, remove obstructions from the channels and tonify Qi and Blood.
Late stage: resolve Dampness, remove obstructions from the channels, move Blood and expel Wind (use insects).

The formulae suggested are outlined below.

(i) Beginning stage

One must distinguish between a Cold- and a Heat-type.

Cold type

Bai Zhu *Rhizoma Atractylodis macrocephalae* 9 g
Cang Zhu *Rhizoma Atractylodis lanceae* 9 g
Qiang Huo *Radix et Rhizoma Notopterygii* 9 g
Du Huo *Radix Angelicae pubescentis* 9 g
Gui Zhi *Ramulus Cinnamomi cassiae* 4.5 g
Fu Zi *Radix Aconiti carmichaeli praeparata* 6 g
Fang Feng *Radix Ledebouriellae sesloidis* 6 g

Explanation

- **Bai Zhu** and **Cang Zhu** drain Dampness.
- **Qiang Huo** and **Du Huo** expel Wind-Dampness and remove obstructions from the channels.
- **Gui Zhi** and **Fu Zi** scatter Cold.
- **Fang Feng** expels Wind.

Heat type

Shi Gao *Gypsum fibrosum* 30 g
Zhi Mu *Rhizoma Anemarrhenae asphodeloidis* 9 g
Huang Qin *Radix Scutellariae baicalensis* 9 g
Yi Yi Ren *Semen Coicis lachryma jobi* 15 g
Gan Cao *Radix Glycyrrhizae uralensis* 9 g
Fang Ji *Radix Stephaniae tetrandae* 9 g
Yin Chen Hao *Herba Artemisiae capillaris* 9 g
Luo Shi Teng *Caulis Trachelospermi jasminoidis* 9 g
Dang Gui *Radix Angelicae sinensis* 9 g

Explanation

- **Shi Gao** and **Zhi Mu** clear Heat.

- **Huang Qin** helps to clear Heat and also dries Dampness.
- **Yi Yi Ren** and **Gan Cao** clear Heat, drain Dampness and stop pain.
- **Fang Ji** and **Yin Chen Hao** clear Heat, resolve Dampness and eliminate swelling.
- **Luo Shi Teng** expels Wind-Dampness and removes obstructions from the channels.
- **Dang Gui** nourishes and moves Blood.

(ii) Middle stage

Dang Shen *Radix Codonopsis pilosulae* 9 g
Huang Qi *Radix Astragali membranacei* 9 g
Dang Gui *Radix Angelicae sinensis* 9 g
Bai Shao *Radix Paeoniae albae* 9 g
Chuan Xiong *Radix Ligustici wallichii* 6 g
Bai Zhu *Rhizoma Atractylodis macrocephalae* 9 g
Qin Jiao *Radix Gentianae macrophyllae* 9 g
Di Long *Pheretima aspergillum* 9 g
Lao Guan Cao *Herba Geranii wilfordii* 12 g
Feng Fang *Polistes mandarinus* 6 g
Xu Duan *Radix Dipsaci* 6 g
Chuan Niu Xi *Radix Cyathulae* 9 g
Hong Zao *Fructus Ziziphi jujubae* 3 dates

Explanation

- **Dang Shen**, **Huang Qi**, **Dang Gui**, **Bai Shao**, **Chuan Xiong** and **Bai Zhu** tonify Qi and Blood and move Blood.
- **Qin Jiao**, **Di Long**, **Lao Guan Cao** and **Feng Fang** expel Wind-Dampness, expel Wind and remove obstructions from the channels.
- **Xu Duan** tonifies the Kidneys and benefits bones.
- **Niu Xi** moves Blood.
- **Hong Zao** harmonizes.

Variations

- If there are Cold symptoms add Gui Zhi *Ramulus Cinnamomi cassiae*.
- If there are Heat symptoms add Huang Qin *Radix Scutellariae baicalensis*.
- If there is contraction of tendons add more insects or animal substances such as Jiang Can *Bombyx batryticatus* or Can Sha *Excrementum Bombycis mori*.

(iii) Late stage

Shu Di Huang *Radix Rehmanniae glutinosae praeparata* 30 g
Gou Ji *Rhizoma Cibotii barometz* 15 g
Huai Niu Xi *Radix Achyranthis bidentatae* 9 g
Bai Shao *Radix Paeoniae albae* 9 g
Gui Zhi *Ramulus Cinnamomi cassiae* 4.5 g
Xi Xin *Herba Asari cum radice* 3 g
Cang Zhu *Rhizoma Atractylodis lanceae* 9 g
Yi Yi Ren *Semen Coicis lachryma jobi* 15 g
Luo Shi Teng *Caulis Trachelospermi jasminoidis* 15 g
Can Sha *Excrementum Bombicis Mori* 6 g
Wu Gong *Scolopendra subspinipes* 1 piece

Explanation

- **Shu Di**, **Gou Ji**, **Huai Niu Xi** and **Bai Shao** nourish Liver and Kidneys and benefit sinews and bones.
- **Gui Zhi** and **Xi Xin** scatter Cold and warm the channels.
- **Cang Zhu** and **Yi Yi Ren** drain Dampness and resolve swelling.
- **Luo Shi Teng** expels Wind-Dampness and removes obstructions from the channels.
- **Can Sha** and **Wu Gong** expel Wind, resolve Dampness, remove obstructions from the channels and stop pain.

Case history

A 36-year-old woman had been suffering from rheumathoid arthritis for 2 years. The acute stage lasted 2 weeks during which she had a fever and her small joints became swollen, hot and painful. After the acute attack, some of the pain and swelling subsided, but never completely. When she came for the consultation two years later her small joints were swollen and sore but not very hot to the touch. In the mornings she ached everywhere including the lower back and she was very stiff. After 1–2 hours, the stiffness and general ache usually subsided except from the hands. Apart from this problem, her periods were regular and the flow was rather scanty. She occasionally experienced tingling of her legs and some floaters in her eyes. Sometimes she sweated at night and experienced some tinnitus. Her tongue was slightly Pale with swollen sides and the root had no spirit. Her pulse was generally Weak, particularly on both Rear positions.

Diagnosis

The original attack 2 years previously was a typical acute attack of Heat Painful Obstruction Syndrome characterized by invasion of Wind, Dampness and Heat in the joints. The condition as it presented at the time of the consultation was characterized by Damp Painful Obstruction Syndrome against an underlying deficiency of Qi and Blood and of Kidney-Qi. It was a type of Sinews-Bones Painful Obstruction Syndrome at the middle-late stage. The Kidney deficiency is evidenced by the back-ache in the mornings, the occasional night-sweating and tinnitus, the lack of spirit on the root of the tongue and the Weak pulse on both Kidney positions. The deficiency of Blood causes the occasional floaters and tingling of the limbs, while the deficiency of Spleen-Qi is shown by the swelling on the sides of the tongue.

Treatment principle

The treatment principle adopted was to tonify Qi and Blood, strengthen Kidney-Yang, benefit sinews and bones and expel Wind-Dampness. She was treated with both acupuncture and herbs.

Acupuncture

The acupuncture points used (with reinforcing method to tonify Qi and Blood and even method to expel Wind-Dampness) were selected from the following:

- **T.B.-5** Waiguan to expel Wind.
- **L.I.-11** Quchi to resolve Dampness and benefit sinews.
- **SP-9** Yinlingquan, **SP-6** Sanyinjiao and **BL-22** Sanjiaoshu to resolve Dampness.
- **Baxie** extra points to expel Wind-Dampness from the fingers.
- **Ren-6** Qihai and **Ren-4** Guanyuan to tonify Qi and Blood in general.
- **ST-36** Zusanli to tonify Spleen-Qi.
- **BL-11** Dashu, Gathering point for bones, to benefit the bones.
- **Du-14** Dazhui and **Du-12** Shenzhu to strengthen the Governing Vessel and the Defensive-Qi in order to expel pathogenic factors.

Herbal treatment

The decoction used was a variation of the combination of the two prescriptions for the middle and late stages of Sinews-Bones Painful Obstruction Syndrome.

Dang Shen *Radix Codonopsis pilosulae* 9 g
Huang Qi *Radix Astragali membranacei* 9 g
Bai Zhu *Rhizoma Atractylodis macrocephalae* 9 g
Dang Gui *Radix Angelicae sinensis* 9 g
Shu Di Huang *Radix Rehmanniae glutinosae praeparata* 30 g
Bai Shao *Radix Paeoniae albae* 9 g
Chuan Xiong *Radix Ligustici wallichii* 6 g
Xu Duan *Radix Dipsaci* 6 g

Gou Ji *Rhizoma Cibotii barometz* 15 g
Gui Zhi *Ramulus Cinnamomi cassiae* 4.5 g
Cang Zhu *Rhizoma Atractylodis lanceae* 9 g
Yi Yi Ren *Semen Coicis lachryma jobi* 15 g
Qin Jiao *Radix Gentianae macrophyllae* 9 g
Can Sha *Excrementum Bombicis Mori* 6 g
Hai Feng Teng *Caulis Piperis* 6 g
Sang Zhi *Ramulus Mori albae* 6 g
Hong Zao *Fructus Ziziphi jujubae* 3 dates

Explanation
- **Dang Shen**, **Huang Qi** and **Bai Zhu** tonify Qi.
- **Dang Gui**, **Shu Di Huang**, **Bai Shao** and **Chuan Xiong**, the Si Wu Tang *Four Substances Decoction*, nourish and harmonize Blood.
- **Xu Duan** and **Gou Ji** tonify Kidney-Yang.
- **Gui Zhi** expels Wind and affects the upper limbs.
- **Cang Zhu** and **Yi Yi Ren** drain Dampness.
- **Qin Jiao**, **Can Sha**, **Hai Feng Teng** and **Sang Zhi** expel Wind-Dampness. Hai Feng Teng and Sang Zhi affect the limbs.
- **Hong Zao** harmonizes.

This patient was treated for over a year with fortnightly acupuncture sessions and daily decoctions, after which she was free of pain and the swelling of her joints subsided.

Treatment of specific parts of the body

Having dealt with the acupuncture and herbal treatment of the various Painful Obstruction Syndrome types according to pathogenic factor (Wind, Cold, Dampness and Heat), we can now discuss the treatment of Painful Obstruction Syndrome according to specific parts of the body. The discussion will concentrate mostly on the acupuncture treatment as this is much more specific than herbal treatment in targeting a specific area of the body. Whilst there are certain herbs that have an affinity for a certain part of the body (e.g. Qiang Huo *Radix et Rhizoma Notopterygii* for the neck and top of the shoulders, Gao Ben *Radix Ligustici sinensis* for the spine, etc.), acupuncture is certainly much more specific and direct to treat individual areas. Quite simply, if a joint is affected, the acupuncture treatment is applied mostly to that joint and can eliminate pathogenic factors directly. For example, if the left wrist is affected, the acupuncture treatment will be applied to that wrist,

directly eliminating Wind-Cold-Damp from that joint. No herbal treatment could be as specific as that, unless, of course, external herbal treatment is applied.

Thus the herbal treatment is based more on the type of pattern (Wind, Cold, Damp or Heat) and underlying condition (Qi-Blood deficiency, deficiency of Liver-Kidneys, Phlegm, stasis of Blood), rather than the part of the body affected. The acupuncture treatment, by its very nature, is very much based on the part of the body affected. However, there are herbs that direct prescriptions to specific parts of the body and the following is a partial list:

- *Neck, top of shoulders:* Qiang Huo *Radix et Rhizoma Notopterygii*, Gao Ben *Rhizoma Ligustici*.
- *Shoulder joint:* Jiang Huang *Rhizoma Curcumae longae*.
- *Spine:* Gao Ben *Rhizoma Ligustici*.
- *Lower back:* Du Huo *Radix Angelicae pubescentis*, Hai Tong Pi *Cortex Erythrinae variegatae*.
- *Leg:* Bi Xie *Radix Dioscoreae hypoglaucae*.
- *Knee:* Niu Xi *Radix Achyranthis bidentatae seu Cyathulae*, Hai Tong Pi *Cortex Erythrinae variegatae*.

Besides single herbs, there are also some empirical prescriptions for specific parts of the body. The following formulae, all for chronic cases, can be used as they are, or the expelling Wind-Dampness herbs contained within them can be extracted to be added to other formulae.

NECK

Ge Gen *Radix Puerariae* 6 g
Wei Ling Xian *Radix Clematidis chinensis* 9 g
Qin Jiao *Radix Gentianae macrophyllae* 6 g
Qiang Huo *Radix et Rhizoma Notopterygii* 6 g
Tou Gu Cao *Herba Speranskiae tuberculatae* 9 g
Ji Xue Teng *Caulis Millettiae seu Caulis Spatholobi* 9 g
Dang Gui *Radix Angelicae sinensis* 9 g
Sheng Di Huang *Radix Rehmanniae glutinosae* 9 g
Bai Shao *Radix Paeoniae albae* 9 g
Xiang Fu *Rhizoma Cyperi rotundi* 6 g

SHOULDER

Qiang Huo *Radix et Rhizoma Notopterygii* 9 g
Gui Zhi *Ramulus Cinnamomi cassiae* 6 g
Sheng Di Huang *Radix Rehmanniae glutinosae* 9 g
Tou Gu Cao *Herba Speranskiae tuberculatae* 9 g
Ji Xue Teng *Caulis Millettiae seu Caulis Spatholobi* 9 g
Dang Gui *Radix Angelicae sinensis* 9 g
Dan Shen *Radix Salviae miltiorrhizae* 6 g
Xiang Fu *Rhizoma Cyperi rotundi* 6 g

LOWER BACK

Dang Gui *Radix Angelicae sinensis* 9 g
Ji Xue Teng *Caulis Millettiae seu Caulis Spatholobi* 12 g
Tou Gu Cao *Herba Speranskiae tuberculatae* 9 g
Lao Guan Cao *Herba Geranii wilfordii* 6 g
Qiang Huo *Radix et Rhizoma Notopterygii* 6 g
Sang Ji Sheng *Ramus Loranthi* 9 g
Xu Duan *Radix Dipsaci* 9 g
Xiang Fu *Rhizoma Cyperi rotundi* 6 g

UPPER LIMBS

Huang Qi *Radix Astragali membranacei* 12 g
Gui Zhi *Ramulus Cinnamomi cassiae* 6 g
Sang Zhi *Ramulus Mori albae* 9 g
Wei Ling Xian *Radix Clematidis chinensis* 9 g
Qin Jiao *Radix Gentianae macrophyllae* 6 g
Qiang Huo *Radix et Rhizoma Notopterygii* 9 g
Dang Gui *Radix Angelicae sinensis* 9 g
Ji Xue Teng *Caulis Millettiae seu Caulis Spatholobi* 9 g
Lao Guan Cao *Herba Geranii wilfordii* 9 g
Bai Shao *Radix Paeoniae albae* 9 g
Jiang Huang *Rhizoma Curcumae* 6 g
Xiang Fu *Rhizoma Cyperi rotundi* 6 g

LOWER LIMBS

Dang Gui *Radix Angelicae sinensis* 9 g
Dan Shen *Radix Salviae miltiorrhizae* 6 g
Qiang Huo *Radix et Rhizoma Notopterygii* 9 g
Lao Guan Cao *Herba Geranii wilfordii* 9 g

Bai Zhu *Rhizoma Atractylodis macrocephalae* 9 g
Huai Niu Xi *Radix Achyranthis bidentatae* 9 g
Mu Gua *Fructus Chaenomelis lagenariae* 6 g
Xiang Fu *Rhizoma Cyperi rotundi* 6 g

The following is a discussion of the acupuncture treatment of specific parts of the body.

NECK AND TOP OF SHOULDERS

Pain in the neck and shoulders is an extremely common complaint in Western patients. The neck is a crucial part of the body which very readily reflects the state of tension and stress typical of the rushed life-style of industrialized countries which causes tensing of the neck muscles and pulling of the head backwards. One only needs to observe the effortless and graceful way in which a toddler bends down to pick up something from the floor to realize the importance of the proper use of the neck. A toddler will bend from his or her knees and straighten up, all the time keeping the neck free and the head forward. Most adults would instinctively pull the head backwards and tighten the neck as they get up from a sitting position.

The situation is of course aggravated further for those who, in their work, have to keep their head fixed in a position of intense concentration for long periods of time. For example, typists, VDU operators, draughtsmen, assemblers of electronic components, and generally workers in many different types of factories using a production line.

AETIOLOGY

In discussing neck pain it is useful to distinguish acute from chronic cases.

Acute neck ache is due either to invasion of Wind-Cold or to sprain. The symptoms are similar in both cases: neck ache with sudden onset, rigidity or stiffness and a limitation of movement in turning the neck from side to side. An underlying Liver pattern (either Liver-Blood deficiency, Liver-Yang rising or Liver-Qi stagnation) is a predisposing factor for this condition. If acute neck ache is due to exposure to climatic factors, it is invariably due to Wind because this attacks the top part of the body and causes stiffness and rigidity.

Chronic neck ache develops as a consequence of repeated acute attacks which are not treated properly. In chronic cases, an underlying Liver pattern is almost always present. In women it is most likely to be Liver-Blood deficiency, in men it is most likely to be Liver-Qi stagnation or Liver-Yang rising, and in the elderly it is more likely to be Liver-Fire or Liver-Wind.

Acute flare-ups of a chronic neck ache are often typically elicited by exposure to wind. It is not unusual to hear patients say that they always get a neck ache during spells of windy weather, and some even say that an East wind will cause it.

TREATMENT

There are three main differences between the treatment of acute or chronic neck ache:

1. in acute cases the needles are manipulated more vigorously, i.e. with a reducing method
2. in acute cases, distal points play a more important role than in chronic cases
3. in chronic cases, it is always necessary to treat any underlying condition that might be contributing to the neck ache.

ACUTE

In acute cases the distal points play a primary role and they are needled with reducing method. The main *distal* points to use are:

– **S.I.-3** Houxi is the main distal point to use when the pain is on the occiput and back of the neck, along the Bladder channel. This point expels Wind and treats the upper part of the Greater Yang channels and is especially used in acute cases.
– **T.B.-5** Waiguan is the distal point to use when the pain is on the side of the neck and it can be used unilaterally on the affected side only.
– **G.B.-39** Xuanzhong is very effective as a

distal point when the pain is on both sides of the neck and the movement of the neck from side to side is restricted. This point should be reduced while the patient slowly moves the neck from side to side. It is very effective in freeing the neck (Fig. 23.3).

The main *local* points to use are:

– **BL-10** Tianzhu if the pain is on the occiput and is bilateral.
– **G.B.-20** Fengchi if the pain is at the base of the neck extending to the top of the shoulders. It is especially indicated if the pain is due to Wind.
– **Du-16** Fengfu is indicated if the pain is due to Wind.
– **G.B.-21** Jianjing is a useful local point to use as neck ache is often associated with (or stems from) muscle tension in the top of the shoulders (trapezius muscle).

Any local point tender on pressure can also be used, and warming the affected area along a channel with a moxa stick is very effective.

CHRONIC

The main *distal* points to use in chronic cases are:

– **BL-60** Kunlun is the main distal point for chronic neck ache. It treats not only the neck,

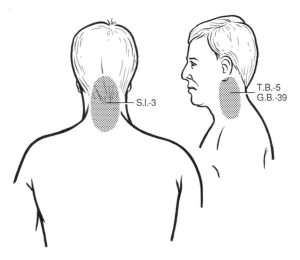

Fig. 23.3   Distal points in acute neck-ache

but also the top of the shoulders and the upper back. It is particularly indicated, of course, if the pain is along the Greater-Yang channels.

– **T.B.-5** Waiguan is used if the pain is unilateral on the side of the neck.
– **T.B.-8** Sanyangluo is used if the area of pain involves two or three of the Yang channels of the arm.
– **P-6** Neiguan is effective in women. It treats the neck by virtue of it being the Connecting point and therefore affecting the Triple Burner channel. It is particularly effective when the neck ache is associated with general nervous tension which causes the neck muscles to tense up.
– **KI-4** Dazhong can be used as a distal point by virtue of it being the Connecting point and therefore in relation with the Bladder channel. It is especially useful when the neck ache is associated with a Kidney-deficiency.
– **ST-40** Fenglong is the Connecting point and can be used for neck ache as a branch of the Stomach Connecting channel separates in the neck and flows to the throat (Fig. 23.4).

The *local* points to use are obviously the same as for acute cases. The main difference is that it is often necessary to use points further down the upper back such as S.I.-9 Jianzhen, S.I.-10 Naoshu, S.I.-11 Tianzong, S.I.-12 Bingfeng, S.I.-

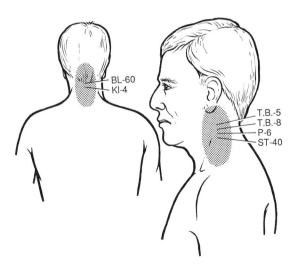

BL-60
KI-4

T.B.-5
T.B.-8
P-6
ST-40

Fig. 23.4 Distal points in chronic neck-ache

13 Quyuan, S.I.-14 Jianwaishu, S.I.-15 Jianzhong-shu and T.B.-15 Tianliao. These points should always be checked for tenderness and needled if they are tender. Of the above points, S.I.-11, S.I.-13 and T.B.-15 are the ones that are most frequently tender. Warming needle or cupping are very effective in removing pain and relaxing the muscles.

SHOULDER JOINT

Pain and stiffness of the shoulder joint is an extremely common complaint both in the West and China. Acupuncture normally gives excellent results in both acute and chronic cases.

AETIOLOGY

1. COLD

Invasion of the shoulder channels by external Cold is one of the most common aetiological factors. Cold contracts muscles and sinews and therefore causes pain and stiffness. Typically, the pain would be aggravated by exposure to cold or when the weather is rainy and damp. The local invasion of Cold leads to stagnation of Qi in the shoulder channels and if the Cold is not expelled, the stagnation can become chronic. This will cause pain and also predispose the channels to further invasion of Cold, thus starting a vicious circle.

2. EXCESSIVE WORK OR EXERCISE

The constant repetition of a movement involving the shoulder joint, either through a particular sport or through work, will, over the years, lead to local stagnation of Qi in the shoulder.

3. ACCIDENTS

Minor accidents cause local stagnation of Qi, while serious ones cause local stasis of Blood. Very often, old accidents which may have long been forgotten predispose the shoulder joint (or any joint) to invasion of Cold later on in life.

4. GALL-BLADDER PROBLEM

In a small number of cases, a problem in the Gall-Bladder (such as Damp-Heat) can affect the Small Intestine and Gall-Bladder channels in the shoulder and cause referred pain in the shoulder joint.

5. LARGE INTESTINE PROBLEM

In an equally small number of cases, a shoulder pain along the Large Intestine channel can be the external manifestation of an organ problem.

TREATMENT

ACUTE

Distal points are primary in the treatment of acute shoulder pain. They are manipulated strongly in order to remove obstructions from the channel involved. After manipulating the distal points, local points can be used. The main distal point for acute shoulder pain and stiffness is ST-38 Tiaokou. This point is needled on the same side as the affected shoulder and is manipulated vigorously for a few minutes while the patient gently rotates the shoulder joint. If movement of the joint is severely impaired, it is preferable that a third person holds the patient's arm by the elbow and gently helps him or her to rotate the shoulder.

If the main area of pain is along the Small Intestine channel, the distal point to use is BL-58 Feiyang, with exactly the same technique as for ST-38.

After manipulating the distal point as described above, local points are used with warming needle if necessary. The choice of local points is made according to the distribution of pain along a certain channel. If the shoulder is stiff, the channel involved can also be identified according to the particular movement that is inhibited. If the patient cannot raise the arm sideways, it indicates that the Large Intestine channel is involved (Fig. 23.5).

If he or she cannot touch the opposite shoulder joint, then the Lung channel is probably affected (Fig. 23.6).

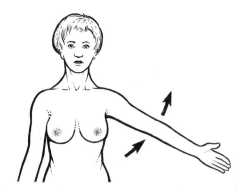

Fig. 23.5   Difficulty in abducting arm (Large Intestine channel)

If he or she cannot twist the arm backwards over the scapula, it denotes involvement of the Small Intestine channel (Fig. 23.7).

With the aid of the above techniques, careful observation of the distribution of pain and pressing the points checking for tenderness, the involved channel can be identified and the local points chosen.

It cannot be overemphasized how important it is to choose the local points according to the involved channel (identified by checking for tenderness on pressure) and not according to preconceived ideas about certain points. For example, L.I.-15 Jianyu is certainly the most important local point for the shoulder joint, but

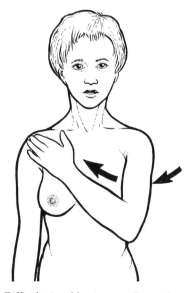

Fig. 23.6   Difficulty in adducting arm (Lung channel)

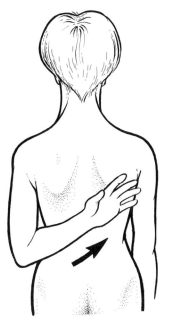

Fig. 23.7 Difficulty in twisting arm backwards (Small Intestine channel)

if only the point T.B.-14 Jianliao is tender on pressure, then the latter should be used and *not* L.I.-15. It is an extremely simple rule, but one that is frequently forgotten in practice.

The main local points for each channel are:

- *Large Intestine:* L.I.-15 Jianyu, L.I.-14 Binao.
- *Small Intestine:* S.I.-9 Jianzhen, S.I.-10 Naoshu, S.I.-11 Tianzong, S.I.-12 Bingfeng, S.I.-13 Quyuan, S.I.-14 Jianwaishu and S.I.-15 Jianzhongshu. Of these, the two most frequently tender points are S.I.-11 and S.I.-13.
- *Triple Burner:* T.B.-14 Jianliao, T.B.-13 Naohui, T.B.-15 Tianliao.
- *Gall-Bladder:* G.B.-21 Jianjing.
- *Lung:* LU-2 Yunmen.
- *Heart:* HE-1 Jiquan.

An important local extra point is **Jianneiling** which is situated half-way between the acromio-clavicular articulation and the anterior axillary fold (Fig. 23.8). This point is very effective when the main area of pain is in the front of the shoulder joint.

The warming needle can be used since this type of pain and stiffness is usually caused by a combination of Wind, Dampness and Cold, with a predominance of Cold.

In my experience, the choice of local points needs to be guided not only by the involvement of the channels, but also by Western anatomical considerations. In order to understand this we need to look at the anatomy of the joints involved in shoulder pain. There are three joints in the shoulder: the scapulo-humeral joint, the acromio-clavicular joint and the sterno-clavicular joint, the first two being the most important ones in shoulder pain (Fig. 23.9).

The scapulo-humeral joint is the shoulder joint proper, i.e. the one that connects the scapula to the arm: this is also the joint that is most involved in shoulder pain and limitation of movement of the arm. Furthermore, the abduction, flexion and rotation of the arm, are all under the control of the scapulo-humeral muscles. It follows that in order to affect the scapulo-humeral joint, it is important to treat the muscles overlying the scapula: hence the importance of the points situated over the scapula, i.e. S.I.-10 Naoshu, S.I.-11 Tianzong, S.I.-12 Bingfeng, S.I.-13 Quyuan and T.B.-15 Tianliao. I find that in pain of the shoulder with limitation of movement, best results are obtained if two or three of the above points are needled with moxa on the needle and that needling only the points on the acromio-clavicular joint (such as L.I.-15 Jianyu and T.B.-14 Jianliao) is not enough: the reason for this is that the joint governing the movement of the arm is not the acromio-clavicular joint but the scapulo-humeral one.

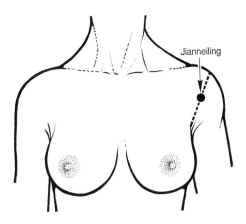

Fig. 23.8 Location of extra point Jianneiling

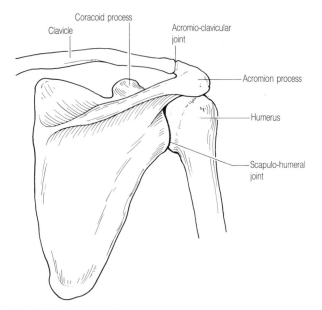

Fig. 23.9   Anatomy of shoulder joints

CHRONIC

In the treatment of chronic shoulder pain, distal points are also used but they are stimulated with less intensity or not at all. The choice of distal points depends on the channel involved:

– *Large Intestine:* L.I.-1 Shangyang or L.I.-4 Hegu. LU-7 Lieque can also be used.
– *Lung:* LU-7 Lieque.
– *Small Intestine:* S.I.-3 Houxi or S.I.-1 Shaoze.
– *Triple Burner:* T.B.-1 Guanchong or T.B.-5 Waiguan.

These distal points are stimulated with moderate intensity and the local points are inserted immediately after the distal ones.

The local points to use are the same as for acute cases. In chronic cases, it is usually important to use the points along the Small Intestine channel if they are tender on pressure. So, even though the patient may not complain of pain in that area, they should always be checked for tenderness on pressure.

Case history

A 58-year-old man had been experiencing pain in both shoulder joints for the previous 4 years. He had

been working as a car mechanic for over 25 years. The pain was aggravated by exposure to cold. The points L.I.-15 Jianyu were tender on pressure. He did not present any other symptoms and was otherwise a very healthy and strong man.

Diagnosis
This an example of Cold Painful Obstruction Syndrome. There is, however, the additional component of stagnation of Qi in the shoulders from over-use of the joints through his work as a car mechanic. This is evidenced by the fact that both shoulders are equally affected. If the pain is due purely to Painful Obstruction Syndrome, usually only one shoulder is affected or, at least, one shoulder is definitely worse than the other.

Treatment principle
The treatment principle adopted was to expel Cold, warm the channels, and move Qi.

Acupuncture
The main points used were:

– **L.I.-15** Jianyu and **S.I.-10** Naoshu with warm needle as a local point to remove obstructions from the channels.
– **L.I.-11** Quchi to benefit tendons.

Six weekly treatments were enough to clear up this problem.

Case history

A 50-year-old woman had been suffering from pain of

the shoulder for the past 14 years. She had had several cortisone injections. The pain was located in the left shoulder joint and it extended up to the neck and down the arm along the Large Intestine channel. At times the pain extended also to the left scapula. The points L.I.-15 Jianyu, T.B.-14 Jianliao, Jianneiling extra-point, S.I.-11 Tianzong, S.I.-9 Jianzhen and S.I.-10 Naoshu were all very tender on pressure. The shoulder was very stiff and the arm difficult to abduct. The pain was aggravated during spells of rainy weather and alleviated by heat. She was overweight and her tongue was Pale-Purplish.

Diagnosis
This is a case of Cold Painful Obstruction Syndrome. She also had an internal condition of Yang deficiency and Internal Cold as shown by the Pale-Purplish tongue. In such chronic cases of shoulder ache it is essential to search for tender points not only around the joint itself, but also the points on the corresponding scapula along the Small Intestine channel, i.e. S.I.-9 Jianzhen, S.I.-10 Naoshu, S.I.-11 Tianzong, S.I.-12 Bingfeng, S.I.-13 Quyuan and S.I.-14 Jianwaishu. T.B.-15 Tianliao should also always be checked for tenderness.

Treatment principle
The treatment principle adopted was to expel Cold, warm the channels and tonify Yang.

Acupuncture
In this case the main points used were:

– **L.I.-15** Jianyu, **G.B.-21** Jianjing and **Jianneiling** extra point as local points.
– **L.I.-1** Shangyang as distal point to remove obstructions from the Large Intestine channel. This was alternated with **T.B.-8** Sanyangluo, meeting point of the three channels of the arm because the pain involved all these three channels.
– A selection of two points out of the following according to tenderness on pressure: **S.I.-9** Jianzhen, **S.I.-10** Naoshu, **S.I.-11** Tianzong, **S.I.-12** Bingfeng, **S.I.-13** Quyuan, **S.I.-14** Jianwaishu and **T.B.-15** Tianliao with warm needle.

The treatment in this case was prolonged and results slow to come due partly to the long duration of the problem and partly to the cortisone injections which usually slow down the results obtained with acupuncture. The problem was however, resolved after 18 fortnightly treatments.

ELBOW

Pain in the elbow is usually caused by a combination of exposure to Damp-Cold and over-exertion, either due to sports or work. By far the most frequent area of pain is on the lateral side of the elbow, i.e. along the Large Intestine channel, but pain can sometimes occur immediately above the tip of the olecranon (i.e. along the Triple Burner channel) or between the olecranon and the medial condyle of the humerus (i.e. along the Small Intestine channel). Occasionally, pain occurs on the medial surface of the arm along the Lung channel.

The pain often radiates upwards or downwards along the Large Intestine channel. In some cases, pain can radiate from about L.I.-11 Quchi downwards along the Large Intestine channel. Numbness and tingling can also be experienced down the arm and fingertips.

TREATMENT

The treatment is practically the same for acute or chronic cases apart of course for the intensity of needle manipulation which, following general principles, would be more vigorous in acute cases.

The main distal points are chosen from the Large Intestine channel and they are either L.I.-1 Shangyang or L.I.-4 Hegu. If the area of pain extends slightly over to the tip of the olecranon, T.B.-5 Waiguan can be used in addition to one of the former. If the area of pain seems to cover both the Large Intestine and Triple Burner channels, T.B.-8 Sanyangluo is selected.

The most important local points are:

– **L.I.-11** Quchi: this is one of the most important local points. In this case, this point functions both as a local and a systemic point since it also benefits sinews in general, thus helping to relieve Painful Obstruction Syndrome.
– **Quyangwei** is an extra point located immediately adjacent to the epicondyle when the elbow is bent (Fig. 23.10). This point is extremely effective especially when used with warming needle.
– **L.I.-12** Zhouliao is used particularly when the elbow pain radiates upwards.
– **T.B.-10** Tianjing is used when the pain is located around the tip of the olecranon.
– **S.I.-8** Xiaohai is used when the pain is located around the medial condyle of the humerus.

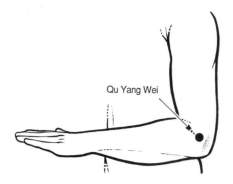

Fig. 23.10   Location of extra point Qu Yang Wei

– **LU-5** Chize relaxes the tendons of the arm and is used when the elbow is stiff. The "ABC of Acupuncture" (AD 259) says: *"When the arm cannot be raised to the head or there is pain in the elbow, needle LU-5"*.[13] The "Illustrated Manual of Acupuncture Points as Shown on the Bronze Man" (AD 1026) says: *"LU-5 can treat Wind-Painful Obstruction Syndrome of the elbow and inability to raise the arm"*.[14]

Results are usually very good with a few treatments. Occasionally, in long-standing cases, results are slow to come. This is especially so if cortisone injections were administered to the elbow as these tend to slow down the effects of acupuncture. In these cases, it might be useful to try and needle the healthy side as well as the affected one. A particularly effective way of doing this is by needling the Connecting point of the affected channel on the opposite side. For example, if the pain occurs along the Large Intestine channel on the left side, L.I.-6 Pianli on the right side would be needled. Other points can simply be used bilaterally. A more specific way of doing this is by reducing the points on the healthy side and reinforcing (especially with warming needle) those on the affected side. The rationale of this treatment lies in the fact that in chronic channel problems, the affected side becomes empty and the healthy side relatively full.

WRIST

Pain in the wrists is common in elderly patients. It is usually due to invasion of Damp-Cold,

aggravated by over-use of the joint (e.g. flute-players).

TREATMENT

The treatment of acute and chronic cases is not significantly different.

In *acute* cases, one needles the distal point first with reducing method and then uses local points. Since the wrist is almost at the extremity of the arm, there are no distal points as such along the channel involved. However, in my experience ST-36 Zusanli can be used as a distal point for Painful Obstruction Syndrome of the wrist, especially if from Dampness. Other distal points can be used according to the corresponding channel of the same polarity and opposite end (see Table 23.1 and Table I.3 in Appendix I). For example, if the Triple Burner channel in the wrist is involved, then one can use a point on the ankle on the Gall Bladder channel, i.e. G.B.-40 Qiuxu. This is due to the relation between the Triple Burner and Gall Bladder channels within the Lesser-Yang system. If the Small Intestine or Large Intestine channel on the wrist is involved, one can use BL-60 Kunlun or ST-41 Jiexi respectively. If the Lung, Pericardium or Heart channel on the wrist is involved, one can use SP-5 Shangqiu, LIV-4 Zhongfeng or KI-3 Taixi respectively. In all these cases the distal point is needled with reducing method and the local points are needled afterwards (while the distal point is retained).

In *chronic* cases, the distal point is needled with even method. Since the pain usually occurs

Table 23.1   Correspondence of points on joints of the upper and lower part of the body

Joint	Arm	Leg
Shoulder		
Large Intestine	L.I.-15 Jianyu	ST-31 Biguan
Triple Burner	T.B.-14 Jianliao	G.B.-30 Huantiao
Small Intestine	S.I.-10 Naoshu	BL-36 Chengfu
Elbow		
Large Intestine	L.I.-11 Quchi	ST-36 Zusanli
Triple Burner	T.B.-10 Tianjing	G.B.-34 Yanglingquan
Small Intestine	S.I.-8 Xiaohai	BL-40 Weizhong
Wrist		
Large Intestine	L.I.-5 Yangxi	ST-41 Jiexi
Triple Burner	T.B.-4 Yangchi	G.B.-40 Qiuxu
Small Intestine	S.I.-5 Yanggu	BL-60 Kunlun

on the Yang surface of the wrist the main local points to use are:

– T.B.-4 Yangchi.
– L.I.-5 Yangxi is especially suitable as it is the River point from which pathogenic factors are deviated to joints.
– S.I.-5 Yanggu is also especially indicated for the same reason as above.

Moxa is applicable if Cold is involved. If the wrist is swollen, it can be tapped with the 7-star hammer (or plum-blossom needle) until it bleeds very slightly and moxa smoke should be directed onto the area.

FINGERS

Pain and swelling of the fingers is a common complaint. It is usually due to Cold or Damp Painful Obstruction Syndrome, and is frequently caused by prolonged exposure to cold water or rain over many years (e.g. farmers or cleaners).

TREATMENT

In *acute* cases only local points are used. The main points are:

– **Baxie** extra points. There are two alternative locations for these points and they are both effective. They are located on the dorsum of the hand, either at the end of the fingers' creases when the hand is fisted, or midway between the end of the creases and the metacarpo-phalangeal articulations (Fig. 23.11). They are needled obliquely towards the palm of the hand.

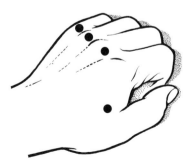

Fig. 23.11   Location of extra points Baxie

– **L.I.-3** Sanjian expels Wind, Cold and Dampness from the fingers. It should be needled at least 0.5 *cun* perpendicularly towards the ulna, i.e. along the palm of the hand. It is very effective and some doctors think that if this point is punctured deeply enough (up to 1 *cun*), there is no need to use the Baxie points.
– **T.B.-3** Zhongzhu also expels Wind, Cold and Dampness from the fingers. It is also effective for Heat Painful Obstruction Syndrome.
– **S.I.-3** Houxi expels Wind from the fingers. Similarly to L.I.-3 Sanjian, it should be needled at least 0.5 *cun* perpendicularly along the palm of the hand.

In *chronic* cases, the above points are also used and they are combined with some adjacent points:

– **T.B.-5** Waiguan is an important adjacent point for Painful Obstruction Syndrome of the fingers. It expels Wind and stimulates the circulation of Qi and Blood in the fingers. One should obtain the needling sensation to radiate downwards towards the fingers.
– **LU-7** Lieque can be used especially when the pain is located mostly along the base of the thumb. This occurs frequently in old people when the invasion of pathogenic factors is combined with a decline of Qi affecting the Lung channel. In young people it occurs in piano or flute players. This point should be needled obliquely downwards and the needling sensation should radiate towards the thumb.
– **S.I.-5** Yanggu is effective in expelling Dampness and is therefore particularly useful when the fingers are swollen.

If the fingers are swollen they can be lightly tapped with the 7-star hammer (or plum-blossom needle) until they bleed slightly and moxa smoke should be directed onto them.

Case history

A 53-year-old woman presented with pain in the fingers which had started two years previously. The fingers were swollen and already deformed. Previously to the pain in the hand, she had also suffered with lower back-ache intermittently. She had been experiencing quite a severe loss of hair for the past year and her knees felt weak.

Her tongue was Pale and tending to be Peeled and her pulse was slightly Floating-Empty.

Diagnosis
The pain in the fingers is clearly due to invasion of Cold and Dampness. It has now turned into chronic Painful Obstruction Syndrome with stagnation of Phlegm in the joints (as evidenced by the bone deformities). Initially, this occurred against a background of Blood deficiency which then began to turn into Yin deficiency (of the Kidneys). The Blood deficiency is apparent from the Pale tongue, whilst the beginning of Yin deficiency is reflected in the falling hair, weak knees and Floating-Empty pulse. This case shows clearly how one can often see in practice borderline cases between Blood and Yin deficiency which happen more frequently in women.

Treatment principle
She was treated with acupuncture and herbs and the treatment was aimed at removing obstruction from the channel, expelling Cold and Dampness, nourishing Blood and Yin.

Acupuncture
The main points used were:

– **L.I.-3** Sanjian and **Baxie** extra points to remove Cold-Dampness from the fingers.
– **T.B.-5** Waiguan to expel Wind.
– **ST-36** Zusanli and **SP-6** Sanyinjiao to nourish Blood.
– **KI-3** Taixi and **BL-23** Shenshu to tonify the Kidneys.

Herbal treatment
The prescription used was a variation of Qin Jiao Si Wu Tang *Gentiana macrophylla Four Substances Decoction*:

Dang Gui *Radix Angelicae sinensis* 6 g
Sheng Di Huang *Radix Rehmanniae glutinosae* 6 g
Bai Shao *Radix Paeoniae albae* 6 g
Chuan Xiong *Radix Ligustici wallichii* 6 g
Qin Jiao *Radix Gentianae macrophyllae* 6 g
Yi Yi Ren *Semen Coicis lachryma jobi* 6 g
Can Sha *Excrementum Bombycis mori* 6 g
Gan Cao *Radix Glycyrrhizae uralensis* 3 g
Ban Xia *Rhizoma Pinelliae ternatae* 6 g
Sang Ji Sheng *Ramus Loranthi* 4 g

Explanation
– Dang Gui, Sheng Di Huang, Bai Shao and Chuan Xiong are a modified version of the *Four Substances Decoction* and will nourish both Blood and Yin since Sheng Di Huang is used instead of Shu Di Huang.
– Qin Jiao and Can Sha expel Wind-Damp.
– Yi Yi Ren expels Dampness.

– Ban Xia was added to resolve Phlegm (in the form of joint deformities).
– Sang Ji Sheng was added to nourish Liver-Blood and simultaneously expel Wind-Damp.

This patient made a gradual improvement and she is still under treatment at the time of writing.

HIP

Pain in the hip is usually due to invasion of Cold and Dampness. From a Western medical viewpoint it may be due to osteoarthritis. In the beginning stages, this can be successfully cured, whilst in the late stages acupuncture cannot effect a cure. The pain is usually unilateral.

TREATMENT

Pain in the hip seldom occurs as an acute episode. It usually develops very gradually over the years.

The main *distal points* to use are:

– **G.B.-41** Zulinqi is the main distal point. It affects the hip and it expels Dampness. It is the Stream point of the Gall-Bladder channel and, as such it expels pathogenic factors from the channel. It is also the opening point of the Girdle Vessel which flows over the hip.
– **G.B.-40** Qiuxu is the Source point of the Gall-Bladder channel which is always involved in hip pain.
– **BL-62** Shenmai is the opening point of the Yang Heel Vessel which also flows over the hip. The Yang Heel Vessel promotes agility and movement and this point is especially useful if the hip is very stiff.
– **SP-3** Taibai can also be used as a distal point as the Spleen channel affects the inner aspect of the hip. It is especially useful if the hip pain radiates to the groin.

The main *local points* to use are:

– **G.B.-30** Huantiao is by far the most important local point. It expels Dampness and removes obstructions from the channel. It should be needled at least 2 inches deep with the patient lying on the opposite side and the leg slightly

bent. Use of the warming needle on this point is very effective.
- **G.B.-29** Juliao is an useful point to use in combination with G.B.-30.
- **SP-12** Chongmen can be used as a local point especially when the pain extends to the groin.

KNEE

As the knees are influenced by the Kidney energy, it is important to differentiate knee pain due to Kidney deficiency from that due to Painful Obstruction Syndrome. When it is due to Kidney deficiency, the knee pain is usually bilateral and develops very gradually over a long period of time. In addition, the knees feel weak and possibly cold, especially if Kidney-Yang is deficient. This type of knee pain is not affected by weather and the knees would not be swollen.

When it is due to invasion of pathogenic factors, the knee pain is more often unilateral (or it is worse on one side) and it starts fairly suddenly. It is definitely affected by weather (usually worsening with rainy or damp weather) and the knee may be swollen (which indicates retention of Dampness).

Painful Obstruction Syndrome of the knee often occurs from a combination of factors, i.e. an invasion of exterior Cold and Dampness and a previous local stagnation of Qi due to an old accident.

Another frequent cause of knee pain is of course local stagnation of Qi and Blood from over-use of the joint. This occurs in brick-layers, joggers, cleaners, etc. In this case, it is not strictly speaking Painful Obstruction Syndrome but it is treated in exactly the same way.

TREATMENT

The treatment of acute and chronic cases is not significantly different so that they can be discussed together. The most important factor to keep in mind when selecting points is to clearly identify the channel involved according to the site of pain. Pain in the knee may occur in the front along the Stomach channel, above the knee, inside the joint itself, on the inner aspect along the Spleen and Liver channels and in the back of the knee in the popliteal crease (Fig. 23.12).

Three distal points can be used for knee pain according to the channel involved:

- **SP-5** Shangqiu is the main one to use. It expels Dampness and, being the River point, it affects joints. It can be used as a general distal point for knee pain, irrespective of the channel involved.
- **G.B.-40** Qiuxu is used as a distal point if the pain is along the Gall Bladder channel.
- **ST-41** Jiexi is used as a distal point if the pain occurs along the Stomach channel.

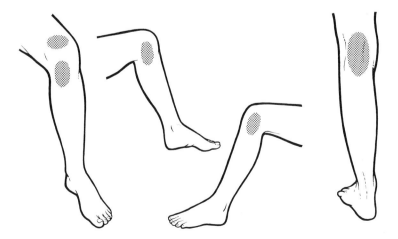

Fig. 23.12 Areas of knee pain

As for local points, it is best to discuss the points according to the area of pain.

PAIN ABOVE THE KNEE (Fig. 23.13)

This usually affects the Stomach channel and there is some swelling indicating retention of Dampness. The main point to use is:

– **ST-34** Liangqiu is the main one to use. It is the Accumulation point of the Stomach channel and, as such, it is a good point to stop pain and remove obstructions from the channel. The use of warming needle is very effective.

PAIN ON THE LATERAL SIDE (Fig. 23.14)

Pain in this area affects the Stomach or Gall Bladder channels. It is usually associated with stiffness of the knee and difficulty in bending. The main points to use are:

– **ST-36** Zusanli is the main one to use. Besides all its other functions, it expels Dampness from the knee.
– **G.B.-34** Yanglingquan is the Gathering point for Sinews and it is therefore very important to use if the knee is stiff.

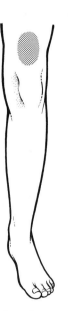

Fig. 23.13   Area of pain above knee

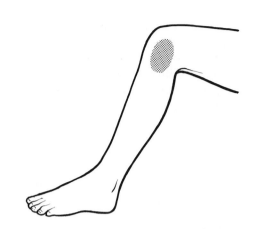

Fig. 23.14   Area of knee pain on the lateral side

– **G.B.-33** Xiyangguan is an useful adjacent point to use which also relaxes the tendons.

PAIN ON THE INNER SIDE (Fig. 23.15)

Pain in this area involves the Spleen or Liver channel. In chronic cases there is often a swelling in this area, especially in women. The main points to use are:

– **SP-9** Yinlingquan is one of the main points to use on the Spleen channel. It must always be needled if the knee is swollen, since this indicates invasion of Dampness, and this point resolves Dampness.
– **LIV-7** Xiguan means "Knee-gate". It is a special point to expel Dampness and Cold from the knee. It also relaxes the tendons and relieves stiffness.

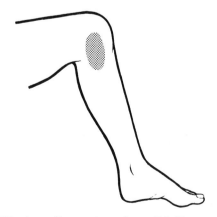

Fig. 23.15   Area of knee pain on the medial side

– **LIV-8** Ququan expels Dampness and nourishes Liver-Blood: it therefore also relieves stiffness by promoting the nourishment of sinews by Liver-Blood. It is particularly important to use in old people with an underlying deficiency of Liver and Kidneys.

Case history

An 82-year-old woman had been suffering from pain and swelling in the medial side of both knees for the past 7 years. Apart from this she felt quite well and the only other problem was poor sleep. Her tongue was Red without coating and with cracks. Her pulse was almost normal and only slightly Fine.

Diagnosis
Even though she has not many symptoms, we can deduce that the pain in the knees is due to invasion of Cold and Dampness (because of the swelling) against a background of Kidney-Yin deficiency, the only other sign of which is the Red and Peeled tongue with cracks.

Treatment principle
The treatment principle adopted was to resolve Dampness, expel Cold, and remove obstructions from the channels. She was treated with acupuncture only.

Acupuncture
The main points used were:

– **LIV-8** Ququan, **SP-6** Sanyinjiao and **KI-3** Taixi to nourish Liver and Kidney Yin. In addition, LIV-8 also functions as a local point.
– **SP-9** Yinlingquan as a local point and to resolve Dampness.
– **LIV-7** Xiguan with warm needle as a local point.

Although the pain in the knees did not disappear entirely, probably on account of her age, it nevertheless decreased dramatically and she was able to walk much more than before.

PAIN INSIDE THE KNEE JOINT

This pain is experienced deep inside the joint. The main points to use are:

– **Xiyan** extra points. These are a pair of points in two depressions medial and lateral to the patellar ligament (Fig. 23.16). "Xiyan" means "knee-eyes". They are called lateral and medial Xiyan, and the lateral one coincides with the point ST-35 Dubi. They are best

needled with the knee slightly flexed after placing a small pad under the patient's knee. They should be needled at least 0.5 inch deep. The warming needle can be used with good results unless the knee feels hot to the touch and is swollen (which denotes Heat Painful Obstruction Syndrome).
– **ST-36** Zusanli, which expels Dampness, can also be used when the pain is felt inside the knee joint.

PAIN AT THE BACK OF THE KNEE

Pain in this area occurs much less frequently than in the front or sides of the knee. It is due to invasion of Dampness in the Bladder channel. The main point is:

– **BL-40** Weizhong which, besides being the local point for pain behind the knee, also expels Dampness, and in particular Damp-Heat.

ANKLE

Pain in the ankle is usually due to invasion of Damp-Cold and to local stagnation of Qi from over-use of the joint. The main points to use are:

– **SP-5** Shangqiu is one of the two main points to use (with G.B.-40 Qiuxu). Besides being a local point, it expels Dampness, and, being the River point, it affects joints. It is usually needled in combination with G.B.-40 Qiuxu.

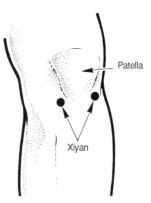

Fig. 23.16 Location of extra points Xiyan

- **G.B.-40** Qiuxu is used if the pain is on the outside of the ankle, and is often used with warming needle.
- **ST-41** Jiexi is used if the pain is on the instep of the foot. It also expels Dampness. It should be needled perpendicularly at least 0.5 inch.

TOES

The main points to use for pain in the toes are:

- **Bafeng** extra points. These are located on the dorsum of the foot, proximal to the margins of the webs. They expel Cold and Dampness from the foot.
- **ST-41** Jiexi is an useful adjacent point to use. It affects all the toes and the needling sensation should radiate downwards towards the toes.
- **SP-3** Taibai is an important point to use particularly for Damp Painful Obstruction Syndrome as it expels Dampness.

In old people, Painful Obstruction Syndrome of the toes often occurs against a background of Yin deficiency. In this case, the patient would have a feeling of heat in the feet, especially at night in bed, sometimes having to hold his or her feet out of the bedcovers. In these cases, it is important to add points which simultaneously nourish Yin and act as adjacent points such as:

- **KI-3** Taixi and **SP-6** Sanyinjiao. For both these points (and particularly for KI-3) the needling sensation should radiate to the toes.

Prognosis and prevention

Both acupuncture and Chinese herbs are extremely effective in treating Painful Obstruction Syndrome. Acupuncture, in particular, is the treatment of choice in this condition giving excellent results in both acute and chronic cases. Acute cases, in fact, can usually be resolved in a few treatments. However, the majority of patients we see with this problem present very chronic conditions. These cases can be treated successfully too, but the more long-standing the condition, the longer it will take to clear.

Osteoarthritis is easier to treat than rheumathoid arthritis but this can also be helped, sometimes even when bone deformities have already set in. In such cases, the treatment may take a very long time and even years.

As for the relative importance of acupuncture and herbs, in general, the more chronic the condition, the more herbs (or patent remedies) are applicable. Herbs are particularly good in chronic cases to resolve Phlegm (and bone deformities), move Blood and nourish Liver and Kidneys.

As for prevention, Painful Obstruction Syndrome is probably the most common affliction of mankind and it affects the elderly in particular as the decline of Qi and Blood and the weakening of Liver and Kidneys makes them prone to invasion of external pathogenic factors. Painful Obstruction Syndrome, however, is not an inevitable consequence of old age and it is possible to take steps to minimize it or prevent it altogether. The two most important areas in life to take care of in order to prevent Painful Obstruction Syndrome, are exercise and diet. Let us look at each of these areas in detail.

EXERCISE

A proper amount of regular exercise is absolutely essential to preserve good health and mobility. Regular exercise stimulates the circulation of Qi and Blood and keeps the sinews supple: both of these effects contribute to prevent invasion of external pathogenic factors. In modern industrial societies, where many people engaged in office work lead very inactive lives, proper exercise is all the more important for good health.

The importance of exercise for health has been recognized in Chinese culture since very early times. An ancient Chinese saying states: *"Running water does not become stale; a door hinge never gets worm-eaten"* (in old China door hinges were made of wood and leather). One of the earliest written references to exercise for health dates back to the Han dynasty and is by the famous doctor Hua Tuo (AD 136–208). He devised five types of exercises based on the imitation of five animals, i.e. tiger, stag, bear, monkey and crane. Each of these five exercises had a specific beneficial effect on the body.

Generally speaking, Chinese culture refers to two types of exercise, one known as "external exercises", the other as "internal exercises". External exercises are aimed at developing muscles and sinews: all Western-type sports, exercises and games can be classified as such. Internal exercises are aimed at developing Qi and "massaging" the internal organs by a coordination or movement, breathing and concentration. *Tai Ji Quan* is an outstanding example of internal exercise. It is gentle yet powerful, it exercises all muscles and sinews, makes the tendons supple, develops Qi, massages the internal organs and quietens the mind.

It is important to realize that physical fitness and health are *not* synonymous. Regular practice of Western-type of exercises such as weight-lifting or jogging may make one fit, but it does not necessarily make one healthy, indeed the opposite may be true as will be explained later.

As far as prevention of Painful Obstruction Syndrome is concerned, both external and internal exercises are beneficial. Indeed, a combination of the two is ideal. Apart from *Tai Ji Quan*, Yoga is also an excellent type of internal exercise that develops suppleness and "massages" the internal organs. Of the external exercises, the only ones which are *not* particularly beneficial are jogging, weight-lifting, squash and aerobic exercises.

Jogging puts a strain on the spine and knees and may be a contributory factor in Painful Obstruction Syndrome of the knees or lower back. Weight-lifting weakens Kidney-Qi: it is a well-known axiom in Chinese Medicine that excessive lifting injures Kidney-Qi and the lower back. Squash is good as an exercise, but, due to its extremely fast pace, it often generates more nervous tension in already tense persons. It is frequent to see in practice tense and stressed businessmen whose idea of relaxation is a frenetic game of squash. Aerobic exercises are simply too strenuous and may lead to injury of the back in weak people.

The Western-type exercises which are more beneficial for prevention of Painful Obstruction Syndrome are walking, tennis and cycling.

DIET

The subject of Chinese principles of diet in health and disease is of course very vast and could fill a volume by itself. I shall limit myself here to a brief discussion about Chinese dietary principles

in the prevention and treatment of Painful Obstruction Syndrome. I shall also limit the discussion to traditional Chinese principles of diet.

Dietary principles for Painful Obstruction Syndrome vary according to the type.

In Cold Painful Obstruction Syndrome, it is essential not to eat too much of the cold-energy foods such as raw vegetables and fruit. It is also imperative not to drink iced drinks. This is because cold-energy foods and cold drinks produce internal Cold which will cause more pain in the joints. Beneficial foods are the warm-energy ones such as meat (in moderation), ginger, eggs, garlic, and spices (in moderation). Ginger, in particular, is beneficial as it is warm in energy, stimulates the circulation and expels Cold. It can be taken as a decoction made by boiling three slices of the fresh root for about 10 minutes and mixed with a small teaspoonful of brown sugar (which also has a warm energy).

A very small amount of alcohol (in the form of wine, brandy, cognac or rice-wine) may be beneficial to those suffering from Cold Painful Obstruction Syndrome. Of course, this does *not* apply to those who regularly drink substantial quantities of alcohol on a daily basis. According to Chinese dietary principles, alcohol can warm the Stomach, expel Cold, expel poisons, stimulate the descending of Qi, prevent epidemic diseases and dispel worry (!). A very small amount of alcohol (say, 5–15 ml a day) can therefore be beneficial to old people suffering from Cold Painful Obstruction Syndrome. Of particular benefit, would be tinctures (i.e. alcoholic cold macerations) of herbs which simultaneously expel Wind-Damp and nourish tendons and bones, such as Wu Jia Pi *Cortex Acanthopanacis radicis*, Ji Xue Teng *Caulis Millettiae seu Caulis Spatholobi* and Sang Ji Sheng *Ramus Loranthi*. Such medicinal wines for Painful Obstruction Syndrome are produced in China and are readily available at Chinese supermarkets in the West.

Patients suffering from Damp Painful Obstruction Syndrome, should not eat Damp-producing foods, such as milk, cheese, butter, cream, ice-cream, peanuts, bananas and any greasy-fried foods.

Those suffering from Wind Painful Obstruction Syndrome should not eat "irritant" foods such as prawns, shrimps, crab, lobster, spinach, rhubarb and mushrooms. They should make a point of eating mild, Blood-nourishing foods such as chicken, hen-soup, rice and carrots.

Those suffering from Heat Painful Obstruction Syndrome should obviously not eat too much of the hot or warm-energy foods such as game, lamb, beef, alcohol, garlic, ginger and spices.

Irrespective of the type of Painful Obstruction Syndrome, patients should also avoid eating sour foods which upset the Liver and increase pain. Examples of sour foods are yoghurt, vinegar, oranges, grapefruit, gooseberries, pickles and rhubarb.

ACUPUNCTURE

Acupuncture can be used to prevent re-occurrence of Painful Obstruction Syndrome once it has been successfully cured. The main guiding rule is to tonify Blood according to the principle that "in order to extinguish Wind one must nourish Blood". In old people it may also be necessary to nourish Yin. If a patient has been treated for Bone Painful Obstruction Syndrome, it is also necessary to use points that tonify Qi and resolve Phlegm (as the bone deformities seen in Bone Painful Obstruction Syndrome are a manifestation of Phlegm).

Apart from these general principles, one can add certain points to prevent Painful Obstruction Syndrome according to its location. The points are treated with 5 direct moxa cones in summertime. They are:

– Upper limbs: L.I.-11 Quchi.
– Lower limbs: ST-36 Zusanli.
– Upper back: BL-43 Gaohuangshu.
– Lower back: BL-23 Shenshu.

END NOTES

1. Shen Jin Ao 1773 The Origin of Complicated Diseases (*Za Bing Yuan Liu Xi Hu* 杂病源流犀烛), cited in Zhang Bo Yu 1986 Internal Medicine (*Zhong Yi Nei Ke Xue* 中医内科学), Shanghai Science Publishing House, Shanghai, p. 269.
2. Chao Yuan Fang AD 610 "Discussion on the Origin of All Illnesses" (*Zhu Bing Yuan Hou Lun* 诸病源候论), cited in Internal Medicine p. 265.
3. Lin Pei Qin 1839 Treatment Strategies for Assorted Syndromes (*Lei Zheng Zhi Cai* 类证治裁), cited in Internal Medicine, p. 269.
4. 1979 The Yellow Emperor's Classic of Internal Medicine — Simple Questions (*Huang Ti Nei Jing Su Wen* 黄帝内经素问), People's Health Publishing House, Beijing. First published *c.* 100 BC, p. 240.
5. Zhang Jie Bin (also called Zhang Jing Yue) 1624 Classic of Categories (*Lei Jing* 类经, cited in Wang Jin Quan 1987 Discussion on Categories of Syndromes from the Yellow Emperor's Classic of Internal Medicine (*Nei Jing Lei Zheng Lun Zhi* 内经类证论治), Shanxi Science Publishing House, Xian, p. 227.
6. Simple Questions, p. 241.
7. Ibid., p. 241.
8. Ibid., p. 243.
9. Li Zhong Xin 1637 Essential Readings from Medical Masters (*Yi Zong Bi Du* 医宗必读), cited in Internal Medicine, p. 265.
10. Cheng Guo Duo 1732 Enlightenment of Medical Theory (*Yi Xue Xin Wu* 医学心悟), cited in Traditional Internal Medicine, p. 266.
11. Shi Yu Guang 1988 Essential Clinical Experience of Famous Contemporary Doctors (*Dang Dai Ming Yi Lin Zheng Jing Hua* 当代名医临证精华), article by Prof. Qiu Mao Liang, Ancient Chinese Medical Texts Publishing House, Beijing, pp. 1–2.
12. Yang Ji Zhou 1984 Compendium of Acupuncture (*Zhen Jiu Da Cheng* 针灸大成), edited by the Chinese Medicine Research Group of the Heilongjiang Province, People's Health Publishing House, Beijing, p. 1084. First published in 1601.
13. Huang Fu Mi AD 259. The ABC of Acupuncture, in: Li Shi Zhen 1985 Clinical Application of Frequently Used Acupuncture Points (*Chang Yong Shu Xue Lin Chuang Fa Hui* 常用输穴临床发挥), People's Health Publishing House, Beijing, p. 41.
14. Wang Wei Yi 1026 Illustrated Manual of Acupuncture Points as shown on the Bronze Man (*Tong Ren Shu Xue Zhen Jiu Tu Jing* 铜人腧穴针灸图经), cited in Clinical Application of Frequently Used Acupuncture Points, p. 41.

Lower back-ache and sciatica 24 腰痛

Lower back-ache and sciatica can be discussed together as they share similar aetiology, pathology and treatment. Of all the musculo-skeletal complaints, back-ache is the most common. The statistics regarding back pain are staggering. It is estimated that at least 50% of people in Western industrialized countries will suffer from back pain at some time of their life. In the UK, approximately one million patients consult their GP for back pain each year.[1] Several million working days are lost each year because of back pain. Chinese medicine, and in particular acupuncture, gives excellent results in the treatment of this complaint.

By "lower" back-ache is meant ache anywhere in the back region (including the buttocks) below the lower border of the rib-cage, which is approximately level with BL-21 Weishu (Fig. 24.1).

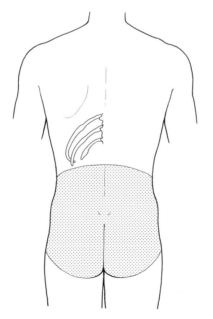

Fig. 24.1 Area of lower back-ache

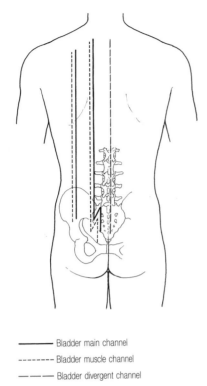

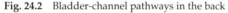
——— Bladder main channel
------- Bladder muscle channel
— — — Bladder divergent channel

Fig. 24.2   Bladder-channel pathways in the back

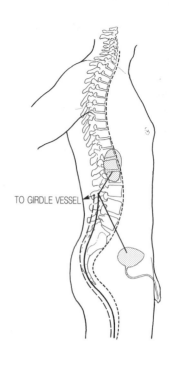

TO GIRDLE VESSEL

——— Kidney main channel
------- Kidney muscle channel
— — — Kidney divergent channel

Fig. 24.3   Kidney's main, muscle- and divergent channels

The lower back area is strongly influenced by the Bladder and Kidney channels (Fig. 24.2):

- The Bladder main channel flows along the back in two lines
- The Bladder muscle-channel follows the muscles alongside the spine
- The Bladder divergent channel flows alongside the spine (Fig. 24.2)
- The Kidney main channel from the perineum flows up along the spine and goes to the kidneys and bladder
- The Kidney muscle-channel flows alongside the anterior aspect of the spine
- The Kidney divergent channel flows upwards with the Bladder channel and, at the level of BL-23 Shenshu, it joins the Girdle Vessel (Fig. 24.3)
- The Governing Vessel, closely related to the Kidneys, of course flows along the spine
- The Penetrating Vessel, also stemming from in between the Kidneys, from the perineum, sends a branch up in the spine to the level of BL-23 Shenshu (Fig. 24.4).

The "Simple Questions" in chapter 17 says: *"The lower back is the residence of the Kidneys . . ."*.[2] In chapter 41 it gives the symptoms and signs of back-ache deriving from each of the channels. The "Prescriptions of the Golden Chest" in chapter 11 describes the effects on the lower back of Wind, Cold and Dampness:

When the Kidneys are affected by Wind there is a feeling of heaviness of the body and cold in the lower back and the patient feels as if sitting in water . . . there is no thirst, urination is normal and appetite is not affected, thus the disease is in the Lower Burner [as opposed to the Kidneys themselves]. This is due to perspiring while working making the clothes wet and cold. If this condition persists for a long time the lower back will ache from Cold and there will be a feeling of heaviness around the waist as if he or she were carrying 1000 coins around his/her waist. In these cases use the Glycyrrhiza-Zingiber-Poria-Atractylodes Decoction.[3]

The "General Treatise on the Aetiology and

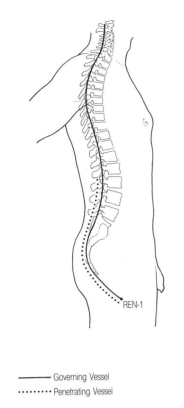

— Governing Vessel
········· Penetrating Vessel

Fig. 24.4 Governing and Penetrating vessels' pathways

Symptomatology of Diseases" (610) describes five causes of lower back-ache, i.e. Kidney deficiency, Wind-Cold invading the back, overexertion, falls and sleeping on damp surfaces.[4] The "Essential Methods of Dan Xi" (1481) describes five types of back-ache, i.e. from Kidney deficiency, Damp-Heat, stasis of Blood, contusion and Phlegm.[5]

Aetiology

1. EXCESSIVE PHYSICAL WORK

Excessive physical work, in particular regularly lifting objects, strains the muscles of the lower back and the Kidneys. Excessive lifting therefore weakens the back in two ways: in a purely physical way, it strains the muscles of the lower back, and in an energetic way, it weakens Kidney-Qi. Thus, it starts a vicious circle as a

deficiency of Kidney-Qi, by itself, leads to a weakening of the back muscles. On the other hand, at the acute stage, excessive physical work also causes local stagnation of Qi and Blood in the back area. This causes intense pain.

This is a common cause of both acute and chronic back-ache in modern societies. In acute cases, excessive physical work is the most common cause of back strain. Excessive physical work may occur in the course of one's occupation, sports or exercises. Examples are excessive lifting by removal men, excessive aerobic exercises, ballet or weight lifting. Particularly in the case of those engaged in ballet from early childhood, the space between the lumbar vertebrae will be found to be abnormally wide.

2. EXCESSIVE SEXUAL ACTIVITY

Excessive sexual activity weakens the back in an energetic sense as it depletes Kidney-Qi and a deficient Kidney-Qi fails to nourish and strengthen the back muscles. This causes only chronic, not acute, back-ache.

3. PREGNANCY AND CHILDBIRTH

Pregnancy and childbirth also weaken the back in two ways: in a purely physical way, they put a strain on the back muscles, and in an energetic sense, they weaken Kidney-Qi which consequently fails to strengthen the back muscles.

However, pregnancy and childbirth are not by themselves a cause of disease. They only become that in women of weak constitution, in those who do not take care or rest after childbirth, or in those who have several children in close succession. In fact, if a woman takes particular care after childbirth having adequate rest and a good, nourishing diet, a weak constitution may even be strengthened.

4. INVASION OF EXTERNAL COLD AND DAMPNESS

Invasion of external Cold and Dampness is an

extremely common cause of back-ache. The area of the back which is the residence of the Original Qi and the Fire of the Gate of Vitality, should be kept warm and protected. Exposure to cold and dampness easily leads to invasion of pathogenic factors in the muscles, sinews and channels of the back.

Although most people in Western industrialized countries have more than adequate clothing and warm housing, invasion of the back muscles by cold and dampness is a common occurrence. This happens either because of wearing insufficient clothes when following the demands of fashion, or because of ignorance as to the effect of climatic factors on our bodies. Examples of exposure to cold and dampness abound: the jogger who jogs in the early morning in cold and damp weather exposing the sweating body to pathogenic factors, the swimmer who does not change out of a wet swimming suit on a windy beach, the woman who dresses inadequately at the slightest ray of sunshine in early spring, the building worker who works outdoors in the rain with his trousers very low on his hips leaving the loins exposed, the enthusiastic DIY expert who, on a sunny day, strips off his shirt and paints the exterior frames of his windows, working bare-chested in the cool shade, etc.

Invasion of Cold and Dampness to the back muscles can cause both acute and chronic back-ache. Prolonged retention of Cold and Dampness in the lower back, on the other hand, will impair and weaken the Kidneys: this leads to a complicated condition of Fullness (of Cold and Dampness) and Emptiness (of the Kidneys) and chronic back-ache. This situation is extremely common.

Occasionally, back-ache, especially sciatica, may be caused by invasion of external Damp-Heat in the Bladder or Gall-Bladder channel, but this is not common.

5. OVERWORK

Overwork in the sense of working long hours without adequate rest over many years depletes Kidney-Yin. This fails to nourish the back and leads to chronic back-ache.

6. INADEQUATE EXERCISE

Apart from the above specific causes of back-ache it is many experts' opinion that the tremendous increase in back problems in Western industrialized societies is due to a *lack* of physical exercise especially for the vast numbers of people engaged in sedentary work. The enormous increase in the number of cars in the past 40 years also means that most people drive a car when in the past they might have walked or ridden a bicycle, as is the case in China, for example. The lack of exercise leads to a weakening of the spine ligaments and joints and therefore predisposes the person to disc problems especially when combined with a poor posture. Thus, although patients should avoid lifting heavy weights and performing excessive exercises (such as aerobic exercises), they should be advised to perform sensible, regular exercises to strengthen the back and keep the muscles and ligaments supple. *Tai Ji Chuan* is an excellent form of exercise which strengthens the Kidneys, keeps the muscles and sinews supple and calms the Mind.

Pathology

The three most common pathological conditions are retention of Cold and Dampness, stagnation of Qi and Blood from sprain, and Kidney deficiency.

RETENTION OF DAMP-COLD

Damp-Cold can cause both acute and chronic back-ache. The pain is worse in the morning and better with light exercise. The pain is also relieved by application of heat and is worse when the weather is cold and damp.

In retention of Damp-Cold there may a prevalence of Cold or Dampness. When Cold predominates there may be stiffness and contraction of the back muscles and the pain is more severe, is aggravated by rest and improved by movement. It also responds to application of heat, such as a hot-water bottle. When Dampness predominates there may be swelling, numbness and a feeling of heaviness.

When caused by Cold and Dampness, lower back-ache is a form of Painful Obstruction Syndrome (see ch. 23).

STAGNATION OF QI AND BLOOD

Stagnation of Qi and Blood is characterized by a severe, stabbing pain which becomes worse with rest and better with light exercise although it would be worse with overexertion. It is tender to touch, does not respond to changes in weather and is much worse standing or sitting. It is also unaffected by the application of heat. There is also marked rigidity and stiffness of the back muscles and inability to flex, extend or turn the waist. Stagnation of Qi and Blood in the back in an acute case is due to sprain. In chronic cases, repeated sprain causes recurrent attacks of back-ache, especially if there is a background of Kidney deficiency.

KIDNEY DEFICIENCY

Kidney deficiency causes chronic back-ache. The pain is dull and comes in bouts. It is definitely better with rest and worse when the person gets overtired. It is also aggravated by sexual activity. If it is caused by a deficiency of Kidney-Yang there may be a cold sensation in the back; this may show a slight but not a significant improvement with the application of heat.

A Kidney deficiency is a cause of chronic back-ache by itself but it also forms the background which facilitates both invasions of Cold-Damp and repeated sprains. Any Kidney deficiency can give rise to back-ache, although that from Kidney-Yang deficiency is more common.

Obviously a back-ache from Kidney deficiency is more common in middle-aged or elderly people. However, young people may also suffer from this type of back-ache and, if they do, it is usually from a hereditary Kidney deficiency. An exception to this is when a child does a lot of physical work (such as children

who need to help their parents on a farm) or exercise (such as ballet) around the time of puberty. This is a vulnerable time from an energetic point of view and excessive exercise at this time of life may seriously weaken the Kidneys and the back.

Some doctors consider a Kidney deficiency to be always the underlying condition in any type of back pain. The "Standards of Diagnosis and Treatment" (1602), for example, says: "[In back-ache], Wind, Dampness, Cold, Heat, sprain, stasis of Blood, stagnation of Qi, accumulations are all the Manifestation; the Root is always Kidney deficiency."[6]

There is considerable interaction among the above three conditions which influence one another. For example, repeated invasions of Cold-Dampness lead to permanent retention of Damp-Cold in the back muscles. This on the one hand weakens the Kidneys as Damp-Cold interferes with the Kidney's transformation of Water and leads to Kidney deficiency, and on the other hand it obstructs the circulation of Qi and Blood in the area and gives rise to stagnation of Qi and Blood.

Diagnosis

This will be discussed under the following headings:

- observation
- interrogation
- palpation
- pulse.

OBSERVATION
FACE COLOUR

- Pale: Kidney-Yang deficiency
- Dark like a beetroot: Kidney-Yin deficiency
- Bluish: stasis of blood, chronic pain.

BACK AND LEGS

- Congested venules at the back of the legs:

stasis of Blood in the Connecting channels of the back
- Sunken muscle on the point KI-3 Taixi: Kidney deficiency.

INTERROGATION

It is first of all very important to establish whether the back-ache is acute or chronic and if it is acute, whether it is an exacerbation of a chronic condition.

A severe, stabbing pain suggests stagnation of Qi and Blood in the area, while a dull ache indicates a Deficiency condition.

If the back-ache improves with light exercise it indicates that it is due to local stagnation, while if it improves with rest it is due to a deficiency of the Kidneys.

If the back-ache is worse at the start of the morning and gets gradually better as the morning goes on, it indicates invasion of Cold. If it is better in the morning on waking up and gradually gets worse during the day, it is due to a deficiency of the Kidneys.

If the back-ache clearly worsens when the weather is cold and damp, then it suggests invasion of external Cold and Dampness. If it is unrelated to the weather, it is either due to sprain or to a Kidney deficiency.

PALPATION

Palpation is absolutely essential for a proper diagnosis of back problems.

If the muscles of the back are stiff, hard and rigid it indicates local stasis of Blood from sprain. If the back or the back of the legs feel cold to touch it indicates Kidney-Yang deficiency.

If the spaces between the lumbar vertebrae are wider than normal it indicates excessive exercise during childhood or puberty and Kidney deficiency.

If the area of pain is rather large it suggests either a Kidney deficiency or invasion of Cold and Dampness. If the area of pain is small it suggests sprain.

Finally, it is essential to find the most tender points on palpation in order to identify the channel involved and the Ah Shi points. This is most important for treatment. The points which are most frequently tender on the back and leg are (Fig. 24.5):

- BL-26 Guanyuanshu
- BL-25 Dachangshu
- BL-54 Zhibian
- Tunzhong extra point
- BL-36 Chengfu
- BL-37 Yinmen.

PULSE

The pulse reflects the condition not only of the internal organs but also of areas of the body. The lower back is reflected on the left Rear position of the pulse. This pulse reflects especially back conditions which affect the Bladder channel in either leg. If this position is Wiry and Floating it may indicate either acute back-ache or an acute exacerbation of a chronic back problem.

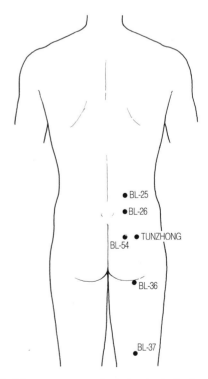

Fig. 24.5   Most common tender points in the back

If the left Rear position is Fine, Deep but also slightly Wiry, it denotes chronic back-ache on a background of Kidney deficiency. If this position is Tight it indicates invasion of Damp-Cold in the Bladder channel.

According to "A Study of the Eight Extraordinary Vessels" by Li Shi Zhen, when the left pulse feels Floating and slightly Wiry in all three positions, it reflects tension in the Governing Vessel and acute back-ache from Wind-Cold.[7]

If the pulse on the left Rear position is Weak-Floating (Soft), Fine and very slightly Wiry it indicates chronic back-ache from Dampness in the back channels.

If the left-Rear position of the pulse is Wiry and the pulse is Rapid, it may denote invasion of Damp-Heat in the back channels.

Of course, any of the above-mentioned pulse pictures may also reflect a pathological condition of the Bladder organ itself rather than a channel problem. However, the absence of Bladder symptoms (urinary difficulty, pain or dribbling) may confirm affection of the channel only.

Finally, something should be said about the distinction between a back pain from a channel problem and one from an actual kidney affliction. For example, if a patient has a dull ache on the right loin, how do we know that this is simply a channel problem causing back-ache and not a condition of the kidney itself?

In acute cases, the differentiation is relatively easy as an actual kidney problem such as acute nephritis would manifest itself with obvious symptoms and signs such as a fever, oedema of the face, scanty-dark urine, malaise and a headache. If the problem were due to kidney stones, this would be very obvious from the severity of the colicky pain and from its gradual migration from the loin to the groin.

In chronic cases, an affection of the kidney itself, such as chronic nephritis, would be manifest from the general malaise, slight oedema of the ankles, exhaustion and the presence of protein in the urine. This can be quickly and easily tested with the diagnostic strips.

Apart from the differentiation according to accompanying symptoms, a back-ache from an actual kidney problem is located higher than one from a channel problem only (Fig. 24.6). However, this is not an absolutely reliable guide as the higher location of the back pain may also be seen in channel problems.

Of course, a chronic back-ache may be associated not with a kidney disease in a Western sense but with a Kidney disharmony in a Chinese sense. This is quite frequent. Thus the patient will complain of chronic back-ache, dizziness, some tinnitus, frequent and pale urination, etc. However, it is not unusual for chronic back-ache to be the only symptom of a Kidney deficiency especially in young or middle-aged people.

Differentiation and treatment

The treatment of back-ache is based on a differentiation between acute and chronic cases rather than a differentiation of patterns. The most important aspects for a successful treatment are not so much a differentiation of patterns but a proper selection of distal and local points with the appropriate manipulation and radiation of

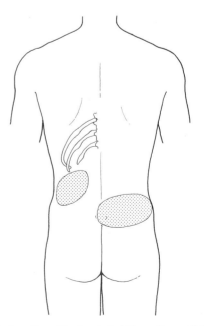

Fig. 24.6   Location of back pain in kidney disease (left) and channel problem (right)

the needling sensation. The choice of points is guided not so much by an identification of patterns as by the location and nature of the pain.

However, there are some differences in approach which depend on the pattern. These are:

INVASION OF COLD AND DAMPNESS

Use the reducing method in acute cases and the even method in chronic cases. Moxa should be used.

STAGNATION OF QI AND BLOOD

Use the reducing method in acute cases and the even method in chronic ones. Unless there are Heat signs, moxa may also be used as it has the effect of relaxing the sinews and spreading Qi thus relieving stagnation of Qi and Blood.

KIDNEY DEFICIENCY

Use the reinforcing method. Moxa should be used if there is deficiency of Kidney-Yang.

By contrast, the herbal treatment must be based on the pattern and the formula for each pattern should be modified according to whether the condition is acute or chronic. In chronic conditions, the formulae should be modified to introduce some tonification.

ACUPUNCTURE

ACUTE CONDITIONS

These are due either to Damp-Cold or to stagnation of Qi and Blood in the area.

DISTAL POINTS

In acute cases distal points are particularly important. They are inserted first and manipulated for some time before inserting the local points.

The choice of distal points depends on the location of the pain. The main ones are:

- **BL-40** Weizhong if the pain is in the lower part of the back, just above the buttock whether unilateral or bilateral.
- **Du-26** Renzhong if the pain is on the midline or starting from the midline and spreading out.
- **BL-10** Tianzhu, same as above. The needling sensation should preferably radiate downwards along the Bladder channel.
- **S.I.-3** Houxi if the pain is unilateral and slightly higher, roughly level with the umbilicus.
- **Yaotongxue** extra point if the pain is unilateral and in the middle part of the back, higher than the level of the umbilicus (Fig. 24.7).
- **BL-58** Feiyang if there is a pain in the leg between the Bladder and Gall-Bladder channel (i.e. not clearly in one channel or the other).
- **BL-62** Shenmai if the pain is unilateral and radiates down to one leg.
- **BL-59** Fuyang if walking is difficult. From this point one should obtain a needling sensation that radiates upwards along the Bladder channel.

The connection between distal points and the

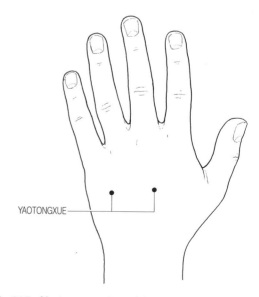

Fig. 24.7　Yaotongxue extra point

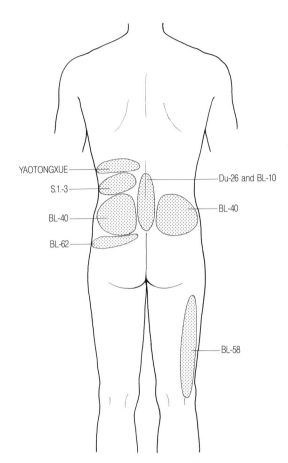

Fig. 24.8 Distal points for acute back-ache

area affected by them is best illustrated by a figure (see Figure 24.8).

The technique used is to insert the distal point or points first, obtain the needling sensation and then manipulate the needle quite vigorously with reducing method while the patient gently flexes and turns the waist. If a third person is available, he or she could help the patient to effect these movements. In most cases this procedure is best carried out while the patient is standing. This is the only example of treatment given while the patient stands. The distal needle or needles are retained for about 15 minutes during which time they can be manipulated at intervals.

After this, the distal needles are removed and the patient lies down for the local points to be needled.

LOCAL POINTS

These are selected according to tenderness on pressure. It is therefore very important to press and try various points systematically.

The local points are needled with reducing method and the needles are then left in place for about 20 minutes during which time they can be manipulated at intervals. An effective way of reducing the points is to adopt the "clock technique", i.e. lifting and thrusting the needle with a circular movement like the hour-hand round the face of a clock. The local points which are most likely to be tender have been mentioned above (Fig. 24.5).

Apart from the Ah Shi points, there are local points which can be needled irrespective of tenderness. These are:

- **Du-3** Yaoyangguan: it strengthens the back and legs. It is especially used if the pain radiates to the leg. To make the needling sensation radiate downwards is difficult, but if it radiates outwards from the point that should be sufficient.
- **Du-4** Mingmen: it tonifies Kidney-Yang and strengthens the back.
- **Du-8** Jinsuo: it relaxes the sinews and relieves stiffness and contraction.
- **Shiqizhuixia**: this is an extremely effective extra point for back-ache in the centre of the lower part of the back.
- **BL-32** Ciliao: this point is used if the pain is over the sacrum. The needling sensation should radiate outwards.

Other points on the Governing Vessel may be chosen according to deviation and rotation of vertebrae. The points on the Governing Vessel may be combined with the corresponding Huatuojiaji points. If a vertebra is rotated it is best to use the Governing Vessel point below it, as well as three pairs of Huatuojiaji points at its level and immediately below and above it (Fig. 24.9).

Case history

A 44-year-old woman complained of an acute back-ache which had started after working in the garden.

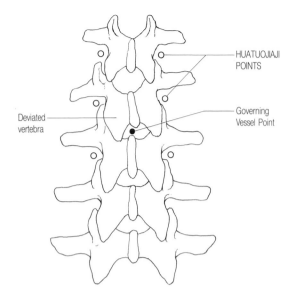

Fig. 24.9 Use of Governing Vessel and Huatuojiaji points for vertebra rotation

HUATUOJIAJI POINTS

Governing Vessel Point

Deviated vertebra

The pain was intense and was centred around the left sacro-iliac area. It radiated downwards to the left buttock and the back of the leg. She had not suffered from any back-ache before.

On examination, the muscles on the left side of her back were in spasm and the whole area felt very stiff. The most tender point was BL-26 Guanyuanshu. She was quite a tense person and her pulse was slightly Rapid and Wiry.

Diagnosis
This is a case of acute back-ache from sprain.

Treatment
She was treated only with acupuncture. The distal points used were:

– **BL-62** Shenmai on the left, **P-7** Daling on the right and **LIV-3** Taichong bilaterally. BL-62 was used to remove obstructions from the Bladder channel on the left side. P-7 was selected to calm the Mind and relax the muscles. LIV-3 was chosen to relax muscles and sinews. These points were reduced and then left in place for 45 minutes, being manipulated again a few times during this period.

The local points, inserted after withdrawing the distal ones, were:

– **BL-26** Guanyuanshu on the left with needle (reducing method) and cupping. The needle was manipulated vigorously applying a lift-thrust reducing technique. It was left in place about 10 minutes, then withdrawn, and cupping was applied to the point for another 10 minutes.
– **Tunzhong**, the extra point lateral to BL-54 Zhibian,

was selected as it was tender on pressure. This was needled at a depth of 2.5 inches and a good needling sensation was obtained radiating down the back of the leg as far as the knee. As a good needling sensation was obtained, no other points were necessary.

This treatment was repeated once more the next day and two sessions were enough to clear up the problem completely. However, as on further analysis it became evident that she had an underlying Kidney-Yin deficiency, the patent remedy Zhi Bo Ba Wei Wan *Anemarrhena-Phellodendron Eight-Ingredient Pill* was prescribed and she was advised to take that only during the winter months. At the time of writing (3 years later), there has not been any recurrence.

Case history

A 45-year-old man complained of acute sprain of the lower back. This was not the first time as he had had several attacks in the previous 10 years. The first attack occurred after lifting a heavy weight: at this time he could not move at all for a week. The present attack had also been elicited by lifting and he experienced a severe pain on the right side around the right sacro-iliac area. The pain radiated down to the buttock and back of the leg. The straight-leg raising test proved positive, i.e. raising his right leg with the knee straight provoked intense pain in the back. This indicates lumbo-sacral nerve-root compression from a prolapsed disc at the level L4-L5.

Diagnosis
This is obvious from the symptoms: from the Chinese viewpoint it is an acute sprain of the lower back, and from the Western perspective it is a herniation of the L4-L5 disc. As he had had repeated attacks over 10 years, this showed that there must also be an underlying deficiency of the Kidneys. His pulse, Weak on both Rear positions, and some of his symptoms such as back-ache after sex, confirmed this.

Treatment
Only acupuncture was administered at his home as he could not move from bed. The distal points used were:

– **BL-62** Shenmai on the right, **HE-7** Shenmen on the left, **KI-4** Dazhong on the left and **LIV-3** Taichong on the right. BL-62 was used to remove obstructions from the Bladder channel on the right side. HE-7 was selected to calm the Mind and relax the nerves. KI-4, Connecting point, was used to simultaneously tonify the Kidneys and invigorate its Connecting channel and therefore the Bladder channel. LIV-3 was chosen to relax the muscles and sinews. The placing of needles unilaterally in this pattern is a very effective and dynamic way of combining points.

– **BL-40** Weizhong on the right was also used as a distal point once he turned over, to remove obstructions from the Bladder channel.
All the distal points were needled with reducing method, except for KI-4, and were left in place for 45 minutes.

The local points were selected according to tenderness:

– **BL-26** Guanyuanshu on the right side, was reduced vigorously and then cupped;
– **BL-23** Shenshu was needled because the attacks recurred repeatedly over 10 years, indicating a Kidney deficiency;
– **Tunzhong** was needled with reducing method at a depth of 2.5".

Ten daily sessions produced a complete remission. He was, however, advised to take more exercise, do stretching exercises for his back, reduce his sexual activity and avoid lifting weights. He was also prescribed the Jin Gui Shen Qi Wan *Golden Chest Kidney-Qi Pill* to tonify Kidney-Yang and strengthen the back.
After this attack, he had other, less severe attacks, which acupuncture cleared up very quickly in one or two sessions.

CHRONIC CONDITIONS

Chronic conditions are always due to a Kidney deficiency which can be combined with retention of Damp-Cold or stagnation of Qi and Blood or even both these conditions.

In chronic conditions local points are primary in relation to distal ones.

DISTAL POINTS

The distal points to use are the same as for acute cases with some additional ones:

– **S.I.-3** Houxi and **BL-62** Shenmai in combination open the Governing Vessel, strengthen the spine and tonify the Kidneys. They are an excellent treatment for chronic back-ache from Kidney deficiency. In a man, needle S.I.-3 on the left and BL-62 on the right. In women, the Governing Vessel is best combined with the Directing Vessel. Thus, in a woman, needle S.I.-3 on the right, BL-62 on the left, LU-7 on the left and KI-6 on the right in this order (Fig. 24.10). Remove the needles

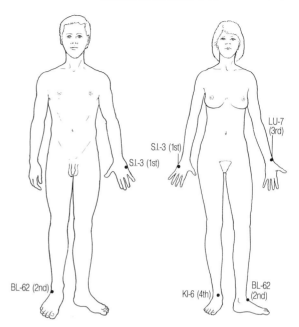

Fig. 24.10   Use of Governing Vessel in men and women

in reverse order. These two treatments are only effective if the back-ache stems from the midline, over the spine. If the ache starts on one side only, then different points should be used.
– **BL-62** Shenmai and **S.I.-3** Houxi, in this order, open the Yang Heel Vessel and may be used if the back-ache radiates outwards towards the hip. In a man, use BL-62 on the left and S.I.-3 on the right, and the opposite in a woman (Fig. 24.11).
– **BL-60** Kunlun is a very important distal point for chronic back-ache. In chronic cases it is the point of choice to replace BL-40 Weizhong, which may sometimes aggravate the back-ache if used in chronic cases. BL-60 also affects the upper part of the back and the neck.
– **KI-4** Dazhong is good if there is an underlying Kidney deficiency as it will simultaneously tonify the Kidneys and affect the Bladder channel by virtue of its being the Connecting point.
– **SP-3** Taibai influences the spine and is good to select in chronic back-ache with obvious scoliosis of the spine. Chapter 4 of the "Simple Questions" says: *"Diseases of the*

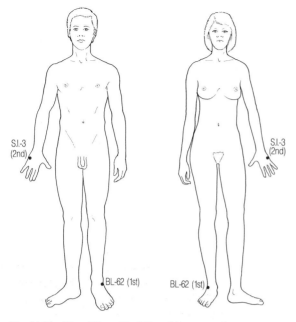

Fig. 24.11   Use of Yang Heel Vessel in men and women

Spleen affect the spine."[8] I use this point quite frequently in these cases with good results.

– **Du-20** Baihui can be used as a distal point to affect the Governing Vessel when the pain is on the lower part of the lumbar spine.

– **HE-7** Shenmen affects the back indirectly because of its relation with the Kidney channel within the Lesser Yin. It also relieves back-ache by calming the Mind and relieving spasm. Strange as it may seem, I use this point very frequently in chronic back-ache (suitably combined with others) with excellent results. It is especially indicated in tense men with a Wiry and Fine pulse. An example of combination of distal points for chronic back-ache stemming from the midline in a man might be:

– S.I.-3 Houxi on the left and BL-62 Shenmai on the right (i.e. the Governing Vessel points), HE-7 Shenmen on the right and SP-3 Taibai on the left (Fig. 24.12). This combination opens the Governing Vessel and removes obstructions from it, strengthens the Kidneys and the spine, expels Wind, calms the Mind, relieves spasm and straightens the spine. After withdrawal of these points, local points could be used. In a woman, the combination would be:

– S.I.-3 Houxi on the right and BL-62 Shenmai on the left (i.e. the Governing Vessel points), LU-7 Lieque on the left and KI-6 on the right (i.e. the Directing Vessel points), HE-7 Shenmen on the right and SP-3 on the left (Fig. 24.12).

In chronic cases it is important to select other points to treat the general condition underlying the back problem. In particular, one must treat the Spleen to affect the back muscles, the Liver to affect the vertebrae ligaments and cartilage and the Kidneys to affect the bones. The combination of Source points with Back-Transporting points would be particularly effective:

– **SP-3** Taibai and **BL-20** Pishu for the Spleen
– **KI-3** Taixi and **BL-23** Shenshu for the Kidneys
– **BL-11** Dashu and **G.B.-39** Xuanzhong for the bones.

LOCAL POINTS

The local points in chronic back-ache are also selected according to tenderness on pressure but **BL-23** Shenshu should be used in *every* case. Other very important local points are:

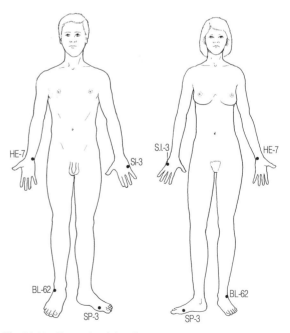

Fig. 24.12   Example of distal points combination in chronic back-ache

- **BL-26** Guanyuanshu
- **Shiqizhuixia**
- **BL-54** Zhibian if the pain radiates to the buttocks
- **Tunzhong**: this is an extra point (Fig. 24.13) lateral to BL-54 half-way between the midline and the edge of the buttock. It is an extremely effective point for pain in the buttocks also when it radiates to the leg. It is more often tender on pressure than BL-54. If the pain radiates down to the leg, a good needling sensation should be obtained, preferably running down the leg
- **Yaoyan**, an extra point in the depression lateral to the interspace between the spinous processes of L4 and L5, is a good local point for chronic back-ache, especially in the lower part. It is often tender on pressure (Fig. 24.13).

If there is Kidney-Yang deficiency, or if there is Cold-Dampness in the back, the moxa box placed on the lower back over, say, BL-26 and Shiqizhuixia, is extremely effective.

Case history

A 54-year-old man had been suffering from back-ache for over 20 years. The ache was across the lower back

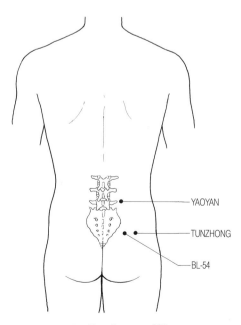

Fig. 24.13 Extra point Tunzhong and Yaoyan

stemming from the midline and was aggravated by work and improved by rest. Other symptoms and signs included night-sweating, depression, a dry mouth at night, insomnia (waking up frequently during the night) and a Red tongue generally without coating except for a sticky-yellow coating on the root.

Diagnosis
This is a very clear case of back-ache from deficiency of Kidney-Yin as all the other manifestations show. There was also some Damp-Heat in the Lower Burner as evidenced by the sticky-yellow coating on the root of the tongue. This would play a part in the pathogenesis of his back-ache.

Treatment principle
The treatment principle was to nourish Kidney-Yin and strengthen the back.

Acupuncture
The main points used were:

- **KI-3** Taixi, **KI-6** Zhaohai and **Ren-4** Guanyuan to nourish Kidney-Yin.
- **BL-23** Shenshu to strengthen the back.
- **BL-26** Guanyuanshu and **Shiqizhuixia** as local points according to tenderness.
- **S.I.-3** and **BL-62** to open the Governing Vessel, tonify the Kidneys, strengthen the back, boost the Will-Power and lift depression.
- **Du-20** Baihui, in combination with the opening points of the Governing Vessel to boost Will-Power and lift depression. It also acts as a distal point for lower back-ache when the ache stems from the midline.

Herbal treatment
Only a patent remedy was used: this was the Zhi Bo Ba Wei Wan *Anemarrhena-Phellodendron Eight-Ingredient Pill* to nourish Kidney-Yin and drain Damp-Heat from the Lower Burner. This pill is particularly good for lower back-ache against a background of Kidney-Yin deficiency since Huang Bo *Cortex Phellodendri* and Zhi Mu *Radix Anemarrhenae asphodeloidis* will act on the Lower Burner and the Bladder channel, thus relieving back-ache.

The back-ache was the first symptom to react to the treatment improving by 90% after a few sessions. All the other symptoms improved only gradually over a period of several months as Yin deficiency can only be supplemented slowly.

Case history

A 63-year-old woman had been suffering from lower back-ache for most of her life. This had started after she contracted polio at the age of 13. Her left leg became paralysed and the resulting limp caused the back-ache. Her knees also ached and her urination was very frequent, also at night, and pale. She also felt very tired and experienced dizziness and tinnitus. She felt easily cold. Her tongue was Pale and Swollen and her pulse was Deep, Slow (60) and Weak, especially on both Rear positions.

Diagnosis
This back-ache was originally due to the paralysis and shortening of one leg from polio. Subsequently, Kidney-Yang deficiency contributed to its development.

Treatment principle
The treatment principle adopted was to tonify and warm the Kidneys and strengthen the back.

Acupuncture
The main points used were:

– **BL-23** Shenshu and **Du-4** Mingmen to tonify and warm Kidney-Yang. The points were needled and warmed with a moxa stick.
– **BL-26** Guanyuanshu, **Du-3** Yaoyangguan and **Shiqizhuixia** as local points to strengthen the lower back. Du-3 was selected because it affects both the lower back and the legs and it would therefore help her knee-ache.
– **BL-60** Kunlun was used as a distal point to strengthen the Bladder channel. This was alternated with **BL-57** Chengshan.
– **ST-36** Zusanli, **SP-6** Sanyinjiao and **KI-7** Fuliu, with warming needle, to tonify and warm Spleen- and Kidney-Yang.

Herbal treatment
Only a patent remedy was used: the Jin Gui Shen Qi Wan *Golden Chest Kidney-Qi Pill* to tonify and warm Kidney-Yang.

This patient's back-ache disappeared after only a few sessions. Acupuncture can sometimes give exceptional results in chronic back-ache even when there are gross structural imbalances. In this case, for example, this patient's left leg was over 1" shorter with a resulting pronounced scoliosis.

SCIATICA

If the pain radiates down to the leg from the back it indicates a more Full condition, usually due to Damp-Cold in the leg channels. Occasionally, it may also be due to Damp-Heat. The pain may also only occur in the leg without affecting the back.

DISTAL POINTS

To select the distal points one must accurately identify the channel involved. The main distal points for sciatica are as follows:

– **BL-40** Weizhong if the pain is on the Bladder channel. This point is better for acute than chronic cases. It should also be kept in mind that this point tends to have a reducing and cooling effect. It is therefore not suitable if there is a deficiency of Kidney-Yang.
– **BL-60** Kunlun if the pain is on the Bladder channel and is chronic.
– **BL-57** Chengshan may be selected as a distal point instead of BL-40 when there is an underlying Kidney-Yang deficiency.
– **BL-58** Feiyang if the pain is in between the Bladder and Gall-Bladder channel.
– **BL-62** Shenmai if the pain starts from around the hip area, radiates to the lateral side of the thigh and then to the back of the lower leg along the Bladder channel.
– **G.B.-41** Zulinqi or **G.B.-40** Qiuxu if the pain occurs along the Gall-Bladder channel.
– **KI-4** Dazhong, Connecting point of the Kidney channel, is a good distal point to choose when there is an underlying Kidney deficiency as it simultaneously tonifies the Kidneys and invigorates its Connecting channel and therefore the Bladder channel.

Obviously any of the above distal points may be used as a local point when the pain extends to the lower leg.

LOCAL POINTS

The main local points are:

– **Tunzhong** if the leg pain starts from the buttock. This point should be inserted at least 2" deep and a good needling sensation obtained preferably radiating down to the leg.
– **BL-36** Chengfu is often a tender point and if so should be selected. Again, the needling sensation should radiate down the leg.
– **BL-37** Yinmen, same as above.
– **G.B.-30** Huantiao is an extremely important point if the leg pain occurs along the Gall-Bladder channel. This point should be needled at least 2.5" deep, with the patient

lying on the opposite side. The needling sensation should preferably radiate all the way down to the ankle. If it does, one does not need to use any other local point. If the needling sensation radiates only as far as the knee, then one can use G.B.-34 Yanglingquan to extend the sensation further to the foot. Moxa on the needle on G.B.-30 is very beneficial.

– **G.B.-31** Fengshi is an important local point for sciatica along the Gall-Bladder channel. Moxa on the needle is very effective.
– **G.B.-34** Yanglingquan is selected if the pain occurs in the lower leg. Apart from its function as a local point, it benefits the sinews and would therefore help to relax the tendons.

Unless there is Damp-Heat in the Bladder or Gall-Bladder channel, moxa is extremely beneficial in sciatica. This is best done with a moxa stick gently heating the area around each needle and especially Tunzhong, BL-36 and BL-37. A good method is also to gently heat the Bladder channel all the way from BL-36 to BL-40 until a red line appears.

HERBAL TREATMENT

As mentioned above, the herbal treatment must be based on the patterns. The main patterns are:

– Damp-Cold invading the back channels
– Damp-Heat invading the back channels
– Stagnation of Qi and Blood in the back
– Kidney deficiency.

The first three patterns can occur in both acute and chronic cases while the fourth one can only occur in chronic conditions. In chronic cases, the formulae for the first three patterns will need to be modified by the introduction of herbs to tonify the Spleen, Liver and Kidneys, depending on the condition of the patient.

Likewise, since patterns are often combined in practice, it is quite common, indeed prevalent, to see conditions characterized by both Fullness and Emptiness. For example, the combination of the pattern of Kidney deficiency with either Damp-Cold or Stagnation of Qi and Blood or

even both is very common. In these cases, one must decide whether the condition is predominantly Full or Empty, select a formula accordingly, and modify it according to actual clinical manifestations.

1. DAMP-COLD INVADING THE BACK CHANNELS

(a) PRESCRIPTION

GAN JIANG LING ZHU TANG Variation
Glycyrrhiza-Zingiber-Poria-Atractylodes Decoction
Zhi Gan Cao *Radix Glycyrrhizae uralensis praeparata* 6 g
Gan Jiang *Rhizoma Zingiberis officinalis* 6 g
Fu Ling *Sclerotium Poriae cocos* 9 g
Bai Zhu *Rhizoma Atractylodis macrocephalae* 9 g
Gui Zhi *Ramulus Cinnamomi cassiae* 3 g
Niu Xi *Radix Achyranthis bidentatae seu Cyathulae* 9 g
Du Zhong *Cortex Eucommiae ulmoidis* 6 g
Sang Ji Sheng *Ramus Loranthi* 6 g
Xu Duan *Radix Dipsaci* 6 g

Explanation

– **Zhi Gan Cao** and **Gan Jiang** expel Cold and warm the Centre.
– **Fu Ling** and **Bai Zhu** dry Dampness and tonify the Spleen, which will, by itself, help to resolve Dampness.
– **Gui Zhi** and **Niu Xi** benefit the channels and sinews and expel Cold.
– **Du Zhong**, **Sang Ji Sheng** and **Xu Duan** tonify Kidney-Yang, strengthen the lower back and benefit sinews and bones.

Variations

– If the Cold signs are very prominent add Fu Zi *Radix Aconiti carmichaeli praeparata*.
– If signs of Dampness are pronounced add Cang Zhu *Rhizoma Atractylodis lanceae*.

(b) PRESCRIPTION

CANG BAI ER CHEN TANG Variation

Grey and White Atractylodes Two Old Decoction
Cang Zhu *Rhizoma Atractylodis lanceae* 6 g
Bai Zhu *Rhizoma Atractylodis macrocephalae* 6 g
Chen Pi *Pericarpium Citri reticulatae* 4.5 g
Ban Xia *Rhizoma Pinelliae ternatae* 9 g
Fu Ling *Sclerotium Poriae cocos* 6 g
Zhi Gan Cao *Radix Glycyrrhizae uralensis prae-parata* 3 g
Sheng Jiang *Rhizoma Zingiberis officinalis recens* 3 slices
Du Huo *Radix Angelicae pubescentis* 6 g

Explanation

This formula is used if there is a predominance of Dampness over Cold.

- The first seven herbs make up the Cang Bai Er Chen Tang, i.e. the Er Chen Tang plus Cang Zhu and Bai Zhu. This formula resolves Dampness.
- **Du Huo** is added to enter the channels of the lower back, thus resolving Dampness from the lower back.

(c) PRESCRIPTION

ER CHEN TANG Variation
Two Old Decoction
Ban Xia *Rhizoma Pinelliae ternatae* 15 g
Chen Pi *Pericarpium Citri reticulatae* 15 g
Fu Ling *Sclerotium Poriae cocos* 9 g
Zhi Gan Cao *Radix Glycyrrhizae uralensis prae-parata* 5 g
Sheng Jiang *Rhizoma Zingiberis officinalis recens* 3 g
Wu Mei *Fructus Pruni mume* 1 prune
Bai Zhu *Rhizoma Atractylodis macrocephalae* 6 g
Bi Xie *Rhizoma Dioscoreae hypoglaucae* 6 g
Bai Jie Zi *Semen Sinapis albae* 4.5 g
Zhu Li *Succus Bambusae* 10 ml

Explanation

This formula is used in overweight people with some oedema of the lower back, usually over the sacrum. The back feels very soft on pressure and does not ache on pressing. The pulse is Slippery.

- The first six herbs constitute the Er Chen Tang which resolves Dampness and Phlegm.
- **Bai Zhu** tonifies the Spleen and resolves Dampness.
- **Bi Xie** resolves Dampness from the Bladder channel.
- **Bai Jie Zi** and **Zhu Li** resolve Cold Phlegm. Zhu Li (bamboo sap) may be added at the end in the cup. If Zhu Li is not available, substitute Zhu Ru.

2. DAMP-HEAT INVADING THE BACK CHANNELS

PRESCRIPTION

SI MIAO SAN Variation
Four Wonderful Powder Variation
Cang Zhu *Rhizoma Atractylodis lanceae* 9 g
Huang Bo *Cortex Phellodendri* 9 g
Niu Xi *Radix Achyranthis bidentatae seu Cyathulae* 9 g
Yi Yi Ren *Semen Coicis lachryma jobi* 9 g
Wei Ling Xian *Radix Clematidis chinensis* 6 g
Hai Tong Pi *Cortex Erythrinae variegatae* 6 g

Explanation

- The first four herbs form the Si Miao San which resolves Damp-Heat in the lower part of the body.
- **Wei Ling Xian** and **Hai Tong Pi** expel Wind-Damp from the channels.

Variations

- If symptoms and signs of Heat are pronounced add Zhi Zi *Fructus Gardeniae jasminoidis*, Ze Xie *Rhizoma Alismatis orientalis* and Mu Tong *Caulis Akebiae*.
- If the Heat part of Damp-Heat has begun to injure Yin fluids, add Zhi Mu *Radix Anemarrhenae asphodeloidis* and Tian Men Dong *Tuber Asparagi cochinchinensis*.

PATENT REMEDY

QIAN JIN ZHI DAI WAN
Thousand Gold Pieces Stopping Leukorrhoea Pill

Da Qing Ye *Folium Isatidis seu Baphicacanthi*
Dang Shen *Radix Codonopsis pilosulae*
Mu Li *Concha Ostreae*
Mu Xiang *Radix Saussureae*
Dang Gui *Radix Angelicae sinensis*
Yan Hu Suo *Rhizoma Corydalis yanhusuo*
Xu Duan *Radix Dipsaci*
Bai Zhu *Rhizoma Atractylodis macrocephalae*
Xiao Hui Xiang *Fructus Foeniculi vulgaris*

Explanation

Although the main use of this pill is to treat leukorrhoea, it can be used to treat acute or sub-acute back-ache and sciatica from Damp-Heat. This remedy, in fact, drains Damp-Heat from the Lower Burner and moves Qi and Blood: both these actions are applicable to treat back-ache and sciatica from Damp-Heat in the Bladder channel.

3. STAGNATION OF QI AND BLOOD

PRESCRIPTION

SHEN TONG ZHU YU TANG Variation
Body-Pain Eliminating Stagnation Decoction
Dang Gui *Radix Angelicae sinensis* 9 g
Chuan Xiong *Radix Ligustici wallichii* 6 g
Tao Ren *Semen Persicae* 9 g
Hong Hua *Flos Carthami tinctorii* 9 g
Mo Yao *Myrrha* 6 g
Wu Ling Zhi *Excrementum Trogopteri* 6 g
Xiang Fu *Rhizoma Cyperi rotundi* 3 g
Niu Xi *Radix Achyranthis bidentatae seu Cyathulae* 9 g
Di Long *Pheretima aspergillum* 6 g
Gan Cao *Radix Glycyrrhizae uralensis* 3 g

Explanation

- **Dang Gui**, **Chuan Xiong**, **Tao Ren** and **Hong Hua** nourish, harmonize and move Blood.
- **Mo Yao** and **Wu Ling Zhi** move Blood, eliminate stasis and stop pain.
- **Xiang Fu** moves Qi and stops pain.
- **Niu Xi** moves Blood, tonifies Liver and Kidneys, benefits sinews and bones and strengthens the lower back.

- **Di Long** expels Wind-Damp and stops pain.
- **Gan Cao** harmonizes.
- **Qiang Huo** and **Qin Jiao** have been eliminated from the original formula which was for pain all over the body. Qiang Huo treats mostly the upper part of the body while the present variation is directed at the lower part.

Variations

- If there is also Damp-Cold in the lower back add Du Huo *Radix Angelicae pubescentis*.
- If there is Kidney-Yang deficiency add Du Zhong *Cortex Eucommiae ulmoidis* and Gou Ji *Rhizoma Cibotii barometz*.

(i) PATENT REMEDY

GU ZHE CUO SHANG SAN
Fracture and Contusion Powder
Ye Zhu Gu *Cranium Suis Scrofae*
Huang Gua Zi *Semen Cucumeris sativae*
Dang Gui *Radix Angelicae sinensis*
Hong Hua *Flos Carthami tinctorii*
Xue Jie *Sangui Draconis*
Da Huang *Rhizoma Rhei*
Ru Xiang *Gummi Olibanum*
Mo Yao *Myrrha*
Di Bie Chong *Eupolyphaga sue opishoplatia*

Explanation

Although this remedy is mostly for fractures and contusions, it can be used for acute back-ache from local stagnation of Qi and Blood.

It is contraindicated in pregnancy and it should be used only for a short time (about one week) as it contains Da Huang which moves downwards and Di Bie Chong which is slightly toxic.

(ii) PATENT REMEDY

DA HUO LUO DAN
Great Invigorating the Connecting Channels Pill

An Xi Xiang *Benzonium*
Bing Pian *Borneol*
Cao Wu Tou *Radix Aconiti carmichaeli*
Chen Xiang *Lignum Aquilariae*
Chi Shao *Radix Paeoniae rubrae*
Chuan Niu Xi *Radix Cyathulae*
Chuan Xiong *Radix Ligustici wallichii*
Da Huang *Rhizoma Rhei*
Dang Gui *Radix Angelicae sinensis*
Di Long *Pheretima aspergillum*
Ding Xiang *Flos Caryophylli*
Cao Dou Kou *Semen Alpiniae katsumadae*
Fang Feng *Radix Ledebouriellae sesloidis*
Fu Ling *Sclerotium Poriae cocos*
Gan Cao *Radix Glycyrrhizae uralensis*
Ge Gen *Radix Puerariae*
Gu Sui Bu *Rhizoma Gusuibu*
Guan Zhong *Radix seu Herba Potentillae*
Gui Ban *Plastrum Testudinis*
Shou Wu *Radix Polygoni multiflori*
Hu Gu *Os Tigris*
Huang Lian *Rhizoma Coptidis*
Huang Qin *Radix Scutellariae baicalensis*
Huo Xiang *Herba Agastachis*
Jiang Can *Bombyx batryticatus*
Ma Huang *Herba Ephedrae*
Mo Yao *Myrrha*
Mu Xiang *Radix Saussureae*
Niu Huang *Calculus Bovis*
Qi She *Agkistrodon acutus*
Qiang Huo *Radix et Rhizoma Notopterygii*
Qing Pi *Pericarpium Citri reticulatae viridae*
Ren Shen *Radix Ginseng*
Rou Gui *Cortex Cinnamomi cassiae*
Ru Xiang *Gummi Olibanum*
She Xiang *Secretio Moschus moschiferi*
Shu Di Huang *Radix Rehmanniae glutinosae praeparatae*
Song Xiang *Resina praeparata Pini*
Tian Ma *Rhizoma Gastrodiae elatae*
Dan Nan Xing *Rhizoma Arisaematis praeparata*
Wei Ling Xian *Radix Clematidis chinensis*
Wu Shao She *Zaocys dhumnades*
Wu Yao *Radix Lynderae strychnifoliae*
Shui Niu Jiao *Cornu Bufali*
Xi Xin *Herba Asari cum radice*
Xiang Fu *Rhizoma Cyperi rotundi*
Xuan Shen *Radix Scrophulariae ningpoensis*
Xue Jie *Sanguis draconis*

Explanation

This remedy moves Qi and Blood, eliminates stasis and expels Wind. Its main use is for the sequelae stage of Wind-stroke, but it can be used for acute or sub-acute back-ache from local stagnation of Qi and Blood.

It is contraindicated in pregnancy and it should be used only for a short time (one or two weeks) as it is a powerful remedy containing many different herbs.

4. KIDNEY DEFICIENCY

(a) PRESCRIPTION

DU HUO JI SHENG TANG
Angelica pubescens-Loranthus Decoction
Du Huo *Radix Angelicae pubescentis* 9 g
Xi Xin *Herba Asari cum radice* 3 g
Fang Feng *Radix Ledebouriellae sesloidis* 6 g
Qin Jiao *Radix Gentianae macrophyllae* 6 g
Sang Ji Sheng *Ramus Loranthi* 6 g
Du Zhong *Cortex Eucommiae ulmoidis* 6 g
Niu Xi *Radix Achyranthis bidentatae* 6 g
Dang Gui *Radix Angelicae sinensis* 6 g
Chuan Xiong *Radix Ligustici wallichii* 6 g
Sheng Di Huang *Radix Rehmanniae glutinosae* 6 g
Bai Shao *Radix Paeoniae albae* 6 g
Ren Shen *Radix Ginseng* 6 g
Fu Ling *Sclerotium Poriae cocos* 6 g
Rou Gui *Cortex Cinnamomi cassiae* 6 g
Gan Cao *Radix Glycyrrhizae uralensis* 6 g

Explanation

This formula, which has already been explained in chapter 23, tonifies the Kidneys and Liver and benefits sinews and bones. It is specific for chronic Painful Obstruction Syndrome of the lower back and knees. However, the formula contains many hot herbs and is primarily for Kidney-Yang deficiency; it would not be at all suitable if there were Kidney-Yin deficiency.

This prescription is also a popular patent remedy and makes a very useful addition to the acupuncture treatment of chronic lower back-ache.

(b) PRESCRIPTION

ZUO GUI WAN
Restoring the Left [Kidney] Pill
Shu Di Huang *Radix Rehmanniae glutinosae prae-parata* 15 g
Shan Yao *Radix Dioscoreae oppositae* 9 g
Shan Zhu Yu *Fructus Corni officinalis* 9 g
Gou Qi Zi *Fructus Lycii chinensis* 9 g
Chuan Niu Xi *Radix Cyathulae* 6 g
Tu Si Zi *Semen Cuscutae* 9 g
Lu Jiao *Cornu Cervi* 9 g
Gui Ban Jiao *Colla Plastri Testudinis* 9 g

Explanation

This formula, which has already been explained in chapters 1 and 9, tonifies Kidney-Yin. Niu Xi and Lu Jiao within the formula strengthen the back.

- To enhance its effect on the lower back add Wu Jia Pi *Cortex Acanthopanacis radicis* and Ji Xue Teng *Caulis Millettiae seu Caulis Spatholobi*.
- If there are pronounced symptoms of Yin deficiency and Empty-Heat add Nu Zhen Zi *Fructus Ligustri lucidi* and Han Lian Cao *Herba Ecliptae prostratae*.
- If there are symptoms of Damp-Cold in the lower back add Du Huo *Radix Angelicae pubescentis*.
- If there are symptoms of Damp-Heat in the lower back add Huang Bo *Cortex Phellodendri* and Bi Xie *Rhizoma Dioscoreae hypoglaucae*.
- If there is stasis of Blood in the back increase the dosage of Niu Xi *Radix Cyathulae*.

(i) PATENT REMEDY

YAO TONG PIAN
Back-ache Tablet
Dang Gui *Radix Angelicae sinensis*
Xu Duan *Radix Dipsaci*
Du Zhong *Cortex Eucommiae ulmoidis*
Gou Qi Zi *Fructus Lycii chinensis*
Bai Zhu *Rhizoma Atractylodis macrocephalae*
Bu Gu Zhi *Fructus Psoraleae corylifoliae*
Niu Xi *Radix Achyranthis bidentatae seu Cyathulae*

Explanation

This tablet tonifies Kidney-Yang and strengthens the lower back. It is for chronic back-ache from Kidney-Yang deficiency.

The tongue presentation appropriate to this remedy is a Pale, Swollen and wet body.

(ii) PATENT REMEDY

DU HUO JI SHENG WAN
Angelica pubescens-Loranthus Pill

Explanation

This pill has the same ingredients and functions as the homonymous prescription above. It is particularly indicated for chronic back-ache from deficiency of Blood and Kidney-Yang in women.

The tongue presentation appropriate to this remedy is a Pale and Thin body.

(iii) PATENT REMEDY

DU ZHONG HU GU WAN
Eucommia-Tiger Bone Pill
Ren Shen *Radix Ginseng*
Bai Zhu *Rhizoma Atractylodis macrocephalae*
Dang Gui *Radix Angelicae sinensis*
Chuan Xiong *Radix Ligustici wallichii*
Ji Xue Teng *Caulis Millettiae seu Caulis Spatholobi*
San Qi *Radix Notoginseng*
Du Zhong *Cortex Eucommiae ulmoidis*
Hu Gu *Os Tigris*
Mu Gua *Fructus Chaenomelis lagenariae*
Yin Yang Huo *Herba Epimedii*
Wu Shao She *Zaocys dhumnades*
Lu Lu Tong *Fructus Liquidambaris taiwanianae*
Cang Zhu *Rhizoma Atractylodis lanceae*
Xun Gu Feng *Rhizoma seu Herba Aristolochiae*
Wei Ling Xian *Radix Clematidis chinensis*
Shi Nan Teng *Ramus Photiniae*
Sang Zhi *Ramulus Mori albae*

Explanation

This pill is similar in effect to remedy (i) above,

but it is stronger and has a more complex action. It tonifies Kidney-Yang, strengthens the back, nourishes and moves Blood, and expels Wind-Dampness. It is therefore suitable for chronic back-ache in the elderly from deficiency of Kidney-Yang and Blood, retention of Cold-Dampness in the lower back and some local stasis of Blood.

The tongue presentation appropriate to this remedy is a Pale-Bluish-Purple and rather Stiff body.

(iv) PATENT REMEDY

JIAN BU HU QIAN WAN
Vigorous Walk [like] Stealthy Tiger Pill
Mu Gua *Fructus Chaenomelis lagenariae*
Huai Niu Xi *Radix Achyranthis bidentatae*
Hu Gu *Os Tigris*
Qin Jiao *Radix Gentianae macrophyllae*
Dang Gui *Radix Angelicae sinensis*
Ren Shen *Radix Ginseng*
Feng Mi *Mel*

Explanation

This pill nourishes Liver- and Kidney-Yin and strengthens sinews and bones. It is suitable for chronic back-ache in the elderly from deficiency of Liver- and Kidney-Yin.

The tongue presentation appropriate to this remedy is a Red body without coating.

(v) PATENT REMEDY

TE XIAO YAO TONG LING
Especially-Effective Back-ache Pill
Du Zhong *Cortex Eucommiae ulmoidis*
Ba Ji Tian *Radix Morindae officinalis*
Chuan Xiong *Radix Ligustici wallichii*
Hong Hua *Flos Carthami tinctorii*
Huai Niu Xi *Radix Achyranthis bidentatae*
Qin Jiao *Radix Gentianae macrophyllae*
Shou Wu *Radix Polygoni multiflori*
Du Huo *Radix Angelicae pubescentis*
Sang Ji Sheng *Ramulus Loranthi*
Dang Gui *Radix Angelicae sinensis*
Wei Ling Xian *Radix Clematidis chinensis*

Explanation

This pill tonifies Kidney-Yang and nourishes and moves Blood. It is suitable for chronic back-ache from deficiency of Kidney-Yang and Blood. It is similar in effect to Du Huo Ji Sheng Wan *Angelica pubescens-Loranthus Pill*: it differs from it in so far as it is less hot in energy and, in a small dose, is suitable also if there is some deficiency of Kidney-Yin.

The tongue presentation appropriate to this remedy is a Pale body.

Prognosis and prevention

Acupuncture can be extremely effective in the treatment of both acute and chronic back-ache, more so than herbal medicine. It sometimes produces extraordinary results in the face of all odds when there are severe structural imbalances in the spine. The duration of the complaint seems to be less relevant in back-ache than in other diseases: many cases of very chronic back-ache of, say, over 20 years' duration are sometimes cleared in a few sessions.

Acute attacks from sprain or invasion of Damp-Cold can be cleared in a few treatments, sometimes even only one. If, however, the acute attack is a recurrence of a chronic problem, the treatment will take much longer: usually about 10–15 sessions.

When the back-ache is accompanied by sciatica it will usually take longer to treat. If the patient's tongue is Red and Peeled and the pulse is Rapid, Slippery and Wiry, the prognosis is poor and the treatment will either be unsuccessful or will take a long time.

Further indications on prognosis must take into account Western diagnosis, distinguishing the four conditions of chronic lower lumbar ligamentous strain, spondylosis, osteoarthritis and disc herniation.

Chronic lower lumbar ligamentous strain and spondylosis respond extremely well to treatment, in the way indicated above.

Severe spinal osteoarthritis obviously reduces the effectiveness of acupuncture which, although it will produce an improvement, may never completely cure it. However, it is important not to attribute excessive importance to a diagnosis of spinal osteoarthritis as this often has no correlation with clinical symptoms. For example, many patients show severe osteoarthritic changes in the spine without suffering any back-ache. Conversely, sometimes very slight degenerative changes in the vertebrae may produce severe pain. This apparent paradox can be explained in the light of the Chinese pathology of back-ache: there are other factors at play, besides spinal osteoarthritis, producing back-ache, i.e. sprain, Damp-Cold and a Kidney deficiency.

Thus, if a patient suffering from chronic back-ache presents with X-rays pronouncing spinal osteoarthritis, it is important always to keep in mind the possibility that such degenerative changes are *not* related to the pain experienced by the patient. This explains how many patients with supposedly fairly severe osteoarthritis of the spine, do respond to acupuncture extremely well. Of course, if severe spinal osteoarthritis *is* the cause of the pain in old people, then acupuncture will be less effective.

As for prolapsed disc, acupuncture can be very effective to treat both acute and chronic cases of disc herniation as the nucleus pulposus can be reabsorbed into the annulus fibrosus. The treatment principle and selection of points do not differ from those indicated above for acute and chronic back-ache. Obviously, in acute cases of disc herniation treatment should be given every day for at least one week. After that, it can be spaced out to every 2–3 days. In that time, the patient should have complete bed-rest.

As for prevention, as indicated above, probably the main underlying cause of chronic back-ache in Western industrialized countries is the *lack* of exercise. Many people lead a very sedentary life and have almost no exercise. In order to prevent back-ache, such people should be encouraged to take regular exercise even if it is only brisk walking. *Tai Ji Chuan* is an excellent form of exercise which gently strengthens the back and keeps all sinews and ligaments supple. Gentle back stretching and twisting exercises are also important.

Those who have a tendency to back sprain should never lift heavy weights as this not only can cause an acute sprain, but also weakens Kidney-Qi. Those who have a tendency to back problems and a Kidney deficiency should also reduce their sexual activity. This applies to men more than women.

It should also be said, with regard to prevention, that *excessive* exercise is also a frequent cause of back problems. In particular excessive jogging or aerobic exercises can cause back sprain. This is more likely to occur to those who start engaging in such activities fairly abruptly in their late 30s or early 40s after a completely sedentary life.

Western differentiation

Lower back-ache can be treated perfectly adequately and successfully according to the Chinese diagnosis and treatment outlined above without any reference to Western medicine. However, it is important for acupuncture practitioners to understand at least the basics of the Western pathology of back pain, if only to be able to communicate with patients and their doctors. Western medical doctors are increasingly referring patients to us.

From a Western medical perspective, the pathology of back pain is not well understood. There are many cases when the pathogenesis of back pain is not clear. Back pain may be caused by very many conditions, the most common of which are:

- Chronic lower lumbar ligamentous strain (ligaments)
- Spondylosis (synovial joints of vertebrae)
- Spinal osteoarthritis (vertebrae)
- Prolapsed lumbar disc (disc).

These four conditions affect each of the main structures of the lumbar spine as indicated above in parentheses, i.e. the ligaments, the zygo-apophysial joints (synovial joints) between vertebrae, the vertebrae themselves, and the discs in between the vertebrae. Figure 24.14 shows the anatomy of two lumbar vertebrae, while figure 24.15 shows the zygo-apophysial joints between two lumbar vertebrae.

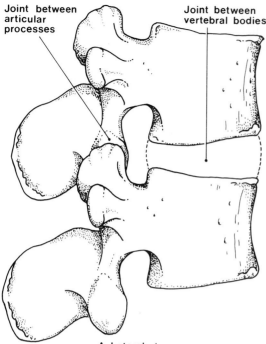

A. Lateral view

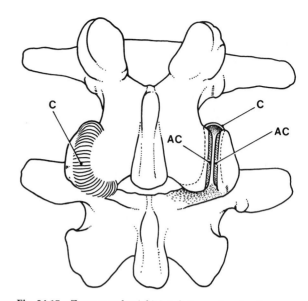

Fig. 24.15 Zygo-apophysial joints between two lumbar vertebrae. Reproduced with permission from "Clinical Anatomy of the Lumbar Spine" by N. Bogduk and L. Twomey, Churchill Livingstone 1987

CHRONIC LOWER LUMBAR LIGAMENTOUS STRAIN

This is a very general term which applies to an ill-defined group of conditions characterized by persistent and recurrent back pain without a recognizable pathology.

It is due to the back muscles failing to protect the ligaments in maintaining posture. The pain is usually better with rest and worse on exercise.

From a Chinese medical perspective, as the problem lies within the muscles and ligaments, it is necessary to treat the Spleen and Liver with points such as SP-3 Taibai and G.B.-34 Yanglingquan. It is interesting to note that the "Simple Questions" says that Spleen diseases influence the spine as mentioned above. This is obviously in the sense that it influences the muscles alongside the spine.

SPONDYLOSIS

This consists in disease (usually ankylosis) of the zygo-apophysial joints between vertebrae (see Fig. 24.12 above).

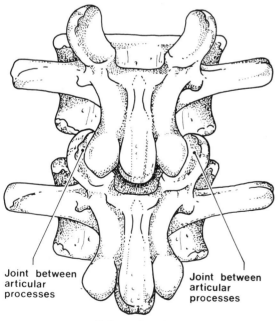

B. Posterior view

Fig. 24.14 Lumbar vertebrae. Reproduced with permission from "Clinical Anatomy of the Lumbar Spine" by N. Bogduk and L. Twomey, Churchill Livingstone 1987

The symptoms consist of back pain which is worse for movement especially extension and tenderness over the affected joint. The movement of the joints is restricted and the muscles alongside the spine are stiff and under spasm.

As this is a condition affecting the synovial joints with their cartilage and ligaments, one would treat the Liver with points such as G.B.-34 Yanglingquan, LIV-8 Ququan, and BL-18 Ganshu.

SPINAL OSTEOARTHRITIS

This consists in degenerative changes of the vertebrae bodies themselves. These changes cause a narrowing of the discs and hypertrophy of bone at the joint margins which leads to the formation of osteophytes (Fig. 24.16). Osteoarthritis of the spine can be very severe without causing any symptoms. In most cases it causes an ache which is worse on exertion and in the morning. There may be a feeling of stiffness when getting up from a sitting position.

As this condition consists in degeneration of the vertebral bodies themselves, one would treat the Kidneys and the bones with KI-3 Taixi, BL-23 Shenshu and BL-11 Dashu.

PROLAPSED LUMBAR DISC

This is the most common cause of nerve-root compression. It is caused by the nucleus pulpo-sus (the ball of collagenous material inside the disc) bursting through the annulus fibrosus (the tough and yet elastic fibrocartilaginous ring constituting the outside of the disc). This condition, illustrated in Figure 24.17, is commonly referred to as "slipped disc". This is of course a misleading term as the disc itself does not move: it is only the central nucleus that bursts through the outer ring.

The most common discs to prolapse are those at L4/5 and L5/S1. The thinnest part of the annulus fibrosus is in the posterolateral region of the disc: thus most prolapses occur in this region where interference with nerve roots is most likely. The nucleus pulposus may also prolapse only partially: this gives rise to pain without nerve root irritation. Prolapse of the nucleus pulposus is more frequent in people in their 30s or early 40s when degeneration of the annulus fibrosus occurs. It is rare later on in life as the nucleus pulposus becomes fibrous and cannot herniate.

The main clinical manifestations of a prolapsed nucleus pulposus are a sudden and severe shooting pain in the back radiating down to either leg (sciatica). The radiation of the pain follows the dermatome distribution (Fig. 24.18).

It is interesting to note that the location of pain in sciatica follows the distribution of the acupuncture channels and not necessarily the dermatomes. We must therefore always base our selection of points on the channel distribution and not the dermatomes. However, in the case of disc prolapse, it is also useful to take the der-

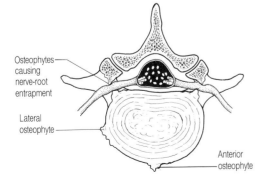

Fig. 24.16 Osteophytes

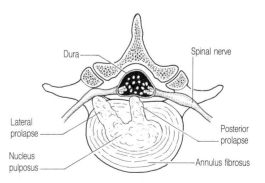

Fig. 24.17 Lateral and posterior disc prolapse

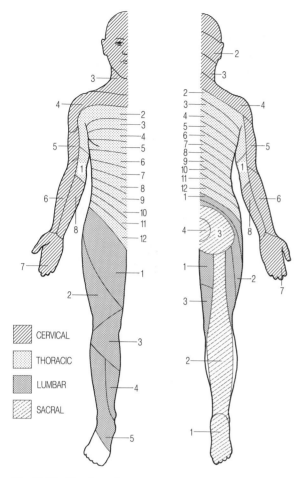

CERVICAL

THORACIC

LUMBAR

SACRAL

Fig. 24.18 The dermatomes

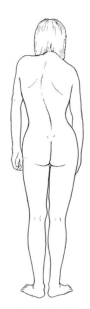

Fig. 24.19 Scoliosis posture in disc herniation

matome distribution into account and use points on the Governing Vessel and their corresponding Huatuojiaji points at the level of the disc lesion and one space below this level. This is because the symptoms and signs arise from the compression of the nerve root of the spinal nerve below the disc. For example, herniation of the disc between L5 and S1 causes symptoms of nerve-root irritation of the S1 spinal nerve.

In acute cases, the back pain is severe and no position is comfortable. The patient instinctively

adopts a posture of scoliosis curving towards the side of the prolapse and movements of the spine are extremely restricted (Fig. 24.19). Straight leg raising is limited on the side of the root irritation and produces intense pain. This test is carried out with the patient supine (face up). Holding the knee straight, lift each leg in turn flexing at the hip. Marked impairment of the leg movement and pain when lifted over 30 degrees indicates lumbo-sacral nerve-root compression. This is further confirmed if more pain is elicited by dorsiflexion of the foot. Numbness of the leg will appear in a dermatome distribution.

The pain deriving from a prolapsed disc is not due to the disc itself but to compression of the nerve root and dura mater. The torn annulus fibrosus can heal and the herniated nucleus pulposus can be reabsorbed.

Disc herniation may persist for months or even years, becoming chronic. The area of pain and other signs may be summarized in Figure 24.20.

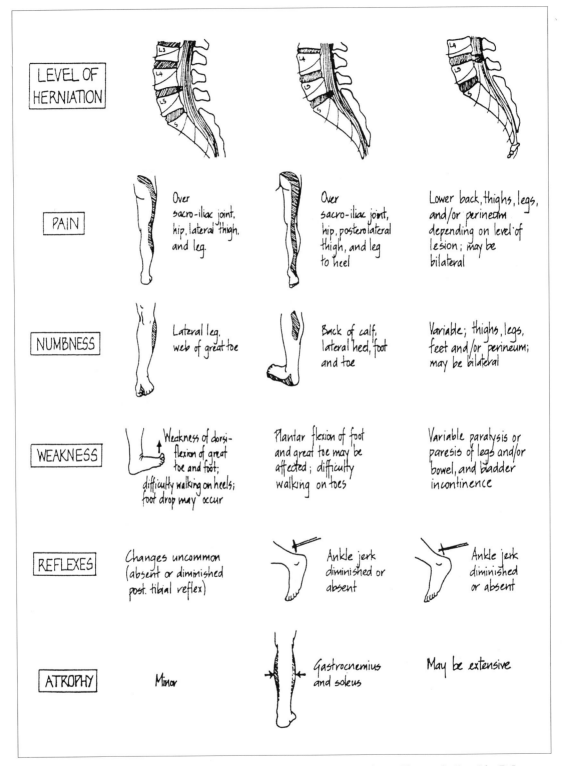

Fig. 24.20 Features of chronic disc herniation. Reproduced with permission from "Close to the Bone" by D. Legge, Sydney College Press 1990

END NOTES

1. Hickling P and Golding J 1984 An Outline of Rheumatology, Wright, Bristol, p. 24.
2. 1979 The Yellow Emperor's Classic of Internal Medicine — Simple Questions (*Huang Ti Nei Jing Su Wen* 黄帝内经素问), People's Health Publishing House, Beijing. First published *c.* 100 BC, p. 100.
3. He Ren 1981 A New Explanation of the Essential Prescriptions of the Golden Chest (*Jin Gui Yao Lue Xin Jie* 金匮要略新解), Zhejiang Science Publishing House, p. 80. The "Essential Prescriptions of the Golden Chest" itself was written by Zhang Zhong Jing and first published *c.* AD 200.
4. Chao Yuan Fang AD 610 General Treatise on the Aetiology and Symptomatology of Diseases (*Zhu Bing Yuan Hou Lun* 诸病源候论), cited in Internal Medicine, p. 245.
5. Zhu Dan Xi 1481 Essential Methods of Dan Xi (*Dan Xi Xin Fa* 丹溪心法), cited in Internal Medicine, p. 245.
6. Wang Ken Tang 1602 Standards of Diagnosis and Treatment (*Zheng Zhi Zhun Sheng* 证治准绳), cited in Internal Medicine, p. 248.
7. Wang Luo Zhen 1985 A Compilation of the Study of the Eight Extraordinary Vessels (*Qi Jing Ba Mai Kao Jiao Zhu* 奇经八脉考校注), Shanghai Science Publishing House, p. 109. The "Study of the Eight Extraordinary Vessels" itself was written by Li Shi Zhen and first published in 1578.
8. Simple Questions, p. 23.

Myalgic encephalomyelitis (post-viral syndrome, chronic Epstein-Barr virus disease)

25

伏邪

From a Western medical perspective, myalgic encephalomyelitis (ME) is a relatively "new" disease. It is not clear what the causative agent might be; indeed, there is no general agreement that it is a separate "disease" at all. Even its name is not generally agreed upon. In fact it is variously called also "Royal-Free disease", "post-viral syndrome", "epidemic neuromyasthenia", "chronic mono", "chronic Epstein-Barr virus disease" and "chronic fatigue syndrome".

"Myalgic" means "pain in the muscles" while "encephalomyelitis" means inflammation of the brain and nerves. The reason that there is no general agreement on the nature and causative agent of this disease is that there is no conclusive test which is specific to ME. Current research, however, does show that ME might be caused by an enterovirus and, specifically, the Coxsackie sub-group of enteroviruses.[1] In the USA, research seems to be more oriented towards the Epstein-Barr virus (the one that causes "glandular fever" or mononucleosis) as a cause of ME. Some doctors restrict the definition of ME to post-viral symptoms with a gradual and insidious onset and accompanied by evidence of persistent infection by enteroviruses. They distinguish this from an acute-onset post-viral syndrome clearly starting after an acute infection. ME symptoms appear either gradually and insidiously without an apparent infection, or after an acute infection. Typically, this can be influenza or an influenza-like infection, a specific infection such as varicella (chicken-pox), or gastroenteritis. The symptoms at this acute stage would include fever, shivering, aches, swollen glands, and fatigue. Various other symptoms may be present depending on the type of infection, such as vomiting, nausea, diarrhoea, earache, dizziness, sore throat or cough.

After an apparent recovery from the above symptoms, the person starts to feel unwell again and various symptoms persist ever after. The main symptoms of ME are pronounced muscle fatigue and ache, poor memory and concentration, exhaustion and a persisting, intermittent, generally flu-like feeling.

From a Chinese medical perspective, the distinction between "true" ME with insidious onset and other types of general post-viral fatigue is irrelevant. Any type of post-viral fatigue, whether ME or not, can be interpreted, diagnosed and treated according to the principles of Chinese medicine. However, in my experience, there is a difference between "true" ME characterized by a persistent viral infection, and post-viral syndrome, characterized by a disharmony of the internal organs following a viral infection. The main way to distinguish these two conditions is in the symptoms of muscle ache and a general flu-like feeling: in "true" ME these are very predominant and persistent. Also, in "true" ME the pulse has a certain Full quality, which may be Slippery or Wiry.

The diagnosis and treatment discussed in this chapter can however be applied to any type of ME or post-viral fatigue syndrome.

Chinese medical books have, since very early times, described the cause, diagnosis and treatment of conditions similar to ME or post-viral syndrome. The three main conditions with which ME can manifest are:

– Residual pathogenic factor
– Latent Heat
– Lesser Yang pattern.

Residual pathogenic factor

One of the main conditions leading to post-viral fatigue is that of "residual pathogenic factor". If external Wind invades the body and is not cleared properly, or if the person fails to rest during an acute invasion of Wind, the pathogenic factor may remain in the Interior (usually either as Heat or Damp-Heat). Here, on the one hand, it continues to produce symptoms and signs, or on the other, predisposes the person to further invasions of exterior pathogenic factors because it obstructs the proper spreading and descending of Lung-Qi. Moreover, it will also tend to weaken Qi and/or Yin, establishing a vicious circle of pathogenic factor and deficiency.

Apart from Heat itself, Damp-Heat is a very frequent residual pathogenic factor after a febrile disease. There are two main reasons for this. First of all, in the course of a febrile disease, the ascending and descending movements of Spleen and Stomach are upset. Thus, because Stomach-Qi cannot descend, turbid fluids are not transformed, and because Spleen-Qi cannot ascend, the clear fluids cannot be transformed: this leads to the formation of Dampness. Secondly, Heat burns the body fluids which can then condense into Dampness. Once formed, Dampness is rather self-perpetuating. In fact, Dampness impairs the Spleen transformation and transportation which in itself leads to more Dampness being formed, thus establishing a vicious circle.

It is therefore important to take special care and rest during or immediately after an invasion of an exterior pathogenic factor. At this time one should rest more than usual, take care not to catch cold, eat simple and bland food and abstain from sex altogether. If not, the pathogenic factor will not be cleared properly and will remain inside, usually either as Heat or Damp-Heat.

Antibiotics are one of the most common causes of residual pathogenic factor in our society. Whilst they do destroy bacteria, from the point of view of Chinese Medicine they tend to "lock" the pathogenic factor in the Interior and do not release the Exterior in the beginning stages of an exterior invasion, nor clear Heat or resolve Phlegm in the later stages. Dr J. H. F. Shen uses an excellent simile to illustrate the effect of antibiotics. If we heard a burglar entering our house in the middle of the night, we could react in one of two different ways: either we could get up, make a noise and scare the burglar off; or, if we had a gun, we could shoot the burglar dead. Killing the burglar clearly gets rid of him but at the cost of creating a bigger problem: the immediate difficulty of being lumbered with a dead body in the house, and the long-term difficulty of trouble with the law. Thus the first option is clearly preferable: the burglar leaves the house before having the opportunity of stealing anything, our property and life are safe and that is the end of the problem. If we take the burglar to symbolize the invasion of an external pathogenic factor, the first option corresponds to the way Chinese medicine works: it gets rid of the pathogenic factor without harming the body. The second option corresponds to the way antibiotics work: they kill the bacteria, but they do not get rid of the pathogenic factor. The body is therefore lumbered with a residual pathogenic factor (the "dead burglar's body"). Furthermore, Chinese medicine gets rid of the pathogenic factor by raising the immune response and strengthening the body resistance. Although antibiotics kill the harmful bacteria, they inevitably kill beneficial bacteria as well and leave the body weakened.

The above is not intended to be a critique of antibiotics but an objective analysis of their mode of action as compared with Chinese medicine. There are many instances when antibiotics *do* need to be used when an infection is advanced, widespread and potentially dangerous. In many cases, however, antibiotics are used unnecessarily and routinely. Furthermore, Chinese herbs can be taken in conjunction with antibiotic therapy if necessary as the two work in different ways. Antibiotics will kill the bacteria, while Chinese herbs will either release the Exterior and expel the pathogenic factor (in the beginning stages) or clear Heat and resolve Phlegm (in the later stages). Indeed, Chinese herbs can also help to counteract the side-effects of antibiotics. These destroy beneficial bacteria and from the Chinese point of view, they injure Stomach-Yin. This can be observed in the partial peeling of the tongue coating that occurs after antibiotic therapy. The addition of some herbs to tonify Stomach-Yin (such as Tai Zi Shen *Radix Pseudostellariae*) can help to counteract the side-effects of antibiotics and restore the intestinal flora.

Latent Heat

Symptoms of ME appearing without an acute infection can be explained as a manifestation of Latent Heat. The "Simple Questions" in chapter 3 says: *"If Cold enters the body in wintertime, it comes out as Heat in springtime."*[2] This means that under certain circumstances, a pathogenic factor (which may be Wind-Cold or Wind-Heat) can enter the body without causing immediate symptoms. It then incubates inside the body for some time, turning into Heat which later emerges towards the Exterior causing a person to feel suddenly very tired with weary limbs, slightly thirsty, hot and irritable. He or she would not sleep well and the urine would be dark. At this time the pulse feels Fine and slightly Rapid and the tongue is Red. This condition is called Latent Heat or Spring Heat, although it can occur in any season and not just in

springtime. Besides causing the above symptoms and signs, Latent Heat will also tend to injure Qi and/or Yin, thus establishing a vicious circle of Heat and deficiency. This process of "incubation" of an exterior pathogenic factor in the Interior to emerge as Heat later, explains many cases of ME. Latent Heat can emerge on the surface by itself, as described above, or it can be "pulled" towards the surface by a new invasion of external Wind. In this case, in addition to the above symptoms of interior Heat, there would also be some exterior symptoms such as shivering, fever, occipital headache, aches and sneezing. The pulse (Fine and Rapid) and tongue (Red), however, clearly point to interior Heat.

Another factor that may draw Latent Heat towards the surface is emotional stress. Especially when this affects the Liver and causes Heat, it may pull Latent Heat outwards.

Thus Latent Heat occurs when an individual suffers an invasion of exterior Wind without developing immediate symptoms and the pathogenic factor goes into the Interior where it turns into Heat and comes out months later. The underlying reason for this is usually a Kidney deficiency. If the body condition and the Kidneys are relatively good, a person will develop symptoms at the time of invasion of external Wind. This is a healthy reaction. If the Kidneys are weakened by overwork and excessive sexual activity, the body's Qi is too weak even to respond to the invading external Wind. This causes the Wind to penetrate into the Interior without the person developing exterior symptoms. Once in the Interior, it incubates and turns into Heat to come out some months later.

The ancient doctors believed in particular that if the Essence is properly guarded and not dissipated, pathogenic factors will not enter the body and Latent Heat will not develop. The "Simple Questions" in chapter 4 says: *"The Essence is the root of the body, if it is guarded and stored Latent Heat will not appear in springtime."*[3] This concept is very important in practice as it implies that resistance to pathogenic factors does not depend only on Lung-Qi (which influences Defensive Qi), but also on Kidney-Qi and Kidney-Essence. In fact, Defensive Qi is spread by the Lungs but it has its root in the Kidneys, specifically Kidney-Yang. Moreover, in chronic, recurrent infections such as ME, Kidney-Qi is very often deficient, leading to a decreased immune response.

Another possible cause of Latent Heat can be immunizations, when attenuated or inert forms of certain pathogenic organisms are injected in the body, by-passing the body's first line of resistance. From a Chinese medical perspective it is as if an external pathogenic factor penetrated the body's Interior directly, completely by-passing the Exterior levels. This is exactly what happens with Latent Heat.

To summarize, the two conditions which can lead to ME can be illustrated with a diagram (Fig. 25.1).

In both the above conditions the underlying cause is overexertion and lack of adequate rest as explained above.

It is important to understand the causes of these conditions so that we can advise patients accordingly. Most people have no idea that special precautions should be taken during and after an invasion of an exterior pathogenic factor.

Lesser Yang pattern

Both residual pathogenic factor and Latent Heat can assume the form of the Lesser Yang pattern (which is part of both the 6-Stage and 4-Level patterns), and though this is not really a third separate way in which ME can manifest itself, it has such special and defined characteristics that it is best discussed separately.

Exterior Wind-Heat (or Wind-Cold) can sometimes lodge itself in an energetic niche which is in between the Interior and Exterior (called Half-Exterior Half-Interior in Chinese). The main clinical manifestations of this pattern are: feeling hot and cold in alternation, fullness of the hypochondriac region, poor appetite, irritability, dry throat, nausea, bitter taste, blurred vision, white-sticky tongue coating on one side only and a Wiry pulse. These symptoms describe the Lesser Yang pattern of the 6 Stages. In the context of the 4 Levels, the pattern of Gall-Bladder Heat (Qi level) is basically the same, the only difference being that it is characterized by more Heat. Thus, there will be a prevalence of heat sensation and the tongue coating will be yellow. From a channel perspective, most of the Lesser Yang manifestations are symptoms of Gall-Bladder channel Heat (fullness of hypochondrium, dry throat, nausea, bitter taste, blurred vision and Wiry pulse).

The Lesser Yang is the hinge between Greater Yang which opens onto the Exterior and Bright Yang which opens onto the Interior. The pathogenic factor, in this case Heat, can remain lodged in between the Exterior and Interior for a long time, months or even years. This happens when the person's body condition is particularly weak at the time of invasion of the exterior pathogenic factor.

Both Wind-Heat and Latent-Heat can manifest with the above Lesser Yang pattern.

To summarize, three factors can give rise to ME:

1. A residual pathogenic factor (usually Heat or Damp-Heat) after an invasion of an exterior pathogenic factor
2. Latent Heat, in the way described above
3. A pathogenic factor lodged between the Exterior and Interior, i.e. Lesser Yang pattern.

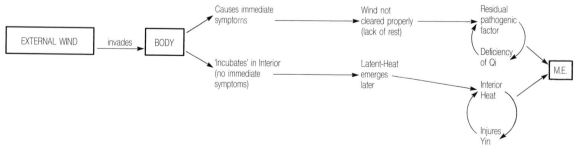

Fig. 25.1 Two conditions leading to ME

Treatment

In all these three cases, it is crucial to diagnose exactly the relative strength of pathogenic factor vs. deficiency of body's Qi. To treat ME properly, it is most important to be able to distinguish whether the predominant aspect is the pathogenic factor (i.e. Excess pattern) or the deficiency of body's Qi (i.e. Deficiency pattern). Of course, almost all cases are characterized by a mixture of Excess (of Heat or Damp-Heat) and Deficiency (usually of Qi and/or Yin). For this reason to treat ME one nearly always needs to combine tonification with expelling, and expelling with tonification. One of these conditions, however, is always predominant and treatment should be clearly aimed at either clearing a pathogenic factor or tonifying the body's Qi. If we tonify when a pathogenic factor is predominant, or if we clear when a deficiency is predominant, the patient will definitely be worse.

One of the main factors which enables us to distinguish whether the condition is predominantly one of Deficiency or Excess is the pulse. Quite simply, if the pulse is very Fine or Weak, Deficiency is predominant; if the pulse is of the Full-type (which could be Wiry or Slippery), an Excess is predominant. Another symptom which allows us to differentiate between a predominantly Deficienct or predominantly Full condition, is the muscle ache: if this is very pronounced, it indicates that the pathogenic factor (Dampness) is predominant.

When the pathogenic factor is between the Exterior and Interior, treatment is aimed at harmonizing the Lesser Yang.

Another important consideration in treating ME is that every effort should be made to treat any new infection the patient might develop during the course of treatment. This is because a new acute viral infection such as a cold or influenza can often undo the work of weeks of treatment. For this reason, it is a good idea to give the patient a supply of Yin Qiao Wan *Lonicera-Forsythia Pill* to take at the first signs of an infection with such symptoms as shivering, a temperature, a sore throat, aches in the muscles, a headache and general lassitude.

Let us now examine the treatment of the various conditions with which ME can manifest itself. The patterns discussed are:

EXCESS CONDITIONS

Damp-Heat in the muscles
Heat lurking in the Interior
Lesser Yang pattern

DEFICIENCY CONDITIONS

Qi Deficiency
Yin Deficiency
Yang Deficiency

EXCESS

1. DAMP-HEAT IN THE MUSCLES

CLINICAL MANIFESTATIONS

Aches in the muscles, tiredness and sleepiness, feeling of heaviness of the body or head, muscle fatigue after even the slightest exertion, no appetite, feeling of oppression of the chest or epigastrium, a sticky taste, lack of concentration, a "muzzy" feeling of the brain, poor concentration and short-term memory, dull headache, a sticky-yellow tongue coating and a Slippery pulse.

If Heat is evident there will be: thirst, dark urine, yellow vaginal discharge, mucus in the stools with burning sensation of the anus on defecation, possibly blood in the stools, possibly night sweating and a sticky-yellow tongue coating.

If Damp-Heat affects the Gall-Bladder and Liver there will be a bitter taste, hypochondrial pain and distension and possibly jaundice. A sticky-yellow tongue coating will be concentrated on the sides.

If Damp-Heat affects the Bladder there will be urinary difficulty, turbid urine and burning on urination. The tongue will have a sticky-yellow tongue coating on the root with red spots.

It is, of course, also possible for Dampness to occur without Heat. In this case the symptoms would be practically the same except that there would be no thirst and the tongue coating would be white.

Dampness can overflow into the space between the skin and muscles and cause the typical muscle ache experienced in ME. It also causes the feeling of heaviness of the muscles, especially in the limbs.

Dampness can also cloud the brain, hence the poor memory and concentration and general muzzy feeling.

The other manifestations are mostly due to Dampness obstructing the Stomach and Spleen.

TREATMENT PRINCIPLE

Resolve Dampness, clear Heat.

ACUPUNCTURE

SP-9 Yinlingquan, SP-6 Sanyinjiao, BL-22 Sanjiaoshu, Ren-12 Zhongwan, Ren-9 Shuifen, L.I.-11 Quchi, SP-3 Taibai, ST-8 Touwei, T.B.-7 Huizong, Du-14 Dazhui: all with reducing or even method.

Explanation

- **SP-9**, **SP-6** and **BL-22** resolve Dampness.
- **Ren-12** and **Ren-9** regulate the transformation of fluids and therefore help to resolve Dampness.
- **L.I.-11** clears Damp-Heat.
- **SP-3** resolves Dampness, especially from the brain.
- **ST-8** is an important local point to resolve Dampness from the head.
- **T.B.-7** relieves pain in the muscles, especially that occurring against a background of Heat.
- **Du-14 Dazhui** clears Heat: this is an important point to use as it is particularly effective in clearing chronic, "hidden", and lingering Heat, such as that which occurs in ME.

HERBAL TREATMENT

(a) Prescription

LIAN PO YIN
Coptis-Magnolia Decoction

Huang Lian *Rhizoma Coptidis* 3 g
Hou Po *Cortex Magnoliae officinalis* 3 g
Shan Zhi Zi *Fructus Gardeniae jasminoidis* 9 g
Dan Dou Chi *Semen Sojae praeparatum* 9 g
Shi Chang Pu *Rhizoma Acori graminei* 3 g
Ban Xia *Rhizoma Pinelliae ternatae* 3 g
Lu Gen *Rhizoma Phragmitis communis* 15 g

Explanation

- **Huang Lian** clears Heat and dries Dampness.
- **Hou Po** fragrantly resolves Dampness and moves Qi (which in itself also helps to resolve Dampness).
- **Zhi Zi** and **Dan Dou Chi** clear Heat. They specifically clear "hidden" Heat, i.e. any Heat remaining in the Interior after an invasion of Wind-Heat or Damp-Heat.
- **Shi Chang Pu** opens the orifices and helps to resolve Dampness. It is said to "awaken" the Spleen and it clears the brain.
- **Ban Xia** resolves Phlegm, harmonizes the Stomach and stops vomiting.
- **Lu Gen** clears Heat and stops nausea and vomiting.

This prescription is excellent to clear Damp-Heat in Stomach and Spleen. It is especially suited to clear lingering Damp-Heat causing chronic tiredness and ache in the muscles. The main symptoms and signs indicating this prescription are a feeling of heaviness, ache and fatigue of the muscles, a muzzy feeling of the head, thirst, a sticky taste, nausea, epigastric fullness, tiredness, lethargy, sleepiness, loose foul-smelling stools, a sticky-yellow tongue coating and a Slippery-Rapid pulse.

This is the best prescription to clear remaining Damp-Heat in the Interior causing symptoms of ME. In practice, the Damp-Heat is bound to be accompanied by a deficiency of the Spleen, and the prescription should be adapted to address this situation. A very simple change would be merely the addition of Bai Zhu *Rhizoma Atractylodis macrocephalae*.

(b) Prescription

ZHI SHI DAO ZHI WAN
Citrus aurantius Eliminating Stagnation Pill

Da Huang *Rhizoma Rhei* 15 g
Zhi Shi *Fructus Citri aurantii immaturus* 12 g
Huang Lian *Rhizoma Coptidis* 6 g
Huang Qin *Radix Scutellariae baicalensis* 6 g
Fu Ling *Sclerotium Poriae cocos* 6 g
Ze Xie *Rhizoma Alismatis orientalis* 6 g
Bai Zhu *Rhizoma Atractylodis macrocephalae* 6 g
Shen Qu *Massa Fermentata Medicinalis* 12 g

Explanation

– **Da Huang** and **Zhi Shi** move downward and eliminate Dampness by purging.
– **Huang Lian** and **Huang Qin** clear Damp-Heat.
– **Fu Ling** and **Ze Xie** drain Dampness.
– **Bai Zhu** and **Shen Qu** tonify the Spleen to resolve Dampness and resolve food accumulation.

While the previous prescription is suitable if the stools are loose, this prescription is used if the stools are dry or normal and there is retention of food. The main symptoms of retention of food are belching, sour regurgitation, poor appetite, foul breath and a thick-sticky yellow tongue coating.

(c) Prescription

HUO PO XIA LING TANG
Agastache-Magnolia-Pinellia-Poria Decoction
Huo Xiang *Herba Agastachis* 6 g
Bai Dou Kou *Fructus Amomi cardamomi* 2 g
Hou Po *Cortex Magnoliae officinalis* 3 g
Fu Ling *Sclerotium Poriae cocos* 9 g
Zhu Ling *Sclerotium Polypori umbellati* 4.5 g
Yi Yi Ren *Semen Coicis lachryma jobi* 12 g
Ze Xie *Rhizoma Alismatis orientalis* 4.5 g
Ban Xia *Rhizoma Pinelliae ternatae* 4.5 g
Dan Dou Chi *Semen Sojae praeparatum* 9 g
Xing Ren *Semen Pruni armeniacae* 9 g

Explanation

This prescription is suited for Dampness without Heat. The main manifestations would be a feeling of heaviness, epigastric fullness, tiredness, chilliness, a sticky-white tongue coating and a Slippery pulse.

– **Huo Xiang**, **Bai Dou Kou**, and **Hou Po** fragrantly resolve Dampness. Fragrant herbs that resolve Dampness do so by affecting the muscles and promoting sweating. This will help to relieve the muscle ache.
– **Fu Ling**, **Zhu Ling**, **Yi Yi Ren** and **Ze Xie** drain Dampness.
– **Ban Xia** helps to drain Dampness by resolving Phlegm.
– **Dan Dou Chi** clears Heat and stops irritability.
– **Xing Ren** helps to drain Dampness by making Lung-Qi descend (and therefore move fluids downwards towards the Bladder and Kidneys).

Variations

The following variations apply to all three previous prescriptions.

– If muscle ache is pronounced add Sha Ren *Fructus seu Semen Amomi* and Pei Lan *Herba Eupatorei fortunei*.
– If symptoms of Dampness are very pronounced add (or increase the dosage of) Fu Ling *Sclerotium Poriae cocos*, Cang Zhu *Rhizoma Atractylodis lanceae*, and Yi Yi Ren *Semen Coicis lachryma jobi*.
– If there is pronounced Qi deficiency together with Dampness (with the pulse being Slippery but Weak), add Huang Qi *Radix Astragali membranacei*.

These three prescriptions can be used (with opportune variations) for several weeks, until symptoms of Dampness have gone or markedly decreased. In particular, one would look for a disappearance of the muscle ache and fatigue, a clearing of the tongue coating and the loss of the slippery quality of the pulse. After clearing Dampness, the treatment principle can be changed to tonify Qi and/or Yin. Thus, a tonifying prescription can be used and adapted by the addition of a few herbs to continue to drain Dampness.

Patent remedy

HUO XIANG ZHENG QI WAN

Agastache Upright Qi Pill
Huo Xiang *Herba Agastachis*
Zi Su Ye *Folium Perillae frutescentis*
Bai Zhi *Radix Angelicae dahuricae*
Ban Xia *Rhizoma Pinelliae ternatae*
Chen Pi *Pericarpium Citri reticulatae*
Bai Zhu *Rhizoma Atractylodis macrocephalae*
Fu Ling *Sclerotium Poriae cocos*
Hou Po *Cortex Magnoliae officinalis*
Da Fu Pi *Pericarpium Arecae catechu*
Jie Geng *Radix Platycodi grandiflori*
Sheng Jiang *Rhizoma Zingiberis officinalis recens*
Da Zao *Fructus Ziziphi jujubae*
Zhi Gan Cao *Radix Glycyrrhizae uralensis prae-parata*

Explanation

This remedy releases the Exterior and resolves Dampness. In conjunction with acupuncture, it is suitable to treat ME and especially muscle aches as the remedy contains three herbs which fragrantly resolve Dampness from the muscles (Huo Xiang, Hou Po and Da Fu Pi).

The tongue presentation appropriate to this remedy is a sticky-white tongue coating.

Case history

A 27-year-old woman contracted what was diagnosed as viral meningitis one year before she came for treatment. At the time of infection she had a high temperature, a severe headache, vomiting, photophobia and neck pain and rigidity. Before this happened she had had vesicles on her feet. These were itchy and filled with fluid and after some weeks they turned into pustules. After the meningitis she felt extremely tired and experienced a feeling of heaviness and ache of the limbs. She also felt hot and thirsty. On interrogation, she said she experienced a sticky taste in her mouth and had an excessive vaginal discharge. She also had some abdominal pain and her stools were always loose. Her memory and concentration were poor and she sweated at night sometimes.

She was quite overweight, her skin was greasy and she spoke very slowly. Her pulse was Slippery and her tongue-body colour was normal, while there was a very sticky-yellow coating all over. The tongue body was Swollen.

She had been treated with acupuncture by another practitioner. Whilst some of the symptoms got better, they both felt that she had not made sufficient improvement. Her practitioner then referred her to me.

Diagnosis
Most of her problems are due to remaining Damp-Heat after the febrile disease (meningitis). The manifestations of Damp-Heat are tiredness, heaviness and ache of the muscles, being overweight, greasy skin (Dampness in the muscles), poor memory and concentration, sticky taste (Dampness in the head), excessive vaginal discharge, pustules on feet (Dampness in the Lower Burner), night sweating, Slippery pulse and sticky tongue coating. Thirst, feeling of heat and the yellow colour of the coating indicate Heat. In this case, Dampness was predominant in relation to Heat. I felt that the main reason she had not improved much was that she had been treated by tonification only. In fact, various signs showed that her body condition was not that deficient: a normal tongue-body colour without cracks and a Slippery pulse that was not Weak. Since the condition was predominantly still an Excess one (being characterized by the presence of Damp-Heat), the treatment should have been aimed at expelling Dampness first.

Treatment principle
The treatment was aimed at expelling Damp-Heat first with herbs only.

Herbal treatment
The prescription used was a variation of Lian-Po Yin *Coptis-Magnolia Decoction*, adapted with the addition of only three herbs to drain Dampness (as this was the main problem rather than Heat) and of Bai Zhu *Rhizoma Atractylodis macrocephalae* to introduce some tonification within the draining. The prescription used thus was:

Huang Lian *Rhizoma Coptidis* 4 g
Hou Po *Cortex Magnoliae officinalis* 4 g
Shi Chang Pu *Rhizoma Acori graminei* 4 g
Lu Gen *Rhizoma Phragmitis communis* 6 g
Ban Xia *Rhizoma Pinelliae ternatae* 6 g
Zhi Zi *Fructus Gardeniae jasminoidis* 3 g
Dan Dou Chi *Semen Sojae praeparatum* 4 g
Fu Ling *Sclerotium Poriae cocos* 4 g
Sha Ren *Fructus seu Semen Amomi* 4 g
Yi Yi Ren *Semen Coicis lachryma jobi* 4 g
Bai Zhu *Rhizoma Atractylodis macrocephalae* 4 g

Four courses (each course being 20 days) of this prescription (with minor variations) produced a nearly complete recovery. This prescription was then followed by two courses of a tonifying prescription (still incorporating some draining Dampness). The prescription was a variation of Liu Jun Zi Tang *Six Gentlemen Decoction*.

Case history

A 53-year-old woman complained of exhaustion, muscle fatigue and ache, a quivering of the muscles, poor memory and concentration, a feeling of muzziness and heaviness of the head and headaches. All these symptoms started after a viral infection 3 years previously. Her pulse was Weak and Fine but also Slippery. Her tongue was slightly Red and Swollen and had a sticky-yellow coating.

Diagnosis
This condition is also due to Damp-Heat, remaining after the viral infection. It is very similar to the previous one, with one difference: this condition is more deficient than the previous one as evidenced by the Weak and Fine pulse. Thus, underlining the condition of Damp-Heat there is a pronounced deficiency of the Spleen. However, in spite of this it is still better to clear the Damp-Heat before tonifying.

Treatment principle
The treatment principle adopted was to resolve Damp-Heat.

Herbal treatment
The prescription used was again a variation of Lian Po Yin *Coptis-Magnolia Decoction*.

Huang Lian *Rhizoma Coptidis* 4 g
Hou Po *Cortex Magnoliae officinalis* 4 g
Shi Chang Pu *Rhizoma Acori graminei* 4 g
Zhi Zi *Fructus Gardeniae jasminoidis* 3 g
Dan Dou Chi *Semen Sojae praeparatum* 5 g
Ban Xia *Rhizoma Pinelliae ternatae* 6 g
Lu Gen *Rhizoma Phragmitis communis* 6 g
Bai Zhu *Rhizoma Atractylodis macrocephalae* 6 g
Huang Qi *Radix Astragali membranacei* 5 g

Bai Zhu *Rhizoma Atractylodis macrocephalae* and Huang Qi *Radix Astragali membranacei* were added to tonify Spleen-Qi. After three courses of this prescription, a variation of Bu Zhong Yi Qi Tang *Tonifying the Centre and Benefiting Qi Decoction* was used with the addition of Ze Xie *Rhizoma Alismatis orientalis*, Yi Yi Ren *Semen Coicis lachryma jobi* and Sha Ren *Fructus seu Semen Amomi* to continue to drain Dampness.

Case history

A 33-year-old man had suffered from exhaustion for the previous 4 years. He felt especially tired after eating, he sweated at night and his limbs felt heavy, tired and achy. He also experienced dull headaches when tired. His tongue was Red, Swollen and had a sticky-yellow coating (Plate 25.1). His pulse was Weak but Slippery and slightly Rapid. All these symptoms had started after a bout of influenza 4 years previously from which he had never recovered.

Diagnosis
This is again a condition of Damp-Heat. In this case Heat is predominant as evidenced by the Red tongue.

Treatment principle
The treatment principle adopted was to clear Heat and resolve Dampness.

Herbal treatment
Again a variation of Lian Po Yin *Coptis-Magnolia Decoction* was used.

Huang Lian *Rhizoma Coptidis* 4 g
Hou Po *Cortex Magnoliae officinalis* 4 g
Shi Chang Pu *Rhizoma Acori graminei* 4 g
Zhi Zi *Fructus Gardeniae jasminoidis* 6 g
Dan Dou Chi *Semen Sojae praeparatum* 5 g
Ban Xia *Rhizoma Pinelliae ternatae* 6 g
Lu Gen *Rhizoma Phragmitis communis* 6 g
Bai Zhu *Rhizoma Atractylodis macrocephalae* 6 g
Huang Qi *Radix Astragali membranacei* 5 g

Bai Zhu and Huang Qi were added to tonify Qi as his pulse was weak. This prescription was repeated for five courses and was then followed by a Qi-tonifying prescription:

Huang Qi *Radix Astragali membranacei* 12 g
Bai Zhu *Rhizoma Atractylodis macrocephalae* 6 g
Fu Ling *Sclerotium Poriae cocos* 6 g
Chai Hu *Radix Bupleuri* 4 g
Qing Hao *Herba Artemisiae apiaceae* 3 g
Zhi Gan Cao *Radix Glycyrrhizae uralensis praeparata* 3 g

This is a simple prescription to tonify Qi with the addition of Chai Hu and Qing Hao to drain any remaining Heat. In fact, this patient had made very good progress but was occasionally still experiencing a sensation of heat and a flu-like feeling typical of ME. Both Chai Hu and Qing Hao are particularly good to clear any lingering, hidden Heat causing heat sensations.

Case history

A 28-year-old woman complained of total lack of energy, aches and fatigue of the muscles for the past 3 months. She also felt cold, her thinking was not clear and her head felt muzzy and heavy. Her glands were swollen and she suffered from constipation, although this had been a problem for a long time. Her stools were not dry. She was pale and spoke with a very quiet voice. Her tongue was Pale with teeth-marks and had small white pin-size vesicles. Her pulse was Slow (60), Slippery and Weak. All her symptoms (except for the constipation) had started after receiving an influenza immunization.

Diagnosis
Most of her symptoms are due to Dampness (without Heat) obstructing the head (muzzy and heavy head, lack of concentration and clarity) and the muscles (tiredness, ache and fatigue of the muscles). The pin-sized white vesicles on the tongue are typical of Dampness. The residual pathogenic factor in this case

followed not an infection but an immunization, which from a Chinese medical perspective is comparable to an infection. This obviously took place on a background of Spleen-Yang deficiency. This is borne out by her cold feeling, the Pale tongue with teeth-marks and the constipation. This was due to Spleen-Yang being unable to move the stools. The fact that the stools are *not* dry and she does not feel thirsty shows that the constipation is due to Yang deficiency and not to Heat. Of course it could also have been due to Blood deficiency (which is a more common cause of chronic constipation in women) but the cold feeling and the tongue point to Yang deficiency.

Treatment principle
The treatment principle was concentrated initially on draining Dampness.

Acupuncture
The main acupuncture points used were:

– **SP-9** Yinlingquan, **SP-6** Sanyinjiao and **BL-22** Sanjiaoshu with even method to drain Dampness.
– **L.I.-4** Hegu, **ST-8** Touwei and **Du-20** Baihui with even method to expel Dampness from the head.

Herbal treatment
The herbal prescription used was a variation of Huo Po Xia Ling Tang *Agastache-Magnolia-Pinellia-Poria Decoction*.

Huo Xiang *Herba Agastachis* 6 g
Bai Dou Kou *Fructus Amomi cardamomi* 2 g
Hou Po *Cortex Magnoliae officinalis* 3 g
Fu Ling *Sclerotium Poriae cocos* 9 g
Zhu Ling *Sclerotium Polypori umbellati* 4.5 g
Yi Yi Ren *Semen Coicis lachryma jobi* 6 g
Ze Xie *Rhizoma Alismatis orientalis* 4.5 g
Ban Xia *Rhizoma Pinelliae ternatae* 4.5 g
Xing Ren *Semen Pruni armeniacae* 9 g
Bai Zhu *Rhizoma Atractylodis macrocephalae* 5 g
Cang Zhu *Rhizoma Atractylodis lanceae* 4 g

This variation of the prescription adds Bai Zhu to tonify the Spleen and Cang Zhu to fragrantly resolve Dampness, and eliminates Dan Dou Chi as there is no Heat.

This prescription was used for three courses and was then followed by two courses of Liu Jun Zi Tang *Six Gentlemen Decoction* to tonify the Spleen.

Case history

A 31-year-old man had suffered from ME ever since he caught a viral infection 2 years previously. He had had another viral infection 2 months before he came for treatment, from which he had not recovered and experienced severe muscle fatigue and ache. His limbs felt heavy and his concentration was poor. He felt exhausted all the time and often dizzy. His stools were loose and his glands swollen. He often felt hot and thirsty and had a pain under the right rib-cage. He also had a constant feeling of fullness in the epigastric area. On interrogation, it transpired that he had also had a herpes-zoster infection 1 year before the viral infection which triggered off the ME.

His tongue was Red and had a thick-sticky-yellow coating which was clearly much thicker on the right side. His pulse was Slippery and Wiry on the left side and Weak on the right.

Diagnosis
Most of his symptoms show very clearly the presence of Damp-Heat. Damp-Heat is present in four areas:

– in the Stomach and Spleen: loose stools, epigastric fullness
– in the muscles: muscle fatigue and ache, weakness of the limbs, tiredness, swelling of glands
– in the Gall-Bladder: sticky-yellow coating on the right side of the tongue, hypochondrial pain
– in the head: dizziness.

In this case Heat is quite evident given the Red colour of his tongue, the thirst and the feeling of heat.

Treatment principle
He was treated with acupuncture and herbs. The principle of treatment was aimed at resolving Dampness and clearing Heat first.

Acupuncture
The main points used were **L.I.-11** Quchi and **SP-9** Yinlingquan to resolve Damp-Heat, **T.B.-6** Zhigou to clear Heat from the Gall-Bladder and any remaining Heat, **Ren-12** Zhongwan and **ST-40** Fenglong to resolve Dampness and Phlegm. Other points used later in the course of treatment were **ST-36** Zusanli, **BL-20** Pishu and **BL-21** Weishu to tonify the Stomach and Spleen once the Dampness was resolved, and **Du-20** Baihui to raise Yang and lift the mood.

Herbal treatment
The herbal prescription used was a variation of Lian Po Yin *Coptis-Magnolia Decoction*:

Huang Lian *Rhizoma Coptidis* 4 g
Hou Po *Cortex Magnoliae officinalis* 4 g
Shi Chang Pu *Rhizoma Acori graminei* 4 g
Lu Gen *Rhizoma Phragmitis communis* 4 g
Ban Xia *Rhizoma Pinelliae ternatae* 6 g
Shan Zhi Zi *Fructus Gardeniae jasminoidis* 3 g
Dan Dou Chi *Semen Sojae praeparatum* 4 g
Fu Ling *Sclerotium Poriae cocos* 4 g
Yi Yi Ren *Semen Coicis lachryma jobi* 4 g
Yin Chen Hao *Herba Artemisiae capillaris* 3 g
Mu Xiang *Radix Saussureae* 3 g
Zhi Gan Cao *Radix Glycyrrhizae uralensis praeparata* 3 g

Explanation
– **Fu Ling** and **Yi Yi Ren** were added to resolve Dampness via urination.
– **Yin Chen Hao** was added to resolve Dampness from the Gall-Bladder.

– **Mu Xiang** was added to move Qi in the hypochondrium being made stagnant by the presence of Dampness.

The combination of acupuncture and herbs produced a marked and gradual improvement. Towards the end of the treatment the herbal prescription was changed so that the emphasis would be on tonifying Qi rather than resolving Dampness. However, within the tonifying-Qi prescription (which was Bu Zhong Yi Qi Tang *Tonifying the Centre and Benefiting Qi Decoction*) herbs were still added to resolve Dampness.

Case history

A 59-year-old woman suffered from exhaustion, weakness and aching of the muscles, weight gain and craving for sweets. All her symptoms had started 5 months previously soon after returning from Thailand. Her tongue was Red with a sticky coating and it was partially peeled in the centre. There were also some Stomach-cracks. Her pulse was Rapid and Slippery.

Diagnosis
This is another case of ME, probably following a viral infection contracted in Thailand. Before this happened she was very healthy and active. Her main presenting pattern is, again, Damp-Heat in the muscles. In her case, the Damp-Heat has not affected the brain, which augurs well for the prognosis. The partially-peeled centre and cracks on the tongue indicate a previous deficiency of Stomach-Qi.

Treatment principle
The treatment principle adopted was to resolve Damp-Heat and tonify Stomach-Qi.

Herbal treatment
Again, the prescription Lian Po Yin *Coptis-Magnolia Decoction* was used with good results. Initially it was used without any variation. After three courses, it was modified with the addition of Tai Zi Shen *Radix Pseudostellariae* to tonify Stomach-Yin, Huang Qi *Radix Astragali membranacei* and Bai Zhu *Rhizoma Atractylodis macrocephalae* to tonify Spleen-Qi to resolve Dampness. After three courses of this prescription the treatment principle was changed to tonify Qi primarily with the Liu Jun Zi Tang *Six Gentlemen Decoction*. After three courses of this prescription her symptoms disappeared and her energy was restored.

2. HEAT LURKING IN THE INTERIOR

CLINICAL MANIFESTATIONS

Muscle fatigue without ache or with only a slight ache, thirst, insomnia, cough with scanty-yellow sputum, tiredness, breathlessness on exertion, loss of weight, dry throat.
Tongue: Red with a yellow coating, redder on the front part.
Pulse: Rapid and slightly Wiry.

This condition appears for only a few months at the beginning of development of ME. After some months, it either gives rise to Damp-Heat (an Excess pattern) or the Heat injures Yin giving rise to Yin deficiency (a Deficiency pattern). However, even in the case of Heat, there is always some Dampness which accounts for the slight ache in the muscles.

The Heat is primarily in the Lungs (hence the cough with scanty yellow sputum and red colour in the front part of the tongue) and Heart (hence the insomnia). This condition develops when interior Heat is not cleared properly after an invasion of Wind-Heat. It then lurks in the Interior for a long time giving rise to the above symptoms.

PRINCIPLE OF TREATMENT

Clear interior Heat.

ACUPUNCTURE

Du-14 Dazhui, T.B.-5 Waiguan, L.I.-11 Quchi, LU-10 Yuji, HE-8 Shaofu, SP-6 Sanyinjiao. All with reducing method except for SP-6 which should be reinforced.

Explanation

– **Du-14** is the main point. It clears Heat and especially Heat which has remained in the Interior for a long time.
– **T.B.-5** and **L.I.-11** clear Heat.
– **LU-10** and **HE-8** clear Lung- and Heart-Heat respectively.
– **SP-6** nourishes Yin, which will help to cool Heat.

HERBAL TREATMENT

Prescription

ZHI SHI ZHI ZI TANG

Citrus aurantium-Gardenia Decoction
Zhi Shi *Fructus Citri aurantii immaturus* 6 g
Zhi Zi *Fructus Gardeniae jasminoidis* 9 g
Dan Dou Chi *Semen Sojae praeparatum* 9 g

Explanation

This is the main prescription to clear remaining Heat after an invasion of Wind-Heat.

- **Zhi Shi** is used to move Qi in the chest.
- **Zhi Zi** clears interior Heat.
- **Dan Dou Chi** clears Heat and calms irritability.

This is obviously a skeleton prescription which should be suitably adapted to the case in question. In the case of Lung-Heat, it could actually be combined with:

XIE BAI SAN
Draining Whiteness Powder
Di Gu Pi *Cortex Lycii chinensis radicis* 9 g
Sang Bai Pi *Cortex Mori albae radicis* 9 g
Zhi Gan Cao *Radix Glycyrrhizae uralensis praeparata* 3 g
Geng Mi *Semen Oryzae sativae* 6 g

Explanation. This prescription specifically clears remaining Lung-Heat after an invasion of Wind-Heat.

- **Di Gu Pi** clears lingering Lung-Heat.
- **Sang Bai Pi** clears Lung-Heat and restores the descending of Lung-Qi.
- **Gan Cao** harmonizes.
- **Geng Mi** clears Heat.

In case of Heart-Heat, the first prescription could be combined with:

DAO CHI SAN
Draining Redness Powder
Sheng Di Huang *Radix Rehmanniae glutinosae* 15 g
Mu Tong *Caulis Akebiae* 3 g
Sheng Gan Cao *Radix Glycyrrhizae uralensis* 6 g
Zhu Ye *Herba Lophatheri gracilis* 3 g

Explanation. This prescription clears Heart-Heat.

- **Sheng Di** clears Heat and cools Blood.

- **Mu Tong** and **Zhu Ye** clear Heart-Heat.
- **Gan Cao** harmonizes and clears Heat.

In case of Stomach-Heat, the first prescription could be combined with:

XIE HUANG SAN
Expelling Yellowness Powder
Shi Gao *Gypsum fibrosum* 15 g
Zhi Zi *Fructus Gardeniae jasminoidis* 6 g
Fang Feng *Radix Ledebouriellae sesloidis* 12 g
Huo Xiang *Herba Agastachis* 21 g
Gan Cao *Radix Glycyrrhizae uralensis* 9 g

Explanation

- **Shi Gao**, pungent-cold, clears Stomach-Heat.
- **Zhi Zi**, bitter-cold, clears Heat.
- **Fang Feng** has an ascending and floating movement and is used to make hidden Heat float towards the Exterior to be cleared. Bitter-cold herbs (such as Zhi Zi) on their own have a clearing and descending movement. Whilst a descending movement is appropriate to clear normal Heat, it is not enough to clear hidden residual Heat, which is the type of Heat this prescription is used for. Furthermore, Fang Feng's ascending movement balances the descending movement of Shi Gao and Zhi Zi, and prevents this from injuring the Spleen.
- **Huo Xiang** fragrantly awakens the Spleen and its ascending-floating movement helps Fang Feng to draw the hidden residual Heat out.
- **Gan Cao** resolves Poison and harmonizes the Middle.

This prescription is specific to clear hidden residual Heat in the Stomach and Spleen after an invasion of Wind-Heat. Its main manifestations are mouth ulcers, foul breath, thirst, dry mouth and lips, a Red tongue and a Rapid pulse.

Patent remedy

QI GUAN YAN KE SOU TAN CHUAN WAN
Bronchial Cough, Phlegm and Dyspnoea Pill
Qian Hu *Radix Peucedani*
Xing Ren *Semen Pruni armeniacae*
Yuan Zhi *Radix Polygalae tenuifoliae*

Sang Ye *Folium Mori albae*
Chuan Bei Mu *Bulbus Fritillariae cirrhosae*
Chen Pi *Pericarpium Citri reticulatae*
Pi Pa Ye *Folium Eriobotryae japonicae*
Kuan Dong Hua *Flos Tussilaginis farfarae*
Dang Shen *Radix Codonopsis pilosulae*
Ma Dou Ling *Fructus Aristolochiae*
Wu Wei Zi *Fructus Schisandrae chinensis*
Sheng Jiang *Rhizoma Zingiberis officinalis recens*
Da Zao *Fructus Ziziphi jujubae*

Explanation

This remedy clears Lung-Heat and mildly tonifies Lung- and Spleen-Qi. Because of these two actions, it is suitable to treat chronic ME from residual Lung-Heat against a background of Qi deficiency.

The tongue presentation appropriate to this remedy is a tongue-body which is Red only in the front part (Lung area).

Case history

A 47-year-old woman had been feeling extremely exhausted for the previous 10 years. She had had acupuncture for a long time but this did not help her consistently. Her other symptoms included: a feeling of heaviness, a feeling of heat, hot feet in bed at night, thirst, slight ache in the muscles, insomnia and scanty-dark urine. Her pulse was Full, Slippery, Rapid (88) and slightly Moving (the Moving pulse is short, rapid, vibrating, and shaped like a bean). Her tongue was Red and redder on the tip.

Diagnosis

I considered this to be a type of ME due to residual Heat, concentrated mostly in the Heart. Over the years, Heat injures the body fluids and condenses them into Dampness. For this reason this patient also had some Damp-Heat although not pronounced (there was only a slight ache of the muscles indicating Dampness). Most of the other symptoms indicated Heart-Heat (insomnia, Red tongue with redder tip, thirst, feeling of heat). The Rapid pulse clearly shows Heat. Its Moving quality indicates shock and fear. On interrogation it emerged that she had had a very troubled childhood having been abused by her father. In this case there were obviously deep emotional reasons underlying her condition besides the viral infections that are usually the cause of ME. She had sought pyschotherapeutic help over the years and was dealing with her past.

Treatment principle

In spite of the long duration of the problem, on the basis of her pulse, I felt that the condition was still one of Excess. The main principle of treatment adopted was therefore to clear Heart-Heat and calm the Mind. Only herbs were used.

Herbal treatment

The prescription selected was a variation of the combination of Dao Chi San *Eliminating Redness Powder* and Zhi Shi Zhi Zi Tang *Citrus aurantium-Gardenia Decoction*:

Sheng Di Huang *Radix Rehmanniae glutinosae* 9 g
Zhu Ye *Herba Lophatheri gracilis* 3 g
Mu Tong *Caulis Akebiae* 2 g
Sheng Gan Cao *Radix Glycyrrhizae uralensis* 3 g
Zhi Zi *Fructus Gardeniae jasminoidis* 4 g
Zhi Shi *Fructus Citri aurantii immaturus* 4 g
Dan Dou Chi *Semen Sojae praeparatum* 6 g
Mu Xiang *Radix Saussureae* 3 g

Mu Xiang was added to move Qi which helps to clear knotted Heat. Mu Xiang also has a powerful effect on the Mind in releasing emotional tension.

This prescription produced a dramatic improvement and was repeated several times with minor variations.

3. LESSER YANG PATTERN

CLINICAL MANIFESTATIONS

There are two types of patterns pertaining to the Lesser Yang channels: one from the 6 Stages (from the "Discussion of Cold-induced Diseases" by Zhang Zhong Jing, *c.* AD 200), and the other from the 4 Levels (from the "Discussion on Warm Diseases" by Ye Tian Shi, 1742). They essentially describe the same pattern, the only difference being that the pattern from the 4 Levels involves more Heat.

6 Stages

Alternation of chills and fever (or feeling of heat), fullness of the costal and hypochondrial regions, poor appetite, irritability, dry throat, nausea, bitter taste, blurred vision, white-slippery tongue coating on one side only and a Wiry pulse.

4 Levels

Alternation of chills and fever (or feeling of

heat), the latter being more marked, bitter taste, thirst, dry throat, fullness and pain of the costal and hypochondrial regions, nausea, Red tongue with yellow coating on one side, Wiry and Rapid pulse.

Explanation

Both these patterns describe a condition where the pathogenic factor occupies an energetic niche said to be in between the Exterior and Interior. Since the Greater-Yang channels open on the Exterior, the Bright-Yang channels open on the Interior, and the Lesser-Yang channels are the hinge between the two, this pattern is called Lesser-Yang pattern. The Yang channels, being Yang and therefore more superficial, represent the boundary between the human body and its environment. Within the Yang, however, there is a difference in energetic depth, the Greater Yang being the most superficial, the Bright Yang the deepest and the Lesser Yang the hinge between the two. These could be graphically represented as a door, its outer surface being the Greater Yang, its inner one the Bright Yang, and the hinges the Lesser Yang (Fig. 25.2).

When the pathogenic factor is in the Lesser Yang (whether within the 6 Stages or 4 Levels) it can somehow "hide" there for a long time and become chronic. This cannot happen when it is in the Greater Yang or Bright Yang, where it is bound either to be expelled or to evolve into a different condition.

The essential symptom indicating that the pathogenic factor is in between the Exterior and Interior, is the alternation of chills and fever (or feeling of heat). This is due to the fact that the pathogenic factor "bounces" in between the Ex-

terior and Interior: the patient feels cold when it is on the Exterior, hot when it is in the Interior. It should be noted, however, that there need not be an actual fever, as it may just be a *feeling* of heat. In fact, the temperature may be normal or in some cases even subnormal, and still the person feels hot. In many cases of ME when patients experience alternation of chills and fever for months or years, the temperature is very often subnormal. When the temperature becomes normal the person feels better.[4]

The Lesser-Yang pattern, characterized by alternation of chills and feeling of heat, is quite commonly seen in patients suffering from ME: as was explained above, this pattern is, in itself, a type of residual pathogenic factor just as Damp-Heat is. The Lesser-Yang pattern can even last for years. The longer it goes on, of course, the more it is associated with some deficiency. In these cases, it is necessary to clear the Lesser Yang *before* tonifying.

Apart from the alternation of chills and heat, another essential sign of this condition is the pulse being Wiry. It may be Wiry only on the left side, or it may be slightly Wiry at the same time as being Fine, but it should have some Wiry quality.

As mentioned above, the Lesser-Yang patterns from the 6 Stages and the 4 Levels are essentially the same. The main difference is that in the 4-Level Lesser Yang pattern there is more Heat (hence the thirst, more pronounced feeling of heat, yellow tongue coating and Rapid pulse).

PRINCIPLE OF TREATMENT

Clear the Lesser Yang.

ACUPUNCTURE

T.B.-5 Waiguan, Du-14 Dazhui. Even method.

Explanation

These two points clear the Lesser Yang and release the pathogenic factor. They should be used several times in succession, obviously combined with some other points according to the condition.

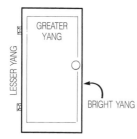

Fig. 25.2   Greater Yang, Bright Yang and Lesser Yang

HERBAL TREATMENT

There are three prescriptions for the Lesser Yang pattern, the first for the one from the 6 Stages, the second and third for the one from the 4 Levels.

6 Stages (predominance of Cold)

Prescription

XIAO CHAI HU TANG
Small Bupleurum Decoction
Chai Hu *Radix Bupleuri* 12 g
Huang Qin *Radix Scutellariae baicalensis* 9 g
Ban Xia *Rhizoma Pinelliae ternatae* 9 g
Ren Shen *Radix Ginseng* 6 g
Zhi Gan Cao *Radix Glycyrrhizae uralensis praeparata* 5 g
Sheng Jiang *Rhizoma Zingiberis officinalis recens* 9 g
Da Zao *Fructus Ziziphi jujubae* 4 dates

Explanation

- **Chai Hu** is the emperor herb and it expels Cold from the Lesser Yang. It clears lightly and it disperses upwards. It expels the pathogenic factor and releases the Exterior.
- **Huang Qin,** minister herb, is bitter and cold and it clears Heat from Lesser Yang. It combines with Chai Hu: one disperses, the other clears, and together they clear the Lesser Yang.
- **Ban Xia**, assistant herb, harmonizes the Stomach and subdues rebellious Qi. It therefore stops nausea and vomiting.
- **Ren Shen** and **Gan Cao**, also assistant herbs, benefit Stomach-Qi, promote fluids, harmonize Nutritive and Defensive Qi and tonify the body's Qi to expel the pathogenic factor.
- **Sheng Jiang** and **Da Zao**, messenger herbs, harmonize the Stomach, benefit Qi and harmonize Nutritive and Defensive Qi.

This prescription is ideal for ME patients who experience recurrent feelings of chills and heat for months or even years. It is particularly indicated since it includes Ren Shen (or Dang Shen) which tonifies Qi, an important treatment aim in ME.

4 Levels (predominance of Heat)

(a) Prescription

HAO QIN QING DAN TANG
Artemisia-Scutellaria Clearing the Gall-Bladder Decoction
Qing Hao *Herba Artemisiae apiaceae* 6 g
Huang Qin *Radix Scutellariae baicalensis* 6 g
Zhu Ru *Caulis Bambusae in Taeniis* 9 g
Ban Xia *Rhizoma Pinelliae ternatae* 5 g
Chen Pi *Pericarpium Citri reticulatae* 5 g
Zhi Ke *Fructus Citri aurantii* 5 g
Fu Ling *Sclerotium Poriae cocos* 9 g
Hua Shi *Talcum* 3 g
Gan Cao *Radix Glycyrrhizae uralensis* 3 g
Qing Dai *Indigo naturalis* 3 g

Explanation

- **Qing Hao** clears Heat in the Lesser Yang.
- **Huang Qin** clears Heat in the Lesser Yang and also clears Gall-Bladder Heat.
- **Zhu Ru** and **Ban Xia** resolve Phlegm.
- **Chen Pi** and **Zhi Ke** free the diaphragm, harmonize the Stomach and subdue rebellious Qi.
- **Fu Ling**, **Hua Shi**, **Gan Cao** and **Qing Dai** clear Damp-Heat and expel Heat via urination.

This prescription is used when the Lesser Yang pattern presents with pronounced Heat and is also characterized by Damp-Heat in the Gall-Bladder. The main manifestations are alternation of chills and heat, the latter being more marked, a bitter taste, a feeling of oppression of the chest, sour regurgitation, nausea, vomiting of sticky-yellow fluid or dry vomiting, fullness and pain of costal and hypochondrial regions, Red tongue with sticky-yellow coating, or with a coating which is half white and half yellow and a Wiry-Slippery-Rapid pulse.

Variations

- In chronic ME cases, both these prescriptions

can be modified by reducing the dosages and adding some Qi or Yin tonics such as Dang Shen *Radix Codonopsis pilosulae*, Huang Qi *Radix Astragali membranacei*, or Mai Men Dong *Tuber Ophiopogonis japonici*.

(b) Prescription

DA YUAN YIN
Extending the Membranes Decoction
Bing Lang *Semen Arecae catechu* 6 g
Hou Po *Cortex Magnoliae officinalis* 3 g
Cao Guo *Fructus Amomi tsaoko* 1.5 g
Zhi Mu *Radix Anemarrhenae asphodeloidis* 3 g
Bai Shao *Radix Paeoniae albae* 3 g
Huang Qin *Radix Scutellariae baicalensis* 3 g
Gan Cao *Radix Glycyrrhizae uralensis* 1.5 g

Explanation

- **Bing Lang**, **Hou Po** and **Cao Guo** fragrantly resolve Dampness and expel the pathogenic factor from the "membranes". This is the anatomical region in between the pleura and diaphragm. It is somewhat analogous to the Lesser Yang.
- **Zhi Mu** nourishes Yin and clears Heat.
- **Bai Shao** helps to nourish Yin. Together with Zhi Mu, it helps to prevent injury of Yin.
- **Huang Qin** clears Heat.
- **Gan Cao** harmonizes.

This prescription is also used for the Lesser-Yang pattern with prevalence of Heat. The main difference from the previous prescription, is that this one is used in cases of pronounced Dampness. The main manifestations would be (besides alternation of chills and heat with prevalence of heat) a feeling of oppression of the chest, nausea or vomiting, headache, irritability, a feeling of fullness of the diaphragm, sighing, a very sticky and dirty tongue coating and a Wiry-Slippery pulse.

Dampness is a very frequent condition associated with the Lesser-Yang pattern in chronic ME and this prescription addresses such a situation.

Patent remedy

XIAO CHAI HU TANG WAN

Small Bupleurum Decoction Pill
Chai Hu *Radix Bupleuri*
Huang Qin *Radix Scutellariae baicalensis*
Ban Xia *Rhizoma Pinelliae ternatae*
Ren Shen *Radix Ginseng*
Zhi Gan Cao *Radix Glycyrrhizae uralensis praeparata*
Sheng Jiang *Rhizoma Zingiberis officinalis recens*
Da Zao *Fructus Ziziphi jujubae*

Explanation

This pill has the same ingredients and functions as the homonymous prescription. It is suitable for ME manifesting with the Lesser Yang pattern, whether within the 6 Stages or 4 Levels.

The tongue presentation appropriate to this remedy is a white coating on one side only.

Case history

An 11-year-old girl had come down with a sore throat and tonsillitis 2 months before she came for treatment. Her tonsils were swollen, inflamed and slightly purulent. During the acute stage she also had a headache and swollen glands. Blood tests had shown a "viral infection similar to glandular fever (mononucleosis)". At the time of her consultation she felt very tired, the tonsils were still swollen albeit not so inflamed, her throat was sore but the glands were not swollen. She still had sharp headaches on the temples and felt hot and cold in alternation. She felt thirsty, irritable and did not sleep well. She occasionally had a pain on the right hypochondral region.

Diagnosis
The original attack was an invasion of Wind-Damp-Heat with some Fire-Poison: the Dampness is shown by the swelling of the glands and the Fire-Poison by the swollen, inflamed, and purulent tonsils.

At the time of her consultation 2 months later, the pathogenic factor had lodged itself in between the Interior and Exterior, giving rise to a Gall-Bladder Heat pattern within the Qi Level. This pattern is almost the same as the Lesser-Yang pattern of the 6 Stages, except that there is more Heat. The symptoms of Gall-Bladder Heat pattern at the Qi Level are: alternation of feeling hot and cold, thirst, irritability, insomnia, hypochondrial pain, sore throat and headache.

Treatment principle
She was treated with herbs only and the principle of treatment adopted was to harmonize the Lesser Yang,

clear Gall-Bladder Heat and expel residual pathogenic factor.

Herbal treatment
The formula chosen was a variation of Hao Qin Qing Dan Tang *Artemisia-Scutellaria Clearing the Gall-Bladder Decoction*:

Chai Hu *Radix Bupleuri* 6 g
Huang Qin *Radix Scutellariae baicalensis* 4 g
Dang Shen *Radix Codonopsis pilosulae* 6 g
Ban Xia *Rhizoma Pinelliae ternatae* 6 g
Qing Hao *Herba Artemisiae apiaceae* 4 g
Zhu Ru *Caulis Bambusae in Taeniis* 4 g
Chen Pi *Pericarpium Citri reticulatae* 3 g
Zhi Ke *Fructus Citri aurantii* 4 g
Hua Shi *Talcum* 6 g
Da Qing Ye *Folium Isatidis seu Baphicacanthi* 6 g
Jin Yin Hua *Flos Lonicerae japonicae* 4 g
Zhi Gan Cao *Radix Glycyrrhizae uralensis praeparata* 3 g

Explanation
– The first 9 herbs are part of the root formula to harmonize the Lesser Yang and clear Gall-Bladder Heat.
– **Qing Dai** was eliminated and replaced with Da Qing Ye as this is better at resolving Fire-Poison from the throat and has anti-viral properties.
– **Jin Yin Hua** was added to resolve Fire-Poison and clear residual Heat.
– **Gan Cao** harmonizes.

This girl was very diligent and cooperative in taking the herbal decoction and after 15 doses of it, all the symptoms of the Lesser Yang pattern went. She still felt quite tired and I prescribed the patent remedy Bu Zhong Yi Qi Wan *Tonifying the Centre and Benefiting Qi Pill* which restored her energy to normal in 1 month.

Case history

A 13-year-old girl had had an influenza-like viral infection 4 months previously. This persisted and was not treated for 1 month, after which she was given antibiotics. These did not alleviate the condition at all and gave her mouth ulcers. When she came for treatment her symptoms and signs were the following: feeling hot and cold in alternation, dry and sore throat, headaches on the temples, umbilical and hypochondrial pain, itchy eyes and poor appetite. Her tongue was Red and slightly peeled in the centre. There was a strip of white coating on the right side. Her pulse was Fine and slightly Wiry.

Diagnosis
This is a clear example of Lesser-Yang pattern. Some of the symptoms are not typical of it (umbilical pain, poor appetite and peeled centre of tongue) but they can be explained by the use of antibiotics. These most probably injured the Yin of Stomach and Intestines which caused the peeling of the centre of the tongue, the lack of appetite and the umbilical pain.

This is a clear case when the antibiotics did not expel the pathogenic factor and weakened the body condition. The pathogenic factor remained "stuck" in between the Exterior and Interior, hence the Lesser-Yang pattern. Without treatment, this condition could go on for months or even years.

Treatment principle
The treatment principle adopted was to harmonize the Lesser Yang and nourish Stomach-Yin. Only herbs were administered.

Herbal treatment
A combination of Xiao Chai Hu Tang *Small Bupleurum Decoction* and Sha Shen Mai Dong Tang *Glehnia-Ophiopogon Decoction* was used. The first was used to clear the Lesser Yang and the second to nourish Stomach-Yin.

Chai Hu *Radix Bupleuri* 6 g
Huang Qin *Radix Scutellariae baicalensis* 4 g
Dang Shen *Radix Codonopsis pilosulae* 4 g
Ban Xia *Rhizoma Pinelliae ternatae* 5 g
Mai Men Dong *Tuber Ophiopogonis japonici* 5 g
Bei Sha Shen *Radix Glehniae littoralis* 5 g
Sang Ye *Folium Mori albae* 3 g
Yu Zhu *Rhizoma Polygonati odorati* 4 g
Tian Hua Fen *Radix Trichosanthis* 4 g
Bian Dou *Semen Dolichoris lablab* 4 g
Tai Zi Shen *Radix Pseudostellariae* 4 g
Zhi Gan Cao *Radix Glycyrrhizae uralensis praeparata* 3 g
Da Zao *Fructus Ziziphi jujubae* 3 dates
Sheng Jiang *Rhizoma Zingiberis officinalis recens* 3 slices

Explanation
The combination of these two prescriptions is ideally suited to this girl's condition. One clears the Lesser Yang, the other nourishes Stomach-Yin. In particular, this prescription also suits her symptoms well because **Sang Ye** will not only soothe the throat but also alleviate the headaches; **Tian Hua Fen** and **Yu Zhu** will moisten dryness; **Bian Dou** will tonify Stomach and Spleen Yin while **Tai Zi Shen** nourishes Stomach-Yin.

This girl needed only 20 days of treatment after which her condition was completely cured.

DEFICIENCY

1. QI DEFICIENCY

CLINICAL MANIFESTATIONS

Tiredness which is worse in the mornings, slight ache in the muscles, muscle fatigue after slight exertion, shortness of breath, weak voice, spontaneous daytime sweating, poor appetite, slight epigastric and abdominal distension, loose stools, Empty pulse, Pale tongue.

- If Heart-Qi is deficient there will be palpitations.
- If Kidney-Qi is deficient there will be frequent urination.

Qi deficiency is the most common eventual outcome of an invasion of Wind complicated by a subsequent residual pathogenic factor. Both Damp-Heat or Heat will impair the ascending of Spleen-Qi and therefore lead, in time, to weakening of Qi.

However, ME is unlikely to manifest purely with a deficiency of Qi as nearly always there will be some residual pathogenic factor (especially Damp-Heat). In treatment, it is necessary to evaluate the relative importance of the deficiency of Qi or the strength of the pathogenic factor. If the condition is predominantly deficient (say, 80%), it should be treated as a deficiency with one of the prescriptions indicated below. These prescriptions, however, should be opportunely adapted to take into account eliminating any residual pathogenic factor.

PRINCIPLE OF TREATMENT

Tonify Qi primarily, expel any remaning pathogenic factor secondarily.

ACUPUNCTURE

ST-36 Zusanli, SP-6 Sanyinjiao, BL-20 Pishu, BL-21 Weishu, Ren-6 Qihai, L.I.-10 Shousanli, LU-9 Taiyuan, HE-5 Tongli, Du-12 Shenzhu, BL-13 Feishu, Du-20 Baihui. All reinforced. Moxa can be used unless there is some Heat or Damp-Heat left.

Explanation

- **ST-36**, **SP-6**, **BL-20** and **BL-21** tonify Stomach and Spleen.
- **LU-9**, **Du-12** and **BL-13** tonify Lung-Qi.
- **HE-5** tonifies Heart-Qi.

- **Ren-6** tonifies Qi in general.
- **L.I.-10** tonifies Qi and is particularly useful, in combination with ST-36 to reduce muscle ache and fatigue in the limbs.
- **Du-20** raises Yang and lifts the mood, a very important consideration in this condition which can last for years and inevitably makes the person depressed.

HERBAL TREATMENT

Prescription

BU ZHONG YI QI TANG
Tonifying the Centre and Benefiting Qi Decoction
Huang Qi *Radix Astragali membranacei* 15 g
Dang Shen *Radix Codonopsis pilosulae* 10 g
Bai Zhu *Rhizoma Atractylodis macrocephalae* 10 g
Zhi Gan Cao *Radix Glycyrrhizae uralensis praeparata* 5 g
Chen Pi *Pericarpium Citri reticulatae* 6 g
Dang Gui *Radix Angelicae sinensis* 10 g
Sheng Ma *Rhizoma Cimicifugae* 3 g
Chai Hu *Radix Bupleuri* 3 g

Explanation

- **Huang Qi**, **Dang Shen**, **Bai Zhu** and **Zhi Gan Cao** tonify and raise Qi.
- **Chen Pi** regulates Qi and prevents the stagnation that may derive from excessive tonification.
- **Dang Gui** tonifies Blood to help to tonify Qi.
- **Sheng Ma** and **Chai Hu** raise Qi.

This prescription is the best to tonify Qi in cases of ME because it is specific to clear any Empty-Heat that may derive from Qi deficiency. This is the role of Chai Hu and Sheng Ma. Historically this prescription was used for extreme Qi deficiency from overwork leading to some Empty-Heat, manifested with a feeling of heat or even a low-grade fever. Patients suffering from ME frequently experience a feeling of heat and Chai Hu is excellent to expel any hidden residual Heat. Besides this, Chai Hu and Sheng Ma also raise Qi, and this is a very beneficial effect in patients with ME who feel extremely tired and have a feeling of heaviness like being pulled down. Finally, the action of raising Qi acts also on a psychological level and this prescription can lift the mood and relieve depression, thus helping recovery.

Variations

- In case of some residual Damp-Heat add: Ze Xie *Rhizoma Alismatis orientalis*, Sha Ren *Fructus seu Semen Amomi* and Huang Qin *Radix Scutellariae baicalensis*.
- In case of residual Dampness without Heat add Fu Ling *Sclerotium Poriae cocos*, Sha Ren *Fructus seu Semen Amomi* and Yi Yi Ren *Semen Coicis lachryma jobi*.
- In case of some remaining Heat add: Huang Qin *Radix Scutellariae baicalensis* (for Lung-Heat), Zhu Ye *Herba Lophatheri gracilis* (for Heart-Heat), or Huang Lian *Rhizoma Coptidis* (for Stomach-Heat).

Patent remedy

BU ZHONG YI QI WAN
Tonifying the Centre and Benefiting Qi Pill
Huang Qi *Radix Astragali membranacei*
Dang Shen *Radix Codonopsis pilosulae*
Zhi Gan Cao *Radix Glycyrrhizae uralensis praeparata*
Bai Zhu *Rhizoma Atractylodis macrocephalae*
Dang Gui *Radix Angelicae sinensis*
Chen Pi *Pericarpium Citri reticulatae*
Sheng Ma *Rhizoma Cimicifugae*
Chai Hu *Radix Bupleuri*
Sheng Jiang *Rhizoma Zingiberis officinalis recens*
Da Zao *Fructus Ziziphi jujubae*

Explanation

This well-known remedy is ideal to treat ME when the condition is predominantly deficient. It will boost the patient's energy as it tonifies Qi; on a mental level, it will lift their mood as it raises Qi, and it will lightly clear any residual Heat due to the presence of Chai Hu and Sheng Ma.

The tongue presentation appropriate to this remedy is a Pale body and the *absence* of a thick-sticky coating.

Case history

A 40-year-old woman had been suffering from what had been diagnosed as ME for the previous 6 years. All her symptoms started after contracting influenza during her second pregnancy. During this acute infection she felt completely exhausted and could hardly walk. She never recovered after this infection and continued to feel exhausted, shivery and experiencing a general flu-like feeling. Her muscles ached and felt very quickly fatigued after the slightest exercise. Her head felt muzzy and her short-term memory was poor. Four years after the initial infection she contracted a new one which severely aggravated her symptoms. She had a pain in the spine and occiput, a numbness of her face, headaches, sore eyes, breathlessness, palpitations, a weakness of the right arm, diarrhoea, and weak legs. She felt shivery and sweated. This condition lasted for 5 months during which time she was in bed most of the time. At the time of her consultation these symptoms had disappeared but she still felt exhausted and shivery and had a flu-like feeling most of the time. The ache in the muscles had subsided while the fatigue remained. Her pulse was extremely Fine, almost Minute and Weak, being almost non-existent on the right Front position (Lungs). Her tongue was Pale, was slightly Swollen and had a midline (Stomach) crack.

Diagnosis
The present condition is very clearly predominantly deficient. There is a very obvious deficiency of Lungs and Spleen. The initial symptoms showed some Dampness, evidenced by the ache in the muscles. The aggravation 4 years later probably led to the exhaustion of Qi.

Treatment principle
The treatment principle in this case is simply to tonify Qi of the Lungs and Spleen.

Acupuncture
The acupuncture treatment consisted in reinforcing **LU-9** Taiyuan, **ST-36** Zusanli, **SP-6** Sanyinjiao, **L.I.-10** Shousanli, **BL-20** Pishu, **BL-13** Feishu, **Du-12** Shenzhu, **BL-21** Weishu and **Du-20** Baihui.

Herbal treatment
The herbal prescription used was a simple variation of Bu Zhong Yi Qi Tang *Tonifying the Centre and Benefiting Qi Decoction*:

Huang Qi *Radix Astragali membranacei* 15 g
Bai Zhu *Rhizoma Atractylodis macrocephalae* 6 g
Dang Shen *Radix Codonopsis pilosulae* 9 g
Mai Men Dong *Tuber Ophiopogonis japonici* 3 g
Chai Hu *Radix Bupleuri* 3 g

At various times during the treatment (over 2 years) she needed to have prescriptions to clear Heat during acute exacerbations of her condition. Sometimes she had the Xiao Chai Hu Tang *Small Bupleurum Decoction* and at other times she had Xie Bai Tang *Draining Whiteness Decoction*. She achieved an almost complete recovery after 2 years.

2. YIN DEFICIENCY

CLINICAL MANIFESTATIONS

These vary according to the organ involved. The three organs which most frequently suffer from Yin deficiency in ME are the Lungs, Stomach and Kidneys. Combinations of two or even all three of these are common.

Lung-Yin Deficiency

Dry throat, dry cough, exhaustion, breathlessness, hoarse voice, feeling of heat in the afternoon, night sweating, 5-palm sweating, malar flush.
Tongue: Red without coating (possibly only in the front part). There may be cracks in the Lung area (see Fig. 12.2 in chapter 12).
Pulse: Fine and Rapid or Floating-Empty.

This pattern frequently occurs after a febrile disease during which Heat dries up the body fluids. In young adults it can happen after glandular fever (mononucleosis), when the Yin is injured by prolonged Heat and gives rise to ME.

Principle of treatment

Nourish Yin, generate fluids, strengthen the Lungs.

Acupuncture

LU-9 Taiyuan, Ren-17 Shanzhong, BL-43 Gaohuangshu, BL-13 Feishu, Du-12 Shenzhu, Ren-12 Zhongwan, ST-36 Zusanli, SP-6 Sanyinjiao, Du-20 Baihui. All with reinforcing method. No moxa.

Explanation

- **LU-9** and **Ren-17** tonify Lung-Yin and Lung-Qi respectively.
- **BL-43** nourishes Lung-Yin and is particularly indicated for chronic conditions.
- **BL-13** and **Du-12** tonify Lung-Qi.
- **Ren-12**, **ST-36** and **SP-6** tonify Stomach and Spleen and generate fluids. In particular, Ren-12 also tonifies the Lungs as the deep pathway of the Lung channel starts at this point.
- **Du-20** clears the brain and lifts mood.

Herbal treatment

Prescription

SHA SHEN MAI DONG TANG
Glehnia-Ophiopogon Decoction
Bei Sha Shen *Radix Glehniae littoralis* 9 g
Mai Men Dong *Tuber Ophiopogonis japonici* 9 g
Yu Zhu *Rhizoma Polygonati odorati* 6 g
Tian Hua Fen *Radix Trichosanthis* 4.5 g
Sang Ye *Folium Mori albae* 4.5 g
Bian Dou *Semen Dolichoris lablab* 4.5 g
Gan Cao *Radix Glycyrrhizae uralensis* 3 g

Explanation

- **Bei Sha Shen** promotes body fluids and nourishes Yin.
- **Mai Men Dong** nourishes Yin of Stomach and Lungs.
- **Yu Zhu** and **Tian Hua Fen** nourish Stomach and Lung Yin, generate fluids and clear Heat.
- **Sang Ye** clears Lung-Heat and stimulates the descending of Lung-Qi.
- **Bian Dou** tonifies Spleen Qi and Yin and is used according to the principle of "strengthening the Earth to promote Metal".

Variations

- In case of cough add Bai Bu *Radix Stemonae* or Kuan Dong Hua *Flos Tussilaginis farfarae*.
- In case of haemoptysis add Bai Mao Gen *Rhizoma Imperatae cylindricae*.
- In case of Empty-Heat add Di Gu Pi *Cortex Lycii chinensis radicis*.

Stomach-Yin Deficiency

Dry mouth, no appetite, tiredness, dry stools, slight epigastric pain, malar flush, thirst with no desire to drink or a desire to drink only in small sips.
Tongue: normal body-colour, midline crack in the centre, rootless coating or no coating in the centre, transversal cracks on the sides indicating

chronic Spleen-Qi and Spleen-Yin deficiency (see Fig. 12.3).
Pulse: Fine-Rapid, Floating-Empty on the right Middle position.

The residual Heat which follows a febrile disease dries up the Stomach fluids and often causes Stomach-Yin deficiency.

Principle of treatment

Nourish Yin, strengthen Stomach and Spleen.

Acupuncture

ST-36 Zusanli, SP-6 Sanyinjiao, Ren-12 Zhongwan, ST-44 Neiting, Du-20 Baihui. All with reinforcing method. If the tongue body is not Red, a little moxa can be used on ST-36.

Explanation

- **ST-36**, **SP-6** and **Ren-12** nourish Stomach-Yin.
- **ST-44** clears Stomach-Heat or Empty-Heat.
- **Du-20** clears the brain and lifts mood.

Herbal treatment

Prescription

YI WEI TANG
Benefiting the Stomach Decoction
Bei Sha Shen *Radix Glehniae littoralis* 9 g
Mai Men Dong *Tuber Ophiopogonis japonici* 9 g
Sheng Di Huang *Radix Rehmanniae glutinosae* 12 g
Yu Zhu *Rhizoma Polygonati odorati* 6 g
Bing Tang *Brown sugar* 3 g

Explanation

- **Bei Sha Shen** and **Mai Men Dong** nourish Stomach Yin.
- **Sheng Di Huang** nourishes Spleen and Kidney Yin.
- **Yu Zhu** nourishes Stomach-Yin and clears Heat.
- **Bing Tang** nourishes the Stomach and harmonizes the Middle.

Kidney-Yin Deficiency

Soreness of the lower back, exhaustion, depression, lack of drive and will-power, weak legs and knees, dizziness, tinnitus, deafness, dry mouth and throat which are worse at night, night sweating, malar flush, disturbed sleep (waking up during the night), thin body.
Tongue: Red without coating.
Pulse: Floating-Empty or Rapid-Fine.

A prolonged fever can injure Kidney-Yin in people who have a pre-existing Kidney weakness. Kidney-Yin deficiency causes the patient to feel completely exhausted. It is a type of exhaustion which cannot be relieved by a short rest but only by regulating one's life and taking proper rest over a long period of time. On a mental level, Kidney-Yin deficiency causes a person to feel depressed, lacking in drive and initiative as the Kidneys are the seat of Will-Power (*Zhi*).

Principle of treatment

Nourish Yin, strengthen the Kidneys and firm Will-Power.

Acupuncture

KI-3 Taixi, LU-7 Lieque, KI-6 Zhaohai, Ren-4 Guanyuan, SP-6 Sanyinjiao, BL-23 Shenshu, BL-52 Zhishi, Du-20 Baihui. All with reinforcing method, no moxa.

Explanation

- **KI-3** is the Source point and it nourishes Kidney-Yin.
- **LU-7** and **KI-6** in combination, open the Directing Vessel, nourish Kidney-Yin and moisten the throat.
- **Ren-4** and **SP-6** nourish Kidney-Yin and benefit fluids.
- **BL-23** and **BL-52** in combination, strengthen Will-Power and can improve drive and determination.
- **Du-20** clears the brain and lifts mood.

Herbal treatment

Prescription

ZUO GUI WAN

Restoring the Left [Kidney] Pill
Shu Di Huang *Radix Rehmanniae glutinosae prae-parata* 12 g
Gou Qi Zi *Fructus Lycii chinensis* 6 g
Shan Yao *Radix Dioscoreae oppositae* 6 g
Gui Ban Jiao *Colla Plastri testudinis* 12 g
Chuan Niu Xi *Radix Cyathulae* 4 g
Shan Zhu Yu *Fructus Corni officinalis* 6 g
Tu Si Zi *Semen Cuscutae* 6 g
Lu Jiao Jiao *Colla Cornu Cervi* 6 g

Explanation

– **Shu Di Huang**, **Gou Qi Zi**, **Shan Yao** and **Gui Ban Jiao** nourish Kidney-Yin.
– **Shan Zhu Yu** is astringent and thus helps to nourish Yin and firms the Essence.
– **Tu Si Zi** and **Lu Jiao Jiao** tonify Kidney-Yang. They are added here according to the principle that, because Kidney-Yin and Kidney-Yang share the same root, a long-term deficiency of one always implies also a slight deficiency of the other. A prescription made entirely of Yin-tonics would be too Yin and sticky: it needs a little Fire to set it in motion, i.e. some Kidney-Yang tonics. Lu Jiao Jiao is chosen here instead of Lu Rong as it tonifies both Kidney-Yang and Blood, it is thus more sticky and Yin than Lu Rong.
– **Niu Xi** directs the prescription to the Lower Burner, i.e. to the Kidneys.

Variations. In all three cases of Yin deficiency, there will most probably be some remaining Damp-Heat or Heat. It is usually best to combine tonification with some expelling.

– In case of residual Damp-Heat add Huang Bo *Cortex Phellodendri* (for Kidney-Yin deficiency), Huang Lian *Rhizoma Coptidis* (for Stomach-Yin deficiency) or Huang Qin *Radix Scutellariae baicalensis* (for Lung-Yin deficiency).
– In case of residual Heat add Zhi Mu *Radix Anemarrhenae asphodeloidis* (for Kidney-Yin deficiency), Shi Hu *Herba Dendrobii* (for Stomach-Yin deficiency), or Di Gu Pi *Cortex Lycii chinensis radicis* (for Lung-Yin deficiency).

Patent remedy
HE CHE DA ZAO WAN

Placenta Great Fortifying Pill
Gui Ban *Plastrum Testudinis*
Shu Di Huang *Radix Rehmanniae glutinosae prae-parata*
Dang Shen *Radix Codonopsis pilosulae*
Huang Bo *Cortex Phellodendri*
Du Zhong *Cortex Eucommiae ulmoidis*
Zi He Che *Placenta hominis*
Niu Xi *Radix Achyranthis bidentatae seu Cyathulae*
Tian Men Dong *Tuber Asparagi cochinchinensis*
Mai Men Dong *Tuber Ophiopogonis japonici*
Fu Ling *Sclerotium Poriae cocos*
Sha Ren *Fructus seu Semen Amomi*

Explanation. This remedy strongly nourishes Yin and Blood and is excellent for chronic ME with Kidney-Yin deficiency. It is particularly suitable because, apart from nourishing Yin, it tonifies Qi with Dang Shen and Kidney-Yang with Du Zhong. This herb has a particularly beneficial action on a mental level to lift mood and strengthen will-power, an important consideration in chronic ME. For this reason, it is preferable to other famous Yin-tonic remedies such as Liu Wei Di Huang Wan *Six-Ingredient Rehmannia Pill*.

3. YANG DEFICIENCY

CLINICAL MANIFESTATIONS

The clinical manifestations depend on the organ involved. The two organs which most commonly suffer from Yang deficiency are the Spleen and Kidneys. The symptoms of Spleen-Yang deficiency are practically the same as those of Spleen-Qi deficiency (see above) with the addition of chilliness. The symptoms and signs of Kidney-Yang deficiency are as follows.

Kidney-Yang Deficiency

Soreness of the lower back, cold knees, sensation of cold in the back, chilliness, weak legs and knees, bright-white complexion, impotence in men, premature ejaculation, lack of sexual desire, lassitude, abundant-clear urination, apathy, oedema of the ankles, infertility.
Tongue: Pale, Swollen, wet.
Pulse: Deep-Weak.

In some cases, the remaining pathogenic factor leads to Yang deficiency. This happens in those who have a pre-existing Yang deficiency.

Treatment principle

Tonify Yang, warm the Kidneys.

Acupuncture

BL-23 Shenshu, Du-4 Mingmen, Ren-4 Guanyuan, KI-3 Taixi, KI-7 Fuliu, BL-52 Zhishi, Du-20 Baihui. All with reinforcing method. Moxa should be used.

Explanation

- **BL-23**, Back-Transporting point of the Kidneys, tonifies Kidney-Yang.
- **Du-4**, with moxa, strongly tonifies the Fire of the Gate of Vitality.
- **Ren-4**, with moxa, tonifies Kidney-Yang (without moxa it can nourish Kidney-Yin).
- **KI-3**, Source point, can tonify both Kidney-Yang or Kidney-Yin.
- **KI-7** tonifies Kidney-Yang and resolves oedema.
- **BL-52**, called the "Room of Will-Power", strengthens the mental aspect of the Kidney, i.e. will-power and determination.
- **Du-20** clears the brain and lifts mood.

Herbal treatment

(a) Prescription

YOU GUI YIN
Restoring the Right [Kidney] Decoction
Shu Di Huang *Radix Rehmanniae glutinosae praeparata* 15 g
Shan Zhu Yu *Fructus Corni officinalis* 3 g
Shan Yao *Radix Dioscoreae oppositae* 6 g
Du Zhong *Cortex Eucommiae ulmoidis* 6 g
Rou Gui *Cortex Cinnamomi cassiae* 3 g
Fu Zi *Radix Aconiti carmichaeli praeparata* 3 g
Gou Qi Zi *Fructus Lycii chinensis* 6 g
Zhi Gan Cao *Radix Glycyrrhizae uralensis praeparata* 3 g

Explanation

- **Shu Di Huang, Shan Zhu Yu, Gou Qi Zi** and

Shan Yao nourish Kidneys, Liver and Spleen.
- **Du Zhong**, **Rou Gui** and **Fu Zi** tonify and warm Kidney-Yang and the Gate of Vitality.
- **Gan Cao** harmonizes.

(b) Prescription

YOU GUI WAN
Restoring the Right [Kidney] Pill
Fu Zi *Radix Aconiti carmichaeli praeparata* 3 g
Rou Gui *Cortex Cinnamomi cassiae* 3 g
Du Zhong *Cortex Eucommiae ulmoidis* 6 g
Shan Zhu Yu *Fructus Corni officinalis* 4.5 g
Tu Si Zi *Semen Cuscutae* 6 g
Lu Jiao Jiao *Colla Cornu Cervi* 6 g
Shu Di Huang *Radix Rehmanniae glutinosae praeparata* 12 g
Shan Yao *Radix Dioscoreae oppositae* 6 g
Gou Qi Zi *Fructus Lycii chinensis* 6 g
Dang Gui *Radix Angelicae sinensis* 4.5 g

Explanation

- **Shu Di Huang, Tu Si Zi, Shan Zhu Yu, Gou Qi Zi** and **Shan Yao** nourish Kidney, Liver and Spleen.
- **Du Zhong, Rou Gui, Fu Zi** and **Lu Jiao Jiao** tonify and warm Kidney-Yang and the Gate of Vitality.
- **Dang Gui** and **Lu Jiao Jiao** nourish Blood.

These two prescriptions are very similar. They differ only in the inclusion of Dang Gui, Tu Si Zi and Lu Jiao Jiao in the second one. As Dang Gui and Lu Jiao Jiao nourish Blood and Tu Si Zi benefits the ovaries, this second prescription is better for women.

Variations

- If there is Damp-Heat in the muscles add Huang Lian *Rhizoma Coptidis*, Sha Ren *Fructus seu Semen Amomi* and Pei Lan *Herba Eupatorei fortunei*.

(i) Patent remedy

REN SHEN LU RONG WAN
Ginseng-Cornu Cervi Pill
Ren Shen *Radix Ginseng*

Du Zhong *Cortex Eucommiae ulmoidis*
Ba Ji Tian *Radix Morindae officinalis*
Huang Qi *Radix Astragali membranacei*
Lu Rong *Cornu Cervi parvum*
Dang Gui *Radix Angelicae sinensis*
Niu Xi *Radix Achyranthis bidentatae seu Cyathulae*
Long Yan Rou *Arillus Euphoriae longanae*

Explanation. This remedy tonifies Qi and Kidney-Yang. It is particularly suitable for chronic ME for the mood-lifting effect of herbs such as Huang Qi and Lu Rong.

The tongue and pulse presentation appropriate to this remedy is a Pale and Swollen tonguebody and a pulse which is Weak and Deep on both Rear positions.

(ii) Patent remedy

GE JIE BU SHEN WAN
Gecko Tonifying the Kidneys Pill
Ge Jie *Gecko*
Lu Rong *Cornu Cervi parvum*
Ren Shen *Radix Ginseng*
Huang Qi *Radix Astragali membranacei*
Du Zhong *Cortex Eucommiae ulmoidis*
Gou Shen *Testis et Penis Canis*
Dong Chong Xia Cao *Sclerotium Cordicipitis chinensis*
Gou Qi Zi *Fructus Lycii chinensis*
Fu Ling *Sclerotium Poriae cocos*
Bai Zhu *Rhizoma Atractylodis macrocephalae*

Explanation. This remedy tonifies Lung- and Kidney-Yang. It is therefore suitable for chronic ME with a deficiency of Lung-Qi and Kidney-Yang, with such symptoms as breathlessness on exertion, a weak voice, a propensity to catching colds, back-ache, frequent-pale urination and a Pale tongue.

Case history

A 59-year-old woman had been diagnosed as having had ME for the previous 4 years. She could not say exactly how it started. Her main symptoms when she came for treatment were: feeling "flat", constipation, "racing feeling" with palpitations, ache and fatigue of muscles after the slightest exertion, exhaustion, "lacking energy and incentive", passing water three times a night, back-ache, dizziness, tinnitus, feeling cold, breathlessness with palpitations, cold hands, flu-like feeling like a "burning coldness", prone to catching colds after a shower or washing hair. Her tongue was Pale, with a slightly peeled centre and a central Stomach crack. Her pulse was generally Weak.

Diagnosis
Most of her symptoms indicate Kidney-Yang deficiency: back-ache, dizziness, tinnitus, feeling cold, lacking incentive, constipation, nocturia. Kidney-Yang is the root of Heart-Yang and deficiency of the former often leads to deficiency of the latter, hence the palpitations with racing feeling and breathlessness. There is also some residual Dampness in the muscles evidenced by the ache, but this is quite secondary in relation to the general deficiency of Yang.

Treatment principle
The main principle of treatment is therefore to tonify Kidney-Yang and only secondarily to resolve Dampness.

Acupuncture
She was given acupuncture to tonify Spleen- and Kidney-Yang and resolve Dampness using mostly **ST-36** Zusanli, **SP-6** Sanyinjiao, **BL-20** Pishu, **BL-21** Weishu to tonify Spleen-Yang (with moxa), **BL-23** Shenshu and **KI-7** Fuliu to tonify Kidney-Yang (with moxa) and **SP-9** Yinlingquan to resolve Dampness.

Herbal treatment
The herbal prescription chosen was a variation of You Gui Yin *Restoring the Right [Kidney] Decoction*:

Shu Di Huang *Radix Rehmanniae glutinosae praeparata* 12 g
Shan Zhu Yu *Fructus Corni officinalis* 4 g
Shan Yao *Radix Dioscoreae oppositae* 6 g
Gou Qi Zi *Fructus Lycii chinensis* 6 g
Du Zhong *Cortex Eucommiae ulmoidis* 6 g
Rou Gui *Cortex Cinnamomi cassiae* 1.5 g
Fu Zi *Radix Aconiti carmichaeli praeparata* 1 g
Rou Cong Rong *Herba Cistanchis* 6 g
Ze Xie *Rhizoma Alismatis orientalis* 3 g
Zhi Gan Cao *Radix Glycyrrhizae uralensis praeparata* 3 g

Explanation
This prescription was altered only with the addition of Rou Cong Rong to tonify Kidney-Yang and move the stools and Ze Xie to moderate the effect of the other herbs all of which are hot in energy.

The combination of acupuncture and herbal therapy produced an immediate improvement which continued gradually and steadily throughout the course of treatment. All her symptoms were relieved after 6 months.

END NOTES

1. Shepherd C 1989 Living with ME, Cedar, William Heinemann Ltd, London, pp. 14–16.
2. 1979 The Yellow Emperor's Classic of Internal Medicine — Simple Questions (*Huang Ti Nei Jing Su Wen* 黄帝内经素问), People's Health Publishing House, Beijing. First published *c.* 100 BC, p. 21.
3. Ibid., p. 24.
4. Smith D 1989 Understanding ME, Robinson Publishing, London, p. 128.

Parkinson's disease 26

震顫性麻痺

Parkinson's disease is a clinical syndrome characterized by impairment of movement, rigidity and tremor, which results from damage to the basal ganglia. Its pathology consists in cellular loss and depigmentation of the substantia nigra. This is accompanied by biochemical changes in the corpus striatum where there is a decrease of dopamine. The substantia nigra and corpus striatum are connected by fibres where dopamine and acetylcholine act as neurotransmitters. In Parkinson's disease there is an imbalance between these two neurotransmitters, with a decrease in dopamine accounting for the impairment of movement, and an increase in acetylcholine accounting for the rigidity and tremor.

The onset of the disease usually occurs between the ages of 50 and 60. The first sign is usually a tremor of the hand. It is a coarse tremor 4 to 8 times per second. Difficulty in movement and rigidity follow the onset of tremor. The face also loses its expressive movements, giving the patient the typical staring look which is diagnostic of this disease. Automatic swinging of the arms when walking is decreased or lost and the patient walks taking small shuffling steps. The handwriting becomes progressively smaller.

The tremor of Parkinson's disease is coarse while that of thyrotoxicosis or alcoholism is finer and more rapid.

In Chinese medicine, Parkinson's disease comes under the symptom of "Convulsions" and is always related to Liver-Wind. The "Principles of Medicine" (1565) says: *"Wind tremors are [caused by] Wind entering the Liver and the Qi of the channels rebelling upwards, this causes tics of the face and tremors of the limbs."*[1] The "Original Theory of Medicine" (Ming dynasty) says:

[Tremors may be caused by:] deficient Qi unable to attract fluids and Blood towards sinews and channels to nourish them; deficient fluids and Blood not nourishing the sinews; Phlegm-Fire obstructing the channels and sinews so that fluids and Blood cannot nourish them; deficient Original Qi facilitating the invasion of pathogenic factors in the channels so that Blood cannot nourish sinews and channels. Although there are many different causes, in all of them there is a deficiency of fluids and Blood not nourishing sinews and channels.[2]

Aetiology and pathology

1. OVERWORK AND EXCESSIVE SEXUAL ACTIVITY

Overwork in the sense of working long hours without adequate rest for several years weakens the Kidneys and particularly Kidney-Yin. When overwork is associated with excessive sexual activity it weakens the Kidneys even more.

A deficient Kidney-Yin fails to nourish Liver-Yin and, in time, this may lead to the development of Liver-Wind which causes tremors. Liver-Yin (and by implication Liver-Blood too) fails to nourish and moisten the sinews: this dryness of the sinews, combined with Liver-Wind, leads to tremors.

2. DIET

Excessive consumption of greasy-fried or sweet foods leads to the formation of Phlegm. With time, Phlegm easily combines with Fire, especially when the person consumes alcohol as well.

Phlegm-Fire on its own would not cause Parkinson's disease but it does so when associated with Liver-Wind, which it often is in old people. Phlegm obstructs the channels and prevents fluids and Blood from nourishing them, hence the tremor.

3. EMOTIONAL STRESS

Anger, frustration and resentment may cause Liver-Yang to rise and, with time, this may lead to Liver-Wind.

Thus, as the quotation from the "Original Theory of Medicine" above shows, in Parkinson's disease the tremor is always due to fluids and Blood not nourishing the channels and sinews.

Differentiation and treatment

ACUPUNCTURE

BODY ACUPUNCTURE

The following points may be used as a general prescription to extinguish Wind: G.B.-20 Fengchi, L.I.-11 Quchi, Xiaochanxue ("Controlling Tremor Point", 1.5 *cun* below HE-3 Shaohai), T.B.-5 Waiguan, G.B.-34 Yanglingquan, LIV-3 Taichong.

Use 30 gauge (0.32 mm diameter) needles with even method and leave needles for ½ hour.

The use of local points on the limb affected by tremor is essential.

Arm: L.I.-11 Quchi, L.I.-10 Shousanli, T.B.-5 Waiguan and L.I.-4 Hegu.
Leg: ST-31 Biguan, G.B.-31 Fengshi, ST-36 Zusanli, G.B.-34 Yanglingquan, ST-41 Jiexi and G.B.-40 Qiuxu.

Other points are chosen according to the prevailing pattern and these will be indicated below.

SCALP ACUPUNCTURE

Use the chorea area on the side opposite the trembling limb (Fig. 26.1). The chorea area is located in relation to the motor area and this, in turn, is located in relation to the midline and the eyebrow-occiput line. The midline is the line from the glabella in between the eyes to the occipital protuberance. Locate the mid-point of the midline: the motor area starts 0.5 cm behind the mid-point and goes to the point of intersection between the eyebrow-occiput line and the hairline. The chorea area is parallel to the motor area and starts 1 cm in front of the mid-point.

One needle is inserted subcutaneously to cover the whole area. If this proves difficult, three needles may be used to cover the chorea line. Electricity with low frequency may be applied to two needles inserted along the chorea area.

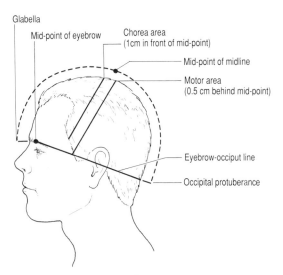

Glabella
Mid-point of eyebrow
Chorea area
(1cm in front of mid-point)
Mid-point of midline
Motor area
(0.5 cm behind mid-point)
Eyebrow-occiput line
Occipital protuberance

Fig. 26.1 Chorea area in scalp acupuncture

ACUPUNCTURE AND HERBAL TREATMENT

The above points, on the body and scalp, are applicable to any type of condition. The choice of other body points and herbal formulae must be based on the identification of patterns.

The main patterns discussed are:

Qi and Blood Deficiency
Phlegm-Heat agitating Wind
Liver- and Kidney-Yin Deficiency.

1. QI AND BLOOD DEFICIENCY

CLINICAL MANIFESTATIONS

Long-standing pronounced tremor of a limb, sallow complexion, staring look, dislike of speaking, occipital stiffness, cramps in the limbs, difficulty in moving, walking uncoordinated, dizziness, blurred vision, sweating, worse with movement.
Tongue: Pale, Swollen with teeth-marks and Quivering.
Pulse: Fine.

TREATMENT PRINCIPLE

Tonify Qi, nourish Blood, invigorate the Connecting channels and extinguish Wind.

ACUPUNCTURE

ST-36 Zusanli, SP-6 Sanyinjiao, Ren-4 Guanyuan, LIV-8 Ququan. Reinforcing method.

Explanation

- **ST-36** and **SP-6** tonify Qi and Blood.
- **Ren-4** nourishes Blood.
- **LIV-8** nourishes Liver-Blood.

HERBAL TREATMENT

Empirical prescription

Huang Qi *Radix Astragali membranacei* 9 g
Dang Shen *Radix Codonopsis pilosulae* 6 g
Dang Gui *Radix Angelicae sinensis* 9 g
Bai Shao *Radix Paeoniae albae* 6 g
Ji Xue Teng *Caulis Millettiae seu Caulis Spatholobi* 6 g
Tian Ma *Rhizoma Gastrodiae elatae* 9 g
Gou Teng *Ramulus Uncariae* 6 g
Zhen Zhu Mu *Concha margaritiferae* 12 g
Ling Yang Jiao *Cornu Antelopis* 4.5 g
Dan Shen *Radix Salviae miltiorrhizae* 4 g

Explanation

- **Huang Qi** and **Dang Shen** tonify Qi.
- **Dang Gui**, **Bai Shao** and **Ji Xue Teng** nourish Blood and expel Wind from the channels.
- **Tian Ma**, **Gou Teng**, **Zhen Zhu Mu** and **Ling Yang Jiao** extinguish Wind.
- **Dan Shen** moves Blood.

Case history

A 51-year-old woman had been suffering from Parkinson's disease for 2 years. Her main problem was a tremor of the head which she tried to stop by bending her head forward. She sometimes felt that her tremor started from the lower back running all the way up the spine to the head. Apart from this she had few other symptoms. She felt tired easily and her vision was sometimes blurred. She had been prescribed anticholinergic drugs which produced side-effects such as a dry mouth and tunnel vision. She was a very tense person with a very strong sense of responsibility probably deriving from a very strict upbringing. Her tongue was Pale and Thin, while her pulse was Choppy.

Diagnosis
Qi and Blood deficiency of the Liver leading to Liver-Wind.

Treatment principle
This patient was treated only with acupuncture and the treatment given was very simple, being aimed at tonifying Qi and Blood, calming the Mind and subduing Liver-Wind.

Acupuncture
The main points used were:

– **ST-36** Zusanli and **SP-6** Sanyinjiao to tonify Qi and Blood.
– **HE-7** Shenmen or **HE-5** Tongli to calm the Mind and relax the nervous system.
– **LIV-3** Taichong and **Du-16** Fengfu to subdue Wind.

After a few months of treatment she was able to stop her drugs and after 1 year she was 90% free of tremor.

2. PHLEGM-HEAT AGITATING WIND

CLINICAL MANIFESTATIONS

Obesity, staring look, dislike of exercise, a feeling of oppression of the chest, dry mouth, sweating, dizziness, spitting of yellow phlegm, stiff neck and back, tremor of a limb which can be stopped.
Tongue: Red with yellow-sticky coating.
Pulse: Wiry-Fine-Rapid.

TREATMENT PRINCIPLE

Resolve Phlegm, clear Heat, extinguish Wind and invigorate the Connecting channels.

ACUPUNCTURE

ST-40 Fenglong, Ren-12 Zhongwan, BL-20 Pishu, SP-6 Sanyinjiao, SP-9 Yinlingquan, LIV-3 Taichong. Even method, except for Ren-12 and BL-20 which should be reinforced.

Explanation

– **ST-40** resolves Phlegm.

– **Ren-12** and **BL-20** tonify the Spleen to resolve Phlegm.
– **SP-6** and **SP-9** help to resolve Phlegm.
– **LIV-3** subdues Wind.

HERBAL TREATMENT

Empirical prescription

Gua Lou *Fructus Trichosanthis* 9 g
Dan Nan Xing *Rhizoma Arisaematis praeparata* 6 g
Zhu Li *Succus Bambusae* 6 g
Gou Teng *Ramulus Uncariae* 6 g
Tian Ma *Rhizoma Gastrodiae elatae* 6 g
Ling Yang Jiao *Cornu Antelopis* 4.5 g
Zhen Zhu Mu *Concha margaritiferae* 12 g
Dan Shen *Radix Salviae miltiorrhizae* 4.5 g
Chi Shao *Radix Paeoniae rubrae* 4 g

Explanation

– **Gua Lou**, **Nan Xing** and **Zhu Li** resolve Phlegm.
– **Gou Teng**, **Tian Ma**, **Ling Yang Jiao** and **Zhen Zhu Mu** extinguish Wind.
– **Dan Shen** and **Chi Shao** move Blood.

Case history

A 53-year-old man had been suffering from Parkinson's disease for 1 year. The first symptoms he experienced were lack of concentration, apathy, tiredness, dizziness, poor sleep and nausea. He was prescribed Valium at that time. A few months later his writing started to become progressively smaller and he developed a tremor of the left hand on lifting things. He also had stiffness of the neck and difficulty in walking. He said he felt as if walking on water. His mouth was dry and his vision was sometimes blurred. He had the typical staring look associated with Parkinson's disease. He was a businessman working long hours in London with a long commuting time to and from work.

His tongue was Red with a sticky-yellow coating and a Heart-crack. His pulse was generally Slippery.

Diagnosis
Phlegm-Heat with Liver-Wind. The signs of Phlegm are blurred vision, lack of concentration, nausea, a Slippery pulse and a sticky tongue coating. Signs of Heat are a dry mouth and a Red tongue. Signs of Liver-Wind are the tremor of his hand, dizziness and the small handwriting.

Treatment principle

This patient was treated with both acupuncture and herbal medicine. The acupuncture treatment was mostly aimed at expelling Wind from the channels whilst the herbal treatment was aimed at resolving Phlegm, clearing Heat and subduing Wind.

Acupuncture

The main points used were:

- **L.I.-11** Quchi, **G.B.-20** Fengchi, **Xiaochanxue**, **T.B.-5** Waiguan and **LIV-3** Taichong to expel Wind from the channels.
- **LIV-8** Ququan to nourish Liver-Yin in order to subdue Liver-Wind.
- **ST-40** Fenglong and **SP-6** Sanyinjiao to resolve Phlegm.
- Scalp acupuncture: chorea area on the right side.

Herbal treatment

The herbal formula used was a variation of Wen Dan Tang *Warming the Gall-Bladder Decoction*:

Zhu Ru *Caulis Bambusae in Taeniis* 6 g
Zhi Shi *Fructus Citri aurantii immaturus* 6 g
Ban Xia *Rhizoma Pinelliae ternatae* 6 g
Chen Pi *Pericarpium Citri reticulatae* 3 g
Fu Ling *Sclerotium Poriae cocos* 4 g
Gou Qi Zi *Fructus Lycii chinensis* 6 g
Tian Ma *Rhizoma Gastrodiae elatae* 6 g
Di Long *Pheretima aspergillum* 4.5 g
Mai Ya *Fructus Hordei vulgaris germinatus* 6 g
Zhi Gan Cao *Radix Glycyrrhizae uralensis praeparata* 3 g
Da Zao *Fructus Ziziphi jujubae* 3 dates
Sheng Jiang *Rhizoma Zingiberis officinalis recens* 3 slices

Explanation

- The first five herbs constitute the Wen Dan Tang which resolves Phlegm-Heat.
- **Gou Qi Zi** nourishes Liver-Yin to subdue Liver-Wind.
- **Tian Ma** and **Di Long** subdue Liver-Wind. Di Long also expels Wind from the channels.
- **Mai Ya** is added as a digestive. I always use one or two digestive herbs when a formula contains insects.
- **Zhi Gan Cao**, **Da Zao** and **Sheng Jiang** harmonize.

This treatment is still being given and the patient is making steady progress. His tremor has diminished by 50% and his movements and walking are much more coordinated.

3. LIVER AND KIDNEY-YIN DEFICIENCY

CLINICAL MANIFESTATIONS

Thin body, dizziness, tinnitus, insomnia, dream-disturbed sleep, headache, night-sweating, men-tal restlessness, sore back and knees, numbness of the limbs, stiff neck and back, tremor of head, clenched teeth and tremor of jaw, long-standing tremor of a limb with marked amplitude, cramps in the limbs, difficulty and clumsiness of walking, staring look, poor memory.
Tongue: Thin, Red without coating, Moving.
Pulse: Fine-Rapid or Floating-Empty.

TREATMENT PRINCIPLE

Nourish Yin, extinguish Wind, invigorate the Connecting channels.

ACUPUNCTURE

Ren-4 Guanyuan, BL-23 Shenshu, KI-3 Taixi, SP-6 Sanyinjiao, BL-18 Ganshu, LIV-8 Ququan, LIV-3 Taichong. All with reinforcing method except for LIV-3 which should be needled with even method.

Explanation

- **Ren-4**, **BL-23**, **KI-3** and **SP-6** nourish Kidney-Yin.
- **BL-18** and **LIV-8** nourish Liver-Yin.
- **LIV-3** subdues Liver-Wind.

HERBAL TREATMENT

Empirical prescription

Sheng Di Huang *Radix Rehmanniae glutinosae* 12 g
Shu Di Huang *Radix Rehmanniae glutinosae praeparata* 12 g
Shou Wu *Radix Polygoni multiflori* 9 g
Xuan Shen *Radix Scrophulariae ningpoensis* 6 g
Gou Teng *Ramulus Uncariae* 6 g
Bai Ji Li *Fructus Tribuli terrestris* 6 g
Ling Yang Jiao *Cornu Antelopis* 4.5 g
Mu Li *Concha Ostreae* 15 g
Dan Shen *Radix Salviae miltiorrhizae* 4.5 g
Chi Shao *Radix Paeoniae rubrae* 4.5 g
Du Zhong *Cortex Eucommiae ulmoidis* 6 g

Explanation

- **Sheng Di**, **Shu Di**, **Shou Wu** and **Xuan Shen** nourish Blood and Yin.
- **Gou Teng**, **Bai Ji Li** and **Ling Yang Jiao** extinguish Wind.
- **Mu Li** nourishes Yin and subdues Wind.
- **Dan Shen** and **Chi Shao** move Blood.
- **Du Zhong** tonifies the Kidneys and expels Wind from the spine.

Case history

A 48-year-old man had been suffering from Parkinson's disease for 3 years. His main symptoms were a tremor of the left hand and blurred vision. He also had the typical staring look of Parkinsonism and his walking was difficult. His tongue was Red with rootless coating and his pulse was Floating-Empty.

Diagnosis
This patient suffered from deficiency of Yin of the Liver with Liver-Wind. The deficiency of Yin was clearly evident from the Red tongue with rootless coating and the Floating-Empty pulse.

Treatment principle
The principle of treatment was to nourish Liver-Yin, subdue Liver-Wind and invigorate the Connecting channels. Acupuncture was mostly used to invigorate the Connecting channels and expel Wind from the channels, while the herbal treatment was used to nourish Liver-Yin and subdue Liver-Wind.

Acupuncture
The main points used were:

- **L.I.-11** Quchi, **Xiaochanxue**, **T.B.-5** Waiguan, **G.B.-20** Fengchi and **L.I.-10** Shousanli with even method to expel Wind from the channels.
- **LIV-8** Ququan, **SP-6** Sanyinjiao and **KI-3** Taixi with reinforcing method to nourish Liver-Yin.
- **LIV-3** Taichong with even method to subdue Liver-Wind.

Herbal treatment
The herbal formula used was a variation of the one mentioned above for Liver- and Kidney-Yin deficiency:

Sheng Di Huang *Radix Rehmanniae glutinosae* 12 g
Shu Di Huang *Radix Rehmanniae glutinosae praeparata* 12 g
Shou Wu *Radix Polygoni multiflori* 9 g
Gou Qi Zi *Fructus Lycii chinensis* 6 g
Sang Ji Sheng *Ramulus Loranthi* 6 g
Gou Teng *Ramulus Uncariae* 6 g
Tian Ma *Rhizoma Gastrodiae elatae* 6 g
Di Long *Pheretima aspergillum* 4.5 g

Bai Ji Li *Fructus Tribuli terrestris* 6 g
Ling Yang Jiao *Cornu Antelopis* 4.5 g
Dan Shen *Radix Salviae miltiorrhizae* 4.5 g
Mai Ya *Fructus Hordei vulgaris germinatus* 6 g
Zhi Gan Cao *Radix Glycyrrhizae uralensis praeparata* 3 g

Explanation
- **Shu Di**, **Sheng Di**, **Shou Wu**, **Gou Qi Zi** and **Sang Ji Sheng** nourish Liver-Yin.
- **Gou Teng**, **Tian Ma**, **Di Long**, **Bai Ji Li** and **Ling Yang Jiao** subdue Liver-Wind. Di Long, in particular, expels Wind from the channels.
- **Dan Shen** moves Blood and calms the Mind.
- **Mai Ya** and **Gan Cao** harmonize.

After one year of treatment there was an improvement of about 70% in the patient's tremor and walking. He felt much better and in general freer in movement.

PATENT REMEDIES

The following patent remedies are suitable for any type of Parkinson's disease as they address the Manifestation, i.e. Liver-Wind, rather than the Root.

(i) PATENT REMEDY

XIAO CHAN WAN
Calming Tremor Pill
Tian Ma *Rhizoma Gastrodiae elatae*
Gou Teng *Ramulus Uncariae*
Zhen Zhu Mu *Concha margaritiferae*
Jiang Can *Bombyx batryticatus*

Explanation

This pill extinguishes Liver-Wind: it treats only the Manifestation and is suitable for any pattern.

(ii) PATENT REMEDY

LING JIAO POWDER
Ling Yang Jiao *Cornu Antelopis*

Explanation

This is not a patent remedy but powdered Ling Yang Jiao. It is often used as an adjuvant to the treatment in order to treat the Manifestation, i.e. extinguish Liver-Wind.

Ling Yang Jiao is salty and cold, enters the Liver, Heart and Lungs: it clears Liver-Fire, brightens the eyes, pacifies the Liver, extinguishes Wind, moves Blood and expels toxins.

The usual dosage is 2–3 g a day taken with hot soup of whatever herbal decoction is being used.

Prognosis and prevention

With a combination of acupuncture and herbal treatment this disease can be controlled and its progress halted at best, but it cannot be completely cured. Best results are obtained in Parkinsonism from Qi and Blood deficiency, second best from Phlegm-Fire and worst from Yin deficiency. The sooner the treatment is started after its onset, the better the results.

In general, the tongue is a good indicator of the prognosis: if it shows advanced signs of Yin deficiency, such as a Red, Thin and dry body with cracks, the prognosis is poor.

Generally speaking, the acupuncture and herbal treatment may be given in conjunction with Western medication. This is based either on anti-cholinergic agents which reduce tremor and/or L-Dopa to improve movement and reduce rigidity. After some weeks of treatment the dosage of the drugs could be reduced but this should be done very gradually.

As for prevention, this is obvious from what was said about the aetiology of this condition. Any person over 50 who suddenly develops symptoms such as dizziness, stiffness, and an increasing difficulty in walking, should immediately change their life-style by working less, never getting exhausted, taking more rest, avoiding emotional stress and reducing sexual activity.

END NOTES

1. Lou Ying 1565 Principles of Medicine (*Yi Xue Gang Mu* 医学纲目), cited in Wang Quan Yan "Observation on the treatment of 35 cases of Parkinson disease with Chinese medicine" in Journal of Chinese Medicine, vol. 27, no. 8, p. 24.

2. Zhu Ji Original Theory of Medicine (*Yi Xue Yuan Li* 医学原理), cited in ibid., p. 24.

Wind-stroke 27

中
风

The term Wind-stroke in Chinese medicine corresponds to four possible Western medical conditions:

- cerebral haemorrhage
- cerebral thrombosis
- cerebral embolism
- spasm of a cerebral vessel.

In Western medicine these four conditions come under the term "cerebro-vascular accident" (CVA), i.e. a pathological state of the blood vessels in the brain. The sudden neurological impairment caused by a CVA is called "apoplexy" in Western medicine and popularly referred to as "stroke".

Cerebral haemorrhage consists in bleeding from an intracerebral artery into the subarachnoid space.

Cerebral thrombosis is the total or partial obstruction of a cerebral artery by a thrombus with consequent infarction and anoxia of the surrounding tissue. A thrombus is a blood clot that forms in the lining of an artery and remains attached to its place of origin.

Cerebral embolism occurs when an embolus detaches from a thrombus and occludes a cerebral artery with consequent infarction and anoxia of the surrounding cerebral tissue. An embolus is a bubble of air or a piece of a thrombus that detaches from it, and travels along the arterial system, eventually occluding an artery.

Spasm of a cerebral vessel occurs when it temporarily contracts. This may also be due to a passing embolus which causes a temporary narrowing or obstruction of its lumen and therefore temporary anoxia of the surrounding cerebral tissue. This condition is the least severe of the four and is usually followed by complete recovery.

Aetiology and pathology

The aetiology of Wind-stroke is very complex as this condition, although it occurs suddenly, "brews up" over many years. There are four main aetiological factors.

1. OVERWORK, EMOTIONAL STRESS AND EXCESSIVE SEXUAL ACTIVITY

Working long hours under stressful conditions without adequate rest, emotional strain and excessive sexual activity, all lead to deficiency of Kidney-Yin. A combination of these three factors is the most common cause of Kidney-Yin deficiency in industrialized societies. Deficiency of Kidney-Yin often leads to deficiency of Liver-Yin and the rising of Liver-Yang. Liver-Yang, especially in the elderly, often gives rise to Liver-Wind. Liver-Wind causes apoplexy, coma, mental cloudiness and paralysis, and the tongue is Moving, Deviated or Stiff. There is also an interaction between internal and external Wind as the latter may stir up the former.

2. IRREGULAR DIET AND PHYSICAL OVERWORK

Eating irregularly or eating excessive amounts of fats, dairy foods, greasy, fried foods and sugar weakens the Spleen and leads to Phlegm, which predisposes to obesity. Eventually, Phlegm often combines with Fire to form Phlegm-Fire. Phlegm causes numbness in the limbs, mental cloudiness, slurred speech or aphasia, and a Swollen tongue with a sticky coating.

3. EXCESSIVE SEXUAL ACTIVITY AND INADEQUATE REST

Excessive sexual activity combined with inadequate rest weakens the Kidney-Essence and leads to Marrow deficiency. Marrow fails to nourish Blood and, eventually this may lead to stasis of Blood. Stasis of Blood causes stiffness and pain in the limbs and a Purple tongue.

4. PHYSICAL OVERWORK AND INADEQUATE REST

Physical overwork, such as excessive lifting or excessive exercise and sport activities, weakens the Spleen, the muscles and the channels. The pre-existing internal Wind exploits the deficiency of Qi and Blood in the channels to penetrate them. On the other hand, exposure to external Wind interacts with the internal Wind in the channels and this leads to paralysis of the limbs.

These four aetiological factors and their interactions are summarized in Figure 27.1.

Thus, the pathology of Wind-stroke may be summarized in only four words:

WIND — PHLEGM — FIRE — STASIS

These are the four pathogenic factors involved in the pathogenesis of Wind-stroke. They may not all be present but there must usually be at least three of them to cause Wind-stroke. Also, they may be present in different degrees of intensity giving rise to many different types of Wind-stroke.

Of course, these are only the pathogenic factors appearing in Wind-stroke. Besides these,

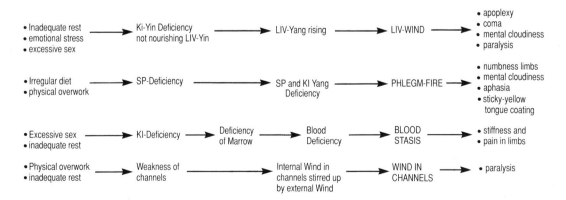

Fig. 27.1   The four aetiological factors in Wind-stroke

Table 27.1 Tongue appearance before Wind-stroke

Pathogenic factor	Tongue appearance
Wind	Stiff, Moving, Deviated, Quivering
Phlegm	Swollen, sticky coating
Fire	Red tongue body
Stasis	Reddish-Purple tongue body

there will also be some deficiency of Qi, Blood, or Yin, especially Kidney- and/or Liver-Yin.

The tongue appearance is an important indicator especially in the prevention of Wind-stroke. The four pathological factors and the way they are reflected on the tongue are summarized in Table 27.1.

The real value of tongue diagnosis in Wind-stroke lies in its preventive role. If an old person's tongue presents an appearance as in the above table, it strongly indicates at least the possibility of Wind-stroke. For example, the tongue may be Reddish-Purple, Stiff and Swollen, indicating Fire, Stasis, Wind and Phlegm, the four pathogenic factors of Wind-stroke.

Differentiation

The most important differentiation in Wind-stroke is between that which attacks the internal organs and channels and that which attacks only the channels. According to this distinction there are two types of Wind-stroke:

- *Severe type* which attacks the internal organs *and* the channels
- *Mild type* which attacks only the channels.

Wind-stroke from attack of the internal organs and channels is characterized by apoplexy, loss of consciousness, possibly coma, aphasia, paralysis and numbness. The distinguishing signs of attack of the internal organs by Wind are loss of consciousness, coma and aphasia.

Wind-stroke from attack of the channels alone is characterized by unilateral paralysis, numbness and slurred speech. There is no loss of consciousness or coma.

Following a severe type attack of Wind to the internal organs, a person who survives will enter the sequelae stage when the clinical manifestations are the same as in a mild type (attack of channels only), i.e. unilateral paralysis (hemiplegia), numbness and slurred speech. Thus, these manifestations may either arise independently from an attack of the channels alone, or they may be the sequelae of an attack of the internal organs.

The severe type (attack of internal organs and channels) is further divided into the Tense (or Closed) type and the Flaccid (or Open) type according to the clinical manifestations, as will be explained shortly.

The mild type (attack of channels alone) is further divided into an attack of the main channels, characterized by hemiplegia and numbness, and an attack of the Connecting channels alone characterized only by numbness.

This is summarized in Table 27.2.

ATTACK OF INTERNAL ORGANS (SEVERE TYPE)

As we have seen, attack of the internal organs and channels by Wind is characterized by apoplexy, loss of consciousness, possibly coma, aphasia, hemiplegia and numbness. The loss of consciousness indicates attack of the internal organs. There are two types of patterns: one called Tense (or Closed) corresponding to collapse of Yin, and the other called Flaccid (or Open) corresponding to collapse of Yang.

Table 27.2 Differentiation of Wind-stroke

Type	Internal organs and channels		Channels	
Manifestations	Apoplexy, coma, aphasia, hemiplegia		Hemiplegia, numbness	
Type	*Tense*	*Flaccid*	*Main*	*Connecting*
Manifestations	Collapse of Yin	Collapse of Yang	Hemiplegia, numbness	Numbness
Sequelae	Hemiplegia, numbness, slurred speech			

TENSE (OR CLOSED) TYPE

This corresponds to collapse of Yin.

CLINICAL MANIFESTATIONS

Sudden collapse, loss of consciousness, coma, clenched teeth, closed fists, lock-jaw, red face and ears, profuse sputum, rattling sound in the throat, coarse breathing, constipation, retention of urine.
Tongue: Red body, Stiff, Deviated, sticky-yellow coating.
Pulse: Wiry-Full-Rapid-Slippery.

FLACCID (OR OPEN) TYPE

This corresponds to collapse of Yang.

CLINICAL MANIFESTATIONS

Sudden collapse, loss of consciousness, coma, hands and mouth open, eyes closed, pale face, oily sweat beads on the forehead, incontinence of stools and urine, cold limbs.
Tongue: Pale, Swollen.
Pulse: Minute-Hidden-Scattered.

The manifestations determining the two types are shown in Table 27.3.

Table 27.3 Differentiation of Tense and Flaccid types in attack of the internal organs

Manifestations	Tense type	Flaccid type
Eyes	Open	Closed
Mouth	Clenched	Open
Hands	Clenched	Relaxed
Sweating	None	Oily sweat on forehead
Urine	Retention	Incontinence
Stools	Constipation	Incontinence
Tongue	Red, Stiff, Deviated, sticky-yellow coating	Pale, Swollen
Pulse	Wiry-Full-Rapid-Slippery	Minute-Hidden-Scattered
Treatment	Rescue Yin	Rescue Yang

SEQUELAE OF ATTACK OF THE INTERNAL ORGANS

Wind-stroke from attack of the internal organs (whether of the Tense or Flaccid type) always leaves sequelae if the patient survives. These consist primarily of:

– hemiplegia
– facial paralysis (deviation of eye and mouth)
– slurred speech
– numbness of limbs.

In prolonged cases there will also be contraction and stiffness of the limbs due to malnourishment of the channels.

ATTACK OF THE CHANNELS ALONE (MILD TYPE)

As we have seen, when only the channels are attacked there is no loss of consciousness or coma, but only unilateral paralysis of the limbs and deviation of eye and mouth. The clinical manifestations of attack of the channels alone are basically the same as during the sequelae stage of attack of the internal organs.

The clinical manifestations vary according to whether the main or Connecting channels are attacked.

ATTACK OF MAIN CHANNELS
CLINICAL MANIFESTATIONS

Facial paralysis, hemiplegia, numbness of limbs, limitation of movement, slurred speech (this is not always present).

ATTACK OF CONNECTING CHANNELS ONLY
CLINICAL MANIFESTATIONS

Unilateral numbness of face and limbs, slurred speech (this is not always present).

Treatment

The discussion of treatment will be structured as follows:

ATTACK OF THE INTERNAL ORGANS

Tense Type
Flaccid Type

ATTACK OF THE CHANNELS ALONE

Hemiplegia
Aphasia (or slurred speech)
Hypertension
Facial paralysis
Incontinence of stools and urine
Dizziness
Stiffness and contraction of the muscles

PATTERNS IN THE SEQUELAE STAGE

Wind-Phlegm
Damp-Phlegm
Stagnation of Qi and Blood
Yin Deficiency with Empty-Heat

ATTACK OF THE INTERNAL ORGANS

At this acute stage it is imperative that Chinese medicine be combined with Western medical treatment in hospital.

The general principles of treatment are:

1. Relieve spasm
2. Induce resuscitation
3. Lower blood pressure.

These are only the general aims of treatment; the more specific aims depend on the differentiation between the Tense and Flaccid types.

The acupuncture points which may be used for the above objectives are:

1. P-6 Neiguan, SP-6 Sanyinjiao, reducing method
2. Du-26 Renzhong, L.I.-4 Hegu, reducing method
3. L.I.-11 Quchi, ST-36 Zusanli, LIV-3 Taichong, KI-3 Taixi, reducing method except for KI-3 which should be reinforced.

Treatment should be given every 6 hours without retention of needles.

TENSE TYPE

TREATMENT PRINCIPLE

Induce resuscitation, relax spasm, clear Heat, subdue Wind, resolve Phlegm, open the orifices.

ACUPUNCTURE

Du-26 Renzhong, Du-20 Baihui, Du-16 Fengfu, G.B.-20 Fengchi, the 12 Well points of the hand, KI-1 Yongquan, P-7 Daling or P-8 Laogong, ST-40 Fenglong. All with reducing method.

Explanation

– **Du-26**, needled oblique upwards, promotes resuscitation.
– **Du-20** (needled horizontally forwards), **Du-16** and **G.B.-20** subdue internal Wind.
– **12 Well points of the hand**, with bleeding method, subdue Wind and clear Heat.
– **KI-1** subdues Wind, lowers blood pressure and relaxes spasm.
– **P-7** or **P-8** open the orifices and clear Heat.
– **ST-40** resolves Phlegm.

Variations

Other points according to symptoms and signs:

– *Lock-jaw:* ST-6 Jiache, ST-7 Xiaguan and L.I.-4 Hegu.
– *Profuse sputum:* Ren-22 Tiantu, ST-40 Fenglong with reducing method.
– *Aphasia:* Ren-23 Lianquan, HE-5 Tongli.

HERBAL TREATMENT

Prescription

LING JIAO GOU TENG TANG Variation
Cornu Antelopis-Uncaria Decoction
Ling Yang Jiao *Cornu Antelopis* 4.5 g
Gou Teng *Ramulus Uncariae* 9 g
Ju Hua *Flos Chrysanthemi morifolii* 9 g
Xia Ku Cao *Spica Prunellae vulgaris* 6 g
Chan Tui *Periostracum Cicadae* 6 g
Bai Shao *Radix Paeoniae albae* 9 g

Gui Ban *Plastrum Testudinis* 15 g
Shi Jue Ming *Concha Haliotidis* 15 g
Sheng Di Huang *Radix Rehmanniae glutinosae* 15 g
Mu Dan Pi *Cortex Moutan radicis* 6 g
Chuan Bei Mu *Bulbus Fritillariae cirrhosae* 12 g
Zhu Ru *Caulis Bambusae in Taeniis* 15 g
Gan Cao *Radix Glycyrrhizae uralensis* 2.5 g

Explanation

– **Ling Yang Jiao**, **Gou Teng**, **Ju Hua**, **Xia Ku Cao** and **Chan Tui** subdue internal Wind and clear Heat.
– **Bai Shao**, **Gui Ban** and **Shi Jue Ming** nourish Yin and sink Yang.
– **Sheng Di** and **Mu Dan Pi** clear Heat and cool Blood.
– **Chuan Bei Mu** and **Zhu Ru** clear Heat and resolve Phlegm.

Variations

– If Phlegm is predominant add Ban Xia *Rhizoma Pinelliae ternatae*, Gua Lou *Semen Trichosanthis* and Dan Nan Xing *Rhizoma Arisaematis praeparata*.
– If there is coma from Phlegm add Yu Jin *Tuber Curcumae* and Shi Chang Pu *Rhizoma Acori graminei*.

(a) Patent remedy

XI HUANG WAN
Rhinoceros-Calculus Bovis Pill
Niu Huang *Calculus Bovis*
She Xiang *Secretio Moschus moschiferi*
Ru Xiang *Gummi Olibanum*
Mo Yao *Myrrha*

Explanation

This pill used to contain rhino horn (hence its name), but this has now been replaced by musk (She Xiang). This remedy opens the orifices, clears Heat, moves Blood and resolves Fire-Poison and can be used for the acute stage of the severe-tense type of Wind-stroke.

(b) Patent remedy

WAN SHI NIU HUANG QING XIN WAN
Wan's Calculus Bovis Clearing the Heart Pill
Niu Huang *Calculus Bovis*
Zhi Zi *Fructus Gardeniae jasminoidis*
Huang Lian *Rhizoma Coptidis*
Huang Qin *Radix Scutellariae baicalensis*
Yu Jin *Tuber Curcumae*
Zhu Sha *Cinnabaris*

Explanation

This remedy opens the orifices and drains Fire. It is suitable for the acute stage of the severe-tense type of Wind-stroke. It is more potent at draining Fire than the previous remedy.

FLACCID TYPE

TREATMENT PRINCIPLE

Recapture Yang, induce resuscitation.

ACUPUNCTURE

Ren-6 Qihai, Ren-4 Guanyuan, Ren-8 Shenque, ST-36 Zusanli, SP-6 Sanyinjiao, P-6 Neiguan, Du-4 Mingmen, BL-23 Shenshu. Reinforcing method and strong moxibustion.

Explanation

– **Ren-6**, **Ren-4** and **Ren-8**, with moxa, recapture Yang. Ren-6 and Ren-4 are best used with moxa cones on a slice of aconite (which is itself a herb to recapture Yang). Moxa cones are applied to Ren-8 after filling the umbilicus with salt.
– **ST-36**, **SP-6** and **P-6** strengthen Heart-Yang to relieve collapse of Yang.
– **Du-4** and **BL-23**, with moxa, strengthen the Fire of the Gate of Vitality also to relieve collapse of Yang.

In some cases the distinction between Tense and Flaccid type may not be clear or the pattern may change from Tense to Flaccid or vice versa.

In such cases, Du-26 Renzhong, ST-36 Zusanli, SP-6 Sanyinjiao, Yintang and P-6 should be needled with even method to induce resuscitation and subdue Wind.

HERBAL TREATMENT

Prescription

SHEN FU TANG and SHENG MAI SAN
Ginseng-Aconitum Decoction and *Generating the Pulse Powder*
Mai Men Dong *Tuber Ophiopogonis japonici* 9 g
Wu Wei Zi *Fructus Schisandrae chinensis* 3 g
Ren Shen *Radix Ginseng* 9 g
Fu Zi *Radix Aconiti carmichaeli praeparata* 6 g

Explanation

- **Mai Dong**, **Wu Wei Zi** and **Ren Shen** tonify Qi and Yin.
- **Fu Zi** recaptures Yang.

Variations

- If there is profuse sweating add Huang Qi *Radix Astragali membranacei*, Long Gu *Os Draconis*, Mu Li *Concha Ostreae* and Shan Zhu Yu *Fructus Corni officinalis*.

ATTACK OF THE CHANNELS ALONE

The treatment for attack of the channels only is exactly the same as for the sequelae stage of attack of the internal organs. During the acute stage of Wind-stroke from attack of the internal organs, Chinese medicine plays only a secondary role to Western medicine; during the sequelae stage, or in attack of the channels alone, Chinese medicine plays a primary role. Acupuncture in particular gives excellent results in the treatment of hemiplegia and facial paralysis. The time factor, however, is very important: best results are obtained if treatment is given within one month of the attack. More than six months after its occurrence treatment becomes increasingly difficult.

Normally paralysis of the leg responds to treatment better than that of the arm, and large joints respond better than small joints.

The general principles of treatment are:

1. Remove obstructions from the channels
2. Subdue Wind and resolve Phlegm
3. Invigorate the Connecting channels
4. Regulate the circulation of Qi and Blood in the channels.

The next section of this chapter deals with the treatment of the following specific symptoms appearing after an attack of the channels:

- Hemiplegia
- Aphasia (or slurred speech)
- Hypertension
- Facial paralysis (deviation of eye and mouth)
- Incontinence of stools and urine
- Dizziness
- Rigidity and contraction of the muscles.

This is followed by a discussion of the treatment of some underlying conditions frequently seen during the sequelae stage of Wind-stroke.

HEMIPLEGIA

Hemiplegia is caused by obstruction of the channels by Wind and Phlegm. Pronounced stiffness of the joints and contraction of the muscles indicates stasis of Blood. The pathogenic factors obstruct the channels against a background of Qi, Blood or Yin deficiency.

Zhu Dan Xi (1281-1358), in his book "The Essential Methods of Dan Xi", makes an interesting distinction according to whether the left or right side is affected:

Wind-stroke is mostly due to Blood deficiency and Phlegm. One must first resolve Phlegm and then nourish and move Blood . . . Hemiplegia is due to Phlegm [in general]: if the left side is affected, it is due to Blood deficiency and stasis; if the right side is affected, it is due to Phlegm, Fire and Qi deficiency.[1]

In treating unilateral paralysis of the limbs, generally more points from Yang channels are selected because Yang corresponds to movement and agility.

In general, the points of the affected (paralysed side) are chosen and they are needled with reducing method if within one month of the stroke, or with even method if more than one month has elapsed. The points are reduced because it is Wind and Phlegm in the channels that cause the paralysis. Relatively thick needles must be used, i.e. at least 0.34 mm in diameter. It is essential to obtain a good needling sensation and it is even better if this propagates down the channel.

Under a different method, the duration of the condition determines the side of needling, distinguishing between a condition of under three months or over three months' duration.

If the Wind-stroke occurred within the last three months, the points of the paralysed side are needled with reducing method and the corresponding points of the healthy side are needled with reinforcing method. This is because in the first few weeks after the stroke, the channels of the affected side are in a Full condition, i.e. they are obstructed by Wind and Phlegm. The channels of the healthy side are in a relatively Empty condition.

If the Wind-stroke occurred more than three months previously, the points of the affected side are needled with reinforcing method and moxa, and the corresponding points of the healthy side with reducing method. This is because, after three months, the pathogenic factors (Wind and Phlegm) in the channels of the paralysed side have moved deeper and also moved on to the healthy side. Also, obstruction of the channels of the affected side by pathogenic factors leads to malnourishment of the channels. Thus, the channels of the affected side are empty in relation to those of the healthy side.

In any case, the points chosen consist of two groups: one of general points to subdue Wind, and one of points to remove obstruction from the channels. The points to subdue Wind in general are:

- **Du-26** Renzhong, **Du-20** Baihui and **BL-7** Tongtian.

The points to remove obstructions from the channels are:

Paralysis of the arm: L.I.-15 Jianyu, T.B.-14 Jianliao, L.I.-11 Quchi, L.I.-10 Shousanli, T.B.-5 Waiguan, L.I.-4 Hegu, T.B.-3 Zhongzhu, S.I.-3 Houxi.

Paralysis of the leg: BL-23 Shenshu, G.B.-30 Huantiao (a very important point for this condition), G.B.-29 Juliao, ST-31 Biguan, G.B.-31 Fengshi, ST-32 Futu, BL-40 Weizhong, G.B.-34 Yanglingquan, ST-36 Zusanli, BL-57 Chengshan, G.B.-39 Xuanzhong, ST-41 Jiexi, BL-60 Kunlun, G.B.-40 Qiuxu.

Only three or four points should be used each time for each limb. The points are also selected according to the joint involved. They should be needled rather deep and intramuscular penetration of two points with one needle is often used. For example:

L.I.-15 Jianyu to L.I.-14 Binao
ST-36 Zusanli to ST-37 Shangjuxu
T.B.-5 Waiguan to P-6 Neiguan
L.I.-11 Quchi to HE-3 Shaohai
G.B.-34 Yanglingquan to SP-9 Yinlingquan
G.B.-39 Xuanzhong to SP-6 Sanyinjiao

Although more Yang points are used, points from the Yin channels should not be overlooked. Yin points are particularly indicated in conditions of more than six months' duration where there is pronounced stiffness and contraction of the limbs.

HERBAL TREATMENT

Treatment principle

Tonify Qi, move Blood, remove obstructions from the channels and invigorate the Connecting channels.

1. Prescription

BU YANG HAI WU TANG
Tonify Yang and Restore the ⁵/₁₀th Decoction
Huang Qi *Radix Astragali membranacei* 18 g
Dang Gui Wei *Radix Angelicae sinensis* ("tails") 6 g
Chuan Xiong *Radix Ligustici wallichii* 3 g
Tao Ren *Semen Persicae* 3 g
Hong Hua *Flos Carthami tinctorii* 3 g
Chi Shao Yao *Radix Paeoniae rubrae* 4.5 g
Di Long *Pheretima aspergillum* 3 g

Explanation

- **Huang Qi** is the emperor herb to strongly tonify Qi. It is used here for stasis of Blood from Qi deficiency.
- **Dang Gui Wei, Chuan Xiong, Tao Ren, Hong Hua** and **Chi Shao** move Blood.
- **Di Long** expels Wind and removes obstructions from the channels.

This formula is for stasis of Blood and Wind in the channels against a background of Qi deficiency.

2. Prescription

DA QIN JIAO TANG Variation
Great Gentiana macrophylla Decoction
Qin Jiao *Radix Gentianae macrophyllae* 9 g
Qiang Huo *Radix et Rhizoma Notopterygii* 6 g
Fang Feng *Radix Ledebouriellae sesloidis* 6 g
Bai Zhi *Radix Angelicae dahuricae* 4 g
Xi Xin *Herba Asari cum radice* 1.5 g
Dang Gui *Radix Angelicae sinensis* 6 g
Sheng Di Huang *Radix Rehmanniae glutinosae* 9 g
Chuan Xiong *Radix Ligustici wallichii* 4 g
Chi Shao Yao *Radix Paeoniae rubrae* 6 g
Bai Zhu *Rhizoma Atractylodis macrocephalae* 6 g
Fu Ling *Sclerotium Poriae cocos* 6 g
Shi Gao *Gypsum fibrosum* 15 g
Huang Qin *Radix Scutellariae baicalensis* 4 g
Bai Fu Zi *Rhizoma Thyphonii gigantei* 3 g
Quan Xie *Buthus Martensi* 1.5 g
Gan Cao *Radix Glycyrrhizae uralensis* 3 g

Explanation

- **Qin Jiao, Qiang Huo, Fang Feng, Bai Zhi** and **Xi Xin** release the Exterior and expel Wind.
- **Sheng Di, Dang Gui, Chuan Xiong** and **Chi Shao** harmonize Blood, according to the principle "harmonize Blood in order to extinguish Wind".
- **Bai Zhu** and **Fu Ling** drain Dampness.
- **Shi Gao** and **Huang Qin** clear Heat.
- **Bai Fu Zi** and **Quan Xie** expel Wind from the channels and invigorate the Connecting channels.

This formula is used for Wind in the channels against a background of Blood deficiency.

3. Prescription

ZHEN GAN XI FENG TANG
Pacifying the Liver and Subduing Wind Decoction
Dai Zhe Shi *Haematitum* 15 g
Long Gu *Os Draconis* 12 g
Mu Li *Concha Ostreae* 12 g
Gui Ban *Plastrum Testudinis* 12 g
Huai Niu Xi *Radix Achyrantis bidentatae* 15 g
Xuan Shen *Radix Scrophulariae ningpoensis* 12 g
Tian Men Dong *Tuber Asparagi cochinchinensis* 12 g
Bai Shao *Radix Paeoniae albae* 12 g
Tian Ma *Rhizoma Gastrodiae elatae* 12 g
Gou Teng *Ramulus Uncariae* 9 g
Ju Hua *Flos Chrysanthemi morifolii* 6 g
Dan Nan Xing *Rhizoma Arisaematis praeparata* 12 g
Zhu Ru *Caulis Bambusae in Taeniis* 6 g
Zhe Bei Mu *Bulbus Fritillariae thunbergii* 6 g
Gan Cao *Radix Glycyrrhizae uralensis* 6 g

Explanation

- **Long Gu, Mu Li, Gui Ban** and **Dai Zhe Shi** subdue Liver-Yang and Liver-Wind
- **Niu Xi** attracts Blood downwards
- **Tian Ma, Gou Teng** and **Ju Hua** subdue Wind
- **Nan Xing, Zhu Ru** and **Bei Mu** resolve Phlegm-Heat.

This prescription is used to expel Wind and Phlegm from the channels in hemiplegia with a background of Yin deficiency.

Variations

- If symptoms of Wind in the channels are pronounced add Quan Xie *Buthus Martensi* and Wu Shao She *Zaocys Dhumnades*.
- If the leg is affected add Sang Ji Sheng *Ramulus Loranthi*.
- If the arm is affected add Gui Zhi *Ramulus Cinnamomi cassiae* and Sang Zhi *Ramulus Mori albae*.
- If the limb is swollen add Fu Ling *Sclerotium Poriae cocos*, Ze Xie *Rhizoma Alismatis orientalis*, Yi Yi Ren *Semen Coicis lachryma jobi* and Fang Ji *Radix Stephaniae tetrandae*.

- If there is slurred speech add Yu Jin *Tuber Curcumae*, Shi Chang Pu *Rhizoma Acori graminei* and Yuan Zhi *Radix Polygalae tenuifoliae*.
- If there is facial paralysis add Bai Fu Zi *Rhizoma Thyphonii gigantei*, Quan Xie *Buthus Martensi* and Jiang Can *Bombyx batryticatus*.
- If numbness is pronounced add Chen Pi *Pericarpium Citri reticulatae*, Ban Xia *Rhizoma Pinelliae ternatae*, Fu Ling *Sclerotium Poriae cocos* and Dan Nan Xing *Rhizoma Arisaematis praeparata*.
- If there is constipation add Huo Ma Ren *Semen Cannabis sativae*, Yu Li Ren *Semen Pruni* and Rou Cong Rong *Herba Cistanchis*.

(a) Patent remedy

REN SHEN ZAI ZAO WAN
Ginseng Renewal Pill
Ren Shen *Radix Ginseng*
Huang Qi *Radix Astragali membranacei*
Shu Di Huang *Radix Rehmanniae glutinosae praeparata*
Shou Wu *Radix Polygoni multiflori*
Gui Ban *Plastrum Testudinis*
Hu Gu *Os Tigris*
Gu Sui Bu *Rhizoma Gusuibu*
Quan Xie *Buthus Martensi*
Di Long *Pheretima aspergillum*
Tian Ma *Rhizoma Gastrodiae elatae*
Jiang Can *Bombyx batryticatus*
Qi She Rou *Agkistrodon*
Sang Ji Sheng *Ramus Loranthi*
Bi Xie *Rhizoma Dioscoreae hypoglaucae*
Song Jie *Lignum Pini nodi*
Wei Ling Xian *Radix Clematidis chinensis*
Ma Huang *Herba Ephedrae*
Xi Xin *Herba Asari cum radice*
Fang Feng *Radix Ledebouriellae sesloidis*
Qiang Huo *Radix et Rhizoma Notopterygii*
Bai Zhi *Radix Angelicae dahuricae*
Ge Gen *Radix Puerariae*
Qing Pi *Pericarpium Citri reticulatae viridae*
Ding Xiang *Flos Caryophylli*
Xuan Shen *Radix Scrophulariae ningpoensis*
Da Huang *Rhizoma Rhei*
Hong Qu *Semen Oryzae cum Monasco*

Huang Lian *Rhizoma Coptidis*
Zhu Sha *Cinnabaris*
Tan Xiang *Lignum Santali albi*
Jiang Huang *Rhizoma Curcumae longae*
Huo Xiang *Herba Agastachis*
Chi Shao *Radix Paeoniae rubrae*
Fu Zi *Radix Aconiti carmichaeli praeparata*
Rou Gui *Cortex Cinnamomi cassiae*
Chuan Xiong *Radix Ligustici wallichii*
Chen Xiang *Lignum Aquilariae*
Wu Yao *Radix Linderae strychnifoliae*
Xiang Fu *Rhizoma Cyperi rotundi*
Xue Jie *Sanguis draconis*
Ru Xiang *Gummi Olibanum*
Mo Yao *Myrrha*
San Qi *Radix Notoginseng*
Dang Gui *Radix Angelicae sinensis*
Chen Pi *Pericarpium Citri reticulatae*
Bai Zhu *Rhizoma Atractylodis macrocephalae*
Fu Ling *Sclerotium Poriae cocos*
Gan Cao *Radix Glycyrrhizae uralensis*
Dou Kou *Semen Alpiniae katsumadai*
Shen Qu *Massa Fermentata Medicinalis*
Niu Huang *Calculus Bovis*
Shui Niu Jiao *Cornu Bufali*
Tian Zhu Huang *Secretio Siliceae Bambusae*
Bing Pian *Borneol*
She Xiang *Secretio Moschus moschiferi*

Explanation

This pill, which has a large number of ingredients, tonifies Qi and Blood, eliminates stagnation, subdues internal Wind and removes obstructions from the channels.

It can be used for the sequelae stage of Windstroke to treat paralysis of a limb and slurred speech or aphasia.

The tongue presentation appropriate to this remedy is a Pale and Stiff body.

(b) Patent remedy

ZAI ZAO WAN
Renewal Pill
Chen Xiang *Lignum Aquilariae*
Hu Gu *Os Tigris*
Ren Shen *Radix Ginseng*

Mo Yao *Myrrha*
She Xiang *Secretio Moschus moschiferi*
Dang Gui *Radix Angelicae sinensis*
Niu Huang *Calculus Bovis*
Shui Niu Jiao *Cornu Bufali*
Huang Qi *Radix Astragali membranacei*
Rou Gui *Cortex Cinnamomi cassiae*
Xue Jie *Sanguis Draconis*
Tian Ma *Rhizoma Gastrodiae elatae*
Hong Hua *Flos Carthami tinctorii*
Wu Shao She *Zaocys Dhumnades*
Sheng Di Huang *Radix Rehmanniae glutinosae*
Bai Dou Kou *Fructus Amomi cardamomi*
Fang Feng *Radix Ledebouriellae sesloidis*
Chuan Xiong *Radix Ligustici wallichii*

Explanation

This remedy eliminates stagnation, moves Blood and subdues Wind. It is used for hemiplegia and facial paralysis following Wind-stroke.

The tongue presentation appropriate to this remedy is a Purple and Stiff body.

(c) Patent remedy

REN SHEN ZAI ZAO WAN (2)
Ginseng Renewal Pill
Chuan Shan Jia *Squama Manitis pentadactylae*
Wu Shao She *Zaocys Dhumnades*
Quan Xie *Buthus Martensi*
Ren Shen *Radix Ginseng*
Hu Po *Succinum*
Hu Gu *Os Tigris*
Tian Ma *Rhizoma Gastrodiae elatae*
Shui Niu Jiao *Cornu Bufali*
Niu Huang *Calculus Bovis*

Explanation

This pill has the same name as remedy (a) above, but it has different ingredients. It is specific to subdue internal Wind after Wind-stroke and is therefore used to treat hemiplegia, facial paralysis and aphasia when internal Wind predominates over Phlegm or stasis of Blood.

The tongue presentation appropriate to this remedy is a Stiff and Deviated body.

(d) Patent remedy

DA HUO LUO DAN
Great Invigorating the Connecting Channels Pill
An Xi Xiang *Benzonium*
Bing Pian *Borneol*
Cao Wu Tou *Radix Aconiti carmichaeli*
Chen Xiang *Lignum Aquilariae*
Chi Shao *Radix Paeoniae rubrae*
Chuan Niu Xi *Radix Cyathulae*
Chuan Xiong *Radix Ligustici wallichii*
Da Huang *Rhizoma Rhei*
Dang Gui *Radix Angelicae sinensis*
Di Long *Pheretima aspergillum*
Ding Xiang *Flos Caryophylli*
Cao Dou Kou *Semen Alpiniae katsumadae*
Fang Feng *Radix Ledebouriellae sesloidis*
Fu Ling *Sclerotium Poriae cocos*
Gan Cao *Radix Glycyrrhizae uralensis*
Ge Gen *Radix Puerariae*
Gu Sui Bu *Rhizoma Gusuibu*
Guan Zhong *Radix seu Herba Potentillae*
Gui Ban *Plastrum Testudinis*
Shou Wu *Radix Polygoni multiflori*
Hu Gu *Os Tigris*
Huang Lian *Rhizoma Coptidis*
Huang Qin *Radix Scutellariae baicalensis*
Huo Xiang *Herba Agastachis*
Jiang Can *Bombyx batryticatus*
Ma Huang *Herba Ephedrae*
Mo Yao *Myrrha*
Mu Xiang *Radix Saussureae*
Niu Huang *Calculus Bovis*
Qi She *Agkistrodon acutus*
Qiang Huo *Radix et Rhizoma Notopterygii*
Qing Pi *Pericarpium Citri reticulatae viridae*
Ren Shen *Radix Ginseng*
Rou Gui *Cortex Cinnamomi cassiae*
Ru Xiang *Gummi Olibanum*
She Xiang *Secretio Moschus moschiferi*
Shu Di Huang *Radix Rehmanniae glutinosae praeparata*
Song Xiang *Resina Pini praeparata*
Tian Ma *Rhizoma Gastrodiae elatae*
Dan Nan Xing *Rhizoma Arisaematis praeparata*
Wei Ling Xian *Radix Clematidis chinensis*
Wu Shao She *Zaocys dhumnades*
Wu Yao *Radix Lynderae strychnifoliae*
Shui Niu Jiao *Cornu Bufali*

Xi Xin *Herba Asari cum radice*
Xiang Fu *Rhizoma Cyperi rotundi*
Xuan Shen *Radix Scrophulariae ningpoensis*
Xue Jie *Sanguis draconis*

Explanation

This pill removes obstructions from the channels, moves Blood and expels Wind-Dampness. It is mainly used for Painful Obstruction Syndrome in the elderly but can also be used for hemiplegia and numbness of the limbs after Wind-stroke.

The tongue presentation appropriate to this remedy is a Purple and Swollen body.

APHASIA (OR SLURRED SPEECH)

The main acupuncture points are:

- **Ren-23** Lianquan to ease the throat and promote speech.
- **HE-5** Tongli to resolve Phlegm and open the orifices. The Heart controls the tongue and speech.
- **KI-6** Zhaohai to benefit the throat.

These points are needled with reducing method if the Wind-stroke occurred within one month and even method if more than a month has elapsed.

HERBAL TREATMENT

Prescription

JIE YU DAN
Relaxing Speech Pill
Tian Ma *Rhizoma Gastrodiae elatae* 6 g
Quan Xie *Buthus Martensi* 1.5 g
Dan Nan Xing *Rhizoma Arisaematis praeparata* 6 g
Bai Fu Zi *Rhizoma Thyphonii gigantei* 3 g
Yuan Zhi *Radix Polygalae tenuifoliae* 6 g
Shi Chang Pu *Rhizoma Acori graminei* 6 g
Mu Xiang *Radix Saussureae* 4 g
Qiang Huo *Radix et Rhizoma Notopterygii* 3 g

Explanation

- **Tian Ma, Quan Xie, Nan Xing** and **Bai Fu Zi**

pacify the Liver, subdue Wind and resolve Phlegm.
- **Yuan Zhi, Chang Pu** and **Mu Xiang** open the orifices.
- **Qiang Huo** expels Wind.

HYPERTENSION

If the blood pressure is raised, it is important to take measures to lower it, as this can be a predisposing factor for further strokes.

A general prescription to lower the blood pressure after a stroke is:

- **L.I.-4** Hegu and **LIV-3** Taichong with reducing method to subdue Liver-Yang and Liver-Wind.
- **KI-3** Taixi with reinforcing method to tonify Kidney- and Liver-Yin.
- **ST-9** Renying as an empirical point to reduce blood pressure.

Another combination of points is ST-36 Zusanli and G.B.-39 Xuanzhong with moxibustion.

Another method to reduce blood pressure consists in tapping the following points with a plum-blossom needle:

- **ST-9** Renying, **P-6** Neiguan and **SP-6** Sanyinjiao.

HERBAL TREATMENT

Prescription

TIAN MA GOU TENG YIN
Gastrodia-Uncaria Decoction
Tian Ma *Rhizoma Gastrodiae elatae* 9 g
Gou Teng *Ramulus Uncariae* 9 g
Shi Jue Ming *Concha Haliotidis* 6 g
Sang Ji Sheng *Ramulus Loranthi* 9 g
Du Zhong *Radix Eucommiae ulmoidis* 9 g
Chuan Niu Xi *Radix Cyathulae* 9 g
Shan Zhi Zi *Fructus Gardeniae jasminoidis* 6 g
Huang Qin *Radix Scutellariae baicalensis* 9 g
Yi Mu Cao *Herba Leonori heterophylli* 9 g
Ye Jiao Teng *Caulis Polygoni multiflori* 9 g
Fu Shen *Sclerotium Poriae cocos* 6 g

Explanation

This formula has already been explained in the chapter on Headaches (ch. 1).

FACIAL PARALYSIS

The facial paralysis following a stroke is called central facial paralysis in Western medicine as it arises from the central nervous system. Peripheral facial paralysis occurring without a stroke is due to injury of the peripheral nerves alone. In facial paralysis following Wind-stroke the nerves above the eyes are not affected, i.e. the movement of the eyebrows and furrowing of the forehead are normal. In peripheral facial paralysis the patient will only be able to move one eyebrow when trying to frown and furrowing of the forehead will not occur on the paralysed side. In other words, the two most prominent signs in facial paralysis following a stroke are deviation of an eye and the mouth.

Although the aetiology of central and peripheral facial paralysis is different, treatment with Chinese medicine is similar for both. Thus, the treatment recommended here for facial paralysis following a stroke applies also to peripheral facial paralysis (Bell's palsy). From a Chinese perspective, facial paralysis following a stroke is due to internal Wind, whilst Bell's palsy is due to external Wind.

On examination, one should ask the patient to close the eyes, bulge the cheeks, grin and whistle in order for the site and extent of paralysis to be ascertained. The eye on the paralysed side will not close completely, the mouth will deviate towards the unaffected side, and the lips on the paralysed side will not move on attempting to grin. This will also provide a guideline for the selection of local points (Fig. 27.2).

The treatment of facial paralysis is based on distal and local points. The distal points are needled with reducing method if the paralysis is of less than one month's duration and even method if it has persisted longer. For very prolonged cases moxa with small cones may be used and also cupping on the cheek with small cups.

Only one distal point and three to five local ones on the paralysed side are normally selected.

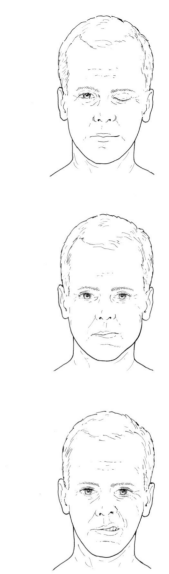

Fig. 27.2   Examination in facial paralysis

DISTAL POINTS

The two most common distal points are **L.I.-4** Hegu or **T.B.-5** Waiguan depending on the channel principally involved.

The combination of **L.I.-4** Hegu and **LIV-3** Taichong called the "Four Gates" expels Wind from the face.

LOCAL POINTS

The most commonly used local points are:

- **G.B.-14** Yangbai horizontal downwards.
- **BL-2** Zanzhu horizontal downwards or towards Yuyao.
- **Yuyao** horizontal towards BL-2 Zanzhu.
- **T.B.-23** Sizhukong towards Yuyao.
- **G.B.-1** Tongziliao towards Yuyao.
- **ST-2** Sibai horizontal downwards.
- **S.I.-18** Quanliao horizontal towards L.I.-20 Yingxiang.
- **L.I.-20** Yingxiang horizontal towards S.I.-18 Quanliao.
- **ST-7** Xiaguan horizontal towards ST-4 Dicang.
- **ST-6** Jiache oblique towards ST-4 Dicang.
- **ST-4** Dicang horizontal towards ST-6 Jiache.
- **L.I.-19** Heliao horizontal towards L.I.-20 Yingxiang.
- **Ren-24** Chengjiang horizontal towards ST-4 Dicang.
- **Du-26** Renzhong horizontal towards L.I.-19 Heliao.

ADJACENT POINTS

- **T.B.-17** Yifeng oblique towards the opposite eye, deep puncture (at least 1 *cun*). Some doctors say that if this point is needled deep enough with a good needling sensation, other local points are unnecessary. They say this point should be used if there is tenderness on the mastoid process.
- **G.B.-20** Fengchi oblique towards the eye on the same side.

An empirical method for the treatment of facial paralysis consists of pricking certain points inside the cheek. These are nine extra points between the rows of teeth arranged in three rows of three points each with 0.2 *cun* between each row and 0.2 *cun* between points in each row (Fig. 27.3).

These points are pricked to cause slight bleeding and then cupping is applied to the cheek (outside). The points are pricked from top to bottom and from left to right.

HERBAL TREATMENT

Prescription

QIAN ZHENG SAN

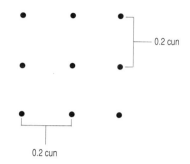

0.2 cun

0.2 cun

Fig. 27.3 Empirical points for facial paralysis

Pulling the Upright Powder
Bai Fu Zi *Rhizoma Thyphonii gigantei* 6 g
Jiang Can *Bombyx batryticatus* 6 g
Quan Xie *Buthus Martensi* 1.5 g

Explanation

- **Bai Fu Zi** expels Wind from the channels, specifically reaches the face, resolves Phlegm and invigorates the Connecting channels.
- **Jiang Can** and **Quan Xie** expel Wind from the channels, resolve Phlegm and resolve paralysis.

In facial paralysis the facial muscles are pulled towards the healthy side, hence the name of the formula, i.e. to pull the muscles of the healthy side straight.

Variations

- If there is a tic add Tian Ma *Rhizoma Gastrodiae elatae*, Gou Teng *Ramulus Uncariae* and Shi Jue Ming *Concha Haliotidis*.

(a) Patent remedy

Both Zai Zao Wan *Renewal Pill* and Ren Shen Zai Zao Wan *Ginseng Renewal Pill*, mentioned above, are suitable to treat facial paralysis following a stroke.

(b) Patent remedy

TIAN MA QU FENG BU PIAN
Gastrodia Expelling Wind and Tonifying Tablet
Tian Ma *Rhizoma Gastrodiae elatae*
Dang Gui *Radix Angelicae sinensis*

Sheng Di Huang *Radix Rehmanniae glutinosae*
Rou Gui *Cortex Cinnamomi cassiae*
Huai Niu Xi *Radix Achyranthis bidentatae*
Du Zhong *Cortex Eucommiae ulmoidis*
Qiang Huo *Radix et Rhizoma Notopterygii*
Bai Fu Zi *Rhizoma Typhonii gigantei*

Explanation

This tablet nourishes Liver and Kidneys and subdues internal Wind. It is particularly good for treating facial paralysis in elderly people with an underlying deficiency of Liver and Kidneys.

The tongue presentation appropriate to this remedy is a Red body without coating.

INCONTINENCE OF STOOLS AND URINE

A general prescription for incontinence of both stools and urine is:

– BL-33 Zhongliao, BL-25 Dachangshu, Ren-6 Qihai, Ren-4 Guanyuan and SP-6 Sanyinjiao.

The needling sensation from BL-33 should propagate to the pelvic cavity and that from Ren-4 and Ren-6 downwards towards the genitals.

In addition to the above points, one can also use Du-4 Mingmen and BL-23 Shenshu to strengthen the Fire of the Gate of Vitality because Kidney-Yang controls both lower orifices (i.e. urethra and anus).

DIZZINESS

Dizziness is a common symptom after a stroke. The results in treating hemiplegia will be better if the dizziness is tackled at the same time. Dizziness after a Wind-stroke is due to Liver-Wind.

The main points to use are:

– LIV-3 Taichong and BL-18 Ganshu, with reducing method, to subdue Liver-Wind.
– BL-23 Shenshu, KI-3 Taixi and Ren-4 Guanyuan, with reinforcing method, to nourish the Kidneys.

– Du-20 Baihui and G.B.-20 Fengchi to subdue internal Wind.

STIFFNESS AND CONTRACTION OF THE MUSCLES

In the late stages of sequelae of Wind-stroke the muscles become rigid and contracted and the joints stiff. Eventually, the lack of movement leads to atrophy of the muscles and malnourishment of tendons and channels. Physiotherapy is an essential part of the treatment in such cases.

Acupuncture points from Yang channels are usually chosen and moxa on needle must be used when there is atrophy of the muscles.

The main points used are:

Shoulder joint

– **L.I.-15** Jianyu oblique towards L.I.-14 Binao.

Elbow joint

– **L.I.-11** Quchi towards HE-3 Shaohai.

Finger joints

– **L.I.-3** Sanjian at least 1 *cun* towards S.I.-3 Houxi.
– **S.I.-3** Houxi at least 1 *cun* towards L.I.-3 Sanjian.

General points to subdue Wind may be added such as:

– L.I.-4 Hegu, LIV-3 Taichong, T.B.-17 Yifeng and G.B.-20 Fengchi.

If the muscles of the lateral side of the leg are contracted and stiff, KI-6 Zhaohai should be reinforced and BL-62 Shenmai reduced, i.e. the Yin Heel Vessel should be tonified and the Yang Heel Vessel sedated. The reverse should be done if the muscles of the medial side of the leg are contracted and stiff.

Although mainly Yang points are chosen, Yin points should not be overlooked. They are especially useful in long-standing cases with malnourishment of channels and sinews and consequent rigidity and stiffness. The main ones are:

- **HE-1** Jiquan for the shoulder joint.
- **LU-5** Chize and **P-3** Quze for the elbow joint.
- **P-6** Neiguan for the finger joints.
- **SP-12** Chongmen for the hip joint.
- **LIV-8** Ququan for the knee joint.
- **SP-5** Shangqiu and **KI-3** Taixi for the toe joints.

HERBAL TREATMENT

Prescription

HUO LUO XIAO LING DAN
Miraculously Effective Invigorating the Connecting Channels Pill
Dang Gui *Radix Angelicae sinensis* 15 g
Dan Shen *Radix Salviae miltiorrhizae* 15 g
Ru Xiang *Gummi Olibanum* 15 g
Mo Yao *Myrrha* 15 g

Explanation

- **Dang Gui** nourishes and moves Blood.
- **Dan Shen**, **Ru Xiang** and **Mo Yao** move Blood. Ru Xiang, in particular, moves Blood in the channels.

Variations

For the treatment of hemiplegia this formula should be adapted by the addition of herbs which simultaneously nourish Blood and invigorate the channels, such as Sang Ji Sheng *Ramulus Loranthi*, Ji Xue Teng *Caulis Millettiae seu Caulis Spatholobi* and Wu Jia Pi *Cortex Acanthopanacis radicis*.

In addition, some herbs which expel Wind from the channels should also be added, such as Sang Zhi *Ramulus Mori albae* or Wei Ling Xian *Radix Clematidis chinensis*.

PATTERNS IN THE SEQUELAE STAGE

After a Wind-stroke attack, besides treating the above symptoms, it is important to attend to the underlying imbalances which caused the stroke in the first place. These imbalances are obviously still present and they predispose the patient to further attacks.

The most common patterns encountered are listed below with their treatment.

WIND-PHLEGM

CLINICAL MANIFESTATIONS

Contraction of limbs, severe dizziness, giddiness, stiffness, a Stiff and Deviated tongue and a Wiry pulse.

TREATMENT PRINCIPLE

Resolve Phlegm and extinguish Wind.

ACUPUNCTURE

- Du-20 Baihui, Du-16 Fengfu and G.B.-20 Fengchi with reducing or even method to subdue Wind.
- ST-40 Fenglong and LU-9 Taiyuan with reducing or even method to resolve Phlegm.

HERBAL TREATMENT

1. Prescription

BAN XIA BAI ZHU TIAN MA TANG
Pinellia-Atractylodes-Gastrodia Decoction
Ban Xia *Rhizoma Pinelliae ternatae* 9 g
Tian Ma *Rhizoma Gastrodiae elatae* 6 g
Bai Zhu *Rhizoma Atractylodis macrocephalae* 15 g
Fu Ling *Sclerotium Poriae cocos* 6 g
Chen Pi *Pericarpium Citri reticulatae* 6 g
Gan Cao *Rhizoma Glycyrrhizae uralensis* 4 g
Sheng Jiang *Rhizoma Zingiberis officinalis recens* 1 slice
Da Zao *Fructus Ziziphi jujubae* 2 pieces

Explanation

This formula has already been explained in the chapter on Headache (ch. 1). It is specific to resolve Phlegm and subdue Wind.

2. Prescription

DING XIAN WAN
Stopping Epilepsy Pill
Tian Ma *Rhizoma Gastrodiae elatae* 9 g
Dan Nan Xing *Rhizoma Arisaematis praeparata* 9 g
Quan Xie *Buthus Martensi* 1.5 g
Jiang Can *Bombyx batryticatus* 4 g
Chuan Bei Mu *Bulbus Fritillariae cirrhosae* 9 g
Ban Xia *Rhizoma Pinelliae ternatae* 9 g
Zhu Li *Succus Bambusae* 10 ml
Fu Ling *Sclerotium Poriae cocos* 6 g
Chen Pi *Pericarpium Citri reticulatae* 4 g
Fu Shen *Sclerotium Poriae cocos pararadicis* 6 g
Shi Chang Pu *Rhizoma Acori graminei* 6 g
Yuan Zhi *Radix Polygalae tenuifoliae* 6 g
Dan Shen *Radix Salviae miltiorrhizae* 6 g
Deng Xin Cao *Medulla Junci effusi* 6 g
Hu Po *Succinum* 6 g
Mai Men Dong *Tuber Ophiopogonis japonici* 6 g
Gan Cao *Radix Glycyrrhizae uralensis* 3 g
Sheng Jiang *Rhizoma Zingiberis officinalis recens* 3 slices

Explanation

– **Tian Ma, Nan Xing, Quan Xie** and **Jiang Can** subdue Wind.
– **Bei Mu, Ban Xia, Zhu Li, Fu Ling** and **Chen Pi** resolve Phlegm.
– **Fu Shen, Chang Pu, Yuan Zhi, Dan Shen, Xin Cao** and **Hu Po** calm the Mind and open the orifices.
– **Mai Dong** nourishes Yin.
– **Gan Cao** and **Sheng Jiang** harmonize.

This prescription is stronger than the previous one, both in resolving Phlegm and subduing Wind.

DAMP-PHLEGM

CLINICAL MANIFESTATIONS

A feeling of heaviness of the body and of oppression of the chest, profuse sputum, a rattling sound in the throat, blurred vision, dizziness, a Swollen tongue with sticky coating and a Slippery pulse.

TREATMENT PRINCIPLE

Tonify the Spleen, drain Dampness and resolve Phlegm.

ACUPUNCTURE

– BL-20 Pishu and Ren-12 Zhongwan with reinforcing method to tonify the Spleen to resolve Phlegm.
– ST-40 Fenglong and SP-6 Sanyinjiao with even method to resolve Phlegm.

HERBAL TREATMENT

1. Prescription

ER CHEN TANG
Two Old Decoction
Ban Xia *Rhizoma Pinelliae ternatae* 15 g
Chen Pi *Pericarpium Citri reticulatae* 15 g
Fu Ling *Sclerotium Poriae cocos* 9 g
Zhi Gan Cao *Radix Glycyrrhizae uralensis praeparata* 5 g
Sheng Jiang *Rhizoma Zingiberis officinalis recens* 3 g
Wu Mei *Fructus Pruni mume* 1 prune

Explanation

This formula has already been explained in chapter 12. It is the most widely used formula to resolve Damp-Phlegm, often added as a unit to other prescriptions.

2. Prescription

WEN DAN TANG
Warming the Gall-Bladder Decoction
Ban Xia *Rhizoma Pinelliae ternatae* 6 g
Fu Ling *Sclerotium Poriae cocos* 5 g
Chen Pi *Pericarpium Citri reticulatae* 9 g
Zhu Ru *Caulis Bambusae in Taeniis* 6 g
Zhi Shi *Fructus Citri aurantii immaturus* 6 g
Zhi Gan Cao *Radix Glycyrrhizae uralensis praeparata* 3 g
Sheng Jiang *Rhizoma Zingiberis officinalis recens* 5 slices
Da Zao *Fructus Ziziphi jujubae* 1 date

Explanation

This formula has already been explained in chapter 9. It is used instead of the previous one if there are symptoms of Heat.

(a) Patent remedy

ER CHEN WAN
Two Old Pill

Explanation

This pill has the same ingredients and functions as the prescription above.

The tongue presentation appropriate to this remedy is a Swollen body with a sticky-white coating.

(b) Patent remedy

BAO JIAN MEI JIAN FEI CHA
Maintaining Vigour and Beauty and Reducing Fat Tea
Qing Cha *Green tea*
Shan Zha *Fructus Crataegi*
Chi Xiao Dou *Semen Phaseoli calcarati*
Mai Ya *Fructus Hordei vulgaris germinatus*
Chen Pi *Pericarpium Citri reticulatae*
Shen Qu *Massa Fermentata Medicinalis*
Jue Ming Zi *Semen Cassiae torae*
Qian Niu Zi *Semen Pharbitidis*
Ze Xie *Rhizoma Alismatis orientalis*
Lai Fu Zi *Semen Raphani sativi*

Explanation

This remedy drains Dampness and relieves retention of food. It can be used to drain Dampness and resolve Phlegm after a stroke.

The tongue presentation appropriate to this remedy is a thick-sticky coating.

STAGNATION OF QI AND BLOOD

CLINICAL MANIFESTATIONS

Hemiplegia, pains in the shoulder and hip, a Purple tongue and a Firm pulse.

TREATMENT PRINCIPLE

Move Qi and regulate Blood.

ACUPUNCTURE

– Ren-17 Shanzhong with even method to move Qi in order to move Blood.
– BL-17 Geshu and SP-10 Xuehai with even method to move Blood.

HERBAL TREATMENT

Prescription

HUO LUO XIAO LING DAN
Miraculously Effective Invigorating the Connecting Channels Pill
Dang Gui *Radix Angelicae sinensis* 15 g
Dan Shen *Radix Salviae miltiorrhizae* 15 g
Ru Xiang *Gummi Olibanum* 15 g
Mo Yao *Myrrha* 15 g

Explanation

This formula has already been explained above.

YIN DEFICIENCY WITH EMPTY-HEAT

CLINICAL MANIFESTATIONS

Feeling of heat in the afternoon and evening, dizziness, tinnitus, night-sweating, five-palm heat, feeling of heaviness of the upper part of the body and weakness of the lower part when walking, a Red tongue without coating and a Floating-Empty and Rapid pulse.

TREATMENT PRINCIPLE

Nourish Yin and clear Empty-Heat.

ACUPUNCTURE

– KI-6 Zhaohai, KI-3 Taixi and Ren-4 Guanyuan to nourish Kidney-Yin, reinforcing method.

- HE-6 Yinxi to clear Empty-Heat, reducing method.
- G.B.-20 Fengchi to subdue Wind.

HERBAL TREATMENT

Prescription

LIU WEI DI HUANG WAN
Six-Ingredient Rehmannia Pill
Shu Di Huang *Radix Rehmanniae glutinosae prae-parata* 24 g
Shan Zhu Yu *Fructus Corni officinalis* 12 g
Shan Yao *Radix Dioscoreae oppositae* 12 g
Ze Xie *Rhizoma Alismatis orientalis* 9 g
Mu Dan Pi *Cortex Moutan radicis* 9 g
Fu Ling *Sclerotium Poriae cocos* 9 g

Explanation

This is a well-known formula to nourish Yin which has been explained previously (ch. 1).

Prognosis and frequency of treatment

Best results are obtained if treatment is given within one month of the Wind-stroke attack and good results if within 3 months. It is difficult to treat Wind-stroke of more than six months' duration and even more difficult if more than a year has elapsed. However, in my experience, it is always worth trying, even if the Wind-stroke occurred more than a year previously.

If the stroke occurred within the last three months, treatment should be given literally every day, including Sundays. If the stroke occurred more than three months previously, treatment may be given every other day. A break of one to two weeks is necessary after one to two months.

Other methods of treatment

Apart from acupuncture and herbal treatment, other techniques can be helpful.

ELECTRICAL ACUPUNCTURE

Electrical stimulation may be used on the limbs to treat hemiplegia. A dense-sparse current is used with low frequency connecting two points on the same limb. The intensity of the current is gradually increased each time the patient's sensation diminishes. If electrical stimulation is used, fewer points need be selected. For example:

- *Arm*: L.I.-10 Shousanli and L.I.-4 Hegu.
- *Leg*: G.B.-30 Huantiao and G.B.-34 Yanglingquan.

The electrical stimulation should be maintained for 20 minutes, every other day. The longer the duration, the stronger the intensity of the current should be.

SCALP ACUPUNCTURE

A complete discussion of scalp acupuncture is beyond the scope of this text and the reader is referred to specialized textbooks.[2] Scalp acupuncture gives good results if given within one month of the stroke. No body points are used when scalp acupuncture is used and this may be alternated with normal body acupuncture.

Scalp acupuncture consists of needling lines rather than points on the skull according to the brain's anatomy. In the case of hemiplegia one would needle the motor line, its upper 1/5 for the leg, middle 2/5 for the arm and lower 2/5 for the face (Fig. 27.4). See also Figure 26.1.

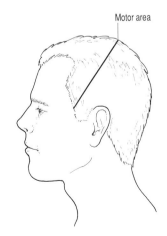

Fig. 27.4   Motor line for scalp acupuncture

This line is needled subcutaneously with one needle to cover the whole section of the line required (according to whether one is treating the arm or the leg). If inserting one needle subcutaneously for its whole length proves difficult, one can use up to three needles each for a shorter distance so that the whole section of that line is covered. The needle (or needles) is retained for 20 minutes and mild electrical stimulation at low frequency may also be applied.

POINT-INJECTION THERAPY

This consists in injecting certain solutions into acupuncture points. In the case of hemiplegia the solutions used are those of Angelica sinensis, Carthamus tinctorius, Vitamin B-6 or Vitamin B-12. The points used are:

- **L.I.-4** Hegu, **L.I.-11** Quchi and **L.I.-15** Jianyu for the arm.
- **ST-31** Biguan, **ST-36** Zusanli, **ST-40** Fenglong and **G.B.-39** Xuanzhong for the leg.

Only one point from each limb is used at any one time. Five doses, each of 1 cm^3 of solution, are injected at intervals of two days.

PHYSIOTHERAPY

This is absolutely essential to aid recovery in the sequelae stage of Wind-stroke. Gentle exercise is also recommended although it should never be carried out to the point of exhaustion.

Prevention

Old people with symptoms of Yin deficiency, Phlegm, Heat and Liver-Yang rising are more prone to be attacked by Wind-stroke. High blood pressure and obesity are also predisposing factors.

If we refer to the four main pathological factors of Wind-stroke, i.e. Wind, Fire, Stasis and Phlegm, it is easy to see that any elderly person who shows symptoms and signs of four or even three of these factors may be prone to Wind-stroke. The presence of these four factors can be observed particularly clearly on the tongue:

- *Wind* makes the tongue Stiff, Deviated, Moving or Quivering or a combination of these.
- *Fire* makes the tongue Red, and *Empty-Fire* makes it Red without a coating.
- *Stasis of Blood* makes the tongue Reddish-Purple.
- *Phlegm* makes the tongue Swollen with a sticky coating.

Thus, if an elderly person has a tongue that presents three or four of the above characteristics, he or she should be treated to prevent the occurrence of Wind-stroke. Action must be taken to subdue Wind, clear Heat, nourish Yin if there is Yin deficiency, move Blood and resolve Phlegm.

Some particular prodromal signs are especially indicative of the possibility of Wind-stroke, including numbness of the first three fingers of one hand and slightly slurred speech.

Other preventive measures can be deduced from analysis of the aetiological factors of Wind-stroke. An old or middle-aged person with some of the above symptoms and tongue signs should take immediate steps to avoid overwork, take adequate rest, reduce sexual activity and avoid eating greasy-fried food and drinking alcohol. Emotionally, it is important to overcome anger, hatred, resentment or repressed animosity which would stir up the rising of Liver-Yang.

When the above symptoms and signs are present, direct moxibustion on G.B.-39 Xuanzhong and ST-36 Zusanli can also be used.

END NOTES

1. Zhu Dan Xi 1481 The Essential Method of Dan Xi (*Dan Xi Xin Fa* 丹溪心法), cited in Internal Medicine, p. 213.

2. Scalp-Needling Therapy 1975, Medicine and Health Publishing Co., Hong Kong.

Atrophy Syndrome 28

痿証

The earliest discussion of Atrophy Syndrome occurs in chapter 44 of the "Simple Questions". There, it is called *Wei Bi*. The Chinese term *Wei* means "withered" and, in Chinese medicine, it refers to a condition characterized by "withering" of muscles and tendons from lack of nourishment. The term *Bi* suggests inability to walk because the foot cannot be lifted properly.

Thus, Atrophy Syndrome is a condition characterized by a weakness of the four limbs, progressively leading to atrophy, a limp state of muscles and tendons, an inability to walk properly and eventually paralysis. This weakness generally occurs without pain. Multiple sclerosis and the paralysis following an attack of poliomyelitis are examples of Atrophy Syndrome.

Aetiology and pathology

The "Simple Questions" in chapter 44 describes five types of Atrophy Syndrome, one for each Yin organ and its related tissue, i.e. Atrophy Syndrome of skin (Lungs), muscles (Spleen), blood vessels (Heart), tendons (Liver) and bones (Kidneys).[1] The book attributes each of these to Heat drying up the body fluids and leading to withering of skin, muscles, blood vessels, sinews and bones. Although this classification of Atrophy Syndrome is not generally followed any longer, it is still significant as, for example, in its beginning stages, Atrophy Syndrome is characterized by injury of skin and muscles (and therefore Lungs and Spleen), and, in the late stages, by deterioration of sinews and bones and therefore of Liver and Kidneys.

The idea of Heat drying up body fluids and injuring muscles and sinews is also important. Poliomyelitis is a case in point as paralysis follows the febrile stage when Heat dries up the fluids and leads to malnourishment of muscles, sinews and channels. It will also be observed that in those suffering from multiple sclerosis, the disease is often aggravated by a febrile disease. However, not every type of Atrophy Syndrome is caused by Heat.

The "Simple Questions" also describes a type of Atrophy Syndrome due to invasion of Dampness in the Bright-Yang channels.[2] This is a very common type of Atrophy Syndrome.

The six main aetiological factors are as follows.

1. WIND-HEAT FROM A WARM DISEASE

A Warm disease is due to invasion of Wind-Heat when the pathogenic factor is particularly virulent and infectious. Although every Warm disease is due to Wind-Heat, not every invasion of Wind-Heat is a Warm disease. Such a disease is due to an infectious pathogenic factor which enters via the nose and mouth, and is particularly strong. Measles and poliomyelitis are examples of Warm diseases (see chapter 34).

Wind-Heat from a Warm disease is therefore particularly strong, invades the body rapidly and has a strong tendency to dry up the body fluids and the Yin. It enters via the nose and mouth and affects the Lungs and Stomach. After the initial stage, it quickly changes into interior Heat burning the Yin of Lungs and Stomach. The drying up of fluids leads to malnourishment of muscles, sinews and channels and therefore paralysis. Poliomyelitis is an example of this pathological process as, in fact, the paralysis appears after the febrile stage.

2. EXTERNAL DAMPNESS

External Dampness is a very important and common aetiological factor especially in the British Isles where the weather is so damp. Chapter 44 of the "Simple Questions" says:

When the air is very moist and the person has a predisposition to Dampness, the moist air will invade the body and settle there. If the person also lives in a damp place, his or her muscles are invaded by Dampness and this will lead to numbness and then Atrophy Syndrome.[3]

Dampness is contracted from living in a damp house, or being exposed to damp weather for long periods; it invades the muscles and sinews and, in time, causes them to wither and become paralysed.

3. DIET

Excessive consumption of dairy foods, greasy foods, or irregular eating may impair the function of the Spleen and lead to the formation of Dampness. If this settles in the muscles, which it has the tendency to do, it will cause numbness and a progressive weakening of the muscles.

4. EXCESSIVE SEXUAL ACTIVITY AND OVERWORK

Excessive sexual activity and working too hard deplete the Kidneys and Liver, and therefore weaken bones and sinews. When these are deprived of the nourishment of the Kidney-Essence and Liver-Blood they become weak and may eventually lead to Atrophy Syndrome.

5. TRAUMAS

Traumas to the head may cause stagnation of Qi and Blood in the area controlling the motor nerves and lead to numbness, tingling and weakness of a limb.

6. SHOCK

Emotional shocks deplete Heart and Spleen. The Spleen controls the muscles and the Heart controls the blood vessels and circulation. When Heart and Spleen are depleted the muscles become weak and circulation of Blood to the limbs is defective. This may cause or contribute to the development of Atrophy Syndrome.

Atrophy Syndrome is never usually caused by a single factor but results from a combination of factors: for example, the invasion of external Dampness together with irregular diet and shock. Another example of combination of factors could be the invasion of external Dampness together with excessive sexual activity, overwork and a trauma.

The main patterns appearing in Atrophy Syndrome are:

1. Heat in the Lungs injuring Yin fluids (Full type)
2. Invasion of Damp-Heat (Full type)

3. Invasion of Cold-Dampness (Full type)
4. Stomach and Spleen deficiency (Empty type)
5. Spleen and Heart collapse (Empty type)
6. Liver and Kidney deficiency (Empty type)
7. Blood stasis in the channels (Full-Empty type).

The pathology of Atrophy Syndrome is characterized by Fullness in its initial stages and either Emptiness or a combination of Fullness and Emptiness in the middle and late stages. Thus the first three of the above patterns usually appear in the beginning stages of the disease and the others in the middle-late stages. The Full patterns inevitably change into Empty patterns with time.

For example:

– Lung-Heat develops into Liver-Kidney deficiency
– Damp-Heat develops into Stomach and Spleen deficiency
– Cold-Dampness develops into Stomach and Spleen deficiency.

The reverse is also possible, i.e. deficient patterns can give rise to Excess ones. For example:

– Stomach-Spleen deficiency may lead to Dampness
– Kidney-Liver deficiency may lead to Blood stasis.

Full and Empty patterns of Atrophy Syndrome are differentiated in Table 28.1.

It is very common, especially in the middle-late stages of the disease, to see a combination of Full and Empty patterns, e.g.:

– Damp-Heat and Stomach-Spleen deficiency
– Cold-Dampness and Stomach-Spleen deficiency
– Stomach-Spleen deficiency and Heart-Spleen collapse
– Stomach-Spleen deficiency and Kidney-Liver deficiency
– Kidney-Liver deficiency and Stasis of Blood in the channels.

There is a correspondence between aetiological factors and patterns as follows:

1. *Wind-Heat in a Warm disease* causes only one pattern, i.e. that of Lung-Heat injuring Yin fluids
2. *External Dampness* leads to Damp-Heat or Cold-Dampness
3. *Irregular diet* causes the patterns of Damp-Heat, Cold-Dampness and Stomach-Spleen deficiency
4. *Excessive sex and overwork* cause the patterns of Kidney-Liver deficiency and Blood stasis in the channels
5. *Trauma* causes the pattern of Blood stasis in the channels
6. *Shock* leads to the pattern of Heart-Spleen collapse.

The relationships between aetiological factors and patterns are illustrated in Figure 28.1.

The symptoms and signs of Atrophy Syndrome may have some similarities with those of

Table 28.1 Differentiation between Full and Empty type of Atrophy Syndrome

	Full	Empty
Duration	Short	Long
Onset	Abrupt onset and rapid development	Gradual onset
History	History of invasion of external Dampness or living in damp place	Developing from Full types or in patients with weak constitution
Main symptoms	Weakness of limbs and difficulty in movement. No atrophy	Very weak limbs, atrophy
Other symptoms	Numbness, pain, even convulsions (e.g. polio)	No pain (except in Blood stasis in the channels)

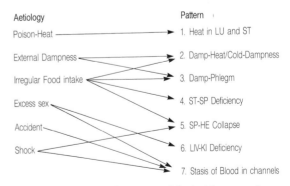

Fig. 28.1 Relationship between aetiological factors and patterns in Atrophy Syndrome

Painful Obstruction Syndrome and Wind-stroke. Although these three conditions have very different pathologies from the point of view of Western medicine, in Chinese medicine there are similarities. In particular, if we consider the beginning-middle stages of Atrophy Syndrome and compare its symptoms to Painful Obstruction Syndrome and Wind-stroke, we see that all three conditions are characterized by obstruction of muscles, sinews and channels by pathogenic factors.

However, there are also differences between Atrophy Syndrome, Painful Obstruction Syndrome and Wind-stroke, and these are summarized in Table 28.2.

Differentiation and treatment

Generally speaking, acupuncture is more relevant than herbal medicine for the treatment of Atrophy Syndrome as it provides a direct and immediate stimulation of Qi and Blood in the channels. Herbal treatment, however, provides a useful adjuvant to the therapy. Before discussing the treatment of individual patterns, we can discuss the general treatment of the channels with acupuncture as this is basically the same for all patterns, except for the differences in needling method used.

The "Simple Questions" in chapter 44 suggests using predominantly points from the Bright-Yang channels (Stomach and Large Intestines).

The main points to stimulate Qi and Blood and eliminate pathogenic factors from the channels in Atrophy Syndrome are:

Arm: L.I.-15 Jianyu, L.I.-14 Binao, L.I.-11 Quchi,

L.I.-10 Shousanli, T.B.-5 Waiguan, L.I.-4 Hegu and S.I.-3 Houxi.
Leg: G.B.-30 Huantiao, G.B.-31 Fengshi, ST-31 Biguan, ST-32 Futu, G.B.-34 Yanglingquan, ST-36 Zusanli, ST-41 Jiexi and G.B.-40 Qiuxu.
Other points: BL-32 Ciliao, Du-3 Yaoyangguan, Du-12 Shenzhu, Du-14 Dazhui and corresponding Huatuojiaji points, ST-30 Qichong.

EXPLANATION

– **L.I.-15** and **L.I.-14** are important local points either to remove obstructions from the channel or to tonify Qi and Blood in the channel. A good needling sensation should be obtained, preferably travelling downwards at least to the elbow.
– **L.I.-11** benefits the sinews.
– **L.I.-10** is an important local point for the lower arm, similar to L.I.-15 for the upper arm. However, it also has general tonic properties somewhat similar to (but weaker than) ST-36 Zusanli.
– **T.B.-5** removes obstructions from the channels and expels Wind. It is therefore also used in the late stages when there are spasms in the muscles. T.B.-5 is indirectly related to the Gall-Bladder (within the Lesser Yang) and it therefore influences the sinews.
– **L.I.-4** and **S.I.-3** are local points to affect the hand and fingers. S.I.-3 also expels Wind and it is therefore useful in the late stages of the disease when spasms of the hand make writing and holding things very difficult.
– **G.B.-30** is a very important point either to tonify Qi and Blood of the channel or to remove obstructions from it. It also has general tonic properties. It must be needled

Table 28.2   Differentiation between Atrophy Syndrome, Painful Obstruction Syndrome and Wind-stroke

	Atrophy Syndrome	Painful Obstruction Syndrome	Wind-stroke
Aetiology	Combination of external and internal	Only external	Internal disharmonies, Wind, Phlegm, Fire, stasis
Location	Muscles, sinews, channels	Joints more than muscles, difficulty in flexing and extending	Hemiplegia, only one side affected, movement of other side is free
Pain	No pain, except late stages with Blood stasis	Local pain of joints very pronounced	Only on movement of joint of affected side in late stages

with the patient lying on the side opposite to the one being needled and it is essential to obtain a good needling sensation, preferably all the way down to the foot, or at least to the knee.

- **G.B.-31** is a local point to stimulate Qi and Blood and also benefit sinews and expel Wind.
- **ST-31** is an important point to tonify Qi and Blood in the channel and, in particular, to facilitate the raising of the leg which is so important when the person has difficulty in walking.
- **ST-32** is a local point for the Stomach channel and it affects blood vessels.
- **G.B.-34** is used for its local as well as its general effect on the sinews.
- **ST-36** is probably the most important point to tonify the channel and tonify Stomach and Spleen in general.
- **ST-41** and **G.B.-40** are used as local points for the foot. In particular, they facilitate the lifting of the foot which is so important when the foot is dropped and dragged along, making walking very difficult.
- **BL-32** and **Du-3** stimulate the circulation of Qi and Blood to the legs.
- **Du-12**, **Du-14** and their corresponding Huatuojiaji points may be chosen to affect the spinal nerves according to the distribution of symptoms. Besides that, Du-12 tonifies Qi in general and Du-14 expels Wind.
- **ST-30** strengthens the Stomach channel and promotes the circulation of nutrient substances from the Stomach to the limbs. Chapter 44 of the "Simple Questions" prescribes the use of the Bright-Yang channel to treat Atrophy Syndrome. It says: *"The Bright Yang is the Sea of the 5 Yin and 6 Yang organs, it irrigates the original sinews which run to the pubic bone and up the spine in the back."*[4] Thus, there are several good reasons for choosing points from the Stomach channel: first, they have general tonic properties as the Stomach is the source of post-natal Qi; secondly, the Bright-Yang channels abound in Qi and Blood; thirdly, the point ST-30 is also a crossing point with the Penetrating Vessel so that reinforcing this point strengthens the Stomach and the Penetrating Vessel, as well

as the so-called "original sinews" which gather around the pubic bone and which go through ST-30 and then up to the spine. In fact, the "Simple Questions" goes on by saying:

The Penetrating Vessel is the Sea of the 12 channels, it irrigates the rivers and valleys [i.e. channels and muscles] and it meets with the Bright Yang at the original sinews, Yin and Yang channels meet here and converge at ST-30 which is on the Bright Yang. The Girdle Vessel and Governing Vessel also converge at this point. Thus when the Bright Yang is deficient the original sinews are weakened, the Girdle Vessel does not fasten and Atrophy Syndrome results.[5]

To sum up, reinforcing the point ST-30 will promote the circulation of nutrient substances from the Stomach downwards to the legs and upwards to the sinews and ligaments alongside the spine.

All the above points can be used according to symptoms in any type of Atrophy Syndrome, irrespective of the pattern. Further choice of points and herbal prescriptions depends of course on the pattern involved.

The patterns discussed are:

- Heat in the Lungs injuring Yin Fluids
- Invasion of Damp-Heat
- Invasion of Cold-Dampness
- Stomach and Spleen Deficiency
- Spleen and Heart Collapse
- Kidney and Liver Deficiency
- Blood Stasis in the Channels.

EXCESS

1. HEAT IN LUNGS INJURING YIN FLUIDS

CLINICAL MANIFESTATIONS

Fever, weakness and flaccidity of limbs which follows after the fever subsides, dry skin, mental restlessness, thirst, cough, dry throat, scanty-dark urine, dry stools.
Tongue: Red, no coating.
Pulse: Fine and Rapid.

These are the manifestations of Lung-Heat injuring Yin following an invasion of Wind-Heat during a Warm disease. Poliomyelitis would be a typical example, but muscular weakness and impairment of walking in children may occur also after other infectious febrile diseases.

TREATMENT PRINCIPLE

Clear Heat, cool Blood and nourish Yin of Lungs and Stomach.

ACUPUNCTURE

Du-14 Dazhui, BL-13 Feishu, LU-1 Zhongfu, LU-5 Chize, ST-44 Neiting, ST-36 Zusanli, SP-6 Sanyinjiao and KI-3 Taixi. Reducing method on all points except the last three which should be reinforced. No moxa. This is an acute condition and treatment should therefore be given every day.

EXPLANATION

- **Du-14** clears Heat.
- **BL-13**, **LU-1** and **LU-5** clear Lung-Heat.
- **ST-44** clears Stomach-Heat.
- **ST-36**, **SP-6** and **KI-3** nourish Yin and promote fluids.

HERBAL TREATMENT

PRESCRIPTION

QING ZAO JIU FEI TANG
Clearing Dryness and Rescuing the Lungs Decoction
Sang Ye *Folium Mori albae* 9 g
Shi Gao *Gypsum fibrosum* 7.5 g
Mai Men Dong *Tuber Ophiopogonis japonici* 3.6 g
Ren Shen *Radix Ginseng* 2 g
Hu Ma Ren (Hei Zhi Ma) *Semen Sesami indici* 3 g
E Jiao *Gelatinum Corii Asini* 2.4 g
Xing Ren *Semen Pruni armeniacae* 2 g
Pi Pa Ye *Folium Eriobotryae japonicae* 3 g
Gan Cao *Radix Glycyrrhizae uralensis* 3 g

Explanation

This formula, which has already been explained

in chapter 8, is specific to clear residual Heat in the Lungs after a Warm disease, nourish Yin after injury from Heat and benefit fluids.

Variations

- To strengthen the channels and benefit sinews in Atrophy Syndrome add Niu Xi *Radix Achyranthis bidentatae seu Cyathulae*, Ji Xue Teng *Caulis Millettiae seu Caulis Spatholobi* and Wu Jia Pi *Cortex Acanthopanacis radicis*.
- If symptoms of Heat are still pronounced add Zhi Mu *Rhizoma Anemarrhenae asphodeloidis*, Lian Qiao *Fructus Forsythiae suspensae* and Jin Yin Hua *Flos Lonicerae japonicae*.
- If there is a cough add Gua Lou *Fructus Trichosanthis*, Sang Bai Pi *Cortex Mori albae radicis* and Pi Pa Ye *Folium Eriobotryae japonicae*.
- If symptoms of dryness are pronounced add Tian Hua Fen *Radix Trichosanthis*, Yu Zhu *Rhizoma Polygonati odorati* and Bai He *Bulbus Lilii*.

(i) PATENT REMEDY

QING FEI YI HUO PIAN
Clearing the Lungs and Eliminating Fire Tablet
Huang Qin *Radix Scutellariae baicalensis*
Shan Zhi Zi *Fructus Gardeniae jasminoidis*
Da Huang *Rhizoma Rhei*
Qian Hu *Radix Peucedani*
Ku Shen *Radix Sophorae flavescentis*
Tian Hua Fen *Radix Trichosanthis*
Jie Geng *Radix Platycodi grandiflori*
Zhi Mu *Radix Anemarrhenae asphodeloidis*

Explanation

This tablet drains Lung-Fire and is suitable to treat an acute febrile episode which is beginning to cause paralysis. This remedy is specific for Lung-Fire at the Qi Level and two conditions for its use are a thick-dry-yellow (or black) tongue coating and dry stools.

(ii) PATENT REMEDY

YANG YIN QING FEI TANG JIAN

Nourishing Yin and Clearing the Lungs Syrup
Mu Dan Pi *Cortex Moutan radicis*
Zhe Bei Mu *Bulbus Fritillariae thunbergii*
Bai Shao *Radix Paeoniae albae*
Xuan Shen *Radix Scrophulariae ningpoensis*
Sheng Di Huang *Radix Rehmanniae glutinosae*
Mai Men Dong *Tuber Ophiopogonis japonici*
Gan Cao *Radix Glycyrrhizae uralensis*
Bo He *Herba Menthae*

Explanation

This remedy is for a stage further than the one outlined above under the previous remedy. It is for the stage when Fire has already begun to dry up the Lung fluids noticeably, paralysis is setting in and symptoms and signs of deficiency of Yin are beginning to appear.

The tongue presentation for this remedy is different than the one for the previous remedy: in this case the tongue is Red, dry and without coating. There may also be constipation, but this is due to lack of fluids in the Intestines rather than to Fire.

2. INVASION OF DAMP-HEAT

CLINICAL MANIFESTATIONS

Constant low-grade fever which does not abate with sweating, weakness, heaviness and swelling of the legs, numbness, a feeling of oppression of the chest and epigastrium, cloudy urine, a feeling of heaviness of the body, yellow complexion, a feeling of heat in the feet.
Tongue: yellow-sticky coating.
Pulse: Slippery and Rapid.

TREATMENT PRINCIPLE

Clear Heat, resolve Dampness.

ACUPUNCTURE

Du-14 Dazhui, L.I.-11 Quchi, SP-9 Yinlingquan, SP-6 Sanyinjiao, BL-22 Sanjiaoshu, ST-36 Zusanli. Reducing method, no moxa. At the acute stage, treatment should be given every day. If this condition appears in middle or late stages of Atrophy Syndrome, it will usually be associated with an underlying deficiency of Stomach and Spleen which should therefore be reinforced.

EXPLANATION

- **Du-14** and **L.I.-11** resolve Damp-Heat.
- **SP-9**, **SP-6** and **BL-22** resolve Dampness, mostly from the Lower Burner.
- **ST-36** is reinforced to strengthen the Spleen and Stomach to resolve Dampness.

HERBAL TREATMENT
PRESCRIPTION

ER MIAO SAN
Two Wonderful Powder
Cang Zhu *Rhizoma Atractylodis lanceae* 9 g
Huang Bo *Cortex Phellodendri* 9 g

Explanation

This formula drains Damp-Heat from the Lower Burner.

Variations

- To strengthen the channels and benefit the sinews in Atrophy Syndrome add Niu Xi *Radix Achyranthis bidentatae seu Cyathulae*, Can Sha *Excrementum Bombycis mori* and Mu Gua *Fructus Chaenomelis lagenariae*.
- If symptoms of Dampness are pronounced add Bi Xie *Rhizoma Dioscoreae hypoglaucae* and Fang Ji *Radix Stephaniae tetrandae*.
- If there is Dampness in the epigastrium and chest (feeling of oppression and heaviness) add Hou Po *Cortex Magnoliae officinalis*.
- If the Heat part of Damp-Heat has begun to injure Yin and the muscles are beginning to waste add Sheng Di Huang *Radix Rehmanniae glutinosae* and Mai Men Dong *Tuber Ophiopogonis japonici*.

- If there is stasis of Blood (pain in the joints and Purple tongue) add Chi Shao *Radix Paeoniae rubrae*, Tao Ren *Semen Persicae* and Hong Hua *Flos Carthami tinctorii*.
- If Damp-Heat is retained for a long time it easily injures Kidney-Yin and this leads to a complicated situation of Fullness (Damp-Heat) and Emptiness (Kidney-Yin deficiency). In this case use a variation of Zhi Bo Di Huang Wan *Anemarrhena-Phellodendron-Rehmannia Pill*.

3. INVASION OF COLD-DAMPNESS

CLINICAL MANIFESTATIONS

Dizziness, a feeling of heaviness, blurred vision, pain in back and shoulders, numbness of the back, weakness, flaccidity and coldness of the limbs.
Tongue: Pale, white-sticky coating.
Pulse: Slippery and Deep.

TREATMENT PRINCIPLE

Resolve Dampness and warm the Spleen.

ACUPUNCTURE

ST-40 Fenglong, SP-9 Yinlingquan, SP-6 Sanyinjiao, ST-8 Touwei, Ren-12 Zhongwan, BL-20 Pishu, ST-36 Zusanli, Du-4 Mingmen. The first three points should be reduced to resolve Dampness, ST-8 should be needled with even method and all the others should be reinforced to strengthen Stomach and Spleen to resolve Dampness. Moxa should be used.

HERBAL TREATMENT

PRESCRIPTION

LIU HE TANG
Six Harmonizing Decoction
Ren Shen *Radix Ginseng* 6 g
Bai Zhu *Rhizoma Atractylodis macrocephalae* 6 g
Sha Ren *Fructus seu Semen Amomi* 3 g

Huo Xiang *Herba Agastachis* 6 g
Hou Po *Cortex Magnoliae officinalis* 2.4 g
Fu Ling *Sclerotium Poriae cocos* 6 g
Bian Dou *Semen Dolichoris lablab* 6 g
Ban Xia *Rhizoma Pinelliae ternatae* 6 g
Xing Ren *Semen Pruni armeniacae* 6 g
Mu Gua *Fructus Chaenomelis lagenariae* 4.5 g
Gan Cao *Radix Glycyrrhizae uralensis* 1.5 g

Explanation

- **Ren Shen** and **Bai Zhu** tonify Spleen-Qi.
- **Sha Ren**, **Huo Xiang** and **Hou Po** fragrantly resolve Dampness and benefit the muscles.
- **Fu Ling** and **Bian Dou** drain Dampness. Bian Dou also mildly tonifies the Spleen.
- **Ban Xia** helps to resolve Dampness by resolving Phlegm.
- **Xing Ren** helps to resolve Dampness by promoting the descending of Qi and therefore helping the draining of Dampness.
- **Mu Gua** resolves Wind-Damp and benefits sinews.
- **Gan Cao** harmonizes.

Variations

- To treat Atrophy Syndrome add herbs to benefit channels such as Ji Xue Teng *Caulis Millettiae seu Caulis Spatholobi* and Wu Jia Pi *Cortex Acanthopanacis radicis* for the lower limbs, and Gui Zhi *Ramulus Cinnamomi cassiae* for the upper limbs.
- If there is pronounced Dampness in the muscles (manifested with numbness and a feeling of heaviness) add Fang Ji *Radix Stephaniae tetrandae* for the upper limbs and Bi Xie *Rhizoma Dioscoreae hypoglaucae* for the legs.

PATENT REMEDY

XIANG SHA LIU JUN ZI WAN
Saussurea-Amomum Six Gentlemen Pill
Dang Shen *Radix Codonopsis pilosulae*
Bai Zhu *Rhizoma Atractylodis macrocephalae*
Fu Ling *Sclerotium Poriae cocos*
Zhi Gan Cao *Radix Glycyrrhizae uralensis praeparata*
Chen Pi *Pericarpium Citri reticulatae*

Ban Xia *Rhizoma Pinelliae ternatae*
Mu Xiang *Radix Saussureae*
Sha Ren *Fructus seu Semen Amomi*

Explanation

This pill tonifies the Spleen and resolves Dampness. Although this is primarily a tonic, and not a Dampness-resolving remedy, it can be used in this case as it contains several herbs which resolve Dampness and Phlegm.

If the symptoms and signs of Dampness and Phlegm are very pronounced, this remedy can be combined with Er Chen Wan *Two Old Pill*.

DEFICIENCY

1. STOMACH AND SPLEEN DEFICIENCY

CLINICAL MANIFESTATIONS

Muscular weakness, a feeling of weakness of the limbs, tiredness, easily fatigued, poor appetite, loose stools, a sallow complexion.
Tongue: Pale.
Pulse: Weak.

This pattern appears in the middle-late stages of Atrophy Syndrome and it may develop from one of the two previous patterns, i.e. those characterized by Dampness. In these cases, the condition will be one of Emptiness (of Stomach and Spleen) with Fullness (Dampness), and the treatment needs to be suitably adapted so that it will simultaneously tonify the Stomach and Spleen and resolve Dampness.

TREATMENT PRINCIPLE

Tonify Stomach and Spleen, strengthen the muscles. If necessary, resolve Dampness.

ACUPUNCTURE

ST-36 Zusanli, SP-3 Taibai, BL-20 Pishu, BL-21 Weishu, Ren-12 Zhongwan. Reinforcing method; moxa is applicable.

EXPLANATION

All these points tonify Stomach and Spleen.

HERBAL TREATMENT

(a) PRESCRIPTION

SHEN LING BAI ZHU SAN
Ginseng-Poria-Atractylodes Powder
Ren Shen *Radix Ginseng* 6 g (or **Dang Shen** *Radix Codonopsis pilosulae* 12 g)
Bai Zhu *Rhizoma Atractylodis macrocephalae* 9 g
Fu Ling *Sclerotium Poriae cocos* 12 g
Zhi Gan Cao *Radix Glycyrrhizae uralensis praeparata* 6 g
Bian Dou *Semen Dolichoris lablab* 12 g
Shan Yao *Radix Dioscoreae oppositae* 12 g
Lian Zi *Semen Nelumbinis nuciferae* 12 g
Sha Ren *Fructus seu Semen Amomi* 4.5 g
Yi Yi Ren *Semen Coicis lachryma jobi* 10 g
Jie Geng *Radix Platycodi grandiflori* 6 g

Explanation

This formula, which has already been explained tonifies Qi, resolves Dampness and stops diarrhoea.

(b) PRESCRIPTION

LIU JUN ZI TANG
Six Gentlemen Decoction
Ren Shen *Radix Ginseng* 10 g
Bai Zhu *Rhizoma Atractylodis macrocephalae* 9 g
Fu Ling *Sclerotium Poriae cocos* 9 g
Zhi Gan Cao *Radix Glycyrrhizae uralensis praeparata* 6 g
Chen Pi *Pericarpium Citri reticulatae* 9 g
Ban Xia *Rhizoma Pinelliae ternatae* 12 g

Explanation

This formula, which has already been explained, tonifies Qi and resolves Dampness. It is suitable if there are marked symptoms of Dampness.

(c) PRESCRIPTION

BU ZHONG YI QI TANG
Tonifying the Centre and Benefiting Qi Decoction
Huang Qi *Radix Astragali membranacei* 12 g
Ren Shen *Radix Ginseng* 9 g
Bai Zhu *Rhizoma Atractylodis macrocephalae* 9 g
Dang Gui *Radix Angelicae sinensis* 6 g
Chen Pi *Pericarpium Citri reticulatae* 6 g
Sheng Ma *Rhizoma Cimicifugae* 3 g
Chai Hu *Radix Bupleuri* 3 g

Explanation

This formula, which has already been explained in chapters 1 and 25, is used if there are symptoms of sinking Qi.

Variations

Any of the above three prescriptions should be modified with the addition of herbs to benefit the channels and sinews.

- If the legs are mostly affected add Ji Xue Teng *Caulis Millettiae seu Caulis Spatholobi* and Niu Xi *Radix Achyranthis bidentatae seu Cyathulae*.
- If the arms are weak add Gui Zhi *Ramulus Cinnamomi cassiae* and Sang Zhi *Ramulus Mori albae*.
- If there is numbness of the limbs add Wei Ling Xian *Radix Clematidis chinensis*.
- If the lower back is weak add Du Zhong *Cortex Eucommiae ulmoidis* and Wu Jia Pi *Cortex Acanthopanacis radicis*.

(i) PATENT REMEDY

BU ZHONG YI QI WAN
Tonifying the Centre and Benefiting Qi Pill

Explanation

This remedy has the same ingredients and functions as the homonymous prescription above.

The tongue presentation appropriate to this remedy is a Pale body.

(ii) PATENT REMEDY

XIANG SHA LIU JUN ZI WAN
Saussurea-Amomum Six Gentlemen Pill

Explanation

This remedy, already explained under the previous pattern above, can be used in this pattern to tonify the Spleen and resolve Dampness.

The tongue presentation appropriate to this remedy is a Pale body with a sticky coating.

It should be remembered that the pattern of Spleen-Qi deficiency is very often combined with that of either Damp-Heat or Cold-Dampness. One has to assess whether the condition is primarily Full or Empty and choose the prescription accordingly to resolve Dampness or tonify Stomach and Spleen. The chosen prescription should then be modified with herbs to tonify the Spleen or resolve Dampness respectively.

2. SPLEEN AND HEART COLLAPSE

CLINICAL MANIFESTATIONS

Muscular weakness of sudden onset after a shock, palpitations, insomnia, poor appetite, white complexion, loose stools.
Tongue: Pale.
Pulse: Weak or slightly Floating-Empty.

This is a condition occurring after a shock which depletes Heart and Spleen suddenly.

TREATMENT PRINCIPLE

Tonify Spleen- and Heart-Qi and nourish Blood.

ACUPUNCTURE

Du-14 Dazhui, HE-5 Tongli, HE-7 Shenmen, BL-15 Xinshu, BL-20 Pishu, ST-36 Zusanli, SP-6 Sanyinjiao, Ren-4 Guanyuan. Reinforcing method; moxa is applicable.

EXPLANATION

- **Du-14**, with direct moxa, tonifies the Heart.
- **HE-5**, **HE-7** and **BL-15** tonify Heart Qi and Blood and calm the Mind.
- **BL-20**, **ST-36** and **SP-6** tonify the Stomach and Spleen and nourish Blood.
- **Ren-4** nourishes Blood and calms the Mind.

HERBAL TREATMENT

PRESCRIPTION

DING ZHI WAN
Settling the Will-Power Pill
Ren Shen *Radix Ginseng* 9 g
Fu Ling *Sclerotium Poriae cocos* 9 g
Shi Chang Pu *Rhizoma Acori graminei* 6 g
Yuan Zhi *Radix Polygalae tenuifoliae* 6 g

Explanation

- **Ren Shen** and **Fu Ling** tonify Spleen-Qi. Fu Ling also calms the Mind.
- **Chang Pu** and **Yuan Zhi** open the Heart's orifices.

This formula is used for the after-effects of shock which leave the Mind unrooted. It tonifies Heart- and Spleen-Qi.

Variations

- To treat Atrophy Syndrome, adopt variations similar to those indicated for the previous pattern.

PATENT REMEDY

GUI PI WAN
Tonifying the Spleen Pill
Dang Shen *Radix Codonopsis pilosulae*
Huang Qi *Radix Astragali membranacei*
Bai Zhu *Rhizoma Atractylodis macrocephalae*
Fu Shen *Sclerotium Poriae cocos pararadicis*
Suan Zao Ren *Semen Ziziphi spinosae*
Yuan Zhi *Radix Polygalae tenuifoliae*
Dang Gui *Radix Angelicae sinensis*
Mu Xiang *Radix Saussureae*

Gan Cao *Radix Glycyrrhizae uralensis*
Long Yan Rou *Arillus Euphoriae longanae*

Explanation

This famous remedy tonifies Spleen- and Heart-Blood and can be used for Atrophy Syndrome from Spleen and Heart Collapse.

The tongue presentation appropriate to this remedy is a Pale and Thin body.

3. KIDNEY AND LIVER DEFICIENCY

CLINICAL MANIFESTATIONS

Weakness and atrophy of leg muscles, sore back, dizziness, tinnitus, blurred vision, dry eyes, dribbling of urine, exhaustion.
Tongue: Red without coating.
Pulse: Fine and Deep.

This consists in deficiency of Yin of the Liver and Kidneys and weakness and malnourishment of sinews and bones. This pattern only appears at the late stages of Atrophy Syndrome and the symptoms and signs develop gradually. It may also develop from any of the above patterns in their late stages.

TREATMENT PRINCIPLE

Nourish Liver and Kidneys, strengthen sinews and bones.

ACUPUNCTURE

BL-18 Ganshu, BL-23 Shenshu, Du-3 Yaoyang-guan, G.B.-34 Yanglingquan, G.B.-39 Xuan-zhong, LIV-8 Ququan, KI-3 Taixi, Ren-4 Guanyuan. Reinforcing method. Although there is Yin deficiency a small amount of moxa on the needle may be used on certain points (the general ones for the channels indicated above) provided there are no Empty-Heat signs.

EXPLANATION

- **BL-18**, **LIV-8**, **BL-23** and **KI-3** tonify Liver and Kidneys.

- **Du-3** tonifies the Kidneys and stimulates the circulation of Qi and Blood to the legs.
- **G.B.-34** and **G.B.-39** nourish sinews and bone-marrow respectively.
- **Ren-4** tonifies Kidney-Yin.

HERBAL TREATMENT

PRESCRIPTION

HU QIAN WAN
Hidden Tiger Pill
Hu Gu *Os Tigris* 6 g
Suo Yang *Herba Cynomorii songarici* 4.5 g
Huai Niu Xi *Radix Achyranthis bidentatae* 6 g
Dang Gui *Radix Angelicae sinensis* 6 g
Huang Bo *Cortex Phellodendri* 15 g
Zhi Mu *Rhizoma Anemarrhenae asphodeloidis* 6 g
Shu Di Huang *Radix Rehmanniae glutinosae praeparata* 6 g
Gui Ban *Plastrum Testudinis* 12 g
Bai Shao *Radix Paeoniae albae* 6 g

EXPLANATION

- **Hu Gu**, **Suo Yang** and **Niu Xi** strengthen bones and sinews. Although Suo Yang is a warm herb it is added because it nourishes the Essence and Marrow.
- **Dang Gui** nourishes Blood and helps the other ingredients to nourish Yin.
- **Huang Bo** and **Zhi Mu** clear Empty-Heat.
- **Shu Di**, **Gui Ban** and **Bai Shao** nourish Yin.

This formula is specific for Atrophy Syndrome from Liver- and Kidney-Yin deficiency. It nourishes Liver- and Kidney-Yin, clears Empty-Heat and strengthens sinews and bones.

VARIATIONS

- If there are also symptoms of Blood deficiency add Huang Qi *Radix Astragali membranacei*, Dang Shen *Radix Codonopsis pilosulae*, Dang Gui *Radix Angelicae sinensis* and Ji Xue Teng *Caulis Millettiae seu Caulis Spatholobi*.

- If the illness is very long-standing and symptoms of Kidney-Yang deficiency appear (such as incontinence of urine) in addition to those of Kidney-Yin deficiency reduce the dosage of Huang Bo and Zhi Mu and add Lu Jiao *Cornu Cervi*, Bu Gu Zhi *Fructus Psoraleae corylifoliae*, Ba Ji Tian *Radix Morindae officinalis* and Rou Gui *Cortex Cinnamomi cassiae*.

(i) PATENT REMEDY

JI XUE TENG QIN GAO PIAN
Millettia Liquid Extract Tablet
Ji Xue Teng *Caulis Millettiae seu Caulis Spatholobi*

Explanation

This remedy nourishes Liver-Blood, moves Blood, strengthens the sinews, and benefits the back and legs. It is suitable for Atrophy Syndrome against a background of Liver-Blood deficiency. It is a mild remedy and can therefore be used for several months.

The tongue presentation appropriate to this remedy is a Pale and Thin body.

(ii) PATENT REMEDY

DU ZHONG HU GU WAN
Eucommia-Tiger Bone Pill
Ren Shen *Radix Ginseng*
Bai Zhu *Rhizoma Atractylodis macrocephalae*
Dang Gui *Radix Angelicae sinensis*
Chuan Xiong *Radix Ligustici wallichii*
Ji Xue Teng *Caulis Millettiae seu Caulis Spatholobi*
San Qi *Radix Notoginseng*
Du Zhong *Cortex Eucommiae ulmoidis*
Hu Gu *Os Tigris*
Mu Gua *Fructus Chaenomelis lagenariae*
Yin Yang Huo *Herba Epimedii*
Wu Shao She *Zaocys dhumnades*
Lu Lu Tong *Fructus Liquidambaris taiwanianae*
Cang Zhu *Rhizoma Atractylodis lanceae*
Xun Gu Feng *Rhizoma seu Herba Aristolochiae*
Wei Ling Xian *Radix Clematidis chinensis*
Shi Nan Teng *Ramus Photiniae*
Sang Zhi *Ramulus Mori albae*

Explanation

This pill tonifies Kidney-Yang, nourishes and moves Blood and strengthens sinews and bones. It is suitable for middle-late stages of Atrophy Syndrome from Kidney-Yang deficiency.

The tongue presentation appropriate to this remedy is a Pale, slightly Purple, and wet body.

4. BLOOD STASIS IN THE CHANNELS

CLINICAL MANIFESTATIONS

Numbness, weakness and pain in the limbs, withered lips, bluish colour of limbs, pain on flexion of limbs.
Tongue: Purple.
Pulse: Deep, Fine and Choppy.

This pattern also appears in the late stages of Atrophy Syndrome and it is the only one characterized by pain. It is often associated with the previous pattern of Liver and Kidney deficiency.

TREATMENT PRINCIPLE

Nourish and move Blood and eliminate stasis.

ACUPUNCTURE

BL-17 Geshu, BL-11 Dashu, SP-10 Xuehai, Du-9 Zhiyang, Du-8 Jinsuo, ST-36 Zusanli and SP-6 Sanyinjiao. Even method on all, except on ST-36 and SP-6 which should be reinforced.

EXPLANATION

- **BL-17** and **SP-10** move Blood and eliminate stasis.
- **BL-11** nourishes Blood.
- **Du-9** and **Du-8** relax the sinews.
- **ST-36** and **SP-6** nourish Blood.

HERBAL TREATMENT

(a) PRESCRIPTION

BU YANG HAI WU TANG

Tonify Yang and Restore the ⁵/₁₀th Decoction
Huang Qi *Radix Astragali membranacei* 18 g
Dang Gui Wei *Radix Angelicae sinensis* ("tails") 6 g
Chuan Xiong *Radix Ligustici wallichii* 3 g
Tao Ren *Semen Persicae* 3 g
Hong Hua *Flos Carthami tinctorii* 3 g
Chi Shao Yao *Radix Paeoniae rubrae* 4.5 g
Di Long *Pheretima aspergillum* 3 g

Explanation

- **Huang Qi** tonifies Qi in order to move Blood.
- **Dang Gui**, **Chuan Xiong**, **Tao Ren**, **Hong Hua** and **Chi Shao** move Blood.
- **Di Long** extinguishes internal Wind and invigorates the channels.

This formula is for stasis of Blood occurring against a background of Qi deficiency. In this case, the tongue would be Pale-Purplish.

(b) PRESCRIPTION

HUO LUO XIAO LING DAN

Miraculously Effective Invigorating the Connecting Channels Pill
Dang Gui *Radix Angelicae sinensis* 15 g
Dan Shen *Radix Salviae miltiorrhizae* 15 g
Ru Xiang *Gummi Olibanum* 15 g
Mo Yao *Myrrha* 15 g

Explanation

- **Dang Gui** nourishes and moves Blood.
- **Dan Shen**, **Ru Xiang** and **Mo Yao** move Blood and eliminate stasis.

This formula is for stasis of Blood affecting the channels, and is therefore well suited to Atrophy Syndrome.

Variations

As the pattern of Stasis of Blood in Atrophy Syndrome usually occurs together with that of Deficiency of Liver and Kidneys, both the above formulae should be modified with the addition of herbs to nourish Liver and Kidneys and benefit sinews and bones, such as: Huai Niu Xi *Radix Achyranthis bidentatae*, Wu Jia Pi *Cortex Acanthopanacis radicis*, Ji Xue Teng *Caulis Millettiae seu Caulis Spatholobi*, Shu Di Huang *Radix Rehmanniae glutinosae praeparata*, and Du Zhong *Cortex Eucommiae ulmoidis*.

– Instead of the above two formulae, the prescription indicated for deficiency of Liver and Kidneys can be used with the addition of herbs to move Blood and eliminate stasis.

PATENT REMEDY

GU ZHE CUO SHANG SAN
Fracture and Contusion Powder
Ye Zhu Gu *Cranium Suis Scrofae*
Huang Gua Zi *Semen Cucumeris sativae*
Dang Gui *Radix Angelicae sinensis*
Hong Hua *Flos Carthami tinctorii*
Xue Jie *Sangui Draconis*
Da Huang *Rhizoma Rhei*
Ru Xiang *Gummi Olibanum*
Mo Yao *Myrrha*
Di Bie Chong *Eupolyphaga sue opishoplatia*

Explanation

This remedy moves Blood and invigorates the channels. It can be used for stasis of Blood in Atrophy Syndrome causing pain and stiffness of the joints. This is a strong remedy which should only be used for a few weeks at a time. As it contains Da Huang which moves downwards, it should be used only if the tongue has a fairly thick coating, or at least it has a coating. If the tongue has no coating, this remedy should not be used.

Prognosis and Western differentiation

In the case of Atrophy Syndrome it is essential for the patient to obtain a Western diagnosis from a neurologist as the prognosis depends very much on the type of disease involved.

First of all, according to Western medicine paralysis may occur either from injury of the spinal or motor nerves, or from injury to the muscles. The Chinese theory of Atrophy Syndrome does not differentiate between these two.

Thus, Atrophy Syndrome could appear in any of the following diseases:

– poliomyelitis
– myasthenia gravis
– motor-neurone disease
– multiple sclerosis
– muscular dystrophy.

1. POLIOMYELITIS

This is an infection caused by a polio-virus. It starts with symptoms of a respiratory infection with fever and a headache. In some cases, after a remission of about a week, the fever starts again and, as it abates, it is followed by the paralysis of a limb.

2. MYASTHENIA GRAVIS

This consists in abnormal fatiguability of muscles. The first symptoms are weakness when chewing, swallowing and speaking. Any muscle can be affected, but those of the shoulders are more frequently involved.

3. MOTOR-NEURONE DISEASE

This is due to damage of motor neurones in the spinal cord or brain stem. It usually appears between the ages of 50 and 70. The main symptoms and signs are weakness and wasting of the muscles. In the bulbar type (when the motor neurones of medulla and pons are affected) the speech is severely impaired and swallowing is difficult.

4. MULTIPLE SCLEROSIS

This disease results in de-myelination of the myelin sheath. See chapter on Multiple Sclerosis (ch. 29).

5. MUSCULAR DYSTROPHY

This causes progressive degeneration of the muscles without involvement of the nervous system. The wasting and weakness are symmetrical and there is no sensory loss.

There are different types of this disease but all of them are genetic and they usually start within the first three years of life.

Acupuncture and Chinese herbs can be very effective in treating the paralysis following an attack of poliomyelitis but only if the treatment is given as early as possible after its onset. They are also effective in treating multiple sclerosis (see chapter 29). Less good results are obtained in the treatment of myasthenia gravis and usually none at all in motor-neurone disease and muscular dystrophy.

However, there are many cases of Atrophy Syndrome which do not correspond to any recognized Western "disease". These cases can usually be helped quite well. For example, the symptoms and signs of Atrophy Syndrome may appear after any febrile disease, not only poliomyelitis. The following case history is an example of such a condition.

Case history

A 52-year-old lady fell ill with a sudden viral infection. She had a high temperature, a very stiff neck and a severe headache. Her symptoms resembled meningitis. After a week in which her temperature remained constantly high, she developed extreme weakness of both arm and leg on the left side. At times she could hardly walk. It was at this time that she sought treatment.

Diagnosis
This was a very clear case of a Warm disease with invasion of Wind-Heat turning into interior Heat which injured the Yin fluids. This led to malnourishment of sinews and channels and therefore to Atrophy Syndrome affecting arm and leg.

Treatment principle
The treatment principle applied was to clear residual Heat in Lungs and Stomach, nourish Yin, benefit fluids and nourish the channels. She was treated only with acupuncture.

Acupuncture
The main points used were:

LU-10 Yuji, **ST-44** Neiting, **L.I.-11** Quchi, **Du-14** Dazhui, **Ren-12** Zhongwan, **SP-6** Sanyinjiao, **ST-36** Zusanli and **KI-3** Taixi. The first four points were reduced to clear Heat, while the others were reinforced to nourish Yin and benefit fluids.

In addition to the above points, other points were reinforced to benefit the channels. These were:

L.I.-10 Shousanli and **T.B.-5** Waiguan for the arm and **ST-31** Biguan and **ST-34** Liangqiu for the leg.

Eight treatments were enough to restore her muscular strength and walking ability to normal.

END NOTES

1. 1979 The Yellow Emperor's Classic of Internal Medicine — Simple Questions (*Huang Ti Nei Jing Su Wen* 黄帝内经素问), People's Health Publishing House, Beijing. First published *c.* 100 BC, p. 246.
2. Ibid., p. 249.
3. Ibid., p. 248.
4. Ibid., p. 249.
5. Ibid., p. 249.

Multiple sclerosis 29

多
发
性
硬
化

Multiple sclerosis is the most common neurological disease in the Northern hemisphere. Its pathology consists in the partial destruction of the myelin sheaths around the spinal cord, brain and optic nerves. The lesions are disseminated at intervals and the many varied symptoms depend on the location of the lesions. Because the lesions can partially heal, this disease goes through characteristic phases of remission and relapse.

In young people the first presenting symptom is often retrobulbar neuritis causing blurred vision, whilst in old people it is weakness of a leg.

As mentioned above, this disease is characterized by many different symptoms according to the location of the lesions in the myelin sheath. These include: blurred vision, weakness and heaviness of one or both legs, jerking of the legs, double vision, vertigo, vomiting, incoordination, a feeling in arms and legs like suffering an electric shock, numbness or tingling of limbs, urgency or hesitancy of urination, impotence. With the progressive degeneration of the myelin sheath there is an increasing incoordination and weakness of the legs and arms. In the late stages there is complete paralysis usually of the spastic type together with urinary incontinence and gross cerebellar disturbance with ataxic gait.

In Chinese medicine, multiple sclerosis is a type of Atrophy Syndrome.

Aetiology and pathology

1. INVASION OF EXTERNAL DAMPNESS

Invasion of external Dampness is an important cause of disease in the beginning stages. External Dampness invades the channels of the legs first and creeps upwards. This is contracted by living in damp places, sitting on damp grass, failing to dry oneself after swimming, being exposed to damp weather when wearing insufficient clothes, or being exposed to foggy weather. Women are particularly prone to invasion of Dampness during their menstrual cycle and after childbirth.

Dampness obstructs the channels and causes a feeling of heaviness in the legs, numbness and tingling.

2. DIET

Excessive consumption of greasy-fried or cold foods impairs the Spleen and leads to the formation of Dampness. Dairy foods such as milk, cheese, butter and cream are one of the most common causes of Dampness in Western countries.

3. EXCESSIVE SEXUAL ACTIVITY

Excessive sexual activity weakens the Kidneys and Liver and is particularly responsible for the manifestations in the middle to late stages of multiple sclerosis, i.e. dizziness, blurred vision, urgency or hesitancy of urination and extreme weakness of the legs.

4. SHOCK

Shock causes a sudden depletion of Heart- and Spleen-Qi. The Spleen influences the muscles, so this depletion deprives the muscles of nourishment, and the Heart controls the circulation of Blood, so it leads to poor circulation of both Qi and Blood to the limbs. Both these factors may cause weakness of the legs, dizziness and vertigo.

In most cases the symptoms in the early stages reflect an invasion of Dampness: they are a feeling of heaviness, numbness and tingling of the limbs. In the middle stages of the disease there is a progressive deficiency of Liver and Kidneys with such symptoms as dizziness, vertigo, blurred vision, progressive weakness of the legs, and urinary hesitancy or urgency. If Liver-Yang develops, there is stiffness of the legs, more severe vertigo and vomiting. In the late stages, with the development of Liver-Wind,

there is tremor and severe spasms of the legs.

Thus the symptoms at the various stages can be summarized as follows (Table 29.1).

Differentiation and treatment

Acupuncture is the treatment of choice for multiple sclerosis.

There are only two basic patterns:

Damp-Phlegm with Spleen Deficiency
Liver and Kidney Deficiency

DAMP-PHLEGM WITH SPLEEN DEFICIENCY
CLINICAL MANIFESTATIONS

Numbness, feeling of heaviness of the legs, tingling, dizziness, tiredness.
Tongue: Swollen with teeth-marks and a sticky coating.
Pulse: Weak and Slippery.

TREATMENT PRINCIPLE

Resolve Dampness, tonify the Spleen and invigorate the Connecting channels.

ACUPUNCTURE

Ren-12 Zhongwan, BL-20 Pishu, SP-9 Yinlingquan, SP-6 Sanyinjiao, ST-40 Fenglong. Reducing or even method depending on how acute the condition is.

EXPLANATION

– **Ren-12** and **BL-20** tonify the Spleen.

Table 29.1   Patterns and symptoms in multiple sclerosis

Beginning stage	Middle stage		Late stage
Dampness Heaviness of legs, dizziness, numbness, tingling	Kidney-Liver deficiency Blurred vision, weakness of legs dizziness, vertigo, urinary hesitancy or urgency	Liver-Yang rising Stiffness of legs, vertigo, vomiting	Liver-Wind Tremor, spasms, paraplegia

- **SP-9** and **SP-6** resolve Dampness.
- **ST-40** resolves Phlegm.

HERBAL TREATMENT

PRESCRIPTION

SI MIAO SAN Variation
Four Wonderful Powder
Cang Zhu *Rhizoma Atractylodis lanceae* 6 g
Huang Bo *Cortex Phellodendri* 9 g
Niu Xi *Radix Achyranthis bidentatae seu Cyathulae* 6 g
Yi Yi Ren *Semen Coicis lachryma jobi* 9 g
Bi Xie *Rhizoma Dioscoreae hypoglaucae* 6 g
Bai Zhu *Rhizoma Atractylodis macrocephalae* 6 g
Du Huo *Radix Angelicae pubescentis* 6 g

Explanation

- **Si Miao San** (first four herbs) resolves Damp-Heat from the Lower Burner and legs.
- **Bi Xie** resolves Dampness from the legs.
- **Bai Zhu** tonifies Spleen-Qi and dries Dampness.
- **Du Huo** expels Wind-Dampness from the Lower Burner and invigorates the Connecting channels.

Variations

- If the condition is very long-standing and Dampness is pronounced add Huo Xiang *Herba Agastachis* and Pei Lan *Herba Eupatorii fortunei*.
- If there is a lot of numbness and tingling add Sha Ren *Fructus seu Semen Amomi* and Wei Ling Xian *Radix Clematidis chinensis*.

Case history

A 45-year-old man had been diagnosed as suffering from multiple sclerosis (MS) only a few months earlier. The first symptoms of his condition were numbness of the left arm, tingling of the limbs and around the mouth, dizziness and a feeling of heaviness of the head and legs. He also felt very tired. His pulse was Slippery but also Weak and his tongue was Swollen with a sticky-yellow coating inside a Stomach-crack.

Diagnosis
This condition was clearly due to Dampness and Phlegm obstructing the channels and also the head. There was also an underlying deficiency of Spleen and Stomach as evidenced by the tiredness, Weak pulse and Stomach-crack on the tongue.

Treatment principle
The principle of treatment applied was to tonify the Spleen and resolve Dampness, as well as remove obstruction from the channels and invigorate the Connecting channels.

Acupuncture
The acupuncture treatment was based mostly on the following points:

- **ST-36** Zusanli, **SP-3** Taibai, **Ren-12** Zhongwan, **BL-20** Pishu and **BL-21** Weishu to tonify Stomach and Spleen. Reinforcing method.
- **SP-9** Yinlingquan, **SP-6** Sanyinjiao, **ST-40** Fenglong and **BL-22** Sanjiaoshu to resolve Dampness. Even method.
- **L.I.-10** Shousanli, **T.B.-5** Waiguan and **ST-31** Biguan to expel Dampness from the channels and invigorate the Connecting channels.
- **LU-7** Lieque and **KI-6** Zhaohai in combination to open the Directing Vessel in order to relieve tingling and numbness around the lips.

Herbal treatment
The herbal formula used was a variation of Si Miao San *Four Wonderful Powder*:

Huang Bo *Cortex Phellodendri* 6 g
Cang Zhu *Rhizoma Atractylodis lanceae* 6 g
Yi Yi Ren *Semen Coicis lachryma jobi* 9 g
Niu Xi *Radix Achyranthis bidentatae seu Cyathulae* 6 g
Bai Zhu *Rhizoma Atractylodis macrocephalae* 6 g
Wei Ling Xian *Radix Clematidis chinensis* 4.5 g
Sha Ren *Fructus seu Semen Amomi* 4 g

Explanation
- The first four herbs resolve Dampness in the Lower Burner.
- **Bai Zhu** tonifies the Spleen and drains Dampness.
- **Wei Ling Xian** and **Sha Ren** eliminate obstructions from the channels, resolve Dampness and invigorate the Connecting channels.

Case history

A 36-year-old woman had been suffering from MS for 3 years. Her main symptoms were a feeling of heaviness of her legs, lack of balance, weakness of the legs, difficulty in walking and urinary incontinence. She had a 2-year-old child and her symptoms improved during the pregnancy. Her tongue was slightly Pale but with a Red tip. It was Swollen and had a Heart-crack. The coating was sticky. Her pulse was Weak and Fine and the Heart position was particularly Weak.

Diagnosis
The main manifestations are clearly those of Dampness invading the Lower Burner and the leg channels. However, the cause of the disease had its roots not only in the Spleen but also the Heart. The Weak Heart pulse and Heart crack on the tongue point to shock injuring both Spleen and Heart. She confirmed that she had suffered a severe shock a year before the onset of her symptoms.

Treatment principle
The treatment principle adopted was to resolve Dampness from the Lower Burner, tonify the Spleen and strengthen the Heart. She was treated primarily with acupuncture.

Acupuncture
The points used were chosen from the following:

- **ST-36** Zusanli, **SP-6** Sanyinjiao, **Ren-12** Zhongwan and **BL-20** Pishu to tonify Stomach and Spleen. Reinforcing method.
- **SP-9** Yinlingquan and **BL-22** Sanyinjiao to resolve Dampness. Even method.
- **HE-5** Tongli to calm the Mind.
- **ST-31** Biguan, **ST-34** Liangqiu, **ST-41** Jiexi and **G.B.-40** Qiuxu to remove obstructions from the channels and invigorate the Connecting channels. The last two points ST-41 and G.B.-40 are particularly good to lift the feet which eliminates stumbling and makes walking much easier.
- **BL-28** Pangguangshu and **BL-32** Ciliao to tonify the Bladder and stop incontinence.

This patient is still being treated; her condition has shown an improvement of some 60% and is now quite stable.

LIVER AND KIDNEY DEFICIENCY

CLINICAL MANIFESTATIONS

Progressive weakness of the legs, weak back and knees, dizziness, poor memory, blurred vision, hesitancy or urgency of urination.

TREATMENT PRINCIPLE

Tonify Kidneys and Liver and strengthen bones and tendons.

ACUPUNCTURE

KI-3 Taixi, Ren-4 Guanyuan, BL-23 Shenshu, SP-6 Sanyinjiao, LIV-8 Ququan, BL-18 Ganshu, S.I.-3 Houxi and BL-62 Shenmai, LIV-3 Taichong, G.B.-20 Fengchi. Reinforcing method except on the last two points which should be needled with even method. Moxa should be used if there is Yang deficiency, otherwise not.

EXPLANATION

- **KI-3**, **Ren-4**, **BL-23** and **SP-6** tonify the Kidneys.
- **LIV-8** and **BL-18** tonify the Liver.
- **S.I.-3** and **BL-62** strengthen the Governing Vessel and the spine.
- **LIV-3** and **G.B.-20** subdue Liver-Wind. G.B.-20 also brightens the eyes in case of blurred or double vision.

HERBAL TREATMENT

PRESCRIPTION

LIU WEI DI HUANG WAN Variation
Six-Ingredient Rehmannia Pill
Shu Di Huang *Radix Rehmanniae glutinosae prae-parata* 24 g
Shan Zhu Yu *Fructus Corni officinalis* 12 g
Shan Yao *Radix Dioscoreae oppositae* 12 g
Ze Xie *Rhizoma Alismatis orientalis* 9 g
Mu Dan Pi *Cortex Moutan radicis* 9 g
Fu Ling *Sclerotium Poriae cocos* 9 g
Du Huo *Radix Angelicae pubescentis* 4 g
Sang Ji Sheng *Ramus Loranthi* 6 g
Ji Xue Teng *Caulis Millettiae seu Caulis Spatholobi* 6 g
Wu Jia Pi *Cortex Acanthopanacis radicis* 6 g
Du Zhong *Cortex Eucommiae ulmoidis* 4.5 g

Explanation

- The formula Liu Wei Di Huang Wan (first six herbs) nourishes Kidney- and Liver-Yin.
- **Du Huo** expels Wind-Damp from the channels of the Lower Burner and invigorates the Connecting channels.
- **Sang Ji Sheng** nourishes Liver-Blood and the tendons.

- **Ji Xue Teng** and **Wu Jia Pi** invigorate the Connecting channels, move Blood and strengthen tendons and bones.
- **Du Zhong** may be added in a small dose, even though it is a Yang tonic, to tonify the lower back and legs and strengthen the spine. The emphasis of the formula as a whole is to nourish Yin, so it is good to include a Yang tonic as Yang corresponds to movement.

Variations

- If there is stasis of Blood evidenced by pain in the limbs add Hong Hua *Flos Carthami tinctorii*, Tao Ren *Semen Persicae* and Niu Xi *Radix Achyranthis bidentatae seu Cyathulae*.
- If there are spasms, add Jiang Can *Bombyx batryticatus* and Di Long *Pheretima aspergillum*.
- If, in a very chronic case, there is a deficiency of both Yin and Yang of the Kidneys (deficiency of Yang appearing later while the tongue is still Red), add Lu Jiao *Cornu Cervi* to tonify Kidney-Yang and strengthen the spine.

(i) PATENT REMEDY

DU HUO JI SHENG WAN
Angelica pubescens-Loranthus Pill
Du Huo *Radix Angelicae pubescentis*
Xi Xin *Herba Asari cum radice*
Fang Feng *Radix Ledebouriellae sesloidis*
Qin Jiao *Radix Gentianae macrophyllae*
Sang Ji Sheng *Ramus Loranthi*
Du Zhong *Radix Eucommiae ulmoidis*
Niu Xi *Radix Achyranthis bidentatae seu Cyathulae*
Dang Gui *Radix Angelicae sinensis*
Chuan Xiong *Radix Ligustici wallichii*
Sheng Di Huang *Radix Rehmanniae glutinosae*
Bai Shao *Radix Paeoniae albae*
Ren Shen *Radix Ginseng*
Fu Ling *Sclerotium Poriae cocos*
Rou Gui *Cortex Cinnamomi cassiae*
Gan Cao *Radix Glycyrrhizae uralensis*

Explanation

This remedy tonifies Liver and Kidneys and expels Wind-Dampness from the back and legs. It is suitable only if there is a deficiency of Kid-

ney-Yang. The tongue presentation appropriate to this remedy, therefore, is a Pale body.

(ii) PATENT REMEDY

DU ZHONG BU TIAN SU
Eucommia Benefiting Heaven Pill
Du Zhong *Cortex Eucommiae ulmoidis*
Gou Qi Zi *Fructus Lycii chinensis*
Huang Qi *Radix Astragali membranacei*
Dang Shen *Radix Codonopsis pilosulae*
Dang Gui *Radix Angelicae sinensis*
Sheng Di Huang *Radix Rehmanniae glutinosae*
Ba Ji Tian *Radix Morindae officinalis*
Shan Zhu Yu *Fructus Corni officinalis*
Rou Cong Rong *Herba Cistanchis*
Lian Zi *Semen Nelumbinis nuciferae*
Bai Zi Ren *Semen Biotae orientalis*

Explanation

This remedy tonifies both Kidney-Yang and Kidney-Yin, nourishes the Liver, and benefits sinews and bones. It is suitable for multiple sclerosis from deficiency of Liver- and Kidney-Yin: the Kidney-Yang tonics within the formula will help the movement of the limbs.

The tongue presentation appropriate to this remedy is a slightly Red body colour with a rootless coating. If the body-colour is very Red and the tongue is completely without coating, this pill is not suitable.

(iii) PATENT REMEDY

LIU WEI DI HUANG WAN
Six-Ingredient Rehmannia Pill
Shu Di Huang *Radix Rehmanniae glutinosae praeparata*
Shan Yao *Radix Dioscoreae oppositae*
Shan Zhu Yu *Fructus Corni officinalis*
Ze Xie *Rhizoma Alismatis orientalis*
Fu Ling *Sclerotium Poriae cocos*
Mu Dan Pi *Cortex Moutan radicis*

Explanation

This pill nourishes Liver- and Kidney-Yin: it will

not have any direct effect on the channels and sinews, but it can be used to nourish Kidney-Yin in conjunction with acupuncture.

The tongue presentation appropriate to this remedy is a Red body with a rootless coating or without coating.

ACUPUNCTURE

Apart from the acupuncture points indicated for the above two patterns, local points on the limbs should be used to remove obstructions from the channels. These are exactly the same as those indicated for the treatment of hemiplegia following Wind-stroke (ch. 27).

In addition to these, it is important to use points on the Governing Vessel and Huatuojiaji points since the myelin sheath lesions are located around the spine. The most frequently used points on the Governing Vessel are Du-3 Yaoyangguan which affects circulation of Qi to the legs, Du-4 Mingmen which tonifies the Fire of the Gate of Vitality and Kidney-Yang, Du-12 Shenzhu, Du-14 Dazhui and Du-20 Baihui. The corresponding Huatuojiaji points may also be used.

In the late stages of multiple sclerosis there may also be stasis of Blood. This is extremely distressing for the patient as, in addition to the paraplegia and spasms, there is also pain in the limbs. In these cases one must use points to move Blood such as BL-17 Geshu and SP-10 Xuehai.

The Extraordinary Vessels are often helpful in the treatment of multiple sclerosis. The Girdle Vessel encircles the leg channels and a dysfunction of this vessel may impair the circulation of Qi and Blood in the leg channels. This vessel is often affected by Dampness, and the patient may feel as if sitting in water, a feeling which those suffering from multiple sclerosis sometimes experience. The Girdle Vessel may also be affected by a deficiency of the Stomach channel so that it cannot bind properly. The "Simple Questions" in chapter 44 says: *"When the Bright Yang channels are deficient, the Girdle Vessel cannot bind and atrophy of the legs may result."*[1] In these cases one can use the Girdle Vessel, i.e. G.B.-41 on the left

for men and right for women and T.B.-5 on the opposite side, together with ST-36 Zusanli to strengthen the Bright Yang and BL-23 Shenshu to strengthen the leg channels. It will be remembered that the Kidney divergent channel intersects the Girdle Vessel at BL-23 Shenshu.

The Governing Vessel is very important in the treatment of multiple sclerosis since it strengthens the Kidneys and the spine. To open it, one needles S.I.-3 Houxi on the left for men and right for women and BL-62 Shenmai on the opposite side. When using the Governing Vessel in women, it is best combined with the Directing Vessel. Thus one would needle S.I.-3 Houxi on the right, BL-62 Shenmai on the left, LU-7 Lieque on the left and KI-6 Zhaohai on the right in this order.

If the muscles on the lateral side of the legs are stiff and tight one may tonify the Yin Heel Vessel and reduce the Yang Heel Vessel, i.e. reinforce KI-6 Zhaohai and reduce BL-62 Shenmai on the same leg. If the muscles of the medial side of the leg are stiff and tight, one may tonify the Yang Heel Vessel and reduce the Yin Heel Vessel, i.e. reinforce BL-62 Shenmai and reduce KI-6 Zhaohai on the same leg. The "Pulse Classic" (AD 280) by Wang Shu He says:

When the Yang Qiao is diseased the muscles of the medial side of the leg are slack and those of the lateral side tight; when the Yin Qiao is diseased the muscles of the medial side of the leg are tight and those of the lateral side slack.[2]

Finally, scalp acupuncture is very useful to treat multiple sclerosis. The motor area should be used, the upper part for the leg and the lower part for the arm (see Fig. 27.4 in chapter 27 on "Wind-stroke"). The technique of needle insertion is the same as that indicated for Parkinson's disease (ch. 26) and Wind-stroke (ch. 27).

Prognosis

Whilst Chinese medicine cannot completely cure this condition, it can offer considerable help in alleviating its symptoms and slowing down its progress. Acupuncture helps considerably in eliminating the feeling of heaviness and tingling of the limbs and in facilitating walking.

The earlier the treatment is started the better the results. If the patient is still walking one can expect some results, but if he or she is permanently in a wheelchair then results will be very poor or non-existent. If treatment is started at the very early stages, the symptoms can be eliminated completely and the progression of the disease halted indefinitely. This is all the more likely to happen if the patient cooperates in changing life style by taking more rest, adjusting the diet, and reducing sexual activity.

Initially, treatment should be carried out 2–3 times a week. After a few weeks it can be spaced out to once a week and then once a fortnight. If a good improvement is obtained, the patient should be seen about once a month thereafter.

END NOTES

1. 1979 The Yellow Emperor's Classic of Internal Medicine — Simple Questions (*Huang Ti Nei Jing Su Wen* 黄帝内经素问), People's Health Publishing House, Beijing. First published *c.* 100 BC, p. 249.
2. Shandong College of Traditional Chinese Medicine 1984 An Explanation of the Pulse Classic (*Mai Jing Jiao Shi* 脉经校释), People's Health Publishing House, Beijing, p. 88. The "Pulse Classic" itself was written by Wang Shu He and first published *c.* AD 280.

Bleeding 30

血
证

This chapter will discuss first the causes and patterns of bleeding and the general approach to treatment, and then the specific treatment of bleeding from various parts of the body. Acupuncture and Chinese herbal medicine are extremely effective in stopping bleeding both in acute and chronic conditions.

Aetiology

1. EXTERNAL PATHOGENIC FACTORS

Wind-Heat, when particularly intense, may injure the Lung's Blood Connecting channels and cause bleeding either from the nose or with coughing.

External Damp-Heat may invade the Intestines or Bladder and injure the Blood Connecting channels there leading to bleeding in the stools or urine.

2. DIET

Excessive consumption of hot foods, or hot-greasy foods and alcohol leads to Heat or Damp-Heat. Heat invades the Blood portion and causes blood to push out of the vessels. This is bleeding from Blood-Heat.

Excessive consumption of greasy foods and dairy products may weaken the Spleen: deficient Spleen-Qi may fail to hold Blood in the vessels leading to bleeding. This is bleeding from Qi deficiency.

3. EMOTIONAL STRAIN

Emotional strain is an important cause of bleeding. Every emotion, when excessive and prolonged, impairs the proper movement of Qi and leads to stagnation of Qi. Stagnant-Qi over a long period of time often leads to Fire. Fire enters the Blood portion and makes the Blood "reckless", causing bleeding.

Bleeding from emotional strain is especially associated with Qi rebelling upwards such as happens in Liver-Fire. In such a case the bleeding would occur upwards, i.e. with vomiting, coughing or from the nose. In more severe cases and in old people with a more complex pathology this may also lead to bleeding upwards in the brain and cause a cerebral haemorrhage.

4. OVERWORK

Overwork is also an extremely common cause of bleeding, especially in chronic cases. Working long hours without adequate rest over many years weakens Spleen-Qi and Kidney-Yin. This may lead to bleeding in two different ways. Both deficient Qi or Yin may fail to hold Blood and cause bleeding. Furthermore, deficiency of Yin over a long period of time leads to Empty-Heat which may agitate the Blood and cause bleeding.

5. CHRONIC ILLNESS AND CHILDBIRTH

A long, chronic illness inevitably causes Spleen deficiency and this may cause bleeding in the way described above.

In women of weak body-condition, childbirth may deplete the Kidneys: this may cause bleeding from Qi or Yin deficiency or from Empty-Heat.

6. AFTERMATH OF A HEAT DISEASE

Wind-Heat has a strong tendency to cause internal dryness as it dries up the body fluids, and also because it may quickly turn into interior Heat. Heat may damage the Blood-Connecting channels and cause bleeding, especially from the lungs, stomach or intestines.

Pathology

There are four main pathological conditions involved in bleeding:

Qi Deficiency
Heat
Empty-Heat
Stasis of Blood.

The first two conditions are the most common ones.

1. QI DEFICIENCY

One of the functions of Qi is to control Blood, holding it in the vessels. If Qi is deficient it may fail to hold Blood in the vessels and lead to bleeding. This is a deficient type of bleeding and is due to Spleen-Qi deficiency. This does not mean, of course, that Qi deficiency always leads to bleeding. Bleeding from Qi deficiency is often (but not exclusively) characterized by a downward movement, i.e. as a form of sinking of Spleen-Qi. Thus, it often causes bleeding from the lower orifices. Typical examples would be excessive menstrual bleeding or bleeding in the stools or urine from deficient Spleen-Qi not holding Blood.

Bleeding from Qi deficiency is characterized by a fresh appearance and bright-red colour of the blood and is of course accompanied by symptoms and signs of Qi deficiency.

2. HEAT

Heat causes bleeding by invading the Blood portion and damaging the Blood-Connecting channels. Heat makes the Blood reckless and causes it to extravasate.

Bleeding from Heat may be upwards or downwards. For example, excessive menstrual bleeding and bleeding in the stools or bladder mentioned above may also be caused by Heat in the Blood. Bleeding upwards is usually typical of Blood-Heat. An example is bleeding from the nose and vomiting or coughing of blood. This type of bleeding is associated with Qi rebelling upwards, "carrying" Fire with it and injuring the Blood-Connecting channels upwards.

In bleeding from Heat the blood may be bright-red or dark-red and the flow is usually profuse.

3. EMPTY-HEAT

Empty-Heat from Yin deficiency leads to bleeding in two ways. First of all, Yin-Qi is a type of Qi and just as deficient Qi fails to hold Blood, so deficient-Yin may also fail to hold Blood. Secondly, Empty-Heat deriving from Yin deficiency may invade the Blood portion rather as Full-Heat makes Blood reckless so that it pushes out of the blood vessels.

Bleeding from Empty-Heat is usually scanty (as there is Yin deficiency and Blood is part of Yin). The colour of the blood is fresh-red or scarlet-red. It may occur in coughing, from the nose, under the skin (petechiae), in the stools, from the uterus or in the urine.

4. STASIS OF BLOOD

Stasis of Blood may also lead to bleeding. This may seem strange as stasis implies congealing of Blood. However, when Blood stagnates in the vessels and the Blood-Connecting channels, it obstructs them so that the new Blood which is continuously formed cannot enter the vessels and leaks out.

Bleeding from Blood stasis is characterized by dark blood with clots and by pain. It may occur from the uterus, intestines, bladder or under the skin.

It is easy for Full conditions causing bleeding to turn into Empty conditions. For example, prolonged loss of blood from Blood-Heat may lead to Blood and Qi deficiency (which, in itself, may be a further cause of bleeding). It may also happen that prolonged bleeding from Blood-Heat leads to Yin deficiency as Blood is part of Yin. Yin deficiency may cause Empty-Heat which may become a further cause of bleeding, thus giving rise to a complex pathological condition.

Treatment

Bleeding *must* always be treated by attending to the underlying cause, i.e. Heat, Empty-Heat, Qi deficiency or Blood stasis and *never* by simply using herbs which stop bleeding.

The principles of treatment of bleeding were outlined in great detail by Dr Tang Zong Hai in his book "A Discussion of Blood Syndromes" (1884). In this book he outlines a fourfold strategy to treat bleeding.[1] The four principles of treatment which are aimed at harmonizing Blood, are:

1. Harmonize Blood
2. Treat the Root-cause of bleeding
3. Astringe
4. Treat Qi.

The first of these aims, in turn, is composed of four steps:

(a) Stop bleeding
(b) Eliminate stasis
(c) Calm Blood
(d) Nourish Blood.

All these four principles of treatment are to be adopted simultaneously in any type of bleeding (Fig. 30.1).

The rationale of the four treatment aims is briefly as follows:

1. *Harmonize Blood*: this is necessary to move, calm and nourish Blood after stopping bleeding.

2. *Treat the Root-cause*: this is essential to treat bleeding. The Root-cause may be Heat, Empty-Heat, Qi deficiency or stasis of Blood as indicated before. Rarely, bleeding may derive from Cold.

3. *Astringe*: this is an adjuvant to the stopping-bleeding method. It consists in the use of astringent herbs which, although they do not stop bleeding by themselves, they help the stopping-bleeding herbs.

4. *Treat Qi*: this consists in either tonifying Qi for bleeding from Spleen-Qi deficiency or subduing rebellious Qi for bleeding upwards (such as epistaxis or haemoptysis).

We can now discuss each of the four treatment aims in detail.

1. HARMONIZE BLOOD

Whatever its cause, bleeding must be treated by

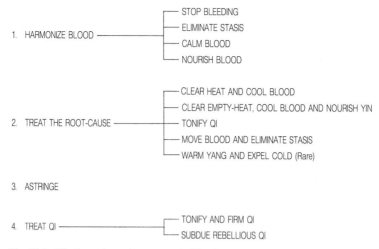

Fig. 30.1 The four aims of treatment in bleeding

harmonizing Blood according to the four steps indicated above, partly to stop the bleeding itself and partly to treat the consequences of blood loss. These four steps are:

- Stop bleeding
- Eliminate stasis
- Calm Blood
- Nourish Blood.

These will now be analysed in detail.

(a) STOP BLEEDING

The first step simply consists in using stopping-bleeding herbs. These herbs stop bleeding from whatever cause. As indicated above, they must *never* be used on their own but must *always* be combined with herbs which treat the underlying cause of bleeding.

Examples of herbs that stop bleeding are:

Pu Huang *Pollen Typhae*
Xian He Cao *Herba Agrimoniae pilosae*
San Qi *Radix Notoginseng*
Bai Ji *Rhizoma Bletillae striatae*
Xiao Ji *Herba Cephalanoplos segeti*
Da Ji *Herba Cirsii japonici*
Di Yu *Radix Sanguisorbae officinalis*
Huai Hua *Flos Sophorae japonicae immaturus*
Qian Cao Gen *Radix Rubiae cordifoliae*
Ce Bai Ye *Cacumen Biotae orientalis*
Ai Ye *Folium Artemisiae*

Ou Jie *Nodus Nelumbinis nuciferae rhizomatis*
Bai Mao Gen *Rhizoma Imperatae cylindricae*
Zao Xin Huang Tu (also called Fu Long Gan) *Terra Flava usta*

Although all these herbs will stop bleeding, they should be carefully selected keeping their auxiliary properties in mind. We can classify the above herbs in three ways to help us select them in a rational way:

- according to their nature (hot or cold)
- according to part of body and organ reached
- according to whether they move Blood or not.

(i) ACCORDING TO THEIR NATURE

Cold: Bai Ji, Da Ji, Xiao Ji, Di Yu, Huai Hua, Qian Cao Gen, Ce Bai Ye and Bai Mao Gen.
Warm: San Qi, Ai Ye and Zao Xin Huang Tu.
Those not mentioned above are neutral in nature.

(ii) ACCORDING TO PART OF BODY AND ORGAN REACHED

Lungs: Xian He Cao, Bai Ji, Ou Jie, Xiao Ji, Ce Bai Ye and San Qi.
Intestines: Di Yu, Huai Hua and San Qi.
Stomach: Bai Ji, Di Yu, Xian He Cao, Ou Jie and Zao Xin Huang Tu.

Nose: Xiao Ji.
Bladder: Xiao Ji, Da Ji, Huai Hua, Bai Mao Gen, Pu Huang and Qian Cao Gen.
Uterus: Pu Huang, Xian He Cao, Di Yu, Qian Cao Gen and Ai Ye.

(iii) ACCORDING TO WHETHER THEY MOVE BLOOD

Since herbs that stop bleeding may have a tendency, by their very nature, to congeal Blood, herbs which stop bleeding *and* move Blood are particularly useful.

Herbs that stop bleeding and move Blood are: Pu Huang, San Qi, and Qian Cao Gen.

Apart from herbs belonging to the category of stopping-bleeding herbs, many herbs from other categories also stop bleeding. These, however, are more selective as they only stop bleeding in conditions pertaining to their particular category. For example, Gan Jiang can stop bleeding only when this is caused by Cold (which is rare), whilst a herb such as Xian He Cao (from the stopping-bleeding category) will stop bleeding from any cause.

Herbs that stop bleeding from categories other than the stopping-bleeding category are:

Expelling Wind-Cold

Jing Jie *Herba seu Flos Schizonepetae tenuifoliae*
Sheng Jiang *Rhizoma Zingiberis officinalis recens*

Expelling Wind-Heat

Chai Hu *Radix Bupleuri*
Sheng Ma *Rhizoma Cimicifugae*
Qing Hao *Herba Artemisiae apiaceae*

Clearing Heat

Huang Qin *Radix Scutellariae baicalensis*
Huang Lian *Rhizoma Coptidis*
Shi Gao *Gypsum fibrosum*
Zhi Zi *Fructus Gardeniae jasminoidis* (an important one)

Cooling Blood

Shui Niu Jiao *Cornu Bufali*

Sheng Di Huang *Radix Rehmanniae glutinosae*
Dan Pi *Cortex Moutan radicis*
Chi Shao *Radix Paeoniae rubrae*

Resolving Fire-Poison

Qing Dai *Indigo naturalis*
Ma Chi Xian *Herba Portulacae oleraceae*

Warming

Gan Jiang *Rhizoma Zingiberis officinalis*

Moving downwards

Da Huang *Rhizoma Rhei*

Resolving Damp-Heat

Hai Jin Sha *Spora Lygodii japonici*
Mu Tong *Caulis Akebiae*

Moving Blood

Pu Huang *Pollen Typhae*
San Qi *Radix Notoginseng*
Niu Xi *Radix Achyranthis bidentatae seu Cyathulae*

Nourishing Blood

E Jiao *Gelatinum Corii Asini*

Tonifying Yang

Du Zhong *Cortex Eucommiae ulmoidis*
Xu Duan *Radix Dipsaci*

Nourishing Yin

Gui Ban *Plastrum Testudinis*
Han Lian Cao *Herba Ecliptae prostratae*

Astringents

Shan Zhu Yu *Fructus Corni officinalis*
Wu Zei Gu *Os Sepiae*
Chi Shi Zhi *Halloysitum rubrum*

Calming the Mind

Long Gu *Os Draconis*

Extinguishing Wind

Bai Shao *Radix Paeoniae albae*

Digestive

Shan Zha *Fructus Crataegi*

(b) ELIMINATE STASIS

This is the second of the four steps to harmonize Blood. This second step is necessary for two reasons. First of all, after bleeding, as the blood leaves the blood vessels, there is always some blood left over in the skin, muscles, the space between skin and muscles, and the Connecting channels. Eliminating stasis will help to get rid of this left-over blood. Secondly, because stopping-bleeding herbs may have the tendency to congeal Blood, it is best to combine them with some moving-Blood herbs.

For this second step, any of the moving Blood herbs may be used such as Hong Hua *Flos Carthami tinctorii* or Chuan Xiong *Radix Ligustici wallichii*. However, the best herbs to use are those that move Blood *and* stop bleeding such as Pu Huang *Pollen Typhae*, San Qi *Radix Notoginseng* and Qian Cao Gen *Radix Rubiae cordifoliae*.

(c) CALM BLOOD

This is the third step in harmonizing Blood. In any type of bleeding the Sea of Blood of the Penetrating Vessel is agitated by rebellious Qi. It is rebellious Qi in the Penetrating Vessel which enters the Blood-Connecting channels and stirs up the Sea of Blood making the Blood reckless and causing it to leave the blood vessels. Thus, in order to prevent recurrence of bleeding, one must not only stop bleeding and move Blood but also "calm" Blood. Thus "calming Blood" means subduing rebellious Qi of the Penetrating Vessel and calming its Sea of Blood.

Herbs that calm the Blood are those which enter the Blood and are cool and absorbing. Examples of calming-Blood herbs are:

Bai Shao *Radix Paeoniae albae*
Sheng Di Huang *Radix Rehmanniae glutinosae*
Han Lian Cao *Herba Ecliptae prostratae*
Mu Dan Pi *Cortex Moutan radicis*

(d) NOURISH BLOOD

This is the last step in harmonizing Blood. After blood loss, whether it be acute and massive or scanty but prolonged, there is naturally a tendency to Blood deficiency. Thus, it is necessary to nourish Blood. Any of the nourishing-Blood herbs are applicable such as Dang Gui *Radix Angelicae sinensis*, Shu Di Huang *Radix Rehmanniae glutinosae praeparata*, or Gou Qi Zi *Fructus Lycii chinensis*.

Thus, in a nutshell, the reasons for adopting these four steps to harmonize Blood in bleeding are as follows:

- *Stop bleeding*: to arrest blood loss
- *Eliminate stasis*: to prevent Blood from congealing
- *Calm Blood*: to prevent recurrence of bleeding
- *Nourish Blood*: to restore the Blood after the blood loss.

The above four steps to harmonize Blood must always be combined with the other three principles of treatment, i.e. to treat the underlying cause of bleeding, to astringe and to treat Qi.

2. TREAT THE ROOT-CAUSE

The underlying cause of bleeding *must* always be identified clearly and be treated accordingly. Bleeding is *never* treated just by the addition of one or two stopping-bleeding herbs.

The main causes of bleeding are:

(a) Heat
(b) Empty-Heat
(c) Qi Deficiency
(d) Stasis of Blood
(e) Yang Deficiency and Cold (this is rare).

(a) HEAT

Some of the herbs used here are those that clear

Heat and drain Fire and some are those that clear Heat and cool Blood.

(i) CLEAR HEAT AND DRAIN FIRE

The most important of all in this category is Shan Zhi Zi *Fructus Gardeniae jasminoidis* especially if charred. Other herbs that help to stop bleeding by clearing Heat are Shi Gao *Gypsum fibrosum*, Huang Qin *Radix Scutellariae baicalensis* and Huang Lian *Rhizoma Coptidis*.

(ii) CLEAR HEAT AND COOL BLOOD

Herbs from this category are the most important ones to stop bleeding from Blood-Heat. The three most important ones are Sheng Di Huang *Radix Rehmanniae glutinosae*, Chi Shao *Radix Paeoniae rubrae*, and Mu Dan Pi *Cortex Moutan radicis*. Di Gu Pi *Cortex Lycii chinensis radicis* also stops bleeding from Blood-Heat especially in the lungs.

(b) EMPTY-HEAT

The two main herbs that stop bleeding by clearing Empty-Heat are Qing Hao *Herba Artemisiae apiaceae* and Han Lian Cao *Herba Ecliptae prostratae*.

(c) QI DEFICIENCY

Any Qi tonic will stop bleeding from Qi deficiency but the most effective one is Huang Qi *Radix Astragali membranacei*. The main formula to stop bleeding from Qi deficiency is Dang Gui Bu Xue Tang *Angelica Tonifying Blood Decoction* which is composed only of Huang Qi and Dang Gui *Radix Angelicae sinensis* in the proportions of 5:1.

(d) STASIS OF BLOOD

Any moving Blood herb can stop bleeding from Blood stasis, but the best are those which move Blood *and* stop bleeding such as Pu Huang *Pollen Typhae*, San Qi *Radix Notoginseng* and Qian Cao Gen *Radix Rubiae cordifoliae*.

(e) YANG DEFICIENCY AND COLD

This is quite a rare cause of bleeding. It occurs when Yang-Qi is deficient and fails to hold Blood. It is rare as internal Cold deriving from Yang deficiency has the tendency to coagulate Blood. The herbs that can stop bleeding by warming the channels are Gan Jiang *Rhizoma Zingiberis officinalis* or toasted Sheng Jiang *Rhizoma Zingiberis officinalis recens*, Ai Ye *Folium Artemisiae* and Zao Xin Huang Tu *Terra Flava usta*.

3. ASTRINGE

To astringe is the third treatment aim in bleeding. Astringent herbs are used as adjuvant to the stopping-bleeding herbs. As they astringe, absorb and retain fluids, they obviously help to stop bleeding.

The main herbs used in this context are Shan Zhu Yu *Fructus Corni officinalis*, Wu Wei Zi *Fructus Schisandrae chinensis*, Bai Shao *Radix Paeoniae albae*, Wu Zei Gu *Os Sepiae*, Lian Zi *Semen Nelumbinis nuciferae* and Chi Shi Zhi *Halloysitum rubrum*.

Three of the stopping-bleeding herbs are also astringent. These are Di Yu *Radix Sanguisorbae officinalis*, Ce Bai Ye *Cacumen Biotae orientalis* and Ou Jie *Nodus Nelumbinis nuciferae rhizomatis*.

4. TREAT QI

"Treating Qi" consists in two separate aims of treatment:

(a) *Tonify and firm Qi* for bleeding from Qi deficiency. The main herbs are Huang Qi *Radix Astragali membranacei*, Ren Shen *Radix Ginseng*, Fu Zi *Radix Aconiti carmichaeli praeparata* (if there is deficiency of Yang), Long Gu *Os Draconis*, Mu Li *Concha Ostreae* and Zhi Gan Cao *Radix*

Glycyrrhizae uralensis praeparata. Included in this aim of treatment is also raising Qi for bleeding downwards from sinking of Spleen-Qi. The two herbs that do this are Chai Hu *Radix Bupleuri* and Sheng Ma *Rhizoma Cimicifugae.*

(b) *Subdue rebellious Qi* for bleeding from Qi rebelling upwards. The main herb is Niu Xi *Radix Achyranthis bidentatae seu Cyathulae* which attracts Blood downwards.

If the above four aims of treatment are followed (including the four steps within the first aim), any formula can be adapted to treat bleeding from any part of the body. From looking at these principles of treatment it may seem that one needs to use very many herbs but this is not the case as some herbs have more than one of the above functions. For example, Bai Shao calms Blood (third step of first aim of treatment) and astringes (third aim of treatment). Sheng Di Huang has three of the above functions: it cools Blood and stops bleeding (second aim of treatment), calms Blood (third step of the first aim of treatment) and nourishes Blood (fourth step of the first aim of treatment). Qian Cao Gen stops bleeding (first step of the first aim of treatment), moves Blood (second step of the first aim of treatment) and cools Blood (second aim of treatment).

We can analyse two stopping-bleeding formulae to illustrate the above principles of treatment.

1. XIAO JI YIN ZI

Cephalanoplos Decoction
Xiao Ji *Herba Cephalanoplos segeti*
Ou Jie *Nodus Nelumbinis nuciferae rhizomatis*
Pu Huang *Pollen Typhae*
Hua Shi *Talcum*
Mu Tong *Caulis Akebiae*
Zhu Ye *Herba Lophatheri gracilis*
Zhi Zi *Fructus Gardeniae jasminoidis*
Sheng Di Huang *Radix Rehmanniae glutinosae*
Dang Gui *Radix Angelicae sinensis*
Gan Cao *Radix Glycyrrhizae uralensis*

This formula treats bleeding in the urine from Blood-Heat affecting the Bladder. The Root-

cause of bleeding in this case is therefore Full-Heat affecting the Blood.

We can now list the herbs from this formula against the principles of treatment outlined above:

1. *Harmonize Blood*
   (a) *Stop bleeding*: Xiao Ji, Ou Jie and Pu Huang
   (b) *Eliminate stasis*: Pu Huang
   (c) *Calm Blood*: Sheng Di Huang
   (d) *Nourish Blood*: Dang Gui and Sheng Di Huang
2. *Treat the Root-cause of bleeding* (in this case Blood-Heat): Sheng Di, Zhi Zi, Mu Tong, Zhu Ye and Hua Shi
3. *Astringe*: Ou Jie
4. *Treat Qi*: Gan Cao.

2. QIAN GEN SAN

Rubia Powder
Qian Cao Gen *Radix Rubiae cordifoliae*
Ce Bai Ye *Cacumen Biotae orientalis*
Huang Qin *Radix Scutellariae baicalensis*
Sheng Di Huang *Radix Rehmanniae glutinosae*
E Jiao *Gelatinum Corii Asini*
Gan Cao *Radix Glycyrrhizae uralensis*

This formula treats epistaxis from Blood-Heat. We can now analyse it according to the aims of treatment.

1. *Harmonize Blood*
   (a) *Stop bleeding*: Qian Cao Gen and Ce Bai Ye
   (b) *Eliminate stasis*: Qian Cao Gen
   (c) *Calm Blood*: Sheng Di Huang
   (d) *Nourish Blood*: E Jiao and Sheng Di Huang
2. *Treat the Root-cause of bleeding* (in this case Blood-Heat): Sheng Di Huang and Huang Qin
3. *Astringe*: Ce Bai Ye
4. *Treat Qi*: Gan Cao.

As for acupuncture, although it *is* effective in stopping bleeding, its points are less specific in their action than the above herbs. Although in order to stop bleeding with acupuncture, one can follow the four-step protocol outlined above, there are no "astringent" points in the same way as herbs, nor are there points which "calm Blood" as such. However, the general principle of treating the Root-cause of bleeding, harmonizing Blood and stopping bleeding is still valid.

As for points which specifically stop bleeding, Accumulation points, and especially those of the Yin channels, can stop bleeding. For example:

LU-6 Kongzui: coughing of blood.
L.I.-7 Wenliu: nosebleed, bleeding gums.
ST-34 Liangqiu: nosebleed, bleeding gums, vomiting of blood.
SP-8 Diji: uterine bleeding.
HE-6 Yinxi: vomiting of blood and epistaxis.
S.I.-6 Yanglao: blood-shot eyes.
BL-63 Jinmen: urinary bleeding.
KI-5 Shuiquan: urinary and uterine bleeding.
P-4 Ximen: vomiting of blood, coughing of blood, bleeding under the skin.
T.B.-7 Huizong: bleeding from ear-drum.
G.B.-36 Waiqiu: not for bleeding.
LIV-6 Zhongdu: urinary and uterine bleeding.
KI-8 Jiaoxin (Accumulation point of the Yin Heel Vessel): bloody leukorrhoea and uterine bleeding.

Other points specifically affect the Sea of Blood and can therefore be used to direct the effect of the treatment to the Blood portion in order to stop bleeding. These points are: **BL-17** Geshu and **SP-10** Xuehai.

The Connecting points, especially those of the Yin channels, can also stop bleeding. This is because these points control the Blood Connecting channels; this is a network of small, capillary-like channels which cover the whole body and spread Blood under the skin. The "Spiritual Axis" in chapter 81 says:

If fluids are harmonized . . . in the Middle Burner, they are transformed into Blood, when Blood is harmonized it first fills and irrigates the Blood Connecting channels, then percolates to the Connecting channels and finally in the main channels.[2]

The Blood Connecting channels are particularly involved in chronic conditions with stasis of Blood. The Connecting points, especially those of the Yin channels, can therefore be used to stop bleeding in chronic cases, particularly if there is some stasis of Blood. For example:

LU-7 Lieque: coughing of blood, nosebleed.

HE-5 Yinxi: coughing or vomiting of blood.
SP-4 Gongsun: bleeding under the skin.
KI-4 Dazhong: uterine or urinary bleeding.
P-6 Neiguan: coughing of blood and bleeding under the skin.
LIV-5 Ligou: urinary or uterine bleeding and bleeding under the skin.

We can now discuss the treatment of specific sites of bleeding. These are:

- Coughing blood
- Blood in stools
- Blood in urine
- Bleeding under the skin (petechiae)
- Bleeding gums.

Profuse menstrual bleeding will be discussed separately in the chapter on Menorrhagia (ch. 32).

Every one of the formulae mentioned for these conditions by definition treats the Root-cause of bleeding (second aim of treatment) and should be modified according to the principles indicated above for the other three aims of treatment. This means harmonizing Blood, astringing and treating Qi. These will be discussed for each formula with herbs to harmonize Blood, astringe and treat Qi specifically applicable to each pattern.

COUGHING BLOOD

This may range from coughing up large amounts of blood to coughing sputum which is only slightly blood-streaked.

The patterns discussed are:

Wind-Dry-Heat
Liver-Fire invading Lungs
Lung-Yin Deficiency with Empty-Heat.

WIND-DRY-HEAT
CLINICAL MANIFESTATIONS

Itchy throat, cough with blood-tinged sputum, nosebleed, dry mouth and nose, aversion to cold.

Tongue: Red on the sides and Front part, dry.
Pulse: Floating-Rapid.

TREATMENT PRINCIPLE

Clear Heat, expel Wind, moisten the Lungs, stop bleeding.

ACUPUNCTURE

LU-11 Shaoshang, L.I.-4 Hegu, BL-12 Fengmen, LU-6 Kongzui, LU-9 Taiyuan, Ren-12 Zhong-wan, SP-6 Sanyinjiao. Reducing method for the first four points and reinforcing on the others. No moxa.

Explanation

– **LU-11**, **L.I.-4** and **BL-12** expel Wind and clear Heat.
– **LU-6**, Accumulation point of the Lungs, stops bleeding from the Lung channel.
– **LU-9**, **Ren-12** and **SP-6** nourish Lung-fluids.

HERBAL TREATMENT

Prescription

SANG XING TANG
Morus-Prunus Decoction
Sang Ye *Folium Mori albae* 9 g
Xing Ren *Semen Pruni armeniacae* 9 g
Dan Dou Chi *Semen Sojae praeparatum* 9 g
Zhi Zi *Fructus Gardeniae jasminoidis* 6 g
Zhe Bei Mu *Bulbus Fritillariae thunbergii* 6 g
Nan Sha Shen *Radix Adenophorae* 6 g
Li Pi *Pericarpium Fructi Pyri* 6 g

Explanation

This formula, which has already been explained in chapter 8, expels Wind-Dry-Heat from the Lung's Defensive-Qi portion.

Variations

– To harmonize Blood (stop bleeding, eliminate

stasis, calm and nourish Blood) add Bai Ji *Rhizoma Bletillae striatae*, Ou Jie *Nodus Nelumbinis nuciferae rhizomatis*, San Qi *Radix Notoginseng*, Bai Shao *Radix Paeoniae albae* and Dang Gui *Radix Angelicae sinensis*.
– If Wind-Heat has begun to injure Yin add Mai Men Dong *Tuber Ophiopogonis japonici* and Tian Hua Fen *Radix Trichosanthis*.

Patent remedy

SANG JU GAN MAO PIAN
Morus-Chrysanthemum Common Cold Tablet
Sang Ye *Folium Mori albae*
Ju Hua *Flos Chrysanthemi morifolii*
Bo He *Herba Menthae*
Xing Ren *Semen Pruni armeniacae*
Jie Geng *Radix Platycodi grandiflori*
Lian Qiao *Fructus Forsythiae suspensae*
Lu Gen *Rhizoma Phragmitis communis*
Gan Cao *Radix Glycyrrhizae uralensis*

Explanation

This tablet has the same ingredients and functions as the formula Sang Ju Yin *Morus-Chrysanthemum Decoction*: it expels Wind-Heat from the Lung's Defensive-Qi portion and restores the descending of Lung-Qi. Although it contains no herbs which stop bleeding, it will do so by treating the Root, i.e. expelling Wind-Heat from the Lungs.

LIVER-FIRE INVADING LUNGS

CLINICAL MANIFESTATIONS

Cough with fresh-red blood in sputum, hypochondrial pain, irritability, propensity to outbursts of anger, a bitter taste.
Tongue: Red with yellow coating.
Pulse: Wiry and Rapid.

TREATMENT PRINCIPLE

Clear Liver-Fire, clear the Lungs, cool Blood and stop bleeding.

ACUPUNCTURE

LIV-2 Xingjian, L.I.-11 Quchi, SP-10 Xuehai, BL-17 Geshu, LU-10 Yuji, LU-6 Kongzui.

Explanation

- **LIV-2** clears Liver-Fire.
- **L.I.-11**, **SP-10** and **BL-17** cool Blood and stop bleeding.
- **LU-10** clears Lung-Heat.
- **LU-6**, Accumulation point, stops bleeding from the Lung channel.

HERBAL TREATMENT

Prescription

XIE BAI SAN and QING DAI SAN
Draining Whiteness Powder and *Indigo Powder*
Di Gu Pi *Cortex Lycii chinensis radicis* 9 g
Sang Bai Pi *Cortex Mori albae radicis* 9 g
Zhi Gan Cao *Radix Glycyrrhizae uralensis praeparata* 3 g
Geng Mi *Semen Oryzae sativae* 6 g
Qing Dai *Indigo naturalis* 9 g
Hai Ge Ke *Concha Cyclinae sinensis* 12 g

Explanation

- The formula Xie Bai San clears Lung-Heat. Di Gu Pi also stops bleeding.
- The formula Qing Dai San clears Liver-Fire and Lung Phlegm-Heat. Qing Dai also stops bleeding.

Variations

- To harmonize Blood (stop bleeding, eliminate stasis, calm and nourish Blood) add Bai Ji *Rhizoma Bletillae striatae*, Ou Jie *Nodus Nelumbinis nuciferae rhizomatis*, San Qi *Radix Notoginseng*, Sheng Di Huang *Radix Rehmanniae glutinosae* and Dang Gui *Radix Angelicae sinensis*.
- To astringe add Wu Wei Zi *Fructus Schisandrae chinensis*.
- To treat Qi add Mu Li *Concha Ostreae* to firm Qi and Niu Xi *Radix Achyranthis bidentatae seu Cyathulae* to conduct Blood downwards.

- If symptoms of Liver-Fire are pronounced add Mu Dan Pi *Cortex Moutan radicis*, Zhi Zi *Fructus Gardeniae jasminoidis* and Huang Qin *Radix Scutellariae baicalensis*.

LUNG-YIN DEFICIENCY WITH EMPTY-HEAT

CLINICAL MANIFESTATIONS

Cough with scanty blood-tinged sputum, dry throat, afternoon fever or feeling of heat, night sweating, 5-palm heat.
Tongue: Red without coating, dry.
Pulse: Floating-Empty.

TREATMENT PRINCIPLE

Nourish Lung-Yin, clear Empty-Heat, stop bleeding.

ACUPUNCTURE

LU-9 Taiyuan, Ren-12 Zhongwan, SP-6 Sanyinjiao, ST-36 Zusanli, KI-3 Taixi, LU-10 Yuji, LU-6 Kongzui. Reducing method on LU-10 and LU-6, reinforcing method for all the other points. No moxa.

Explanation

- **LU-9** nourishes Lung-Yin.
- **Ren-12**, **SP-6** and **ST-36** strengthen Earth to nourish Metal. The Stomach is also the origin of fluids, so that tonifying these points will benefit fluids and Yin.
- **KI-3** nourishes Yin.
- **LU-10** clears Lung-Heat.
- **LU-6** stops bleeding.

HERBAL TREATMENT

Prescription

BAI HE GU JIN TANG
Lilium Consolidating Metal Decoction
Bai He *Bulbus Lilii* 15 g

Mai Dong *Tuber Ophiopogonis japonici* 9 g
Xuan Shen *Radix Scrophulariae ningpoensis* 9 g
Sheng Di Huang *Radix Rehmanniae glutinosae* 9 g
Shu Di Huang *Radix Rehmanniae glutinosae praeparata* 9 g
Dang Gui *Radix Angelicae sinensis* 6 g
Bai Shao *Radix Paeoniae albae* 9 g
Jie Geng *Radix Platycodi grandiflori* 6 g
Chuan Bei Mu *Bulbus Fritillariae cirrhosae* 6 g
Gan Cao *Radix Glycyrrhizae uralensis* 3 g

Explanation

This formula, which has already been explained in chapter 5, nourishes Lung-Yin and clears Heat.

– To harmonize Blood (stop bleeding, eliminate stasis, calm and nourish Blood) add Bai Ji *Rhizoma Bletillae striatae*, Ou Jie *Nodus Nelumbinis nuciferae rhizomatis* and San Qi *Radix Notoginseng*. No addition is necessary to calm and nourish Blood as the formula already contains Sheng Di Huang and Dang Gui.
– To astringe add Wu Wei Zi *Fructus Schisandrae chinensis*. This will also help to nourish Lung-Yin.
– To treat Qi add Mu Li *Concha Ostreae*. This will also help to nourish Yin.
– If the symptoms of Empty-Heat are pronounced add Qing Hao *Herba Artemisiae apiaceae* and Di Gu Pi *Cortex Lycii chinensis radicis*, both of which also help to stop bleeding.

Case history

A 65-year-old woman had been suffering from breathlessness for many years. She had had TB of the lungs 40 years earlier. Her main problem at the time of consultation was breathlessness on exertion, general exhaustion and coughing of blood-specked sputum. She also suffered from night-sweating, a dry throat and a feeling of heat in the afternoon. She was very prone to cold which immediately affected her chest and caused bronchitis with the expectoration of profuse yellow-greenish sputum. She was overweight. Her tongue was slightly Red, Swollen and with a rootless coating in the front part. Her pulse was Slippery.

Diagnosis
This patient suffered from two conditions causing

rather contradictory signs. In fact, there are clear symptoms of Lung-Yin deficiency: night-sweating, dry throat, breathlessness, feeling of heat in the evening and cough with blood-tinged sputum. However, the tongue and the pulse show a different condition. Although the tongue has a rootless coating in the front part which does show Lung-Yin deficiency, in this condition it should be Thin rather than Swollen. The pulse should be Floating-Empty rather than Slippery. These two findings are due to the fact that there is also Spleen-Qi deficiency leading to Phlegm. This is also confirmed by the expectoration of profuse sputum when she has bronchitis and her being overweight.

Treatment principle
The treatment principle adopted was to nourish Lung-Yin, clear Lung Empty-Heat, tonify Spleen-Qi and resolve Phlegm. This patient was treated only with acupuncture.

Acupuncture
The main points (all with reinforcing method except those to resolve Phlegm) were selected from the following:

– **Ren-12** Zhongwan, **ST-36** Zusanli and **SP-6** Sanyinjiao to tonify the Spleen and resolve Phlegm. Ren-12 also tonifies the Lungs.
– **LU-9** Taiyuan to nourish Lung-Yin.
– **BL-13** Feishu, **BL-43** Gaohuangshu and **Du-12** Shenzhu to strengthen the Lungs. BL-43 is particularly indicated to nourish Lung-Yin in chronic conditions.
– **LU-10** Yuji, with even method, to clear Lung Empty-Heat and stop bleeding from the lungs.
– **ST-40** Fenglong, with even method, to resolve Phlegm.

The bleeding from the lungs stopped after 6 treatments but she was treated for over 2 years to strengthen the Lungs and Spleen on a long-term basis.

BLOOD IN THE STOOLS

The darker the blood, the higher the site of bleeding in the alimentary canal. Thus, very dark blood in the stools may indicate bleeding from the stomach, while fresh-red blood denotes bleeding from the intestines. The most common conditions to cause blood in the stools are peptic ulcer, diverticulitis, ulcerative colitis and carcinoma of the bowel. Any patient over 40 who regularly presents with blood in the stools should undergo a thorough Western diagnosis to exclude the possibility of carcinoma of the bowel. Of course, one must also exclude the most obvious cause of bleeding, i.e. haemorrhoids.

From the Chinese point of view, the colour of the blood is interpreted in terms of the underlying pattern rather than the site of bleeding. Thus, fresh-red blood or fresh but slightly dark blood indicates that the bleeding is caused by Blood-Heat. Fresh-red and very profuse blood indicates Qi deficiency, while very dark blood indicates stasis of Blood.

The patterns discussed are:

Damp-Heat in the Intestines
Stomach and Spleen Deficiency

DAMP-HEAT IN THE INTESTINES

CLINICAL MANIFESTATIONS

Fresh blood (either bright-red or slightly dark-red) in the stools, loose and frequent stools with mucus, abdominal pain.
Tongue: Red with a yellow-sticky coating on the root with red spots.
Pulse: Slippery-Rapid.

TREATMENT PRINCIPLE

Clear Heat, resolve Dampness, stop bleeding.

ACUPUNCTURE

SP-9 Yinlingquan, SP-6 Sanyinjiao, Ren-10 Xiawan, ST-25 Tianshu, BL-25 Dachangshu, BL-20 Pishu, BL-22 Sanjiaoshu, ST-37 Shangjuxu, L.I.-11 Quchi and SP-10 Xuehai. Reinforcing method on BL-20, even method on all the others.

Explanation

– **SP-9**, **SP-6** and **BL-22** resolve Damp-Heat from the Lower Burner.
– **Ren-10** helps to resolve Dampness in the Lower Burner.
– **ST-25**, and **BL-25**, Front-Collecting and Back-Transporting point of the Large Intestine respectively, clear Heat, resolve Dampness and stop diarrhoea.

– **BL-20** tonifies the Spleen to resolve Dampness.
– **ST-37** stops chronic diarrhoea.
– **L.I.-11** and **SP-10** cool Blood and stop bleeding. L.I.-11 also resolves Damp-Heat from the Large Intestine.

HERBAL TREATMENT

Prescription

DI YU SAN
Sanguisorba Powder
Di Yu *Radix Sanguisorbae officinalis* 9 g
Qian Cao Gen *Radix Rubiae cordifoliae* 6 g
Huang Qin *Radix Scutellariae baicalensis* 6 g
Huang Lian *Rhizoma Coptidis* 4.5 g
Zhi Zi *Fructus Gardeniae jasminoidis* 6 g
Fu Ling *Sclerotium Poriae cocos* 6 g

Explanation

This formula is specific for bleeding from the Intestine caused by Damp-Heat.

Variations

– To harmonize Blood (stop bleeding, eliminate stasis, calm and nourish Blood) add Bai Shao *Radix Paeoniae albae* and Dang Gui *Radix Angelicae sinensis*. No addition is necessary to stop bleeding or move Blood as Di Yu, Qian Cao Gen and Zhi Zi stop bleeding and Qian Cao Gen also moves Blood.
– To astringe add Lian Zi *Semen Nelumbinis nuciferae* which also stops diarrhoea.
– To treat Qi add Sheng Ma *Rhizoma Cimicifugae* to raise Qi.
– If the condition is very chronic and there are signs of Spleen deficiency add Bai Zhu *Rhizoma Atractylodis macrocephalae*.
– If the abdominal pain is severe add Yan Hu Suo *Rhizoma Corydalis yanhusuo*.

STOMACH AND SPLEEN DEFICIENCY

CLINICAL MANIFESTATIONS

Profuse fresh blood in the stools, slight abdominal pain, pale face, exhaustion, depression, loose and frequent stools with mucus.

Tongue: Pale with swollen sides.
Pulse: Weak.

TREATMENT PRINCIPLE

Strengthen the Spleen, warm the Centre, stop bleeding.

ACUPUNCTURE

Ren-12 Zhongwan, Ren-6 Qihai, ST-25 Tianshu, SP-6 Sanyinjiao, BL-20 Pishu, BL-21 Weishu, ST-36 Zusanli, ST-37 Shangjuxu, SP-10 Xuehai, Du-20 Baihui.

Explanation

- **Ren-12, BL-20, BL-21**, and **ST-36** tonify Stomach and Spleen.
- **Ren-6** and **ST-25** tonify Qi and stop diarrhoea. Moxa on ginger may be used on Ren-6.
- **SP-6** resolves Dampness from the Lower Burner.
- **ST-37** stops chronic diarrhoea.
- **SP-10** stops bleeding.
- **Du-20**, with direct moxa, raises Qi.

HERBAL TREATMENT

Prescription

LI ZHONG WAN
Regulating the Centre Pill
Ren Shen *Radix Ginseng* 6 g (or **Dang Shen** *Radix Codonopsis pilosulae* 12 g)
Bai Zhu *Rhizoma Atractylodis macrocephalae* 9 g
Gan Jiang *Rhizoma Zingiberis officinalis* 5 g
Zhi Gan Cao *Radix Glycyrrhizae uralensis praeparata* 6 g

Explanation

This formula, which has already been explained in chapter 12, tonifies Spleen-Qi and Spleen-Yang and stops abdominal pain. Gan Jiang stops bleeding from Qi and Yang deficiency.

Variations

- To harmonize Blood (stop bleeding, eliminate stasis, calm and nourish Blood) add one or two of the following herbs: Zao Xin Huang Tu *Terra Flava usta*, Xian He Cao *Herba Agrimoniae pilosae*, San Qi *Radix Notoginseng*, Bai Shao *Radix Paeoniae albae,* or Dang Gui *Radix Angelicae sinensis.*
- To astringe add Lian Zi *Semen Nelumbinis nuciferae.*
- To treat Qi add Sheng Ma *Rhizoma Cimicifugae* to raise Qi.

Case history

A 60-year-old man had been suffering from blood in the stools for 2 years. He had no abdominal pain and his bowel movements were loose and very frequent. The blood was fresh-red and haemorrhoids were excluded as a cause of bleeding. He felt very tired most of the time and felt the cold very much. Even in summertime on a hot day when he came for his consultation he had a jumper and a jacket on. His tongue was Pale, Swollen and had a white-sticky coating. His pulse was generally Weak, especially so on the right-Middle position.

Diagnosis
This is a clear condition of Spleen-Yang deficiency with some internal Cold and the bleeding is due to Spleen-Qi not holding Blood.

Treatment Principle
The treatment principle adopted was to tonify and warm Spleen-Yang and expel Cold. This patient was treated only with herbs.

Herbal treatment
The formula used was a combination of Li Zhong Wan *Regulating the Centre Pill* and Gui Pi Tang *Tonifying the Spleen Decoction.* The former tonifies Spleen-Yang and expels Cold and the latter tonifies the Spleen function of holding Blood. The latter prescription which also calms the Mind, fitted the case well as, during the consultation, it transpired that the problem had started after a deep emotional upset with his son.

Ren Shen *Radix Ginseng* 6 g
Bai Zhu *Rhizoma Atractylodis macrocephalae* 9 g
Gan Jiang *Rhizoma Zingiberis officinalis* 5 g
Zhi Gan Cao *Radix Glycyrrhizae uralensis praeparata* 3 g
Huang Qi *Radix Astragali membranacei* 9 g
Fu Ling *Sclerotium Poriae cocos* 6 g
Suan Zao Ren *Semen Ziziphi spinosae* 4 g
Yuan Zhi *Radix Polygalae tenuifoliae* 4 g
Dang Gui *Radix Angelicae sinensis* 6 g

Mu Xiang *Radix Saussureae* 3 g
Xian He Cao *Herba Agrimoniae pilosae* 6 g
Pu Huang *Pollen Typhae* 4 g
Bai Shao *Radix Paeoniae albae* 9 g

Explanation
– Long Yan Rou was eliminated as the patient did not suffer from insomnia, and Fu Shen was substituted for Fu Ling for the same reason.
– **Xian He Cao** was added to stop bleeding.
– **Pu Huang** was added to move Blood.
– **Bai Shao** calms and nourishes Blood.

If we analyse this prescription, we can see that the four aims of treatment to stop bleeding are fulfilled:

1. *Harmonize Blood*
   Stop bleeding: Xian He Cao
   Move Blood: Pu Huang
   Calm Blood: Bai Shao
   Nourish Blood: Dang Gui
2. *Treat the Root-Cause*: Huang Qi, Ren Shen and Bai Zhu (tonify Qi)
3. *Astringe*: Suan Zao Ren
4. *Treat Qi*: Huang Qi (raise Qi).

This patient's condition improved gradually over 1 year after which his bleeding stopped and he felt much better in general.

BLOOD IN THE URINE

This consists in bleeding in the urine without pain on micturition. If there is pain on micturition, refer to Blood Painful Urinary Syndrome (ch. 20).

Blood in the urine may range from profuse frank blood, to microscopic traces of which are invisible to the naked eye.

The patterns discussed are:

Bladder Heat
Kidney Yin Deficiency with Empty-Heat
Deficient Spleen not controlling Blood
Kidney-Qi not Firm

BLADDER HEAT

CLINICAL MANIFESTATIONS

Scanty-dark urine with fresh blood, mental restlessness, thirst, insomnia, red face, tongue ulcers, bitter taste.
Tongue: Red with redder tip, yellow coating with red spots on the root.

Pulse: Rapid, slightly Overflowing, Wiry on the left Rear position.

This consists in Bladder-Heat deriving from Small-Intestine Heat and Heart-Fire.

TREATMENT PRINCIPLE

Clear Heat from the Bladder and Small Intestine, drain Heart-Fire, calm the Mind, cool Blood and stop bleeding.

ACUPUNCTURE

HE-8 Shaofu, S.I.-2 Qiangu, BL-66 Tonggu, Ren-3 Zhongji, BL-28 Pangguangshu, L.I.-11 Quchi, SP-10 Xuehai, BL-63 Jinmen. Reducing method.

Explanation

– **HE-8** drains Heart-Fire.
– **S.I.-2** clears Small Intestine Heat.
– **BL-66** clears Bladder-Heat.
– **Ren-3** and **BL-28**, Front-Collecting and Back-Transporting points of the Bladder respectively, clear Bladder-Heat.
– **L.I.-11** and **SP-10** cool Blood and stop bleeding.
– **BL-63**, Accumulation point, stops bleeding from the Bladder channel.

HERBAL TREATMENT

Prescription

XIAO JI YIN ZI
Cephalanoplos Decoction
Xiao Ji *Herba Cephalanoplos segeti* 30 g
Ou Jie *Nodus Nelumbinis nuciferae rhizomatis* 6 g
Pu Huang *Pollen Typhae* 9 g
Hua Shi *Talcum* 15 g
Mu Tong *Caulis Akebiae* 9 g
Zhu Ye *Herba Lophatheri gracilis* 9 g
Zhi Zi *Fructus Gardeniae jasminoidis* 9 g
Sheng Di Huang *Radix Rehmanniae glutinosae* 30 g
Dang Gui *Radix Angelicae sinensis* 6 g
Gan Cao *Radix Glycyrrhizae uralensis* 6 g

Explanation

This formula, which has already been explained above as an example of the application of the four aims of treatment in stopping bleeding, is specific to stop bleeding in the urine from Blood-Heat.

This prescription needs no variation to stop bleeding as it already contains all the ingredients according to the four aims of treatment indicated above.

Patent remedy

TE XIAO PAI SHI WAN
Especially-Effective Discharging Stones Pill
Jin Qian Cao *Herba Desmodii styracifolii*
Hai Jin Sha *Spora Lygodii japonici*
Bai Zhi *Radix Angelicae dahuricae*
Chuan Xin Lian *Herba Andrographis paniculatae*
Chuan Niu Xi *Radix Cyathulae*
Wu Hua Guo Gen *Radix Fici*
Huang Lian *Rhizoma Coptidis*
Da Huang *Rhizoma Rhei*
Niu Da Li *Radix Millettiae speciosae*
San Qi *Radix Notoginseng*
Hu Po *Succinum*

Explanation

This remedy drains Damp-Heat from the Bladder and expels urinary stones. It is suitable to treat the Root-cause of bleeding from the Bladder when this is due to Bladder-Heat or Damp-Heat. It can be combined with the patent remedy YUNNAN TE CHAN TIAN QI PIAN *Yunnan Specially-Prepared Notoginseng Tablet* (containing only San Qi) to treat the Manifestation, i.e. stop bleeding. This remedy is contraindicated in pregnancy.

The tongue presentation appropriate to this remedy is a Red body with a yellow coating all over and a thicker, sticky-yellow coating with red spots on the root.

KIDNEY YIN DEFICIENCY WITH EMPTY-HEAT

CLINICAL MANIFESTATIONS

Scanty-dark urine with blood, dizziness, tinni-tus, back-ache, exhaustion, feeling of heat in the afternoon, night sweating.
Tongue: Red without coating.
Pulse: Floating-Empty.

TREATMENT PRINCIPLE

Nourish Kidney-Yin, clear Empty-Heat, cool Blood, stop bleeding.

ACUPUNCTURE

KI-3 Taixi, KI-6 Zhaohai, Ren-4 Guanyuan, SP-6 Sanyinjiao, KI-5 Shuiquan, Ren-3 Zhongji, BL-28 Pangguangshu, KI-2 Rangu, SP-10 Xuehai. Reinforcing method on KI-3, KI-6, Ren-4 and SP-6 and even method on the others.

Explanation

- **KI-3**, **KI-6**, **Ren-4** and **SP-6** nourish Kidney-Yin.
- **KI-5** Shuiquan, Accumulation point, stops urinary bleeding.
- **Ren-3** and **BL-28** clear Bladder-Heat.
- **KI-2** clears Kidney Empty-Heat.
- **SP-10** cools Blood and stops bleeding.

HERBAL TREATMENT

Prescription

ZHI BO DI HUANG WAN
Anemarrhena-Phellodendron-Rehmannia Pill
Shu Di Huang *Radix Rehmanniae glutinosae praeparata* 24 g
Shan Zhu Yu *Fructus Corni officinalis* 12 g
Shan Yao *Radix Dioscoreae oppositae* 12 g
Ze Xie *Rhizoma Alismatis orientalis* 9 g
Fu Ling *Sclerotium Poriae cocos* 9 g
Mu Dan Pi *Cortex Moutan radicis* 9 g
Zhi Mu *Radix Anemarrhenae asphodeloidis* 9 g
Huang Bo *Cortex Phellodendri* 9 g

Explanation

This formula, which has already been explained,

is specific to nourish Kidney-Yin and clear Empty-Heat.

Variations

– To harmonize Blood (stop bleeding, eliminate stasis, calm and nourish Blood) add Xiao Ji *Herba Cephalanoplos segeti*, Qian Cao Gen *Radix Rubiae cordifoliae*, Sheng Di Huang *Radix Rehmanniae glutinosae* and Gou Qi Zi *Fructus Lycii chinensis*.
– To astringe: it is not necessary to add an astringent as the formula already has Shan Zhu Yu.
– To treat Qi add Mu Li *Concha Ostreae*.
– If symptoms of Empty-Heat are very pronounced add Han Lian Cao *Herba Ecliptae prostratae* and Qing Hao *Herba Artemisiae apiaceae* which also stop bleeding.

Patent remedy

ZHI BO BA WEI WAN
Anemarrhena-Phellodendron Eight-Ingredient Pill
Shu Di Huang *Radix Rehmanniae glutinosae prae-parata*
Shan Zhu Yu *Fructus Corni officinalis*
Shan Yao *Radix Dioscoreae oppositae*
Ze Xie *Rhizoma Alismatis orientalis*
Fu Ling *Sclerotium Poriae cocos*
Mu Dan Pi *Cortex Moutan radicis*
Zhi Mu *Radix Anemarrhenae asphodeloidis*
Huang Bo *Cortex Phellodendri*

Explanation

This pill has the same ingredients and functions as the formula Zhi Bo Di Huang Wan above (the two names are interchangeable). It is suitable to treat chronic bleeding in the urine caused by Bladder Damp-Heat occurring against a background of Kidney-Yin deficiency. As for the previous remedy, it could be combined with the tablet Yunnan Te Chan Tian Qi Pian to treat the Manifestation, i.e. stop bleeding.

The tongue presentation appropriate to this remedy is a Red body without coating, but with a sticky-yellow coating with red spots on the root.

Case history

A 75-year-old man had been suffering from bleeding in the urine for 3 months. There was no pain on urination and the blood was dark, sometimes with tiny clots. He felt generally hot and his mouth felt very dry and hot. His tongue was Red, dry, and nearly completely peeled. His pulse was Floating-Empty.

Diagnosis
Although this patient had relatively few symptoms, the tongue showed very clearly a deficiency of Kidney-Yin with Empty-Heat. This was the cause of the bleeding from the urinary tract. I advised him to seek a Western diagnosis as should always be done in a man over 50 with this symptom which can indicate cancer of the bladder. However, he steadfastly refused to go to hospital for tests. I agreed to treat him and used a variation of Zhi Bo Ba Wei Tang *Anemarrhena-Phellodendron Eight-Ingredient Decoction*:

Sheng Di Huang *Radix Rehmanniae glutinosae* 6 g
Shan Zhu Yu *Fructus Corni officinalis* 3 g
Shan Yao *Radix Dioscoreae oppositae* 6 g
Ze Xie *Rhizoma Alismatis orientalis* 4 g
Fu Ling *Sclerotium Poriae cocos* 6 g
Mu Dan Pi *Cortex Moutan radicis* 6 g
Zhi Mu *Radix Anemarrhenae asphodeloidis* 4 g
Huang Bo *Cortex Phellodendri* 4 g
Xiao Ji *Herba Cephalanoplos segeti* 6 g
Pu Huang *Pollen Typhae* 4 g
Dang Gui *Radix Angelicae sinensis* 6 g
Mu Li *Concha Ostreae* 12 g

Explanation
– The first eight herbs constitute the root formula (exchanging Sheng Di for Shu Di to nourish Yin more) to nourish Kidney-Yin and clear Empty-Heat from the Bladder.
– **Xiao Ji** was added to stop bleeding from the urinary tract.
– **Pu Huang** was added to move Blood and stop bleeding.
– **Dang Gui** was added to nourish Blood.
– **Mu Li** was added to firm Qi.

If we analyse this prescription, we can see that the four aims of treatment to stop bleeding are fulfilled:

1. *Harmonize Blood*
   Stop bleeding: Xiao Ji
   Move Blood: Pu Huang
   Calm Blood: Sheng Di
   Nourish Blood: Dang Gui
2. *Treat the Root-Cause*: The root-formula (nourish Yin and clear Empty-Heat)
3. *Astringe*: Shan Zhu Yu
4. *Treat Qi*: Mu Li (firm Qi).

This prescription stopped the bleeding almost

immediately. However, bleeding recurred after 3 months; again, I used a similar formula and again the bleeding stopped, only to start again after 2 months. At this point I was almost certain this patient had carcinoma of the bladder. It also became clear that he himself suspected this but he still refused to undergo tests. It gradually became obvious that he was so tired of life that he wanted to die. He, in fact, died 4 months later.

DEFICIENT SPLEEN NOT CONTROLLING BLOOD

CLINICAL MANIFESTATIONS

Chronic bleeding in the urine, tiredness, pale face, no appetite, depression.
Tongue: Pale.
Pulse: Weak.

TREATMENT PRINCIPLE

Tonify the Spleen to control Blood, stop bleeding.

ACUPUNCTURE

ST-36 Zusanli, SP-6 Sanyinjiao, Ren-12 Zhongwan, BL-20 Pishu, BL-21 Weishu, Ren-6 Qihai, SP-10 Xuehai, BL-63 Jinmen, BL-23 Shenshu, BL-28 Pangguangshu, Du-20 Baihui. Reinforcing method. Moxa may be used.

Explanation

- **ST-36**, **SP-6**, **Ren-12**, **BL-20** and **BL-21** tonify Stomach and Spleen.
- **Ren-6** consolidates Qi in the lower abdomen to stop bleeding.
- **SP-10** stops bleeding.
- **BL-63** stops bleeding from the Bladder channel.
- **BL-23** and **BL-28** strengthen the Bladder to stop bleeding.
- **Du-20** with direct moxa, raises Qi.

HERBAL TREATMENT

Prescription

GUI PI TANG

Tonifying the Spleen Decoction
Ren Shen *Radix Ginseng* 6 g (or **Dang Shen** *Radix Codonopsis pilosulae* 12 g)
Huang Qi *Radix Astragali membranacei* 15 g
Bai Zhu *Rhizoma Atractylodis macrocephalae* 12 g
Dang Gui *Radix Angelicae sinensis* 3 g
Fu Shen *Sclerotium Poriae cocos* 9 g
Suan Zao Ren *Semen Ziziphi spinosae* 9 g
Long Yan Rou *Arillus Euphoriae longanae* 12 g
Yuan Zhi *Radix Polygalae tenuifoliae* 9 g
Mu Xiang *Radix Saussureae* 6 g
Zhi Gan Cao *Radix Glycyrrhizae uralensis praeparata* 4 g
Sheng Jiang *Rhizoma Zingiberis officinalis recens* 3 slices
Hong Zao *Fructus Ziziphi jujubae* 5 dates

Explanation

This prescription, which has already been explained in chapters 9 and 11, is specific to stop bleeding from Spleen-Qi deficiency.

Variations

- To harmonize Blood (stop bleeding, eliminate stasis, calm and nourish Blood) add Xiao Ji *Herba Cephalanoplos segeti*, Hong Hua *Flos Carthami tinctorii* and Bai Shao *Radix Paeoniae albae*. There is no need to add any herb to nourish Blood as the formula already contains Dang Gui.
- To astringe: there is no need to add an astringent as the formula already contains Suan Zao Ren.
- To treat Qi add Sheng Ma *Rhizoma Cimicifugae* and Chai Hu *Radix Bupleuri* to raise Qi.

Patent remedy

GUI PI WAN
Tonifying the Spleen Pill

Explanation

This pill has the same ingredients and functions as the homonymous prescription. It is suitable to treat bleeding due to Spleen-Qi not holding Blood from any source. In order to treat the

Manifestation, i.e. stop bleeding, it could be combined with the tablet Yunnan Te Chan Tian Qi Pian.

The tongue presentation appropriate to this remedy is a Pale and Thin body.

KIDNEY-QI NOT FIRM

CLINICAL MANIFESTATIONS

Chronic bleeding in the urine with pale blood, dizziness, tinnitus, exhaustion, depression, sore back.
Tongue: Pale and Swollen.
Pulse: Weak.

TREATMENT PRINCIPLE

Tonify Kidney-Yang, stop bleeding.

ACUPUNCTURE

BL-23 Shenshu, BL-28 Pangguangshu, BL-20 Pishu, BL-17 Geshu, SP-10 Xuehai, KI-3 Taixi. Reinforcing method. Moxa may be used.

Explanation

- **BL-23**, **BL-28** and **BL-20** tonify the Kidneys, Bladder and Spleen. Tonifying the Spleen helps to hold Blood.
- **BL-17** and **SP-10** stop bleeding.
- **KI-3**, with moxa, tonifies Kidney-Yang.

HERBAL TREATMENT

Prescription

WU BI SHAN YAO WAN
Incomparable Dioscorea Pill
Shan Yao *Radix Dioscoreae oppositae* 15 g
Rou Cong Rong *Herba Cistanchis* 9 g
Tu Si Zi *Semen Cuscutae* 9 g
Ba Ji Tian *Radix Morindae officinalis* 6 g
Du Zhong *Cortex Eucommiae ulmoidis* 6 g
Shu Di Huang *Radix Rehmanniae glutinosae praeparata* 9 g

Shan Zhu Yu *Fructus Corni officinalis* 6 g
Niu Xi *Radix Achyranthis bidentatae seu Cyathulae* 6 g
Wu Wei Zi *Fructus Schisandrae chinensis* 4.5 g
Chi Shi Zhi *Halloysitum rubrum* 6 g
Ze Xie *Rhizoma Alismatis orientalis* 6 g
Fu Shen *Sclerotium Poriae cocos pararadicis* 6 g

Explanation

This formula, which has already been explained in chapter 20, tonifies Kidney-Yang and reduces urination.

Variations

- To harmonize Blood (stop bleeding, eliminate stasis, calm and nourish Blood) add Xiao Ji *Herba Cephalanoplos segeti*, Pu Huang *Pollen Typhae*, Bai Shao *Radix Paeoniae albae* and Dang Gui *Radix Angelicae sinensis*.
- To astringe: no addition is necessary as the formula already contains Shan Zhu Yu, Wu Wei Zi and Chi Shi Zhi.
- To treat Qi add Sheng Ma *Rhizoma Cimicifugae* to raise Qi.

BLEEDING UNDER THE SKIN (PETECHIAE)

Bleeding under the skin consists of bruising and is common in old people. In young people, it occurs in leukaemia. Bleeding under the skin also occurs at the Blood-Level stage of an acute febrile disease when it indicates Blood-Heat.

The patterns discussed are:

Blood-Heat
Yin Deficiency with Empty-Heat
Deficient Qi not holding Blood

BLOOD-HEAT

CLINICAL MANIFESTATIONS

Bright-purple spots under the skin, bleeding from other sites such as nose, intestines or bladder, mental restlessness, fever at night, thirst.

Tongue: Red without coating, red points all over.
Pulse: Rapid and Fine.

This represents the Blood-Level stage of an acute febrile disease indicating Blood-Heat. It is always a serious condition. However, it may also occur as a chronic condition in old people with Blood-Heat usually deriving from Liver-Fire. In such cases there will be no fever.

TREATMENT PRINCIPLE

Cool Blood, expel Poison, stop bleeding.

ACUPUNCTURE

L.I.-11 Quchi, SP-10 Xuehai, KI-2 Rangu, LIV-3 Taichong, SP-6 Sanyinjiao, SP-4 Gongsun. Reducing method.

Explanation

- **L.I.-11** and **SP-10** cool the Blood and stop bleeding.
- **KI-2** and **LIV-3** cool the Blood. LIV-3 also subdues Wind which is likely to appear at the Blood Level of a febrile disease.
- **SP-6** cools Blood and nourishes Yin.
- **SP-4** controls the Blood Connecting channels and stops bleeding under the skin.
- **LIV-5** also stops bleeding under the skin.

HERBAL TREATMENT

Prescription

XI JIAO DI HUANG TANG
Cornu Bufali-Rehmannia Decoction
Shui Niu Jiao *Cornu Bufali* 30 g
Sheng Di Huang *Radix Rehmanniae glutinosae* 30 g
Chi Shao *Radix Paeoniae rubrae* 12 g
Mu Dan Pi *Cortex Moutan radicis* 9 g

Explanation

- **Shui Niu Jiao** is specific to cool Blood at the Blood Level of febrile diseases. It also stops bleeding.
- **Sheng Di Huang** cools Blood and stops bleeding.
- **Chi Shao** and **Dan Pi** cool and move Blood and stop bleeding.

Variations

- To harmonize Blood (stop bleeding, eliminate stasis, calm and nourish Blood) add Qian Cao Gen *Radix Rubiae cordifoliae* (both to stop bleeding and move Blood), Di Yu *Radix Sanguisorbae officinalis* and Gou Qi Zi *Fructus Lycii chinensis*. There is no need to add any herb to calm Blood as the formula already contains Sheng Di Huang.
- To astringe add Shan Zhu Yu *Fructus Corni officinalis*.
- To treat Qi add Mu Li *Concha Ostreae*.
- If Blood-Heat is very pronounced add Zi Cao *Radix Lithospermi seu Arnebiae*.

Patent remedy

LIAN QIAO BAI DU PIAN
Forsythia Expelling Poison Tablet
Lian Qiao *Fructus Forsythiae suspensae*
Jin Yin Hua *Flos Lonicerae japonicae*
Fang Feng *Radix Ledebouriellae sesloidis*
Bai Xian Pi *Cortex Dictami dasycarpi Radicis*
Chan Tui *Periostracum Cicadae*
Chi Shao *Radix Paeoniae rubrae*
Da Huang *Rhizoma Rhei*
Huang Qin *Radix Scutellariae baicalensis*
Zhi Zi *Fructus Gardeniae jasminoidis*

Explanation

This remedy expels Wind-Heat, drains Interior Heat and resolves Fire-Poison. It also clears Heat from the skin: this makes it suitable to treat bleeding under the skin caused by Blood-Heat.

It is contraindicated in pregnancy. The tongue presentation appropriate to this remedy is a Red body with a yellow coating.

YIN DEFICIENCY WITH EMPTY-HEAT

CLINICAL MANIFESTATIONS

Scarlet-red spots under the skin, bleeding from

other sites such as nose or gums, malar flush, mental restlessness, dry mouth, 5-palm heat, feeling of heat in the afternoon, night sweating. Tongue: Red, no coating, red points all over. Pulse: Floating-Empty and slightly Rapid.

This is a chronic condition in old people with Yin deficiency of the Kidneys and Empty-Heat agitating the Blood.

TREATMENT PRINCIPLE

Nourish Yin, clear Empty-Heat, stop bleeding.

ACUPUNCTURE

KI-3 Taixi, KI-6 Zhaohai, Ren-4 Guanyuan, SP-6 Sanyinjiao, KI-2 Rangu, LIV-3 Taichong, L.I.-11 Quchi, SP-10 Xuehai. Reducing or even method, except on the first four points which should be reinforced. No moxa.

Explanation

- **KI-3**, **KI-6**, **Ren-4** and **SP-6** nourish Yin.
- **KI-2** and **LIV-3** cool Blood.
- **L.I.-11** and **SP-10** cool Blood and stop bleeding.

HERBAL TREATMENT

Prescription

QIAN GEN SAN
Rubia Powder
Qian Cao Gen *Radix Rubiae cordifoliae* 9 g
Ce Bai Ye *Cacumen Biotae orientalis* 9 g
Huang Qin *Radix Scutellariae baicalensis* 6 g
Sheng Di Huang *Radix Rehmanniae glutinosae* 12 g
E Jiao *Gelatinum Corii Asini* 9 g
Gan Cao *Radix Glycyrrhizae uralensis* 3 g

Explanation

This formula has already been analysed above as an example of the application of the four aims of treatment to stop bleeding.

It stops bleeding from Empty-Heat agitating the Blood.

Variations

This formula needs no variations to stop bleeding as it already contains herbs according to the four aims of treatment.

- If there are pronounced signs of Empty-Heat add Han Lian Cao *Herba Ecliptae prostratae* and Qing Hao *Herba Artemisiae apiaceae*, both of which also stop bleeding.

Patent remedy

ZHI BO BA WEI WAN
Anemarrhena-Phellodendron Eight-Ingredient Pill

Explanation

This pill, already mentioned above, is suitable to treat bleeding from Empty-Heat against a background of Yin deficiency combined with Yunnan Te Chan Tian Qi Pian to treat the Manifestation, i.e. stop bleeding.

The tongue presentation appropriate to this remedy, in this condition, is a Red, dry, cracked and peeled body.

DEFICIENT QI NOT HOLDING BLOOD

CLINICAL MANIFESTATIONS

Pale-red spots under the skin, exhaustion, depression, pale face, no appetite.
Tongue: Pale.
Pulse: Weak.

TREATMENT PRINCIPLE

Tonify Spleen-Qi to control Blood.

ACUPUNCTURE

ST-36 Zusanli, SP-6 Sanyinjiao, Ren-12 Zhongwan, BL-20 Pishu, BL-21 Weishu, Ren-6 Qihai, SP-10 Xuehai, LU-9 Taiyuan, SP-4 Gongsun.

Explanation

- **ST-36**, **SP-6**, **Ren-12**, **BL-20** and **BL-21** tonify Stomach and Spleen.
- **Ren-6** consolidates Qi in the lower abdomen to stop bleeding.
- **SP-10** stops bleeding.
- **LU-9** tonifies Qi.
- **SP-4** stops bleeding under the skin.

HERBAL TREATMENT

Prescription

GUI PI TANG
Tonifying the Spleen Decoction
Ren Shen *Radix Ginseng* 6 g (or **Dang Shen** *Radix Codonopsis pilosulae* 12 g)
Huang Qi *Radix Astragali membranacei* 15 g
Bai Zhu *Rhizoma Atractylodis macrocephalae* 12 g
Dang Gui *Radix Angelicae sinensis* 3 g
Fu Shen *Sclerotium Poriae cocos pararadicis* 9 g
Suan Zao Ren *Semen Ziziphi spinosae* 9 g
Long Yan Rou *Arillus Euphoriae longanae* 12 g
Yuan Zhi *Radix Polygalae tenuifoliae* 9 g
Mu Xiang *Radix Saussureae* 6 g
Zhi Gan Cao *Radix Glycyrrhizae uralensis praeparata* 4 g
Sheng Jiang *Rhizoma Zingiberis officinalis recens* 3 slices
Hong Zao *Fructus Ziziphi jujubae 5* dates

Explanation

This formula has already been explained above under "Blood in the urine" and its variations to stop bleeding are the same.

Patent remedy

GUI PI WAN
Tonifying the Spleen Pill

Explanation

As mentioned above, this pill can be used to treat the Root in bleeding from Spleen-Qi not holding Blood. It can be combined with Yunnan Te Chan Tian Qi Pian to treat the Manifestation,

i.e. stop bleeding.

The tongue presentation appropriate to this remedy is a Pale and Thin body.

BLEEDING GUMS

The patterns discussed are:

Stomach-Heat
Stomach Yin Deficiency with Empty-Heat
Stomach and Spleen Deficiency

STOMACH-HEAT

CLINICAL MANIFESTATIONS

Profuse bleeding, painful and swollen gums, frontal headache, thirst.
Tongue: Red with dry-yellow coating.
Pulse: Rapid, Overflowing on the right Middle position.

TREATMENT PRINCIPLE

Clear Stomach-Heat, cool Blood, stop bleeding.

ACUPUNCTURE

L.I.-4 Hegu, L.I.-11 Quchi, L.I.-7 Wenliu, ST-21 Liangmen, ST-34 Lianqiu, ST-44 Neiting. Reducing method. No moxa.

Explanation

- **L.I.-4** clears Stomach-Heat and affects the Stomach channel on the face.
- **L.I.-11** clears Heat and cools Blood.
- **L.I.-7**, Accumulation points, stops bleeding along the Large Intestine channel area.
- **ST-21** clears Stomach Heat.
- **ST-34**, Accumulation point, stops bleeding from the Stomach channel area.
- **ST-44** clears Stomach Heat and affects the Stomach channel on the face.

HERBAL TREATMENT

Prescription

YU NU JIAN
Jade Woman Decoction

Shi Gao *Gypsum fibrosum* 30 g
Zhi Mu *Radix Anemarrhenae asphodeloidis* 4.5 g
Shu Di Huang *Radix Rehmanniae glutinosae prae-parata* 9 g
Mai Men Dong *Tuber Ophiopogonis japonici* 6 g
Niu Xi *Radix Achyranthis bidentatae seu Cyathulae* 4.5 g

Explanation

– **Shi Gao** and **Zhi Mu** clear Stomach-Heat.
– **Shu Di** and **Mai Dong** prevent injury of Yin from Heat.
– **Niu Xi** attracts Heat downwards. It also has the function of attracting Blood downwards to stop bleeding from the gums, a sign which this formula is designed to treat.

Variations

– To harmonize Blood (stop bleeding, eliminate stasis, calm and nourish Blood) add Di Yu *Radix Sanguisorbae officinalis*, San Qi *Radix Notoginseng* and Bai Shao *Radix Paeoniae albae*. There is no need to add any herb to nourish Blood as the formula already contains Shu Di Huang.
– To astringe add Lian Zi *Semen Nelumbinis nuciferae*.
– To treat Qi: there is no need to add any herb for Qi as the formula contains Niu Xi which attracts Blood downwards.
– If Stomach-Heat has turned into Stomach-Fire manifesting with constipation, dry stools, abdominal pain and mental restlessness add Da Huang *Rhizoma Rhei*.

Patent remedy

NIU HUANG JIE DU PIAN
Calculus Bovis Resolving Poison Tablet
Da Huang *Rhizoma Rhei*
Shi Gao *Gypsum fibrosum*
Huang Qin *Radix Scutellariae baicalensis*
Jie Geng *Radix Platycodi grandiflori*
Gan Cao *Radix Glycyrrhizae uralensis*
Bing Pian *Borneol*
Niu Huang *Calculus Bovis*

Explanation

This tablet drains Stomach-Fire. It is therefore suitable to treat the Root in bleeding from Stomach-Fire, but only in acute cases as it is not appropriate for long-term use. It is contraindicated in pregnancy.

The tongue presentation appropriate to this remedy is a Dark-Red body with a yellow coating and red points around the centre.

STOMACH YIN DEFICIENCY WITH EMPTY-HEAT

CLINICAL MANIFESTATIONS

Slight bleeding from the gums, mental restlessness, gums diseased, loose teeth.
Tongue: Red without coating in the centre.
Pulse: Floating-Empty on the right Middle position.

TREATMENT PRINCIPLE

Nourish Stomach-Yin, clear Empty-Heat, cool Blood and stop bleeding.

ACUPUNCTURE

ST-36 Zusanli, SP-6 Sanyinjiao, Ren-12 Zhongwan, ST-44 Neiting, L.I.-4 Hegu, ST-34 Liangqiu, L.I.-11 Quchi, SP-10 Xuehai. Reinforcing method on the first three and even method on the others. No moxa.

Explanation

– **ST-36**, **SP-6** and **Ren-12** nourish Stomach-Yin.
– **ST-44** and **L.I.-4** clear Stomach-Heat or Empty-Heat and affect the Stomach channel on the face.
– **ST-34** stops bleeding from the Stomach channel.
– **L.I.-11** and **SP-10** cool Blood and stop bleeding.

HERBAL TREATMENT

Prescription

QING WEI SAN

Clearing the Stomach Powder
Huang Lian *Rhizoma Coptidis* 5 g
Sheng Di Huang *Radix Rehmanniae glutinosae* 12 g
Mu Dan Pi *Cortex Moutan radicis* 9 g
Dang Gui *Radix Angelicae sinensis* 6 g
Sheng Ma *Rhizoma Cimicifugae* 6 g

Explanation

This formula, which has already been explained in chapter 1, clears Heat and cools Blood within the Stomach.

Variations

– To harmonize Blood (stop bleeding, eliminate stasis, calm and nourish Blood) add Di Yu *Radix Sanguisorbae officinalis* and San Qi *Radix Notoginseng*. No addition is necessary to calm and nourish Blood as the formula already contains Sheng Di Huang and Dang Gui.
– To astringe add Lian Zi *Semen Nelumbinis nuciferae*.
– To treat Qi add Niu Xi *Radix Achyranthis bidentatae seu Cyathulae* to conduct Blood downwards.
– If the symptoms of Stomach-Yin deficiency are pronounced add Mai Men Dong *Tuber Ophiopogonis japonici* and Tai Zi Shen *Radix Pseudostellariae heterophyllae*.
– If there are pronounced symptoms of dryness from Yin deficiency and Empty-Heat add Tian Hua Fen *Radix Trichosanthis* and Yu Zhu *Rhizoma Polygonati odorati*.

STOMACH AND SPLEEN DEFICIENCY

CLINICAL MANIFESTATIONS

Chronic but slight bleeding from the gums, pale gums and lips, tiredness, poor appetite, loose stools.
Tongue: Pale.
Pulse: Weak.

TREATMENT PRINCIPLE

Tonify Stomach and Spleen to hold Blood.

ACUPUNCTURE

ST-36 Zusanli, SP-6 Sanyinjiao, Ren-12 Zhongwan, BL-20 Pishu, BL-21 Weishu, L.I.-4 Hegu, ST-34 Liangqiu, BL-17 Geshu. Reinforcing method except on ST-34 and BL-17 which should be needled with even method.

Explanation

– **ST-36**, **SP-6**, **Ren-12**, **BL-20** and **BL-21** tonify Stomach and Spleen.
– **L.I.-4** is used to affect the Stomach channel on the face.
– **ST-34** and **BL-17**, in combination, stop bleeding from the Stomach channel.

HERBAL TREATMENT

Prescription

GUI PI TANG
Tonifying the Spleen Decoction

Explanation

This formula has already been explained above in this chapter. It is specific to stop bleeding from Spleen deficiency.

Variations

– To harmonize Blood (stop bleeding, eliminate stasis, calm and nourish Blood) add Ou Jie *Nodus Nelumbinis nuciferae rhizomatis*, San Qi *Radix Notoginseng* and Bai Shao *Radix Paeoniae albae*. There is no need to add any herb to nourish Blood as the formula already contains Dang Gui.
– To astringe add Lian Zi *Semen Nelumbinis nuciferae*.
– To treat Qi: there is no need to add any herb for this as the formula contains Huang Qi and Ren Shen.

Patent remedy

GUI PI WAN
Tonifying the Spleen Pill

Explanation

This pill, already mentioned in this chapter, is suitable to treat the Root in bleeding from Spleen-Qi not holding Blood.

The tongue presentation appropriate to this remedy is a Pale and Thin body.

Prognosis and prevention

Both acupuncture and herbs are effective in treating bleeding, although herbal medicine is slightly more so.

Acute bleeding can be stopped very effectively with a combination of acupuncture and herbal medicine. The patent remedy YUNNAN BAI YAO *Yunnan White Medicine* (containing San Qi *Radix Notoginseng* and other undisclosed ingredients) is very effective in stopping acute bleeding. In very severe bleeding, the small red pill contained inside the bottle of Yunnan Bai Yao should be taken.

Chronic bleeding is probably better treated with herbs and also responds to treatment well.

As for prevention, two things are particularly important for any patient who has been cured of bleeding. The first is to avoid the excessive consumption of hot-energy foods such as lamb, beef, spices, curry, and alcohol. This is because hot foods may create Heat in the Blood and this may push the blood out of the vessels. This precaution applies even when the bleeding of which the patient has been cured was of the deficient type, i.e. from Spleen-Qi not holding Blood. The second factor to keep in mind is overwork: this depletes Yin and leads to Empty-Heat. Both the deficiency of Yin-Qi and the Empty-Heat may lead to bleeding.

END NOTES

1. Pei Zheng Xue 1979 A Commentary on the Discussion of Blood Syndromes (*Xue Zheng Lun Ping Shi* 血证论评释), People's Health Publishing House, Beijing, pp. 6 and 7. The "Discussion of Blood Syndromes" itself by Tang Zong Hai was first published in 1884.

2. 1981 Spiritual Axis (*Ling Shu Jing* 灵枢经), People's Health Publishing House, Beijing. First published *c.* 100 BC, p. 153.

Dysmenorrhoea 31

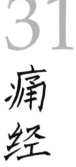

Dysmenorrhoea indicates pain occurring before, during or after menstruation. The pain may occur in the lower abdomen or sacral region.

From the point of view of Chinese medicine the Liver, Penetrating Vessel and Directing Vessel are responsible for the physiology of menstruation. For a normal period to occur, Blood must be abundant and move adequately. Proper movement of Blood relies on the free flow of Liver-Qi.

Four different phases may be identified during each menstrual cycle.

- *During menstruation* Blood is moving, for which it relies on Liver-Qi and Liver-Blood
- *After menstruation* Blood and Yin are empty
- *During mid-cycle* Blood and Yin gradually fill up in the Penetrating and Directing Vessels
- *Before menstruation* Yang rises to prepare to move Blood during the period. Liver-Qi moves in preparation to move Blood during the period (see Fig. 31.1)

Thus, a proper movement of Liver-Qi and Liver-Blood is essential for a pain-free period. If Liver-Qi stagnates it may cause pain especially before the period, while if Liver-Blood stagnates it will cause pain during the period. Stagnation is therefore the most important pathological condition causing dysmenorrhoea.

Aetiology and pathology

1. EMOTIONAL STRAIN

Emotional strain is a very important aetiological factor in dysmenorrhoea. Anger, frustration, resentment, hatred may all lead to Liver-Qi stagnation. In women, Liver-Qi stagnation causes Blood to stagnate in the uterus and therefore leads to painful periods.

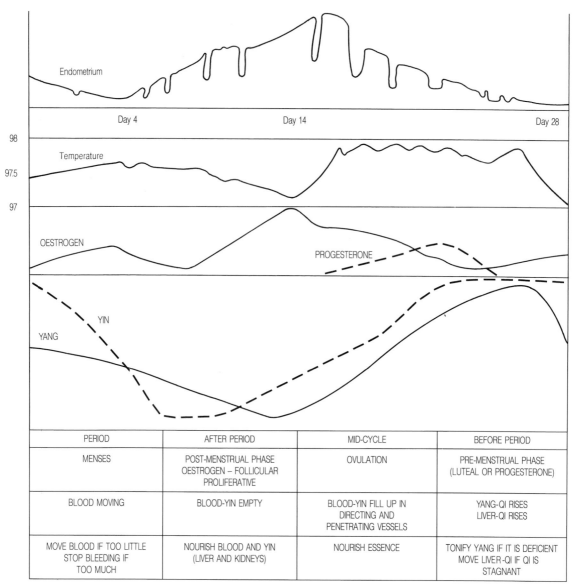

Fig. 31.1   The four phases of the menstrual cycle

PERIOD	AFTER PERIOD	MID-CYCLE	BEFORE PERIOD
MENSES	POST-MENSTRUAL PHASE OESTROGEN – FOLLICULAR PROLIFERATIVE	OVULATION	PRE-MENSTRUAL PHASE (LUTEAL OR PROGESTERONE)
BLOOD MOVING	BLOOD-YIN EMPTY	BLOOD-YIN FILL UP IN DIRECTING AND PENETRATING VESSELS	YANG-QI RISES LIVER-QI RISES
MOVE BLOOD IF TOO LITTLE STOP BLEEDING IF TOO MUCH	NOURISH BLOOD AND YIN (LIVER AND KIDNEYS)	NOURISH ESSENCE	TONIFY YANG IF IT IS DEFICIENT MOVE LIVER-QI IF QI IS STAGNANT

2. COLD AND DAMPNESS

Excessive exposure to cold and dampness, especially when this occurs during the puberty years, may cause Cold to invade the uterus. Cold contracts and causes stasis of Blood in the uterus and therefore painful periods.

Women are particularly prone to invasion of Cold in the uterus during and soon after the period when the uterus and Blood are in a rela- tively weakened state. At this time therefore, they should take particular care not to be ex- posed to cold and dampness.

Women with a pre-existing condition of Yang deficiency are obviously more prone to invasion of external Cold.

3. OVERWORK, CHRONIC ILLNESS

Physical overwork or a chronic illness leads to

deficiency of Qi and Blood especially of Stomach and Spleen. Deficiency of Blood leads to malnourishment of the Penetrating and Directing Vessels so that the Blood has no force to move properly thus causing relative stagnation and pain.

4. EXCESSIVE SEXUAL ACTIVITY, CHILDBIRTH

The Liver and Kidneys are weakened by excessive sexual activity (which affects women somewhat less than men), too many childbirths too close together, and sexual activity starting too early. A deficiency of Liver and Kidneys induces emptiness of the Penetrating and Directing Vessels so that they cannot move Qi and Blood properly, thus causing dysmenorrhoea.

Thus, stagnation of Qi and/or Blood, which may arise by itself or be caused by Cold in the uterus, is the most important factor in dysmenorrhoea. Even in Deficiency-types of dysmenorrhoea from Blood or Liver/Kidney deficiency, there is an element of stagnation as the deficient Blood fails to move properly.

Diagnosis

TIME OF ONSET

Pain before and during the period is usually of the Full type, while pain after the period is of the Empty type.

PRESSURE

If the pain is made worse by pressure it indicates Fullness, while if the patient gets relief from pressing the lower abdomen it indicates Emptiness.

HEAT-COLD

If the pain is relieved by the application of heat (such as a hot-water bottle) it indicates either a Cold condition or stasis of Blood from Cold. It should be kept in mind, however, that this sign is not always indicative of dysmenorrhoea from Cold as other conditions, such as stagnation of Qi or Blood, may also be alleviated by the application of a hot-water bottle. If the pain is aggravated by heat, it indicates Blood-Heat.

CHARACTER OF PAIN

- Pain better after passing clots: stasis of Blood
- Pain with pronounced feeling of distension: stagnation of Qi
- Burning pain: Blood-Heat
- Cramping pain: Cold in the uterus
- Stabbing pain, not moving: stasis of Blood
- Pulling pain: stasis of Blood
- Bearing-down pain before the period: stasis of Blood
- Bearing-down pain after the period: Kidney deficiency.

LOCATION OF PAIN

- Pain both sides of lower abdomen: Liver channel
- Pain on sacrum: Kidney channel, deficiency.

CYCLE

If the cycle is prolonged and the menstrual blood is dark and clotted it indicates stasis of Blood. If the menstrual blood is red with small dark clots it indicates Cold in the uterus.

If the cycle is short, the period is heavy and the blood is bright-red, it indicates Blood-Heat.

Differentiation and treatment

The most important differentiation is that between Full and Empty types of dysmenorrhoea. Full types are much more common and clinically more important as they are characterized by more intense pain than Empty types. Moreover, even in Empty types of dysmenorrhoea there is an element of stasis of Blood as deficient Blood fails to move properly. For this reason, even for Empty types of dysmenorrhoea, some Blood-moving herbs are added to the prescription used.

The general principle of treatment is to regulate Qi and Blood in the Penetrating and Directing Vessels. On the basis of the main pattern, the treatment principle also includes moving Qi, moving Blood, scattering Cold, clearing Heat or tonifying.

The treatment principle is often changed according to the time of the menstrual cycle. During the period one concentrates on treating the Manifestation, i.e. move Blood and stop pain. At other times of the cycle one treats the Root, i.e. according to the main pattern. In particular, if there is a deficiency, this is best treated during the two weeks or thereabouts following the period.

The patterns discussed are:

EXCESS

Stagnation of Qi and Blood
Stagnation of Cold
Damp-Heat

DEFICIENCY

Qi and Blood Deficiency
Kidney and Liver Deficiency

EXCESS TYPES

1. STAGNATION OF QI AND BLOOD

CLINICAL MANIFESTATIONS

Lower abdominal pain during, or one to two days before the period, a feeling of distension of the abdomen and breasts, hesitant start to the period, menstrual blood dark with clots, pain relieved after passing clots, pre-menstrual tension and irritability.

Tongue: Purple.
Pulse: Choppy or Wiry.

– Stagnation of Qi: more pronounced distension of abdomen and breasts, menstrual blood not so dark, tongue not too Purple.
– Stasis of Blood: more pain than distension, pain very intense, menstrual blood dark with clots, tongue definitely Purple.

TREATMENT PRINCIPLE

Move Qi and Blood, eliminate stasis, stop pain.

ACUPUNCTURE

LIV-3 Taichong, Ren-6 Qihai, G.B.-34 Yanglingquan, SP-8 Diji, ST-29 Guilai, SP-10 Xuehai, SP-6 Sanyinjiao, LU-7 Lieque and KI-6 Zhaohai, SP-4 Gongsun and P-6 Neiguan. Reducing or even method.

Explanation

– **LIV-3** moves Qi and Blood and stops pain.
– **Ren-6** moves Qi in the lower abdomen.
– **G.B.-34**, in combination with Ren-6, moves Qi in the lower abdomen.
– **SP-8** regulates Blood in the uterus and stops pain.
– **ST-29** regulates Blood in the uterus.
– **SP-10** moves Blood.
– **SP-6** helps to move Blood and stop pain.
– **LU-7** and **KI-6** open the Directing Vessel and regulate Qi in the uterus.
– **SP-4** and **P-6** open the Penetrating Vessel and regulate Blood in the uterus.

HERBAL TREATMENT

Stagnation of Qi

Prescription

XIAO YAO SAN Variation
Free and Easy Wanderer Powder
Bo He *Herba Menthae* 3 g
Chai Hu *Radix Bupleuri* 9 g

Dang Gui *Radix Angelicae sinensis* 9 g
Bai Shao *Radix Paeoniae albae* 12 g
Bai Zhu *Rhizoma Atractylodis macrocephalae* 9 g
Fu Ling *Sclerotium Poriae cocos* 15 g
Gan Cao *Radix Glycyrrhizae uralensis* 6 g
Sheng Jiang *Rhizoma Zingiberis officinalis recens* 3 slices
Wu Yao *Radix Linderae strychnifoliae* 6 g
Xiang Fu *Rhizoma Cyperi rotundi* 6 g
Zhi Ke *Fructus Citri aurantii* 6 g
Yan Hu Suo *Rhizoma Corydalis yanhusuo* 6 g

Explanation

The first eight herbs constitute the Xiao Yao San which moves Qi and is specific for menstrual problems, especially from emotional strain.

- **Wu Yao**, **Xiang Fu**, **Zhi Ke** and **Yan Hu Suo** move Qi more strongly and stop pain.

Stasis of Blood

(a) Prescription

TAO HONG SI WU TANG Variation
Persica-Carthamus Four Substances Decoction
Dang Gui *Radix Angelicae sinensis* 9 g
Chuan Xiong *Radix Ligustici wallichii* 6 g
Shu Di Huang *Radix Rehmanniae glutinosae praeparata* 12 g
Bai Shao *Radix Paeoniae albae* 9 g
Tao Ren *Semen Persicae* 6 g
Hong Hua *Flos Carthami tinctorii* 6 g
Yan Hu Suo *Rhizoma Corydalis yanhusuo* 6 g
Xiang Fu *Rhizoma Cyperi rotundi* 6 g
Chuan Niu Xi *Radix Cyathulae* 6 g

Explanation

The first six herbs constitute the Tao Hong Si Wu Tang which moves Blood.

- **Yan Hu Suo**, **Xiang Fu** and **Niu Xi** move Qi and Blood in the lower abdomen and stop pain.

(b) Prescription

GE XIA ZHU YU TANG
Eliminating Stasis below the Diaphragm Decoction

Dang Gui *Radix Angelicae sinensis* 9 g
Chuan Xiong *Radix Ligustici wallichii* 3 g
Chi Shao *Radix Paeoniae rubrae* 6 g
Hong Hua *Flos Carthami tinctorii* 9 g
Tao Ren *Semen Persicae* 9 g
Wu Ling Zhi *Excrementum Trogopteri* 9 g
Yan Hu Suo *Rhizoma Corydalis yanhusuo* 3 g
Xiang Fu *Rhizoma Cyperi rotundi* 3 g
Zhi Ke *Fructus Citri aurantii* 5 g
Wu Yao *Radix Linderae strychnifoliae* 6 g
Mu Dan Pi *Cortex Moutan radicis* 6 g
Gan Cao *Radix Glycyrrhizae uralensis* 9 g

Explanation

This formula, which has already been explained in chapter 17, is specific to move Blood in the lower abdomen. It is stronger than the previous one and is therefore selected when pain is more intense.

Case history

A 29-year-old woman had been suffering from dysmenorrhoea ever since her periods started. The pain occurred during the period and the menstrual blood was dark with some clots. The period started hesitantly and there was not much distension. The pain was alleviated by the application of a hot-water bottle.

She also suffered from thrush with itching of the vagina and a white-sticky discharge. She felt generally tired and her stools were loose. She had a lower back-ache, her memory was poor and she felt always cold. Her tongue was Pale and her pulse was Slow (68) and Weak on the Liver and right Kidney positions.

Diagnosis
My diagnosis was dysmenorrhoea from mild stasis of Blood occurring against a background of Liver and Kidney deficiency. The tiredness, cold feeling, back-ache, poor memory and tongue and pulse all pointed to Liver and Kidney deficiency. Besides this, she also suffered from Spleen deficiency (loose stools) and Dampness in the Lower Burner (vaginal itching and discharge).

Treatment principle
This case is given here as an example of wrong principle of treatment adopted. Since I came to the conclusion that the main aspect of the condition was a Deficiency (of Liver, Kidneys and Spleen) with only a mild and secondary Excess (stasis of Blood and Dampness in the Lower Burner), I adopted the

principle of tonifying and warming the Kidneys and nourishing the Liver.

Herbal treatment
I therefore chose a variation of the formula You Gui Wan *Restoring the Right [Kidney] Pill*:

Shu Di Huang *Radix Rehmanniae glutinosae praeparata* 9 g
Shan Yao *Radix Dioscoreae oppositae* 6 g
Shan Zhu Yu *Fructus Corni officinalis* 3 g
Tu Si Zi *Semen Cuscutae* 6 g
Gou Qi Zi *Fructus Lycii chinensis* 6 g
Du Zhong *Cortex Eucommiae ulmoidis* 4 g
Dang Gui *Radix Angelicae sinensis* 6 g
Lu Jiao Jiao *Colla Cornu Cervi* 6 g
Bai Zhu *Rhizoma Atractylodis macrocephalae* 6 g
Fu Ling *Sclerotium Poriae cocos* 6 g
Xiang Fu *Rhizoma Cyperi rotundi* 4 g
Yi Mu Cao *Herba Leonori heterophylli* 4 g
Zhi Gan Cao *Radix Glycyrrhizae uralensis praeparata* 3 g

Explanation
The first 8 herbs constitute a variation of You Gui Wan to tonify and warm the Kidneys and nourish the Liver.

- **Bai Zhu** and **Fu Ling** were added to tonify the Spleen.
- **Xiang Fu** and **Yi Mu Cao** were added to move Qi and Blood and stop pain.

After 10 packets of this decoction, she was no better at all. I therefore reassessed the diagnosis and principle of treatment and came to the conclusion that, although there was a pronounced deficiency, it would be better to eliminate pathogenic factors first. I did this by giving her 10 packets of a decoction to resolve Dampness first, and then 10 packets of a decoction to move Blood and eliminate stasis. The first decoction was a variation of Si Miao San *Four Wonderful Powder*:

Cang Zhu *Rhizoma Atractylodis lanceae* 4 g
Huang Bo *Cortex Phellodendri* 4 g
Niu Xi *Radix Achyranthis bidentatae seu Cyathulae* 4 g
Yi Yi Ren *Semen Coicis lachryma jobi* 9 g
Dang Gui *Radix Angelicae sinensis* 6 g
Bai Zhu *Rhizoma Atractylodis macrocephalae* 6 g
Fu Ling *Sclerotium Poriae cocos* 6 g
Hong Hua *Flos Carthami tinctorii* 4 g
Tao Ren *Semen Persicae* 6 g
Tu Si Zi *Semen Cuscutae* 4 g

Explanation
The first four herbs represent the Si Miao San.

- **Bai Zhu** and **Fu Ling** were added to tonify the Spleen.
- **Hong Hua** and **Tao Ren** were added to move Blood, eliminate stasis and stop pain.
- **Dang Gui** and **Tu Si Zi** were added to nourish Liver and Kidneys.

She improved considerably after this decoction which was then followed by a variation of Ge Xia Zhu Yu Tang *Eliminating Stasis below the Diaphragm Decoction* to move Blood and eliminate stasis:

Wu Ling Zhi *Excrementum Trogopteri* 4 g
Dang Gui *Radix Angelicae sinensis* 6 g
Chuan Xiong *Radix Ligustici wallichii* 4 g
Tao Ren *Semen Persicae* 4 g
Hong Hua *Flos Carthami tinctorii* 4 g
Chi Shao *Radix Paeoniae rubrae* 4 g
Wu Yao *Radix Linderae strychnifoliae* 4 g
Yan Hu Suo *Rhizoma Corydalis yanhusuo* 4 g
Xiang Fu *Rhizoma Cyperi rotundi* 4 g
Gan Cao *Radix Glycyrrhizae uralensis* 3 g
Zhi Ke *Fructus Citri aurantii* 4 g
Bai Zhu *Rhizoma Atractylodis macrocephalae* 6 g
Tu Si Zi *Semen Cuscutae* 6 g

This is a variation of Ge Xia Zhu Yu Tang with the addition of Bai Zhu to tonify the Spleen and Tu Si Zi to tonify the Kidneys.

After 20 packets of this decoction she was much better and her periods were painless. Even though neither of the above two formulae is tonifying, she had more energy. After 20 packets of this last decoction, the treatment principle reverted to the original one of tonifying Kidneys and Liver with You Gui Wan. This time, she felt well on it.

This case history is given to illustrate the importance of adopting a correct principle of treatment: even if the diagnosis is correct, adoption of the wrong principle of treatment will not yield results. This case also shows the importance, in mixed Excess and Deficieny conditions, of eliminating pathogenic factors *before* tonifying: this approach is particularly important when herbs are used and not so much if only acupuncture is used.

2. STAGNATION OF COLD

CLINICAL MANIFESTATIONS

Lower abdominal pain before or after the period, pain more central, pain relieved by the application of heat, menstrual blood rather scanty and bright-red with dark clots, feeling cold, sore back.
Tongue: Pale-Bluish or Bluish-Purple.
Pulse: Deep and Choppy or Deep and Wiry.

TREATMENT PRINCIPLE

Warm the uterus, expel Cold, move Blood.

ACUPUNCTURE

Ren-4 Guanyuan, Ren-6 Qihai, ST-29 Guilai, SP-8 Diji, SP-6 Sanyinjiao, ST-36 Zusanli. Reducing method except on ST-36 which should be reinforced. Moxa must be used.

Explanation

- **Ren-4**, with moxa, warms the uterus.
- **Ren-6**, with moxa, moves Qi and expels Cold from the lower abdomen.
- **ST-29** moves Blood.
- **SP-8** and **SP-6** move Blood and stops pain.
- **ST-36** tonifies Qi and helps to scatter Cold.

HERBAL TREATMENT

Empty Cold

(a) Prescription

WEN JING TANG
Warm the Menses Decoction
Wu Zhu Yu *Fructus Evodiae rutaecarpae* 9 g
Gui Zhi *Ramulus Cinnamomi cassiae* 9 g
Sheng Jiang *Rhizoma Zingiberis officinalis recens* 6 g
Dang Gui *Radix Angelicae sinensis* 9 g
Chuan Xiong *Radix Ligustici wallichii* 4.5 g
Bai Shao *Radix Paeoniae albae* 9 g
Dang Shen *Radix Codonopsis pilosulae* 12 g
Mai Men Dong *Tuber Ophiopogonis japonici* 6 g
E Jiao *Gelatinum Corii Asini* 9 g
Mu Dan Pi *Cortex Moutan radicis* 4.5 g
Ban Xia *Rhizoma Pinelliae ternatae* 6 g
Zhi Gan Cao *Radix Glycyrrhizae uralensis praeparata* 3 g

Explanation

- **Wu Zhu Yu**, **Gui Zhi** and **Sheng Jiang** warm the uterus and expel Cold.
- **Dang Gui**, **Chuan Xiong** and **Bai Shao** nourish and move Blood.
- **Dang Shen** tonifies Qi to nourish Blood. It is necessary to nourish Blood as the obstruction of the uterus by Cold prevents new Blood from taking its proper place in the uterus.
- **Mai Men Dong** and **E Jiao** nourish Blood and Yin.
- **Mu Dan Pi** clears any Empty-Heat which might arise from Blood deficiency.
- **Ban Xia** harmonizes the uterus via the Stomach channel to which it is connected.
- **Gan Cao** harmonizes.

(b) Prescription

AI FU NUAN GONG WAN
Artemisia-Cyperus Warming the Uterus Pill
Ai Ye *Folium Artemisiae* 9 g
Wu Zhu Yu *Fructus Evodiae rutaecarpae* 4.5 g
Rou Gui *Cortex Cinnamomi cassiae* 4.5 g
Xiang Fu *Rhizoma Cyperi rotundi* 9 g
Dang Gui *Radix Angelicae sinensis* 9 g
Chuan Xiong *Radix Ligustici wallichii* 6 g
Bai Shao *Radix Paeoniae albae* 6 g
Huang Qi *Radix Astragali membranacei* 6 g
Sheng Di Huang *Radix Rehmanniae glutinosae* 9 g
Xu Duan *Radix Dipsaci* 6 g

Explanation

- **Ai Ye**, **Wu Zhu Yu** and **Rou Gui** warm the uterus and expel Cold.
- **Xiang Fu** moves Qi in the lower abdomen.
- **Dang Gui**, **Chuan Xiong** and **Bai Shao** nourish and move Blood.
- **Huang Qi** tonifies Qi in order to help to produce more Blood.
- **Sheng Di Huang** nourishes Blood and Yin.
- **Xu Duan** tonifies the Kidneys to help to nourish Blood.

The above two formulae are similar in action. The main difference between the two is that the former is applicable when the obstruction of Cold in the uterus leads to a deficiency of Blood and Yin with some symptoms of Empty-Heat such as a malar flush and a feeling of heat. Thus, the first formula, Wen Jing Tang, addresses the situation when the deficiency of Blood is a consequence of Cold obstructing the uterus. The latter formula, Ai Fu Nuan Gong Wan, is for a situation when it is the deficiency of Yang and Blood that leads to internal Cold.

Variations

These variations apply to both formulae.

- If symptoms of Cold are very pronounced add (or increase if already in the formula) Fu Zi *Radix Aconiti carmichaeli praeparata* and Ai Ye *Folium Artemisiae*.
- If there is Dampness as well as Cold add Cang Zhu *Rhizoma Atractylodis lanceae* and Fu Ling *Sclerotium Poriae cocos*.

Patent remedy

TONG JING WAN
Dysmenorrhoea Pill
Shu Di Huang *Radix Rehmanniae glutinosae praeparata*
Dang Gui *Radix Angelicae sinensis*
Dan Shen *Radix Salviae miltiorrhizae*
Xiang Fu *Rhizoma Cyperi rotundi*
Shan Zha *Fructus Crataegi*
Bai Shao *Radix Paeoniae albae*
Yan Hu Suo *Rhizoma Corydalis yanhusuo*
Wu Ling Zhi *Excrementum Trogopteri*
Chuan Xiong *Radix Ligustici wallichii*
Hong Hua *Flos Carthami tinctorii*
Mu Xiang *Radix Saussureae*
Qing Pi *Pericarpium Citri reticulatae viridae*
Rou Gui *Cortex Cinnamomi cassiae*
Gan Jiang *Rhizoma Zingiberis officinalis*
Yi Mu Cao *Herba Leonori heterophylli*

Explanation

This remedy nourishes Blood, moves Qi and Blood and warms the Lower Burner. It is therefore suitable for dysmenorrhoea deriving from deficiency of Yang and Empty Cold in the uterus.

The tongue presentation appropriate to this remedy is a Pale-Purplish body.

Case history

A 42-year-old woman had been suffering from painful periods for 15 years. Her cycle was short, with a period coming every 21–25 days. She experienced severe pain during the period and the blood was red with small dark clots. She felt cold in general, but especially so during the period. She also suffered from back-ache and dizziness. Her tongue was Pale and slightly Swollen. Her pulse was very Slow (52), Choppy, Weak on the left Rear position and had no wave.

Diagnosis

The dysmenorrhoea itself is due to Cold obstructing the uterus. This is Cold of the Empty type as is clearly shown by the Weak and Choppy pulse. Besides this, there is an underlying deficiency of Kidney-Yang as shown by the Slow and Weak pulse on the left-Rear position, Pale and Swollen tongue, dizziness, cold feeling and back-ache and some deficiency of Qi and Blood as evidenced by the Choppy pulse.

Treatment principle

The treatment principle adopted was to tonify and warm Kidney-Yang, scatter internal Cold, nourish Blood and stop pain. She was treated with both acupuncture and herbs.

Acupuncture

The acupuncture points, used with even method to scatter Cold and reinforcing method to tonify the Kidneys and nourish Blood, were selected from the following:

- **LU-7** Lieque and **KI-6** Zhaohai to open the Directing Vessel, regulate Qi and Blood in the uterus and stop pain.
- **ST-29** Guilai, with moxa, to regulate Blood, scatter Cold and stop pain.
- **Ren-6** Qihai and **Ren-4** Guanyuan, with moxa, to tonify Qi and Blood and tonify Kidney-Yang.
- **BL-23** Shenshu, with needle and moxa, to tonify and warm Kidney-Yang.
- **SP-6** Sanyinjiao and **ST-36** Zusanli to tonify Qi and Blood.

Herbal treatment

The formula used was a variation of Ai Fu Nuan Gong Wan *Artemisia-Cyperus Warming the Uterus Pill*:

Ai Ye *Folium Artemisiae* 9 g
Wu Zhu Yu *Fructus Evodiae rutaecarpae* 4.5 g
Rou Gui *Cortex Cinnamomi cassiae* 3 g
Xiang Fu *Rhizoma Cyperi rotundi* 6 g
Dang Gui *Radix Angelicae sinensis* 9 g
Chuan Xiong *Radix Ligustici wallichii* 6 g
Bai Shao *Radix Paeoniae albae* 9 g
Huang Qi *Radix Astragali membranacei* 6 g
Sheng Di Huang *Radix Rehmanniae glutinosae* 9 g
Xu Duan *Radix Dipsaci* 6 g
Wu Yao *Radix Linderae strychnifoliae* 6 g
Yan Hu Suo *Rhizoma Corydalis yanhusuo* 6 g

Explanation

- The first ten herbs constitute the root formula which scatters Cold, warms the Uterus, tonifies Qi and Blood and tonifies and warms Kidney-Yang.
- **Wu Yao** and **Yan Hu Suo** move Qi and Blood and stop pain.

This patient was treated with acupuncture every two weeks and took the above decoction, with slight variations, for 6 months. After this time, her cycle became regular and the menstrual pain was reduced by 80%.

Full Cold

Prescription

SHAO FU ZHU YU TANG
Lower Abdomen Eliminating Stasis Decoction
Xiao Hui Xiang *Fructus Foeniculi vulgaris* 6 g
Gan Jiang *Rhizoma Zingiberis officinalis* 2 g
Rou Gui *Cortex Cinnamomi cassiae* 1.5 g
Yan Hu Suo *Rhizoma Corydalis yanhusuo* 6 g
Mo Yao *Myrrha* 6 g
Pu Huang *Pollen Typhae* 6 g
Wu Ling Zhi *Excrementum Trogopteri* 4.5 g
Dang Gui *Radix Angelicae sinensis* 9 g
Chuan Xiong *Radix Ligustici wallichii* 4.5 g
Chi Shao Yao *Radix Paeoniae rubrae* 6 g

Explanation

- **Xiao Hui Xiang**, **Gan Jiang** and **Rou Gui** warm the uterus and expel Cold.
- **Yan Hu Suo**, **Mo Yao**, **Pu Huang** and **Wu Ling Zhi** move Blood and stop pain.
- **Dang Gui**, **Chuan Xiong** and **Chi Shao** nourish and move Blood.

Variations

- If there is Dampness add Cang Zhu *Rhizoma Atractylodis lanceae* and Fu Ling *Sclerotium Poriae cocos*.

3. DAMP-HEAT

CLINICAL MANIFESTATIONS

Hypogastric pain before the period and sometimes on mid-cycle, burning sensation extending to the sacrum, feeling of heat, menstrual blood red with small clots, vaginal discharge, scanty-dark urine.
Tongue: Red, sticky-yellow tongue coating.
Pulse: Slippery.

TREATMENT PRINCIPLE

Clear Heat, resolve Dampness, eliminate stasis.

ACUPUNCTURE

SP-9 Yinlingquan, SP-6 Sanyinjiao, LU-7 Lieque and KI-6 Zhaohai, Ren-3 Zhongji, ST-28 Shuidao, BL-32 Ciliao, BL-22 Sanjiaoshu. Reducing method.

Explanation

- **SP-9** and **SP-6** resolve Dampness in the Lower Burner. SP-6 also moves Blood.
- **LU-7** and **KI-6** open the Directing Vessel and regulate the uterus.
- **Ren-3** and **ST-28** resolve Dampness from the Lower Burner and uterus.
- **BL-32** resolves Dampness in the uterus.
- **BL-22** promotes the transformation of fluids and resolves Dampness from the Lower Burner.

HERBAL TREATMENT

(a) Prescription

QING RE TIAO XUE TANG
Clearing Heat and Regulating Blood Decoction
Mu Dan Pi *Cortex Moutan radicis* 6 g
Sheng Di Huang *Radix Rehmanniae glutinosae* 9 g
Huang Lian *Rhizoma Coptidis* 4.5 g
Dang Gui *Radix Angelicae sinensis* 9 g
Bai Shao *Radix Paeoniae albae* 9 g
Chuan Xiong *Radix Ligustici wallichii* 6 g
Hong Hua *Flos Carthami tinctorii* 6 g
Tao Ren *Semen Persicae* 6 g
E Zhu *Rhizoma Curcumae zedoariae* 6 g
Xiang Fu *Rhizoma Cyperi rotundi* 6 g
Yan Hu Suo *Rhizoma Corydalis yanhusuo* 6 g

Explanation

- **Dan Pi** and **Sheng Di** clear Heat and cool Blood.
- **Huang Lian** resolves Damp-Heat.
- **Dang Gui** and **Bai Shao** harmonize Blood.
- **Chuan Xiong**, **Hong Hua**, **Tao Ren** and **E Zhu** move Blood.
- **Xiang Fu** and **Yan Hu Suo** move Qi and stop pain.

(b) Prescription

Empirical prescription
Qu Mai *Herba Dianthi* 6 g
Bian Xu *Herba Polygoni avicularis* 6 g
Mu Tong *Caulis Akebiae* 4.5 g
Che Qian Zi *Semen Plantaginis* 6 g
Huang Qin *Radix Scutellariae baicalensis* 6 g
Chi Shao *Radix Paeoniae rubrae* 6 g
Di Gu Pi *Cortex Lycii chinensis radicis* 6 g
Chuan Lian Zi *Fructus Meliae toosendan* 4.5 g
Yan Hu Suo *Rhizoma Corydalis yanhusuo* 9 g
Zhi Gan Cao *Radix Glycyrrhizae uralensis praeparata* 3 g

Explanation

- **Qu Mai**, **Bian Xu**, **Mu Tong** and **Che Qian Zi** drain Dampness via urination.
- **Huang Qin** resolves Damp-Heat.
- **Chi Shao** and **Di Gu Pi** clear Heat and cool Blood.
- **Chuan Lian Zi** and **Yan Hu Suo** move Qi and stop pain.
- **Gan Cao** harmonizes.

DEFICIENCY TYPES

1. QI AND BLOOD DEFICIENCY

CLINICAL MANIFESTATIONS

Dull hypogastric pain towards the end of or after the period, dragging sensation in the lower abdomen, pain relieved by pressure and massage, scanty bleeding, pale complexion, tiredness, slight dizziness, loose stools.

TREATMENT PRINCIPLE

Tonify Qi, strengthen the Spleen, nourish Blood.

ACUPUNCTURE

Ren-4 Guanyuan, Ren-6 Qihai, ST-36 Zusanli, SP-6 Sanyinjiao, SP-8 Diji, BL-20 Pishu. Reinforcing method. Moxa is applicable.

Explanation

- **Ren-4** nourishes Blood and the uterus.
- **Ren-6** tonifies and moves Qi in the lower abdomen.
- **ST-36** and **SP-6** tonify Qi, strengthen the Spleen and nourish Blood.
- **SP-8** stops pain.
- **BL-20** strengthens the Spleen and nourishes Blood.

HERBAL TREATMENT

(a) Prescription

SHENG YU TANG
Sage-like Healing Decoction
Ren Shen *Radix Ginseng* 12 g
Huang Qi *Radix Astragali membranacei* 18 g
Dang Gui *Radix Angelicae sinensis* 15 g
Chuan Xiong *Radix Ligustici wallichii* 8 g
Shu Di Huang *Radix Rehmanniae glutinosae praeparata* 18 g
Bai Shao *Radix Paeoniae albae* 12 g

Explanation

- **Ren Shen** and **Huang Qi** tonify Qi.
- **Dang Gui**, **Chuan Xiong**, **Shu Di** and **Bai Shao** nourish and move Blood.

(b) Prescription

BA ZHEN YI MU TANG
Eight Precious Leonorus Decoction
Dang Gui *Radix Angelicae sinensis* 10 g
Chuan Xiong *Radix Ligustici wallichii* 5 g
Bai Shao *Radix Paeoniae albae* 8 g
Shu Di Huang *Radix Rehmanniae glutinosae praeparata* 15 g
Ren Shen *Radix Ginseng* 3 g
Bai Zhu *Rhizoma Atractylodis macrocephalae* 10 g
Fu Ling *Sclerotium Poriae cocos* 8 g
Zhi Gan Cao *Radix Glycyrrhizae uralensis praeparata* 5 g
Yi Mu Cao *Herba Leonori heterophylli* 9 g

Explanation

This is the Ba Zhen Tang *Eight Precious Decoction*,

which has already been explained in chapter 17, with the addition of Yi Mu Cao *Herba Leonori heterophylli* to move Blood and stop pain.

(c) Prescription

SHI QUAN DA BU TANG
Ten Complete Great Tonification Decoction
Ba Zhen Tang *Eight Precious Decoction* plus:
Huang Qi *Radix Astragali membranacei* 8 g
Rou Gui *Cortex Cinnamomi cassiae* 4 g

Explanation

This formula is used if there are symptoms of Cold.

Variations

– As even in a Deficiency-type of dysmenorrhea there is always an element of stagnation, in order to move Qi and Blood and stop pain add Xiang Fu *Rhizoma Cyperi rotundi* and Yan Hu Suo *Rhizoma Corydalis yanhusuo*.

(i) Patent remedy

BA ZHEN YI MU WAN
Eight Precious Leonorus Pill

Explanation

This pill has the same ingredients and functions as the homonymous prescription above. It is suitable for dysmenorrhoea from deficiency of Qi and Blood.

The tongue presentation appropriate to this remedy is a Pale and Thin body.

(ii) Patent remedy

SHI QUAN DA BU WAN
Ten Complete Great Tonification Pill

Explanation

This pill has the same ingredients and functions as the homonymous prescription above. It is suitable for dysmenorrhoea from deficiency of Yang and Blood with internal Cold.

The tongue presentation appropriate to this remedy is a Pale, Thin and wet body.

2. KIDNEY- AND LIVER-YIN DEFICIENCY

CLINICAL MANIFESTATIONS

Dull hypogastric pain towards the end of or after the period, sore back, dizziness, scanty bleeding, pain relieved by pressure and massage, tinnitus, blurred vision, exhaustion.
Tongue: Red without coating.
Pulse: Floating-Empty.

TREATMENT PRINCIPLE

Nourish Yin, benefit the Kidneys, nourish the Liver.

ACUPUNCTURE

BL-23 Shenshu, BL-18 Ganshu, Ren-4 Guanyuan, SP-6 Sanyinjiao, KI-3 Taixi, ST-36 Zusanli. Reinforcing method. A small amount of moxa may be used if the tongue is not too Red.

Explanation

– **BL-23** and **BL-18** tonify Kidneys and Liver.
– **Ren-4** nourishes Yin and tonifies the Kidneys and the uterus.
– **SP-6** and **KI-3** nourish the Kidneys and Liver and regulate Blood.
– **ST-36** tonifies Qi and Blood and regulates the uterus Connecting channel.

HERBAL TREATMENT

Prescription

TIAO GAN TANG
Regulating the Liver Decoction
Dang Gui *Radix Angelicae sinensis* 9 g
Bai Shao *Radix Paeoniae albae* 9 g

Shan Yao *Radix Dioscoreae oppositae* 12 g
E Jiao *Gelatinum Corii Asini* 9 g
Shan Zhu Yu *Fructus Corni officinalis* 6 g
Ba Ji Tian *Radix Morindae officinalis* 9 g
Zhi Gan Cao *Radix Glycyrrhizae uralensis prae-*
parata 3 g

Explanation

- **Dang Gui** and **Bai Shao** nourish and move Blood.
- **Shan Yao** tonifies Stomach and Kidneys.
- **E Jiao** nourishes Blood.
- **Shan Zhu Yu** nourishes Liver-Yin.
- **Ba Ji Tian** tonifies Kidney-Yang and Kidney-Essence.
- **Gan Cao** harmonizes.

Case history

A 33-year-old woman had been suffering from painful periods for 10 years. The pain occurred during the period and the blood was bright-red and rather scanty. She felt cold in general and colder during the period. She had had 4 miscarriages. She also suffered from back-ache, dizziness, tinnitus, poor memory, a dry mouth at night and night-sweating. Her urination was frequent and occasionally it dribbled. She felt always very tired and her knees ached. Her tongue was of a normal colour but without spirit on the root. Her pulse was generally Weak and, on the left side, very Fine and Empty at the deep level.

Diagnosis
This is a complicated condition characterized by a deficiency of both Kidney-Yin and Kidney-Yang. The symptoms of Kidney-Yin deficiency are: dizziness, tinnitus, dry mouth at night, night-sweating, poor memory, tongue root without spirit and pulse Empty at the deep level. The symptoms of Kidney-Yang deficiency are: feeling cold, achy knees, and frequent and dribbling urination. The miscarriages were due to the Kidney deficiency. Thus, this is a Deficiency type of dysmenorrhoea.

Treatment principle
The treatment principle adopted was to nourish Kidney-Yin and warm and tonify Kidney-Yang. The emphasis was put on nourishing Kidney-Yin as when both Yin and Yang are deficient, it is important to nourish the substance first (Kidney-Yin) rather than the function (Kidney-Yang). The very Fine pulse which is also Empty at the deep level also indicates the importance of nourishing the Yin primarily.

However, secondary tonification of Kidney-Yang should not be overlooked.

Herbal treatment
The formula used was a variation of Tiao Gan Tang *Regulating the Liver Decoction*:

Dang Gui *Radix Angelicae sinensis* 9 g
Bai Shao *Radix Paeoniae albae* 9 g
Shan Yao *Radix Dioscoreae oppositae* 6 g
E Jiao *Gelatinum Corii Asini* 6 g
Shan Zhu Yu *Fructus Corni officinalis* 6 g
Ba Ji Tian *Radix Morindae officinalis* 4 g
Zhi Gan Cao *Radix Glycyrrhizae uralensis praeparata* 3 g
Chi Shao *Radix Paeoniae rubrae* 6 g
Yi Mu Cao *Herba Leonori heterophylli* 6 g
Gou Ji *Rhizoma Cibotii barometz* 4 g
Gou Qi Zi *Fructus Lycii chinensis* 9 g
Sheng Di Huang *Radix Rehmanniae glutinosae* 12 g

Explanation
- The first seven herbs constitute the Tiao Gan Tang which nourishes Liver and Kidneys.
- **Chi Shao** and **Yi Mu Cao** move Blood and stop pain.
- **Gou Ji** was added to tonify Kidney-Yang and strengthen the back and knees.
- **Gou Qi Zi** was added to nourish Liver-Yin.
- **Sheng Di Huang** was added to nourish Kidney-Yin.

This patient was treated with this decoction (with slight variations) for 6 months, producing a cure in the dysmenorrhoea. After a further 6 months of treatment with the same decoction taken on alternate weeks, she conceived and delivered a healthy baby.

Prognosis

Both acupuncture and Chinese herbs either singly or in combination give excellent results in dysmenorrhoea and the overwhelming majority of cases can be cured. The Empty types are easier to treat than the Full types. Of the Full types, the one from Damp-Heat is the most difficult to treat while the one from stagnation of Qi and Blood is the easiest. Of course, in many patients there is a mixed condition of Deficiency and Excess, in which case one concentrates on treating the stagnation in the two weeks before the periods and the Deficiency in the two weeks after. In some cases, it is better to eliminate pathogenic factors before tonifying: see case history above (p. 739).

In any menstrual problem, it takes a minimum of three menstrual cycles to regulate Blood and the Directing and Penetrating Vessels. Three months is therefore the very minimum time for the treatment to be successful.

If dysmenorrhoea is due to endometriosis (see below) the treatment will take considerably longer than for functional dysmenorrhoea.

Western differentiation

Western medicine differentiates *primary* from *secondary* dysmenorrhoea.

Primary dysmenorrhoea starts during adolescence and is not associated with any organic disorder. From the Chinese point of view, this is often due to invasion of Cold in the uterus when young girls are exposed to cold during puberty either because they often play outdoor games during cold and wet winters, or because they have been engaged in physical work (such as farming) outdoors.

Secondary dysmenorrhoea starts later in life and may be associated (although not necessarily) with organic diseases such as endometriosis, pelvic inflammatory disease or myomas.

ENDOMETRIOSIS

In endometriosis ectopic endometrium is implanted in adjacent pelvic organs such as ovaries, fallopian tubes, pelvic ligaments, vagina, sigmoid colon, rectum, ureters or bladder. Endometriosis is on the increase and it has become the commonest cause of secondary dysmenorrhoea. Other symptoms apart from painful periods with the pain radiating to the rectum or perineum may include menorrhagia and dyspareunia (pain on intercourse).

Some Chinese doctors say that if no results are obtained in a case of dysmenorrhoea, one should suspect endometriosis.

MYOMA

Myomas do not usually cause pain. However, if there is torsion they may cause dysmenorrhoea.

Dysmenorrhoea due to myomas may be helped even if the myomas cannot be dissolved. Regulating Blood and eliminating stasis will help the dysmenorrhoea and will make the abdomen feel more comfortable in general in spite of the myomas.

Very small myomas (up to about 2 cm in diameter) may be dissolved with acupuncture and Chinese herbs. If the diagnosis of myomas is definitely confirmed, then the formulae used should include strong herbs which "break" Blood such as E Zhu *Rhizoma Curcumae zedoariae*, Ze Lan *Herba Lycopi lucidi* and San Leng *Rhizoma Sparganii*. A particularly good formula for myomas from stasis of Blood is Gui Zhi Fu Ling Tang *Ramulus Cinnamomi-Poria Decoction* which contains Gui Zhi *Ramulus Cinnamomi cassiae*, Fu Ling *Sclerotium Poriae cocos*, Tao Ren *Semen Persicae*, Chi Shao *Radix Paeoniae rubrae* and Mu Dan Pi *Cortex Moutan radicis*.

MITTELSCHMERZ

Mittelschmerz consists of pain in mid-cycle. It is probably due to the rupture of a follicular cyst. The pain occurs in either lateral region of the lower abdomen and does not usually last more than 24 hours.

From the Chinese point of view, it is often due to Dampness.

Menorrhagia and metrorrhagia

32

崩
漏

Menorrhagia indicates excessive menstrual flow while metrorrhagia indicates bleeding outside the normal menstrual period. The average blood loss during a period is about 80 ml and any loss over this amount is considered as "excessive period". About 78% of the blood loss occurs within the first two days.

In Chinese medicine, a distinction is made between two slightly different pathological conditions. "Excessive periods" indicates heavy blood loss during the proper period time (about five days), with the periods coming at regular intervals. "Flooding" (in Chinese called *ben lou*, *ben* meaning "bursting through" and *lou* meaning "leaking") indicates a sudden and profuse bleeding which may or may not occur during the proper period time, while the periods are irregular. Thus, *ben lou* may indicate the period coming early with sudden flooding or trickling for a long time after the proper period time.

In general, the pathology of "excessive periods" and "flooding" is the same and the two conditions may be discussed together, although "flooding" is a more serious condition.

Aetiology and pathology

1. EMOTIONAL STRAIN

Any emotion may lead to stagnation of Qi and this to Fire. Fire usually affects the Liver and, as this stores Blood, it may cause Blood-Heat. Heat makes the Blood reckless and causes it to burst out of the blood vessels. This is a major cause of bleeding in gynaecological problems.

Emotional problems may also cause bleeding in a different way, by leading to stagnation of Qi which will, in time, cause stasis of Blood. Stasis of Blood in the uterus prevents new blood from taking its place and it therefore leaks out.

2. OVERWORK AND EXCESSIVE SEXUAL ACTIVITY

Overwork and excessive sexual activity weaken Liver and Kidney Yin. Deficiency of

Yin over a long period of time gives rise to Empty-Heat which may affect the Blood. Empty-Heat may also make the Blood reckless in the same way as Blood-Heat, causing blood to burst out of the vessels.

Deficiency of Kidney-Yin may also cause excessive menstrual bleeding by itself, without Empty-Heat, as Kidney-Yin fails to hold Blood.

3. PHYSICAL OVERWORK, CHRONIC ILLNESS

Physical overwork and chronic illness weaken the Spleen which fails to control Blood so that this leaks out. This is another major cause of excessive menstrual bleeding.

4. CHILDBIRTH

Excessive loss of blood at childbirth can weaken the Kidneys and Liver which fail to hold Blood and therefore cause bleeding.

On the other hand, stasis of Blood often occurs after childbirth in women who have a tendency to stagnation. Stasis of Blood in the uterus may cause bleeding in the way described above.

As for pathology, there are four major causes of bleeding:

  Blood-Heat
  Blood Empty-Heat
  Qi Deficiency
  Blood stasis.

Blood-Heat is characterized by profuse bleeding with bright-red or dark-red blood. It may cause both menorrhagia and metrorrhagia.

Blood Empty-Heat is characterized by lesser bleeding or by prolonged spotting after the end of the proper period. The colour of the blood is red or scarlet red.

Qi deficiency may cause flooding at the beginning of the period or prolonged spotting after the period. The blood is pale-red. Qi deficiency should be understood here in a broad sense as including Yang-Qi or Yin-Qi deficiency. Thus it is not only Spleen deficiency which causes defi-

cient bleeding, but also Spleen-Yang, Kidney-Yang or Kidney-Yin deficiency.

Blood stasis causes excessive blood loss during the period and also some blood loss before the proper period time. The blood is dark with dark clots.

Excessive menstrual bleeding often leads to complex pathological conditions as the excessive bleeding over many years itself becomes a pathogenic factor. For example, excessive bleeding from Blood-Heat may eventually lead to Blood and Yin deficiency. This, in turn, leads to Empty-Heat which, itself, becomes a further cause of bleeding. Excessive bleeding from Qi deficiency will eventually also cause Blood deficiency. As Blood is the mother of Qi, blood loss will further weaken Qi thus perpetuating the condition.

Differentiation and treatment

The treatment strategy of menorrhagia and metrorrhagia is largely based on the general principles outlined in the chapter on "Bleeding" (ch. 30). These were first advanced in the book "Discussion of Blood Syndromes" by Dr Tang Zong Hai (1884). As will be remembered, Dr Tang adopts a four-fold strategy, i.e.:

1. Harmonize Blood
2. Treat the Root-cause of bleeding
3. Astringe
4. Treat Qi.

The first of these treatment aims, in turn, is composed of four steps:

(a) Stop bleeding
(b) Eliminate stasis
(c) Calm Blood
(d) Nourish Blood.

Let us now analyse these four treatment aims to stop bleeding with particular reference to gynaecology.

1. HARMONIZE BLOOD

In a nutshell, the reasons for adopting the above

four steps to harmonize Blood in bleeding are as follows:

- *Stop bleeding:* to arrest blood loss
- *Eliminate stasis:* to prevent Blood from congealing
- *Calm Blood:* to prevent recurrence of bleeding
- *Nourish Blood:* to restore the Blood after the blood loss.

These four treatment aims to harmonize Blood are all the more important in gynaecology as Blood is obviously central to all women's gynaecological complaints.

(a) STOP BLEEDING

Examples of herbs that stop bleeding especially from the uterus are:

Pu Huang *Pollen Typhae*
Xian He Cao *Herba Agrimoniae pilosae*
Di Yu *Radix Sanguisorbae officinalis*
Qian Cao Gen *Radix Rubiae cordifoliae*
Ai Ye *Folium Artemisiae*

(b) ELIMINATE STASIS

Eliminating stasis is necessary to prevent Blood from congealing when stopping-bleeding herbs are used.

As the proper movement and circulation of Blood is extremely important to women's physiology and stopping-bleeding herbs may have a tendency to congeal Blood, herbs which simultaneously stop bleeding *and* move Blood are particularly useful. These are:

Pu Huang *Pollen Typhae*
San Qi *Radix Notoginseng*
Qian Cao Gen *Radix Rubiae cordifoliae*

Apart from these three, many other moving-Blood herbs are used in menorrhagia, for example Chuan Xiong *Radix Ligustici wallichii*, Yi Mu Cao *Herba Leonori heterophylli*, Hong Hua *Flos Carthami tinctorii* and Tao Ren *Semen Persicae*.

(c) CALM BLOOD

In bleeding, especially from Blood-Heat, the Blood is reckless and bursts out of the blood vessels. "Calming" Blood means that it will stay in the vessels.

Examples of calming-Blood herbs are:

Bai Shao *Radix Paeoniae albae*
Sheng Di Huang *Radix Rehmanniae glutinosae*
Han Lian Cao *Herba Ecliptae prostratae*
Mu Dan Pi *Cortex Moutan radicis*

(d) NOURISH BLOOD

Nourishing Blood is necessary to restore it to replace the Blood lost in bleeding.

The main herbs which nourish Blood are of course Dang Gui *Radix Angelicae sinensis* and Shu Di Huang *Radix Rehmanniae glutinosae praeparata*. E Jiao *Gelatinum Corii Asini* is also very important as it nourishes Blood *and* stops bleeding.

2. TREAT THE ROOT-CAUSE OF BLEEDING

The Root-cause of bleeding in menorrhagia is:

Blood-Heat
Blood Empty-Heat
Qi Deficiency
Stasis of Blood
Deficiency of Yang and Cold (this is quite rare).

(a) BLOOD-HEAT

Herbs are chosen from the clearing Heat and Draining Fire and especially the clearing Heat and cooling Blood categories:

(i) CLEAR HEAT AND DRAIN FIRE

The most important of all in this category is Shan Zhi Zi *Fructus Gardeniae jasminoidis* especially if charred. Other herbs that help to stop bleeding by clearing Heat are Shi Gao *Gypsum fibrosum*, Huang Qin *Radix Scutellariae baicalensis* and Huang Lian *Rhizoma Coptidis*.

(ii) CLEAR HEAT AND COOL BLOOD

Herbs from this category are the most important

ones to stop bleeding from Blood-Heat in gynae-cology. The three most important ones are Sheng Di Huang *Radix Rehmanniae glutinosae*, Chi Shao *Radix Paeoniae rubrae* and Mu Dan Pi *Cortex Moutan radicis*.

(b) EMPTY-HEAT

The two main herbs that stop bleeding by clear-ing Empty-Heat are Qing Hao *Herba Artemisiae apiaceae* and Han Lian Cao *Herba Ecliptae prostratae*. Han Lian Cao is the more important one in gynaecology and is often used in conjunc-tion with Nu Zhen Zi *Fructus Ligustri lucidi*.

(c) QI DEFICIENCY

Any Qi tonic will stop bleeding from Qi defi-ciency but the most effective one is Huang Qi *Radix Astragali membranacei*. The main formula to stop bleeding from Qi deficiency in gynaecology is Dang Gui Bu Xue Tang *Angelica Tonifying Blood Decoction* which is composed only of Huang Qi and Dang Gui *Radix Angelicae sinensis* in the proportions of 5:1.

(d) STASIS OF BLOOD

Any moving-Blood herb can stop bleeding from Blood stasis, but the best are those which move Blood *and* stop bleeding such as Pu Huang *Pollen Typhae*, San Qi *Radix Notoginseng* and Qian Cao Gen *Radix Rubiae cordifoliae*. Other herbs particularly used in gynaecology to move Blood are Yi Mu Cao *Herba Leonori heterophylli* and Hong Hua *Flos Carthami tinctorii* and Tao Ren *Semen Persicae* in combination.

(e) YANG DEFICIENCY AND COLD

Yang deficiency is quite a rare cause of bleeding in gynaecology and it is a type of Qi-deficiency bleeding. It occurs when Yang-Qi is deficient and fails to hold Blood. It is rare as internal Cold deriving from Yang deficiency has the tendency

to coagulate Blood. The main herb to stop bleed-ing from the uterus by warming is Ai Ye *Folium Artemisiae*.

3. ASTRINGE

The main astringent herbs used in this context in gynaecology are Shan Zhu Yu *Fructus Corni officinalis* and Bai Shao *Radix Paeoniae albae*.

One of the stopping-bleeding herbs used in gynaecology is also astringent: this is Di Yu *Radix Sanguisorbae officinalis*.

4. TREAT QI

Treating Qi includes *tonifying and firming Qi* for bleeding from Qi deficiency. The main herbs used in gynaecology for this purpose are Huang Qi *Radix Astragali membranacei*, Ren Shen *Radix Ginseng*, Fu Zi *Radix Aconiti carmichaeli praeparata* (if there is deficiency of Yang), Mu Li *Concha Ostreae* and Zhi Gan Cao *Radix Glycyrrhizae uralensis praeparata*.

Also included in this strategy of treatment is raising Qi for bleeding downwards from sinking of Spleen-Qi. The two herbs that do this are Chai Hu *Radix Bupleuri* and Sheng Ma *Rhizoma Cimicifugae*.

In gynaecology, excessive bleeding may occur not only from Spleen-Qi sinking but often also from Kidney-Qi sinking. In this case the main herb to use is Xu Duan *Radix Dipsaci*.

The patterns examined are:

EXCESS

Blood-Heat
Blood Empty-Heat
Stasis of Blood
Damp-Heat in the Uterus

DEFICIENCY

Spleen not holding Blood
Kidney-Yang Deficiency
Kidney-Yin Deficiency

EXCESS CONDITIONS

1. BLOOD-HEAT

CLINICAL MANIFESTATIONS

Flooding suddenly, often before the proper time, or trickling of blood for a long time after the end of the proper period, blood bright-red or dark-red, thirst, red face, agitation, feeling of heat, dark urine, constipation.
Tongue: Red with a yellow coating.
Pulse: Rapid-Overflowing.

TREATMENT PRINCIPLE

Clear Heat, cool Blood, stop bleeding.

ACUPUNCTURE

SP-4 Gongsun and P-6 Neiguan, L.I.-11 Quchi, SP-10 Xuehai, SP-8 Diji, SP-1 Yinbai, KI-5 Shuiquan, SP-6 Sanyinjiao. Reducing method, no moxa.

Explanation

- **SP-4** and **P-6** open the Penetrating Vessel which is the Sea of Blood and controls all the Blood Connecting channels. In bleeding, Blood bursts out of the Blood Connecting channels.
- **L.I.-11** and **SP-10** cool Blood and stop bleeding.
- **SP-8**, Accumulation point, stops bleeding from the uterus.
- **SP-1** is an empirical point to stop uterine bleeding.
- **KI-5** cools Blood in the uterus.
- **SP-6** cools and moves blood.

HERBAL TREATMENT

Prescription

QING RE ZHI BEN TANG
Clearing Heat and Stopping Flooding Decoction
Shan Zhi Zi *Fructus Gardeniae jasminoidis* 9 g

Huang Qin *Radix Scutellariae baicalensis* 9 g
Huang Bo *Cortex Phellodendri* 6 g
Sheng Di Huang *Radix Rehmanniae glutinosae* 24 g
Mu Dan Pi *Cortex Moutan radicis* 9 g
Di Yu *Radix Sanguisorbae officinalis* 12 g
Ce Bai Ye *Cacumen Biotae orientalis* 12 g
Chun Gen Bai Pi *Cortex Ailanthi altissimae* 12 g
Gui Ban *Plastrum Testudinis* 15 g
Bai Shao *Radix Paeoniae albae* 24 g

Explanation

- **Zhi Zi**, **Huang Qin** and **Huang Bo** clear Heat.
- **Sheng Di** and **Mu Dan Pi** cool Blood.
- **Di Yu**, **Ce Bai Ye** and **Chun Gen Bai Pi** stop bleeding. Di Yu also cools Blood.
- **Gui Ban** and **Bai Shao** nourish Yin and calm Blood.

We can analyse this prescription in the light of the four aims of treatment to stop bleeding outlined above.

1. **Harmonize blood**
   (a) *Stop bleeding*
       Ce Bai Ye, Di Yu and Chun Gen Bai Pi
   (b) *Eliminate stasis*
       Mu Dan Pi
   (c) *Calm Blood*
       Sheng Di and Bai Shao
   (d) *Nourish Blood*
       Bai Shao
2. **Treat the Root-cause**
   Zhi Zi, Huang Qin and Huang Bo to clear Heat and Sheng Di and Dan Pi to cool Blood
3. **Astringe**
   Di Yu
4. **Treat Qi**
   Gui Ban to firm Qi.

(i) Patent remedy

LONG DAN XIE GAN WAN
Gentiana Draining the Liver Pill
Long Dan Cao *Radix Gentianae scabrae*
Huang Qin *Radix Scutellariae baicalensis*
Shan Zhi Zi *Fructus Gardeniae jasminoidis*
Ze Xie *Rhizoma Alismatis orientalis*
Mu Tong *Caulis Akebiae*

Che Qian Zi *Semen Plantaginis*
Sheng Di Huang *Radix Rehmanniae glutinosae*
Dang Gui *Radix Angelicae sinensis*
Chai Hu *Radix Bupleuri*
Gan Cao *Radix Glycyrrhizae uralensis*

Explanation

This pill drains Liver-Fire and is suitable to stop bleeding when Blood-Heat is caused by Liver-Fire. However, it should be noted that it treats only the Root, i.e. Blood-Heat from Liver-Fire, not the Manifestation. In order to treat this as well, it could be combined with the remedy Yunnan Bai Yao (see below).

The tongue presentation appropriate to this remedy is a Red body with redder sides, possibly with red points on them, and a yellow coating.

(ii) Patent remedy

YUNNAN BAI YAO
Yunnan White Medicine
San Qi *Radix Notoginseng*
Other ingredients not disclosed

Explanation

This well-known remedy stops bleeding, and calms, moves and nourishes Blood. It can be used to treat the Manifestation, i.e. stop bleeding from any part of the body. It is particularly effective for menorrhagia. Each bottle contains a small red pill which can be taken in case of acute, profuse bleeding.

2. BLOOD EMPTY-HEAT

CLINICAL MANIFESTATIONS

Sudden flooding outside the time of proper period or trickling for many days after the period, blood fresh-red and rather watery, mental restlessness, feeling of heat in the evening, malar flush, scanty-dark urine, dry stools.
Tongue: Red without coating.
Pulse: Floating-Empty.

TREATMENT PRINCIPLE

Clear Empty-Heat, cool Blood, nourish Yin, stop bleeding.

ACUPUNCTURE

KI-2 Rangu, LIV-3 Taichong, KI-5 Shuiquan, SP-1 Yinbai, SP-6 Sanyinjiao, SP-8 Diji, Ren-4 Guanyuan, L.I.-11 Quchi, SP-10 Xuehai. Reducing method except on Ren-4 which should be reinforced.

Explanation

- **KI-2** and **LIV-3** cool Blood. KI-2 also clears Empty-Heat.
- **KI-5** cools Blood and stops bleeding from the uterus.
- **SP-1** stops uterine bleeding.
- **SP-6** cools Blood.
- **SP-8** stops uterine bleeding.
- **Ren-4** nourishes Yin.
- **L.I.-11** and **SP-10** cool Blood and stop bleeding.

HERBAL TREATMENT

BAO YIN JIAN Variation
Protecting Yin Decoction
Sheng Di Huang *Radix Rehmanniae glutinosae* 24 g
Shu Di Huang *Radix Rehmanniae glutinosae praeparata* 15 g
Bai Shao *Radix Paeoniae albae* 12 g
Shan Yao *Radix Dioscoreae oppositae* 12 g
Huang Qin *Radix Scutellariae baicalensis* 9 g
Huang Bo *Cortex Phellodendri* 9 g
Xu Duan *Radix Dipsaci* 6 g
Gan Cao *Radix Glycyrrhizae uralensis* 3 g
Han Lian Cao *Herba Ecliptae prostratae* 9 g
Qing Hao *Herba Artemisiae apiaceae* 6 g
Di Yu *Radix Sanguisorbae officinalis* 9 g
Qian Cao Gen *Radix Rubiae cordifoliae* 6 g

Explanation

The first eight herbs constitute the Bao Yin Jian.

- **Sheng Di**, **Shu Di**, **Bai Shao** and **Shan Yao** nourish Yin. Sheng Di and Bai Shao also calm Blood. Sheng Di also cools Blood and stops bleeding. Shu Di and Bai Shao also nourish Blood.
- **Huang Qin** and **Huang Bo** clear Heat.
- **Xu Duan** is added even though it tonifies Kidney-Yang to firm Qi, stop bleeding and strengthen the Kidneys.
- **Gan Cao** harmonizes.
- **Han Lian Cao** and **Qing Hao** clear Empty-Heat and stop bleeding.
- **Di Yu** cools Blood, stops bleeding and astringes.
- **Qian Cao Gen** cools Blood, stops bleeding and moves Blood.

Patent remedy

ZHI BO BA WEI WAN
Anemarrhena-Phellodendron Eight-Ingredient Pill
Shu Di Huang *Radix Rehmanniae glutinosae praeparata*
Shan Zhu Yu *Fructus Corni officinalis*
Shan Yao *Radix Dioscoreae oppositae*
Ze Xie *Rhizoma Alismatis orientalis*
Fu Ling *Sclerotium Poriae cocos*
Mu Dan Pi *Cortex Moutan radicis*
Zhi Mu *Radix Anemarrhenae asphodeloidis*
Huang Bo *Cortex Phellodendri*

Explanation

This pill nourishes Kidney-Yin and clears Empty-Heat. It is suitable to treat the Root in menorrhagia from Kidney Empty-Heat affecting the Blood.

The tongue presentation appropriate to this remedy is a Red body without coating except for a yellow coating on the root.

3. STASIS OF BLOOD
CLINICAL MANIFESTATIONS

Period is hesitant starting and stopping, period seems to stop then starts again with a flood, trickling for a long time after the period, pain before the period, blood dark with clots, abdominal distension, dark complexion.
Tongue: Bluish-Purple or Reddish-Purple.
Pulse: Choppy.

TREATMENT PRINCIPLE

Move Blood, eliminate stasis, stop bleeding.

ACUPUNCTURE

LIV-3 Taichong, T.B.-6 Zhigou, LIV-1 Dadun, SP-8 Diji, SP-4 Gongsun and P-6 Neiguan, ST-30 Qichong, SP-12 Chongmen, SP-10 Xuehai, SP-6 Sanyinjiao. Reducing method.

Explanation

- **LIV-3** stimulates the free flow of Liver-Qi and moves Blood.
- **T.B.-6** stimulates the free flow of Liver-Qi.
- **LIV-1** moves Liver-Blood and stops bleeding.
- **SP-8** stops uterine bleeding.
- **SP-4** and **P-6** open the Penetrating Vessel which controls the Sea of Blood and the Blood Connecting channels. The Penetrating Vessel's opening points also move Blood and subdue rebellious Qi.
- **ST-30** and **SP-12**, points on the Penetrating Vessel, move Blood. The *"chong"* in the name of both these points refers to *"Chong Mai"*, i.e. the Penetrating Vessel.
- **SP-10** moves Blood and stops bleeding.
- **SP-6** moves Blood.

HERBAL TREATMENT
Prescription

TAO HONG SI WU TANG and SHI XIAO SAN Variation
Persica-Carthamus Four Substances Decoction and Breaking into a Smile Powder
Dang Gui *Radix Angelicae sinensis* 9 g
Chuan Xiong *Radix Ligustici wallichii* 6 g
Shu Di Huang *Radix Rehmanniae glutinosae praeparata* 12 g

Bai Shao *Radix Paeoniae albae* 9 g
Tao Ren *Semen Persicae* 6 g
Hong Hua *Flos Carthami tinctorii* 6 g
Pu Huang *Pollen Typhae* 9 g
Wu Ling Zhi *Excrementum Trogopteri* 9 g
Qian Cao Gen *Radix Rubiae cordifoliae* 6 g
San Qi *Radix Notoginseng* 6 g

Explanation

The first six herbs constitute the Tao Hong Si Wu Tang which nourishes and moves Blood.

- **Pu Huang** and **Wu Ling Zhi** constitute the Shi Xiao San which moves Blood and stops pain. Pu Huang also stops bleeding.
- **Qian Cao Gen** and **San Qi** are added because they move Blood *and* stop bleeding.

Variations

- If the stasis of Blood derives from Cold in the uterus (tongue Bluish-Purple) add Ai Ye *Folium Artemisiae* and Fu Zi *Radix Aconiti carmichaeli praeparata*.
- If the stasis of Blood derives from Heat (tongue Reddish-Purple) add Sheng Di Huang *Radix Rehmanniae glutinosae*, Mu Dan Pi *Cortex Moutan radicis* and Di Yu *Radix Sanguisorbae officinalis*.

(i) Patent remedy

DANG GUI PIAN
Angelica Tablet
Dang Gui *Radix Angelicae sinensis*

Explanation

This tablet nourishes and moves Blood and is suitable to treat menorrhagia from Blood stasis only in fairly mild cases.

The tongue presentation appropriate to this remedy is a body which is only slightly Purple on the sides.

(ii) Patent remedy

AN TAI WAN
Calming the Foetus Pill

Dang Gui *Radix Angelicae sinensis*
Bai Shao *Radix Paeoniae albae*
Huang Qin *Radix Scutellariae baicalensis*
Bai Zhu *Rhizoma Atractylodis macrocephalae*
Chuan Xiong *Radix Ligustici wallichii*

Explanation

This remedy nourishes and moves Blood. Although it is primarily used for threatened miscarriage, it can also be used for menorrhagia from stasis of Blood, but only for mild cases.

(iii) Patent remedy

JIN GU DIE SHANG WAN
Muscle and Bone Traumatic Injury Pill
San Qi *Radix Notoginseng*
Xue Jie *Sanguis Draconis*
Dang Gui *Radix Angelicae sinensis*
Ru Xiang *Gummi Olibanum*
Mo Yao *Myrrha*
Hong Hua *Flos Carthami tinctorii*

Explanation

This remedy moves Blood and eliminates stasis. Although it is primarily used for traumatic injuries, it can be used to treat menorrhagia from Blood stasis. It treats not only the Root, i.e. stasis of Blood, but also the Manifestation as it contains San Qi which simultaneously moves Blood and stops bleeding.

The tongue presentation appropriate to this remedy is a Reddish-Purple body.

(iv) Patent remedy

YUNNAN BAI YAO
Yunnan White Medicine
San Qi *Radix Notoginseng*

Explanation

This remedy nourishes, calms, cools and moves Blood and stops bleeding. It is suitable to treat menorrhagia from Blood stasis as it both moves Blood and stops bleeding.

(v) Patent remedy

TONG JING WAN

Penetrating Menses Pill
E Zhu *Rhizoma Curcumae zedoariae*
San Leng *Rhizoma Sparganii*
Chi Shao *Radix Paeoniae rubrae*
Hong Hua *Flos Carthami tinctorii*
Chuan Xiong *Radix Ligustici wallichii*
Dang Gui *Radix Angelicae sinensis*
Dan Shen *Radix Salviae miltiorrhizae*

Explanation

This remedy strongly moves Blood and eliminates stasis. It is suitable for menorrhagia from
Blood stasis to treat the Root only. As it does not
treat the Manifestation, it should be combined
with another remedy to stop bleeding, such as
Yunnan Bai Yao.

The tongue presentation appropriate to this
remedy is a very Purple tongue body with
purple spots.

4. DAMP-HEAT IN THE UTERUS

CLINICAL MANIFESTATIONS

Menstrual bleeding could be either scanty or
abundant, bleeding on mid-cycle, blood sticky,
yellow-brownish discharge appearing before
bleeding starts, no clots, feeling of heaviness,
dragging sensation in the lower abdomen, burning pain in the lower abdomen, pain in the
joints, a feeling of oppression of the chest, irritability, scanty-dark urine, burning on urination,
vaginal discharge.
Tongue: Sticky-yellow coating.
Pulse: Slippery.

TREATMENT PRINCIPLE

Clear Heat, resolve Dampness, cool Blood, stop
bleeding.

ACUPUNCTURE

SP-4 Gongsun and P-6 Neiguan, L.I.-11 Quchi,
SP-10 Xuehai, SP-8 Diji, SP-1 Yinbai, KI-5
Shuiquan, SP-6 Sanyinjiao, SP-9 Yinlingquan,
Ren-3 Zhongji, BL-22 Sanjiaoshu, BL-32 Ciliao.
Reducing method, no moxa.

Explanation

- **SP-4** and **P-6** open the Penetrating Vessel
  which is the Sea of Blood and controls all the
  Blood Connecting channels. In bleeding,
  Blood bursts out of the Blood Connecting
  channels.
- **L.I.-11** and **SP-10** cool Blood and stop
  bleeding.
- **SP-8**, Accumulation point, stops bleeding
  from the uterus.
- **SP-1** is an empirical point to stop uterine
  bleeding.
- **KI-5** cools Blood in the uterus and stops
  uterine bleeding.
- **SP-6** cools and moves Blood.
- **SP-9** and **Ren-3** resolve Damp-Heat in the
  Lower Burner.
- **BL-22** and **BL-32** promote the transformation
  of fluids and resolve Damp-Heat from the
  uterus.

HERBAL TREATMENT

Prescription

QING RE LI SHI TANG Variation
Clearing Heat and Resolving Dampness Decoction
Bi Xie *Rhizoma Dioscoreae hypoglaucae* 12 g
Qu Mai *Herba Dianthi* 12 g
Shan Zhi Zi *Fructus Gardeniae jasminoidis*
(charred) 9 g
Huang Qin *Radix Scutellariae baicalensis* 9 g
Huang Lian *Rhizoma Coptidis* 6 g
Zhi Mu *Radix Anemarrhenae asphodeloidis* 9 g
Mu Dan Pi *Cortex Moutan radicis* 6 g
Ou Jie *Nodus Nelumbinis nuciferae rhizomatis* 15 g
Xian He Cao *Herba Agrimoniae pilosae* 12 g

Explanation

- **Bi Xie** and **Qu Mai** drain Dampness via
  urination.
- **Zhi Zi**, **Huang Qin** and **Huang Lian** drain
  Damp-Heat. Zhi Zi, especially charred, also
  stops bleeding.

- **Zhi Mu** clears Heat.
- **Mu Dan Pi** cools Blood and stops bleeding.
- **Ou Jie**, astringent, helps to stop bleeding.
- **Xian He Cao**, substituted for Bai Mao Gen from the original prescription, stops uterine bleeding.

DEFICIENCY CONDITIONS

1. SPLEEN NOT HOLDING BLOOD

CLINICAL MANIFESTATIONS

Flooding at the beginning of the period which then stops and goes on with a trickle for a long time after the period proper, pale and watery blood, pale face, tiredness, slight dizziness, no appetite, loose stools.
Tongue: Pale, teeth-marks.
Pulse: Weak.

TREATMENT PRINCIPLE

Tonify Qi, strengthen the Spleen, nourish Blood, stop bleeding.

ACUPUNCTURE

Ren-6 Qihai, Ren-12 Zhongwan, ST-36 Zusanli, SP-6 Sanyinjiao, BL-20 Pishu, BL-21 Weishu, Du-20 Baihui. Reinforcing method, moxa may be used.

Explanation

- **Ren-6** tonifies Qi and stops bleeding from Qi sinking.
- **Ren-12**, **ST-36**, **SP-6**, **BL-20**, and **BL-21** tonify Spleen-Qi.
- **Du-20** raises Qi and stops bleeding from sinking Qi.

HERBAL TREATMENT

(a) Prescription

GU BEN ZHI BEN TANG

Consolidating the Root and Stopping Menorrhagia Decoction
Huang Qi *Radix Astragali membranacei* 15 g
Ren Shen *Radix Ginseng* 12 g
Bai Zhu *Rhizoma Atractylodis macrocephalae* 18 g
Shu Di Huang *Radix Rehmanniae glutinosae praeparata* 9 g
Dang Gui *Radix Angelicae sinensis* 6 g
Pao Jiang *Rhizoma Zingiberis officinalis recens* (fried) 6 g

Explanation

- **Huang Qi**, **Ren Shen** and **Bai Zhu** tonify and raise Qi.
- **Shu Di** and **Dang Gui** nourish Blood and firm Qi. They are also included so that the formula enters the Blood portion to stop bleeding.
- **Pao Jiang** warms the channels and stops bleeding.

(b) Prescription

DANG GUI BU XUE TANG
Angelica Tonifying Blood Decoction
Huang Qi *Radix Astragali membranacei* 30 g
Dang Gui *Radix Angelicae sinensis* 6 g

Explanation

This is a very simple formula to stop bleeding from Qi deficiency which may be added to other formulae.

- **Huang Qi** tonifies and raises Qi.
- **Dang Gui** enters the Blood portion and directs the formula to the Blood so that it stops bleeding from Qi deficiency.

(c) Prescription

GUI PI TANG
Tonifying the Spleen Decoction
Ren Shen *Radix Ginseng* 6 g or **Dang Shen** *Radix Codonopsis pilosulae* 12 g
Huang Qi *Radix Astragali membranacei* 15 g
Bai Zhu *Rhizoma Atractylodis macrocephalae* 12 g
Dang Gui *Radix Angelicae sinensis* 6 g
Fu Shen *Sclerotium Poriae cocos pararadicis* 9 g

Suan Zao Ren *Semen Ziziphi spinosae* 9 g
Long Yan Rou *Arillus Euphoriae longanae* 12 g
Yuan Zhi *Radix Polygalae tenuifoliae* 9 g
Mu Xiang *Radix Saussureae* 3 g
Zhi Gan Cao *Radix Glycyrrhizae uralensis praeparata* 4 g
Sheng Jiang *Rhizoma Zingiberis officinalis recens* 3 slices
Hong Zao *Fructus Ziziphi jujubae* 5 dates

Explanation

This formula, which has already been explained in chapters 9 and 12, is very frequently used to stop bleeding from Qi deficiency. It is selected in preference to the previous two when there is also a deficiency of Heart-Blood causing insomnia, anxiety and forgetfulness.

Patent remedy

GUI PI WAN
Tonifying the Spleen Pill
Dang Shen *Radix Codonopsis pilosulae*
Huang Qi *Radix Astragali membranacei*
Bai Zhu *Rhizoma Atractylodis macrocephalae*
Fu Shen *Sclerotium Poriae cocos pararadicis*
Suan Zao Ren *Semen Ziziphi spinosae*
Yuan Zhi *Radix Polygalae tenuifoliae*
Dang Gui *Radix Angelicae sinensis*
Mu Xiang *Radix Saussureae*
Gan Cao *Radix Glycyrrhizae uralensis*
Long Yan Rou *Arillus Euphoriae longanae*

Explanation

This remedy tonifies Spleen-Qi and Spleen-Blood and, as it contains herbs which enter the Blood portion, it is specific to bolster the Spleen's function of holding Blood. It is therefore very frequently used for menorrhagia from Spleen-Qi not holding Blood.

The tongue presentation appropriate to this remedy is a Pale and Thin body.

2. KIDNEY-YANG DEFICIENCY
CLINICAL MANIFESTATIONS

Prolonged bleeding with a trickle for a long time after the proper period, periods coming late, blood pale, feeling cold, sore back, cold limbs, pale complexion, weak knees, pale urine.
Tongue: Pale and Swollen.
Pulse: Deep and Weak.

TREATMENT PRINCIPLE

Tonify and warm the Kidneys, consolidate the Penetrating Vessel, stop bleeding.

ACUPUNCTURE

Ren-6 Qihai, BL-23 Shenshu, Ren-4 Guanyuan, ST-30 Qichong, KI-7 Fuliu, ST-36 Zusanli, SP-6 Sanyinjiao. Reinforcing method, moxa must be used.

A prescription which is specific to raise Qi and consolidate the Penetrating Vessel to hold Blood is: SP-1 Yinbai with moxa cones, BL-20 Pishu, SP-6 Sanyinjiao, Du-20 Baihui, Ren-6 Qihai and Ren-4 Guanyuan, all with reinforcing method.

Explanation

- **Ren-6** tonifies Qi and stops bleeding.
- **BL-23** and **Ren-4**, with moxa, tonify and warm Kidney-Yang and consolidate the Penetrating Vessel.
- **ST-30**, with moxa, consolidates the Penetrating Vessel.
- **KI-7** tonifies Kidney-Yang.
- **ST-36** and **SP-6** tonify Qi and Blood.

HERBAL TREATMENT
Prescription

YOU GUI WAN
Restoring the Right [Kidney] Pill
Fu Zi *Radix Aconiti carmichaeli praeparata* 3 g
Rou Gui *Cortex Cinnamomi cassiae* 3 g
Du Zhong *Cortex Eucommiae ulmoidis* 6 g
Shan Zhu Yu *Fructus Corni officinalis* 4.5 g
Tu Si Zi *Semen Cuscutae* 6 g
Lu Jiao Jiao *Colla Cornu Cervi* 6 g
Shu Di Huang *Radix Rehmanniae glutinosae praeparata* 12 g

Shan Yao *Radix Dioscoreae oppositae* 6 g
Gou Qi Zi *Fructus Lycii chinensis* 6 g
Dang Gui *Radix Angelicae sinensis* 4.5 g

Explanation

This formula, which has already been explained in chapters 1 and 25, tonifies and warms Kidney-Yang. It is suitable to stop bleeding as Fu Zi can stop bleeding from Yang deficiency and Cold, Shan Zhu Yu is astringent and will help to stop bleeding, Lu Jiao Jiao will nourish and calm Blood and Dang Gui enters the Blood portion to direct the formula to the Blood and stop bleeding.

Variations

– To enhance the stopping-bleeding effect, add Xian He Cao *Herba Agrimoniae pilosae*.

Patent remedy

BU XUE TIAO JING PIAN
Tonifying Blood and Regulating Menses Tablet
Xiang Fu *Rhizoma Cyperi rotundi*
Jin Ying Zi *Fructus Rosae laevigatae*
Ji Xue Teng *Caulis Millettiae seu Caulis Spatholobi*
Sang Ji Sheng *Ramus Loranthi*
Shang Cang Zi *Fructus Litseae*
Gang Nian *Herba Rhodomyrti*
Qian Jin Ba *Radix Moghaniae*
Yi Mu Cao *Herba Leonori heterophylli*
Gao Liang Jiang *Rhizoma Alpiniae officinari*
Wu Hua Guo Gen *Radix Fici*
Ai Ye *Folium Artemisiae*
Ji Cai *Herba Houttuyniae cordatae*
Dang Shen *Radix Codonopsis pilosulae*
Bai Zhu *Rhizoma Atractylodis macrocephalae*
Zhi Gan Cao *Radix Glycyrrhizae uralensis praeparata*
E Jiao *Gelatinum Corii Asini*
Rou Gui *Cortex Cinnamomi cassiae*
Bai Bei Ye *Herba Baipo*

Explanation

This remedy nourishes Blood, tonifies Kidney-Yang and moves Qi and Blood. It is suitable to treat menorrhagia occurring against a background of Blood and Kidney-Yang deficiency.

The tongue presentation appropriate to this remedy is a Pale body.

Case history

A 50-year-old woman had been suffering from heavy menstrual bleeding for 18 months. The menstrual blood was bright-red with small dark clots. Her period was very painful and she felt very cold during it. Her uterus was prolapsed. She also suffered from back-ache, dizziness, exhaustion, poor memory and frequency of urination. Her tongue was slightly Pale and Swollen and her pulse was Deep and Weak, particularly so on both Rear positions.

Diagnosis
This is a rather complex condition. There is definitely a deficiency of Spleen- and Kidney-Yang: this is evident from the prolapse of the uterus (Spleen-Qi sinking), the cold feeling, back-ache, dizziness, poor memory, Deep-Weak pulse and Pale tongue. The heavy menstrual bleeding is caused by such deficient Spleen- and Kidney-Qi not holding Blood. However, the painful period and small dark clots indicate that there is also internal Cold in the uterus. This presumably originated from the Kidney-Yang deficiency.

Treatment principle
This patient was being treated with acupuncture by another practitioner who referred her to me for herbal treatment. The treatment principle adopted was to scatter Cold and warm the uterus and tonify and warm Spleen- and Kidney-Yang.

Herbal treatment
One could have chosen the formula indicated above, i.e. You Gui Wan *Restoring the Right [Kidney] Pill* to tonify and warm Kidney-Yang. However, the condition is characterized by both Deficiency (of Spleen- and Kidney-Yang) and Excess (Cold in the uterus), I decided to place the emphasis on expelling Cold first. I often find in practice that it is preferable to eliminate the Excess before tonifying the Deficiency. I therefore selected a variation of Ai Fu Nuan Gong Wan *Artemisia Cyperus Warming the Uterus Pill* (see chapter 31):

Ai Ye *Folium Artemisiae* 6 g
Wu Zhu Yu *Fructus Evodiae rutaecarpae* 4.5 g
Rou Gui *Cortex Cinnamomi cassiae* 3 g
Xiang Fu *Rhizoma Cyperi rotundi* 6 g
Dang Gui *Radix Angelicae sinensis* 9 g
Chuan Xiong *Radix Ligustici wallichii* 6 g
Bai Shao *Radix Paeoniae albae* 9 g
Huang Qi *Radix Astragali membranacei* 9 g
Sheng Di Huang *Radix Rehmanniae glutinosae* 9 g

Xu Duan *Radix Dipsaci* 6 g
Xian He Cao *Herba Agrimoniae pilosae* 6 g
Shu Di Huang *Radix Rehmanniae glutinosae praeparata* 9 g
Shan Zhu Yu *Fructus Corni officinalis* 4 g
Chai Hu *Radix Bupleuri* 3 g
Sheng Ma *Rhizoma Cimicifugae* 3 g

Explanation
- The first ten herbs constitute the root formula which scatters Cold from the uterus, nourishes Blood and tonifies Kidney-Yang.
- **Xian He Cao** was added to stop bleeding.
- **Shu Di Huang** was added to strengthen the Kidneys.
- **Shan Zhu Yu** was added to nourish the Liver and Kidneys and also as an astringent to help to stop bleeding.
- **Chai Hu** and **Sheng Ma** were added to raise sinking Spleen-Qi.

As the main problem was the heavy menstrual bleeding, the formula was modified to stop bleeding according to the four aims of treatment outlined in the "Discussion on Blood Syndromes" (ch. 30):

1. Harmonize Blood
   (a) Stop bleeding: Xian He Cao
   (b) Eliminate stasis: Chuan Xiong
   (c) Calm Blood: Bai Shao, Sheng Di Huang
   (d) Nourish Blood: Dang Gui, Shu Di Huang
2. Treat the Root-cause of bleeding (Yang deficiency): Xu Duan, Rou Gui
3. Astringe: Shan Zhu Yu
4. Treat Qi (raise Spleen-Qi): Huang Qi, Chai Hu, Sheng Ma.

This patient was treated with this formula (with slight variations) for 6 months, after which the period became much lighter and less painful.

Case history

A 29-year-old woman had been suffering from constant uterine bleeding for 1 year. She bled every day, with the bleeding getting heavier around the period at which time the blood became dark with clots and she experienced period pain. During the other time of the month the bleeding was like a daily trickle. Her other symptoms and signs included exhaustion, back-ache, dizziness, tinnitus, slight night-sweating, feeling very cold, nocturia, blurred vision, numbness of the limbs and poor memory.

Her tongue was Pale and with teethmarks. Her pulse was Choppy and Weak on the right-Rear and left-Middle position.

Diagnosis
This is a clear condition of deficiency of Kidneys and

Liver with a secondary stasis of Liver-Blood. The primary deficiency is that of Kidney-Yang (as indicated by the Pale tongue) even though there is some overlapping Kidney-Yin deficiency (night-sweating): in women, an overlap of Kidney-Yang and Kidney-Yin deficiency is very common.

Treatment principle
The treatment principle adopted was to tonify the Kidneys and nourish and move Liver-Blood. She was treated with both acupuncture and herbs.

Acupuncture
The acupuncture treatment included a selection of the following points:

- **LU-7** Lieque on the right and **KI-6** Zhaohai on the left to open and regulate the Directing Vessel.
- **ST-36** Zusanli and **SP-6** Sanyinjiao to tonify Qi in general.
- **SP-8** Diji to stop bleeding.
- **Ren-4** Guanyuan, **BL-23** Shenshu and **KI-3** Taixi to nourish the Kidneys.

Herbal treatment
The herbal formula used was a variation of Gui Pi Tang *Tonifying the Spleen Decoction*:

Huang Qi *Radix Astragali membranacei* 9 g
Bai Zhu *Rhizoma Atractylodis macrocephalae* 6 g
Dang Shen *Radix Codonopsis pilosulae* 6 g
Fu Ling *Sclerotium Poriae cocos* 6 g
Long Yan Rou *Arillus Euphoriae longanae* 6 g
Suan Zao Ren *Semen Ziziphi spinosae* 3 g
Mu Xiang *Radix Saussureae* 3 g
Dang Gui *Radix Angelicae sinensis* 9 g
Yi Mu Cao *Herba Leonori heterophylli* 4 g
Sheng Di Huang *Radix Rehmanniae glutinosae* 6 g
Bai Shao *Radix Paeoniae albae* 6 g
Xian He Cao *Herba Agrimoniae pilosae* 6 g
Ai Ye *Folium Artemisiae* 4 g
Xu Duan *Radix Dipsaci* 6 g
Chi Shao *Radix Paeoniae rubrae* 4 g
Hong Zao *Fructus Ziziphi jujubae* 3 dates

Explanation
The prescription can be explained in the light of the four aims of treatment outlined above:

1. **Harmonize Blood**
   (a) *Nourish Blood*
       Dang Gui, Sheng Di Huang
   (b) *Move Blood*
       Yi Mu Cao, Chi Shao
   (c) *Calm Blood*
       Sheng Di Huang, Bai Shao
   (d) *Stop bleeding*
       Xian He Cao, Ai Ye
2. **Treat the Root** (deficiency of Kidneys and Liver)
   Sheng Di Huang, Dang Gui, Xu Duan
3. **Astringe**
   Suan Zao Ren

4. **Treat Qi**
Dang Shen, Huang Qi, Bai Zhu to tonify and raise Qi.

The bleeding stopped almost immediately for 20 days out of a 28-day cycle; during the other 8 days the amount of bleeding was much decreased. After four months of treatment her periods were restored to complete normality.

3. KIDNEY-YIN DEFICIENCY

CLINICAL MANIFESTATIONS

Trickling of blood after the period proper, late cycle, fresh-red and watery blood, dizziness, tinnitus, weak knees, feeling of heat in the evening, night-sweating, hot flushes, malar flush, mental restlessness.
Tongue: Red without coating.
Pulse: Floating-Empty.

This pattern is more common in women towards the beginning of the menopause.

TREATMENT PRINCIPLE

Nourish Yin, strengthen the Kidneys, stop bleeding.

ACUPUNCTURE

Ren-6 Qihai, BL-23 Shenshu, Ren-4 Guanyuan, KI-3 Taixi, ST-36 Zusanli, SP-6 Sanyinjiao, KI-2 Rangu. Reinforcing method on all points except KI-2 which should be needled with even method. No moxa.

Explanation

– **Ren-6** tonifies Qi and stops bleeding.
– **BL-23** and **Ren-4** tonify the Kidneys and consolidate the Penetrating Vessel.
– **KI-3** tonifies the Kidneys.
– **ST-36** and **SP-6** tonify Qi and Blood.
– **KI-2** clears Empty-Heat from the Kidneys.

HERBAL TREATMENT

(a) Prescription

ZUO GUI YIN Variation

Restoring the Left [Kidney] Pill
Shu Di Huang *Radix Rehmanniae glutinosae praeparata* 15 g
Shan Yao *Radix Dioscoreae oppositae* 9 g
Shan Zhu Yu *Fructus Corni officinalis* 9 g
Gou Qi Zi *Fructus Lycii chinensis* 9 g
Tu Si Zi *Semen Cuscutae* 9 g
Lu Jiao Jiao *Colla Cornu Cervi* 9 g
Gui Ban Jiao *Colla Plastri Testudinis* 9 g
Nu Zhen Zi *Fructus Ligustri lucidi* 9 g
Han Lian Cao *Herba Ecliptae prostratae* 9 g

Explanation

This formula, already explained in chapter 13, nourishes Kidney-Yin.

– **Niu Xi** has been removed from the original prescription as it pulls Qi downwards and is therefore not suitable for uterine bleeding.
– **Nu Zhen Zi** and **Han Lian Cao** nourish Kidney-Yin and clear Empty-Heat. Han Lian Cao also stops bleeding.

Other herbs in the original prescription make it suitable to stop bleeding: Shan Zhu Yu is astringent and will help to stop bleeding and Lu Jiao Jiao and Gui Ban Jiao calm Blood and stop bleeding.

(b) Prescription

LIANG DI TANG and ER ZHI WAN
Two "Di" Decoction and *Two Solstices Pill*
Sheng Di Huang *Radix Rehmanniae glutinosae* 18 g
Di Gu Pi *Cortex Lycii chinensis radicis* 9 g
Xuan Shen *Radix Scrophulariae ningpoensis* 12 g
Mai Men Dong *Tuber Ophiopogonis japonici* 9 g
Bai Shao *Radix Paeoniae albae* 12 g
E Jiao *Gelatinum Corii Asini* 9 g
Nu Zhen Zi *Fructus Ligustri lucidi* 12 g
Han Lian Cao *Herba Ecliptae prostratae* 9 g

Explanation

These two formulae are selected if the symptoms of Empty-Heat are pronounced, i.e. feeling of heat in the evening, malar flush, hot flushes and Red tongue without any coating.

The first six herbs constitute the Liang Di Tang and the last two the Er Zhi Wan.

- **Sheng Di Huang** and **Di Gu Pi** cool Blood, clear Empty-Heat and nourish Yin. They both also stop bleeding. Sheng Di also calms Blood.
- **Xuan Shen** and **Mai Dong** help the first two herbs to nourish Yin.
- **Bai Shao** and **E Jiao** nourish Blood, which helps to nourish Yin. Bai Shao is also astringent and calms Blood.
- **Nu Zhen Zi** and **Han Lian Cao** nourish Yin and clear Empty-Heat. Han Lian Cao also stops bleeding.

Patent remedy

YONG SHENG HE E JIAO
Eternally Vigorous Combination Donkey Skin Glue
E Jiao *Gelatinum Corii Asini*
Dang Gui *Radix Angelicae sinensis*
Huang Qi *Radix Astragali membranacei*
Mai Men Dong *Tuber Ophiopogonis japonici*
Fu Ling *Sclerotium Poriae cocos*
Shu Di Huang *Radix Rehmanniae glutinosae prae-parata*
Rice wine
Sugar
Sesame oil

Explanation

This remedy tonifies the Kidneys and nourishes Blood. It is suitable to treat menorrhagia from Kidney-Yang deficiency as it contains herbs which stop bleeding, such as E Jiao.

The tongue presentation appropriate to this remedy is a Pale body.

Case history

A 39-year-old woman had been suffering from very heavy periods for 8 years, following the birth of her third child. The periods started with a flood, lasted up to 10 days and the blood was bright-red. There was no pain and the cycle was regular. She felt always very tired and she often sweated at night, especially during her periods. She felt easily thirsty. She also had a lower back-ache and occasionally tinnitus.

Her tongue was slightly Red, cracked and without coating on the root. Her pulse was Rapid and Overflowing but Empty.

Diagnosis

This is a complex condition. The excessive menstrual bleeding is caused by three factors: deficient Spleen-Qi and Kidney-Yin failing to hold Blood, and Empty-Heat agitating Blood. The Spleen-Qi deficiency is evidenced by the tiredness and by the bleeding in a sudden flood (bleeding from Kidney-Yin deficiency only would be a trickle at the end of the period). The Kidney-Yin deficiency is evident from the back-ache, tinnitus, thirst and night-sweating. The Empty-Heat is evident from the Red colour of the tongue without coating and the Rapid and Overflowing-Empty pulse.

Treatment principle

The treatment principle adopted was to tonify Spleen-Qi, nourish Kidney-Yin, clear Empty-Heat and stop bleeding. This patient was treated only with acupuncture.

Acupuncture

The points used (with reinforcing method except for those to clear Empty-Heat which were needled with even method) were selected from the following:

- **LU-7** Lieque and **KI-6** Zhaohai to regulate the Directing Vessel and tonify the uterus.
- **Ren-6** Qihai, **Ren-12** Zhongwan, **ST-36** Zusanli and **SP-6** Sanyinjiao to tonify Spleen-Qi.
- **Du-20** Baihui to raise Qi in order to hold Blood.
- **KI-3** Taixi to nourish Kidney-Yin.
- **KI-2** Rangu to clear Empty-Heat.
- **SP-8** Diji, Accumulation point, to stop uterine bleeding.
- **BL-20** Pishu and **BL-23** Shenshu to tonify Spleen and Kidneys.

This patient was treated once a week for the 2 weeks after her period and twice a week for the two weeks before her period. The period started to decrease in amount after two months and after 6 months it went back to normal.

Prognosis and prevention

Both acupuncture and herbs give good results in menorrhagia and metrorrhagia. Treatment with herbs is slightly more successful especially for the Deficiency-type conditions.

The most difficult to treat is that from Kidney-Yin deficiency and the easiest is that from Blood-Heat.

Obviously, if the uterine bleeding has an organic cause such as carcinoma of the cervix or uterus, myoma or endometrial polyp, results will be much worse (see below). In the case of carcinoma of the cervix or uterus the prognosis is the worst as, by the time bleeding appears, the carcinoma is quite advanced. Bleeding from myomas or polyps can be stopped but it will necessarily take much longer than in functional bleeding.

As for prevention, any woman who has a tendency to, or has been cured of, menorrhagia should take certain precautions. She should avoid overwork as this depletes the Kidneys and may lead to bleeding from Kidney-Qi not holding Blood, or from Kidney Empty-Heat agitating the Blood.

She should avoid excessive sexual activity as this also depletes the Kidneys and may lead to menorrhagia in one of the two ways described above. She should abstain from spicy foods and alcohol (except occasionally) as these can create Blood-Heat which very easily causes bleeding.

Finally, she should avoid emotional stress (if at all possible) as this may lead to Fire and therefore bleeding from Blood-Heat.

Western differentiation

Menorrhagia and metrorrhagia may be either functional or organic. Practitioners of Chinese medicine need to be particularly aware of the possible organic causes of uterine bleeding, which are:

Carcinoma of the cervix
Endometriosis
Carcinoma of the uterus
Myomas
Endometrial polyps

CARCINOMA OF THE CERVIX

Carcinoma of the cervix is more common in women over 30. Bleeding is one of the first symptoms and it typically occurs in between periods. Bleeding may also be noticed after coitus, severe exertion or straining for defecation. The contact bleeding after coitus or pelvic examination is especially characteristic. Unfortunately,

when bleeding does occur, the disease is already quite advanced.

Other symptoms may include a blood-tinged vaginal discharge and bladder irritability. The three symptoms and signs of sacral pain, unilateral lymphoedema and unilateral ureteral obstruction indicate a very advanced stage of the condition.

ENDOMETRIOSIS

Endometriosis has already been described in the chapter on "Dysmenorrhoea" (ch. 31). Symptoms include painful periods with the pain radiating to the rectum or perineum, menorrhagia and dyspareunia (pain on intercourse).

CARCINOMA OF THE UTERUS

Carcinoma of the uterus usually occurs after menopause with roughly 75% of women being post-menopausal, 15% perimenopausal and 10% still menstruating. This disease seems to be more common in women who have no children or only one child.

Abnormal uterine bleeding is the most important symptom of this disease often with a bloody vaginal discharge. In fact, this type of discharge and bleeding in a woman after the menopause should always be investigated and diagnosed by a gynaecologist and *never* treated as just functional bleeding.

MYOMAS

Myomas are the most common cause of prolonged or excessive menstrual bleeding. They are usually painless and a mass would only be felt if the myoma is quite large.

ENDOMETRIAL POLYPS

Endometrial polyps cause bleeding only when they protrude into the cervical canal. The bleeding usually occurs in between periods and is scanty.

Pre-menstrual tension 33

行
经
前
症
状

The term pre-menstrual tension broadly describes some emotional and physical symptoms occurring before the periods. These may include depression, sadness, irritability, crying, propensity to outbursts of anger, clumsiness, distension of abdomen and breasts, and insomnia. These symptoms can vary in intensity from very mild to extremely serious when a woman can actually injure a member of her family or some other person. They can also vary in duration ranging from one day to two weeks before the period. Rarely, these symptoms may be experienced *after* the period.

Aetiology and pathology

1. EMOTIONAL STRAIN

Emotional strain is the most important aetiological factor for pre-menstrual tension. Anger, frustration, and resentment may all, in the long run, cause stagnation of Liver-Qi which is a major cause of pre-menstrual tension.

2. DIET

Excessive consumption of dairy products and greasy foods leads to the formation of Phlegm. If stagnation of Liver-Qi leads to Fire, this combines with Phlegm to form Phlegm-Fire which accumulates in the chest and breasts and obstructs the Mind's orifices. This results in breast distension, a feeling of oppression in the chest and severe mental changes.

3. OVERWORK AND EXCESSIVE SEXUAL ACTIVITY

Overwork and excessive sexual activity weaken Kidney- and Liver-Yin and when these are deficient they can cause stagnation of Liver-Qi.

Thus the most important thing to establish is whether the pre-menstrual tension derives from a Full or Empty condition. If the stagnation of Liver-Qi arises independently from emotional problems it is a purely Full condition. In this case the pulse will be Wiry, either in all positions or only on the left. If it is secondary to a deficiency of Liver-Blood, Liver-Yin or Liver- and Kidney-Yin, the condition is primarily Empty. In such a case the pulse will be Fine and Weak at least on one side.

In women, Liver-Qi stagnation often derives from Liver-Blood or Liver-Yin deficiency. In fact, Liver-Qi and Liver-Blood-Yin are the Yang and Yin aspects of the Liver. Liver-Blood and Liver-Yin are the root and the material basis of Liver-Qi. If Liver-Blood/Yin are deficient, Liver-Qi is deprived of its root and stagnates.

If it is due to Phlegm-Fire, pre-menstrual tension is of the Full type.

Differentiation and treatment

The patterns examined are:

EXCESS

Liver-Qi stagnation
Phlegm-Fire harassing upwards

DEFICIENCY

Liver-Blood Deficiency
Liver- and Kidney-Yin Deficiency
Spleen- and Kidney-Yang Deficiency

EXCESS

1. STAGNATION OF LIVER-QI

CLINICAL MANIFESTATIONS

Abdominal and breast distension before the period, irritability, clumsiness, moodiness, depression, hypochondrial pain and distension.

Tongue: in light cases the tongue body may be unchanged. In chronic cases the sides may be Red.
Pulse: Wiry all over or only on the left.

TREATMENT PRINCIPLE

Soothe the Liver, eliminate stagnation, calm the Mind, settle the Ethereal Soul.

ACUPUNCTURE

LIV-3 Taichong, G.B.-34 Yanglingquan, G.B.-41 Zulinqi, SP-6 Sanyinjiao, T.B.-6 Zhigou, P-6 Neiguan. Reducing or even method.

Explanation

- **LIV-3** and **G.B.-34** soothe the Liver and eliminate stagnation. G.B.-34 specifically treats the hypochondrial region.
- **G.B.-41** is used if the breast distension is very pronounced and the breasts are also painful.
- **SP-6** helps to soothe the Liver and calm the Mind.
- **T.B.-6** moves Liver-Qi and affects the lateral side of the upper body.
- **P-6** moves Liver-Qi, calms the Mind and settles the Ethereal Soul. It also affects the chest and breasts and is a very important point for this condition.

HERBAL TREATMENT

(a) Prescription

XIAO YAO SAN
Free and Easy Wanderer Powder
Bo He *Herba Menthae* 3 g
Chai Hu *Radix Bupleuri* 9 g
Dang Gui *Radix Angelicae sinensis* 9 g
Bai Shao *Radix Paeoniae albae* 12 g
Bai Zhu *Rhizoma Atractylodis macrocephalae* 9 g
Fu Ling *Sclerotium Poriae cocos* 15 g
Gan Cao *Radix Glycyrrhizae uralensis* 6 g

Sheng Jiang *Rhizoma Zingiberis officinalis recens* 3 slices

Explanation

This formula, which has already been explained in chapters 1 and 12, is very widely used for pre-menstrual tension from Liver-Qi stagnation. This prescription is suitable also if there is some deficiency of Liver-Blood and the pulse is not too Wiry.

(b) Prescription

YUE JU WAN
Gardenia-Ligusticum Pill
Cang Zhu *Rhizoma Atractylodis lanceae* 6 g
Chuan Xiong *Radix Ligustici wallichii* 6 g
Xiang Fu *Rhizoma Cyperi rotundi* 6 g
Zhi Zi *Fructus Gardeniae jasminoidis* 6 g
Shen Qu *Massa Fermentata Medicinalis* 6 g

Explanation

This formula, which has already been explained in chapter 12, is selected if the stagnation of Qi is more intense, there is some Heat and the pulse is definitely Wiry in all positions. It is very effective for emotional depression.

(c) Prescription

CHAI HU SU GAN TANG
Bupleurum Soothing the Liver Decoction
Chai Hu *Radix Bupleuri* 6 g
Bai Shao *Radix Paeoniae albae* 4.5 g
Zhi Ke *Fructus Citri aurantii* 4.5 g
Zhi Gan Cao *Radix Glycyrrhizae uralensis prae-parata* 1.5 g
Chen Pi *Pericarpium Citri reticulatae* 6 g

Xiang Fu *Rhizoma Cyperi rotundi* 4.5 g
Chuan Xiong *Radix Ligustici wallichii* 4.5 g

Explanation

This formula, which has already been explained in chapter 16, is selected if the stagnation of Liver-Qi is severe and there is breast and abdominal pain as well as distension.

Table 33.1 compares and contrasts the above three formulae for pre-menstrual tension from Qi stagnation.

Variations

The following are variations applying to all three previous decoctions.

- If the breast distension is very pronounced add Qing Pi *Pericarpium Citri reticulatae viridae* and Yu Jin *Tuber Curcumae*.
- If abdominal distension is pronounced add (or increase) Xiang Fu *Rhizoma Cyperi rotundi*.
- If there is mental depression add He Huan Pi *Cortex Albizziae julibrissin*.
- If there is irritability and propensity to outbursts of anger add Suan Zao Ren *Semen Ziziphi spinosae*.
- If there is irritability, restlessness and insomnia add Long Chi *Dens Draconis* and Zhen Zhu Mu *Concha margaritiferae*.
- If there is a headache before each period add Tian Ma *Rhizoma Gastrodiae elatae*, Gou Teng *Ramulus Uncariae* and Fang Feng *Radix Ledebouriellae sesloidis*.
- If there is pronounced water retention add Zhu Ling *Sclerotium Polypori umbellati*, Yi Yi Ren *Semen Coicis lachryma jobi*, Ze Xie *Rhizoma Alismatis orientalis* and Gui Zhi *Ramulus Cinnamomi cassiae*.

Table 33.1 Comparison of Xiao Yao San, Yue Ju Wan and Chai Hu Su Gan Tang for pre-menstrual tension

	Xiao Yao San	Yue Ju Wan	Chai Hu Su Gan Tang
Symptoms and signs	Distension of abdomen and breasts, irritability and weepiness	Depression, gloomy feeling	Pain in abdomen and breasts
Tongue	Body-colour could be normal or even Pale on the sides	Red, or Red only on the sides, yellow coating	Slightly Red sides
Pulse	Choppy or Weak on the right and slightly Wiry-Fine on the left	Wiry on both sides	Slightly Wiry only on the left

Patent remedy

XIAO YAO WAN
Free and Easy Wanderer Pill
Chai Hu *Radix Bupleuri*
Bo He *Herba Menthae*
Dang Gui *Radix Angelicae sinensis*
Bai Shao *Radix Paeoniae albae*
Bai Zhu *Rhizoma Atractylodis macrocephalae*
Fu Ling *Sclerotium Poriae cocos*
Zhi Gan Cao *Radix Glycyrrhizae uralensis prae-parata*
Sheng Jiang *Rhizoma Zingiberis officinalis recens*

Explanation

This well-known pill has the same ingredients and functions as the homonymous prescription above. It is specific for pre-menstrual tension deriving from stagnation of Liver-Qi against a background of Liver-Blood deficiency.

The tongue presentation appropriate to this remedy is a slightly Pale and Thin body with slightly Red sides. The pulse presentation is a pulse which is slightly Wiry on the left side and Weak-Choppy on the right, or a pulse which is Fine all over and slightly Wiry on the left.

(ii) Patent remedy

YUE JU WAN
Gardenia-Ligusticum Pill
Xiang Fu *Rhizoma Cyperi rotundi*
Cang Zhu *Rhizoma Atractylodis lanceae*
Shan Zhi Zi *Fructus Gardeniae jasminoidis*
Chuan Xiong *Radix Ligustici wallichii*
Shen Qu *Massa Fermentata Medicinalis*

Explanation

This remedy, with the same ingredients and functions as the homonymous prescription above, is excellent for pre-menstrual tension with mental depression deriving from Liver-Qi stagnation and some Heat.

The tongue presentation appropriate to this remedy is a Red body with redder sides or a normal body with Red sides. The pulse picture appropriate to this remedy is a Wiry and Full pulse on all positions.

(iii) Patent remedy

SHU GAN WAN
Pacifying the Liver Pill
Chuan Lian Zi *Fructus Meliae toosendan*
Jiang Huang *Rhizoma Curcumae longae*
Chen Xiang *Lignum Aquilariae*
Yan Hu Suo *Rhizoma Corydalis yanhusuo*
Mu Xiang *Radix Saussureae*
Bai Dou Kou *Fructus Amomi cardamomi*
Bai Shao *Radix Paeoniae albae*
Fu Ling *Sclerotium Poriae cocos*
Zhi Ke *Fructus Citri aurantii*
Chen Pi *Pericarpium Citri reticulatae*
Sha Ren *Fructus seu Semen Amomi*
Hou Po *Cortex Magnoliae officinalis*

Explanation

This remedy pacifies the Liver and eliminates stagnation. It is suitable to treat pre-menstrual tension from stagnation of Liver-Qi.

The tongue presentation appropriate to this remedy is a normal body-colour with Red or Purple sides. The pulse picture appropriate to this remedy is a Wiry pulse. This remedy differs from the previous one in so far as it is purely for stagnation of Liver-Qi without Heat. Also, Yue Ju Wan is better to treat mental depression.

2. PHLEGM-FIRE HARASSING UPWARDS

CLINICAL MANIFESTATIONS

Agitation, depression, slightly manic behaviour, aggressiveness, a feeling of oppression of the chest, a red face, blood-shot eyes.
Tongue: Red with a sticky-yellow coating.
Pulse: Overflowing-Slippery-Rapid.

TREATMENT PRINCIPLE

Clear Heat, resolve Phlegm, calm the Mind, settle the Ethereal Soul.

ACUPUNCTURE

P-7 Daling, ST-40 Fenglong, ST-8 Touwei, Du-24

Shenting, L.I.-11 Quchi, SP-9 Yinlingquan, SP-4 Gongsun and P-6 Neiguan, Ren-12 Zhongwan, BL-20 Pishu. Reducing or even method on all except for Ren-12 and BL-20 which should be reinforced.

Explanation

- **P-7** and **ST-40** resolve Phlegm and calm the Mind.
- **ST-8** and **Du-24** calm the Mind and resolve Phlegm from the head.
- **L.I.-11** clears Heat.
- **SP-9** helps to resolve Phlegm.
- **SP-4** and **P-6** regulate the Penetrating Vessel and subdue rebellious Qi.
- **Ren-12** and **BL-20** tonify the Spleen to resolve Phlegm.

Special empirical treatment

If there is mastitis, which is likely to occur especially with this pattern, look for a bright-red rash on the upper back between C-7 and D-12, with macular spots which do not stick out on touch, and which do not change colour on finger pressure. Prick all the spots with a triangular needle and bleed them slightly.

HERBAL TREATMENT

(a) Prescription

SHENG TIE LUO YIN
Frusta Ferri Decoction
Sheng Tie Luo *Frusta Ferri* 60 g
Dan Nan Xing *Rhizoma Arisaematis praeparata* 9 g
Zhe Bei Mu *Bulbus Fritillariae thunbergii* 9 g
Xuan Shen *Radix Scrophulariae ningpoensis* 9 g
Tian Men Dong *Tuber Asparagi cochinchinensis* 9 g
Mai Men Dong *Tuber Ophiopogonis japonici* 9 g
Lian Qiao *Fructus Forsythiae suspensae* 9 g
Dan Shen *Radix Salviae miltiorrhizae* 12 g
Fu Ling *Sclerotium Poriae cocos* 12 g
Chen Pi *Pericarpium Citri reticulatae* 6 g
Shi Chang Pu *Rhizoma Acori graminei* 6 g
Yuan Zhi *Radix Polygalae tenuifoliae* 6 g
Zhu Sha *Cinnabaris* 1.8 g

Explanation

This formula clears Heat, resolves Phlegm and subdues Liver-Yang. It is appropriate in this case to treat the Liver because of the influence it has on the menstrual function. Phlegm harassing upwards is often associated with Liver-Yang or Liver-Wind rising. Note that the original formula contains Zhu Sha which is toxic and can therefore be omitted.

- **Sheng Tie Luo** subdues Liver-Yang.
- **Nan Xing** and **Bei Mu** resolve Phlegm.
- **Xuan Shen**, **Tian Dong** and **Mai Dong** nourish Yin.
- **Lian Qiao** clears Heat.
- **Dan Shen** enters the Pericardium and it helps to subdue Liver-Yang, calm the Mind and settle the Ethereal Soul.
- **Fu Ling** and **Chen Pi** help to resolve Phlegm.
- **Shi Chang Pu**, **Yuan Zhi** and **Zhu Sha** calm the Mind and open the Mind's orifices.

(b) Prescription

WEN DAN TANG Variation
Warming the Gall-Bladder Decoction
Ban Xia *Rhizoma Pinelliae ternatae* 6 g
Fu Ling *Sclerotium Poriae cocos* 5 g
Chen Pi *Pericarpium Citri reticulatae* 9 g
Zhu Ru *Caulis Bambusae in Taeniis* 6 g
Zhi Shi *Fructus Citri aurantii immaturus* 6 g
Zhi Gan Cao *Radix Glycyrrhizae uralensis praeparata* 3 g
Sheng Jiang *Rhizoma Zingiberis officinalis recens* 5 slices
Da Zao *Fructus Ziziphi jujubae* 1 date
Qing Pi *Pericarpium Citri reticulatae viridae* 6 g
Xiang Fu *Rhizoma Cyperi rotundi* 6 g
He Huan Pi *Cortex Albizziae julibrissin* 6 g

Explanation

This formula, which has already been explained in chapter 9, resolves Phlegm-Heat from the chest area and calms the Mind.

- The first eight herbs constitute Wen Dan Tang.
- **Qing Pi** moves Liver-Qi and relieves breast distension.

- **Xiang Fu** moves Liver-Qi and relieves abdominal distension.
- **He Huan Pi** moves Liver-Qi, subdues Liver-Yang, calms the Mind and lifts depression.

Variations

These variations are applicable to both formulae.

- If Phlegm is very pronounced add (or increase the dosage of) Ban Xia *Rhizoma Pinelliae ternatae* and Gua Lou *Fructus Trichosanthis*. Gua Lou specifically affects the breasts.
- If the breasts are very swollen add Zhu Ling *Sclerotium Polypori umbellati*, Yi Yi Ren *Semen Coicis lachryma jobi* and Lu Lu Tong *Fructus Liquidambaris taiwanianae*.
- If the breast distension is very pronounced add Qing Pi *Pericarpium Citri reticulatae viridae* and Yu Jin *Tuber Curcumae*.
- If abdominal distension is pronounced add (or increase) Xiang Fu *Rhizoma Cyperi rotundi*.
- If there is mental depression add He Huan Pi *Cortex Albizziae julibrissin*.
- If there is irritability and propensity to outbursts of anger add Suan Zao Ren *Semen Ziziphi spinosae*.
- If there is irritability, restlessness and insomnia add Long Chi *Dens Draconis* and Zhen Zhu Mu *Concha margaritiferae*.

DEFICIENCY

1. LIVER-BLOOD DEFICIENCY

CLINICAL MANIFESTATIONS

Depression and weepiness before the period, slight abdominal and breast distension, scanty periods, tiredness, poor memory, poor sleep, slight dizziness and a dull-pale complexion.
Tongue: Pale, possibly only on the sides.
Pulse: Choppy or Fine and possibly slightly Wiry on the left.

TREATMENT PRINCIPLE

Nourish Liver-Blood, move Liver-Qi.

ACUPUNCTURE

Ren-4 Guanyuan, LU-7 Lieque and KI-6 Zhaohai, SP-6 Sanyinjiao, ST-36 Zusanli, G.B.-34 Yanglingquan, P-6 Neiguan, Ren-6 Qihai, LIV-8 Ququan, BL-20 Pishu, BL-18 Ganshu. Reinforcing method except for G.B.-34, P-6 and Ren-6 which should be needled with even method. Moxa can be used.

Explanation

- **Ren-4** nourishes Blood and regulates the Directing Vessel.
- **LU-7** and **KI-6** regulate the Directing Vessel and move Qi.
- **SP-6** and **ST-36** nourish Blood. SP-6 also moves Liver-Qi and calms the Mind.
- **G.B.-34** moves Liver-Qi.
- **P-6** moves Liver-Qi, calms the Mind and settles the Ethereal Soul.
- **Ren-6**, in combination with G.B.-34, moves Qi in the lower abdomen.
- **LIV-8** and **BL-18** nourish Liver-Blood.
- **BL-20** tonifies the Spleen to produce Blood.

HERBAL TREATMENT

(a) Prescription

XIAO YAO SAN
Free and Easy Wanderer Powder
Bo He *Herba Menthae* 3 g
Chai Hu *Radix Bupleuri* 9 g
Dang Gui *Radix Angelicae sinensis* 9 g
Bai Shao *Radix Paeoniae albae* 12 g
Bai Zhu *Rhizoma Atractylodis macrocephalae* 9 g
Fu Ling *Sclerotium Poriae cocos* 15 g
Gan Cao *Radix Glycyrrhizae uralensis* 6 g
Sheng Jiang *Rhizoma Zingiberis officinalis recens* 3 slices

Explanation

This formula, which has already been explained above, moves Liver-Qi and nourishes Liver-Blood. It can therefore be used for this pattern increasing the dosage of Dang Gui and adding some herbs to nourish Liver-Blood such as Shu

Di Huang *Radix Rehmanniae glutinosae praeparata* and Gou Qi Zi *Fructus Lycii chinensis.*

(b) Prescription

BA ZHEN TANG Variation
Eight-Precious Decoction
Dang Gui *Radix Angelicae sinensis* 10 g
Chuan Xiong *Radix Ligustici wallichii* 5 g
Bai Shao *Radix Paeoniae albae* 8 g
Shu Di Huang *Radix Rehmanniae glutinosae praeparata* 15 g
Ren Shen *Radix Ginseng* 3 g
Bai Zhu *Rhizoma Atractylodis macrocephalae* 10 g
Fu Ling *Sclerotium Poriae cocos* 8 g
Zhi Gan Cao *Radix Glycyrrhizae uralensis praeparata* 5 g
Qing Pi *Pericarpium Citri reticulatae viridae* 4.5 g
Chai Hu *Radix Bupleuri* 6 g
He Huan Pi *Cortex Albizziae julibrissin* 9 g

Explanation

The main formula, which has already been explained in chapter 17, nourishes Qi and Blood.

- **Qing Pi** moves Liver-Qi and affects the breasts.
- **Chai Hu** moves Liver-Qi.
- **He Huan Pi** moves Liver-Qi, subdues Liver-Yang and lifts depression.

(i) Patent remedy

XIAO YAO WAN
Free and Easy Wanderer Pill

Explanation

This remedy, already explained above, can be used for pre-menstrual tension from deficiency of Liver-Blood as, besides pacifying the Liver, it nourishes Liver-Blood.

The tongue and pulse presentation appropriate to this remedy, in the context of this pattern, is a Pale tongue body and a Choppy pulse which is slightly Wiry on the left.

(ii) Patent remedy

BA ZHEN WAN

Eight Precious Pill
Dang Gui *Radix Angelicae sinensis*
Chuan Xiong *Radix Ligustici wallichii*
Bai Shao *Radix Paeoniae albae*
Shu Di Huang *Radix Rehmanniae glutinosae praeparata*
Ren Shen *Radix Ginseng*
Bai Zhu *Rhizoma Atractylodis macrocephalae*
Fu Ling *Sclerotium Poriae cocos*
Zhi Gan Cao *Radix Glycyrrhizae uralensis praeparata*

Explanation

This remedy nourishes Qi and Blood and, in particular, Liver-Blood. It can be used to treat pre-menstrual tension from deficiency of Liver-Blood, and, if the condition is severe, can be combined with the previous remedy Xiao Yao Wan.

The tongue and pulse presentation appropriate to this remedy is a Pale and Thin body and a Choppy pulse.

Case history

A 37-year-old woman had been suffering from pre-menstrual tension for 8 years. It had started when she suffered post-natal depression following the birth of her first child . She had another bout of post-natal depression after the birth of her second child. During the pre-menstrual period she was very irritable, irrational, and cried a lot. On a physical level, she had a pronounced feeling of distension of the breasts and abdomen. Apart from her pre-menstrual problem, she also suffered from constipation, headaches, insomnia, excessive dreaming and palpitations. Her pulse was Fine in general, slightly Wiry only on the left-Middle position (Liver) and Weak on the left-Front position (Heart). Her tongue was Pale and slightly Thin but also slightly Red on the sides.

Diagnosis
This is a condition of both Deficiency and Excess. There is a deficiency of Liver-Blood manifesting with constipation, excessive dreaming, Pale tongue and Fine pulse. This deficiency has also induced a deficiency of Heart-Blood manifesting with insomnia and palpitations. The deficiency of Blood most probably started with the loss of blood occurring after childbirth and was the original cause of post-natal depression. The deficiency of Liver-Blood, over the years, gave rise to stagnation of Liver-Qi and therefore the pre-menstrual tension. The fact that,

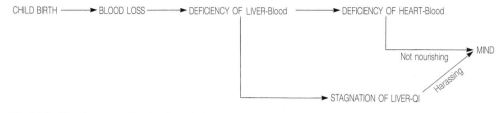

Fig. 33.1   Development of patient's pathology

besides feeling irritable before the periods, she also wept a lot, indicates a Deficiency condition. The development of her condition is represented diagrammatically in Figure 33.1.

Treatment principle
The principle of treatment adopted was to nourish Liver- and Heart-Blood, pacify the Liver, eliminate stagnation, calm the Mind and settle the Ethereal Soul. She was treated with acupuncture and patent remedies.

Acupuncture
The acupuncture points used (with reinforcing method to nourish Liver- and Heart-Blood and even method to pacify the Liver) were selected from the following:

– **LIV-3** Taichong and **G.B.-34** Yanglingquan to pacify the Liver and eliminate stagnation.
– **P-7** Daling to pacify the Liver, calm the Mind and settle the Ethereal Soul.
– **P-6** Neiguan on the right and **SP-4** Gongsun on the left to open the Yin Linking Vessel, nourish Blood and calm the Mind.
– **ST-36** Zusanli and **SP-6** Sanyinjiao to tonify Qi and Blood.
– **BL-20** Pishu, **BL-15** Xinshu and **BL-18** Ganshu to nourish Liver- and Heart-Blood.

She was treated once a week.

Herbal treatment
The patent remedies used were Xiao Yao Wan *Free and Easy Wanderer Pill* to pacify the Liver and eliminate stagnation and Bai Zi Yang Xin Wan *Biota Nourishing the Heart Pill* to nourish Liver and Heart-Blood and calm the Mind.

By the end of 9 months this patient's condition showed about 80% improvement.

Case history

A 35-year-old woman suffered from pre-menstrual tension, complaining of breast distension, irritability and depression. She also suffered from severe abdominal distension and, on a mental level, she lacked confidence and a sense of direction in life, could not concentrate, found it difficult to take decisions, and feared change. She also complained of poor memory, insomnia, blurred vision, dizziness, and numbness of feet. Her tongue was Pale on the sides and the pulse was Fine and slightly Wiry on the left side and Choppy on the right.

Diagnosis
This is a clear case of stagnation of Liver-Qi which is secondary to Liver-Blood deficiency. She had many symptoms of Liver-Blood deficiency: poor memory and concentration, blurred vision, insomnia, dizziness, numbness, Pale tongue, and Fine and Choppy pulse. Also on a mental level, many of her problems were due to deficient Liver-Blood not rooting the Ethereal Soul: lack of confidence, lack of a sense of direction in life, fear of change, depression. Fear was a marked aspect of her mental make-up, and it should be remembered here that this emotion is not always due to the Kidneys as it can also be related to a Liver-Blood deficiency (see chapter 9 on Mental-emotional problems). The pre-menstrual symptoms were characteristic of Liver-Qi stagnation.

Treatment principle
The treatment principle adopted was to nourish Liver-Blood, root the Ethereal Soul and move Liver-Qi. She was treated with acupuncture and patent remedies.

Acupuncture
The acupuncture points were selected from the following:

– **P-6** Neiguan, on the right, to regulate the Liver, calm the Mind and settle the Ethereal Soul.
– **LIV-3** Taichong, on the left, to pacify the Liver, eliminate stagnation, and settle the Ethereal Soul.
– **ST-36** Zusanli, **SP-6** Sanyinjiao, **LIV-8** Ququan (all bilateral) and **Ren-4** Guanyuan to nourish Liver-Blood.
– **Du-20** Baihui to clear the brain and lift mood.

Herbal treatment
The patent remedy used was Xiao Yao Wan *Free and Easy Wanderer Pill*.

This patient made a complete recovery in 9 months and felt much better mentally. In particular, it was interesting to note that she acquired a sense of direction in her life, by taking a new training course and embarking on a new, satisfying career.

2. LIVER- AND KIDNEY-YIN DEFICIENCY

CLINICAL MANIFESTATIONS

Slight breast distension and irritability before the period and occasionally after it, sore back and knees, dizziness, blurred vision, poor memory, insomnia, dry eyes and throat, 5-palm heat.
Tongue: Red without coating.
Pulse: Floating-Empty.

TREATMENT PRINCIPLE

Nourish Liver- and Kidney-Yin and move Liver-Qi.

ACUPUNCTURE

LIV-8 Ququan, Ren-4 Guanyuan, SP-6 Sanyinjiao, LIV-3 Taichong. Reinforcing method on all except LIV-3 which should be needled with even method.

Explanation

- **LIV-8** nourishes Liver-Yin.
- **Ren-4** nourishes Liver- and Kidney-Yin.
- **SP-6** nourishes Liver- and Kidney-Yin and calms the Mind.
- **LIV-3** moves Liver-Qi.

HERBAL TREATMENT

Prescription

YI GUAN JIAN Variation
One Linking Decoction
Bei Sha Shen *Radix Glehniae littoralis* 10 g
Mai Men Dong *Tuber Ophiopogonis japonici* 10 g
Dang Gui *Radix Angelicae sinensis* 10 g
Sheng Di Huang *Radix Rehmanniae glutinosae* 30 g
Gou Qi Zi *Fructus Lycii chinensis* 12 g
Chuan Lian Zi *Fructus Meliae toosendan* 5 g
Mei Gui Hua *Flos Rosae rugosae* 6 g
Fu Shou *Fructus Citri sarcodactylis* 6 g

Explanation

The first six herbs constitute the Yi Guan Jian which nourishes Liver-Yin.

- **Mei Gui Hua** and **Fu Shou** move Liver-Qi without damaging Yin.

Variations

- If Liver- and Kidney-Yin deficiency leads to Liver-Yang rising add Tian Ma *Rhizoma Gastrodiae elatae*, Gou Teng *Ramulus Uncariae* and Shi Jue Ming *Concha Haliotidis*.
- If there is mental restlessness and insomnia add Suan Zao Ren *Semen Ziziphi spinosae* and Ye Jiao Teng *Caulis Polygoni multiflori*.

Patent remedy

QI JU DI HUANG WAN
Lycium-Chrysanthemum-Rehmannia Pill
Gou Qi Zi *Fructus Lycii chinensis*
Ju Hua *Flos Chrysanthemi morifolii*
Shu Di Huang *Radix Rehmanniae glutinosae praeparata*
Shan Yao *Radix Dioscoreae oppositae*
Shan Zhu Yu *Fructus Corni officinalis*
Ze Xie *Rhizoma Alismatis orientalis*
Fu Ling *Sclerotium Poriae cocos*
Mu Dan Pi *Cortex Moutan radicis*

Explanation

This remedy nourishes Liver- and Kidney-Yin and subdues Liver-Yang. It can be used for premenstrual tension with irritability deriving from Liver-Yang rising against a background of Liver-Yin deficiency.

The tongue and pulse presentation appropriate to this remedy is a Red tongue body without coating and a Floating-Empty pulse.

Case history

A 40-year-old woman had been suffering from premenstrual tension for 7 years. Before the period she felt depressed and irritable and had a headache on the vertex. Her periods were regular, lasted 3 days, were rather scanty and not painful. Apart from this, she suffered from constipation, back-ache, a feeling of heat and dry mouth in the evening, sore eyes, and blurred vision. Her hair was dry and had been falling out. Her tongue was slightly Red with a rootless coating. Her pulse was Weak on the left-Rear position.

Diagnosis
This is a clear condition of Liver-Yin deficiency leading to some stagnation of Liver-Qi causing the pre-menstrual tension. The symptoms of Liver-Yin deficiency are a feeling of heat and dry mouth at night, sore eyes, blurred vision and dry and falling hair. There is also some deficiency of Kidney-Yin as evidenced by the back-ache.

Treatment principle
The treatment principle adopted was to nourish Liver-Yin, pacify the Liver, eliminate stagnation, calm the Mind and settle the Ethereal Soul. As she was receiving acupuncture from another practitioner who referred her to me for herbal treatment she was treated only with herbs.

Herbal treatment
The decoction used was a variation of Yi Guan Jian *One Linking Decoction* which nourishes Liver-Yin:

Mai Men Dong *Tuber Ophiopogonis japonici* 6 g
Bei Sha Shen *Radix Glehniae littoralis* 6 g
Gou Qi Zi *Fructus Lycii chinensis* 9 g
Sheng Di Huang *Radix Rehmanniae glutinosae* 9 g
Dang Gui *Radix Angelicae sinensis* 9 g
Chuan Lian Zi *Fructus Meliae toosendan* 4 g
Xiang Fu *Rhizoma Cyperi rotundi* 6 g
Bai Shao *Radix Paeoniae albae* 9 g
Ju Hua *Flos Chrysanthemi morifolii* 6 g
Zhi Gan Cao *Radix Glycyrrhizae uralensis praeparata* 3 g

Explanation
– **Mai Dong**, **Sha Shen**, **Gou Qi Zi**, **Sheng Di** and **Dang Gui** nourish Liver-Yin.
– **Chuan Lian Zi** and **Xiang Fu** pacify the Liver and eliminate stagnation.
– **Bai Shao** nourishes Liver-Yin and pacifies the Liver.
– **Ju Hua** subdues Liver-Yang (headache) and calms the Mind.
– **Gan Cao** harmonizes.

This patient made a gradual improvement over 6 months after which she had no signs of pre-menstrual tension.

3. SPLEEN- AND KIDNEY-YANG DEFICIENCY

CLINICAL MANIFESTATIONS

Slight pre-menstrual tension with depression and weeping, slight abdominal and breast dis-tension, tiredness, sore back, feeling cold, frequent and pale urination, low sexual desire.
Tongue: Pale and Swollen.
Pulse: Deep and Weak.

TREATMENT PRINCIPLE

Tonify Yang, strengthen the Kidneys.

ACUPUNCTURE

BL-23 Shenshu, BL-20 Pishu, Ren-4 Guanyuan, ST-36 Zusanli, SP-6 Sanyinjiao, KI-3 Taixi, LU-7 Lieque and KI-6 Zhaohai. Reinforcing method, moxa should be used.

Explanation

– **BL-23** and **BL-20** tonify Kidneys and Spleen.
– **Ren-4**, with direct moxa, tonifies Kidney-Yang.
– **ST-36** and **SP-6** tonify Qi and Blood.
– **KI-3**, with moxa, tonifies Kidney-Yang.
– **LU-7** and **KI-6** open the Directing Vessel, regulate the uterus and tonify the Kidneys.

HERBAL TREATMENT

Prescription

YOU GUI WAN
Restoring the Right [Kidney] Pill
Fu Zi *Radix Aconiti carmichaeli praeparata* 3 g
Rou Gui *Cortex Cinnamomi cassiae* 3 g
Du Zhong *Cortex Eucommiae ulmoidis* 6 g
Shan Zhu Yu *Fructus Corni officinalis* 4.5 g
Tu Si Zi *Semen Cuscutae* 6 g
Lu Jiao Jiao *Colla Cornu Cervi* 6 g
Shu Di Huang *Radix Rehmanniae glutinosae prae-parata* 12 g
Shan Yao *Radix Dioscoreae oppositae* 6 g
Gou Qi Zi *Fructus Lycii chinensis* 6 g
Dang Gui *Radix Angelicae sinensis* 4.5 g

Explanation

This formula, which has already been explained

in chapters 1 and 25, tonifies Kidney-Yang. It is particularly suited to this pattern as it also contains Shu Di Huang, Dang Gui and Gou Qi Zi which nourish Blood and benefit the Directing Vessel.

Variations

- If the symptoms of Liver-Qi stagnation are pronounced and there is breast distension add Qing Pi *Pericarpium Citri reticulatae viridae*.
- If there is abdominal distension add Xiang Fu *Rhizoma Cyperi rotundi*.

Patent remedy

YOU GUI WAN
Restoring the Right [Kidney] Pill
This remedy has the same ingredients and functions as the homonymous prescription above.

The tongue presentation appropriate to this remedy is a Pale and wet body.

Case history

A 33-year-old woman had been suffering from pre-menstrual tension for 4 years. Before the period she was depressed and anxious. The period itself was painful, the menstrual blood had some small dark clots and she felt very cold during it. Other symptoms included a general cold feeling, back-ache, achy knees, dizziness, tinnitus, urgent and slightly dribbling urination, poor memory, numbness of the limbs, restless sleep and tiredness. Her tongue was Pale but had slightly Red sides. The root of the tongue had no spirit. Her pulse was generally Weak, particularly on the Rear positions.

Diagnosis
This patient has clear symptoms of Kidney-Yang deficiency: back-ache, cold feeling, achy knees, dizziness, tinnitus, poor memory, dribbling urination, Pale tongue and pulse Weak on the Kidney positions. There is also some deficiency of Blood evidenced by the numbness of limbs and restless sleep. The deficiency of the Kidneys leads to Liver deficiency and stagnation of Liver-Qi which causes the pre-menstrual tension.

Treatment principle
The treatment principle adopted was to tonify and warm Kidney-Yang, nourish and pacify the Liver,

eliminate stagnation, calm the Mind and settle the Ethereal Soul. As she had been referred by a fellow acupuncturist for herbal treatment, I treated her only with herbs.

Herbal treatment
I started by using a variation of the decoction You Gui Wan *Restoring the Right [Kidney] Pill*:

Fu Zi *Radix Aconiti carmichaeli praeparata* 3 g
Rou Gui *Cortex Cinnamomi cassiae* 2 g
Du Zhong *Cortex Eucommiae ulmoidis* 6 g
Shan Zhu Yu *Fructus Corni officinalis* 4.5 g
Tu Si Zi *Semen Cuscutae* 6 g
Lu Jiao Jiao *Colla Cornu Cervi* 6 g
Shu Di Huang *Radix Rehmanniae glutinosae praeparata* 12 g
Shan Yao *Radix Dioscoreae oppositae* 6 g
Gou Qi Zi *Fructus Lycii chinensis* 6 g
Dang Gui *Radix Angelicae sinensis* 6 g
Xiang Fu *Rhizoma Cyperi rotundi* 6 g
Bai Shao *Radix Paeoniae albae* 6 g

Explanation
- All the herbs, except for the last two, make up the You Gui Wan which tonifies Kidney-Yang and nourishes Liver-Blood.
- **Xiang Fu** was added to move Liver-Qi and eliminate stagnation.
- **Bai Shao** nourishes and pacifies the Liver and calms the Mind.

After taking this prescription for 3 weeks, she said that, although she had more energy, she felt angry, still had pre-menstrual tension, did not sleep well and was confused. I concluded that the treatment emphasis should have been, as is often the case, on eliminating first rather than tonifying. In this case, the premature tonification had probably created more stagnation affecting the Mind and Ethereal Soul, hence the anger, insomnia and mental confusion. I therefore changed the treatment principle to concentrate on pacifying the Liver, eliminating stagnation, calming the Mind, opening the orifices and settling the Ethereal Soul, and chose to use a variation of Xiao Yao San *Free and Easy Wanderer Powder*:

Bo He *Herba Menthae* 3 g
Chai Hu *Radix Bupleuri* 9 g
Dang Gui *Radix Angelicae sinensis* 9 g
Bai Shao *Radix Paeoniae albae* 12 g
Bai Zhu *Rhizoma Atractylodis macrocephalae* 9 g
Fu Ling *Sclerotium Poriae cocos* 15 g
Gan Cao *Radix Glycyrrhizae uralensis* 6 g
Sheng Jiang *Rhizoma Zingiberis officinalis recens* 3 slices
Shu Di Huang *Radix Rehmanniae glutinosae praeparata* 9 g
Xiang Fu *Rhizoma Cyperi rotundi* 6 g
He Huan Pi *Cortex Albizziae julibrissin* 6 g
Shi Chang Pu *Rhizoma Acori graminei* 6 g

Explanation
- The first 8 herbs constitute the Xiao Yao San which pacifies the Liver and nourishes Liver-Blood.
- **Shu Di** was added to tonify the Kidneys.
- **Xiang Fu**, **He Huan Pi** and **Chang Pu** pacify the Liver, eliminate stagnation, lift depression and open the orifices.

This decoction had a much better effect, improving the pre-menstrual tension, calming her and dispelling the confusion. She continued to be treated with variations of this decoction for about 3 months, after which the treatment principle was changed again to tonify Kidney-Yang primarily. After another 4 months, she felt much better all round and her pre-menstrual tension had gone.

Prognosis

Both acupuncture and herbs, singly or in combination, give excellent results for pre-menstrual tension. It could be said that there is hardly a case that cannot be helped, although those caused by Phlegm-Fire harassing upwards will take longest to treat. As with all menstrual problems, it will take a minimum of 3 menstrual periods to regulate the cycle completely, although some improvement can often be seen even after one month.

Common cold and influenza 34 感冒

Common cold and influenza are viral infections of the upper respiratory tract. The common cold may be caused by a variety of viruses including the adenovirus, echovirus, parainfluenza virus, respiratory syncytial virus and rhinovirus. Influenza may be caused by the influenza viruses A, B or C.

In Chinese medicine both the common cold and influenza correspond to invasions of exterior Wind which may manifest as Wind-Cold, Wind-Heat, Wind-Damp-Heat or Wind-Dry-Heat. However, Wind-Cold and Wind-Heat are the two most common types and, broadly speaking, they are also the two types which encompass most exterior manifestations.

The "Discussion of Cold-induced Diseases" by Zhang Zhong Jing provided the earliest framework for the diagnosis and treatment of diseases from exterior Wind-Cold. Although this famous classic does also discuss invasions of Wind-Heat and their treatment, a comprehensive theory of exterior diseases from Wind-Heat was not developed until the late 1600s by the School of Warm Diseases (*Wen Bing*). Thus, the two schools of thought which form the pillars for the diagnosis and treatment of exterior diseases in Chinese medicine are separated by about 15 centuries: they are the School of Cold-induced Diseases (School of *Shang Han*) based on the "Discussion of Cold-induced Diseases" ("*Shang Han Lun*") by Zhang Zhong Jing (*c.* AD 220) and the School of Warm Diseases (*Wen Bing* School) which started in the late 1600s and early 1700s. The main advocates of this school were Wu You Ke (1582–1652), Ye Tian Shi (1667–1746) and Wu Ju Tong (1758–1836).

What does "Warm disease" mean? This is my own translation of the Chinese term *wen bing*. The above-mentioned doctors from this school of thought introduced important innovations to the theory of Wind in Chinese medicine. The School of Warm Diseases postulates that some exterior pathogenic factors go beyond the natural characters of "Wind"; they are so virulent and strong that, no matter how strong a person's body's Qi may be, men, women and children fall ill by the dozen. More importantly, for the first time in the history of Chinese medicine, these doctors recognized that some external pathogenic factors are *infectious*. This is an extremely important innovative idea in Chinese medicine and one that preceded the introduction of Western medicine into China. Previously, it was believed that a person fell ill from an exterior disease because of a relative imbalance between an external pathogenic factor and the body's Qi. The doctors of the School of Warm Diseases, on the contrary, realized that some pathogenic factors, although still falling under the category of "Wind", are infectious. Indeed, some, called "epidemic evils", are so infectious that entire communities fall ill.

A further innovative idea stemming from this school was that the pathogenic factors causing Warm diseases, all of them falling under the category of Wind-Heat, enter via the nose and mouth, rather than via the skin as happens for Wind-Cold.

The essential characteristics of Warm diseases therefore are:

1. They manifest with the general symptoms and signs of Wind-Heat in the early stages (Wind-Heat is intended here in a broad sense as it may also manifest as Damp-Heat, Summer-Heat, Winter-Heat, Spring-Heat and Dry-Heat)
2. There is always a fever
3. They are infectious
4. The Wind-Heat penetrates via the nose and mouth
5. The pathogenic factor is particularly strong.

Thus, although all pathogenic factors contemplated by the School of Warm Diseases fall under the broad definition of Wind-Heat, not all diseases caused by Wind-Heat are Warm diseases. Some of the exterior diseases that start with symptoms of Wind-Heat are Warm diseases (with all the above-mentioned characteristics) and some are not. Examples of Warm diseases are measles, chicken-pox, German measles, poliomyelitis, smallpox, scarlet fever, whooping cough or meningitis. Examples of Wind-Heat diseases which are *not* Warm diseases are common cold (of the Wind-Heat type), influenza, glandular fever (mononucleosis) and any non-specific upper-respiratory infection manifesting with symptoms of Wind-Heat. This is a very important consideration in practice: it is possible to stop diseases from "simple" Wind-Heat at the early stages, but although true Warm diseases may be alleviated in the initial stages, they may not be entirely stopped.

In theory, as Wind is the pathogenic factor in the early stages of any exterior disease (whether Warm disease or not), by releasing the Exterior and expelling Wind we may stop any exterior invasion at its beginning. Although this is possible for simple invasions of Wind-Heat, it is not possible for Warm diseases. Thus, for example, if a child is infected with the *Bordetella pertussis* bacterium (causing whooping cough), we will not be able to stop the disease completely in its beginning stages.

In the initial stages all exterior diseases manifest with similar symptoms of Wind-Cold or Wind-Heat and at this point it is not possible to tell whether the patient is suffering a simple invasion of Wind-Heat or a Warm disease. It is important to treat them according to the principle of treatment of exterior diseases as, even though Warm diseases may not be stopped completely in the beginning stage, Chinese medicine can alleviate the symptoms, shorten the course of the disease and prevent complications.

Common cold and influenza are simple invasions of Wind which can be stopped in the initial stages. Since common colds and influenza are relatively mild and self-limiting diseases, why does the theory of their diagnosis and treatment have such a prominent place in Chinese medicine? Chinese medicine views these diseases differently from Western medicine, believing that if external Wind is allowed to penetrate the Interior, it can trigger many different diseases; it is therefore important to eliminate the pathogenic factor as early as possible. Simple invasions of Wind-Heat can be stopped at the initial stage; Warm diseases can be alleviated, their course shortened and any complications avoided.

The treatment of exterior invasions is also important because they can have very serious consequences in children and the elderly. In children, many serious diseases start with symptoms of invasion of Wind-Heat: in the initial stages one does not know what disease it might be and it is therefore important to treat the manifestations early. For example, measles, diphtheria, whooping cough, poliomyelitis, acute nephritis, scarlet fever and meningitis may all manifest with symptoms of Wind-Heat in the beginning stage. In the elderly, exterior Wind may easily penetrate the Interior causing bronchitis and pneumonia which is often fatal in old age.

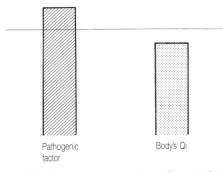

Fig. 34.1 Imbalance between exterior pathogenic factors and body's Qi

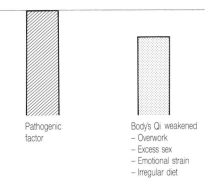

Fig. 34.2 External invasion in a weakened body condition

Infection from the common cold or influenza virus takes place through the upper respiratory tract and may occur in any season but it is more frequent in Winter or Spring. From the Chinese point of view, they can manifest with symptoms either of Wind-Cold or Wind-Heat.

Aetiology and pathology

An invasion of an exterior pathogenic factor is due to a temporary and relative imbalance between it and the body's Qi (Fig. 34.1).

This imbalance may occur either because the body's Qi is *temporarily* and *relatively* weak or because the pathogenic factor is very strong. I have stressed "temporarily" and "relatively" because the body's Qi is not weak in absolute terms but only in relation to an external pathogenic factor at a particular time. The body's Qi may be temporarily and relatively weak due to overwork, excessive sexual activity, irregular diet and emotional stress or a combination of these. When the body is thus weakened, even a mild pathogenic factor may cause an external invasion of Wind (Fig. 34.2).

On the other hand, a particularly strong pathogenic factor may cause an exterior invasion of Wind no matter how strong the body's Qi is. Someone who falls through the ice while crossing a frozen lake in Finland in the middle of winter, will suffer an invasion of Wind no matter how strong the body condition is (Fig. 34.3)!

"Wind" indicates both an aetiological factor and a pathological condition. As an aetiological factor, it literally refers to climatic influences and especially sudden changes of weather to which the body cannot adapt. As a pathological condition, "Wind" refers to a complex of symptoms and signs manifesting as Wind-Cold or Wind-Heat. In clinical practice, this is the most important aspect of the concept of Wind. Thus, the diagnosis of "Wind" invasion is made not on the basis of the history (no need to ask the patient whether he or she has been exposed to wind), but on the basis of the symptoms and signs. If a person has all the symptoms and signs of "Wind" (aversion to cold, shivering, fever, sneezing, runny nose, headache and a Floating pulse), then the condition is one of exterior Wind, no matter what climate that person has been exposed to in the previous days or hours. Indeed, there are also chronic conditions which

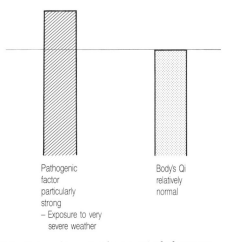

Fig. 34.3 External invasion by a particularly strong pathogenic factor

manifest with symptoms of "Wind" and are treated as such even though they have no relation to climatic factors. For example, allergic rhinitis (due to house-dust mites or pollen) manifests with symptoms and signs of "Wind" and is treated as such.

Common cold and influenza may manifest primarily with symptoms of Wind-Cold or Wind-Heat. These are the two major types of Wind and most other types may be treated by modifying basic formulae for Wind-Cold or Wind-Heat.

THE SIX STAGES

The symptomatology of Wind-Cold was discussed by Zhang Zhong Jing in the "Discussion of Cold-induced Diseases" (c. AD 220) where he first elaborated the theory of the 6 Stages. These are:

- *Greater Yang*
  Wind-Cold with prevalence of Cold
  Wind-Cold with prevalence of Wind
- *Bright Yang*
  Channel pattern (Stomach-Heat)
  Organ pattern (Stomach-Fire)
- *Lesser Yang*
- *Greater Yin*
- *Lesser Yin*
- *Terminal Yin.*

The first stage, Greater Yang, is the only Exterior one. At this stage Wind-Cold is on the Exterior and only the Lung's Defensive-Qi portion is affected, not the Interior. The Lung's dispersing and descending of Qi is impaired and the external Wind is lodged in the space between skin and muscles impairing the circulation of Defensive-Qi.

The essential symptoms of the Greater Yang stage are:

- aversion to cold and shivering
- occipital headache and/or stiff neck
- Floating pulse.

"Aversion to cold" indicates the typical cold feeling and shivering which comes on as a wave in the beginning stages of a cold or influenza. It is characteristic in so far as it is not relieved by covering oneself. Most people who experience a bad cold or flu shiver even in bed under the blankets.

The occipital headache or stiffness is due to the obstruction of Defensive-Qi circulation in the Greater Yang channels (Small Intestine and Bladder) which flow in that area.

The Floating pulse reflects the rushing of Defensive Qi towards the Exterior to fight the pathogenic factor.

Besides these three cardinal symptoms there are many others such as a runny nose, sneezing, possibly a fever, a cough, body aches, itchy throat, etc. All these are due to the impairment of the dispersing and descending of Qi by the Lungs and by the obstruction to the circulation of Defensive-Qi in the muscles.

THE FOUR LEVELS

The symptomatology of Wind-Heat was elaborated in detail by the School of Warm Diseases mentioned above. In particular, Ye Tian Shi (1667–1746) formulated the theory of the 4 Levels to describe the symptomatology of invasions of Wind-Heat. The 4 Levels are:

- *Defensive-Qi Level*
  Wind-Heat
  Damp-Heat
  Summer-Heat
  Wind-Dry-Heat
- *Qi Level*
  Lung-Heat
  Stomach-Heat
  Stomach and Intestines Dry-Heat
  Gall-Bladder Heat
  Stomach and Spleen Damp-Heat
- *Nutritive-Qi Level*
  Heat in Pericardium
  Heat in Nutritive Qi
- *Blood Level*
  Heat Victorious agitates Blood
  Heat Victorious stirs Wind
  Empty-Wind agitates in the Interior
  Collapse of Yin
  Collapse of Yang.

The first Level concerns the exterior stage of an invasion of Wind-Heat, the other three Levels describe pathological conditions which arise when the pathogenic factor penetrates the Interior and turns into Heat. The four Levels represent different levels of energetic depth, the first being the Exterior and the other three being the Interior. The interesting part of this theory is the distinction, within the Interior, of three different levels, the Qi Level being the most superficial (within the Interior) and the Blood Level the deepest.

The Defensive-Qi Level of the 4 Levels broadly corresponds to the Greater Yang Stage of the 6 Stages. The former deals with Wind-Heat and the latter with Wind-Cold. Although the clinical manifestations are different, they share common features as they are both characterized by an invasion of an exterior pathogenic factor, the impairment of the Lung's dispersing and descending of Qi and the obstruction of Defensive-Qi in the space between the skin and muscles. For this reason, in this chapter I shall refer to both the Greater Yang Stage of the 6 Stages and the Defensive-Qi Level of the 4 Levels as "Defensive-Qi Level".

The main symptoms of invasion of Wind-Heat are aversion to cold, shivering, fever, sore throat, swollen tonsils, headache and body-aches, sneezing, cough, runny nose with yellow discharge, slightly dark urine, slightly Red sides of the tongue and a Floating-Rapid pulse. It is worth noting that in Wind-Heat too there is aversion to cold as this is due to Wind-Heat obstructing the Defensive-Qi which therefore fails to warm the muscles.

Table 34.1 compares the manifestations and pathology of invasions of Wind-Cold and Wind-Heat.

Thus, common cold and influenza will always start with manifestations similar to the Greater Yang stage of the 6 Stages or the Defensive-Qi level of the 4 Levels depending on whether the pathogenic factor is Wind-Cold or Wind-Heat. If the pathogenic factor is not expelled at the beginning stages, it will change into Heat and penetrate into the Interior.

Once the pathogenic factor penetrates into the Interior, the body's Qi carries on its fight against it in the Interior: this causes a high fever and a feeling of heat, in marked contrast to the aversion to cold and the shivering which occur when the body's Qi fights the pathogenic factor on the Exterior. At the exterior level, the internal organs are not affected and it is only the Lung's Defensive-Qi portion which is involved. When the pathogenic factor becomes interior, the organs are affected and especially the Lungs and/or Stomach (see below).

This stage of development in the pathology of these diseases is crucial as, if the pathogenic factor is not cleared, it may either penetrate more deeply and cause serious problems (at the Nutritive-Qi or Blood Level) or give rise to residual Heat which is often the cause of chronic post-viral fatigue syndromes. Table 34.2 compares and contrasts the Defensive-Qi and Qi levels of the 4 Levels.

Table 34.1   Comparison of Wind-Cold and Wind-Heat

	Wind-Cold	Wind-Heat
Pathology	Wind-Cold obstructing Defensive Qi	Wind-Heat injuring Defensive Qi and impairing the descending of Lung-Qi
Penetration of pathogenic factor	Via skin	Via nose and mouth
Fever	Light	High
Aversion to cold	Pronounced	Slight
Body aches	Severe	Slight
Thirst	None	Slight
Urine	Pale	Slightly dark
Headache	Occipital	Whole head
Sweating	No sweating or slight sweating on head	Slight sweating
Tongue	No change	Slightly Red on the sides and/or front
Pulse	Floating-Tight	Floating-Rapid
Treatment	Pungent-warm herbs to cause sweating	Pungent-cool herbs to release the Exterior

Table 34.2   Comparison of Defensive-Qi and Qi levels

Level	Eight principles diff.	Internal organs diff.	Body's Qi condition	Location
Defensive Qi	Exterior, Hot, Full	Not affected	Relatively strong	Body's Qi fights on the Exterior
Qi	Interior, Hot, Full	Affected	Relatively strong	Body's Qi fights in the Interior

In the Interior, the main patterns appearing will be either the Bright Yang pattern of the 6 Stages or, more commonly, one of the Qi-Level patterns within the 4 Levels. In general, at the Qi Level, either the Stomach or Lung or both are affected. Wu Ju Tong clearly explained why this should be:

Exterior Wind-Heat penetrates via the mouth and nose, the mouth opens into the Stomach and the nose opens into the Lungs; if Wind-Heat is not expelled [while it is] in the Upper Burner, it will penetrate into the Middle Burner.[1]

The various patterns for both the 6 Stages and 4 Levels at the Qi level are illustrated in Figure 34.4.

The Bright Yang channel and Bright Yang organ patterns of the Bright Yang Stage are exactly the same as Stomach-Heat and Stomach and Intestines Dry Heat of the Qi Level respectively. For this reason, in this chapter I shall refer to both the Bright Yang Stage of the 4 Stages and the Qi Level of the 4 Levels as "Qi Level".

The Lesser Yang pattern of the 6 Stages is nearly (but not quite) the same as the Gall-Bladder Heat pattern of the 4 Levels.

Table 34.3 illustrates the differences between the four Levels.

To put the Four Levels in a nutshell one could say:

– Defensive-Qi Level: aversion to cold
– Qi Level: aversion to heat
– Nutritive-Qi Level: irritability, fever at night
– Blood Level: bleeding and maculae.

In this chapter I will discuss the symptomatology and treatment of common cold and influenza not only in the initial stages, but also in their second stage, i.e. Qi Level. It is important to be able to differentiate and treat patterns of the Qi Level because in most acupuncture practices we are more likely to see patients after the initial invasion of Wind when the pathogenic factor is at the Qi Level. I shall not discuss the Nutritive-Qi or Blood Levels as we are unlikely to ever see patients at this stage.

I will discuss the following exterior patterns:

1. Wind-Cold
2. Wind-Heat
3. Wind-Damp-Heat
4. Wind-Dry-Heat.

In addition to these I will discuss the treatment of some of the interior patterns at the Qi Level:

1. Lung-Heat
2. Lung Phlegm-Heat
3. Stomach-Heat
4. Stomach and Intestines Dry-Heat
5. Gall-Bladder Heat

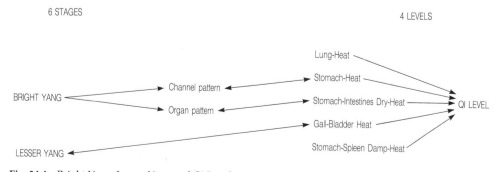

Fig. 34.4   Bright Yang, Lesser Yang and Qi Level patterns

Table 34.3 Comparison of Four levels

Symptoms	Defensive-Qi Level	Qi Level	Nutritive-Qi and Blood Levels
Fever	Slight, aversion to cold	High, aversion to heat	High, at night
Thirst	Slight	Intense	Dry mouth, no desire to drink
Mental state	Unchanged, in children slight irritability	Generally mind clear, if fever is high: delirium	Irritability, delirium, restlessness, coma
Sweating	None or slight	Profuse	None or at night
Tongue	Slightly Red on the sides and/or front	Red body, yellow, brown or black coating	Red, no coating
Pulse	Floating	Rapid, Full	Rapid-Fine or Floating-Empty and Rapid
Pathology	Exterior pattern	Interior pattern, body's Qi strong	Interior pattern, body's Qi weak

6. Lesser Yang pattern
7. Stomach and Spleen Damp-Heat.

The ideal is of course to stop an invasion of an exterior pathogenic factor at the beginning stages. This is not always possible for various reasons: our treatment may not always be the right one, the patient may not take care during the acute invasion, the unnecessary use of antibiotics may aggravate and prolong the condition or the disease may be a Warm disease which cannot be halted completely at the beginning stage in any case. Finally, we may not see the patient until the pathogenic factor is already in the Interior.

Even if, for any of the above reasons, we cannot stop the invasion at the exterior stage, it is still important to stop it at the Qi Level as at this level the condition can become chronic and lead to the development of post-viral fatigue syndromes or myalgic encephalomyelitis (ME).

Differentiation and treatment

The treatment principle of common cold and influenza must be solidly based on the differentiation between Defensive-Qi and Qi Levels. At the Defensive-Qi Level it is imperative to release the Exterior and expel Wind. At the Qi Level, the treatment principle is to clear Qi. In greater detail, the principles of treatment of the two levels are as follows:

1. *DEFENSIVE-QI LEVEL* (or Greater Yang Stage): release the Exterior, expel Wind and restore the dispersing and descending of Lung-Qi. This is achieved by using pungent and floating herbs which release the Exterior. In addition to this:

(a) *Wind-Cold:* expel Wind-Cold with pungent-warm herbs. Examples: Ma Huang *Herba Ephedrae* and Gui Zhi *Ramulus Cinnamomi cassiae.* The representative formula is Ma Huang Tang *Ephedra Decoction.*

(b) *Wind-Heat:* expel Wind and clear Heat with pungent-cool herbs. Examples: Sang Ye *Folium Mori albae,* Bo He *Herba Menthae* and Ju Hua *Flos Chrysanthemi morifolii.* The representative formulae are Yin Qiao San *Lonicera-Forsythia Powder* and Sang Ju Yin *Morus-Chrysanthemum Decoction.*

(c) *Wind-Damp-Heat:* expel Wind, resolve Dampness, clear Heat and harmonize the Centre with herbs which fragrantly resolve Dampness and release the Exterior. Examples: Huo Xiang *Herba Agastachis,* Pei Lan *Herba Eupatorii fortunei,* Cao Guo *Fructus Amomi Tsaoko* and Zi Su Ye *Folium Perillae frutescentis.* The representative formula is Huo Xiang Zheng Qi San *Agastache Upright Qi Powder.*

(d) *Wind-Dry-Heat:* expel Wind, nourish fluids and clear Heat with pungent-cool and sweet-cool herbs. Examples: Sang Ye *Folium Mori albae* and Tian Hua Fen *Radix Trichosanthis.* The representative formula is Sang Xing Tang *Morus-Prunus Decoction.*

2. QI LEVEL: clear Heat at the Qi Level. In addition to this:

(a) *Lung-Heat:* clear Lung-Heat, restore the descending of Lung-Qi and stop cough and asthma with pungent-cold herbs and sinking herbs. Examples: Shi Gao *Gypsum fibrosum* and Xing Ren *Semen Pruni armeniacae*. The representative formula is Ma Xing Shi Gan Tang *Ephedra-Prunus-Gypsum-Glycyrrhiza Decoction*.

(b) *Stomach-Heat:* clear Stomach-Heat and promote the descending of Stomach-Qi with pungent-cold herbs. Examples: Shi Gao *Gypsum fibrosum* and Zhi Mu *Radix Anemarrhenae asphodeloidis*. The representative formula is Bai Hu Tang *White Tiger Decoction*.

(c) *Stomach and Intestines Dry-Heat:* drain Stomach-Fire by purging and nourish fluids if necessary. Examples: Da Huang *Rhizoma Rhei* and Mang Xiao *Mirabilitum*. The representative formula is one of the three variations of Cheng Qi Tang *Conducting Qi Decoction*.

(d) *Gall-Bladder Heat:* harmonize the Lesser Yang and clear Gall-Bladder Heat with bitter-cold and pungent-cool herbs. Examples: Chai Hu *Radix Bupleuri* and Huang Qin *Radix Scutellariae baicalensis*. The representative formula is Hao Qin Qing Dan Tang *Artemisia apiacea-Scutellaria Clearing the Gall-Bladder Decoction* and the Xiao Chai Hu Tang *Small Bupleurum Decoction*.

(e) *Stomach and Spleen Damp-Heat:* clear Heat, resolve Dampness, restore the descending of Stomach-Qi and harmonize the Centre with bitter-cold herbs to make Qi descend, pungent-cool herbs to open Qi, fragrantly-resolving Dampness herbs and bland herbs which drain Dampness. Examples: Huang Lian *Rhizoma Coptidis*, Zi Su Ye *Folium Perillae frutescentis*, Hou Po *Cortex Magnoliae officinalis*, Cang Zhu *Rhizoma Atractylodis lanceae*, Fu Ling *Sclerotium Poriae cocos* and Yi Yi Ren *Semen Coicis lachryma jobi*. The representative formula is Lian Po Yin *Coptis-Magnolia Decoction*.

DEFENSIVE-QI LEVEL

1. WIND-COLD, PREVALENCE OF COLD

CLINICAL MANIFESTATIONS

Aversion to cold, shivering, no fever or very low fever, no sweating, occipital headache, stiff neck, body-aches, slight cough, runny nose with white discharge, sneezing.
Tongue: no change in the initial stages.
Pulse: Floating-Tight.

This is the classical Greater Yang pattern with prevalence of Cold. The absence of sweating indicates the prevalence of Cold. This pattern is an Excess pattern occurring in people with a relatively strong body's Qi.

TREATMENT PRINCIPLE

Release the Exterior, expel Wind, scatter Cold, restore the dispersing and descending of Lung-Qi.

ACUPUNCTURE

LU-7 Lieque, L.I.-4 Hegu, BL-12 Fengmen, G.B.-20 Fengchi, Du-16 Fengfu, BL-13 Feishu, L.I.-20 Yingxiang, Du-23 Shangxing, Du-20 Baihui, KI-7 Fuliu. Reducing method, cupping on BL-12. Direct moxa can be used after withdrawing the needles; for example, on BL-12 or BL-13. Some doctors reinforce the points first and then reduce them in order to summon the Defensive Qi first and then expel the pathogenic factor. They use this method both for Wind-Cold and Wind-Heat.

Explanation

- **LU-7**, **L.I.-4** and **BL-12** are the three most important points to expel Wind-Cold. Cupping on BL-12 is extremely effective. In most cases, just these three points are sufficient to clear the condition. Other points may be selected according to symptoms and signs.
- **G.B.-20** and **Du-16** expel Wind and are selected if the headache and stiff neck are pronounced.
- **BL-13** restores the dispersing and descending of Lung-Qi and is selected if the cough is pronounced.

– **L.I.-20** and **Du-23** expel Wind and clear the nose and are used if sneezing and runny nose are pronounced.
– **Du-20** expels Wind and relieves headache.
– **KI-7** is used in conjunction with L.I.-4 to cause sweating. It should be reinforced while L.I.-4 should be reduced.

HERBAL TREATMENT

(a) Prescription

MA HUANG TANG
Ephedra Decoction
Ma Huang *Herba Ephedrae* 6 g
Gui Zhi *Ramulus Cinnamomi cassiae* 4 g
Xing Ren *Semen Pruni armeniacae* 9 g
Zhi Gan Cao *Radix Glycyrrhizae uralensis praeparata* 3 g

Explanation

This is the classical formula from the "Discussion of Cold-induced Diseases" for the Greater Yang pattern with prevalence of Cold.

– **Ma Huang**, pungent, warm and scattering, is the emperor herb to release the Exterior, expel Wind, scatter Cold and restore the dispersing and descending of Lung-Qi.
– **Gui Zhi**, minister herb, assists Ma Huang in releasing the Exterior and expelling Wind-Cold.
– **Xing Ren**, assistant herb, helps the first two herbs to restore the descending of Lung-Qi and stops cough.
– **Zhi Gan Cao**, messenger herb, harmonizes the other herbs and, being sweet, tempers the scattering effect of Ma Huang.

(b) Prescription

JING FANG JIE BIAO TANG
Schizonepeta-Ledebouriella Releasing the Exterior Decoction
Jing Jie *Herba seu Flos Schizonepetae tenuifoliae* 9 g
Fang Feng *Radix Ledebouriellae sesloidis* 9 g
Zi Su Ye *Folium Perillae frutescentis* 6 g
Qian Hu *Radix Peucedani* 9 g
Jie Geng *Radix Platycodi grandiflori* 6 g

Explanation

– **Jing Jie** and **Fang Feng** expel Wind-Cold and release the Exterior. Fang Feng will also relieve body aches and headache.
– **Zi Su Ye** releases the Exterior and harmonizes the Centre.
– **Qian Hu** and **Jie Geng** restore the descending of Lung-Qi and stop cough.

This formula is selected if body aches, rather than cough and sneezing, are pronounced.

(c) Prescription

CHUAN XIONG CHA TIAO SAN
Ligusticum-Green Tea Regulating Powder
Chuan Xiong *Radix Ligustici wallichii* 6 g
Qiang Huo *Radix et Rhizoma Notopterygii* 6 g
Bai Zhi *Radix Angelicae dahuricae* 6 g
Jing Jie *Herba seu Flos Schizonepetae tenuifoliae* 6 g
Xi Xin *Herba Asari cum radice* 3 g
Fang Feng *Radix Ledebouriellae sesloidis* 6 g
Bo He *Herba Menthae* 3 g
Gan Cao *Radix Glycyrrhizae uralensis* 3 g
Qing Cha (Green Tea) *Folia Cameliae*

Explanation

This formula, which has already been explained in the chapter on "Headaches" (ch. 1), is specific to relieve a headache from exterior Wind-Cold. It also releases the Exterior but its action in this respect is weaker than the previous two formulae.

Variations

These variations apply to all three formulae.

– If body aches are pronounced add (or increase if already in the prescription) Qiang Huo *Radix et Rhizoma Notopterygii* and Du Huo *Radix Angelicae pubescentis*.
– If the headache is pronounced add Gao Ben *Rhizoma et Radix Ligustici sinensis*, Bo He *Herba Menthae* and Chuan Xiong *Radix Ligustici wallichii*.
– If runny nose and sneezing are pronounced add Bai Zhi *Radix Angelicae dahuricae*, Xin Yi

Hua *Flos Magnoliae liliflorae* and Cang Er Zi *Fructus Xanthii*.

- If common cold occurs in summertime add Xiang Ru *Herba Elsholtziae splendentis* which expels Summer-Heat but also deals with invasion of Wind-Cold in summertime. It is called "the Ma Huang of summertime". If Ma Huang Tang is used, either replace Ma Huang with Xiang Ru (which of course turns it into a different formula as the emperor herb cannot be replaced in a prescription) or reduce the dosage of Ma Huang and add Xiang Ru.

(i) Patent remedy

TONG XUAN LI FEI WAN
Penetrating Dispersing and Regulating the Lungs Pill

Ma Huang *Herba Ephedrae*
Zhi Ke *Fructus Citri aurantii*
Jie Geng *Radix Platycodi grandiflori*
Fu Ling *Sclerotium Poriae cocos*
Qian Hu *Radix Peucedani*
Huang Qin *Radix Scutellariae baicalensis*
Chen Pi *Pericarpium Citri reticulatae*
Gan Cao *Radix Glycyrrhizae uralensis*
Ban Xia *Rhizoma Pinelliae ternatae*
Xing Ren *Semen Pruni armeniacae*
Zi Su Ye *Folium Perillae frutescentis*

Explanation

This remedy releases the Exterior, expels Wind-Cold and restores the dispersing and descending of Lung-Qi. It is particularly indicated if there is a cough and frequent sneezing with a profuse white nasal discharge.

Pills or tablets which release the Exterior and expel Wind are more effective if taken with freshly boiled fresh ginger.

(ii) Patent remedy

CHUAN XIONG CHA TIAO WAN
Ligusticum-Green Tea Regulating Pill

Explanation

This remedy has the same ingredients and indi-cations as the above-mentioned decoction of the same name.

Case history

A 42-year-old man was under treatment for asthma when he caught a cold. His symptoms included shivering, an occipital headache, sneezing, a cough and breathlessness. His pulse was Floating. His tongue was usually very Swollen and his asthma was due to Damp-Phlegm obstructing the Lungs.

Diagnosis
This is a clear example of invasion of Wind-Cold over a pre-existing condition of Lung-Qi and Spleen-Qi deficiency with Phlegm.

Treatment principle
The principle of treatment adopted was to release the Exterior, restore the dispersing and descending of Lung-Qi and expel Wind-Cold.

Herbal treatment
The formula used was a variation of Ma Huang Tang *Ephedra Decoction*:

Ma Huang *Herba Ephedrae* 9 g
Gui Zhi *Ramulus Cinnamomi cassiae* 4 g
Xing Ren *Semen Pruni armeniacae* 6 g
Zhi Gan Cao *Radix Glycyrrhizae uralensis praeparata* 3 g
Bai Qian *Radix et Rhizoma Cynanchii stautoni* 6 g
Qian Hu *Radix Peucedani* 6 g
Pi Pa Ye *Folium Eriobotryae japonicae* 6 g

Explanation
- The first four herbs constitute the Ma Huang Tang which releases the Exterior, restores the dispersing and descending of Lung-Qi and expels Wind-Cold.
- **Bai Qian** and **Qian Hu** restore the descending of Lung-Qi, stop cough and resolve Phlegm.
- **Pi Pa Ye** restores the descending of Lung-Qi and stops cough.
- These last three herbs were added to restore the descending of Lung-Qi to ensure that his asthma would not deteriorate as a consequence of the invasion of Wind-Cold.

This formula cleared the cold in two days.

2. WIND-COLD, PREVALENCE OF WIND

CLINICAL MANIFESTATIONS

Aversion to cold, shivering, no fever or very low fever, slight sweating, occipital headache, stiff neck, body aches, slight cough, runny nose with white discharge, sneezing.
Tongue: no change in the initial stages.
Pulse: Floating-Slow.

This is a classical pattern of the Greater Yang when there is prevalence of Wind. It occurs when the body's Qi is relatively weak and Defensive Qi and Nutritive Qi are not harmonized. The deficient Nutritive Qi fails to hold fluids in and causes slight sweating.

TREATMENT PRINCIPLE

Release the Exterior, expel Wind-Cold and harmonize Nutritive and Defensive Qi.

ACUPUNCTURE

LU-7 Lieque, L.I.-4 Hegu, BL-12 Fengmen (with cupping), ST-36 Zusanli, G.B.-20 Fengchi, Du-16 Fengfu, BL-13 Feishu, L.I.-20 Yingxiang, Du-23 Shangxing, BL-18 Ganshu. Reducing method on all points, even method on ST-36 and BL-18 Ganshu.

Explanation

- **LU-7**, **L.I.-4** and **BL-12** are the three most important points to expel Wind-Cold. Cupping on BL-12 is extremely effective. In most cases, just these three points are sufficient to clear the condition. Other points may be selected according to symptoms and signs and these have already been explained under the previous pattern.
- **ST-36** harmonizes Nutritive and Defensive Qi.
- **BL-18**: some doctors use this point to nourish Nutritive Qi and Blood and therefore harmonize Nutritive and Defensive Qi.

HERBAL TREATMENT

Prescription

GUI ZHI TANG
Ramulus Cinnamomi Decoction
Gui Zhi *Ramulus Cinnamomi cassiae* 9 g
Bai Shao *Radix Paeoniae albae* 9 g
Sheng Jiang *Rhizoma Zingiberis officinalis recens* 9 g

Da Zao *Fructus Ziziphi jujubae* 3 dates
Zhi Gan Cao *Radix Glycyrrhizae uralensis praeparata* 6 g

Explanation

- **Gui Zhi** releases the Exterior and expels Wind-Cold.
- **Bai Shao** tonifies the Nutritive Qi. Together with Gui Zhi, they harmonize Defensive and Nutritive Qi.
- **Sheng Jiang** assists Gui Zhi in expelling Wind-Cold.
- **Da Zao** assists Bai Shao in tonifying the Nutritive Qi. Together with Sheng Jiang, they harmonize Defensive and Nutritive Qi.
- **Gan Cao** harmonizes.

Variations

- If there is a pronounced stiffness of the neck and other muscles add Ge Gen *Radix Puerariae*. This makes the Gui Zhi Jia Ge Gen Tang *Ramulus Cinnamomi Decoction plus Pueraria*.
- If there is cough and breathlessness add Hou Po *Cortex Magnoliae officinalis* and Xing Ren *Semen Pruni armeniacae*. This makes the Gui Zhi Jia Hou Po Xing Zi Tang *Ramulus Cinnamomi Decoction plus Magnolia and Prunus*.

3. WIND-HEAT

CLINICAL MANIFESTATIONS

Aversion to cold, shivering, fever, slight sweating, runny nose with yellow discharge, headache, body-aches, cough, sore throat, swollen tonsils, slight thirst, slightly dark urine.
Tongue: slightly Red on the sides and/or front.
Pulse: Floating-Rapid.

TREATMENT PRINCIPLE

Release the Exterior, expel Wind-Heat and restore the dispersing and descending of Lung-Qi.

ACUPUNCTURE

L.I.-4 Hegu, L.I.-11 Quchi, T.B.-5 Waiguan, BL-12 Fengmen (with cupping), BL-13 Feishu, Du-14 Dazhui, LU-11 Shaoshang, G.B.-20 Fengchi, Du-16 Fengfu. Reducing method.

Explanation

– **L.I.-4**, **L.I.-11** and **T.B.-5** are the three main points to expel Wind-Heat. Other points are selected according to symptoms and signs.
– **BL-12** releases the Exterior and expels Wind.
– **BL-13** stimulates the dispersing and descending of Lung-Qi and stops cough.
– **Du-14** is selected if symptoms of Heat are pronounced (e.g. high fever). It should be needled obliquely downwards and one should preferably obtain a strong needling sensation propagating downwards.
– **LU-11**, with bleeding method, expels Wind-Heat and soothes the throat and is selected if the throat and tonsils are sore, swollen and inflamed.
– **G.B.-20** and **Du-16** expel Wind and are selected if the headache is severe.

HERBAL TREATMENT

(a) Prescription

YIN QIAO SAN
Lonicera-Forsythia Powder
Jin Yin Hua *Flos Lonicerae japonicae* 9 g
Lian Qiao *Fructus Forsythiae suspensae* 9 g
Jie Geng *Radix Platycodi grandiflori* 6 g
Niu Bang Zi *Fructus Arctii lappae* 9 g
Bo He *Herba Menthae* 6 g
Jing Jie *Herba seu Flos Schizonepetae tenuifoliae* 5 g
Zhu Ye *Herba Lophatheri gracilis* 4 g
Dan Dou Chi *Semen Sojae praeparatum* 5 g
Gan Cao *Radix Glycyrrhizae uralensis* 5 g

Explanation

– **Jin Yin Hua** and **Lian Qiao** expel Wind-Heat, release the Exterior and resolve Fire-Poison. This last function makes them suitable to treat an inflamed throat and tonsils.

– **Jie Geng** and **Niu Bang Zi** circulate Lung-Qi, expel Wind-Heat and soothe the throat.
– **Bo He** and **Jing Jie** help to release the Exterior and expel Wind. Bo He also relieves headache.
– **Zhu Ye** clears Heat.
– **Dan Dou Chi** expels Wind-Heat and relieves the irritability deriving from Wind-Heat, especially in children.
– **Gan Cao** resolves Poison and harmonizes.

This formula is the most effective for treating mild to moderate cases of invasion of Wind-Heat. It is excellent to treat sore and swollen throat and tonsils and is particularly effective for children. It should be used at the earliest possible time in the initial stages of an invasion of Wind-Heat. If there is any doubt whether the condition is one of Wind-Cold or Wind-Heat, it is preferable to treat it as Wind-Heat with the Yin Qiao San.

Traditionally, this formula was taken as a powder with freshly and lightly boiled lotus root. If it is used as a decoction, it should be simmered only for a short time (under 15 minutes) in order that it enter the Upper Burner and go to the Exterior. If it is boiled for too long it will enter the Middle Burner. Wu Ju Tong, the creator of this formula, said: *"Treat the Upper Burner like a feather, very lightly but not so as to raise it."*[2]

In mild cases it should be taken twice a day. In severe cases it can be taken four times a day.

(b) Prescription

SANG JU YIN
Morus-Chrysanthemum Decoction
Sang Ye *Folium Mori albae* 6 g
Ju Hua *Flos Chrysanthemi morifolii* 3 g
Bo He *Herba Menthae* 3 g
Xing Ren *Semen Pruni armeniacae* 6 g
Jie Geng *Radix Platycodi grandiflori* 6 g
Lian Qiao *Fructus Forsythiae suspensae* 6 g
Lu Gen *Rhizoma Phragmitis communis* 6 g
Gan Cao *Radix Glycyrrhizae uralensis* 3 g

Explanation

– **Sang Ye** and **Ju Hua** release the Exterior, expel Wind-Heat and restore the descending

of Lung-Qi. Sang Ye also soothes the throat and stops cough. Ju Hua benefits the eyes which may be affected in invasions of Wind-Heat.
- **Bo He** helps to expel Wind-Heat.
- **Xing Ren** and **Jie Geng** restore the descending of Lung-Qi, soothe the throat and stop cough.
- **Lian Qiao** expels Wind-Heat and resolves Fire-Poison. It will help the sore and swollen throat and tonsils.
- **Lu Gen** clears Heat and benefits fluids. It therefore prevents injury of Lung- and Stomach-fluids by Heat.
- **Gan Cao** harmonizes and resolves Fire-Poison.

This formula is similar to the previous one but it is better at restoring the descending of Lung-Qi and stopping cough. It is milder in action than the Yin Qiao San. Table 34.4 compares and contrasts Yin Qiao San and Sang Ju Yin.

(i) Patent remedy

YIN QIAO JIE DU WAN (or PIAN)
Lonicera-Forsythia Expelling Poison Pill (or Tablet)

Explanation

This pill has all the same ingredients, functions and applications as the decoction. It is extremely effective to release the Exterior, expel Wind-Heat and resolve Fire-Poison. Due to its latter function, it is very effective for swollen glands and an inflamed throat and tonsils.

It should be a stand-by in any household, especially those with children. If there is any doubt

Table 34.4 Comparison of Yin Qiao San and Sang Ju Yin

Yin Qiao San	Sang Ju Yin
Not so good at restoring the descending of Lung-Qi	Better at restoring the descending of Lung-Qi
Strong action in expelling Wind-Heat	Less strong in expelling Wind-Heat
Resolves Fire-Poison	Resolves Fire-Poison only mildly
For severe cases	For milder cases
Better for releasing the Exterior and treating body aches	Not so good for treating body aches
Not so good for cough	Specific to treat cough

whether the invasion is one of Wind-Cold or Wind-Heat, it can still be used due to its expelling-Wind action and also because, at least in children, Wind-Heat is more common than Wind-Cold. If the condition later turns out to be more clearly caused by Wind-Cold, change to a different pill.

The tongue presentation appropriate to this remedy is slightly Red sides and/or front: in children the same areas frequently have red points in invasions of Wind-Heat.

(ii) Patent remedy

SANG JU GAN MAO PIAN
Morus-Chrysanthemum Common Cold Tablet

Explanation

This remedy has the same ingredients and indications as the above-mentioned decoction Sang Ju Yin. It is used if cough and sore throat are the predominant symptoms.

The tongue presentation appropriate to this remedy is slightly Red front.

(iii) Patent remedy

GAN MAO DAN
Common Cold Pill
Jin Yin Hua *Flos Lonicerae japonicae*
Lian Qiao *Fructus Forsythiae suspensae*
Shan Zhi Zi *Fructus Gardeniae jasminoidis*
Lu Gen *Rhizoma Phragmitis communis*
Chi Shao *Radix Paeoniae rubrae*
Bai Mao Gen *Rhizoma Imperatae cylindricae*
Dan Dou Chi *Semen Sojae praeparatum*
Bo He *Herba Menthae*
Sang Ye *Folium Mori albae*
Jing Jie *Herba seu Flos Schizonepetae tenuifoliae*
Zi Wan *Radix Asteris tatarici*
Jie Geng *Radix Platycodi grandiflori*
Chen Pi *Pericarpium Citri reticulatae*

Explanation

This pill releases the Exterior, expels Wind-Heat and resolves Fire-Poison. It is similar to the Yin Qiao Pill but stronger in its action.

The tongue presentation appropriate to this remedy is Red sides and/or front.

Case history

A 6-year-old boy had come down with an upper-respiratory infection the day before the consultation. His symptoms included a fever, a cough, shivering, a sore throat, swollen tonsils, a headache and a rash. This consisted of small, sparse, red papules. His tongue was Red in the front part, with red points in the front and sides (Plate 34.1).

Diagnosis
This is an invasion of Wind-Heat with some symptoms of Fire-Poison (the swollen tonsils). The rash indicates invasion of the Lung's Defensive-Qi portion by Wind-Heat. The position of red points on the front and sides of the tongue clearly shows the location of the pathogenic factor on the Exterior.

Treatment principle
The principle of treatment adopted was to expel Wind-Heat, release the Exterior, restore the descending of Lung-Qi and resolve Fire-Poison. This boy was treated with herbs only which, with some patience and imagination from his mother, he was able to drink.

Herbal treatment
The formula used was a variation of Yin Qiao San *Lonicera-Forsythia Powder* and the dosages used were not much lower than those used for an adult. The reason for this approach is that children will rarely finish each dose of a decoction and therefore the dose a child takes is accordingly a reduced one.

Jin Yin Hua *Flos Lonicerae japonicae* 6 g
Lian Qiao *Fructus Forsythiae suspensae* 6 g
Jie Geng *Radix Platycodi grandiflori* 4 g
Niu Bang Zi *Fructus Arctii lappae* 6 g
Bo He *Herba Menthae* 4 g
Jing Jie *Herba seu Flos Schizonepetae tenuifoliae* 5 g
Zhu Ye *Herba Lophatheri gracilis* 4 g
Dan Dou Chi *Semen Sojae praeparatum* 5 g
Gan Cao *Radix Glycyrrhizae uralensis* 3 g
Kuan Dong Hua *Flos Tussilaginis farfarae* 4 g
Huang Qin *Radix Scutellariae baicalensis* 4 g
Da Qing Ye *Folium Isatidis seu Baphicacanthi* 6 g

Explanation
- The first 9 herbs constitute the Yin Qiao San which releases the Exterior, expels Wind-Heat and resolves Fire-Poison.
- **Kuan Dong Hua** restores the descending of Lung-Qi and stops cough.
- **Huang Qin** clears interior Heat. This herb was added first of all to enhance the clearing-Heat effect of the prescription and secondly because Wind-Heat has the tendency to turn into interior Heat

fairly rapidly, especially in children. I therefore often add this herb which clears interior Heat, to expelling Wind-Heat prescriptions, especially in children.
- **Da Qing Ye** was added to resolve Fire-Poison from the throat. From a Western point of view, it has antibacterial and antiviral properties.

This formula cleared up the problem in 2 days.

Case history

A 51-year-old woman who was being treated for a chronic herpes infection, caught an acute infection manifesting with symptoms of Wind-Heat. Her main symptoms included shivering, a temperature, a sore throat, very swollen and purulent tonsils, a headache, aches in the body, and a cough. Her tongue was Red in the front part with a thick yellow coating and red points. Her pulse was Floating and slightly Rapid.

Diagnosis
This is a severe invasion of Wind-Heat with symptoms of Fire-Poison as well. Apart from the symptoms, the definitely Red colour of the tongue with red points and thick yellow coating indicate the severity of the attack. In exterior conditions, the thickness of the coating accurately reflects the intensity of the pathogenic factor.

Treatment principle
The treatment principle adopted was to release the Exterior, expel Wind-Heat, restore the descending of Lung-Qi and resolve Fire-Poison.

Herbal treatment
The prescription used was a variation of Yin Qiao San *Lonicera-Forsythia Powder*:

Jin Yin Hua *Flos Lonicerae japonicae* 9 g
Lian Qiao *Fructus Forsythiae suspensae* 9 g
Jie Geng *Radix Platycodi grandiflori* 4 g
Niu Bang Zi *Fructus Arctii lappae* 6 g
Bo He *Herba Menthae* 4 g
Jing Jie *Herba seu Flos Schizonepetae tenuifoliae* 5 g
Zhu Ye *Herba Lophatheri gracilis* 9 g
Dan Dou Chi *Semen Sojae praeparatum* 5 g
Gan Cao *Radix Glycyrrhizae uralensis* 3 g
Da Qing Ye *Folium Isatidis seu Baphicacanthi* 6 g
She Gan *Rhizoma Belamcandae chinensis* 4 g
Huang Qin *Radix Scutellariae baicalensis* 4 g

Explanation
- The first nine herbs constitute the root formula which releases the Exterior, expels Wind-Heat and resolves Fire-Poison.
- **Da Qing Ye** and **She Gan** resolve Fire-Poison from the throat and were added to strengthen this particular action within the formula.
- **Huang Qin** was added to clear Heat as severe Wind-Heat easily turns into interior Heat.

Most of the symptoms went after 2 days of taking this decoction twice a day. After 3 days she was left with dizziness, a yellow nasal discharge and sinus pain, a feeling of heaviness of the head, a dry cough and tiredness. Her tongue went back to a normal colour although it still had a thin, dry yellow coating. These are symptoms of dryness in the Lungs with some residual Lung-Heat: a very common outcome of a severe invasion of Wind-Heat. I prescribed a variation of the formula Qing Zao Jiu Fei Tang *Clearing Dryness and Rescuing the Lungs Decoction*:

Sang Ye *Folium Mori albae* 9 g
Shi Gao *Gypsum fibrosum* 7.5 g
Mai Men Dong *Tuber Ophiopogonis japonici* 3.6 g
Ren Shen *Radix Ginseng* 2 g
Hu Ma Ren (Hei Zhi Ma) *Semen Sesami indici* 3 g
Xing Ren *Semen Pruni armeniacae* 2 g
Pi Pa Ye *Folium Eriobotryae japonicae* 3 g
Gan Cao *Radix Glycyrrhizae uralensis* 3 g
Bai Zhi *Radix Angelicae dahuricae* 3 g
Jin Yin Hua *Flos Lonicerae japonicae* 4 g
Zhi Zi *Fructus Gardeniae jasminoidis* 4 g
Dan Dou Chi *Semen Sojae praeparatum* 4 g

Explanation
- The first eight herbs constitute the root formula which moistens Dryness, clears residual Lung-Heat and nourishes Lung-Yin. E Jiao was omitted.
- **Bai Zhi** and **Jin Yin Hua** were added to resolve Fire-Poison from the sinuses.
- **Zhi Zi** and **Dan Dou Chi** clear residual Heat.

After four doses of this decoction the problem was completely resolved.

4. WIND-DAMP-HEAT

CLINICAL MANIFESTATIONS

Aversion to cold, shivering, fever, a feeling of heaviness of the head and body, nausea, vomiting, swollen glands, headache, feeling worse in the afternoon, a feeling of oppression of the chest and epigastrium, a sticky taste.
Tongue: sticky-yellow coating.
Pulse: Slippery and Floating.

This corresponds to the beginning stages of an invasion of Wind-Heat combined with exterior Dampness. Because Wind-Heat affects the Upper Burner and Dampness more the Middle Burner, besides the usual symptoms there is also nausea, a sticky taste and a feeling of oppression of the epigastrium. Obstruction of the muscles by Dampness causes the feeling of heaviness.

TREATMENT PRINCIPLE

Release the Exterior, expel Wind-Heat and resolve Dampness.

ACUPUNCTURE

L.I.-4 Hegu, L.I.-11 Quchi, SP-9 Yinlingquan, Ren-13 Shangwan, T.B.-5 Waiguan, Du-14 Dazhui, LU-11 Shaoshang. Reducing method.

Explanation

- **L.I.-4** and **L.I.-11** release the Exterior, expel Wind-Heat and resolve Damp-Heat.
- **SP-9** resolves Damp-Heat.
- **Ren-13** resolves Dampness, harmonizes the Centre and subdues rebellious Stomach-Qi.
- **T.B.-5** expels Wind-Heat.
- **Du-14** clears Heat and is selected if Heat is pronounced (high fever).
- **LU-11**, with bleeding method, expels Wind-Heat and treats inflamed tonsils.

HERBAL TREATMENT

(a) Prescription

HUO PO XIA LING TANG
Agastache-Magnolia-Pinellia-Poria Decoction
Huo Xiang *Herba Agastachis* 6 g
Hou Po *Cortex Magnoliae officinalis* 3 g
Bai Dou Kou *Fructus Amomi cardamomi* 2 g
Fu Ling *Sclerotium Poriae cocos* 9 g
Yi Yi Ren *Semen Coicis lachryma jobi* 12 g
Zhu Ling *Sclerotium Polypori umbellati* 4.5 g
Ze Xie *Rhizoma Alismatis orientalis* 4.5 g
Ban Xia *Rhizoma Pinelliae ternatae* 4.5 g
Xing Ren *Semen Pruni armeniacae* 9 g
Dan Dou Chi *Semen Sojae praeparatum* 9 g

Explanation

- **Huo Xiang**, **Hou Po** and **Bai Dou Kou** fragrantly resolve Dampness.
- **Fu Ling**, **Yi Yi Ren**, **Zhu Ling** and **Ze Xie** drain Dampness via urination.

- **Ban Xia** helps to resolve Dampness by resolving Phlegm and harmonizing the Stomach.
- **Xing Ren** helps to resolve Dampness by restoring the descending of Qi.
- **Dan Dou Chi** releases the Exterior, expels Wind-Heat and relieves the irritability deriving from Wind-Heat.

(b) Prescription

HUO XIANG ZHENG QI SAN
Agastache Upright Qi Powder
Huo Xiang *Herba Agastachis* 9 g
Zi Su Ye *Folium Perillae frutescentis* 3 g
Bai Zhi *Radix Angelicae dahuricae* 3 g
Ban Xia *Rhizoma Pinelliae ternatae* 6 g
Chen Pi *Pericarpium Citri reticulatae* 6 g
Bai Zhu *Rhizoma Atractylodis macrocephalae* 6 g
Fu Ling *Sclerotium Poriae cocos* 3 g
Hou Po *Cortex Magnoliae officinalis* 6 g
Da Fu Pi *Pericarpium Arecae catechu* 3 g
Jie Geng *Radix Platycodi grandiflori* 6 g
Sheng Jiang *Rhizoma Zingiberis officinalis recens* 3 slices
Da Zao *Fructus Ziziphi jujubae* 3 dates
Zhi Gan Cao *Radix Glycyrrhizae uralensis praeparata* 3 g

Explanation

This formula, which has already been explained in chapter 18, resolves Dampness and releases the Exterior. The previous formula is better at releasing the Exterior, while this one is better at resolving Dampness.

The key patterns for the use of this formula are exterior invasion of Wind-Cold with interior retention of Dampness in the Stomach. The main symptoms are aversion to cold, fever, nausea, vomiting and diarrhoea. It is also frequently used for food poisoning or any seasonal infection which affects the Stomach and Spleen causing vomiting and diarrhoea.

(i) Patent remedy

HUO XIANG ZHENG QI WAN
Agastache Upright Qi Pill

Explanation

This remedy has the same ingredients and indications as the homonymous prescription above. An invaluable patent remedy which should also be stocked in any household, it is also extremely useful when travellers find a change of climate, food and water causes nausea, vomiting, and diarrhoea.

The tongue presentation appropriate to this remedy is a sticky-white coating.

(ii) Patent remedy

SHEN QU CHA
Massa Fermentata Tea
Qing Hao *Herba Artemisiae apiaceae*
Huang Qin *Radix Scutellariae baicalensis*
Xiang Ru *Herba Elsholtziae splendentis*
Qiang Huo *Radix et Rhizoma Notopterygii*
Du Huo *Radix Angelicae pubescentis*
Qing Pi *Pericarpium Citri reticulatae viridae*
Hu Po *Succinum*
Cao Guo *Fructus Amomi Tsaoko*
Mu Gua *Fructus Chaenomelis lagenariae*
Jie Geng *Radix Platycodi grandiflori*
Shan Yao *Radix Dioscoreae oppositae*
Fu Ling *Sclerotium Poriae cocos*
Gan Cao *Radix Glycyrrhizae uralensis*
Shen Qu *Massa Fermentata Medicinalis*

Explanation

This remedy, which comes in small blocks of dried powdered medicine, can either be decocted for a short time or infused as tea. It releases the Exterior and resolves Dampness and may be used both for Wind-Cold or Wind-Heat, especially for common cold in summertime with some symptoms of Dampness such as nausea, epigastric fullness and diarrhoea.

Case history

An 8-year-old girl was brought by her mother complaining of shivering, vomiting, a dull frontal headache, epigastric fullness and general malaise. These symptoms had appeared 2 days earlier. Her tongue had a sticky coating and a few red points around the centre.

Diagnosis
This is an external invasion of Damp-Heat (with the former being more predominant than the latter) at the Defensive-Qi Level. Defensive-Qi Level is indicated by the shivering.

Treatment principle
The treatment principle adopted was to release the Exterior, resolve Dampness, restore the descending of Stomach-Qi and clear Heat.

Herbal treatment
The formula used was a variation of Huo Xiang Zheng Qi San *Agastache Upright Qi Powder*:

Huo Xiang *Herba Agastachis* 6 g
Zi Su Ye *Folium Perillae frutescentis* 3 g
Ban Xia *Rhizoma Pinelliae ternatae* 6 g
Chen Pi *Pericarpium Citri reticulatae* 3 g
Fu Ling *Sclerotium Poriae cocos* 6 g
Hou Po *Cortex Magnoliae officinalis* 4 g
Da Fu Pi *Pericarpium Arecae catechu* 3 g
Sheng Jiang *Rhizoma Zingiberis officinalis recens* 3 slices
Da Zao *Fructus Ziziphi jujubae* 3 dates
Zhi Gan Cao *Radix Glycyrrhizae uralensis praeparata* 3 g

Explanation
This is the root formula which resolves Dampness at the Defensive-Qi Level and restores the descending of Stomach-Qi. Bai Zhi *Radix Angelicae dahuricae*, Bai Zhu *Rhizoma Atractylodis macrocephalae* and Jie Geng *Radix Platycodi grandiflori* were eliminated as they did not correspond to her symptoms.

She took this formula as a decoction for 5 days, after which the problem was cleared.

5. WIND-DRY-HEAT

CLINICAL MANIFESTATIONS

Aversion to cold, fever, slight sweating, dryness of nose, mouth and throat, dry cough.
Tongue: slightly Red in the front, dry.
Pulse: Floating.

This pattern occurs in places with a very dry climate such as Arizona or New Mexico. However, it may also occur when someone who has been invaded by Wind is subsequently in a very dry, centrally-heated house or work place.

TREATMENT PRINCIPLE

Release the Exterior, expel Wind, restore the descending of Lung-Qi, benefit fluids.

ACUPUNCTURE

LU-7 Lieque, L.I.-4 Hegu, LU-11 Shaoshang, Ren-12 Zhongwan, SP-6 Sanyinjiao, KI-6 Zhaohai. Reducing method on the first three points and reinforcing on the others.

Explanation

- **LU-7, L.I.-4** and **LU-11** release the Exterior and expel Wind-Heat. LU-11 is bled if there is a sore throat.
- **Ren-12, SP-6** and **KI-6** promote fluids. KI-6 in particular soothes the throat.

HERBAL TREATMENT

Prescription

SANG XING TANG
Morus-Prunus Decoction
Sang Ye *Folium Mori albae* 3 g
Dan Dou Chi *Semen Sojae praeparatum* 3 g
Xing Ren *Semen Pruni armeniacae* 4.5 g
Zhe Bei Mu *Bulbus Fritillariae thunbergii* 3 g
Bei Sha Shen *Radix Glehniae littoralis* 6 g
Li Pi *Fructus Pyri* 3 g
Zhi Zi *Fructus Gardeniae jasminoidis* 3 g

Explanation

- **Sang Ye** and **Dan Dou Chi** release the Exterior, expel Wind-Heat and stop cough.
- **Xing Ren** restores the descending of Lung-Qi.
- **Zhe Bei Mu**, **Sha Shen** and **Li Pi** moisten the Lungs and benefit fluids.
- **Zhi Zi** clears Heat.

In the context of invasions of Wind at the Defensive-Qi level, we can now briefly discuss the treatment of certain symptoms which may be due to either Wind-Cold or Wind-Heat.

HOARSE VOICE

Hoarseness may be caused either by Wind-Cold or Wind-Heat and is due to obstruction of the Lung's Defensive-Qi portion by Wind. The Lung is sometimes compared to a bell: it should be empty and give a clear ringing sound, reflected in a clear and loud voice. If the bell is filled up it cannot ring: similarly, when the Lungs are obstructed by a pathogenic factor the voice may be affected and become hoarse or it may be lost completely.

The points to use, all with reducing method, are:

- **Ren-23** Lianquan to benefit the throat.
- **Du-14** Dazhui to clear Heat and expel Wind.
- **L.I.-11** Quchi and **L.I.-4** Hegu to expel Wind-Heat.
- **LU-7** Lieque to promote the descending of Lung-Qi and clear the throat.
- **HE-5** Tongli to benefit the throat.

ACUTE TONSILLITIS

Acute tonsillitis is caused by Wind-Heat and, if severe, Fire-Poison. The points to be used, all with reducing method, are:

- **L.I.-11** Quchi, **L.I.-4** Hegu and **ST-44** Neiting to expel Wind-Heat and clear Stomach-Heat (which often causes tonsillitis).
- **Ren-22** Tiantu, **LU-11** Shaoshang and **LU-10** Yuji to expel Wind-Heat, resolve Fire-Poison and soothe the throat. If there is a temperature bleed LU-11. If the fever is high add Du-14 Dazhui.

SORE THROAT

A sore throat is usually due to Wind-Heat. The points to use, all with reducing method, are:

- **LU-11** Shaoshang and **L.I.-4** Hegu to expel Wind-Heat and benefit the throat.
- **ST-43** Xiangu to clear Stomach-Heat which often causes sore throat, especially in children.

QI LEVEL

1. LUNG-HEAT

CLINICAL MANIFESTATIONS

High fever, feeling of heat, cough, breathless-ness, coughing of yellow sputum, thirst, restless-ness, sweating.
Tongue: Red with yellow coating.
Pulse: Overflowing and Rapid.

This pattern occurs when the external Wind-Heat changes into interior Heat and enters the Lungs. From a Western point of view, acute bronchitis following a common cold or influenza is an example of such a pattern.

TREATMENT PRINCIPLE

Clear Lung-Heat, prevent injury of Yin by Heat.

ACUPUNCTURE

LU-10 Yuji, LU-5 Chize, LU-1 Zhongfu, Du-14 Dazhui, SP-6 Sanyinjiao. Reducing method.

Explanation

- **LU-10** clears Lung-Heat.
- **LU-5** resolves Phlegm-Heat from the Lungs.
- **LU-1** clears Lung-Heat.
- **Du-14** clears Heat.
- **SP-6** stops sweating and prevents injury of Yin by Heat.

HERBAL TREATMENT

Prescription

MA XING SHI GAN TANG
Ephedra-Prunus-Gypsum-Glycyrrhiza Decoction
Ma Huang *Herba Ephedrae* 5 g
Xing Ren *Semen Pruni armeniacae* 9 g
Shi Gao *Gypsum fibrosum* 18 g
Zhi Gan Cao *Radix Glycyrrhizae uralensis prae-parata* 6 g

Explanation

This formula is used for a combined condition of Greater Yang and Bright Yang pattern. However, by reducing the dosage of Ma Huang and increasing that of Shi Gao, it can be used to treat Lung-Heat at the Qi Level.

- **Shi Gao** clears Lung-Heat.
- **Xing Ren** restores the descending of Lung-Qi and stops cough and breathlessness.
- **Ma Huang** restores the descending of Lung-Qi and stops breathlessness.
- **Gan Cao** harmonizes.

(i) Patent remedy

ZHI SOU DING CHUAN WAN
Stopping Cough and Calming Breathlessness Pill

Explanation

This remedy has the same ingredients and indications as Ma Xing Shi Gan Tang explained above.

The tongue presentation appropriate to this remedy is a yellow coating.

(ii) Patent remedy

MA XING ZHI KE PIAN
Ephedra-Prunus Cough Tablet
Ma Huang *Herba Ephedrae*
Xing Ren *Semen Pruni armeniacae*
Shi Gao *Gypsum fibrosum*
Gan Cao *Radix Glycyrrhizae uralensis*
Jie Geng *Radix Platycodi grandiflori*
Chen Pi *Pericarpium Citri reticulatae*
Hua Shi *Talcum*
Feng Mi *Mel*

Explanation

This remedy is based on the above decoction Ma Xing Shi Gan Tang with similar indications. It clears Lung-Heat and restores the descending of Lung-Qi. It is therefore suitable to treat cough, breathlessness, chest pain and fever following an invasion of Wind.

Compared to the previous remedy, it is better at treating cough.

2. LUNG PHLEGM-HEAT

CLINICAL MANIFESTATIONS

High fever, feeling of heat, restlessness, thirst, vomiting after drinking, cough, breathlessness, pain in the chest, coughing of profuse amounts of yellow-sticky sputum, a feeling of oppression of the chest, nausea, dry stools, dark urine.
Tongue: Red with a sticky-yellow coating.
Pulse: Slippery and Rapid.

This pattern is similar to the previous one in so far as there is Lung-Heat but also Phlegm-Heat.

TREATMENT PRINCIPLE

Clear Lung-Heat, resolve Phlegm, restore the descending of Lung-Qi and prevent injury of Yin.

ACUPUNCTURE

LU-5 Chize, LU-1 Zhongfu, ST-40 Fenglong, Ren-22 Tiantu, P-6 Neiguan, SP-6 Sanyinjiao, Du-14 Dazhui. Reducing method except on SP-6 which should be reinforced.

Explanation

- **LU-5** resolves Phlegm-Heat from the Lungs.
- **LU-1** clears Lung-Heat.
- **ST-40** resolves Phlegm.
- **Ren-22** resolves Phlegm and stimulates the descending of Lung-Qi.
- **P-6** opens the chest.
- **SP-6** helps to clear Heat by nourishing Yin.
- **Du-14** clears Heat and is used if there is a high fever.

HERBAL TREATMENT

(a) Prescription

QING QI HUA TAN TANG
Clearing Qi and Resolving Phlegm Decoction
Dan Nan Xing *Rhizoma Arisaematis praeparata* 12 g
Gua Lou *Fructus Trichosanthis* 9 g
Huang Qin *Radix Scutellariae baicalensis* 9 g
Zhi Shi *Fructus Citri aurantii immaturus* 9 g
Chen Pi *Pericarpium Citri reticulatae* 9 g

Fu Ling *Sclerotium Poriae cocos* 9 g
Xing Ren *Semen Pruni armeniacae* 9 g
Fa Ban Xia *Rhizoma Pinelliae ternatae* 12 g

Explanation

This is the typical formula to resolve Phlegm-Heat in the Lungs at the Qi Level in the course of a febrile disease.

– **Nan Xing**, **Gua Lou** and **Ban Xia** resolve Phlegm.
– **Huang Qin** clears Lung-Heat.
– **Zhi Shi** and **Xing Ren** restore the descending of Lung-Heat.
– **Chen Pi** and **Fu Ling** assist the other herbs to resolve Phlegm.

(b) Prescription

XIAO XIAN XIONG TANG JIA ZHI SHI
Small Sinking [Qi of the] Chest Decoction plus Fructus Citri aurantii immaturus
Huang Lian *Rhizoma Coptidis* 6 g
Ban Xia *Rhizoma Pinelliae ternatae* 12 g
Gua Lou *Fructus Trichosanthis* 30 g
Zhi Shi *Fructus Citri aurantii immaturus* 9 g

Explanation

This formula, which is derived from the book "Differentiation of Warm Diseases" by Wu Ju Tong, is specific for Phlegm-Heat in the Lungs at the Qi level. Compared to the previous one, this formula is used when Heat is more evident and when there is a pronounced feeling of oppression of the chest.

– **Huang Lian** and **Ban Xia** are coordinated in this formula. Huang Lian is a bitter herb used to make the Qi of the chest descend to relieve cough and breathlessness. Ban Xia is a pungent herb to open up Qi in the chest and make it move. Besides this, Ban Xia will resolve Phlegm and Huang Lian will help to resolve Phlegm by drying Dampness.
– **Gua Lou** resolves Phlegm-Heat.
– **Zhi Shi** makes Qi descend in the chest and thus helps to resolve Phlegm.

Variations

These variations apply to both above formulae.

– If signs of injury of Lung-Yin are beginning to show add Mai Men Dong *Tuber Ophiopogonis japonici* and Zhi Mu *Radix Anemarrhenae asphodeloidis*.

(i) Patent remedy

QING QI HUA TAN WAN
Clearing Qi and Resolving Phlegm Pill

Explanation

This remedy has the same ingredients and indications as the above-mentioned decoction. This pill is very useful for an acute chest infection following a cold or flu with a cough with profuse yellow sputum, fever, some chest pain and thirst.

The tongue presentation appropriate to this remedy is a Red body with a sticky-yellow coating.

(ii) Patent remedy

QING FEI YI HUO PIAN
Clearing the Lungs and Eliminating Fire Tablet
Huang Qin *Radix Scutellariae baicalensis*
Shan Zhi Zi *Fructus Gardeniae jasminoidis*
Da Huang *Rhizoma Rhei*
Qian Hu *Radix Peucedani*
Ku Shen *Radix Sophorae flavescentis*
Tian Hua Fen *Radix Trichosanthis*
Jie Geng *Radix Platycodi grandiflori*
Zhi Mu *Radix Anemarrhenae asphodeloidis*

Explanation

This tablet contains Da Huang and is therefore suitable to clear Lung-Heat when it is combined with some Stomach-Fire drying up the stools in the Intestines and causing constipation. This is an essential condition for the selection of this remedy. The patient should therefore be constipated (or have dry stools) and the tongue should have a thick-dry-yellow (or even black) coating.

Case history

A 7-year-old boy caught a cold which manifested with such symptoms as shivering, a fever, a cough, a sore throat and a headache (invasion of Wind-Heat). However, his mother brought him to me 5 days after the above symptoms had begun: by the time he came for consultation his symptoms had changed. He felt mostly hot, thirsty, irritable, had a bad cough productive of yellow sputum and a temperature. His tongue was Red all over with red points in the front and centre (Plate 34.2).

Diagnosis
Originally, this was an invasion of Wind-Heat; at the time of consultation it had moved on to the Qi Level. The main two symptoms indicating this were the feeling of heat with thirst, and the overall red colour of the tongue with the extension of red points to the centre. Specifically, it was Phlegm-Heat in the Lungs at the Qi Level and also Stomach-Heat (indicated by the thirst, irritability and red points in the centre of the tongue).

Treatment principle
The treatment principle adopted was to clear Lung-Heat, resolve Phlegm and restore the descending of Lung-Qi.

Herbal treatment
The formula used was a variation of Qing Qi Hua Tan Tang *Clearing Qi and Resolving Phlegm Decoction*:

Dan Nan Xing *Rhizoma Arisaematis praeparata* 6 g
Gua Lou *Fructus Trichosanthis* 6 g
Huang Qin *Radix Scutellariae baicalensis* 4 g
Zhi Shi *Fructus Citri aurantii immaturus* 4 g
Chen Pi *Pericarpium Citri reticulatae* 3 g
Fu Ling *Sclerotium Poriae cocos* 6 g
Xing Ren *Semen Pruni armeniacae* 6 g
Ban Xia *Rhizoma Pinelliae ternatae* 6 g
Shi Gao *Gypsum fibrosum* 12 g
Zhi Mu *Radix Anemarrhenae asphodeloidis* 6 g
Dan Dou Chi *Semen Sojae praeparatum* 6 g

Explanation
- The first eight herbs constitute the root formula which clears Lung-Heat, resolves Phlegm and restores the descending of Lung-Qi.
- **Shi Gao** and **Zhi Mu** clear Stomach-Heat at the Qi Level.
- **Dan Dou Chi** clears Heat and calms irritability in children.

This boy's problem was cleared in 5 days.

3. STOMACH-HEAT

CLINICAL MANIFESTATIONS

High fever, intense thirst, feeling of heat, restlessness, profuse sweating, coarse breathing.
Tongue: Red with dry-yellow coating.
Pulse: Overflowing or Big.

This is the classical pattern of Stomach-Heat at the Qi Level and is identical with the Bright Yang channel pattern of the 6 Stages. It is often summarized as the "Four Bigs", i.e. high fever, intense thirst, profuse sweating and Big pulse.

As a stage following an exterior invasion of Wind, it is more common in children than adults.

TREATMENT PRINCIPLE

Clear Stomach-Heat, prevent injury of Yin.

ACUPUNCTURE

ST-44 Neiting, L.I.-11 Quchi, Du-14 Dazhui. Reducing method.

Explanation

- **ST-44** clears Stomach-Heat.
- **L.I.-11** and **Du-14** clear Heat.

HERBAL TREATMENT

Prescription

BAI HU TANG
White Tiger Decoction
Shi Gao *Gypsum fibrosum* 30 g
Zhi Mu *Radix Anemarrhenae asphodeloidis* 15 g
Gan Cao *Radix Glycyrrhizae uralensis* 4.5 g
Geng Mi *Semen Oryzae sativae* 9 g

Explanation

This is the classical formula for this pattern of Stomach-Heat as opposed to Stomach-Fire. Although very similar in nature, Heat and Fire differ in some respects. Heat is somewhat more superficial than Fire and it needs to be *cleared* with pungent-cold herbs such as Shi Gao. The pungent taste of this herb will push Heat outwards towards the surface, thus ridding the body of it. In the case of Stomach-Heat, Bai Hu Tang is the classical prescription to clear it. Fire, on the contrary, is deeper within the body and is knotted up in the Interior. Fire is also more drying than Heat and it therefore dries up the stools in the Intestines. Thus, it needs to be *drained* by purging with herbs such as Da Huang *Rhizoma Rhei*. The classical prescription to drain Stomach-Fire by purging is Cheng Qi Tang *Conducting Qi Decoction* (see next pattern).

Wu Ju Tong lists four contra-indications against the use of Bai Hu Tang:

(i) pulse not Overflowing
(ii) pulse Deep
(iii) no thirst
(iv) no sweating.

- **Shi Gao** is pungent and cold and clears Stomach-Heat.
- **Zhi Mu** helps Shi Gao to clear Stomach-Heat.
- **Gan Cao** and **Geng Mi** (brown rice) harmonize and benefit fluids to relieve thirst and prevent injury of Yin.

Variations

- If there are signs of the beginning of injury of Stomach-Yin add Lu Gen *Rhizoma Phragmitis communis*, Tian Hua Fen *Radix Trichosanthis* and Mai Men Dong *Tuber Ophiopogonis japonici*.
- If there are bleeding and sore gums add Sheng Ma *Rhizoma Cimicifugae* and Huang Lian *Rhizoma Coptidis*.

4. STOMACH AND INTESTINES DRY-HEAT

CLINICAL MANIFESTATIONS

High fever which is worse in the afternoon, constipation, dry stools, a burning feeling in the anus, abdominal pain and fullness which is worse with pressure, restlessness, thirst, a faint feeling, delirium.
Tongue: Red with very dry-thick yellow, brown or black coating.
Pulse: Deep, Full and Rapid.

This is the classical pattern of Stomach-Fire

as opposed to Stomach-Heat of the previous pattern. Fire lies deeper within the body and dries up fluids in the Intestines, hence the constipation and abdominal pain and fullness. Stomach-Fire is treated by purging.

As a stage following an exterior invasion of Wind, it is more common in children than adults.

TREATMENT PRINCIPLE

Drain Stomach-Fire by purging, benefit fluids.

ACUPUNCTURE

L.I.-11 Quchi, ST-25 Tianshu, SP-15 Daheng, ST-44 Neiting, ST-45 Lidui, BL-25 Dachangshu, T.B.-8 Sanyangluo and KI-6 Zhaohai. Reducing method.

Explanation

- **L.I.-11** clears Stomach and Intestines Heat.
- **ST-25** and **SP-15** regulate the Intestines, clear Stomach-Heat and promote the bowel movement.
- **ST-44** and **ST-45** clear Stomach-Heat; ST-45 is particularly indicated if there is mental restlessness.
- **BL-25** drains Stomach-Fire by promoting the bowel movement.
- **T.B.-8** and **KI-6** promote the bowel movement in Heat diseases.

HERBAL TREATMENT

Prescription

TIAO WEI CHENG QI TANG
Regulating the Stomach Conducting Qi Decoction
Da Huang *Rhizoma Rhei* 12 g
Mang Xiao *Mirabilitum* 9 g
Zhi Gan Cao *Radix Glycyrrhizae uralensis praeparata* 6 g

Explanation

This is one of the three Conducting Qi Decoctions for Stomach-Fire at the Qi level with constipation but without much abdominal pain or fullness.

- **Da Huang** drains Stomach-Fire by purging.
- **Mang Xiao** helps Da Huang to purge.
- **Zhi Gan Cao** harmonizes and tempers the purging action of Da Huang.

Variations

- If there are signs of injury of Yin add Sheng Di Huang *Radix Rehmanniae glutinosae* and Mai Men Dong *Tuber Ophiopogonis japonici*.
- If there is abdominal pain and fullness use Da Cheng Qi Tang *Great Conducting Qi Decoction* instead of the above formula. Da Cheng Qi Tang contains Da Huang, Mang Xiao, Hou Po *Cortex Magnoliae officinalis* and Zhi Shi *Fructus Citri aurantii immaturus*.

5. GALL-BLADDER HEAT

CLINICAL MANIFESTATIONS

Alternation of feeling hot and cold, more hot than cold, bitter taste, thirst, dry throat, irritability, hypochondrial pain, nausea, feeling of fullness in the epigastrium.
Tongue: Red, yellow coating on the right side.
Pulse: Wiry-Rapid.

This is similar to the Lesser Yang pattern of the 6 Stages (see below) with more Heat signs in the Gall-Bladder channel together with some Phlegm-Heat and Damp-Heat.

TREATMENT PRINCIPLE

Clear Gall-Bladder Heat and harmonize the Lesser Yang.

ACUPUNCTURE

T.B.-5 Waiguan, G.B.-41 Zulinqi, G.B.-43 Xiaxi, L.I.-11 Quchi, Du-14 Dazhui, BL-22 Sanjiaoshu. Reducing method.

Explanation

- **T.B.-5** and **G.B.-41** harmonize the Lesser Yang.
- **G.B.-43** clears Gall-Bladder Heat.
- **L.I.-11** and **Du-14** clear Heat.
- **BL-22** resolves Dampness which frequently accompanies this pattern.

HERBAL TREATMENT

Prescription

HAO QIN QING DAN TANG
Artemisia apiacea-Scutellaria Clearing the Gall-Bladder Decoction
Qing Hao *Herba Artemisiae apiaceae* 6 g
Huang Qin *Radix Scutellariae baicalensis* 6 g
Zhu Ru *Caulis Bambusae in Taeniis* 9 g
Ban Xia *Rhizoma Pinelliae ternatae* 5 g
Chen Pi *Pericarpium Citri reticulatae* 5 g
Fu Ling *Sclerotium Poriae cocos* 9 g
Zhi Ke *Fructus Citri aurantii* 5 g
Hua Shi *Talcum* 3 g
Gan Cao *Radix Glycyrrhizae uralensis* 3 g
Qing Dai *Indigo naturalis* 3 g

Explanation

Apart from the first two herbs which regulate the Lesser Yang, this formula clears Gall-Bladder Heat and resolves Phlegm-Heat and Damp-Heat by combining Wen Dan Tang *Warming the Gall-Bladder Decoction* (Zhu Ru, Zhi Ke, Ban Xia, Fu Ling and Chen Pi) which resolves Phlegm-Heat and Bi Yu San *Jasper Powder* (Hua Shi, Gan Cao, Qing Dai) which drains Damp-Heat.

- **Qing Hao** and **Huang Qin** regulate the Lesser Yang. Qing Hao releases the Exterior of the Lesser Yang and Huang Qin clears the Interior of the Lesser Yang.
- **Zhu Ru** resolves Phlegm-Heat and eliminates turbidity.
- **Ban Xia**, **Chen Pi** and **Fu Ling** resolve Dampness and Phlegm.
- **Zhi Ke** moves Qi.
- **Hua Shi**, **Gan Cao** and **Qing Dai** help to resolve Damp-Heat.

6. LESSER YANG PATTERN

CLINICAL MANIFESTATIONS

Alternation of feeling cold and hot, more cold than hot, bitter taste, dry throat, blurred vision, hypochondrial pain, no thirst, irritability, vomiting.
Tongue: white coating on the right side.
Pulse: Wiry and Fine.

This is the Lesser Yang pattern of the 6 Stages. It differs from the previous pattern in so far as there is more cold than heat and not so much Phlegm or Dampness.

Both this pattern and the previous one may appear in the course of post-viral fatigue syndromes.

TREATMENT PRINCIPLE

Harmonize the Lesser Yang, clear the Gall-Bladder.

ACUPUNCTURE

T.B.-5 Waiguan, G.B.-41 Zulinqi, Du-13 Taodao, ST-36 Zusanli. Reducing method except on ST-36 which should be reinforced.

Explanation

– The first three points harmonize the Lesser Yang.
– **ST-36** is reinforced to tonify the Nutritive Qi to help to expel the pathogenic factor.

HERBAL TREATMENT

Prescription

XIAO CHAI HU TANG
Small Bupleurum Decoction
Chai Hu *Radix Bupleuri* 12 g
Huang Qin *Radix Scutellariae baicalensis* 9 g
Ban Xia *Rhizoma Pinelliae ternatae* 9 g
Ren Shen *Radix Ginseng* 6 g

Zhi Gan Cao *Radix Glycyrrhizae uralensis praeparata* 5 g
Sheng Jiang *Rhizoma Zingiberis officinalis recens* 9 g
Da Zao *Fructus Ziziphi jujubae* 4 dates

Explanation

This is the classical prescription to harmonize the Lesser Yang from the "Discussion of Cold-induced Diseases".

– **Chai Hu** releases the Exterior of the Lesser Yang.
– **Huang Qin** clears the Interior of the Lesser Yang. The two together harmonize the Lesser Yang.
– **Ban Xia** harmonizes the Stomach and stops nausea and vomiting.
– **Ren Shen** tonifies Qi.
– **Zhi Gan Cao** harmonizes.
– **Sheng Jiang** helps Chai Hu to release the Exterior of the Lesser Yang.
– **Da Zao** harmonizes.

Patent remedy

XIAO CHAI HU TANG WAN
Small Bupleurum Decoction Pill

Explanation

This remedy has the same ingredients and indications as the above decoction.

7. STOMACH AND SPLEEN DAMP-HEAT

CLINICAL MANIFESTATIONS

Continuous fever which decreases after sweating but then returns, a feeling of heaviness of the body and head, a feeling of oppression of the chest and epigastrium, nausea, loose stools, a sticky taste.
Tongue: Red with a sticky-yellow coating.
Pulse: Slippery and Rapid.

This type of pattern is a frequent outcome of an invasion of Wind-Heat when it reaches the

Qi level. Damp-Heat in the Centre may easily become chronic in the form of residual pathogenic factor, giving rise to some forms of post-viral fatigue syndromes.

TREATMENT PRINCIPLE

Resolve Dampness, harmonize the Stomach, strengthen the Spleen.

ACUPUNCTURE

SP-9 Yinlingquan, SP-6 Sanyinjiao, Ren-12 Zhongwan, Ren-13 Shangwan, Ren-10 Xiawan, ST-36 Zusanli, BL-20 Pishu. Reducing method on all points except the last two which should be reinforced.

Explanation

– **SP-9** and **SP-6** resolve Dampness.
– **Ren-12** resolves Dampness.
– **Ren-13** subdues rebellious Stomach-Qi.
– **Ren-10** stimulates the descending of Stomach-Qi.
– **ST-36** and **BL-20** tonify the Spleen to resolve Dampness.

HERBAL TREATMENT

(a) Prescription

LIAN PO YIN
Coptis-Magnolia Decoction
Huang Lian *Rhizoma Coptidis* 3 g
Hou Po *Cortex Magnoliae officinalis* 3 g
Shan Zhi Zi *Fructus Gardeniae jasminoidis* 9 g
Dan Dou Chi *Semen Sojae praeparatum* 9 g
Shi Chang Pu *Rhizoma Acori graminei* 3 g
Ban Xia *Rhizoma Pinelliae ternatae* 3 g
Lu Gen *Rhizoma Phragmitis communis* 15 g

Explanation

This formula is for Damp-Heat in the Centre, with Heat being pronounced.

– **Huang Lian** and **Hou Po** are coordinated: the

former is bitter and makes Qi descend, the latter is pungent and opens Qi. The combination of the two drains Dampness from the Centre.
– **Zhi Zi** and **Dan Dou Chi**, which form a prescription by themselves called Zhi Zi Chi Tang *Gardenia-Soja Decoction*, are specific to clear residual Heat and relieve irritability deriving from Heat.
– **Chang Pu** opens the orifices and separates clear from turbid: this helps to resolve Dampness and relieve the feeling of fullness in the head.
– **Ban Xia** helps to resolve Dampness by resolving Phlegm.
– **Lu Gen** clears Stomach-Heat and relieves thirst.

(b) Prescription

LEI SHI FANG XIANG HUA ZHUO FA
Fragrant Formula to Resolve Turbidity by the Lei's Clan
Huo Xiang *Herba Agastachis* 3 g
Pei Lan *Herba Eupatorii fortunei* 3 g
Chen Pi *Pericarpium Citri reticulatae* 4.5 g
Ban Xia *Rhizoma Pinelliae ternatae* 4.5 g
Da Fu Pi *Pericarpium Arecae catechu* 3 g
Hou Po *Cortex Magnoliae officinalis* 2 g
Bo He *Herba Menthae* 3 g

Explanation

This formula is used if there is Dampness without much Heat.

– **Huo Xiang** and **Pei Lan** fragrantly resolve Dampness.
– **Chen Pi, Ban Xia, Da Fu Pi** and **Hou Po** resolve Dampness and move Qi in the Centre.
– **Bo He** directs the herbs to the Middle Burner.

(c) Prescription

FU LING PI TANG
Poria Skin Decoction
Fu Ling Pi *Cortex Poriae cocos* 15 g
Yi Yi Ren *Semen Coicis lachryma jobi* 15 g
Zhu Ling *Sclerotium Polypori umbellati* 9 g

Tong Cao *Medulla Tetrapanacis papyriferi* 9 g
Da Fu Pi *Pericarpium Arecae catechu* 9 g
Zhu Ye *Herba Lophatheri gracilis* 6 g

Explanation

This formula is selected if Damp-Heat spreads to the Lower Burner and affects urination.

- **Fu Ling Pi** drains Dampness, resolves oedema and promotes urination.
- **Yi Yi Ren**, **Zhu Ling** and **Tong Cao** resolve Dampness via urination.
- **Da Fu Pi** fragrantly resolves Dampness.
- **Zhu Ye** clears Heat and benefits urination.

(d) Prescription

BAI HU JIA CANG ZHU TANG
White Tiger Decoction plus Rhizoma Atractylodis lanceae
Shi Gao *Gypsum fibrosum* 30 g
Zhi Mu *Radix Anemarrhenae asphodeloidis* 15 g
Gan Cao *Radix Glycyrrhizae uralensis* 4.5 g
Geng Mi *Semen Oryzae sativae* 9 g
Cang Zhu *Rhizoma Atractylodis lanceae* 12 g

Explanation

This formula, a variation of Bai Hu Tang which clears Stomach-Heat, is used if there is a marked prevalence of Heat over Dampness.

Variations

The following variations apply to all four previous formulae.

- If Dampness affects the head causing a pronounced feeling of heaviness and muzziness of the head add (or increase) Shi Chang Pu *Rhizoma Acori graminei*, Yuan Zhi *Radix Polygalae tenuifoliae* and Bai Zhi *Radix Angelicae dahuricae*.
- If symptoms of Heat are pronounced add (or increase) Zhi Zi *Fructus Gardeniae jasminoidis* and Huang Qin *Radix Scutellariae baicalensis*.
- If there is ache in the muscles add (or increase) Pei Lan *Herba Eupatorii fortunei*, Sha Ren *Fructus seu Semen Amomi* and Bai Dou Kou *Fructus Amomi cardamomi*.

- If the urine is dark add Ze Xie *Rhizoma Alismatis orientalis*, Che Qian Zi *Semen Plantaginis* and Yi Yi Ren *Semen Coicis lachryma jobi*.
- If there are symptoms of Phlegm add Ban Xia *Rhizoma Pinelliae ternatae* and Gua Lou *Fructus Trichosanthis*.

Case history

A 42-year-old man presented with acute diarrhoea with foul-smelling stools, a feeling of heaviness, a slight temperature, a feeling of fullness of the epigastrium and poor appetite. His pulse was Slippery and slightly Rapid and his tongue was Red with a sticky-yellow coating. I had successfully treated this patient the year before for chronic ulcerative colitis.

Diagnosis
This is a clear example of Damp-Heat in the Stomach and Intestines at the Qi Level. He was obviously prone to this due to the previous problem in the Intestines.

Treatment principle
The treatment principle adopted was to restore the descending of Stomach-Qi and ascending of Spleen-Qi, resolve Dampness and clear Heat.

Herbal treatment
The formula used was a variation of Lian Po Yin *Coptis-Magnolia Decoction*:

Huang Lian *Rhizoma Coptidis* 4 g
Hou Po *Cortex Magnoliae officinalis* 6 g
Ban Xia *Rhizoma Pinelliae ternatae* 6 g
Lu Gen *Rhizoma Phragmitis communis* 6 g
Zhi Zi *Fructus Gardeniae jasminoidis* 4 g
Dan Dou Chi *Semen Sojae praeparatum* 6 g
Shi Chang Pu *Rhizoma Acori graminei* 6 g
Qin Pi *Cortex Fraxini* 6 g
Bai Tou Weng *Radix Pulsatillae chinensis* 6 g
Huang Bo *Cortex Phellodendri* 6 g
Ge Gen *Radix Puerariae* 6 g
Shan Zha *Fructus Crataegi* 6 g
Shen Qu *Massa Fermentata Medicinalis* 6 g
Zhi Gan Cao *Radix Glycyrrhizae uralensis praeparata* 3 g

Explanation
- The first seven herbs constitute the Lian Po Yin which resolves Damp-Heat from Stomach and Spleen.
- **Qin Pi**, **Bai Tou Weng** and **Huang Bo** resolve Damp-Heat and Fire-Poison from the Intestines.
- **Ge Gen** clears Heat and stops diarrhoea.
- **Shan Zha** and **Shen Qu** resolve food accumulation. Shan Zha also stops diarrhoea.
- **Gan Cao** harmonizes.

This patient reported a remarkable improvement even after only one dose and required a daily decoction for 10 days to clear the problem completely.

Prognosis and prevention

The combination of acupuncture and herbal medicine is very effective in treating exterior invasions of Wind. The beauty of Chinese medicine in the treatment of colds and influenza is that, if the treatment is absolutely right, the Exterior is released and the pathogenic factor expelled completely. It also shortens the course of the disease and prevents complications and injury of Qi or Yin. The use of antibiotics during exterior invasion of Wind or at the Qi level, should definitely be discouraged. Although the common cold and influenza are caused by viruses against which antibiotics are ineffective, they are often prescribed for secondary bacterial infections of the throat or tonsils, for example. In many cases, the use of antibiotics in these conditions leads to the development of a residual pathogenic factor, also because they weaken Stomach-Qi which is the source of Qi and Blood of the body, so that the body's defences are enfeebled rather than strengthened. Of course, in some situations intervention with antibiotic therapy is necessary, as when Chinese medicine might be too slow to act. For example, if a small child develops pneumonia following influenza it is obviously important to administer antibiotics to act quickly and prevent injury of Yin from Heat or the development of Wind from Heat. Moreover, a small child with pneumonia will have a very high temperature and probably delirium so that it would be very difficult to administer herbs in any case.

At the Defensive-Qi Level, acupuncture is as effective as herbal medicine, but treatment definitely needs to be given every day and, in severe cases, even twice a day. Thus, treatment with herbs or patent remedies is easier as it can be carried out by the patient himself or herself at home.

At the Qi level, herbal medicine (with herbs or patent remedies) is more effective than acupuncture, especially in the case of Fire which needs draining by purging. For example, to treat Stomach-Fire affecting the Intestines and causing constipation and abdominal pain, herbal medicine is more effective and more reliable than acupuncture.

It is essential that the patient be advised to take care and rest during an invasion of Wind. He or she should also avoid sexual activity at this time. Not taking care and overworking when the body is attacked by pathogenic Wind is the most common cause for the progression of the pathogenic factor into the Interior and, moreover, for the development of residual Heat. Residual Heat or Damp-Heat is one of the causes of the development of post-viral fatigue syndromes.

If a person is particularly prone to colds and flu due to a deficiency of the Defensive Qi, one can tonify, with moxa, the following points:

– BL-12 Fengmen, BL-13 Feishu, Du-12 Shenzhu and ST-36 Zusanli.

This treatment should be given three times a week for a month and the best time to administer it is between the middle of August and middle of September.

In addition to acupuncture, one can use the Yu Ping Feng San *Jade Wind Screen Powder* to tonify the Defensive Qi.

END NOTES

1. Nanjing College of Traditional Chinese Medicine — Warm Diseases Research Group 1959 Teaching Reference Material on the School of Warm Diseases (*Wen Bing Xue Jiao Xue Can Kao Zi Liao* 温病学教学参考资料), Jiangsu People's Publishing House, p. 49.
2. Ibid., p. 50.

Appendix I
The combination of acupuncture points

The art of acupuncture consists in selecting the right points and combining them in a harmonious way. The lists of acupuncture points which have been given for each pattern in this book are not formulae or prescriptions; they merely set out possible points from which to choose. For each treatment, some points have to be selected from the given lists and combined in a meaningful way. A successful acupuncture treatment depends on many factors among which are:

1. a correct diagnosis ("correct" within the type of acupuncture used, be it Chinese, Korean, 5-Element, Japanese, etc.)
2. a correct plan of treatment
3. a correct choice of points
4. a balanced combination of points.

In this chapter I will discuss point 4 above, i.e. how points are to be combined once a correct diagnosis has been made, a proper principle of treatment has been determined, and the appropriate points have been selected.

Combining points in a safe, effective and harmonious way is a very important part of an acupuncture treatment. The actions of the points, given in the previous chapters for each pattern, are only one of the guidelines in their selection. Using points according to their action brings into play the particular nature of the individual point, while combining points in a harmonious way brings into play the channel system as a whole, and harmonizes Yin and Yang, Top and Bottom, Left and Right, and Front and Back. When points are combined well, the patient has an unmistakable feeling: it may be one of relaxation, elation, alertness, peacefulness or a combination of all these. Ideally, the patient should experience any of the above feelings during and after every treatment. When points are combined well the patient may feel during treatment as if the points are connected among themselves and a needling sensation propagates from one to another. One particular patient said that the points *felt as if forming a circle, as if they were connected*. Another felt as if *a cool liquid was moving into her hands*. Another patient said that during the session she went *into a very deep space*.

As for the feeling experienced after an acupuncture treatment, this is described by patients in many different ways: "I feel brighter", "I feel deeply relaxed", "I feel more awake", "I feel like I had a shower", "I feel more grounded", "I feel spaced out", "I feel like I have been plugged in", "I feel very light", "I feel very heavy", "I feel like I am floating", "I feel like giggling", "I feel euphoric", "I feel like I could dance", etc. In order to observe the patient's reactions and sensations during the treatment, it is important to see one patient at a time or, at least, to allow for spending enough time with the patient; otherwise we will miss their reactions and comments and we will not be able to learn as much. I observe the patient while the needles are retained and, when necessary, I will occasionally change the point combinations during the treatment. For example, during one session I observed that a patient who is normally very relaxed during the treatment, on this occasion looked slightly uncomfortable and restless. I asked her about this and she said she felt a sensation of constriction in the chest and throat. On examining the point prescription used I came to the conclusion that it was unbalanced in so far as all the points were on the legs and torso with none on the arms: on my inserting P-6 Neiguan and withdrawing Ren-12 Zhongwan, her feeling of constriction in the chest and throat disappeared within seconds.

In a few, unusual cases it is necessary to observe the patient very closely during the treatment as their reactions change very rapidly. For example, a patient I was treating for ME (postviral fatigue syndrome) during the acupuncture session felt her head clearing almost immediately and she felt brighter in general: this feeling came over in a wave but disappeared after only a few minutes, being replaced by a feeling of general tiredness and heaviness. On inserting Du-20 Baihui, the wave of well-being returned, only to disappear again after a few minutes. During subsequent sessions I therefore decided to follow her sensations very closely and withdrew the needles only a few minutes after the wave of well-being appeared. This approach produced much better results in this case.

There are of course very many ways of choosing points: according to the 5 Elements, according to pathogenic factors, according to seasons, according to soreness, according to the theory of open points, according to their actions, according to indications, according to the theory of the 5 Transporting points, and many others.

Furthermore, there are many national variations in the style of acupuncture so that, for example, Japanese and Korean acupuncture are quite different from Chinese acupuncture.

However, it could be said that all the different ways of choosing points can be narrowed down to two basic variations: selecting a point according to its particular action, function, nature or quality, or selecting a point according to its position and dynamics within the channel system.

The former approach emphasizes the role of the point in isolation from the channels, while the latter emphasizes the role of the point within the channel system. For example, one can use LIV-2 Xingjian for its action of draining Liver-Fire, or one can select it to draw Qi downwards within the Liver channel: the former approach relies on an intrinsic quality of LIV-2 in draining Fire ("because" it is the Fire point), while the latter approach makes use of the point's dynamics within the channel. When LIV-2 is used in this way to draw Qi downwards, the fact that it is the Fire point is irrelevant, as the point is seen not in isolation but in relation to the channel's flow of Qi.

The Chinese stress on needle manipulation (present in all acupuncture classics) is based on viewing points in isolation, e.g. ST-40 Fenglong (needled with reducing method) to resolve Phlegm.

These two ways of looking at a point, in isolation or in relation to the channel's flow of Qi, have developed in parallel ever since the very early times of Chinese medicine. In fact, while the "Yellow Emperor's Classic of Internal Medicine" (c. 100 BC) mentions at least 160 points and often refers to their "action", the early Han dynasty's text "Prescriptions for 52 Diseases" excavated from Ma Wang Dui's tomb mentions only channels and not points.

To look at a point in isolation and to look at it in relation to the flow of Qi within the channel are not mutually exclusive methods; indeed, the best results are obtained when the two approaches are combined. For example, returning to the above instance, if we wanted to draw Qi downwards within the Liver channel, we could select LIV-1 Dadun, LIV-2 Xingjian or LIV-3

Taichong with equally good results. If the patient has symptoms of Liver-Fire, then LIV-2 is the best choice: by selecting this point we are combining the two approaches, i.e. seeing the point in isolation ("LIV-2 drains Liver-Fire"), and seeing a point's action within the flow of Qi in the channel (i.e. LIV-2 draws Qi downwards not because of a special quality but because of its position within the channel).

In fact, it is good if there is more than one reason for selecting a point: this will make the treatment more powerful and will allow the number of points used to be reduced.

However, selecting a point according to its energetic action and its dynamics within the channel's flow of Qi, needs to be integrated with yet other factors. One of these is selecting the point according to its target area. Most distal points affect a certain area and this needs to be taken into account especially when treating pain. For example, to return to the three points mentioned above, LIV-1, LIV-2 and LIV-3, all stimulate the downward flow of Qi within the Liver channel, but they affect different areas: LIV-1 affects the Lower Burner (particularly urinary passages), LIV-2 affects the eyes and LIV-3 affects the top of the head or face. Thus, if we are using the Liver channel to treat a Liver-related eye problem, LIV-2 would be the best point to use. If, moreover, the patient's eye problem is caused by Liver-Fire, there is an additional reason for choosing LIV-2 as it drains Liver-Fire. Thus, in this example, we are using LIV-2 for three different reasons related to three different viewpoints:

1. because it stimulates the downward movement of Qi within the Liver channel
2. because it affects the eyes
3. because it drains Liver-Fire.

Finally, selecting a point according to the above criteria is still not enough. The next and final step is to combine different acupuncture points from different channels in a harmonious, effective, safe and powerful way. To return to the above example of a patient with an eye problem from Liver-Fire, using LIV-2 only may not be enough and it may need to be combined with other points. This may be necessary either to balance LIV-2 energetically or to treat another symptom. For example, if the patient, besides having an eye problem from Liver-Fire, also suffers from dry mouth and restless sleep from the same cause, we may combine LIV-2 with L.I.-4 Hegu. This combination would be particularly desirable for several reasons:

1. from the point of view of energetic action, L.I.-4 calms the Mind
2. from the point of view of target area, L.I.-4 affects the mouth, thus relieving thirst and dry mouth
3. from the point of view of channel dynamics, L.I.-4 also draws Qi downwards
4. from the point of view of combination of points, L.I.-4 combines well with LIV-2 for three reasons:
   (a) they combine Top and Bottom
   (b) they combine Yin and Yang
   (c) they combine two heavenly stems (this will be explained later).

Thus, to summarize, there are basically four different factors in the selection of points:

1. the energetic action of the point (e.g. draining Liver-Fire)
2. the dynamics of the flow of Qi in the channel (e.g. drawing Qi downwards)
3. the area of the body affected by the point
4. the combination of points from different channels.

Point 1 above has already been discussed in the "Foundations of Chinese Medicine" and will not be repeated here.[1] Points 2, 3 and 4 will be discussed in detail below.

Dynamics of Qi flow in the channels

Qi flows in the channels due to a difference of energetic potential between the chest and the head, the chest being the area of minimum potential and the head the area of maximum potential. On its course from the chest to the head, Qi flows via the fingers, and on its course from the head back to the chest it flows via the toes (see Fig. 1.2 in chapter 1, "Headache"). The area around the fingers and the toes has special energetic significance as Qi is more superficial and changes polarity (from Yin to Yang and vice versa) in these areas. It is for these two reasons that the points around fingers and toes are more dynamic than others and they tend to draw Qi downwards. For example, HE-9 Shaochong can draw Heart-Qi downwards calming the Mind, and KI-1 can subdue rising Empty-Heat within the Kidney channel, also calming the Mind.

The question of Qi flow within the channel will be discussed from five perspectives:

1. order of insertion of needles
2. order of withdrawal of needles
3. distal and local points
4. rising and descending of Qi
5. arm and leg channels.

ORDER OF INSERTION OF NEEDLES

As soon as a needle is inserted it *initially* sends a rush of Qi upwards: for this reason it is best to insert the needles from top to bottom. This approach applies particularly to points on the limbs and not so much to those on the torso. This is because points on the torso are less dynamic and would not send such a rush of Qi upwards as points on the limbs do. There is one exception, for practical reasons, to insertion of needles from top to bottom: if a head point is used in a new patient, it is best to insert this last, as when one is experiencing acupuncture for the first time it may be quite unnerving to start by having a needle in the head.

The order of needle insertion can be further differentiated according to Fullness or Emptiness. If a Full condition is being treated, it is best to insert needles from top to bottom as this will have the effect of draining pathogenic factors. For example, if a patient is suffering from a Full condition of the Stomach such as retention of food, one could insert the following points in this order: L.I.-4 Hegu, P-6 Neiguan, Ren-11 Jianli, ST-36 Zusanli.

If an Empty condition is being treated and the patient's pulse is very Weak and Fine, a different approach could be used whereby the needles are inserted from bottom to top. This has a reinforcing effect on Qi and causes a rush of Qi upwards

much like a container of water being filled from the bottom. In this case, however, the needles should be inserted with a longer interval between each other, say about 1-2 minutes. The time gap between each needle's insertion is important as the patient might otherwise develop a headache. For example, if a patient is being treated for a Deficiency-type Stomach condition one could insert the following points in this order: SP-6 Sanyinjiao, ST-36 Zusanli, Ren-12 Zhongwan and L.I.-4 Hegu.

However, this is not to say that inserting needles from top to bottom has an automatic reducing effect.

Another exception to the rule of inserting needles from top to bottom is when a distal point is used first to clear obstructions from a channel in acute cases. This technique makes use precisely of the above-mentioned upward rush of Qi to remove obstructions from a channel. For example, in acute sprain of the shoulder joint, the distal point ST-38 Tiaokou is needled first and manipulated vigorously to clear stagnation from the shoulder channels. Other points are inserted later.

ORDER OF WITHDRAWAL OF NEEDLES

In general, needles are withdrawn from top to bottom, but the order of withdrawal may be changed according to Fullness or Emptiness.

In Full conditions characterized by Qi rebelling upwards or stagnating horizontally, it is best to withdraw needles from top to bottom: this has the effect of promoting the downward flow of Qi. Examples of conditions characterized by Qi rebelling upwards are cough (Lung-Qi rebelling upwards), hypochondrial pain (Liver-Qi stagnating horizontally), severe giddiness (Liver-Qi rebelling upwards), etc.

In Empty conditions, especially those characterized by sinking of Qi, it is best to withdraw the needles from the bottom towards the top: this has the effect of promoting the lifting of Qi. Examples of conditions characterized by sinking Qi are prolapses and severe Qi deficiency with a dragging-down feeling. For example, if a patient is being treated for severe exhaustion, mental depression and a dragging-down feeling, one might select Du-20 Baihui to raise Qi, Du-26

Renzhong, P-6 Neiguan, ST-36 Zusanli and KI-3 Taixi. Needles should then be withdrawn from the bottom starting with KI-3 and finishing with Du-20.

DISTAL AND LOCAL POINTS

Distal points are the points on the arms below the elbows and on the legs below the knees; local points are those on the head and trunk. As explained above, the distal points, being on the lower arm and leg, are more dynamic than the local points on the trunk. Whilst distal points should always be used in both acute and chronic cases, local points need not be used in every case. The most common approach, however, is to combine distal with local points.

In acute cases, the distal points have the effect of removing obstructions from the channel and expelling pathogenic factors and they are therefore usually needled with reducing method. The local points have the function of supporting the eliminating action of the distal points and focusing it on the desired area: they are usually

needled with even method. For example, in treating an acute sprain of the lower back with bilateral pain on the lower back, one might choose BL-40 Weizhong as a distal point (needled with reducing method) and BL-26 Guanyuanshu as a local point (needled with even method). Sometimes distal points are needled before inserting the local ones. The example of ST-38 Tiaokou for acute sprain of the shoulder has already been given above. To give another example, in acute sprain of the lower back with pain on the midline, the distal point Du-26 Renzhong is selected and manipulated vigorously before inserting the local points.

In chronic cases, distal and local points simply reinforce each other's function.

The following is a list of the main distal and local points according to areas (Table I.1). This table lists points from different channels and the choice of which point to use has to be guided by other factors, chiefly a proper identification of the channel involved.

As mentioned above, the points in Table I.1

Table I.1 Distal and local points according to areas

Area/organ	Local points	Distal points
Face	Yintang	L.I.-4 Hegu, ST-44 Neiting
Temples	Taiyang, G.B.-8 Shuaigu	T.B.-3 Zhongzhu, T.B.-5 Waiguan, G.B.-43 Xiaxi
Occiput	G.B.-20 Fengchi, BL-10 Tianshu	S.I.-3 Houxi, BL-65 Shugu
Vertex	Du-20 Baihui	LIV-3 Taichong
Eye	BL-1 Jingming, ST-1 Chengqi, Yuyao	L.I.-4 Hegu, LIV-2 Taichong, HE-5 Tongli, S.I.-6 Yanglao, T.B.-3 Zhongzhu
Nose	Yintang, Yingxiang, Bitong	LU-7 Lieque, L.I.-4 Hegu
Teeth	ST-4 Dicang, ST-6 Jiache, ST-7 Xiaguan	L.I.-4 Hegu (upper), ST-44 Neiting (lower)
Ear	T.B.-17 Yifeng, S.I.-19 Tinggong, G.B.-2 Tinghui, T.B.-21 Ermen	T.B.-2 Yemen, T.B.-3 Zhongzhu, T.B.-5 Waiguan, G.B.-43 Xiaxi
Tongue	Ren-23 Lianquan	P-8 Laogong, HE-5 Tongli, KI-6 Zhaohai
Throat	Ren-22 Tiantu	L.I.-4 Hegu, LU-11 Shaoshang, KI-6 Zhaohai
Lungs	LU-1 Zhongfu, BL-13 Feishu, Ren-17 Shanzhong, Ren-22 Shanzhong	LU-7 Lieque, LU-5 Chize
Heart	BL-15 Xinshu, BL-14 Jueyinshu, Ren-14 Juque, Ren-15 Jiuwei	P-6 Neiguan, HE-7 Shenmen, P-5 Jianshi, P-4 Ximen
Stomach	BL-21 Weishu, Ren-12 Zhongwan	P-6 Neiguan, ST-36 Zusanli, SP-4 Gongsun
Liver	BL-18 Ganshu, LIV-14 Qimen	LIV-3 Taichong, G.B.-34 Yanglingquan
Gall-Bladder	G.B.-19 Danshu, G.B.-24 Riyue	G.B.-34 Yanglingquan, Dannangxue
Intestines	BL-25 Dachangshu, ST-25 Tianshu	ST-36 Zusanli, SP-6 Sanyinjiao, ST-37 Shangjuxu, ST-39 Xiajuxu
Bladder	Ren-3 Zhongji, BL-28 Pangkuangshu, Ren-2 Qugu, BL-32 Ciliao	SP-6 Sanyinjiao, BL-63 Jinmen
Urethra	Ren-2 Qugu, BL-34 Xialiao	LIV-5 Ligou, BL-63 Jinmen
Anus	Du-1 Changqiang, BL-54 Zhibian, G.B.-30 Huantiao	BL-57 Chengshan, BL-58 Feiyang

are from different channels and their choice has to be further guided by the identification of patterns and channel involved. For example, two of the distal points indicated for the throat are LU-11 Shaoshang and KI-6 Zhaohai: LU-11 would be selected in sore throat from acute invasions of Wind-Heat, while KI-6 would be chosen for a dry throat from Yin deficiency. As another example, the distal points indicated in the table for the Heart are P-4 Ximen, P-5 Jianshi, P-6 Neiguan and HE-7 Shenmen: P-4 would be chosen if there were an irregular heart beat, P-5 if Phlegm were obstructing the Heart, P-6 in Heart-Qi deficiency, and HE-7 for Heart-Blood deficiency.

RISING AND DESCENDING OF QI

An awareness of the rising and descending movement of Qi in the channels is essential to give a balanced acupuncture treatment. Many pathological conditions are due to a derangement in the direction of movement of Qi. The Qi of certain organs naturally descends while that of others naturally ascends.

Organs whose Qi descends are the Stomach, Lungs, Heart and Kidneys; the only organ whose Qi normally ascends is the Spleen. The Liver is different in so far as its Qi spreads in all directions. If Qi ascends when it should descend or vice versa, it is called rebellious Qi.

Symptoms of rebellious Qi in each organ are as follows:

Stomach: hiccups, belching, nausea, vomiting, sour regurgitation.
Lungs: cough, breathlessness, asthma.
Heart: palpitations, bitter taste, anxiety, breathlessness.
Kidneys: asthma, urinary retention.
Spleen: loose stools, diarrhoea, prolapse of an organ, dragging-down sensation.
Liver: headaches, dizziness, tinnitus, irritability, bitter taste, shouting, sighing, hypochondrial distension and pain, abdominal pain, hypogastric distension and pain.

The main points which stimulate the descending of Qi in each channel are:

Stomach: Ren-13 Shangwan, Ren-10 Xiawan, ST-34 Liangqiu, ST-44 Neiting, ST-45 Lidui, L.I.-4 Hegu.
Lungs: LU-7 Lieque, LU-5 Chize, LU-1 Zhongfu.
Heart: HE-5 Tongli, HE-8 Shaofu, Ren-15 Jiuwei.
Kidneys: KI-7 Fuliu, KI-1 Yongquan, Ren-4 Guanyuan.
Liver: LIV-14 Qimen, LIV-3 Taichong, LIV-2 Xingjian, LIV-1 Dadun.

The main points which stimulate the ascending of Qi of the Spleen are: Ren-12 Zhongwan, Ren-6 Qihai, Du-20 Baihui, BL-20 Pishu.

ARM AND LEG CHANNELS

As will be remembered, Qi circulates in the channel system due to a difference of potential between the chest (minimum potential) and the head (maximum potential). The cycle of Qi flow in the 12 channels can be broken down into three cycles of 4 channels each (see Fig. 1.3 in chapter 1, "Headache"). In each of these 4-channel cycles, Qi flows from a Yin organ in the chest to the fingertips, then in a Yang channel up to the head, then into another Yang channel downwards to the toes and finally in a Yin channel back to the chest and to a Yin organ (see Fig. 1.2 in chapter 1, "Headache"). To take the first 4-channel cycle, Qi flows from the Lung organ into the Lung channel ending at the fingertips, then into the Large Intestine channel up to the head; from here Qi flows into the Stomach channel down to the toes and from here into the Spleen channel to return to the chest area and flow into the Spleen organ. Thus, in the first two channels of the cycle (Lung and Large Intestine channels), Qi flows *upwards*, and in the second two channels, Stomach and Spleen, Qi flows *downwards*. "Downwards" here means that they flow towards the area of minimum potential: this should not be confused with the fact that, looking at the human body, these channels flow towards the top.

It should also be noted that, while the Yin channels are not joined directly and superficially (although they obviously are joined internally), the Yang channels are joined directly and superficially on the head.

The implications of all this are as follows:

1. The leg-channels' distal points are stronger than the arm-channels' distal points. This is because the leg-channels' distal points are at a stage of the cycle when Qi is flowing downwards towards the area of minimum potential: these points therefore have a stronger clearing movement and are more powerful than the arm-channels' distal points. For example, if one were treating a problem of the gums or mouth (be it gum ulcers, toothache, herpes simplex, etc.), one could use L.I.-4 Hegu or ST-44 Neiting: the latter point has a stronger effect than the former. Of course, one can also use both points to have an even stronger effect.

2. Because the Yang channels, one arm channel flowing upwards (e.g. Large Intestine) and one leg channel flowing downwards (e.g. Stomach), communicate directly and superficially on the head, their points are particularly good to harmonize Above-Below and regulate the ascending and descending of Qi. For example, L.I.-4 Hegu regulates the ascending and descending of Qi, especially in combination with ST-36 Zusanli. Another example is the combination of T.B.-6 Zhigou and G.B.-34 Yanglingquan to harmonize the Lesser Yang and regulate the ascending and descending in the Three Burners.

3. It is important to balance arm and leg points: an example of this was given earlier at the beginning of the chapter. In asthma, it is especially important to balance leg with arm points and pay attention to using enough arm points. This is because all points send an initial rush of Qi upwards and the "column" of Qi rushing upwards is that much higher in leg points. For example, an asthmatic patient felt a tightness of the chest during the session. The points used were LU-7 Lieque on the right, KI-6 Zhaohai on the left (Directing Vessel's opening points), ST-40 Fenglong and SP-6 Sanyinjiao bilaterally. I concluded that there were not enough arm points; on insertion of P-6 Neiguan the tight feeling of the chest cleared immediately.

4. Because the Yang channels are joined directly and superficially, the arm and the leg channel within each cycle could be considered as one channel, e.g. Large Intestine and Stomach channels (Bright Yang), Small Intestine and Bladder channels (Greater Yang) and Triple Burner and Gall-Bladder channels (Lesser Yang). This means that the points on the related Yang channels are somewhat interchangeable and they affect a common area covered by the two channels. For example, L.I.-4 Hegu and ST-44 Neiting (affecting the face, gums and mouth), S.I.-3 Houxi and BL-60 Kunlun (affecting the occiput) and T.B.-5 Waiguan and G.B.-43 Xiaxi (affecting the temples).

The close connection between arm and leg paired Yang channels and the fact that they affect a common area, makes for many possible combinations of points which harmonize Top and Bottom. The following combinations, all of which harmonize the rising and descending of Qi, are given as examples:

1. BRIGHT YANG

(a) *L.I.-4 Hegu and ST-36 Zusanli* to harmonize the rising and descending of Qi and regulate digestion; this combination affects the Stomach and epigastrium.

(b) *L.I.-4 Hegu and ST-44 Neiting* to harmonize the rising and descending of Qi: this combination affects the face, gums and mouth.

(c) *L.I.-10 Shousanli and ST-36 Zusanli* to harmonize the rising and descending of Qi and strengthen the Bright Yang channels: this combination has a general tonic effect (as L.I.-10 has a tonic effect somewhat similar to ST-36) and invigorates the channels. It is good to invigorate the channels in ME (post-viral fatigue syndrome) and Atrophy Syndrome.

(d) *L.I.-11 Quchi and ST-43 Xiangu* to benefit sinews and expel Wind-Damp-Heat in Heat Painful Obstruction Syndrome.

2. GREATER YANG

(a) *S.I.-3 Houxi and BL-60 Kunlun* to harmonize the rising and descending of Qi and expel Wind: this combination affects the upper back, back of the neck and occiput.

(b) *S.I.-6 Yanglao and BL-66 Tonggu* to harmonize the rising and descending of Qi and expel Wind from the Greater-Yang channels: this combination affects the eyes.

3. LESSER YANG

(a) *T.B.-6 Zhigou and G.B.-31 Fengshi* to harmonize the Lesser Yang, expel Wind, regulate Qi and eliminate stagnation: this combination affects the sides of the body and is good for herpes zoster from Wind-Heat.

(b) *T.B.-4 Yangchi and G.B.-40 Qiuxu* harmonize the Lesser Yang channels and regulate the rising and descending of Qi. This combination affects the temples and is good for Lesser Yang headaches. It also strengthens the Gall-Bladder's mental aspect, i.e. determination and the capacity of taking decisions.

The combination of points from an arm and a leg Yang channel is also used in the Yang Extraordinary Vessels as their opening and coupled points are all points from paired arm and leg Yang channels:

Governing Vessel: S.I.-3 Houxi and BL-62 Shenmai
Yang Heel Vessel: BL-62 Shenmai and S.I.-3 Houxi
Yang Linking Vessel: T.B.-5 Waiguan and G.B.-41 Zulinqi
Girdle Vessel: G.B.-41 Zulinqi and T.B.-5 Waiguan.

Target area of points

Besides taking into account the action of the points and the dynamics of the flow of Qi in the channels, when selecting distal points, it is important also to consider the area of body affected by the point. This is determined by general principles and by experience. The general principle is that, the further a point is along the channel, the farther its influence is exerted. This means that a point at the extremity of a channel will generally affect the opposite extremity (Fig. I.1). With some exceptions, this principle only works one way, i.e. the distal

points of arms and legs affect the top extremity of the channel and not vice versa. As mentioned, there are exceptions to this principle, e.g. the use of Du-20 Baihui for haemorrhoids. Thus, as an example, any point on the Triple Burner channel may affect the general area of the Lesser Yang channels, but if we want to affect the temples, then T.B.-3 Zhongzhu or T.B.-5 Waiguan would be better, while T.B.-1 Guanchong, being at the very extremity of the channel, would affect the opposite end, i.e. the ear.

The following is a partial list of areas affected by various distal points on each channel.

LUNG (Fig. I.2)

Nose: LU-7 Lieque

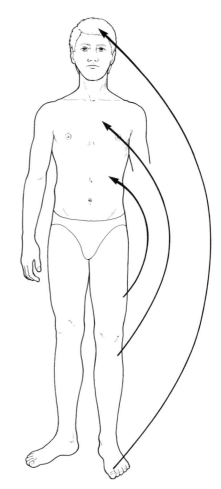

Fig. I.1   General principle of targeting of points

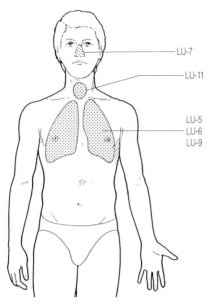

Fig. I.2   Target areas of Lung-channel's distal points

Throat: LU-11 Shaoshang
Lungs: LU-5 Chize, LU-6 Kongzui, LU-9 Taiyuan.

LARGE INTESTINE (Fig. I.3)

Eye: L.I.-14 Binao.

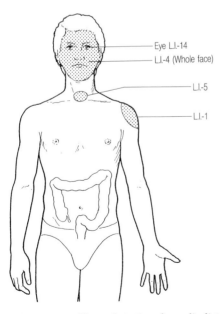

Fig. I.3   Target areas of Large Intestine-channel's distal points

Face, mouth: L.I.-4 Hegu.
Shoulder: L.I.-1 Shangyang.
Throat: L.I.-5 Yangxi.

STOMACH (Fig. I.4)

Face, mouth: ST-44 Neiting.
Mind: ST-40 Fenglong, ST-25 Tianshu.
Throat: ST-41 Jiexi.
Stomach: ST-36 Zusanli, ST-42 Chongyang, ST-40 Fenglong.
Heart (rhythm): ST-36 Zusanli, ST-40 Fenglong.
Lower abdomen: ST-34 Liangqiu.

SPLEEN (Fig. I.5)

Lips: SP-1 Yinbai.

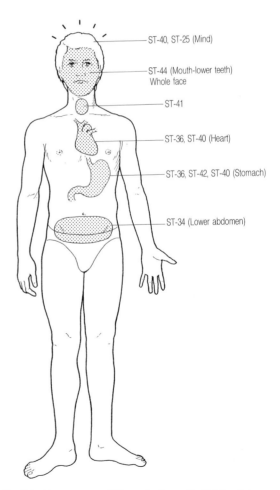

Fig. I.4   Target areas of Stomach-channel's distal points

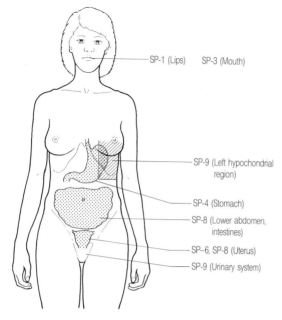

Fig. I.5   Target areas of Spleen-channel's distal points

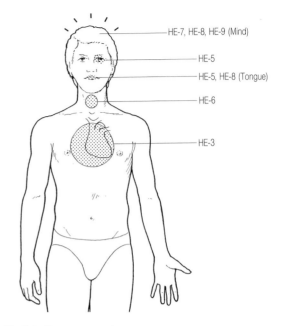

Fig. I.6   Target areas of Heart-channel's distal points

Mouth: SP-3 Taibai.
Left hypochondrial region: SP-9 Yinlingquan.
Stomach: SP-4 Gongsun.
Lower abdomen: SP-8 Diji, SP-6 Sanyinjiao.
Uterus: SP-8 Diji.
Urinary system: SP-9 Yinlingquan.

HEART (Fig. I.6)

Tongue: HE-5 Tongli, HE-8 Shaofu.
Throat: HE-6 Yinxi.
Chest: HE-3 Shaohai.

SMALL INTESTINE (Fig. I.7)

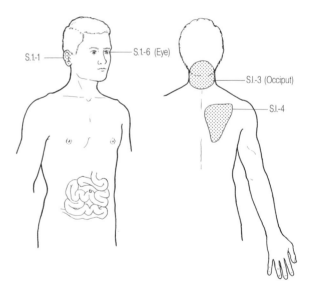

Fig. I.7   Target areas of Small Intestine-channel's distal points

Ear: S.I.-1 Shaoze.
Eye: S.I.-6 Yanglao.
Neck, occiput: S.I.-3 Houxi.
Scapula: S.I.-4 Wangu.

BLADDER (Fig. I.8)

Eye: BL-67 Zhiyin, BL-66 Tonggu.

Top of head: BL-66 Tonggu.
Occiput: BL-65 Shugu.
Upper back: BL-60 Kunlun.
Lower back: BL-40 Weizhong.
Anus: BL-57 Chengshan, BL-58 Feiyang.

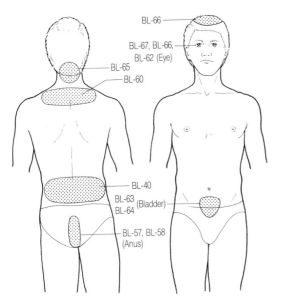

Fig. I.8   Target areas of Bladder-channel's distal points

KIDNEYS (Fig. I.9)

Eye: KI-6 Zhaohai.
Tongue: KI-1 Yongquan.
Throat: KI-6 Zhaohai.
Chest: KI-7 Fuliu, KI-9 Zhubin.
Umbilical area: KI-5 Shuiquan.
Urinary system: KI-10 Yingu.

PERICARDIUM (Fig. I.10)

Mind: P-7 Daling, P-6 Neiguan.
Tongue: P-8 Laogong.
Throat: P-8 Laogong.
Heart: P-6 Neiguan, P-5 Jianshi.
Chest: P-6 Neiguan.

TRIPLE BURNER (Fig. I.11)

Ear: T.B.-2 Yemen.
Temples: T.B.-3 Zhongzhu, T.B.-5 Waiguan.
Neck, top of shoulders: T.B.-8 Sanyangluo.
Shoulder joint: T.B.-1 Guanchong, T.B.-8 Sanyangluo.
Sides of body: T.B.-6 Zhigou.
Uterus: T.B.-4 Yangchi.

GALL-BLADDER (Fig. I.12)

Eye: G.B.-44 Zuqiaoyin.
Ear: G.B.-43 Xiaxi.
Temple: G.B.-43 Xiaxi.
Neck: G.B.-39 Xuanzhong.
Shoulder: G.B.-34 Yanglingquan.

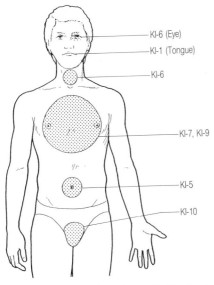

Fig. I.9   Target areas of Kidney-channel's distal points

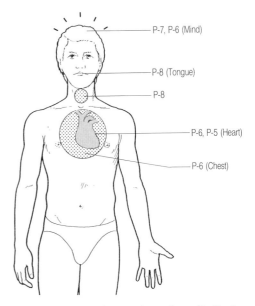

Fig. I.10   Target areas of Pericardium-channel's distal points

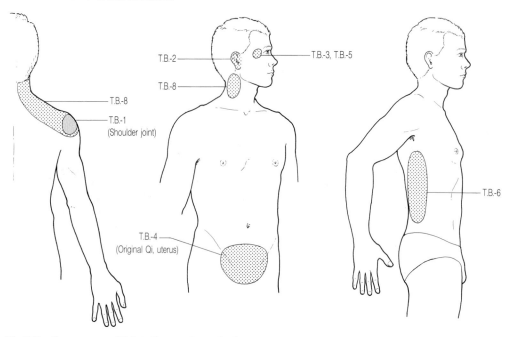

Fig. I.11 Target areas of Triple Burner-channel's distal points

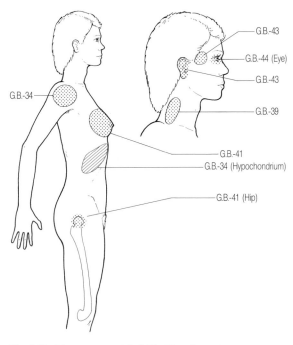

Fig. I.12 Target areas of Gall-Bladder-channel's distal points

Breast: G.B.-41 Zulinqi.
Hypochondrial region: G.B.-34 Yanglingquan.
Hip: G.B.-41 Zulinqi.

LIVER (Fig. I.13)

Eye: LIV-2 Xingjian.
Top of head: LIV-3 Taichong.
Throat: LIV-3 Taichong.
Hypochondrial region: LIV-3 Taichong.
Lower abdomen: LIV-4 Zhongfeng.
Hypogastric region: LIV-8 Ququan, LIV-6 Zhongdu.
Urinary system: LIV-5 Ligou, LIV-6 Zhongdu, LIV-1 Dadun.

Combination of acupuncture points

As mentioned above, a correct and harmonious combination of points in one treatment is an essential part of the art of acupuncture. If we choose points only according to their actions,

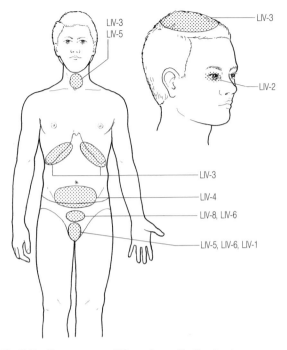

Fig. I.13 Target areas of Liver-channel's distal points

even if our choice is correct from that point of view, it will not be enough to give a balanced treatment. As the points given in all the previous chapters were selected only according to their action, this section of the book should be integrated with the points given with each pattern in order to select a balanced combination of points.

We can discuss the combination of points according to five different points of view:

– Distal and local points
– Top-Bottom
– Yin-Yang
– Back-Front
– Left-Right.

The combination of distal and local points has already been discussed above, so we need to discuss the remaining four aspects.

BALANCING TOP AND BOTTOM

Balancing Top and Bottom areas of the body is an important part of a harmonious acupuncture treatment. As we have seen before, every time

we insert a needle in the body there is an initial rush of Qi upwards: for this reason, a proper balance of points on the upper and lower parts of the body ensures a smooth flow of Qi during the treatment.

Also, as we have seen, the first two channels in a 4-channel cycle (in the upper part of the body) have an ascending potential, while the second two channels (in the lower part of the body) have a descending potential. Thus, balancing points from the Top and Bottom achieves an equalization of flow of Qi in the channels.

Examples of combination of points from arm and leg Yang channels within the same cycle (e.g. Large Intestine and Stomach) have already been given above: these represent one way of balancing Top and Bottom. Obviously combining points from the Top and Bottom also applies to arm and leg Yin channels within the same cycle (e.g. Lung and Spleen) and to points from different channels.

The following are examples of combinations of points from arm and leg Yin channels within the same cycle.

LUNG AND SPLEEN CHANNELS (GREATER YIN)

– *LU-9 Taiyuan and SP-6 Sanyinjiao* to nourish Lung-Yin and moisten dryness.
– *LU-7 Lieque and SP-9 Yinlingquan* to open the Water passages and treat urinary retention or pain on urination.

HEART AND KIDNEY CHANNELS (LESSER YIN)

– *HE-7 Shenmen and KI-3 Taixi*, both Source points, to harmonize Heart and Kidneys, nourish Heart- and Kidney-Yin and calm the Mind.
– *HE-6 Yinxi and KI-7 Fuliu* to harmonize Heart and Kidneys, nourish Heart-Yin and stop night-sweating.
– *HE-7 Shenmen and KI-9 Zhubin* to harmonize Heart and Kidneys, nourish the Kidneys,

relieve oppression of the chest and calm the Mind. This combination is very calming.

PERICARDIUM AND LIVER (TERMINAL YIN)

- *P-6 Neiguan* and *LIV-3 Taichong* to harmonize the Terminal Yin, move Liver-Qi, open the chest, release suppressed emotions and settle the Ethereal Soul. This is an excellent combination of points.
- *P-7 Daling* and *LIV-3 Taichong* to harmonize the Terminal Yin, calm the Mind and settle the Ethereal Soul.

The following are examples of combinations of points from both Yang and Yin channels or unrelated Yang and unrelated Yin channels.

- *P-6 Neiguan* and *ST-36 Zusanli* to harmonize the Middle Burner and subdue rebellious Stomach-Qi. This combination is very effective in a variety of Stomach problems, but especially those characterized by rebellious Stomach-Qi deriving from emotional problems.
- *L.I.-4 Hegu* and *LIV-3 Taichong* (both Source points and called the "four gates") to harmonize Top and Bottom, regulate the ascending and descending of Qi, expel Wind from the face, calm the Mind and settle the Ethereal Soul.
- *T.B.-4 Yangchi* and *ST-42 Chongyang* to tonify the three Burners, strengthen the Stomach and regulate the uterus. This last function is due to the Triple Burner's role as the avenue through which the Original Qi emerges from between the Kidneys (chapter 66 of the "Classic of Difficulties").[2] Also, the term *chong* within the name of the point ST-42 Chongyang refers to the *Chong Mai*, i.e. the Penetrating Vessel which emerges from the uterus, and indicates that this extraordinary vessel goes through this point.
- *P-6 Neiguan* and *ST-40 Fenglong* to regulate the Middle Burner, subdue rebellious Stomach-Qi, resolve Phlegm, calm the Mind and harmonize the rising and descending of Qi. This combination is excellent for Excess patterns of the Stomach characterized by

rebellious Stomach-Qi and not necessarily by Phlegm. It also has a powerful calming effect and is very good in Stomach problems deriving from emotional problems. This combination also treats sprain of the rib muscles. It may be compared with the combination P-6 and ST-36 mentioned above: the combination of P-6 and ST-40 is better for Excess patterns, while P-6 and ST-36 is better for Deficiency patterns.

- *L.I.-4 Hegu* and *LIV-2 Xingjian* to regulate the rising and descending of Qi, clear Heat, drain Fire, calm the Mind and benefit the eyes. This combination, similar in effect to the Four Gates (L.I.-4 and LIV-3), is excellent to treat eye problems deriving from Liver-Fire against a background of Liver-related emotional problems.
- *LU-7 Lieque* and *BL-63 Jinmen* to open the Water passages, promote urination and stop urinary pain. This combination is used in retention of urine or Painful-Urination Syndrome with Dampness obstructing the Water passages.
- *LU-7 Lieque* and *KI-7 Fuliu* to stimulate the descending of Lung-Qi and the Kidney's grasping of Qi. This combination is good to treat asthma from Lung and Kidney deficiency.
- *HE-5 Tongli* and *SP-3 Taibai* to stimulate the Mind and Intellect and strengthen memory and concentration. This combination is good to strengthen memory and concentration in patients with Heart- and Spleen-Blood deficiency. It may also be used to boost memory and concentration in students before an exam: in this case it should be combined with BL-15 Xinshu, BL-20 Pishu and Du-20 Baihui.

Although balancing Top and Bottom is a very important part of a harmonious acupuncture treatment, there are situations when the dynamics of the channel system are exploited to draw Qi upwards or downwards by needling only the top or bottom half of the body. For example, if there is Fullness above and Emptiness below from a deficiency of Kidney-Yin and flaring up of Heart Empty-Heat (red face, insomnia, anxiety, dizziness, back-ache, night-sweating, etc.), one might deliberately choose an unbalanced point prescription, i.e. only KI-1 Yongquan to draw Qi downwards and subdue Empty-Heat.

On the other hand, in prolapse of the uterus from sinking Spleen-Qi, one might choose only a point on the top of the body, e.g. Du-20 Baihui to raise Qi.

Finally, another case when balancing of Top and Bottom is *not* used is when one uses only a distal point in acute sprains. For example, Du-26 Renzhong for acute sprain of the lower back, or ST-38 Tiaokou for acute sprain of the shoulder.

BALANCING YIN AND YANG

Balancing points according to their Yin or Yang character is very important. The Yin or Yang character of a point is in relation with the Yin-Yang dynamics of the channel system. As we have seen, within each 4-channel cycle (Fig. 1.2 in chapter 1, "Headache"), the Yin channels are the beginning and end of the cycle (e.g. Lung and Spleen channels), i.e. the phases of preparation and recuperation. The Yang channels (e.g. Large Intestine and Stomach channels) are in the middle of the cycle, i.e. the phase of activity and dispersal. Furthermore, only the Yang channels reach the head which is the area of maximum potential. In keeping with the principle that Yang corresponds to activity and Yin to inertia, the number of points in the channels reflects the nature of Yin channels as phases of preparation and recuperation, and that of Yang channels as phases of activity and dispersal: in fact, there are more than twice as many Yang points (218) as compared to Yin points (91), excluding the Governing and Directing Vessels. If we include the points of these two extraordinary vessels, the proportion is about the same, i.e. 246 Yang against 115 Yin points.

If we look at the whole cycle of 12 channels (Fig. 1.3 in chapter 1, "Headache"), we can see the flow of Yin and Yang within 24 hours and find an explanation for the names of Bright Yang, Lesser Yin, etc. In the three 4-channel cycles, the flow of Yin and Yang within 24 hours is such that there is maximum Yin ("Greater Yin") and average Yang energy ("Bright Yang") in the first cycle (morning), maximum Yang ("Greater Yang") and minimum Yin energy ("Lesser Yin") in the middle cycle (midday), and average Yin ("Terminal Yin") and minimum Yang energy ("Lesser Yang") in the third cycle (evening).

The implication of all this in practice is that it is important to balance Yin with Yang points in order to equalize the flow of Yin and Yang in the channels. As Yang points exceed Yin ones, it is especially important not to use an excessive number of Yang points without balancing them with Yin ones. Using too many Yang points may make the patient edgy and nervous, while using too many Yin points may make him or her tired. As Yin points may be used to tonify Yang organs or energies (e.g. LU-9 Taiyuan can tonify the Defensive Qi), and Yang points can tonify Yin organs (ST-36 Zusanli to tonify the Spleen), this gives us greater freedom in the choice of points when we are trying to balance Yin and Yang.

Balancing Yin and Yang can be seen from different points of view:

1. Balancing externally-internally paired channels (e.g. Lung and Large Intestine)
2. Balancing unrelated Yin and Yang channels (e.g. Lung and Stomach)
3. Balancing of Connecting and Source points
4. Balancing Yin and Yang according to heavenly stems.

1. BALANCING POINTS OF EXTERNALLY-INTERNALLY PAIRED CHANNELS

The following are some examples of balancing of Yin and Yang points from externally-internally paired channels:

– *LU-9 Taiyuan and L.I.-4 Hegu*, both Source points, to balance Yin and Yang, tonify the Lungs, strengthen the Defensive Qi, consolidate the Exterior and stop sweating.
– *LU-11 Shaoshang and L.I.-4 Hegu* to expel Wind-Heat and relieve sore throat.
– *ST-36 Zusanli and SP-4 Gongsun* to regulate the Middle Burner and subdue rebellious Stomach-Qi in Excess patterns of the Stomach.

- *HE-7 Shenmen* and *S.I.-5 Yanggu* to nourish the Heart, calm the Mind and open the Mind's orifices. This combination is particularly good to give clarity to the Mind and help the patient to make decisions by discriminating between choices.
- *LIV-3 Taichong* and *G.B.-34 Yanglingquan* to move Liver-Qi, eliminate stagnation and settle the Ethereal Soul. This combination is excellent to move Liver-Qi deriving from emotional problems and causing moodiness and depression on a mental level and distension on a physical level.
- *SP-8 Diji, SP-6 Sanyinjiao, ST-28 Shuidao* and *ST-29 Guilai* to resolve Dampness and eliminate stasis from the Lower Burner, stop pain and arrest uterine bleeding. This combination treats the gynaecological system in women especially in Full patterns.
- *LU-3 Tianfu* and *L.I.-4 Hegu* to treat epistaxis.[3]
- *ST-45 Lidui* and *SP-1 Yinbai* to calm the Mind. This combination is used for insomnia and restless sleep with nightmares.[4]
- *HE-6 Yinxi* and *S.I.-3 Houxi* to stop night-sweating from Heart-Yin deficiency.[5]
- *KI-8 Jiaoxin* and *BL-55 Heyang* to tonify Qi to hold Blood. This combination is used to stop excessive uterine bleeding from Qi deficiency.[6]
- *G.B.-30 Huantiao, LIV-2 Xingjian* and *G.B.-31 Fengshi* to treat Painful Obstruction Syndrome with pain in the lower back and leg.[7]
- *LU-5 Chize* and *L.I.-11 Quchi* to clear Lung-Heat and stimulate the descending of Lung-Qi. This combination can be used to clear Lung-Heat in acute conditions with a cough, a fever and expectoration of profuse, sticky, yellow sputum.
- *ST-36 Zusanli* and *SP-6 Sanyinjiao* to tonify Stomach- and Spleen-Qi and Qi and Blood in general. This simple combination is excellent to tonify Qi and Blood in general, especially in women. The effect is enhanced by the use of moxa on the needles.
- *ST-39 Xiajuxu* and *SP-6 Sanyinjiao* to stop lower abdominal pain.
- *BL-63 Jinmen* and *KI-10 Yingu* to open the Water passages and stop urinary pain. This combination can be used for Damp Painful-Urination Syndrome causing slight urinary

retention and burning on urination occurring against a background of Kidney-Yin deficiency.
- *P-6 Neiguan* and *T.B.-6 Zhigou* to regulate Qi, eliminate stagnation in the Three Burners, open the chest and calm the Mind. This combination can be used for stagnation of Liver-Qi, deriving from emotional stress and affecting the hypochondrium and chest and causing a feeling of oppression of the chest and sighing. This combination can also be used for sprain of the rib muscles.
- *T.B.-3 Zhongzhu* and *P-6 Neiguan* to move Qi, eliminate stagnation, open the Mind's orifices, calm the Mind and lift mood. This combination is very good to treat mental depression and confusion deriving from long-standing, suppressed emotional problems.
- *T.B.-3 Zhongzhu* and *P-7 Daling* to move Qi, eliminate stagnation, open the Mind's orifices, calm the Mind, settle the Ethereal Soul and lift mood. This combination is similar in its effect to the previous one. The main difference is that this combination is more calming whereas the previous one is more moving.
- *G.B.-43 Xiaxi* and *LIV-3 Taichong* to subdue Liver-Yang. This combination is very good to treat temporal headaches from Liver-Yang: LIV-3 subdues Liver-Yang, while G.B.-43 affects the temporal area.

2. BALANCING UNRELATED YIN AND YANG CHANNELS

The following are examples of combination of unrelated Yin and Yang channels.

- *LU-9 Taiyuan* and *ST-36 Zusanli* to tonify Lung- and Stomach-Qi and Qi in general. The Stomach is the origin of Food Qi (*Gu Qi*) and the Lungs govern the Gathering Qi (*Zong Qi*): the combination of these two channels therefore powerfully tonifies Qi.
- *L.I.-11 Quchi* and *SP-10 Xuehai* to clear Heat and cool Blood. This combination is excellent to cool Blood in skin diseases.
- *ST-36 Zusanli, KI-3 Taixi* and *SP-6 Sanyinjiao* to nourish Stomach- and Kidney-Yin.

- *ST-36 Zusanli and P-6 Neiguan* to harmonize the Middle Burner and subdue rebellious Stomach-Qi: this combination has already been mentioned in connection with balancing Top and Bottom.
- *ST-40 Fenglong and P-6 Neiguan* to regulate the Middle Burner, subdue rebellious Stomach-Qi, resolve Phlegm, calm the Mind and harmonize the rising and descending of Qi: this combination has already been mentioned above in connection with balancing Top and Bottom.
- *ST-40 Fenglong and P-5 Jianshi* to resolve Phlegm from the Heart, calm the Mind and open the Mind's orifices. This combination can be used when the Mind is obstructed by Phlegm and the person is confused: in severe cases this can lead to mania or schizophrenia.
- *SP-5 Shangqiu and G.B.-40 Qiuxu* to treat Painful Obstruction Syndrome or sprain of the ankle.
- *HE-7 Shenmen and G.B.-40 Qiuxu* to tonify Heart- and Gall-Bladder-Qi, calm the Mind and strengthen the Gall-Bladder's capacity for taking decisions.
- *S.I.-4 Wangu and LIV-3 Taichong* to move Liver-Qi in the hypochondrium and scapula. This combination is good when stagnation of Liver-Qi causes a pain in the hypochondrium extending to the scapula.
- *S.I.-1 Shaoze and LIV-3 Taichong* to move Liver-Qi in the breast. This combination is good when stagnation of Liver-Qi affects the breast causing pre-menstrual distension or retention of milk in nursing mothers.
- *BL-63 Jinmen and LIV-6 Zhongdu* to stop urinary pain related to the Liver channel.
- *L.I.-4 Hegu and KI-7 Fuliu* to regulate sweating. This combination of points can either stimulate sweating (by reinforcing KI-7 and reducing L.I.-4) or stop sweating (by reinforcing L.I.-4 and reducing KI-7).

3. BALANCING OF CONNECTING AND SOURCE POINTS

Balancing Connecting and Source points is an important aspect of the general principle of balancing Yin and Yang.

This consists in selecting first the Source point of the channel treating the main condition and then, the Connecting point of its related channel in order to boost the effect of the Source point. For example, if one is treating Lung-Yin deficiency and the Source point LU-9 Taiyuan is selected, L.I.-6 Pianli can be added to strengthen the effect of LU-9. Thus, the Source point is used as a primary point and the Connecting point as a secondary one.

The following are some of the most important and frequently-used combinations of Source and Connecting points.

- *L.I.-4 Hegu and LU-7 Lieque* to restore the descending of Lung-Qi, and release or consolidate the Exterior. This combination is often used to release the Exterior in invasions of Wind-Cold. However, it can also be used in interior conditions to restore the descending of Lung-Qi, consolidate the Exterior and strengthen the Defensive Qi. Also, on a mental level, this combination settles the Corporeal Soul and has a releasing effect on repressed emotions.
- *P-6 Neiguan and T.B.-4 Yangchi* to regulate the Three Burners, move Liver-Qi and calm the Mind. This is a very good combination to indirectly move Liver-Qi and calm the Mind. It particularly affects and relaxes the muscles of the top of the shoulders and neck and therefore relieves headaches in that area.
- *ST-40 Fenglong and SP-3 Taibai* to tonify the Spleen and resolve Phlegm. This combination is very good especially in Stomach conditions with Phlegm; it also resolves Phlegm from the brain due to the distal position of SP-3 near the end of the channel (and therefore affecting the other extremity).
- *G.B.-37 Guangming and LIV-3 Taichong* to brighten the eyes in Liver patterns.
- *KI-4 Dazhong and BL-64 Jinggu* to treat sciatica (using BL-64 on the affected side and KI-4 on the other).

4. BALANCING YIN AND YANG ACCORDING TO HEAVENLY STEMS

Each channel is associated with a heavenly stem,

Yang channels with Yang stems and Yin channels with Yin stems as follows:

1. Gall-Bladder
2. Liver
3. Small Intestine
4. Heart
5. Stomach
6. Spleen
7. Large Intestine
8. Lungs
9. Bladder
10. Kidneys.

Balancing Yin and Yang points according to heavenly stems simply means balancing points of channel 1 with 6, 2 with 7, 3 with 8, etc. as follows:

Gall-Bladder — Spleen
Small Intestine — Lungs
Stomach — Kidneys
Large Intestine — Liver
Bladder — Heart

It will be noticed that this essentially consists in balancing a Yang-channel's points with those from the Yin channel which is controlled by it in the Controlling cycle of the 5 Elements.

This method stresses the importance of balancing Yang points with Yin ones, rather than the other way round. For example, if one uses several points from the Gall-Bladder channel in one treatment it would be wise to balance them with one or two from the Spleen channel; but if one uses several points from the Spleen channel it is not necessary to balance them with points from the Gall-Bladder channel. The explanation for this is in the 5-Element Controlling cycle and in the theory of Yin-Yang: it is necessary to balance Yang-channel points (Yang corresponding to activity and, in disease, to an "attack" or "invasion") with those of the Yin channel which is controlled by it to prevent the Yang channel from over-acting on the Yin one.

For example, suppose one is treating a patient with sciatica occurring along the Gall-Bladder channel. One selects G.B.-30 Huantiao, G.B.-29 Juliao, G.B.-31 Fengshi and G.B.-34 Yanglingquan. It might be a good idea to balance these four Gall-Bladder points with perhaps one on the Spleen channel, say SP-3 Taibai or SP-6 Sanyinjiao. It is even better if the Spleen point can be chosen according to the condition of the patient rather than just for the sake of balancing the Gall-Bladder points. For example, say that the patient with sciatica also suffers from insomnia from Blood deficiency, then SP-6 Sanyinjiao would be a good choice to balance the Gall-Bladder points as it would not only perform a balancing function but also treat insomnia.

Another example could be that of a patient with chronic shoulder inflammation with pain radiating down to the arm being treated with L.I.-15 Jianyu, L.I.-14 Binao, L.I.-11 Quchi and L.I.-4 Hegu. As four Large Intestine points are being used, it might be necessary to balance these with a point of the Liver channel: LIV-3 Taichong might be an especially suitable choice as this point would also relax the inflamed shoulder's sinews.

In the previous example when Large Intestine points are balanced with SP-6 Sanyinjiao, this point could be used on the opposite side: this would achieve the effect of balancing Top and Bottom, Yin and Yang, the Heavenly Stems, and Left and Right. It would therefore be a very harmonious combination.

Another example of balancing according to the Heavenly Stems could be that of a patient being treated for sciatica along the Bladder channel with BL-54 Zhibian, BL-36 Chengfu, BL-37 Yinmen and BL-40 Weizhong: these Bladder points could be balanced with a point from the Heart channel such as, say, HE-7 Shenmen. This would be all the more indicated if the patient is tense and anxious. In fact, especially in men, the point HE-7 Shenmen has an excellent effect in relaxing the muscles of the back (see chapter 24 on "Lower Back-ache").

Finally, balancing Yin and Yang points is especially necessary when several points of the same polarity are used, as in the examples given above. This is particularly necessary, as mentioned above, when several Yang points from the same channel are used in one treatment.

BALANCING BACK AND FRONT

Balancing Back and Front is another aspect of

balancing of Yin and Yang but it is best discussed separately. Balancing Back and Front has two aspects:

Balancing Back-Transporting with Front-Collecting points
Balancing Governing with Directing Vessel

1. BALANCING BACK-TRANSPORTING WITH FRONT-COLLECTING POINTS

The Back-Transporting points are mentioned in various chapters of the "Yellow Emperor's Classic of Internal Medicine". Chapter 51 of the "Spiritual Axis" lists the Back-Transporting points of the five Yin organs.[8] Chapter 59 and others of the "Simple Questions" discuss the Back-Transporting points of the Yang organs; in all, the "Yellow Emperor's Classic" lists 10 Back-Transporting points, leaving out BL-22 Sanjiaoshu, first mentioned in the "ABC of Acupuncture" (AD 282), and BL-14 Jueyinshu, first mentioned in the "1000 Golden Ducats Prescriptions" (AD 652).

The Back-Transporting points are points where Qi gathers and infuses to the internal organs. Because these points are on the Yang side of the body and, furthermore, on the Bladder channel which pertains to the Greater Yang and which circulates Defensive Qi over the whole back, they can be used, with moxa, to warm the internal organs.

The Front-Collecting points are points where the Qi of the internal organs gathers. They are all on the Yin side of the body and can be used to clear Heat. Traditionally, the Back-Transporting points, Yang in character, were used for Yin diseases ("Yin" meaning chronic, Cold, Deficiency or Yin-organ disease), and the Front-Collecting points, Yin in character, for Yang diseases ("Yang" meaning acute, Heat, Excess or Yang-organ disease). Chapter 67 of the "Classic of Difficulties" in fact says:

Yin diseases reach the Yang and Yang diseases reach the Yin; for this reason, the Front-Collecting points are on the Yin surface and the Back-Transporting points on the Yang surface.[9]

The implication of this statement is that as Yin diseases reach the Yang, the Back-Transporting points are used to treat them, and, as Yang diseases reach the Yin, the Front-Collecting points are used to treat them. However, this is by no means an absolute rule and both sets of points can be used for Yin or Yang diseases, intended in the broad meaning indicated above.

Combining Back-Transporting with Front-Collecting points will balance Yin with Yang, and Nutritive with Defensive Qi. This combination provides a particularly strong treatment of the internal organs in chronic conditions. For example, the combination of Ren-12 Zhongwan with BL-21 Weishu, respectively Front-Collecting and Back-Transporting points of the Stomach, provides a strong tonification of the Stomach (if needled with reinforcing method or used with moxa).

If treatment is given fairly frequently, say, 2–3 times a week, then Back-Transporting points can be alternated with Front-Collecting points on alternate sessions, as the use of both sets of points in each session would be too strong. If treatment is given more infrequently, say, fortnightly or less, then Back-Transporting and Front-Collecting points could be combined in one session.

Back-Transporting points are best used with a short retention of needles of, say, about 10 minutes or less, or with moxa only. If needles are left in these points for longer, they may tend to have a reducing effect and make the patient very tired. In a Deficiency condition, if one is in doubt, it is best to use the Back-Transporting points with moxa only (unless of course, there are signs of Heat or Empty-Heat).

There are also two other ways of combining the Back-Transporting and Front-Collecting points: the former can be combined with the Source points and the latter with the Sea points.

Combining Back-Transporting with the Source points of the same organ specifically treats the Yin organs, chronic diseases and Deficiency conditions. For example, BL-13 Feishu with LU-9 Taiyuan, or BL-18 Ganshu with LIV-3 Taichong.

Combining Front-Collecting with Sea points of the same organ specifically treats the Yang organs, acute diseases and Excess conditions. It should be borne in mind that by Sea point of the Large Intestine, Small Intestine and Triple

Burner is meant their Lower Sea points, i.e. ST-37 Shangjuxu, ST-39 Xiajuxu and BL-39 Weiyang. A full listing of these points is given in Table I.2.

The polarity of Back-Front and specifically Back-Transporting points against Front-Collecting points can also be made use of in correcting the ill effects of a treatment. For example, supposing too many Back-Transporting points have been used, or maybe they have been left in for too long and the patient feels very tired after the treatment, then this effect can be corrected by using one or two points in the front and specifically some Front-Collecting points.

2. BALANCING GOVERNING AND DIRECTING VESSELS

Balancing points from the Governing and Directing Vessels is a very important aspect of Yin-Yang and Back-Front balancing. The Governing Vessel governs all the Yang channels while the Directing vessel governs all the Yin channels: thus points on these two channels acquire special importance in balancing Front and Back.

These two channels are also particularly suited for combining as their pathways arise from the same area between the Kidneys and cross over internally so that they could be seen as one circuit. As these two vessels flow upwards from Ren-1 Huiyin but also downwards internally, combining their points also regulates the ascending and descending of Qi.

Table I.2 Combination of Front-Collecting and Sea points

Channel	Front-Collecting points	Sea points
Lungs	LU-1 Zhongfu	LU-3 Chize
Large intestine	ST-25 Tianshu	ST-37 Shangjuxu
Stomach	Ren-12 Zhongwan	ST-36 Zusanli
Spleen	LIV-13 Zhangmen	SP-9 Yinlingquan
Heart	Ren-14 Juque	HE-3 Shaohai
Small intestine	Ren-4 Guanyuan	ST-39 Xiajuxu
Bladder	Ren-3 Zhongji	BL-40 Weizhong
Kidneys	G.B.-25 Jingmen	KI-10 Yingu
Pericardium	Ren-17 Shanzhong	P-3 Quze
Triple burner	Ren-5 Shimen	BL-39 Weiyang
Gall-Bladder	G.B.-24 Riyue	G.B.-34 Yanglingquan
Liver	LIV-14 Qimen	LIV-8 Ququan

Finally, as these two vessels both flow upwards to the head and the Governing Vessel flows into the brain, combining their points also has a very powerful and important mental effect which can be either excitatory or calming.

The following are examples of combination of points from the Governing and Directing Vessels.

- *Du-19 Houding and Ren-15 Jiuwei* to calm the Mind. Du-19 calms the Mind and extinguishes (internal) Wind while Ren-15 calms the Mind and nourishes the Heart. This combination has a powerful calming effect as Ren-15 nourishes and Du-19 calms. Ren-15 will also relieve anxiety manifesting with a feeling of oppression in the chest.
- *Du-20 Baihui and Ren-15 Jiuwei* to calm the Mind and lift mood. This combination can simultaneously calm the Mind with Ren-15 and improve the mood and lift depression with Du-20. It is an excellent combination for mental depression with anxiety.
- *Du-14 Dazhui and Ren-4 Guanyuan*, both with direct moxa cones, to tonify and warm Yang. Du-14, with moxa, warms all the Yang channels and the Bladder, while Ren-4, with moxa, tonifies and warms Kidney-Yang which is the foundation for all the Yang energies of the body. Thus this combination tonifies the Bladder and Kidney-Yang and Yang Qi in general.
- *Du-16 Fengfu and Ren-24 Chengjiang* to treat occipital headache.[10]
- *Du-20 Baihui and Ren-12 Zhongwan* to tonify the Stomach and Spleen and lift mood. This combination is good to lift depression occurring against a background of deficiency of Stomach and Spleen.
- *Du-24 Shenting and Ren-4 Guanyuan* to nourish the Kidneys, strengthen the Original Qi and calm the Mind. This combination calms the Mind by nourishing Kidney-Yin and strengthening the Original Qi. It is suitable for severe anxiety occurring against a background of Kidney-Yin deficiency. It is particularly indicated for anxiety as it roots Qi in the Lower Burner and draws it

downwards away from the head and the Heart where it harasses the Mind.

- *Yintang and Ren-4 Guanyuan* to calm the Mind and nourish the Kidneys: this combination is similar to the previous one as it roots Qi in the Lower Burner by nourishing the Kidneys and strengthening the Original Qi. Whilst the previous combination is better for anxiety and worrying, this one is better for insomnia.
- *Du-20 Baihui and Ren-4 Guanyuan* to calm the Mind, nourish the Kidneys, strengthen the Original Qi and lift mood. This combination lifts mood and relieves depression by nourishing Kidney-Yin and strengthening the Original Qi. It is suitable for depression and anxiety occurring against a background of Kidney-Yin deficiency.
- *Du-20 Baihui and Ren-6 Qihai* to tonify and raise Qi. Ren-6 tonifies Qi in general while Du-20 raises Qi: the combination of these two points is excellent to tonify and raise Qi in case of prolapses. However, its use need not be confined to such conditions; it also has a powerful mood-lifting effect in depression.

BALANCING LEFT AND RIGHT

Balancing Left and Right provides one of the most interesting options in treatment. The polarity Left-Right surfaces in many aspects of Chinese medicine.

Left and Right are two aspects of the Yang-Yin polarity, Left corresponding to Yang and Right to Yin. There are several "reasons" (if they can be called such) for this. One is related to a myth about the origin of the left-right imbalance in the ancient Chinese cosmos. According to ancient Chinese views, the sky was like an inverted bowl rotating on its own axis above the earth. According to legends, a mythical being called Kong Kong tore a hole in the sky and tilted it towards the East so that the sun shone less in the North-West. This meant that there was a predominance of Heaven (the sky) in the East (=Left) and a predominance of Earth in the West (=Right). Thus, the following polarity was established:

Yang = Heaven = East = Left
Yin = Earth = West = Right.

Chapter 6 of the "Simple Questions" establishes the cardinal points and their reference to Left-Right: *"The Sage stands facing South . . ."*.[11] Thus, he has the East to his left and the West to his right.[12] Hence the following polarity:

South = East = Left = Yang
North = West = Right = Yin.

In chapter 5, the same book confirms the East-West (and Left-Right) imbalance created by the mythical Kong Kong and applies it to the human body:

. . . Right and Left are two aspects of Yin-Yang . . . Heaven is lesser in the North and West [and therefore Right] . . . for this reason the right ear and eye [belonging to Heaven] are not as good as the left ones. Earth is lesser in the South and East [and therefore Left] . . . for this reason the left hand and foot [belonging to Earth] are not as good as the right ones . . . Therefore when pathogenic factors attack the body the right side of the top part, and the left side of the lower part of the body will suffer more severely . . .[13]

The Left-Right polarity is also defined by the energetic sphere of the Extraordinary Vessels. The Governing and Directing Vessels flowing along the midline of the body, the former along the back and the latter along the front, divide it into left and right sides. The Yang Heel and Yin Heel Vessels, associated with the Governing and Directing Vessels respectively, harmonize Left and Right. Thus, there is a correspondence between Back and Left (Governing Vessel and Yang Heel Vessel) and between Front and Right (Directing Vessel and Yin Heel Vessel). The Governing and Directing Vessels represent the earliest embryological separation of left and right sides of the body for, as soon as a spermatozoon penetrates the ovum, it defines the median plane of Governing and Directing Vessels and therefore divides the body into left and right sides. As both the Governing and Directing Vessels originate from the Kidneys and these are considered in Chinese medicine to be the only organ with two separate viscera (the lungs being seen as one viscus) on left and right sides, balancing Left and Right is also an important aspect of balancing Kidney-Yin and Kidney-Yang.

The Chinese correspondence between Back and Left (Yang) and Front and Right (Yin) seems to be confirmed by recent discoveries in palaeontology. According to these theories the ancestor of all vertebrates (500 million years ago) was *Cothurnocystis elizae*, which was strikingly asymmetrical between left and right. Its own ancestor, which lived on the sea bed, had been perfectly symmetrical between left and right. For some reason, it flipped on its right side which became its front, so that its left side became its back.[14] This means that all animals that evolved from *Cothurnocystis elizae*-like organisms, including vertebrates such as Man, have a left and a right that were originally their back and front respectively. As mentioned earlier, the human embryo determines left and right sides early in development: this has to be done if organs are to end up functioning correctly in the appropriate sides of the body.

Left and right sides are never energetically identical as there is always an imbalance between them. The ancient Chinese cosmology, as we have seen, attributed this to a "lack of Heaven" on the right side and a "lack of Earth" on the left side. The Left-Right imbalance can be easily seen on the face in the difference between the left and right eyes and ears, and in the left testicle's being lower than the right, one kidney's being placed higher than the other, the difference in function between left and right sides of the brain, etc.

Furthermore, Left is traditionally associated with Yang and the male element, Right with Yin and the female element. In fact, if we look at the cycle of the 12 Earthly Branches corresponding to the daily cycle of 24 hours, conception was thought to occur at the Earthly Branch *Si* (6th Branch). If we start from the 1st Branch *Zi*, the male element needs to go through 30 Branches (in order to be a multiple of 10) moving towards the left, and the female element needs to go through 20 Branches moving towards the right, in both cases counting the starting Branch (Fig. I.14). Furthermore, according to ancient Chinese ideas, pregnancy lasted 10 (lunar)

months and, if we take each Branch to correspond to a month, the female embryo moves towards the right from the Branch *Si* to the Branch *Shen* (this branch corresponding to female, Autumn and the number 7), and the male embryo moves towards the left from the Branch *Si* to the Branch *Yin* (this branch corresponding to male, Spring and the number 8). The correspondence between left and male and that between right and female are used in the balancing of opening points of the Extraordinary Vessels and can be used for the Left-Right balancing of other channels as well. This will be explained shortly.

Left-Right balancing will be discussed from the following points of view:

Connecting channels
Extraordinary Vessels
Divergent channels
Main channels
    Arm and leg channels of same polarity
    Exteriorly-interiorly related channels
    Other channels
Channel problems

1. CONNECTING CHANNELS

The Connecting point of the affected channel can sometimes be needled on the opposite side. This

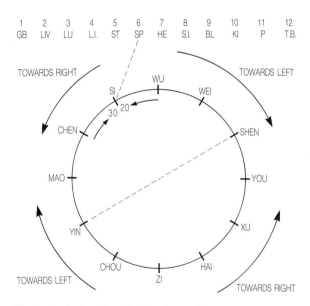

Fig. I.14 Cycle of Earthly Branches and conception

technique is used mostly in acute painful conditions due to invasion of a channel by external pathogenic factors. When a pathogenic factor invades a Connecting channel on one side, it does so because there is a temporary and relative deficiency of Qi in the channel of that side whilst the other side is in a state of relative Excess (due to the imbalance of Qi between one side and the other). Thus to needle a distal point on the affected side with reducing method would further weaken the channel. For this reason, it is necessary to needle (with reducing method) the Connecting point of the opposite side, and local points on the affected side.

For example, in case of invasion of Cold in the Connecting channel of the Large Intestine on the right side causing a pain in the arm extending to the shoulder and jaw, we can needle (with reducing method) L.I.-6 Pianli on the left side and local points (with moxa on needle) on the right side.

Chapter 63 of the "Simple Questions" deals with what it calls "reverse needling":

When the pathogenic factor invades the Connecting channels the left side is in Excess while the disease [i.e. pathogenic factor] is on the right and vice versa.[15]

It further says:

When the pathogenic factor resides in the Kidney Connecting channel . . . needle the left side if the disease is on the right [and vice versa] . . .[16]

In chronic cases the problem is quite different as the pathogenic factor has penetrated into the main channels and the Connecting channels are relatively empty. In this case, local points on one side can be balanced by the Connecting point of the related channel on the opposite side, needled with reinforcing method. For example, if there is a chronic pain from invasion of Cold in the Large Intestine channel on the right side, we can needle (with moxa on needle) local points of the Large Intestine channel on the right side and balance them with the Connecting point of the Lung channel (LU-7 Lieque) on the left side.

2. EXTRAORDINARY VESSELS

The Extraordinary Vessels' opening points are

a prime example of Left-Right balancing. In particular, the Extraordinary Vessels play an important role in balancing the circulation of Qi between Left and Right: this role belongs especially to the Governing Vessel, the Directing Vessel, the Yang Heel Vessel and the Yin Heel Vessel. These four vessels balance Yin and Yang between Left and Right.

The opening points of the Extraordinary Vessels are usually crossed over according to gender: in a man, the opening point (inserted first) is used on the left side and the coupled point on the right side. For example, if the Governing Vessel is used in a man, one would needle S.I.-3 first on the left side and BL-62 Shenmai afterwards on the right. In a woman the reverse is used: the opening point is inserted first on the right side and the coupled point on the left. For example, if the Directing Vessel is used in a woman, LU-7 Lieque is needled first on the right, and KI-6 Zhaohai on the left.

The opening points of the Extraordinary Vessels can be combined with other points, also needled unilaterally. This creates a particularly dynamic combination. For example, if we were treating a man suffering from a deficiency of the Kidneys causing a chronic lower back-ache on the midline, insomnia and anxiety, we could use the opening points of the Governing Vessel, HE-7 Shenmen to calm the Mind and KI-4 Taixi to nourish the Kidneys and strengthen Will-Power. These points could be combined in this way: S.I.-3 Houxi on the left, BL-62 Shenmai on the right, HE-7 Shenmen on the right and KI-4 Dazhong on the left. This particular combination is very powerful and very balanced as it harmonizes Left and Right, Top and Bottom, Yin and Yang, and Greater Yang with Lesser Yin. KI-4 Dazhong, Connecting point, is used in preference to KI-3 Taixi as the Connecting point will also affect the Bladder channel and therefore the back-ache. Other examples of the combination of the Extraordinary Vessels' opening points with other channels' points will be given shortly below.

3. DIVERGENT CHANNELS

One of the functions of the divergent channels is

to harmonize Left and Right. It will be remembered that all the divergent channels start near articulations such as feet, hands, knees, hips and shoulders. From there, they all enter their respective and other organs and re-emerge around the neck; in this area, the Yin divergent channels join their related Yang divergent channel (see Fig. 1.4 in chapter 1, "Headache"), while the Yang divergent channels rejoin their main channel. Thus, in the end, all divergent channels join the Yang main channels around the neck and head. Furthermore, the Yang divergent channels join interiorly-exteriorly related Yin and Yang organs internally (e.g. the Bladder divergent channel joins with both the bladder and the kidney organs). Figure I.15 shows the pathways of the Kidney and Bladder Divergent channels as an example.

Thus, divergent channels harmonize not only Yin and Yang but also Left and Right because they all, in the end, join the Yang main channels in the neck area: in fact, the Yang channels all join in the head superficially and converge at Du-20 Baihui; they play an important role in balancing the circulation of Qi between Left and Right.

Painful symptoms which move from one side to the other (as often happens in migraines) indicate affliction of the divergent channels. In such cases, it is necessary to needle the opposite side (i.e. the side opposite to where the pain is) usually needling the Well point. For example, if a migraine headache occurring on the Gall-Bladder channel normally moves from one side to the other and the patient is seen during an acute attack with pain on the left side, then one can needle the Well point of the right side, i.e. G.B.-44 Zuqiaoyin as a distal point and local points on the affected side. The pain will temporarily move to the right side and then go.

4. MAIN CHANNELS

Using points unilaterally, balancing them between Left and Right, presents us with the opportunity of creating very interesting and balanced combinations of points. Needling points unilaterally, balancing Left and Right has several advantages:

(a) it makes for a particularly dynamic effect
(b) it balances Left and Right
(c) it allows us to reduce the total number of points used.

Far from reducing the effect of the treatment, using points unilaterally makes the treatment more dynamic and powerful: it is like applying a force to the tangents of two opposite poles of a circle, making it spin (Fig. I.16).

Since using points unilaterally and balanced between Left and Right has a particularly dynamic effect, I generally use in this way points which are intended to move Qi or Blood and I use bilaterally those to tonify Qi and Blood, although not exclusively so. For example, if a woman patient presented with symptoms of insomnia, anxiety, and pre-menstrual tension

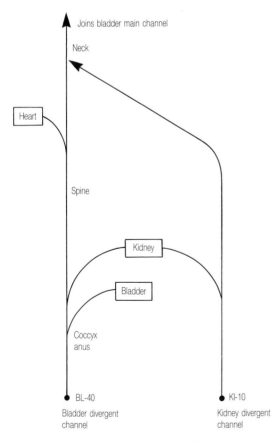

Fig. I.15 Pathways of Kidney and Bladder Divergent channels

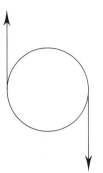

Fig. I.16 Effect of unilateral needling

due to stagnation of Liver-Qi from emotional problems occurring against a background of Qi and Blood deficiency, one could needle P-6 Neiguan on the right and LIV-3 Taichong on the left to move Liver-Qi, calm the Mind and settle the Ethereal Soul, and ST-36 Zusanli and SP-6 Sanyinjiao, both bilaterally, to tonify Qi and Blood.

When needling unilaterally, the laterality can be chosen according to various criteria:

(a) according to painful side: needle distal and local points on the painful side and balance them with some points on the other side (e.g. L.I.-15, L.I.-11 and L.I.-4 on the right and LIV-3 on the left)

(b) according to gender and Top-Bottom: needle an arm-channel point on the left for men and right for women and a leg-channel point on the other side (e.g. P-6 Neiguan on the right in women and left in men, and LIV-3 on the opposite side)

(c) according to Yin-Yang: needle a Yin point on the left (the Yang side) and a Yang point on the right (the Yin side).

Unilateral needling can be discussed from four points of view:

(a) Arm and leg channels of the same polarity
(b) Exteriorly-interiorly related channels
(c) Other channels
(d) Channel problems.

(a) ARM AND LEG CHANNELS OF THE SAME POLARITY

Arm and leg channels of the same polarity are those of Greater Yang (Small Intestine and Bladder), Greater Yin (Lung and Spleen), etc. Since the channels within each of these pairs are closely connected, unilateral needling is particularly effective. Examples of combination of Yang arm and leg channels have already been given above, so they will be discussed here only briefly. In addition, I will give some examples of unilateral needling of points from Yin arm and leg channels.

(i) Bright Yang

– *L.I.-4 Hegu and ST-36 Zusanli* to harmonize the rising and descending of Qi and regulate digestion. L.I.-4 could be used on the right in a woman and on the left in a man, with ST-36 on the opposite side, as explained above.

– *L.I.-4 Hegu and ST-44 Neiting* to harmonize the rising and descending of Qi, with the same laterality as above.

– *L.I.-10 Shousanli and ST-36 Zusanli* to harmonize the rising and descending of Qi and strengthen the Bright Yang channels. It also tonifies Stomach- and Spleen-Qi, invigorates the channels and strengthens the limbs. This combination is useful to tonify Qi and the limbs in patients suffering from ME (post-viral fatigue syndrome).

– *L.I.-11 Quchi and ST-43 Xiangu* to benefit sinews and expel Wind-Damp-Heat in Heat Painful Obstruction Syndrome.

(ii) Greater Yang

– *S.I.-3 Houxi and BL-60 Kunlun* to harmonize the rising and descending of Qi and expel Wind. Needle S.I.-3 on the right in a woman and on the left in a man, and BL-62 on the opposite side.

– *S.I.-6 Yanglao and BL-66 Tonggu* to harmonize the rising and descending of Qi and expel Wind from the Greater-Yang channels. Needle with the same laterality as above.

(iii) Lesser Yang

– *T.B.-6 Zhigou and G.B.-31 Fengshi* to harmonize the Lesser Yang, expel Wind,

regulate Qi and eliminate stagnation. Needle
T.B.-6 on the right for a woman and on the
left for a man, and G.B.-31 on the opposite
side.
- *T.B.-4 Yangchi and G.B.-40 Qiuxu* harmonize
the Lesser Yang channels and regulate the
rising and descending of Qi. Needle with the
same laterality as above.

(iv) Greater Yin

- *LU-9 Taiyuan and SP-3 Taibai*, both Source
points, to tonify Qi. Needle LU-9 on the right
for a man and on the left for a woman.
- *LU-5 Chize and SP-10 Xuehai* to cool Blood,
especially in chronic skin diseases. LU-5
clears Heat and affects the skin (by virtue of
the Lung governing the skin) and SP-10 cools
Blood. Needle LU-5 on the right in a woman
and the left in a man, and SP-10 on the
opposite side.

(v) Terminal Yin

- *P-6 Neiguan and LIV-3 Taichong* to move Liver-
Qi, eliminate stagnation deriving from
repressed emotions, calm the Mind and settle
the Ethereal Soul. Needle P-6 on the right in a
woman and on the left in a man, and LIV-3 on
the opposite side. The left-right unilateral
needling of these two points produces
particularly good results.
- *P-7 Daling and LIV-3 Taichong* to move Liver-
Qi, eliminate stagnation deriving from
emotional stress (especially the breaking-up
of relationships), calm the Mind and settle the
Ethereal Soul. Use with the same laterality as
above.
- *P-3 Quze and LIV-3 Taichong* to clear Heat and
cool Blood in skin diseases.

(vi) Lesser Yin

- *HE-7 Shenmen and KI-3 Taixi* to harmonize
Heart and Kidneys and calm the Mind.
Needle HE-7 on the right in women and on
the left in men, and KI-3 on the opposite side.
- *HE-6 Yinxi and KI-7 Fuliu* to nourish Heart-
Yin and Kidney-Yin and stop night-sweating.
Needle with the same laterality as above.

(b) EXTERIORLY-INTERIORLY RELATED CHANNELS

The exteriorly-interiorly related channels are
Lung and Large Intestine, Stomach and Spleen,
etc. needling points of these channels unilaterally balancing Left and Right also balances Yin
and Yang. These points could be further balanced by needling Yin points on the Yang side
(i.e. left) and Yang points on the Yin side (i.e.
right). Examples of such combinations have already been given above and will only be listed
here:

- *LU-7 Lieque and L.I.-4 Hegu* to release the Exterior and expel Wind.
- *LU-5 Chize and L.I.-11 Quchi* to clear Heat and cool Blood in skin diseases.
- *LU-9 Taiyuan and L.I.-4 Hegu.*
- *LU-11 Shaoshang and L.I.-4 Hegu.*
- *ST-36 Zusanli and SP-4 Gongsun.*
- *HE-7 Shenmen and S.I.-5 Yanggu.*
- *LIV-3 Taichong and G.B.-34 Yanglingquan.*
- *SP-8 Diji, SP-6 Sanyinjiao, ST-28 Shuidao and ST-29 Guilai.*
- *LU-3 Tianfu and L.I.-4 Hegu.*[17]
- *ST-45 Lidui and SP-1 Yinbai.*[18]
- *HE-6 Yinxi and S.I.-3 Houxi.*[19]
- *KI-8 Jiaoxin and BL-55 Heyang.*[20]
- *G.B.-30 Huantiao, LIV-2 Xingjian and G.B.-31 Fengshi.*[21]
- *LU-5 Chize and L.I.-11 Quchi.*
- *ST-36 Zusanli and SP-6 Sanyinjiao.*
- *ST-39 Xiajuxu and SP-6 Sanyinjiao.*
- *BL-63 Jinmen and KI-10 Yingu.*
- *P-6 Neiguan and T.B.-6 Zhigou.*
- *T.B.-3 Zhongzhu and P-6 Neiguan.*
- *T.B.-3 Zhongzhu and P-7 Daling.*
- *G.B.-43 Xiaxi and LIV-3 Taichong.*

(c) OTHER CHANNELS

Unilateral needling, balancing Left and Right,
can be applied to any channel, combining it
with any of the principles discussed so far. For
example, Left-Right balancing can be combined
with Yin-Yang, Top-Bottom or Heavenly Stem
balancing. Combination of Left-Right can be
achieved in several ways:

- combining points of same polarity on the same half of the body
- combining points of different polarity on the same half of the body
- combining points of same polarity in different halves of the body
- combining points of different polarity in different halves of the body.

A few examples will be given for each of these; more examples will be given within the case histories shortly. In all the following examples, one point is used on one side and the other on the opposite side.

(i) Left-Right combining of points of same polarity on same half of the body

- *LU-7 Lieque and P-6 Neiguan* to settle the Corporeal Soul and Ethereal Soul and lift mood. This combination is excellent for emotional problems, such as sadness and grief, affecting the Lungs (and therefore Corporeal Soul), the Liver (and therefore Ethereal Soul) and the Heart. These two points have a dynamic, centrifugal effect, and, on the emotional level, they help the patient to express his or her emotions and get in touch with his or her sadness and grief. They affect the Ethereal Soul, which is housed in the Liver, via the Pericardium to which the Liver is related. It is particularly effective in those cases when sadness has affected the Liver as well as the Lungs.
- *LU-7 Lieque and HE-7 Shenmen* to settle the Corporeal Soul and calm the Mind. These two points have a balanced, co-ordinated effect, as LU-7 brings emotions out and HE-7 calms them down. The combination is therefore suitable in emotional problems such as worry and grief affecting Lungs and Heart and causing anxiety.
- *L.I.-4 Hegu and S.I.-5 Yanggu* to calm the Mind and subdue rebellious Qi. This combination is particularly useful in those who are anxious and confused about choosing the direction to take in life.
- *ST-36 Zusanli and G.B.-34 Yanglingquan* to tonify Stomach-Qi and move Liver-Qi. This combination is used in conditions characterized by deficiency of Stomach- and Spleen-Qi and stagnant Liver-Qi invading the Stomach and causing bad digestion, epigastric distension and nausea.
- *KI-3 Taixi (with reinforcing method) and LIV-3 Taichong (with reducing method)* to nourish the Kidneys and subdue Liver-Yang or Liver-Wind.
- *KI-2 Rangu and LIV-3 Taichong* to cool Blood. This combination can be used in a wide variety of Liver-related problems deriving from Blood-Heat, such as menorrhagia or skin diseases.

(ii) Left-Right combining of points of different polarity on same half of the body

- *LU-7 Lieque and S.I.-5 Yanggu* to settle the Corporeal Soul and calm the Mind. This combination is useful to treat emotional problems such as worry affecting Lungs and Heart; in particular, it helps the person to see issues clearly and make choices.
- *G.B.-34 Yanglingquan and LIV-3 Taichong* to move Liver-Qi, calm the Mind and settle the Ethereal Soul. This combination is excellent to move Liver-Qi on a physical level (hypochondrial or abdominal distension), and on an emotional level (moodiness, depression, pre-menstrual tension). It can be suitably combined with local points to target the area affected: Ren-12 Zhongwan for the epigastrium, LIV-14 Qimen for the hypochondrium and Ren-6 Qihai for the lower abdomen.

(iii) Left-Right combining of points of same polarity in different halves of the body

- *S.I.-5 Yanggu and G.B.-40 Qiuxu*: this combination has a marked mental effect in helping the person to discriminate between choices (with S.I.-5) and find the strength to act upon the chosen course (G.B.-40). The unilateral, Left-Right needling of these two points adds a dynamic dimension to the combination contributing to its moving effect on the mental level, thus helping the person to resolve an indecision which may have been going on for a long time.

– *HE-7 Shenmen and LIV-3 Taichong* to calm the Mind and settle the Ethereal Soul. This combination has a powerful calming effect and is suitable for anxiety and worry related to Heart and Liver patterns.

(iv) Left-Right combining of points of different polarity in different halves of the body

These combinations will balance Top and Bottom, Yin and Yang, and Left and Right.

– *LU-9 Taiyuan and ST-36 Zusanli* to tonify Lung- and Stomach-Qi.
– *L.I.-4 Hegu and LIV-3 Taichong*: this combination has already been explained above and it also represents a balancing according to the Heavenly Stems.
– *L.I.-4 Hegu and KI-7 Fuliu*: this combination, explained previously, regulates sweating.
– *HE-7 Shenmen and G.B.-40 Qiuxu* to calm the Mind and strengthen Will-Power. This combination is effective in helping a person to gain the strength to act on decisions: it is indicated when the indecision (or rather the inability to act on a decision) causes great mental anguish.
– *P-6 Neiguan and ST-36 Zusanli* to regulate the Middle Burner and calm the Mind. This combination is effective for Empty-type Stomach patterns especially if caused by emotional problems.
– *P-6 Neiguan and ST-40 Fenglong* to regulate the Middle Burner, resolve Phlegm and calm the Mind. This combination is effective for Full-type Stomach patterns deriving from emotional stagnation. It is also very effective for bruising of the rib muscles.

(d) CHANNEL PROBLEMS

When treating painful channel syndromes, it is often useful to balance the points on the affected side with one or two points on the opposite side. This may be necessary or desirable to balance Top with Bottom, or Yin with Yang, or the Heavenly Stems, or simply to treat another condition.

We can therefore distinguish six possible situations for balancing the points treating a painful channel problem with one or two points on the opposite side:

(i)   balancing the affected channel with its related opposite-limb channel of the same polarity (e.g. Large Intestine with Stomach)
(ii)   balancing according to the Heavenly Stems
(iii) balancing with an appropriate Gathering point
(iv)   balancing according to accompanying pattern
(v)   balancing according to the Connecting points
(vi)   balancing according to duration in Wind-stroke.

(i) Balancing the affected channel with its related, opposite-limb channel of the same polarity

This means balancing Large Intestine with Stomach, Lungs with Spleen, etc. For example, supposing we are treating a patient with a chronic shoulder problem on the right side using L.I.-15 Jianyu, Jianneiling, L.I.-11 Quchi and L.I.-4 Hegu on the right side, we could balance these points with ST-36 Zusanli on the left side. Another example could be that of G.B.-30 Huantiao, G.B.-31 Fengshi and G.B.-34 Yanglingquan all on the left side to treat sciatica on that side, balanced by T.B.-6 Zhigou on the right side.

The Left-Right balancing of points in treating channel problems can be used according to the correspondence of joints between shoulder and hip, elbow and knee, and wrist and ankle. Bearing in mind this correspondence between joints and arm-leg channels of the same polarity, the local points on one joint can be balanced by the use of a point of its related, opposite-limb channel of the same polarity on the corresponding joint on the opposite half of the body and on the opposite side. An example will make this clearer. Assuming we are treating tennis elbow on the right side with L.I.-12 Zhouliao, L.I.-11 Quchi and L.I.-10 Shousanli on the right, we can balance these points with ST-36 Zusanli on the left side. We choose this point because it is on the related channel of the same polarity and, in the correspondence of joints, the knee corresponds to the elbow. The use of ST-36 will not only balance the treatment but also boost its effectiveness as ST-36 assumes the role of distal point. By using ST-36 on the opposite side we are also balancing Top and Bottom. Another example: assuming we are treating a patient with a sprained wrist and we use T.B.-5 Waiguan, T.B.-4 Yangchi and T.B.-3 Zhongzhu on the left side, we can needle G.B.-40 Qiuxu on the right side, based on the correspondence between wrist and ankle.

Bearing in mind the above correspondence between joints and related leg-arm channels of the same polarity, we can build up a table of corresponding points (Table I.3).

(ii) Balancing according to the Heavenly Stems

This method which has already been described can be used to balance points treating a channel problem. For example, if we are using S.I.-8 Xiaohai, S.I.-7 Zhizheng and S.I.-3 Houxi to treat a painful elbow on one side, we can balance these points with a Lung-channel point on the opposite side, e.g. LU-9 Taiyuan.

Table I.3 Correspondence of joint points on upper and lower parts of the body

Joint	Arm	Leg
Shoulder		*Hip*
Large Intestine	L.I.-15 Jianyu	ST-31 Biguan
Triple Burner	T.B.-14 Jianliao	G.B.-30 Huantiao
Small Intentine	S.I.-10 Naoshu	BL-36 Chengfu
Lung	LU-2 Yunmen	SP-12 Congmen
Heart	HE-1 Jiquan	KI-11 Henggu
Pericardium	P-2 Tianquan	LIV-11 Yinlian
Elbow		*Knee*
Large Intestine	L.I.-11 Quchi	ST-36 Zusanli
Triple Burner	T.B.-10 Tianjing	GB-34 Yanglingquan
Small Intestine	S.I.-8 Xiaohai	BL-40 Weizhong
Lung	LU-5 Chize	SP-9 Yinlingquan
Heart	HE-3 Shaohai	KI-10 Yingu
Pericardium	P-3 Quze	LIV-8 Ququan
Wrist		*Ankle*
Large Intestine	L.I.-5 Yangxi	ST-41 Jiexi
Triple Burner	T.B.-4 Yangchi	G.B.-40 Quixu
Small Intestine	S.I.-5 Yanggu	BL-60 Kunlun
Lung	LU-9 Taiyuan	SP-5 Shangqiu
Heart	HE-6 Yinxi	KI-5 Shuiquan
Pericardium	P-7 Daling	LIV-4 Zhongfeng

(iii) Balancing with an appropriate Gathering point

Points on one side treating a channel problem can be balanced with an appropriate Gathering point on the opposite side. For example, if we are using L.I.-15 Jianyu, L.I.-14 Binao and L.I.-11 Quchi for a shoulder problem characterized by inflammation of the tendons, we can balance these points with G.B.-34 Yanglingquan, Gathering point for sinews, on the opposite side.

(iv) Balancing according to accompanying pattern

The balancing point on the side opposite the one where the channel problem is can be chosen according to an accompanying syndrome or an underlying condition. For example, if we are using L.I.-15 Jianyu, L.I.-11 Quchi and L.I.-4 Hegu on one side and the patient also suffers from stagnation of Liver-Qi, we could balance these points with LIV-3 Taichong on the opposite side: this would simultaneously treat the stagnation of Liver-Qi and balance Left and Right, Top and Bottom and Yin and Yang.

As an another example, if we are treating a patient suffering from chronic Painful Obstruction Syndrome of one hand with swollen joints with T.B.-4 Yangchi and L.I.-3 Sanjian on one side, and the tongue is Swollen with a sticky coating, we could balance these points with SP-9 Yinlingquan and ST-40 Fenglong on the opposite side to help to resolve Dampness and Phlegm.

As another example, if we are treating a patient with tennis elbow with L.I.-11 Quchi and L.I.-10 Shousanli on one side, and this patient also suffers from Spleen-Qi deficiency, we could balance these points with ST-36 Zusanli on the opposite side. Bearing in mind the correspondences mentioned in point (i) above, this would also help the elbow. If the same patient suffered from Kidney-deficiency, we could select KI-3 Taixi instead.

(v) Balancing according to the Connecting points

This has already been mentioned before. In acute

cases, the local points on one side can be balanced with the Connecting point of the same channel on the opposite side. For example: L.I.-11 Quchi, L.I.-10 Shousanli and L.I.-4 Hegu on one side and L.I.-6 Pianli (Connecting point on the opposite side).

In chronic cases the local points on one side can be balanced with the Connecting point of the interiorly-exteriorly related channel on the opposite side. For example: T.B.-14 Jianliao, T.B.-13 Naohui and T.B.-5 Waiguan on one side with P-6 Neiguan on the opposite side.

(vi) Balancing according to duration in Wind-stroke

In treating paralysis following Wind-stroke sometimes the healthy side is needled in conjunction with the paralysed side. This has already been mentioned in the chapter on Wind-stroke (ch. 27) and will only be briefly mentioned here in connection with balancing Left and Right.

In treating paralysis, the duration of the condition can determine the side of needling. If the Wind-stroke occurred within the previous three months, the points of the paralysed side are needled with reducing method and the corresponding points of the healthy side are needled with reinforcing method. If the Wind-stroke occurred more than three months previously, the points of the affected side are needled with reinforcing method and moxa, and the corresponding points of the healthy side with reducing method. For an explanation of the reasoning behind this technique, see chapter 27.

Case histories

The following are case histories illustrating examples of combinations of points according to the principles given above. As these case histories are given mostly to illustrate point combinations, the emphasis will be on description of the treatment rather than the diagnosis.

Only one or two treatment sessions are described as an illustrative example on the applica-

tion of the principle of combination of points: obviously in each case, several sessions were necessary.

WOMAN, 47

This woman had been suffering from palpitations for 9 months. She felt her heart racing and missing beats and had a fluttering sensation just below the heart region. ECG tests showed no abnormality in the heart. Apart from this, she had no other symptoms and she felt generally quite well. Her periods had stopped 1 year before. Her tongue was very Pale and her pulse was very Weak on the right Kidney and on the Stomach position.

Her palpitations were due to a Yang deficiency of Stomach and Kidneys. Both these organs have an influence on the Heart and particularly on the heart's rate. The Stomach influences the Heart via the Great Connecting channel of the Stomach which flows from the Stomach to the left ventricle of the heart: the beat which can be felt on the apex of the heart is called "Xuli" in Chinese medicine and is actually thought of as the beating of this channel. The Kidneys provide Water and Fire as the foundation of the Heart and a Kidney deficiency very often affects the Heart: it is not by chance that the palpitations started after her periods stopped and her Kidney energy declined.

The points used were the following (Fig. I.17):

- P-4 Ximen on the right and ST-40 Fenglong on the left to regulate the Heart's rhythm and the Great Connecting channel of the Stomach which, as explained above, is responsible for the beating of the heart. Such a combination balances Yin and Yang, Top and Bottom, and Left and Right. Points of these two channels combine particularly well as they both flow to the Stomach.
- ST-36 Zusanli, SP-6 Sanyinjiao and KI-3 Taixi, all bilateral, to tonify the Stomach, Qi and Blood and Kidney-Yang (moxa was used on KI-3).

The first two points were used unilaterally to have a more moving and calming effect,

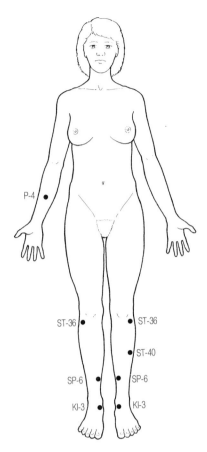

Fig. I.17   Point prescription for woman, 47

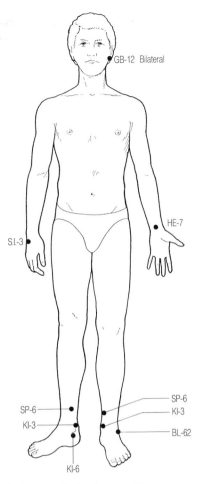

Fig. I.18   Point prescription for man, 54

while the tonifying points were used bilaterally. During the treatment she felt a tingling sensation around the points and a profound relaxing feeling.

MAN, 54

This man complained of dizziness and poor memory following two serious accidents to his head. He was also very tense and suffered from insomnia and slight impotence. His pulse was slightly Wiry, especially on both Front positions, and Weak on both Kidney positions.

The points used were the following (Fig. I.18):

- *BL-62 Shenmai on the left and S.I.-3 Houxi on the right* to open the Yang Heel Vessel. This extraordinary vessel was used because it affects the brain and removes obstructions

from the head. It would therefore eliminate the stagnation in the brain caused by the traumas. It is also indicated when both Front positions of the pulse are Wiry.[22]

- *HE-7 Shenmen on the left and KI-6 Zhaohai on the right* to harmonize Heart and Kidneys and calm the Mind. This combination of points from two arm-leg channels of the same polarity, balances Left and Right, and Top and Bottom. These points were used unilaterally to make the combination more moving and calming. In terms of indications, HE-7 would help his sleep and KI-6 the impotence. These two points are also balanced with the opening points of the Yang Heel Vessel as their positions cross over on the limbs; furthermore these two combinations will balance Greater Yang (S.I.-3 and BL-62) with Lesser Yin (HE-7 and KI-6), i.e. the utmost and most exterior Yang with the utmost and most interior Yin. Finally, KI-6 was chosen also to co-ordinate with the Yang Heel Vessel as this vessel removes Excess Yang from the head and KI-6 brings Yin to it.

– *SP-6 Sanyinjiao and KI-3 Taixi* bilaterally, to nourish the Kidneys. These were used bilaterally as they are tonifying. In terms of indications, SP-6 would also help the insomnia.
– *G.B.-12 Wangu*, bilaterally, as a local point to eliminate stagnation from the head and help the insomnia.

A subsequent treatment consisted of:

– *BL-62 Shenmai on the left and S.I.-3 Houxi on the right* to open the Yang Heel Vessel.
– *HE-7 Shenmen on the left and KI-6 Zhaohai on the right* to harmonize Heart and Kidneys and calm the Mind.
– *SP-6 Sanyinjiao and KI-3 Taixi* bilaterally, to nourish the Kidneys. In terms of indications, SP-6 would also help the insomnia.
– *Yintang* to calm the Mind and promote sleep.

WOMAN, 45

This patient suffered from exhaustion and stiffness of the neck. These were due to long-standing emotional problems (sadness and grief) depleting Qi and Blood. The main patterns were deficiency of Stomach-, Lung- and Spleen-Qi and Blood deficiency.

The points used were (Fig. I.19):

– *Ren-12 Zhongwan* to tonify Stomach and Spleen.
– *LU-7 Lieque on the right and P-7 Daling on the left* to calm the Mind and settle the Corporeal Soul. This combination of points is particularly good for emotional problems such as sadness and grief affecting the Lungs and Heart. LU-7 has a centrifugal movement bringing out repressed emotions or allowing the person to get in touch with his or her grief, and P-7 has a centripetal movement,

calming the Mind. These points were used unilaterally to make the combination simultaneously more moving and more calming.
– *ST-36 Zusanli and SP-6 Sanyinjiao*, bilaterally, to tonify Qi and Blood and strengthen Stomach and Spleen.

A subsequent treatment, when she complained of stiffness of the neck, consisted of the following combination:

– *Ren-12 Zhongwan* to tonify the Stomach and Spleen.
– *LU-7 Lieque on the right and P-7 on the left* for the same reasons as above.
– *T.B.-5 Waiguan on the right and G.B.-39 Xuanzhong on the left*, to benefit the sinews, expel Wind and relieve stiffness of the neck. This combination of two points from related

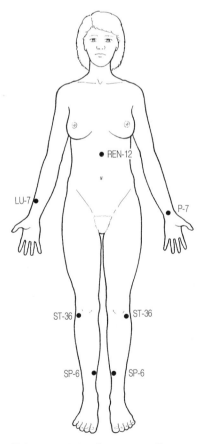

Fig. I.19 Point prescription for woman, 45

arm-leg channels of the same polarity balances Left and Right, and Top and Bottom. The Lesser Yang channels are particularly indicated to relieve stiffness of the neck and shoulders not only because they affect the area of stiffness but also because they benefit sinews.

- *ST-36 Zusanli and SP-6 Sanyinjiao*, bilaterally, for the same reasons as above.

During this treatment she felt extremely relaxed and said she felt as if she was floating. For yet another treatment the following points were used:

- *Ren-12 Zhongwan*
- *ST-36 Zusanli and SP-6 Sanyinjiao*
- *Du-20 Baihui* to raise Qi and lift mood.
- *T.B.-8 Sanyangluo on the right and G.B.-39 Xuanzhong on the left* to regulate the Lesser Yang, benefit the sinews and relieve stiffness of the neck. This combination balances Left and Right and Top and Bottom. The point T.B.-8 relaxes all the Yang channels in the neck area and is excellent for stiffness of this area. After the treatment she said she felt as if she had had a neck massage.

MAN, 41

This patient suffered from "irritable bowel syndrome" with symptoms of distension, flatulence and loose stools. He was a very tense person with a stressful job. The main patterns involved were Liver-Qi stagnation and Spleen-Qi deficiency.

The points used in one treatment were (Fig. I.20):

- *SP-4 Gongsun on the left and P-6 Neiguan on the right* to open the Penetrating Vessel and regulate the Middle and Lower Burner. This extraordinary vessel is indicated in Full patterns of the Stomach and Intestines.
- *Ren-6 Qihai* to move Qi in the lower abdomen. This point targets the action of the previous two to the lower abdomen.
- *HE-7 Shenmen on the left and LIV-3 Taichong on the right* to calm the Mind, settle the Ethereal

Soul and move Liver-Qi. This combination balances Top and Bottom, and Left and Right. It is particularly good to calm anxious persons down as it settles both the Mind and the Ethereal Soul. The unilateral use, one on the right, the other on the left, is particularly effective, and it also crosses over the opening points of the Penetrating Vessel (SP-4 and P-6).

GIRL, 13

This girl suffered from food intolerance, being unable to eat several common foods which caused a rash. She also suffered from eczema. The main pattern was Stomach-Heat.

The points selected for the first treatment were:

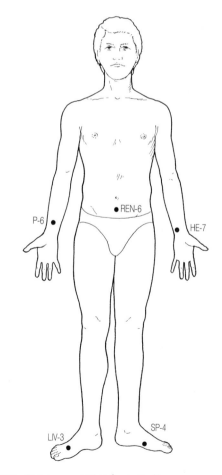

Fig. I.20 Point prescription for man, 41

– *L.I.-4 Hegu on the right and ST-44 Neiting on the left* to clear Stomach-Heat. This combination of points from related arm-leg channels of the same polarity, balances Left and Right, and Top and Bottom. The points were used unilaterally to make the effect more dynamic in clearing Heat; also, being the first treatment, and given the young age of the patient, it allows us to reduce the number of needles.
– *Ren-12 Zhongwan* to regulate the Middle Burner.

After 8 treatments and some herbal decoctions, her food intolerance was completely cured and she was able to eat foods which were previously impossible.

WOMAN, 73

This patient had been suffering from trigeminal neuralgia affecting the right side of the face. This occurred against a background of Kidney-Yin deficiency, which it very often does in the elderly.

The points used were:

– *L.I.-4 Hegu on the right and LIV-3 Taichong on the left* to expel Wind (as trigeminal neuralgia is a manifestation of Wind) from the face. The points were used unilaterally to make the combination more dynamic in expelling Wind; L.I.-4 was needled on the right side as that was the side affected by the neuralgia.
– *SP-6 Sanyinjiao and KI-3 Taixi*, bilaterally, to nourish Kidney-Yin.

During the treatment she felt a tingling around the needles and a flutter over the face.

WOMAN 47

This patient suffered from menopausal hot flushes, insomnia, palpitations, night-sweating, dizziness and tinnitus. The main pattern was Heart and Kidneys not harmonized.

The main points used were (Fig. I.21):

– *LU-7 Lieque on the right and KI-6 Zhaohai on the left* to open the Directing Vessel, regulate Qi and Blood in the uterus and nourish the Kidneys. It is essential to use this extraordinary vessel in menopausal problems.
– *HE-6 Yinxi on the left and KI-7 Fuliu on the right* to harmonize Heart and Kidneys, nourish Heart-Yin and stop night-sweating. This combination of points from related arm-leg channels of the same polarity, balances Left and Right, and Top and Bottom.
– *ST-36 Zusanli and SP-6 Sanyinjiao*, bilaterally, to tonify Blood and the Kidneys.
– *Du-24 Shenting and Ren-15 Jiuwei* to calm the Mind. These two points balance the Directing and Governing Vessels.

During the treatment she went into a deep state of relaxation and fell fast asleep.

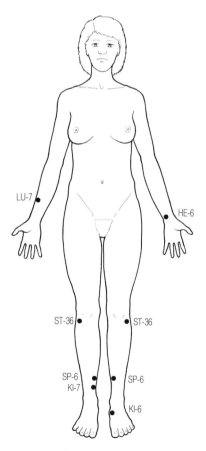

Fig. I.21   Point prescription for woman, 47

WOMAN, 45

This patient suffered from irregular periods and excessive uterine bleeding: these problems started with the onset of the menopause. She also had emotional stress related to relationship difficulties. The main pattern was deficiency of Liver and Kidneys.

The points used in one treatment were:

- *LU-7 Lieque on the right and KI-6 Zhaohai on the left* to open the Directing Vessel, regulate the uterus and nourish the Kidneys. This extraordinary vessel is very important in menopausal problems.
- *P-7 Daling on the left and KI-3 Taixi on the right* to calm the Mind, settle the Ethereal Soul and tonify the Kidneys. This combination balances Left and Right, and Top and Bottom: the points are used with the above laterality to cross over with the opening points of the Directing Vessel (LU-7 on the right and KI-6 on the left). P-7 is particularly useful in emotional stress deriving from relationship difficulties.
- *Ren-4 Guanyuan and KI-13 Qixue* to nourish the Kidneys, tonify the uterus, strengthen the Original Qi and benefit the Essence.
- *ST-36 Zusanli and SP-6 Sanyinjiao* to tonify Qi and Blood and strengthen Qi to hold Blood.

During the treatment she said that she "felt like circuits in her body rather than individual points". She had had several other sessions before so that she was quite an experienced and particularly sensitive patient.

WOMAN, 43

This patient also suffered from menopausal problems with hot flushes and night-sweating. Her tongue however, was very Pale and, apart from the night-sweating, she felt generally cold and her pulse was Slow and Wiry. She was a very tense person.

The main patterns were Kidney-Yang deficiency and stagnation of Liver-Qi from emotional stress.

The points used in one session were:

- *LU-7 Lieque on the right and KI-6 Zhaohai on the left* to open the Directing Vessel, tonify the uterus and nourish the Kidneys.
- *HE-6 Yinxi on the left and KI-7 Fuliu on the right* to harmonize Heart and Kidneys and stop night-sweating. This combination of points from two related arm-leg channels of the same polarity, balances Left and Right, and Top and Bottom. They were used with this laterality to cross over with LU-7 and KI-6.
- *Ren-4 Guanyuan with direct moxa cones* to tonify Kidney-Yang, strengthen the Original Qi, tonify the uterus and benefit the Essence.
- *ST-36 Zusanli on the left and SP-6 Sanyinjiao on the right* to tonify Qi and Blood and nourish the Kidneys. This combination, although tonifying, was used with unilateral points to make it more moving, as her pulse was not too empty.

Although she was an extremely tense person, she fell into a state of deep relaxation during the treatment and, in fact, only one treatment was enough to cure her night-sweating.

WOMAN, 63

This patient suffered from mild Damp Painful Obstruction Syndrome of the left hand with some pain, stiffness and swelling. She mostly sought treatment for preventive purposes. Apart from the Damp Painful Obstruction Syndrome, the main pattern was Kidney deficiency.

The points used for two sessions were:

- *LU-7 Lieque on the right and KI-6 Zhaohai on the left* to open the Directing Vessel and nourish the Kidneys.
- *T.B.-4 Yangchi on the left and KI-7 Fuliu on the right* to expel Wind-Dampness from the hand and tonify the Kidneys. This combination balances Left and Right, Yin and Yang, and Top and Bottom.

During the first session she felt a "stirring sensation" and the second time a "pulsing sensation" below the umbilicus.

WOMAN, 39

This patient suffered a brownish pigmentation of the skin, abdominal pain and distension, throbbing headaches on the temples, heavy periods with clotting and pain, constipation, blurred vision, dizziness, poor memory and pre-menstrual tension. Her tongue was Pale and Thin and her pulse was Choppy.

All her problems were Liver-related and all stemmed originally from Liver-Blood deficiency: this gave rise to Liver-Yang rising (throbbing headaches), stagnation of Liver-Qi and Liver-Blood (pre-menstrual tension, painful periods with clotting, abdominal distension and pain, and constipation) and Blood-Heat (brown pigmentation). The symptoms of Liver-Blood deficiency were poor memory, blurred vision, tiredness, dizziness, Pale-Thin tongue and Choppy pulse.

During one session the following points were used:

– *LU-7 Lieque on the right and KI-6 Zhaohai on the left* to open the Directing Vessel, regulate the uterus, move Qi in the lower abdomen and nourish Liver and Kidneys.
– *P-6 Neiguan on the left and LIV-3 Taichong on the right* to move Liver-Qi and Liver-Blood and eliminate stagnation. This combination of points from two related arm-leg channels of the same polarity, balances Left and Right and Top and Bottom. These points were used unilaterally to make the combination more moving and the points were crossed over with LU-7 and KI-6.
– *LIV-8 Ququan, ST-36 Zusanli and SP-6 Sanyinjiao*, bilaterally, to tonify Blood and nourish the Liver. These points were used bilaterally because they are tonifying.

During the session she said she felt very relaxed and as if she "had been plugged in".

MAN, 37

This patient suffered from an urticaria-like red and itchy rash all over the body. This was due to Wind-Heat affecting the Blood. This occurred against a background of Stomach-Yin deficiency,

his tongue being completely Peeled with a Stomach crack in the centre.

The points used in one session were:

– *T.B.-6 Zhigou on the right and G.B.-31 Fengshi on the left* to expel Wind-Heat. This combination of points from two related arm-leg channels of the same polarity, balances Left and Right, and Top and Bottom. It is excellent to clear Wind-Heat in the Blood causing rashes.
– *L.I.-11 Quchi on the left and SP-10 Xuehai on the right* to cool the Blood in the skin. This combination harmonizes Left and Right, Yin and Yang, and Top and Bottom.
– *ST-36 Zusanli and SP-6 Sanyinjiao*, bilaterally, to nourish Stomach-Yin.

WOMAN, 22

This patient suffered from an acute aggravation of chronic eczema of the Damp-Heat type.

The points used were similar to the ones used for the previous patient:

– *T.B.-6 Zhigou on the right and G.B.-31 Fengshi on the left* to expel Wind and clear Heat.
– *L.I.-11 Quchi on the left and SP-10 Xuehai on the right* to cool Blood in the skin.
– *SP-9 Yinlingquan*, bilaterally, to resolve Damp-Heat.

WOMAN, 32

This patient sought treatment mostly for mental-emotional problems. She was at a time of life marked by confusion about issues, relationships and goals, and suffered from a lack of determination in acting on her decisions. Thus, the problem was twofold: on the one hand, she could not distinguish clearly between issues leading to indecision, and on the other hand, even if she did come to any decision, she did not have the courage to act on it. This situation caused her great anxiety. In terms of patterns, there was a Spleen and Kidney deficiency.

The points used in one session were:

– *S.I.-5 Yanggu on the right and G.B.-40 Qiuxu on*

the left: the first point helps to distinguish issues clearly and the latter to summon the courage to act on decisions. This combination balances Left and Right, and Top and Bottom. The unilateral use of the points enhances their moving effect which is particularly important in this case on a mental level to unblock the situation.

- *ST-36 Zusanli on the right and KI-3 Taixi on the left* to tonify the Kidneys and the Spleen. These points were used unilaterally, even though they are tonifying, to enhance the moving effect on a mental level.
- *Du-24 Shenting and Ren-15 Jiuwei* were used to calm the Mind. This combination harmonizes Yin and Yang, Back and Front, and Directing and Governing Vessels.

She had three sessions (using the same points) and after the treatment she took some important decisions regarding her relationships and career, something which she had been trying to do for years.

MAN, 47

This patient suffered from chronic lower back-ache on the midline. At the time of consultation he had sprained his right knee. The main pattern was Kidney deficiency.

The points used in this session were:

- *ST-34 Liangqiu, ST-35 Dubi, ST-36 Zusanli and SP-9 Yinlingquan*, all on the right side, to benefit sinews of the knee and eliminate stagnation.
- *S.I.-3 Houxi on the left and BL-62 Shenmai on the right* to open the Governing Vessel, tonify the Kidneys and strengthen the back.
- *KI-3 Taixi on the left*, to tonify the Kidneys. Using this point on the side opposite the sprained knee achieves the purpose of balancing Left and Right, Yin and Yang and the Heavenly Stems (Stomach and Kidney).

MAN, 56

This patient suffered from exhaustion, back-ache, depression and impotence. His tongue was Red and Peeled, except on the root where it had a sticky-yellow coating. The main patterns were deficiency of Kidney-Yin with Damp-Heat in the Lower Burner.

The points used in one session were:

- *S.I.-3 Houxi on the left and BL-62 Shenmai on the right* to open the Governing Vessel, tonify the Kidneys, strengthen the spine and lift mood. This extraordinary vessel has a strengthening effect on the Mind and Will-Power when these are affected by a Kidney deficiency. This vessel was therefore used to treat the back-ache and the Will-Power, even though there was a deficiency of Kidney-Yin.
- *Ren-4 Guanyuan and Du-20 Baihui* to nourish Kidney-Yin and lift mood. This combination balances Front and Back, Directing and Governing Vessels, and Yin and Yang. It is effective in relieving depression occurring against a background of Kidney deficiency.
- *ST-36 Zusanli and KI-3 Taixi*, bilaterally, to tonify Qi and nourish the Kidneys. This combination balances Yin and Yang.
- *SP-9 Yinlingquan*, bilaterally, to drain Damp-Heat in the Lower Burner. This, in addition to the deficiency of Kidney-Yin, can be a contributory factor in causing impotence.
- *BL-23 Shenshu and BL-52 Zhishi*, bilaterally, to nourish the Kidneys, strengthen Will-Power and lift mood. This combination is excellent to affect the mental aspect of the Kidneys, i.e. Will-Power which encompasses drive and determination, and thus lift depression.

This patient fell fast asleep while the front points were being retained and reported that the back points woke him up and made his brain feel much brighter.

WOMAN, 54

This patient complained of a back-ache on the left side extending to the loin just below the 12th rib: this pain had started 3 weeks earlier. Her spine showed a pronounced deviation to one side in the lumbar area and her left leg was shorter than the right. Her pulse was Firm (i.e.

Wiry at a deep level), especially Wiry on both Rear positions, and slightly Overflowing on the Heart position.

The points used in one session were as follows:

- KI-6 Zhaohai on the right and LU-7 Lieque on the left to open the Yin Heel Vessel and absorb excess Yin. This condition is evidenced by the Firm quality of the pulse which indicates stagnation in the Interior at the Yin level. The Yin Heel Vessel also harmonizes Left and Right and corrects structural imbalances between left and right: it is therefore often indicated in musculo-skeletal problems characterized by such imbalances, as it was in this case with a deviation of the lumbar vertebrae and a difference in length between right and left leg. The use of the Yin Heel Vessel is also indicated by the Wiry quality on both Rear positions, according to the "Study on the Eight Extraordinary Vessels" by Li Shi Zhen.[23]
- HE-6 Yinxi on the right and KI-2 Rangu on the left to harmonize Heart and Kidneys. This combination of points from two related arm-leg channels of the same polarity harmonizes Left and Right, and Top and Bottom. These two points were selected on the basis not of any particular pattern, but purely of the presenting energetic imbalance as mirrored by the pulse. The Overflowing quality on the Heart pulse and the Wiry one on the Kidney pulse show a breakdown of interaction between Heart and Kidneys with an accumulation of Qi in the lower part (causing the back-ache) and an "escape" of Qi in the upper part. HE-6, Accumulation point, was selected to remove obstructions, which is one of the functions of such points, and KI-2, Spring point, was chosen because the Spring points drain Qi downwards. Both Accumulation and Spring points are particularly dynamic points and the combination of the two makes for a particularly moving treatment in energetic terms. The unilateral use of the points enhances their moving effect.
- SP-6 Sanyinjiao, bilaterally, was used to provide some tonification to balance the other points which are strongly moving.

During the treatment she felt a vibration in the loin region. After this first treatment, the back-ache went from the loin region and was confined to the sacro-iliac region. I repeated the same points as above adding:

- BL-23 Shenshu, bilaterally, to strengthen the back.
- BL-26 Guanyuanshu and BL-40 Weizhong, both on the left, to remove obstructions from the back channels on the left side.

Her back-ache was completely gone after these two treatments and her pulse became much more balanced.

MAN, 58

This man suffered from impotence and anxiety. He was a very tense person and his tension aggravated his impotence, while his sexual inadequacy made him more tense, thus establishing a self-perpetuating vicious circle. His pulse was very Wiry and Full but slightly Weak on both Rear positions and his tongue had a very Red tip. The main patterns were Heart-Fire, stagnation of Liver-Qi and some Kidney deficiency.

The points used in one session were:

- S.I.-3 Houxi on the left and BL-62 Shenmai on the right to open the Governing Vessel and strengthen the Kidneys.
- HE-7 Shenmen on the right and LIV-3 Taichong on the left to calm the Mind, settle the Ethereal Soul and relieve stagnation of Liver-Qi.
- KI-3 Taixi bilaterally to tonify the Kidneys.

WOMAN, 70

This patient suffered from chronic sinusitis and constipation. Her tongue had a very sticky-white coating and her pulse was Slippery. The main patterns were retention of Dampness affecting the sinuses, against a background of Spleen-Qi deficiency and retention of food.

The points used in one session were:

- *SP-4 Gongsun on the right and P-6 Neiguan on the left* to open the Penetrating Vessel, regulate the Spleen and relieve retention of food.
- *L.I.-4 Hegu on the right and ST-40 Fenglong on the left* to regulate the ascending and descending of Qi in the Bright Yang channels (to help the sinuses) and resolve Dampness.
- *Yintang* as a local point to free the sinuses.
- *ST-36 Zusanli and SP-6 Sanyinjiao* to tonify Stomach and Spleen to resolve Dampness.

WOMAN, 25

This woman complained of painful periods with dark-clotted menstrual blood and back-ache. She did not have any other symptoms and her pulse was Weak on the left Rear position and slightly Overflowing on the Heart position. Her tongue had a Heart crack and a Red tip with red points.

The main patterns were Heart-Fire from emotional stress and a constitutional Kidney deficiency.

The points used in one session were:

- *P-7 Daling on the right and LIV-3 Taichong on the left* to calm the Mind and settle the Ethereal Soul.
- *ST-36 Zusanli on the left and KI-3 Taixi (with warm needle) on the right* to tonify Kidney-Yang.
- *SP-6 Sanyinjiao bilaterally* to nourish the Kidneys and calm the Mind.

END NOTES

1. Maciocia G 1991 The Foundations of Chinese Medicine, Churchill Livingstone, Edinburgh.
2. Nanjing College of Traditional Chinese Medicine 1979 A Revised Explanation of the Classic of Difficulties (*Nan Jing Jiao Shi* 难经校释), People's Health Publishing House, Beijing. First published *c.* AD 100, p. 144.
3. Gao Wu 1529 Gathering of Eminent Acupuncturists (*Zhen Jiu Ju Ying* 针灸聚英), cited in Chen You Bang 1990 Chinese Acupuncture Therapy (*Zhong Guo Zhen Jiu Zhi Liao Xue* 中国针灸治疗学), China Science Publishing House, Shanghai, p. 215.
4. Ibid.
5. Ibid.
6. Ibid.
7. Li Chan 1575 The ABC of Chinese Medicine (*Yi Xue Ru Men* 医学入门), cited in Chinese Acupuncture Therapy, p. 215.
8. 1981 Spiritual Axis (*Ling Shu Jing* 灵枢经), People's Health Publishing House, Beijing. First published *c.* 100 BC, p. 100.
9. A Revised Explanation of the Classic of Difficulties, p. 145.
10. Wang Guo Rui 1329 The Jade Dragon Classic of Spiritual Acupuncture from Bian Que (*Bian Que Shen Ying Zhen Jiu Yu Long Jing* 扁鹊神应针灸玉龙经), cited in Chinese Acupuncture Therapy, p. 216.
11. 1979 The Yellow Emperor's Classic of Internal Medicine — Simple Questions (*Huang Ti Nei Jing Su Wen* 黄帝内经素问*)*, People's Health Publishing House, Beijing. First published *c.* 100 BC, p. 49.
12. In the Southern hemisphere a person facing South would have the sun on his/her back. The position outlined in the "Yellow Emperor's Classic of Internal Medicine" should therefore be reversed with the person facing North so that the sun is in the front and the shade in the back. However, this means that the polarity Yin-Yang for Right-Left needs to be reversed as the East (Yang) would be on the right side and West (Yin) on the left.
13. Simple Questions, p. 44.
14. Jefferies R P S 1991 Two types of bilateral symmetry in the Metazoa: chordate and bilaterian, Natural History Museum, London.
15. Simple Questions, p. 344.
16. Ibid., p. 345.
17. Gathering of Eminent Acupuncturists in Chinese Acupuncture Therapy, p. 215.
18. Ibid.
19. Ibid.
20. Ibid.
21. The ABC of Chinese Medicine in Chinese Acupuncture Therapy, p. 215.
22. Wang Luo Zhen 1985 A Compilation of "A Study of the Eight Extraordinary Vessels" (*Qi Jing Ba Mai Kao Jiao Zhu* 奇经八脉考校注), Shanghai Science Publishing House, Shanghai. First published in 1578 by Li Shi Zhen, p. 109.
23. Ibid., p. 110.

Appendix II
Identification of patterns according to the Six Stages

Greater Yang stage

GREATER YANG CHANNEL PATTERN

ATTACK OF COLD

Aversion to cold, shivering, sneezing, cough, runny nose with a white-watery discharge, no fever or slight fever, severe occipital stiffness and ache, no sweating, no thirst.
Tongue: body colour unchanged, thin-white coating.
Pulse: Floating-Tight.

ATTACK OF WIND

Aversion to wind, shivering, slight sweating, no fever or slight fever, slight aches, slight headache, no thirst.
Tongue: body colour unchanged, thin-white coating.
Pulse: Floating-Slow.

GREATER YANG PATTERN: COMPARISON OF ATTACK OF COLD AND WIND

Common symptoms: Floating Pulse, headache, aversion to cold.

	Attack of Cold	*Attack of Wind*
Sweating	No sweating	Slight sweating
Aches	Pronounced	Slight
Headache	Severe	Less severe
Chilliness	Pronounced	Slight
Pulse	Floating-Tight	Floating-Slow

GREATER YANG ORGAN PATTERN

ACCUMULATION OF WATER

Fever, aversion to cold, retention of urine, thirst, difficult urination, vomiting of fluids soon after drinking.
Tongue: yellow coating on the root.
Pulse: Floating-Rapid.

ACCUMULATION OF BLOOD

Feeling of distension-fullness-urgency in the hypogastrium, difficult urination, slight incontinence of urine, blood in the urine, mental restlessness.
Tongue: Red with a yellow coating on the root.
Pulse: Deep-Choppy.

Bright Yang stage

General clinical manifestations
High fever, profuse sweating, aversion to heat, thirst and Overflowing pulse.

BRIGHT YANG CHANNEL PATTERN

High fever, profuse sweating, aversion to heat, thirst with a desire to drink cold water, red face, restlessness.
Tongue: Red with a yellow coating.
Pulse: Overflowing-Rapid.

BRIGHT YANG ORGAN PATTERN

High fever which is worse in the afternoon, profuse sweating, constipation, thirst with a desire to drink cold water, fullness and pain in the abdomen which becomes worse on pressure, restlessness and irritability, in severe cases delirium.
Tongue: Red with a dry, yellow or black coating.
Pulse: Deep-Full-Rapid.

Lesser Yang stage

Alternation of feeling cold and hot, a bitter taste, a dry throat, blurred vision, a feeling of distension-fullness of the hypochondrium and chest, no desire to drink or eat, irritability, vomiting, nausea.
Tongue: white coating on one side only.
Pulse: Wiry-Fine.

Greater Yin stage

Abdominal fullness, vomiting, no appetite, diarrhoea, no thirst.
Tongue: Pale, white coating.
Pulse: Slow-Deep-Fine.

Lesser Yin stage

COLD TRANSFORMATION

Chilliness, lying with body curled up, aversion to cold, listlessness, desire to sleep, cold limbs, diarrhoea, no thirst or desire for warm liquids, pale-abundant urination.
Tongue: Pale.
Pulse: Deep-Weak.

HEAT TRANSFORMATION

Feeling of heat, irritability, insomnia, dry mouth and throat especially at night, dark-scanty urine.
Tongue: Red without coating.
Pulse: Fine-Rapid.

Terminal Yin

Persistent thirst, a feeling of upward disturbance of the heart, pain and heat sensation in the heart and chest, a feeling of hunger but without desire to eat, cold limbs, diarrhoea, vomiting, vomiting of round worms.
Tongue: yellow coating in the front and white coating on the root.
Pulse: Wiry-Fine.

Appendix III
Identification of patterns according to the Four Levels

Defensive-Qi Level

WIND-HEAT

Fever, slight aversion to cold, sore throat, swollen and inflamed tonsils, headache, slight sweating, body aches, runny nose with a yellow discharge, a slight thirst.
Tongue: tip and sides slightly Red, thin-yellow or thin-white coating.
Pulse: Floating-Rapid.

SUMMER-HEAT

Fever, slight aversion to cold, no sweating, headache, a feeling of heaviness, an uncomfortable sensation in the epigastrium, irritability, thirst.
Tongue: Red with a white-sticky coating.
Pulse: Weak-Floating (Soft), Rapid.

DAMP-HEAT

Aversion to cold, fever which is worse in the afternoon, headache as if the head were wrapped, a feeling of heaviness and oppression of the chest and epigastrium, a sticky taste, no thirst.
Tongue: white-sticky coating.
Pulse: Weak-Floating, Slow.

DRY-HEAT

Fever, slight aversion to cold, slight sweating, dryness of skin, mouth, nose and throat, a sore throat, dry cough.

Tongue: Red, dry, thin-white coating.
Pulse: Floating-Rapid.

Qi Level

LUNG HEAT (HEAT IN CHEST AND DIAPHRAGM)

High fever, no aversion to cold, aversion to heat, breathlessness, cough with thin-yellow or rusty-coloured and purulent sputum, thirst.
Tongue: Red, thick-yellow coating.
Pulse: Slippery-Rapid.

STOMACH HEAT

High fever, no aversion to cold, aversion to heat, profuse sweating, severe thirst with desire for cold drinks, coarse breathing.
Tongue: Red, dry-yellow coating.
Pulse: Overflowing-Big-Rapid.
("4 Bigs": big fever, big sweating, big thirst, big pulse).

INTESTINES DRY-HEAT

High fever in the afternoon, constipation, burning sensation in anus, abdominal distention-fullness-pain which is worse on pressure, irritability, faint feeling.
Tongue: Red, yellow-thick-dry or grey-black coating with prickles.
Pulse: Deep-Full-Rapid.

GALL-BLADDER HEAT (HEAT IN LESSER YANG)

Alternating hot and cold feeling, more hot than cold, a bitter taste, thirst, a dry throat, hypochondrial pain which is worse on pressure, nausea, a feeling of fullness of the epigastrium.
Tongue: Red, yellow-sticky coating on one side only.
Pulse: Wiry-Rapid.

STOMACH AND SPLEEN DAMP-HEAT

Continuous fever which decreases with sweating and then starts again, a feeling of heaviness of the body and head, a feeling of oppression of the chest and abdomen, nausea, loose stools.
Tongue: yellow-sticky coating.
Pulse: Weak-Floating, Rapid.

Nutritive-Qi Level

HEAT IN NUTRITIVE-QI PORTION

Fever at night, dry mouth but no desire to drink, insomnia, mental restlessness, aphasia, spots on skin (maculae).
Tongue: Deep-Red without coating.
Pulse: Fine-Rapid.

HEAT IN PERICARDIUM

Mental confusion with delirium or aphasia, high fever, body hot but hands and feet cold.
Tongue: Deep-Red without coating.
Pulse: Fine-Rapid.

Blood Level

HEAT VICTORIOUS MOVES BLOOD

High fever, irritability, manic behaviour, spots under the skin (maculae), vomiting blood, epistaxis, blood in stools, blood in urine.
Tongue: Deep-Red without coating, dry.
Pulse: Wiry, Rapid.

HEAT VICTORIOUS STIRS WIND

High fever, fainting, limbs twitching, rigidity of neck, opisthotonos, eyeballs turning up, clenching of teeth.
Tongue: Deep-Red without coating.
Pulse: Wiry, Rapid.

EMPTY WIND AGITATES IN THE INTERIOR

Tremor and twitching of limbs, convulsions, low-grade fever, emaciation, face "floating"-red, listlessness.
Tongue: Red without coating, dry.
Pulse: Fine, slightly Wiry, Rapid.

COLLAPSE OF YIN

Low-grade fever, night sweating, irritability, in-somnia, a dry mouth with a desire to sip fluids, 5-palm heat, malar flush.
Tongue: Deep-Red without coating, dry.
Pulse: Fine-Rapid.

COLLAPSE OF YANG

Chilliness, aversion to cold, cold limbs, bright-white face, sweating, no thirst, backache, weak back.
Tongue: Pale-Swollen.
Pulse: Minute.

Appendix IV Prescriptions

AI FU NUAN GONG WAN
Artemisia-Cyperus Warming the Uterus Pill
Ai Ye *Folium Artemisiae* 9 g
Wu Zhu Yu *Fructus Evodiae rutaecarpae* 4.5 g
Rou Gui *Cortex Cinnamomi cassiae* 4.5 g
Xiang Fu *Rhizoma Cyperi rotundi* 9 g
Dang Gui *Radix Angelicae sinensis* 9 g
Chuan Xiong *Radix Ligustici wallichii* 6 g
Bai Shao *Radix Paeoniae albae* 6 g
Huang Qi *Radix Astragali membranacei* 6 g
Sheng Di Huang *Radix Rehmanniae glutinosae* 9 g
Xu Duan *Radix Dipsaci* 6 g

AN SHEN DING ZHI WAN
Calming the Mind and Settling the Will-Power Pill
Ren Shen *Radix Ginseng* 9 g
Fu Ling *Sclerotium Poriae cocos* 12 g
Fu Shen *Sclerotium Poriae cocos pararadicis* 9 g
Long Chi *Dens Draconis* 15 g
Yuan Zhi *Radix Polygalae tenuifoliae* 6 g
Shi Chang Pu *Rhizoma Acori graminei* 8 g

BA XIAN CHANG SHOU WAN
Eight Immortals Longevity Pill
Shu Di Huang *Radix Rehmanniae glutinosae praeparata* 24 g
Shan Zhu Yu *Fructus Corni officinalis* 12 g
Shan Yao *Radix Dioscoreae oppositae* 12 g
Ze Xie *Rhizoma Alismatis orientalis* 9 g
Mu Dan Pi *Cortex Moutan radicis* 9 g
Fu Ling *Sclerotium Poriae cocos* 9 g
Mai Men Dong *Tuber Ophiopogonis japonici* 9 g
Wu Wei Zi *Fructus Schisandrae chinensis* 6 g

BA ZHEN TANG
Eight Precious Decoction
Dang Gui *Radix Angelicae sinensis* 10 g
Chuan Xiong *Radix Ligustici wallichii* 5 g
Bai Shao *Radix Paeoniae albae* 8 g
Shu Di Huang *Radix Rehmanniae glutinosae praeparata* 15 g
Ren Shen *Radix Ginseng* 3 g
Bai Zhu *Rhizoma Atractylodis macrocephalae* 10 g
Fu Ling *Sclerotium Poriae cocos* 8 g
Zhi Gan Cao *Radix Glycyrrhizae uralensis praeparata* 5 g

BA ZHEN YI MU TANG
Eight Precious Leonorus Decoction
Dang Gui *Radix Angelicae sinensis* 10 g
Chuan Xiong *Radix Ligustici wallichii* 5 g
Bai Shao *Radix Paeoniae albae* 8 g
Shu Di Huang *Radix Rehmanniae glutinosae praeparata* 15 g
Ren Shen *Radix Ginseng* 3 g
Bai Zhu *Rhizoma Atractylodis macrocephalae* 10 g
Fu Ling *Sclerotium Poriae cocos* 8 g
Zhi Gan Cao *Radix Glycyrrhizae uralensis praeparata* 5 g
Yi Mu Cao *Herba Leonori heterophylli* 9 g

BA ZHENG TANG
Eight Corrections Powder
Bian Xu *Herba Polygoni avicularis* 6 g
Che Qian Zi *Semen Plantaginis* 9 g
Qu Mai *Herba Dianthi* 6 g
Mu Tong *Caulis Akebiae* 6 g
Hua Shi *Talcum* 9 g
Da Huang *Rhizoma Rhei* 6 g
Zhi Zi *Fructus Gardeniae jasminoidis* 6 g
Zhi Gan Cao *Radix Glycyrrhizae uralensis praeparata* 6 g

BAI HE GU JIN TANG
Lilium Consolidating Metal Decoction
Bai He *Bulbus Lilii* 15 g
Mai Men Dong *Tuber Ophiopogonis japonici* 9 g
Xuan Shen *Radix Scrophulariae ningpoensis* 9 g
Sheng Di Huang *Radix Rehmanniae glutinosae* 9 g
Shu Di Huang *Radix Rehmanniae glutinosae praeparata* 9 g
Dang Gui *Radix Angelicae sinensis* 6 g
Bai Shao *Radix Paeoniae albae* 9 g
Jie Geng *Radix Platycodi grandiflori* 6 g
Chuan Bei Mu *Bulbus Fritillariae cirrhosae* 6 g
Gan Cao *Radix Glycyrrhizae uralensis* 3 g

BAI HU JIA CANG ZHU TANG
White Tiger Decoction plus Rhizoma Atractylodis lanceae
Shi Gao *Gypsum fibrosum* 30 g
Zhi Mu *Radix Anemarrhenae asphodeloidis* 15 g
Gan Cao *Radix Glycyrrhizae uralensis* 4.5 g
Geng Mi *Semen Oryzae sativae* 9 g
Cang Zhu *Rhizoma Atractylodis lanceae* 12 g

BAI HU JIA GUI ZHI TANG
White Tiger Ramulus Cinnamomi Decoction
Shi Gao *Gypsum fibrosum* 30 g
Zhi Mu *Radix Anemarrhenae asphodeloidis* 9 g
Gan Cao *Radix Glycyrrhizae uralensis* 3 g
Geng Mi *Semen Oryzae sativae* 6 g
Gui Zhi *Ramulus Cinnamomi cassiae* 5 g

BAI HU TANG
White Tiger Decoction
Shi Gao *Gypsum fibrosum* 30 g
Zhi Mu *Radix Anemarrhenae asphodeloidis* 15 g
Gan Cao *Radix Glycyrrhizae uralensis* 4.5 g
Geng Mi *Semen Oryzae sativae* 9 g

BAI TOU WENG TANG
Pulsatilla Decoction
Bai Tou Weng *Radix Pulsatillae chinensis* 15 g
Huang Bo *Cortex Phellodendri* 12 g
Huang Lian *Rhizoma Coptidis* 4 g
Qin Pi *Cortex Fraxini* 12 g

BAI ZI YANG XIN WAN
Biota Nourishing the Heart Pill
Bai Zi Ren *Semen Biotae orientalis* 120 g
Fu Shen *Sclerotium Poriae cocos pararadicis* 30 g
Gou Qi Zi *Fructus Lycii chinensis* 90 g
Shu Di Huang *Radix Rehmanniae glutinosae praeparata* 60 g
Dang Gui *Radix Angelicae sinensis* 30 g
Xuan Shen *Radix Scrophulariae ningpoensis* 60 g
Mai Men Dong *Tuber Ophiopogonis japonici* 30 g
Shi Chang Pu *Rhizoma Acori graminei* 30 g
Gan Cao *Radix Glycyrrhizae uralensis* 15 g

BAN XIA BAI ZHU TIAN MA TANG
Pinellia-Atractylodes-Gastrodia Decoction

Ban Xia *Rhizoma Pinelliae ternatae* 9 g
Tian Ma *Rhizoma Gastrodiae elatae* 6 g
Bai Zhu *Rhizoma Atractylodis macrocephalae* 15 g
Fu Ling *Sclerotium Poriae cocos* 6 g
Chen Pi *Pericarpium Citri reticulatae* 6 g
Gan Cao *Rhizoma Glycyrrhizae uralensis* 4 g
Sheng Jiang *Rhizoma Zingiberis officinalis recens* 1 slice
Da Zao *Fructus Ziziphi jujubae* 2 pieces

BAN XIA HOU PO TANG
Pinellia-Magnolia Decoction
Ban Xia *Rhizoma Pinelliae ternatae* 12 g
Hou Po *Cortex Magnoliae officinalis* 9 g
Su Ye *Folium Perillae frutescentis* 6 g
Fu Ling *Sclerotium Poriae cocos* 12 g
Sheng Jiang *Rhizoma Zingiberis officinalis recens* 9 g

BAO HE WAN
Preserving and Harmonizing Pill
Shan Zha *Fructus Crataegi* 9 g
Shen Qu *Massa Fermentata Medicinalis* 6 g
Lai Fu Zi *Semen Raphani sativi* 6 g
Ban Xia *Rhizoma Pinelliae ternatae* 6 g
Chen Pi *Pericarpum Citri reticulatae* 3 g
Fu Ling *Sclerotium Poriae cocos* 6 g
Lian Qiao *Fructus Forsythiae suspensae* 6 g

BAO YIN JIAN Variation
Protecting Yin Decoction
Sheng Di Huang *Radix Rehmanniae glutinosae* 24 g
Shu Di Huang *Radix Rehmanniae glutinosae prae-parata* 15 g
Bai Shao *Radix Paeoniae albae* 12 g
Shan Yao *Radix Dioscoreae oppositae* 12 g
Huang Qin *Radix Scutellariae baicalensis* 9 g
Huang Bo *Cortex Phellodendri* 9 g
Xu Duan *Radix Dipsaci* 6 g
Gan Cao *Radix Glycyrrhizae uralensis* 3 g

BEI MU GUA LOU SAN
Fritillaria-Trichosanthes Powder
Chuan Bei Mu *Bulbus Fritillariae cirrhosae* 5 g
Gua Lou *Fructus Trichosanthis* 3 g
Tian Hua Fen *Radix Trichosanthis* 2.5 g
Fu Ling *Sclerotium Poriae cocos* 2.5 g
Chen Pi *Pericarpium Citri reticulatae* 2.5 g
Jie Geng *Radix Platycodi grandiflori* 2.5 g

BI XIE FEN QING YIN
Dioscorea Separating the Clear Decoction
Bi Xie *Rhizoma Dioscoreae hypoglaucae* 12 g
Yi Zhi Ren *Fructus Alpiniae oxyphyllae* 9 g
Wu Yao *Radix Linderae strychnifoliae* 9 g
Shi Chang Pu *Rhizoma Acori graminei* 9 g

BI XIE SHEN SHI TANG
Dioscorea Draining Dampness Decoction
Bi Xie *Rhizoma Dioscoreae hypoglaucae* 6 g
Yi Yi Ren *Semen Coicis lachryma jobi* 12 g
Huang Bo *Cortex Phellodendri* 6 g
Fu Ling *Sclerotium Poriae cocos* 6 g
Mu Dan Pi *Cortex Moutan radicis* 6 g
Ze Xie *Rhizoma Alismatis orientalis* 6 g
Hua Shi *Talcum* 12 g
Mu Tong *Caulis Akebiae* 3 g

BU FEI TANG
Tonifying the Lungs Decoction
Ren Shen *Radix Ginseng* 9 g
Huang Qi *Radix Astragali membranacei* 12 g
Shu Di Huang *Radix Rehmanniae glutinosae prae-parata* 12 g
Wu Wei Zi *Fructus Schisandrae chinensis* 6 g
Zi Wan *Radix Asteris tatarici* 9 g
Sang Bai Pi *Cortex Mori albae radicis* 6 g

BU GAN TANG
Tonifying the Liver Decoction
Shu Di Huang *Radix Rehmanniae glutinosae prae-parata* 12 g
Dang Gui *Radix Angelicae sinensis* 10 g
Bai Shao *Radix Paeoniae albae* 12 g
Chuan Xiong *Radix Ligustici wallichii* 8 g
Mu Gua *Fructus Chaenomelis lagenariae* 6 g
Zhi Gan Cao *Radix Glycyrrhizae uralensis prae-parata* 3 g
Mai Men Dong *Tuber Ophiopogonis japonici* 6 g
Suan Zao Ren *Semen Ziziphi spinosae* 3 g

BU QI CONG MING TANG
Tonifying Qi Clear Hearing Decoction
Huang Qi *Radix Astragali membranacei* 12 g
Ren Shen *Radix Ginseng* 9 g
Sheng Ma *Rhizoma Cimicifugae* 3 g
Ge Gen *Radix Puerariae* 3 g
Man Jing Zi *Fructus Viticis* 3 g
Bai Shao *Radix Paeoniae albae* 6 g

Huang Bo *Cortex Phellodendri* 6 g
Zhi Gan Cao *Radix Glycyrrhizae uralensis prae-parata* 3 g

BU QI YI SHEN TANG

Tonify Qi and Benefit the Kidneys Decoction
Dang Shen *Radix Codonopsis pilosulae* 30 g
Huang Qi *Radix Astragali membranacei* 15 g
Fu Zi *Radix Aconiti carmichaeli praeparata* 10 g
Yin Yang Huo *Herba Epimedii* 9 g
Chai Hu *Radix Bupleuri* 6 g
Chi Shao *Radix Paeoniae rubrae* 12 g
Chuan Xiong *Radix Ligustici wallichii* 6 g
Yi Mu Cao *Herba Leonori heterophylli* 9 g
Da Huang *Radix Rhei* 3 g
San Qi *Radix Notoginseng* 3 g

BU YANG HAI WU TANG

Tonify Yang and Restore the 5/10th Decoction
Huang Qi *Radix Astragali membranacei* 18 g
Dang Gui Wei *Radix Angelicae sinensis* ("tails") 6 g
Chuan Xiong *Radix Ligustici wallichii* 3 g
Tao Ren *Semen Persicae* 3 g
Hong Hua *Flos Carthami tinctorii* 3 g
Chi Shao Yao *Radix Paeoniae rubrae* 4.5 g
Di Long *Pheretima aspergillum* 3 g

BU ZHONG YI QI TANG

Tonifying the Centre and Benefiting Qi Decoction
Huang Qi *Radix Astragali membranacei* 12 g
Ren Shen *Radix Ginseng* 9 g
Bai Zhu *Rhizoma Atractylodis macrocephalae* 9 g
Dang Gui *Radix Angelicae sinensis* 6 g
Chen Pi *Pericarpium Citri reticulatae* 6 g
Sheng Ma *Rhizoma Cimicifugae* 3 g
Chai Hu *Radix Bupleuri* 3 g

CANG BAI ER CHEN TANG

Grey and White Atractylodes Two Old Decoction
Cang Zhu *Rhizoma Atractylodis lanceae* 6 g
Bai Zhu *Rhizoma Atractylodis macrocephalae* 6 g
Chen Pi *Pericarpium Citri reticulatae* 4.5 g
Ban Xia *Rhizoma Pinelliae ternatae* 9 g
Fu Ling *Sclerotium Poriae cocos* 6 g
Zhi Gan Cao *Radix Glycyrrhizae uralensis prae-parata* 3 g
Sheng Jiang *Rhizoma Zingiberis officinalis recens* 3 slices

CANG ER BI DOU YAN FANG

Xanthium Sinusitis Formula
Cang Er Zi *Fructus Xanthii* 9 g
Huang Qin *Radix Scutellariae baicalensis* 9 g
Pu Gong Ying *Herba cum Radice Taraxaci mong-olici* 6 g
Ge Gen *Radix Puerariae* 9 g
Jie Geng *Radix Platycodi grandiflori* 6 g
Bai Zhi *Radix Angelicae dahuricae* 3 g
Che Qian Zi *Semen Plantaginis* 9 g
Gan Cao *Radix Glycyrrhizae uralensis* 3 g

CANG ER ZI SAN

Xanthium Powder
Cang Er Zi *Fructus Xanthii* 7.5 g
Xin Yin Hua *Flos Magnoliae liliflorae* 15 g
Bai Zhi *Radix Angelicae dahuricae* 30 g
Bo He *Herba Menthae* 1.5 g

CHAI GE JIE JI TANG

Bupleurum-Pueraria Relaxing the Tendons Decoction
Ge Gen *Radix Puerariae* 9 g
Chai Hu *Radix Bupleuri* 6 g
Qiang Huo *Radix et Rhizoma Notopterygii* 3 g
Bai Zhi *Radix Angelicae dahuricae* 3 g
Huang Qin *Radix Scutellariae baicalensis* 6 g
Shi Gao *Gypsum fibrosum* 5 g
Jie Geng *Radix Platycodi grandiflori* 3 g
Bai Shao *Radix Paeoniae albae* 6 g
Gan Cao *Radix Glycyrrhizae uralensis* 3 g

CHAI HU SU GAN TANG

Bupleurum Soothing the Liver Decoction
Chai Hu *Radix Bupleuri* 6 g
Bai Shao *Radix Paeoniae albae* 4.5 g
Zhi Ke *Fructus Citri aurantii* 4.5 g
Zhi Gan Cao *Radix Glycyrrhizae uralensis prae-parata* 1.5 g
Chen Pi *Pericarpium Citri reticulatae* 6 g
Xiang Fu *Rhizoma Cyperi rotundi* 4.5 g
Chuan Xiong *Radix Ligustici wallichii* 4.5 g

CHEN XIANG JIANG QI SAN

Aquilaria Subduing Qi Powder
Chen Xiang *Lignum Aquilariae* 3g
Sha Ren *Fructus seu Semen Amomi* 4g
Xiang Fu *Rhizoma Cyperi rotundi* 6 g
Zhi Gan Cao *Radix Glycyrrhizae uralensis prae-parata* 3 g

Sheng Jiang *Rhizoma Zingiberis officinalis recens* 3 slices

CHEN XIANG SAN
Aquilaria Powder
Chen Xiang *Lignum Aquilariae* 9 g
Shi Wei *Folium Pyrrosiae* 6 g
Hua Shi *Talcum* 6 g
Dong Kui Zi *Semen Abutiloni seu Malvae* 6 g
Dang Gui *Radix Angelicae sinensis* 6 g
Wang Bu Liu Xing *Semen Vaccariae segetalis* 6 g
Bai Shao *Radix Paeoniae albae* 6 g
Chen Pi *Pericarpium Citri reticulatae* 4.5 g
Gan Cao *Radix Glycyrrhizae uralensis* 3 g

CHENG SHI BI XIE YIN
Dioscorea Decoction of the Cheng Clan
Bi Xie *Rhizoma Dioscoreae hypoglaucae* 9 g
Shi Chang Pu *Rhizoma Acori graminei* 6 g
Che Qian Zi *Semen Plantaginis* 6 g
Huang Bo *Cortex Phellodendri* 6 g
Fu Ling *Sclerotium Poriae cocos* 9 g
Bai Zhu *Rhizoma Atractylodis macrocephalae* 6 g
Lian Zi *Semen Nelumbinis nuciferae* 6 g
Dan Shen *Radix Salviae miltiorrhizae* 4.5 g

CHENG YANG LI LAO TANG
Assisting Yang and Regulating Tiredness Decoction
Ren Shen *Radix Ginseng* 9 g
Huang Qi *Radix Astragali membranacei* 9 g
Wu Wei Zi *Fructus Schisandrae chinensis* 4.5 g
Zhi Gan Cao *Radix Glycyrrhizae uralensis praeparata* 3 g
Gui Zhi *Ramulus Cinnamomi cassiae* 4.5 g
Sheng Jiang *Rhizoma Zingiberis officinalis recens* 3 slices
Bai Zhu *Rhizoma Atractylodis macrocephalae* 6 g
Chen Pi *Pericarpium Citri reticulatae* 3 g
Dang Gui *Radix Angelicae sinensis* 6 g
Da Zao *Fructus Ziziphi jujubae* 3 dates

CHU SHI WEI LING TANG
Eliminating Dampness Stomach "Ling" Decoction
Cang Zhu *Rhizoma Atractylodis lanceae* 6 g
Hou Po *Cortex Magnoliae officinalis* 4 g
Mu Tong *Caulis Akebiae* 2 g
Zhu Ling *Sclerotium Polypori umbellati* 6 g
Ze Xie *Rhizoma Alismatis orientalis* 6 g
Hua Shi *Talcum* 6 g

Yi Yi Ren *Semen Coicis lachryma jobi* 12 g
Shan Zhi Zi *Fructus Gardeniae jasminoidis* 4 g

CHUAN BI TANG
Eliminating Painful Obstruction Syndrome Decoction
Qiang Huo *Radix et Rhizoma Notopterygii* 6 g
Du Huo *Radix Angelicae pubescentis* 6 g
Qin Jiao *Radix Gentianae macrophyllae* 6 g
Hai Feng Teng *Caulis Piperis* 3 g
Gui Zhi *Ramulus Cinnamomi cassiae* 3 g
Dang Gui *Radix Angelicae sinensis* 6 g
Chuan Xiong *Radix Ligustici wallichii* 3 g
Ru Xiang *Resina Olibani* 3 g
Mu Xiang *Radix Saussureae* 3 g
Sang Zhi *Ramus Mori albae* 6 g
Gan Cao *Radix Glycyrrhizae uralensis* 3 g

CHUAN XIONG CHA TIAO SAN
Ligusticum-Green Tea Regulating Powder
Chuan Xiong *Radix Ligustici wallichii* 6 g
Qiang Huo *Radix et Rhizoma Notopterygii* 6 g
Bai Zhi *Radix Angelicae dahuricae* 6 g
Jing Jie *Herba seu Flos Schizonepetae tenuifoliae* 6 g
Xi Xin *Herba Asari cum radice* 3 g
Fang Feng *Radix Ledebouriellae sesloidis* 6 g
Bo He *Herba Menthae* 3 g
Gan Cao *Radix Glycyrrhizae uralensis* 3 g
Qing Cha (Green Tea) *Folia Cameliae*

CI ZHU WAN
Magnetitum-Cinnabar Pill
Ci Shi *Magnetitum* 6 g
Zhu Sha *Cinnabaris* 3 g
Shen Qu *Massa Fermentata Medicinalis* 9 g

DA BU YIN JIAN
Great Tonifying Yin Decoction
Shu Di Huang *Radix Rehmanniae glutinosae praeparata* 15 g
Shan Yao *Radix Dioscoreae oppositae* 12 g
Shan Zhu Yu *Fructus Corni officinalis* 9 g
Gou Qi Zi *Fructus Lycii chinensis* 12 g
Dang Gui *Radix Angelicae sinensis* 9 g
Dang Shen *Radix Codonopsis pilosulae* 12 g
Du Zhong *Cortex Eucommiae ulmoidis* 9 g
Zhi Gan Cao *Radix Glycyrrhizae uralensis praeparata* 6 g

DA CHAI HU TANG
Big Bupleurum Decoction
Chai Hu *Radix Bupleuri* 15 g
Huang Qin *Radix Scutellariae baicalensis* 9 g
Ban Xia *Rhizoma Pinelliae ternatae* 9 g
Bai Shao *Radix Paeoniae albae* 9 g
Da Huang *Rhizoma Rhei* 6 g
Zhi Shi *Fructus Citri aurantii immaturus* 9 g
Sheng Jiang *Rhizoma Zingiberis officinalis recens* 15 g
Da Zao *Fructus Ziziphi jujubae* 5 dates

DA CHENG QI TANG
Great Conducting Qi Decoction
Da Huang *Rhizoma Rhei* 12 g
Mang Xiao *Mirabilitum* 9 g
Hou Po *Cortex Magnoliae officinalis* 15 g
Zhi Shi *Fructus Citri aurantii immaturus* 12 g

DA HUANG FU ZI TANG
Rheum-Aconitum Decoction
Da Huang *Rhizoma Rhei* 9 g
Fu Zi *Radix Aconiti carmichaeli praeparata* 9 g
Xi Xin *Herba Asari cum radice* 3 g

DA JIAN ZHONG TANG
Major Strengthening the Centre Decoction
Chuan Jiao *Pericarpium Zanthoxyli bungeani* 3 g
Gan Jiang *Rhizoma Zingiberis officinalis* 4.5 g
Ren Shen *Radix Ginseng* 6 g
Yi Tang *Saccharum granorum* 12 g

DA QI QI TANG
Big Seven Qi Decoction
Qing Pi *Pericarpium Citri reticulatae viridae* 6 g
Chen Pi *Pericarpium Citri reticulatae* 4.5 g
Xiang Fu *Rhizoma Cyperi rotundi* 6 g
Jie Geng *Radix Platycodi grandiflori* 3 g
Huo Xiang *Herba Agastachis* 6 g
Rou Gui *Cortex Cinnamomi cassiae* 3 g
Yi Zhi Ren *Fructus Alpiniae oxyphyllae* 6 g
San Leng *Rhizoma Sparganii* 6 g
E Zhu *Rhizoma Curcumae zedoariae* 6 g
Zhi Gan Cao *Radix Glycyrrhizae uralensis praeparata* 3 g
Sheng Jiang *Rhizoma Zingiberis officinalis recens* 3 slices
Da Zao *Fructus Ziziphi jujubae* 3 dates

DA QIN JIAO TANG
Great Gentiana macrophylla Decoction
Qin Jiao *Radix Gentianae macrophyllae* 9 g
Dang Gui *Radix Angelicae sinensis* 6 g
Gan Cao *Radix Glycyrrhizae uralensis* 6 g
Qiang Huo *Radix et Rhizoma Notopterygii* 3 g
Fang Feng *Radix Ledebouriellae sesloidis* 3 g
Bai Zhi *Radix Angelicae dahuricae* 3 g
Shu Di Huang *Radix Rehmanniae glutinosae praeparata* 3 g
Fu Ling *Sclerotium Poriae cocos* 3 g
Shi Gao *Gypsum fibrosum* 6 g
Chuan Xiong *Radix Ligustici wallichii* 6 g
Bai Shao *Radix Paeoniae albae* 6 g
Du Huo *Radix Angelicae pubescentis* 6 g
Huang Qin *Radix Scutellariae baicalensis* 3 g
Sheng Di Huang *Radix Rehmanniae glutinosae* 3 g
Bai Zhu *Rhizoma Atractylodis macrocephalae* 3 g
Xi Xin *Herba Asari cum radice* 1.5 g

DA YUAN YIN
Extending the Membranes Decoction
Bing Lang *Semen Arecae catechu* 6 g
Hou Po *Cortex Magnoliae officinalis* 3 g
Cao Guo *Fructus Tsaoko* 1.5 g
Zhi Mu *Radix Anemarrhenae asphodeloidis* 3 g
Bai Shao *Radix Paeoniae albae* 3 g
Huang Qin *Radix Scutellariae baicalensis* 3 g
Gan Cao *Radix Glycyrrhizae uralensis* 1.5 g

DAI DI DANG SAN
Surrogate Keeping out Powder
Da Huang *Rhizoma Rhei* 9 g
Mang Xiao *Mirabilitum* 6 g
Tao Ren *Semen Persicae* 6 g
Dang Gui *Radix Angelicae sinensis* 6 g
Sheng Di Huang *Radix Rehmanniae glutinosae* 12 g
Shan Jia *Squama Manitis pentadactylae* 6 g
Rou Gui *Cortex Cinnamomi cassiae* 3 g

DAI GE SAN
Indigo-Concha Cyclinae Powder
Qing Dai *Indigo naturalis* 6 g
Hai Ge Ke *Concha Cyclinae sinensis* 12 g

DAN SHEN YIN
Salvia Decoction

Dan Shen *Radix Salviae miltiorrhizae* 30 g
Tan Xiang *Lignum Santali albi* 5 g
Sha Ren *Fructus seu Semen Amomi* 5 g

DANG GUI BU XUE TANG
Angelica Tonifying Blood Decoction
Huang Qi *Radix Astragali membranacei* 30 g
Dang Gui *Radix Angelicae sinensis* 6 g

DANG GUI LONG HUI WAN
Angelica-Gentiana-Aloe Pill
Dang Gui *Radix Angelicae sinensis* 30 g
Long Dan Cao *Radix Gentianae scabrae* 15 g
Lu Hui *Herba Aloes* 15 g
Shan Zhi Zi *Fructus Gardeniae jasminoidis* 6 g
Huang Lian *Rhizoma Coptidis* 4 g
Huang Bo *Cortex Phellodendri* 6 g
Huang Qin *Radix Scutellariae baicalensis* 6 g
Da Huang *Rhizoma Rhei* 9 g
Mu Xiang *Radix Saussureae* 5 g
She Xiang *Secretio Moschus moschiferi* 1.5 g
Qing Dai *Indigo naturalis* 6 g

DANG GUI SI NI TANG
Angelica Four Rebellious Decoction
Dang Gui *Radix Angelicae sinensis* 12 g
Bai Shao *Radix Paeoniae albae* 9 g
Gui Zhi *Ramulus Cinnamomi cassiae* 9 g
Xi Xin *Herba Asari cum radice* 1.5 g
Zhi Gan Cao *Radix Glycyrrhizae uralensis praeparata* 5 g
Da Zao *Fructus Ziziphi jujubae* 8 pieces
Mu Tong *Caulis Akebiae* 3 g

DAO CHI SAN
Eliminating Redness Powder
Sheng Di Huang *Radix Rehmanniae glutinosae* 15 g
Mu Tong *Caulis Akebiae* 3 g
Sheng Gan Cao *Radix Glycyrrhizae uralensis* 6 g
Zhu Ye *Herba Lophateri gracilis* 3 g

DAO TAN TANG
Conducting Phlegm Decoction
Ban Xia *Rhizoma Pinelliae ternatae* 6 g
Dan Nan Xing *Rhizoma Arisaematis praeparata* 3 g
Zhi Shi *Fructus Citri aurantii immaturus* 3 g
Fu Ling *Sclerotium Poriae cocos* 3 g

Chen Pi *Pericarpium Citri reticulatae* 3 g
Zhi Gan Cao *Radix Glycyrrhizae uralensis praeparata* 2 g
Sheng Jiang *Rhizoma Zingiberis officinalis recens* 3 g

DI PO TANG
Earth Corporeal Soul Decoction
Mai Men Dong *Tuber Ophiopogonis japonici* 9 g
Bai Shao *Radix Paeoniae albae* 9 g
Wu Wei Zi *Fructus Schisandrae chinensis* 3 g
Xuan Shen *Radix Scrophulariae ningpoensis* 9 g
Mu Li *Concha Ostreae* 9 g
Ban Xia *Rhizoma Pinelliae ternatae* 9 g
Gan Cao *Radix Glycyrrhizae uralensis* 3 g

DI TAN TANG
Washing Away Phlegm Decoction
Ban Xia *Rhizoma Pinelliae ternatae* 8 g
Dan Nan Xing *Rhizoma Arisaematis praeparata* 8 g
Zhu Ru *Caulis Bambusae in Taeniis* 2 g
Chen Pi *Pericarpium Citri reticulatae* 6 g
Fu Ling *Sclerotium Poriae cocos* 6 g
Zhi Shi *Fructus Citri aurantii immaturus* 6 g
Shi Chang Pu *Rhizoma Acori graminei* 3 g
Ren Shen *Radix Ginseng* (**Dang Shen** *Radix Codonopsis pilosulae*) 3 g
Zhi Gan Cao *Radix Glycyrrhizae uralensis praeparata* 2 g
Sheng Jiang *Rhizoma Zingiberis officinalis recens* 3 slices
Da Zao *Fructus Ziziphi jujubae* 3 dates

DI YU SAN
Sanguisorba Powder
Di Yu *Radix Sanguisorbae officinalis* 9 g
Qian Cao Gen *Radix Rubiae cordifoliae* 6 g
Huang Qin *Radix Scutellariae baicalensis* 6 g
Huang Lian *Rhizoma Coptidis* 4.5 g
Zhi Zi *Fructus Gardeniae jasminoidis* 6 g
Fu Ling *Sclerotium Poriae cocos* 6 g

DING CHUAN SAN
Stopping Breathlessness Powder
Hong Shen *Radix Ginseng* 6 g
Ge Jie *Gecko* 6 g
Bei Sha Shen *Radix Glehniae littoralis* 6 g
Wu Wei Zi *Fructus Schisandrae chinensis* 4 g

Mai Dong *Tuber Ophiopogonis japonici* 6 g
Chen Pi *Pericarpium Citri reticulatae* 3 g
Zi He Che *Placenta hominis* 9 g

DING CHUAN TANG
Stopping Breathlessness Decoction
Ma Huang *Herba Ephedrae* 9 g
Huang Qin *Radix Scutellariae baicalensis* 6 g
Sang Bai Pi *Cortex Mori albae radicis* 9 g
Xing Ren *Semen Pruni armeniacae* 9 g
Ban Xia *Rhizoma Pinelliae ternatae* 9 g
Kuan Dong Hua *Flos Tussilaginis farfarae* 9 g
Su Zi *Fructus Perillae frutescentis* 6 g
Bai Guo *Semen Ginkgo bilobae* 9 g
Gan Cao *Radix Glycyrrhizae uralensis* 3 g

DING XIAN WAN
Stopping Epilepsy Pill
Tian Ma *Rhizoma Gastrodiae elatae* 9 g
Dan Nan Xing *Rhizoma Arisaematis praeparata* 9 g
Quan Xie *Buthus Martensi* 1.5 g
Jiang Can *Bombyx batryticatus* 4 g
Chuan Bei Mu *Bulbus Fritillariae cirrhosae* 9 g
Ban Xia *Rhizoma Pinelliae ternatae* 9 g
Zhu Li *Succus Bambusae* 10 ml
Fu Ling *Sclerotium Poriae cocos* 6 g
Chen Pi *Pericarpium Citri reticulatae* 4 g
Fu Shen *Sclerotium Poriae cocos pararadicis* 6 g
Shi Chang Pu *Rhizoma Acori graminei* 6 g
Yuan Zhi *Radix Polygalae tenuifoliae* 6 g
Dan Shen *Radix Salviae miltiorrhizae* 6 g
Deng Xin Cao *Medulla Junci effusi* 6 g
Hu Po *Succinum* 6 g
Mai Men Dong *Tuber Ophiopogonis japonici* 6 g
Gan Cao *Radix Glycyrrhizae uralensis* 3 g
Sheng Jiang *Rhizoma Zingiberis officinalis recens* 3 slices

DING ZHI WAN
Settling the Will-Power Pill
Ren Shen *Radix Ginseng* 9 g
Fu Ling *Sclerotium Poriae cocos* 6 g
Shi Chang Pu *Rhizoma Acori graminei* 6 g
Yuan Zhi *Radix Polygalae tenuifoliae* 6 g

DU HUO JI SHENG TANG
Angelica pubescens-Loranthus Decoction
Du Huo *Radix Angelicae pubescentis* 9 g
Xi Xin *Herba Asari cum radice* 3 g

Fang Feng *Radix Ledebouriellae sesloidis* 6 g
Qin Jiao *Radix Gentianae macrophyllae* 6 g
Sang Ji Sheng *Ramus Loranthi* 6 g
Du Zhong *Radix Eucommiae ulmoidis* 6 g
Niu Xi *Radix Achyranthis bidentatae seu Cyathulae* 6 g
Dang Gui *Radix Angelicae sinensis* 6 g
Chuan Xiong *Radix Ligustici wallichii* 6 g
Sheng Di Huang *Radix Rehmanniae glutinosae* 6 g
Bai Shao *Radix Paeoniae albae* 6 g
Ren Shen *Radix Ginseng* 6 g
Fu Ling *Sclerotium Poriae cocos* 6 g
Rou Gui *Cortex Cinnamomi cassiae* 6 g
Gan Cao *Radix Glycyrrhizae uralensis* 6 g

ER CHEN TANG
Two Old Decoction
Ban Xia *Rhizoma Pinelliae ternatae* 15 g
Chen Pi *Pericarpium Citri reticulatae* 15 g
Fu Ling *Sclerotium Poriae cocos* 9 g
Zhi Gan Cao *Radix Glycyrrhizae uralensis praeparata* 5 g
Sheng Jiang *Rhizoma Zingiberis officinalis recens* 3 g
Wu Mei *Fructus Pruni Mume* one prune

ER LONG ZUO CI WAN
Pill for Deafness that is Kind to the Left [Kidney]
Shu Di Huang *Radix Rehmanniae glutinosae praeparata* 24 g
Shan Zhu Yu *Fructus Corni officinalis* 12 g
Shan Yao *Radix Dioscoreae oppositae* 12 g
Ze Xie *Rhizoma Alismatis orientalis* 9 g
Mu Dan Pi *Cortex Moutan radicis* 9 g
Fu Ling *Sclerotium Poriae cocos* 9 g
Ci Shi *Magnetitum* 24 g
Shi Chang Pu *Rhizoma Acori graminei* 9 g
Wu Wei Zi *Fructus Schisandrae chinensis* 6 g

ER SHEN SAN
Hai Jin Sha *Spora Lygodii japonici* 9 g
Hua Shi *Talcum* 9 g

ER ZHI WAN
Two Solstices Pill
Nu Zhen Zi *Fructus Ligustri lucidi* 12 g
Han Lian Cao *Herba Ecliptae prostratae* 9 g

FANG FENG TANG
Ledebouriella Decoction

Fang Feng *Radix Ledebouriellae sesloidis* 6 g
Ma Huang *Herba Ephedrae* 3 g
Qin Jiao *Radix Gentianae macrophyllae* 3 g
Xing Ren *Semen Pruni armeniacae* 2 g
Ge Gen *Radix Puerariae* 3 g
Rou Gui *Cortex Cinnamomi cassiae* 1.5 g
Fu Ling *Sclerotium Poriae cocos* 3 g
Dang Gui *Radix Angelicae sinensis* 3 g
Huang Qin *Radix Scutellariae baicalensis* 2 g
Gan Cao *Radix Glycyrrhizae uralensis* 2 g
Sheng Jiang *Rhizoma Zingiberis officinalis recens* 3 slices
Da Zao *Fructus Ziziphi jujubae* 3 dates

FU LING PI TANG
Poria Skin Decoction
Fu Ling Pi *Cortex Poriae cocos* 15 g
Yi Yi Ren *Semen Coicis lachryma jobi* 15 g
Zhu Ling *Sclerotium Polypori umbellati* 9 g
Tong Cao *Medulla Tetrapanacis papyriferi* 9 g
Da Fu Pi *Pericarpium Arecae catechu* 9 g
Zhu Ye *Herba Lophatheri gracilis* 6 g

GAN CAO XIE XIN TANG
Glycyrrhiza Draining the Heart Decoction
Ban Xia *Rhizoma Pinelliae ternatae* 9 g
Gan Jiang *Rhizoma Zingiberis officinalis* 6 g
Huang Qin *Radix Scutellariae baicalensis* 6 g
Huang Lian *Rhizoma Coptidis* 3 g
Zhi Gan Cao *Radix Glycyrrhizae uralensis praeparata* 12 g
Da Zao *Fructus Ziziphi jujubae* 4 dates

GAN JIANG LING ZHU TANG
Glycyrrhiza-Zingiber-Poria-Atractylodes Decoction
Zhi Gan Cao *Radix Glycyrrhizae uralensis praeparata* 6 g
Gan Jiang *Rhizoma Zingiberis officinalis* 6 g
Fu Ling *Sclerotium Poriae cocos* 9 g
Bai Zhu *Rhizoma Atractylodis macrocephalae* 9 g

GAN MAI DA ZAO TANG
Glycyrrhiza-Triticum-Ziziphus Decoction
Fu Xiao Mai *Semen Tritici aestivi levis* 15 g
Gan Cao *Radix Glycyrrhizae uralensis* 9 g
Da Zao *Fructus Ziziphi jujubae* 7 dates

GAO LIN TANG
Sticky Painful-Urination Syndrome Decoction

Shan Yao *Radix Dioscoreae oppositae* 12 g
Qian Shi *Semen Euryales ferocis* 6 g
Sheng Di Huang *Radix Rehmanniae glutinosae* 9 g
Long Gu *Os Draconis* 12 g
Mu Li *Concha Ostreae* 12 g
Bai Shao *Radix Paeoniae albae* 6 g
Dang Shen *Radix Codonopsis pilosulae* 6 g

GE GEN QIN LIAN TANG
Pueraria-Scutellaria-Coptis Decoction
Ge Gen *Radix Puerariae* 9 g
Huang Qin *Radix Scutellariae baicalensis* 9 g
Huang Lian *Rhizoma Coptidis* 4.5 g
Zhi Gan Cao *Radix Glycyrrhizae uralensis praeparata* 3 g

GE XIA ZHU YU TANG
Eliminating Stasis below the Diaphragm Decoction
Dang Gui *Radix Angelicae sinensis* 9 g
Chuan Xiong *Radix Ligustici wallichii* 3 g
Chi Shao *Radix Paeoniae rubrae* 6 g
Hong Hua *Flos Carthami tinctorii* 9 g
Tao Ren *Semen Persicae* 9 g
Wu Ling Zhi *Excrementum Trogopteri* 9 g
Yan Hu Suo *Rhizoma Corydalis yanhusuo* 3 g
Xiang Fu *Rhizoma Cyperi rotundi* 3 g
Zhi Ke *Fructus Citri aurantii* 5 g
Wu Yao *Radix Linderae strychnifoliae* 6 g
Mu Dan Pi *Cortex Moutan radicis* 6 g
Gan Cao *Radix Glycyrrhizae uralensis* 9 g

GU BEN ZHI BENG TANG
Consolidating the Root and Stopping Menorrhagia Decoction
Huang Qi *Radix Astragali membranacei* 15 g
Ren Shen *Radix Ginseng* 12 g
Bai Zhu *Rhizoma Atractylodis macrocephalae* 18 g
Shu Di Huang *Radix Rehmanniae glutinosae praeparata* 9 g
Dang Gui *Radix Angelicae sinensis* 6 g
Pao Jiang *Rhizoma Zingiberis officinalis recens* (fried) 6 g

GUA LOU XIE BAI BAN XIA TANG
Trichosanthes-Allium-Pinellia Decoction
Gua Lou *Fructus Trichosanthis* 12 g
Xie Bai *Bulbus Allii* 12g
Ban Xia *Rhizoma Pinelliae ternatae* 12 g
Bai Jiu White rice wine 30 ml

GUA LOU XIE BAI BAI JIU TANG
Trichosanthes-Allium-White Wine Decoction
Gua Lou *Fructus Trichosanthis* 12 g
Xie Bai *Bulbus Allii* 12 g
Bai Jiu White rice wine 30 ml

GUI FU LI ZHONG TANG
Cinnamomum-Aconitum Regulating the Centre Decoction
Gan Jiang *Rhizoma Zingiberis officinalis* 9 g
Ren Shen *Radix Ginseng* 9 g
Bai Zhu *Rhizoma Atractylodis macrocephalae* 9 g
Zhi Gan Cao *Radix Glycyrrhizae uralensis praeparata* 3 g
Rou Gui *Cortex Cinnamomi cassiae* 3 g
Fu Zi *Radix Aconiti carmichaeli praeparata* 6 g

GUI PI TANG
Tonifying the Spleen Decoction
Ren Shen *Radix Ginseng* 6 g or **Dang Shen** *Radix Codonopsis pilosulae* 12 g
Huang Qi *Radix Astragali membranacei* 15 g
Bai Zhu *Rhizoma Atractylodis macrocephalae* 12 g
Dang Gui *Radix Angelicae sinensis* 6 g
Fu Shen *Sclerotium Poriae cocos pararadicis* 9 g
Suan Zao Ren *Semen Ziziphi spinosae* 9 g
Long Yan Rou *Arillus Euphoriae longanae* 12 g
Yuan Zhi *Radix Polygalae tenuifoliae* 9 g
Mu Xiang *Radix Saussureae* 3 g
Zhi Gan Cao *Radix Glycyrrhizae uralensis praeparata* 4 g
Sheng Jiang *Rhizoma Zingiberis officinalis recens* 3 slices
Hong Zao *Fructus Ziziphi jujubae* 5 dates

GUI SHAO XI CAO TANG
Angelica-Paeonia-Siegesbeckia Decoction
Dang Gui *Radix Angelicae sinensis* 15 g
Chi Shao *Radix Paeoniae rubrae* 15 g
Bai Shao *Radix Paeoniae albae* 15 g
Xi Xian Cao *Herba Siegesbeckiae orientalis* 30 g
Qin Jiao *Radix Gentianae macrophyllae* 10 g
Wei Ling Xian *Radix Clematidis chinensis* 15 g
Di Long *Lumbricus* 10 g
Fang Feng *Radix Ledebouriellae sesloidis* 10 g
Sheng Di Huang *Radix Rehmanniae glutinosae* 30 g
Ru Xiang *Resina Olibani* 6 g
Mo Yao *Resina Myrrhae* 6 g
Sang Zhi *Ramulus Mori albae* 15 g

GUI SHEN TANG
Restoring the Mind Decoction
Ren Shen *Radix Ginseng* 15 g
Bai Zhu *Rhizoma Atractylodis macrocephalae* 30 g
Ba Ji Tian *Radix Morindae officinalis* 30 g
Fu Shen *Sclerotium Poriae cocos pararadicis* 15 g
Zi He Che *Placenta hominis* 6 g
Ban Xia *Rhizoma Pinelliae ternatae* 9 g
Chen Pi *Pericarpium Citri reticulatae* 3 g
Bai Jie Zi *Semen Sinapis albae* 9 g
Shi Chang Pu *Rhizoma Acori graminei* 3 g
Zhu Sha *Cinnabaris* 3 g
Mai Men Dong *Tuber Ophiopogonis japonici* 6 g
Bai Zi Ren *Semen Biotae orientalis* 6 g
Zhi Gan Cao *Radix Glycyrrhizae uralensis praeparata* 3 g

GUI ZHI FU LING WAN
Ramulus Cinnamomi-Poria Pill
Gui Zhi *Ramulus Cinnamomi cassiae* 9 g
Fu Ling *Sclerotium Poriae cocos* 9 g
Chi Shao *Radix Paeoniae rubrae* 9 g
Mu Dan Pi *Cortex Moutan radicis* 9 g
Tao Ren *Semen Persicae* 9 g

GUI ZHI FU ZI TANG
Ramulus Cinnamomi-Aconitum Decoction
Fu Zi *Radix Aconiti carmichaeli praeparata* 3 g
Gui Zhi *Ramulus Cinnamomi cassiae* 6 g
Gan Cao *Radix Glycyrrhizae uralensis* 3 g
Sheng Jiang *Rhizoma Zingiberis officinalis recens* 3 slices
Da Zao *Fructus Ziziphi jujubae* 3 dates

GUI ZHI GAN CAO LONG GU MU LI TANG
Ramulus Cinnamomi-Glycyrrhiza-Os Draconis-Ostrea Decoction
Gui Zhi *Ramulus Cinnamomi cassiae* 9 g
Zhi Gan Cao *Radix Glycyrrhizae uralensis praeparata* 18 g
Long Gu *Os Draconis* 30 g
Mu Li *Concha Ostreae* 30 g

GUI ZHI JIA HOU PO XING ZI TANG
Ramulus Cinnamomi Decoction plus Magnolia and Prunus
Gui Zhi *Ramulus Cinnamomi cassiae* 9 g
Bai Shao *Radix Paeoniae albae* 9 g
Zhi Gan Cao *Radix Glycyrrhizae uralensis praeparata* 6 g

Sheng Jiang *Rhizoma Zingiberis officinalis recens* 9 g
Da Zao *Fructus Ziziphi jujubae* 3 dates
Hou Po *Cortex Magnoliae officinalis* 4 g
Xing Ren *Semen Pruni armeniacae* 6 g

GUI ZHI REN SHEN TANG
Ramulus Cinnamomi-Ginseng Decoction
Gui Zhi *Ramulus Cinnamomi cassiae* 12 g
Zhi Gan Cao *Radix Glycyrrhizae uralensis prae-parata* 12 g
Ren Shen *Radix Ginseng* 15 g
Bai Zhu *Rhizoma Atractylodis macrocephalae* 9 g
Gan Jiang *Rhizoma Zingiberis officinalis* 9 g

GUI ZHI TANG
Ramulus Cinnamomi Decoction
Gui Zhi *Ramulus Cinnamomi cassiae* 9 g
Bai Shao *Radix Paeoniae albae* 9 g
Sheng Jiang *Rhizoma Zingiberis officinalis recens* 9 g
Da Zao *Fructus Ziziphi jujubae* 3 dates
Zhi Gan Cao *Radix Glycyrrhizae uralensis prae-parata* 6 g

GUN TAN WAN
Chasing away Phlegm Pill
Da Huang *Rhizoma Rhei* 15 g
Mang Xiao *Mirabilitum* 3 g
Huang Qin *Radix Scutellariae baicalensis* 15 g
Chen Xiang *Lignum Aquilariae* 3 g

HAO QIN QING DAN TANG
Artemisia apiacea-Scutellaria Clearing the Gall-Bladder Decoction
Qing Hao *Herba Artemisiae apiaceae* 6 g
Huang Qin *Radix Scutellariae baicalensis* 6 g
Zhu Ru *Caulis Bambusae in Taenis* 9 g
Ban Xia *Rhizoma Pinelliae ternatae* 5 g
Chen Pi *Pericarpium Citri reticulatae* 5 g
Zhi Ke *Fructus Citri aurantii* 5 g
Fu Ling *Sclerotium Poriae cocos* 9 g
Hua Shi *Talcum* 3 g
Gan Cao *Radix Glycyrrhizae uralensis* 3 g
Qing Dai *Indigo naturalis* 3 g

HE CHE DA ZAO WAN
Placenta Great Fortifying Pill
Zi He Che *Placenta hominis* 1 placenta

Shu Di Huang *Radix Rehmanniae glutinosae prae-parata* 60 g
Sheng Di Huang *Radix Rehmanniae glutinosae* 45 g
Gou Qi Zi *Fructus Lycii chinensis* 45 g
Tian Men Dong *Tuber Asparagi cochinchinensis* 20 g
Wu Wei Zi *Fructus Schisandrae chinensis* 20 g
Dang Gui *Radix Angelicae sinensis* 20 g
Niu Xi *Radix Achyranthis bidentatae seu Cyathulae* 20 g
Du Zhong *Cortex Eucommiae ulmoidis* 30 g
Suo Yang *Herba Cynomorii songarici* 20 g
Rou Cong Rong *Herba Cistanchis* 20 g
Huang Bo *Cortex Phellodendri* 20 g

HU QIAN WAN
Hidden Tiger Pill
Hu Gu *Os Tigris* 6 g
Suo Yang *Herba Cynomorii songarici* 4.5 g
Niu Xi *Radix Achyranthis bidentatae seu Cyathulae* 6 g
Dang Gui *Radix Angelicae sinensis* 6 g
Huang Bo *Cortex Phellodendri* 15 g
Zhi Mu *Radix Anemarrhenae asphodeloidis* 6 g
Shu Di Huang *Radix Rehmanniae glutinosae prae-parata* 6 g
Gui Ban *Plastrum Testudinis* 12 g
Bai Shao *Radix Paeoniae albae* 6 g

HUA GAI SAN
Glorious Lid Decoction
Ma Huang *Herba Ephedrae* 6 g
Xing Ren *Semen Pruni armeniacae* 9 g
Su Zi *Fructus Perillae frutescentis* 9 g
Sang Bai Pi *Cortex Mori albae radicis* 6 g
Chen Pi *Pericarpium Citri reticulatae* 6 g
Fu Ling *Sclerotium Poriae cocos* 9 g
Gan Cao *Radix Glycyrrhizae uralensis* 3 g

HUA GAN JIAN
Transforming the Liver Decoction
Chen Pi *Pericarpium Citri reticulatae* 6 g
Qing Pi *Pericarpium Citri reticulatae viridae* 4 g
Bai Shao *Radix Paeoniae albae* 9 g
Mu Dan Pi *Cortex Moutan radicis* 6 g
Shan Zhi Zi *Fructus Gardeniae jasminoidis* 6 g
Ze Xie *Rhizoma Alismatis orientalis* 6 g
Zhe Bei Mu *Bulbus Fritillariae thunbergii* 6 g

HUA JI WAN
Resolving Blood Masses Pill
San Leng *Rhizoma Sparganii* 6 g
E Zhu *Rhizoma Curcumae zedoariae* 6 g
Wu Ling Zhi *Excrementum Trogopteri* 6 g
Su Mu *Lignum Sappan* 4.5 g
Xiang Fu *Rhizoma Cyperi rotundi* 6 g
Bing Lang *Semen Arecae catechu* 6 g
Xiong Huang *Realgar* 1.5 g
Wa Leng Zi *Concha Arcae* 15 g
A Wei *Herba Ferulae assafoetidae* 6 g
Hai Fu Shi *Pumice* 15 g

HUANG LIAN E JIAO TANG
Coptis-Gelatinum Corii Asini Decoction
Huang Lian *Rhizoma Coptidis* 3 g
Huang Qin *Radix Scutellariae baicalensis* 9 g
Bai Shao *Radix Paeoniae albae* 9 g
Ji Zi Huang *Egg yolk* 2 yolks
E Jiao *Gelatinum Corii Asini* 9 g

HUANG LIAN WEN DAN TANG
Coptis Warming the Gall-Bladder Decoction
Huang Lian *Rhizoma Coptidis* 4.5 g
Ban Xia *Rhizoma Pinelliae ternatae* 6 g
Fu Ling *Sclerotium Poriae cocos* 5 g
Chen Pi *Pericarpium Citri reticulatae* 9 g
Zhu Ru *Caulis Bambusae in Taeniis* 6 g
Zhi Shi *Fructus Citri aurantii immaturus* 6 g
Zhi Gan Cao *Radix Glycyrrhizae uralensis praeparata* 3 g
Sheng Jiang *Rhizoma Zingiberis officinalis recens* 5 slices
Da Zao *Fructus Ziziphi jujubae* 1 date

HUANG QI JIAN ZHONG TANG
Astragalus Strengthening the Centre Decoction
Huang Qi *Radix Astragali membranacei* 9 g
Bai Shao *Radix Paeoniae albae* 18 g
Gui Zhi *Ramulus Cinnamomi cassiae* 9 g
Zhi Gan Cao *Radix Glycyrrhizae uralensis praeparata* 6 g
Sheng Jiang *Rhizoma Zingiberis officinalis recens* 10 g
Da Zao *Fructus Ziziphi jujubae* 12 dates
Yi Tang *Saccharum granorum* 30 g

HUANG QI TANG
Astragalus Decoction
Huang Qi *Radix Astragali membranacei* 9 g
Chen Pi *Pericarpium Citri reticulatae* 4.5 g
Huo Ma Ren *Semen Cannabis sativae* 6 g
Feng Mi *Mel* 1 teaspoonful

HUANG QIN TANG
Scutellaria Decoction
Huang Qin *Radix Scutellariae baicalensis* 9 g
Bai Shao *Radix Paeoniae albae* 9 g
Zhi Gan Cao *Radix Glycyrrhizae uralensis praeparata* 3 g
Da Zao *Fructus Ziziphi jujubae* 4 dates

HUANG QIN QING FEI YIN
Scutellaria Clearing the Lungs Decoction
Huang Qin *Radix Scutellariae baicalensis* 9 g
Di Gu Pi *Cortex Lycii chinensis radicis* 6 g
Sang Bai Pi *Cortex Mori albae radicis* 6 g
Geng Mi *Semen Oryzae sativae* 6 g
Gan Cao *Radix Glycyrrhizae uralensis* 3 g

HUO LUO XIAO LING DAN
Miraculously Effective Invigorating the Connecting Channels Pill
Dang Gui *Radix Angelicae sinensis* 15 g
Dan Shen *Radix Salviae miltiorrhizae* 15 g
Ru Xiang *Gummi Olibanum* 15 g
Mo Yao *Myrrha* 15 g

HUO PO XIA LING TANG
Agastache-Magnolia-Pinellia-Poria Decoction
Huo Xiang *Herba Agastachis* 6 g
Bai Dou Kou *Fructus Cardamomi rotundi* 2 g
Hou Po *Cortex Magnoliae officinalis* 3 g
Fu Ling *Sclerotium Poriae cocos* 9 g
Zhu Ling *Sclerotium Polypori umbellati* 4.5 g
Yi Yi Ren *Semen Coicis lachryma jobi* 12 g
Ze Xie *Rhizoma Alismatis orientalis* 4.5 g
Ban Xia *Rhizoma Pinelliae ternatae* 4.5 g
Dan Dou Chi *Semen Sojae praeparatum* 9 g
Xing Ren *Semen Pruni armeniacae* 9 g

HUO XIANG ZHENG QI SAN
Agastache Upright Qi Powder
Huo Xiang *Herba Agastachis* 9 g
Zi Su Ye *Folium Perillae frutescentis* 3 g
Bai Zhi *Radix Angelicae dahuricae* 3 g
Ban Xia *Rhizoma Pinelliae ternatae* 6 g
Chen Pi *Pericarpium Citri reticulatae* 6 g

Bai Zhu *Rhizoma Atractylodis macrocephalae* 6 g
Fu Ling *Sclerotium Poriae cocos* 3 g
Hou Po *Cortex Magnoliae officinalis* 6 g
Da Fu Pi *Pericarpium Arecae catechu* 3 g
Jie Geng *Radix Platycodi grandiflori* 6 g
Sheng Jiang *Rhizoma Zingiberis officinalis recens* 3 slices
Da Zao *Fructus Ziziphi jujubae* 3 dates
Zhi Gan Cao *Radix Glycyrrhizae uralensis praeparata* 3 g

JI CHUAN JIAN
Benefit the River Decoction
Dang Gui *Radix Angelicae sinensis* 9 g
Niu Xi *Radix Achyranthis bidentatae seu Cyathulae* 6 g
Rou Cong Rong *Herba Cistanchis* 6 g
Ze Xie *Rhizoma Alismatis orientalis* 4.5 g
Zhi Ke *Fructus Citri aurantii* 3 g
Sheng Ma *Rhizoma Cimicifugae* 1.5 g

JIA JIAN YU ZHU TANG
Variation of Polygonatum Decoction
Yu Zhu *Rhizoma Polygonati odorati* 12 g
Dan Dou Chi *Semen Sojae praeparatum* 9 g
Cong Bai *Herba Allii fistulosi* 15 g
Bo He *Herba Menthae* 6 g
Jie Geng *Radix Platycodi grandiflori* 6 g
Bai Wei *Radix Cynanchi* 6 g
Gan Cao *Radix Glycyrrhizae uralensis* 3 g
Da Zao *Fructus Ziziphi jujubae* 3 g

JIA WEI GUA LOU XIE BAI TANG
Trichosanthes-Allium Decoction Variation
Gua Lou *Fructus Trichosanthis* 15 g
Xie Bai *Bulbus Allii* 9 g
Chi Shao *Radix Paeoniae rubrae* 6 g
Hong Hua *Flos Carthami tinctorii* 6 g
Chuan Xiong *Radix Ligustici wallichii* 6 g
Jiang Huang *Rhizoma Curcumae longae* 6 g

JIA WEI SI JUN ZI TANG
Four Gentlemen Decoction Variation
Ren Shen *Radix Ginseng* 9 g
Huang Qi *Radix Astragali membranacei* 9 g
Bai Zhu *Rhizoma Atractylodis macrocephalae* 6 g
Zhi Gan Cao *Radix Glycyrrhizae uralensis praeparata* 3 g
Fu Ling *Sclerotium Poriae cocos* 6 g
Bian Dou *Semen Dolichoris lablab* 6 g

JIA WEI WU LIN SAN
Augmented Five Painful-Urination Syndrome Powder
Fu Ling *Sclerotium Poriae cocos* 12 g
Dang Gui *Radix Angelicae sinensis* 6 g
Gan Cao *Radix Glycyrrhizae uralensis* 3 g
Chi Shao *Radix Paeoniae rubrae* 9 g
Zhi Zi *Fructus Gardeniae jasminoidis* 9 g
Sheng Di Huang *Radix Rehmanniae glutinosae* 12 g
Ze Xie *Rhizoma Alismatis orientalis* 6 g
Che Qian Zi *Semen Plantaginis* 9 g
Hua Shi *Talcum* 9 g
Mu Tong *Caulis Akebiae* 6 g

JIA WEI XIANG SU SAN
New Cyperus-Perilla Powder
Zi Su Ye *Folium Perillae frutescentis* 5 g
Jing Jie *Herba seu Flos Schizonepetae tenuifoliae* 3 g
Fang Feng *Radix Ledebouriellae sesloidis* 3 g
Qin Jiao *Radix Gentianae macrophyllae* 3 g
Man Jing Zi *Fructus Viticis* 3 g
Xiang Fu *Rhizoma Cyperi rotundi* 4 g
Chuan Xiong *Radix Ligustici wallichii* 1.5 g
Chen Pi *Pericarpium Citri reticulatae* 4 g
Gan Cao *Radix Glycyrrhizae uralensis* 2.5 g

JIA WEI XIAO YAO SAN
Free and Easy Wanderer Powder
Bo He *Herba Menthae* 3 g
Chai Hu *Radix Bupleuri* 9 g
Dang Gui *Radix Angelicae sinensis* 9 g
Bai Shao *Radix Paeoniae albae* 12 g
Bai Zhu *Rhizoma Atractylodis macrocephalae* 9 g
Fu Ling *Sclerotium Poriae cocos* 15 g
Gan Cao *Radix Glycyrrhizae uralensis* 6 g
Sheng Jiang *Rhizoma Zingiberis officinalis recens* 3 slices
Mu Dan Pi *Cortex Moutan radicis* 6 g
Shan Zhi Zi *Fructus Gardeniae jasminoidis* 6 g

JIE YU DAN
Relaxing Speech Pill
Tian Ma *Rhizoma Gastrodiae elatae* 6 g
Quan Xie *Buthus Martensi* 1.5 g
Dan Nan Xing *Rhizoma Arisaematis praeparata* 6 g
Bai Fu Zi *Rhizoma Thyphonii gigantei* 3 g
Yuan Zhi *Radix Polygalae tenuifoliae* 6 g
Shi Chang Pu *Rhizoma Acori graminei* 6 g

Mu Xiang *Radix Saussureae* 4 g
Qiang Huo *Radix et Rhizoma Notopterygii* 3 g

JIN GUI SHEN QI WAN
Golden Chest Kidney-Qi Pill
Fu Zi *Radix Aconiti carmichaeli praeparata* 3 g
Gui Zhi *Ramulus Cinnamomi cassiae* 3 g
Shu Di Huang *Radix Rehmanniae glutinosae praeparata* 24 g
Shan Zhu Yu *Fructus Corni officinalis* 12 g
Shan Yao *Radix Dioscoreae oppositae* 12 g
Ze Xie *Rhizoma Alismatis orientalis* 9 g
Mu Dan Pi *Cortex Moutan radicis* 9 g
Fu Ling *Sclerotium Poriae cocos* 9 g

JIN LING ZI SAN
Fructus Meliae toosendan Powder
Jin Ling Zi (Chuan Lian Zi) *Fructus Meliae toosendan* 30 g
Yan Hu Suo *Rhizoma Corydalis yanhusuo* 30 g

JING FANG JIE BIAO TANG
Schizonepeta-Ledebouriella Releasing the Exterior Decoction
Jing Jie *Herba seu Flos Schizonepetae tenuifoliae* 9 g
Fang Feng *Radix Ledebouriellae sesloidis* 9 g
Zi Su Ye *Folium Perillae frutescentis* 6 g
Qian Hu *Radix Peucedani* 9 g
Jie Geng *Radix Platycodi grandiflori* 6 g

JU HUA CHA TIAO SAN
Chrysanthemum-Green Tea Regulating Powder
Chuan Xiong Cha Tiao San prescription plus:
Ju Hua *Flos Chrysanthemi morifolii* 6 g
Jiang Can *Bombix batryticatus* 6 g

KUAN XIONG WAN
Opening the Chest Pill
Gao Liang Jiang *Rhizoma Alpiniae officinari* 6 g
Yan Hu Suo *Rhizoma Corydalis yanhusuo* 6 g
Tan Xiang *Lignum Santali albi* 6 g
Bi Ba *Fructus Piperis longi* 6 g
Xi Xin *Herba Asari cum radice* 1.5 g
Bing Pian *Borneol* 3 g

LEI SHI FANG XIANG HUA ZHUO FA
Fragrant Formula to Resolve Turbidity by the Lei's Clan
Huo Xiang *Herba Agastachis* 3 g

Pei Lan *Herba Eupatorii fortunei* 3 g
Chen Pi *Pericarpium Citri reticulatae* 4.5 g
Ban Xia *Rhizoma Pinelliae ternatae* 4.5 g
Da Fu Pi *Pericarpium Arecae catechu* 3 g
Hou Po *Cortex Magnoliae officinalis* 2 g
Bo He *Herba Menthae* 3 g

LI ZHONG WAN
Regulating the Centre Pill
Ren Shen *Radix Ginseng* 6 g or **Dang Shen** *Radix Codonopsis pilosulae* 12 g
Bai Zhu *Rhizoma Atractylodis macrocephalae* 9 g
Gan Jiang *Rhizoma Zingiberis officinalis* 5 g
Zhi Gan Cao *Radix Glycyrrhizae uralensis praeparata* 6 g

LIAN PO YIN
Coptis-Magnolia Decoction
Huang Lian *Rhizoma Coptidis* 3 g
Hou Po *Cortex Magnoliae officinalis* 3 g
Shan Zhi Zi *Fructus Gardeniae jasminoidis* 9 g
Dan Dou Chi *Semen Sojae praeparatum* 9 g
Shi Chang Pu *Rhizoma Acori graminei* 3 g
Ban Xia *Rhizoma Pinelliae ternatae* 3 g
Lu Gen *Rhizoma Phragmitis communis* 15 g

LIANG DI TANG
Two "Di" Decoction
Sheng Di Huang *Radix Rehmanniae glutinosae* 18 g
Di Gu Pi *Cortex Lycii chinensis radicis* 9 g
Xuan Shen *Radix Scrophulariae ningpoensis* 12 g
Mai Men Dong *Tuber Ophiopogonis japonici* 9 g
Bai Shao *Radix Paeoniae albae* 12 g
E Jiao *Gelatinum Corii Asini* 9 g

LIANG FU WAN
Alpinia-Cyperus Pill
Gao Liang Jiang *Rhizoma Alpiniae officinari* 6 g
Xiang Fu *Rhizoma Cyperi rotundi* 6 g

LING GAN WU WEI JIANG XIN TANG
Poria-Glycyrrhiza-Schisandra-Zingiber-Asarum Decoction
Fu Ling *Sclerotium Poriae cocos* 12 g
Zhi Gan Cao *Radix Glycyrrhizae uralensis praeparata* 9 g
Gan Jiang *Rhizoma Zingiberis officinalis* 9 g
Xi Xin *Herba Asari cum radice* 9 g
Wu Wei Zi *Fructus Schisandrae chinensis* 6 g

LING GUI FU PING TANG
Poria-Cinnamomum-Spirodela Decoction
Fu Ling *Sclerotium Poriae cocos* 9 g
Gui Zhi *Ramulus Cinnamomi cassiae* 6 g
Fu Ping *Herba Lemnae seu Spirodelae* 9 g
Xing Ren *Semen Pruni armeniacae* 9 g
Ze Xie *Rhizoma Alismatis orientalis* 9 g
Ban Xia *Rhizoma Pinelliae ternatae* 9 g
Zhi Gan Cao *Radix Glycyrrhizae uralensis prae-parata* 3 g

LING GUI ZHU GAN TANG
Poria-Ramulus Cinnamomi-Atractylodes-Glycyrrhiza Decoction
Fu Ling *Sclerotium Poriae cocos* 12 g
Gui Zhi *Ramulus Cinnamomi cassiae* 9 g
Bai Zhu *Rhizoma Atractylodis macrocephalae* 6 g
Zhi Gan Cao *Radix Glycyrrhizae uralensis prae-parata* 3 g

LING JIAO GOU TENG TANG
Cornu Antelopis-Uncaria Decoction
Ling Yang Jiao *Cornu Antelopis* 4.5 g
Gou Teng *Ramulus Uncariae* 9 g
Sang Ye *Folium Mori albae* 6 g
Ju Hua *Flos Chrysanthemi morifolii* 9 g
Bai Shao *Radix Paeoniae albae* 9 g
Sheng Di Huang *Radix Rehmanniae glutinosae* 15 g
Fu Shen *Sclerotium Poriae cocos pararadicis* 9 g
Chuan Bei Mu *Bulbus Fritillariae cirrhosae* 12 g
Zhu Ru *Caulis Bambusae in Taenis* 15 g
Gan Cao *Radix Glycyrrhizae uralensis* 2.5 g

LIU HE TANG
Six Harmonizing Decoction
Ren Shen *Radix Ginseng* 6 g
Bai Zhu *Rhizoma Atractylodis macrocephalae* 6 g
Sha Ren *Fructus seu Semen Amomi* 3 g
Huo Xiang *Herba Agastachis* 6 g
Hou Po *Cortex Magnoliae officinalis* 2.4 g
Fu Ling *Sclerotium Poriae cocos* 6 g
Bian Dou *Semen Dolichoris lablab* 6 g
Ban Xia *Rhizoma Pinelliae ternatae* 6 g
Xing Ren *Semen Pruni armeniacae* 6 g
Mu Gua *Fructus Chaenomelis lagenariae* 4.5 g
Gan Cao *Radix Glycyrrhizae uralensis* 1.5 g

LIU JUN ZI TANG
Six Gentlemen Decoction
Ren Shen *Radix Ginseng* 10 g
Bai Zhu *Rhizoma Atractylodis macrocephalae* 9 g
Fu Ling *Sclerotium Poriae cocos* 9 g
Zhi Gan Cao *Radix Glycyrrhizae uralensis prae-parata* 6 g
Chen Pi *Pericarpium Citri reticulatae* 9 g
Ban Xia *Rhizoma Pinelliae ternatae* 12 g

LIU MO TANG
Six Ground-Herbs Decoction
Mu Xiang *Radix Saussureae* 6 g
Wu Yao *Radix Linderae strychnifoliae* 6 g
Chen Xiang *Lignum Aquilariae* 4.5 g
Da Huang *Rhizoma Rhei* 6 g
Bing Lang *Semen Arecae catechu* 6 g
Zhi Shi *Fructus Citri aurantii immaturus* 6 g

LIU WEI DI HUANG WAN
Six-Ingredient Rehmannia Pill
Shu Di Huang *Radix Rehmanniae glutinosae prae-parata* 24 g
Shan Zhu Yu *Fructus Corni officinalis* 12 g
Shan Yao *Radix Dioscoreae oppositae* 12 g
Ze Xie *Rhizoma Alismatis orientalis* 9 g
Mu Dan Pi *Cortex Moutan radicis* 9 g
Fu Ling *Sclerotium Poriae cocos* 9 g

LONG DAN BI YUAN FANG
Gentiana "Nose Pool" Formula
Long Dan Cao *Radix Gentianae scabrae* 6 g
Huang Qin *Radix Scutellariae baicalensis* 6 g
Xia Ku Cao *Spica Prunellae vulgaris* 6 g
Yu Xing Cao *Herba Houttuyniae cordatae* 9 g
Ju Hua *Flos Chrysanthemi morifolii* 6 g
Bai Zhi *Radix Angelicae dahuricae* 6 g
Cang Er Zi *Fructus Xanthii* 6 g
Huo Xiang *Herba Agastachis* 4.5 g
Yi Yi Ren *Semen Coicis lachryma jobi* 15 g
Che Qian Zi *Semen Plantaginis* 6 g
Jie Geng *Radix Platycodi grandiflori* 6 g

LONG DAN XIE GAN TANG
Gentiana Draining the Liver Decoction
Long Dan Cao *Radix Gentianae scabrae* 6 g
Huang Qin *Radix Scutellariae baicalensis* 9 g
Shan Zhi Zi *Fructus Gardeniae jasminoidis* 9 g
Ze Xie *Rhizoma Alismatis orientalis* 9 g
Mu Tong *Caulis Akebiae* 9 g
Che Qian Zi *Semen Plantaginis* 9 g

Sheng Di Huang *Radix Rehmanniae glutinosae* 12 g
Dang Gui *Radix Angelicae sinensis* 9 g
Chai Hu *Radix Bupleuri* 9 g
Gan Cao *Radix Glycyrrhizae uralensis* 3 g

LU JIAO JIAO TANG
Colla Cornu Cervi Decoction
Lu Jiao Jiao *Colla Cornu Cervi* 9 g
Lu Jiao Shuang *Cornu Cervi deglutinatum* 6 g
Shu Di Huang *Radix Rehmanniae glutinosae praeparata* 12 g
Niu Xi *Radix Achyranthis bidentatae seu Cyathulae* 6 g
Fu Ling *Sclerotium Poriae cocos* 6 g
Tu Si Zi *Semen Cuscutae* 6 g
Ren Shen *Radix Ginseng* 6 g
Dang Gui *Radix Angelicae sinensis* 6 g
Bai Zhu *Rhizoma Atractylodis macrocephalae* 6 g
Du Zhong *Cortex Eucommiae ulmoidis* 6 g
Gui Ban *Plastrum Testudinis* 12 g

MA HUANG FU ZI XI XIN TANG
Ephedra-Aconitum-Asarum Decoction
Ma Huang *Herba Ephedrae* 6 g
Fu Zi *Radix Aconiti carmichaeli praeparata* 9 g
Xi Xin *Herba Asari cum radice* 6 g

MA HUANG LIAN QIAO CHI XIAO DOU TANG
Ephedra-Forsythia-Phaseolus Decoction
Ma Huang *Herba Ephedrae* 9 g
Xing Ren *Semen Pruni armeniacae* 6 g
Sang Bai Pi *Cortex Mori albae radicis* 6 g
Lian Qiao *Fructus Forsythiae suspensae* 6 g
Chi Xiao Dou *Semen Phaseoli calcarati* 9 g
Zhi Gan Cao *Radix Glycyrrhizae uralensis praeparata* 3 g
Sheng Jiang *Rhizoma Zingiberis officinalis recens* 3 slices
Da Zao *Fructus Ziziphi jujubae* 3 dates

MA HUANG TANG
Ephedra Decoction
Ma Huang *Herba Ephedrae* 6 g
Gui Zhi *Ramulus Cinnamomi cassiae* 4 g
Xing Ren *Semen Pruni armeniacae* 9 g
Zhi Gan Cao *Radix Glycyrrhizae uralensis praeparata* 3 g

MA XING SHI GAN TANG
Ephedra-Prunus-Gypsum-Glycyrrhiza Decoction
Ma Huang *Herba Ephedrae* 5 g
Xing Ren *Semen Pruni armeniacae* 9 g
Shi Gao *Gypsum fibrosum* 18 g
Zhi Gan Cao *Radix Glycyrrhizae uralensis praeparata* 6 g

MA ZI REN WAN
Cannabis Pill
Huo Ma Ren *Semen Cannabis sativa* 9 g
Da Huang *Rhizoma Rhei* 6 g
Xing Ren *Semen Pruni armeniacae* 4.5 g
Zhi Shi *Fructus Citri aurantii immaturus* 6 g
Hou Po *Cortex Magnoliae officinalis* 4.5 g
Bai Shao *Radix Paeoniae albae* 4.5 g

MAI MEN DONG TANG
Ophiopogon Decoction
Mai Men Dong *Tuber Ophiopogonis japonici* 60 g
Ban Xia *Rhizoma Pinelliae ternatae* 9 g
Ren Shen *Radix Ginseng* 6 g
Zhi Gan Cao *Radix Glycyrrhizae uralensis praeparata* 4 g
Geng Mi *Semen Oryzae sativae* 6 g
Da Zao *Fructus Ziziphi jujubae* 3 dates

MAI WEI DI HUANG WAN (BA XIAN CHANG SHOU WAN)
Ophiopogon-Schisandra-Rehmannia Pill (Eight Immortals Longevity Pill)
Shu Di Huang *Radix Rehmanniae glutinosae praeparata* 24 g
Shan Zhu Yu *Fructus Corni officinalis* 12 g
Shan Yao *Radix Dioscoreae oppositae* 12 g
Ze Xie *Rhizoma Alismatis orientalis* 9 g
Mu Dan Pi *Cortex Moutan radicis* 9 g
Fu Ling *Sclerotium Poriae cocos* 9 g
Mai Men Dong *Tuber Ophiopogonis japonici* 6 g
Wu Wei Zi *Fructus Schisandrae chinensis* 6 g

PI SHEN SHUANG BU TANG
Decoction Tonifying both Spleen and Kidneys
Dang Shen *Radix Codonopsis pilosulae* 12 g
Bai Zhu *Rhizoma Atractylodis macrocephalae* 12 g
Fu Ling *Sclerotium Poriae cocos* 15 g
Zhi Gan Cao *Radix Glycyrrhizae uralensis praeparata* 6 g

Du Zhong *Cortex Eucommiae ulmoidis* 9 g
Tu Si Zi *Semen Cuscutae* 12 g
Shan Zhu Yu *Fructus Corni officinalis* 6 g
Shu Di Huang *Radix Rehmanniae glutinosae praeparata* 12 g

PING WEI SAN
Balancing the Stomach Powder
Cang Zhu *Rhizoma Atractylodis lanceae* 9 g
Chen Pi *Pericarpium Citri reticulatae* 6 g
Hou Po *Cortex Magnoliae officinalis* 6 g
Zhi Gan Cao *Radix Glycyrrhizae uralensis praeparata* 3 g
Sheng Jiang *Rhizoma Zingiberis officinalis recens* 3 g
Da Zao *Fructus Ziziphi jujubae* 3 dates

QI JU DI HUANG WAN
Lycium-Chrysanthemum-Rehmannia Pill
Gou Qi Zi *Fructus Lycii chinensis* 9 g
Ju Hua *Flos Chrysanthemi morifolii* 6 g
Shu Di Huang *Radix Rehmanniae glutinosae praeparata* 24 g
Shan Zhu Yu *Fructus Corni officinalis* 12 g
Shan Yao *Radix Dioscoreae oppositae* 12 g
Ze Xie *Rhizoma Alismatis orientalis* 9 g
Mu Dan Pi *Cortex Moutan radicis* 9 g
Fu Ling *Sclerotium Poriae cocos* 9 g

QI WEI DU QI TANG
Seven-Ingredient Capital Qi Decoction
Wu Wei Zi *Fructus Schisandrae chinensis* 6 g
Shu Di Huang *Radix Rehmanniae glutinosae praeparata* 24 g
Shan Zhu Yu *Fructus Corni officinalis* 12 g
Shan Yao *Radix Dioscoreae oppositae* 12 g
Ze Xie *Rhizoma Alismatis orientalis* 9 g
Mu Dan Pi *Cortex Moutan radicis* 9 g
Fu Ling *Sclerotium Poriae cocos* 9 g

QIAN GEN SAN
Rubia Powder
Qian Cao Gen *Radix Rubiae cordifoliae* 9 g
Ce Bai Ye *Cacumen Biotae orientalis* 9 g
Huang Qin *Radix Scutellariae baicalensis* 6 g
Sheng Di Huang *Radix Rehmanniae glutinosae* 12 g
E Jiao *Gelatinum Corii Asini* 6 g
Gan Cao *Radix Glycyrrhizae uralensis* 3 g

QIAN ZHENG SAN
Pulling the Upright Powder
Bai Fu Zi *Rhizoma Thyphonii gigantei* 6 g
Jiang Can *Bombyx batryticatus* 6 g
Quan Xie *Buthus Martensi* 1.5 g

QIANG HUO SHENG SHI TANG
Notopterygium Dispelling Dampness Decoction
Qiang Huo *Radix et Rhizoma Notopterygii* 6 g
Du Huo *Radix Angelicae pubescentis* 6 g
Fang Feng *Radix Ledebouriellae sesloidis* 6 g
Gao Ben *Rhizoma Ligustici sinensis* 6 g
Chuan Xiong *Radix Ligustici wallichii* 3 g
Man Jing Zi *Fructus Viticis* 6 g
Zhi Gan Cao *Radix Glycyrrhizae uralensis praeparata* 3 g

QIN JIAO SI WU TANG
Gentiana macrophylla Four Substances Decoction
Dang Gui *Radix Angelicae sinensis* 6 g
Sheng Di Huang *Radix Rehmanniae glutinosae* 6 g
Bai Shao *Radix Paeoniae albae* 6 g
Chuan Xiong *Radix Ligustici wallichii* 6 g
Qin Jiao *Radix Gentianae macrophyllae* 6 g
Yi Yi Ren *Semen Coicis lachryma jobi* 6 g
Can Sha *Excrementum Bombycis mori* 6 g
Gan Cao *Radix Glycyrrhizae uralensis* 3 g

QING DAI SAN
Indigo Powder
Qing Dai *Indigo naturalis* 9 g
Hai Ge Ke *Concha Cyclinae sinensis* 12 g

QING GAN TOU DING TANG
Clearing the Liver and Penetrating the Crown (of the head) Decoction
Ling Yang Jiao *Cornu Antelopis* 4.5 g
Shi Jue Ming *Concha Haliotidis* 12 g
Chan Tui *Periostracum Cicadae* 4.5 g
Sang Ye *Folium Mori albae* 6 g
Bo He *Herba Menthae* 3 g
Xia Ku Cao *Spica Prunellae vulgaris* 6 g
Mu Dan Pi *Cortex Moutan radicis* 4.5 g
Xuan Shen *Radix Scrophulariae ningpoensis* 3 g
Jie Geng *Radix Platycodi grandiflori* 3 g
Chen Pi *Pericarpium Citri reticulatae* 3 g

QING JIN HUA TAN TANG
Clearing Metal and Resolving Phlegm Decoction

Huang Qin *Radix Scutellariae baicalensis* 9 g
Zhi Zi *Fructus Gardeniae jasminoidis* 6 g
Zhi Mu *Radix Anemarrhenae asphodeloidis* 6 g
Zhe Bei Mu *Bulbus Fritillariae thunbergii* 6 g
Gua Lou *Fructus Trichosanthis* 9 g
Sang Bai Pi *Cortex Mori albae radicis* 6 g
Chen Pi *Pericarpium Citri reticulatae* 4.5 g
Fu Ling *Sclerotium Poriae cocos* 6 g
Jie Geng *Radix Platycodi grandiflori* 4.5 g
Mai Men Dong *Tuber Ophiopogonis japonici* 6 g
Gan Cao *Radix Glycyrrhizae uralensis* 3 g

QING QI HUA TAN TANG
Clearing Qi and Resolving Phlegm Decoction
Dan Nan Xing *Rhizoma Arisaematis praeparata* 12 g
Gua Lou *Fructus Trichosanthis* 9 g
Huang Qin *Radix Scutellariae baicalensis* 9 g
Zhi Shi *Fructus Citri aurantii immaturus* 9 g
Chen Pi *Pericarpium Citri reticulatae* 9 g
Fu Ling *Sclerotium Poriae cocos* 9 g
Xing Ren *Semen Pruni armeniacae* 9 g
Ban Xia *Rhizoma Pinelliae ternatae* 12 g

QING RE LI SHI TANG
Clearing Heat and Resolving Dampness Decoction
Bi Xie *Rhizoma Dioscoreae hypoglaucae* 12 g
Qu Mai *Herba Dianthi* 12 g
Shan Zhi Zi *Fructus Gardeniae jasminoidis* (charred) 9 g
Huang Qin *Radix Scutellariae baicalensis* 9 g
Huang Lian *Rhizoma Coptidis* 6 g
Zhi Mu *Radix Anemarrhenae asphodeloidis* 9 g
Mu Dan Pi *Cortex Moutan radicis* 6 g
Ou Jie *Nodus Nelumbinis neciferae rhizomatis* 15 g
Bai Mao Gen *Rhizoma Imperatae cylindricae* 30 g

QING RE SHEN SHI TANG
Clearing Heat and Draining Dampness Decoction
Huang Qin *Radix Scutellariae baicalensis* 3 g
Huang Bo *Cortex Phellodendri* 3 g
Ku Shen *Radix Sophorae flavescentis* 3 g
Bai Xian Pi *Cortex Radicis Dictami dasycarpi* 3 g
Ban Lan Gen *Radix Isatidis seu Baphicacanthi* 5 g
Sheng Di Huang *Radix Rehmanniae glutinosae* 5 g
Fu Ling *Sclerotium Poriae cocos* 3 g
Hua Shi *Talcum* 5 g
Zhu Ye *Herba Lophateri gracilis* 3 g

QING RE TIAO XUE TANG
Clearing Heat and Regulating Blood Decoction
Mu Dan Pi *Cortex Moutan radicis* 6 g
Sheng Di Huang *Radix Rehmanniae glutinosae* 9 g
Huang Lian *Rhizoma Coptidis* 4.5 g
Dang Gui *Radix Angelicae sinensis* 9 g
Bai Shao *Radix Paeoniae albae* 9 g
Chuan Xiong *Radix Ligustici wallichii* 6 g
Hong Hua *Flos Carthami tinctorii* 6 g
Tao Ren *Semen Persicae* 6 g
E Zhu *Rhizoma Curcumae zedoariae* 6 g
Xiang Fu *Rhizoma Cyperi rotundi* 6 g
Yan Hu Suo *Rhizoma Corydalis yanhusuo* 6 g

QING RE ZHI BENG TANG
Clearing Heat and Stopping Flooding Decoction
Shan Zhi Zi *Fructus Gardeniae jasminoidis* 9 g
Huang Qin *Radix Scutellariae baicalensis* 9 g
Huang Bo *Cortex Phellodendri* 6 g
Sheng Di Huang *Radix Rehmanniae glutinosae* 24 g
Mu Dan Pi *Cortex Moutan radicis* 9 g
Di Yu *Radix Sanguisorbae officinalis* 12 g
Ce Bai Ye *Cacumen Biotae orientalis* 12 g
Chun Gen Bai Pi *Cortex Ailanthi altissimae* 12 g
Gui Ban *Plastrum Testudinis* 15 g
Bai Shao *Radix Paeoniae albae* 24 g

QING WEI SAN
Clearing the Stomach Powder
Huang Lian *Rhizoma Coptidis* 5 g
Sheng Di Huang *Radix Rehmanniae glutinosae* 12 g
Mu Dan Pi *Cortex Moutan radicis* 9 g
Dang Gui *Radix Angelicae sinensis* 6 g
Sheng Ma *Rhizoma Cimicifugae* 6 g

QING YING TANG
Clearing Nutritive Qi Decoction
Shui Niu Jiao *Cornu Bufali* 9 g
Sheng Di Huang *Radix Rehmanniae glutinosae* 12 g
Xuan Shen *Radix Scrophulariae ningpoensis* 9 g
Zhu Ye *Herba Lophatheri gracilis* 3 g
Mai Men Dong *Tuber Ophiopogonis japonici* 9 g
Dan Shen *Radix Salviae miltiorrhizae* 6 g
Huang Lian *Rhizoma Coptidis* 5 g
Jin Yin Hua *Flos Lonicerae japonicae* 9 g
Lian Qiao *Fructus Forsythiae suspensae* 6 g

QING ZAO JIU FEI TANG
Clearing Dryness and Rescuing the Lungs Decoction
Sang Ye *Folium Mori albae* 9 g
Shi Gao *Gypsum fibrosum* 7.5 g
Mai Men Dong *Tuber Ophiopogonis japonici* 3.6 g
Ren Shen *Radix Ginseng* 2 g
Hu Ma Ren (Hei Zhi Ma) *Semen Sesami indici* 3 g
E Jiao *Gelatinum Corii Asini* 2.4 g
Xing Ren *Semen Pruni armeniacae* 2 g
Pi Pa Ye *Folium Eriobotryae japonicae* 3 g
Gan Cao *Radix Glycyrrhizae uralensis* 3 g

REN SHEN BAI DU SAN
Ginseng Expelling Poison Powder
Ren Shen *Radix Ginseng* 9 g
Fu Ling *Sclerotium Poriae cocos* 9 g
Zhi Gan Cao *Radix Glycyrrhizae uralensis praeparata* 3 g
Qiang Huo *Radix et Rhizoma Notopterygii* 3 g
Du Huo *Radix Angelicae pubescentis* 6 g
Chuan Xiong *Radix Ligustici wallichii* 6 g
Sheng Jiang *Rhizoma Zingiberis officinalis recens* 3 slices
Chai Hu *Radix Bupleuri* 6 g
Bo He *Herba Menthae* 3 g
Qian Hu *Radix Peucedani* 9 g
Zhi Ke *Fructus Citri aurantii* 6 g
Jie Geng *Radix Platycodi grandiflori* 4 g

REN SHEN GE JIE SAN
Ginseng-Gecko Powder
Ge Jie *Gecko* 9 g
Zhi Gan Cao *Radix Glycyrrhizae uralensis praeparata* 9 g
Ren Shen *Radix Ginseng* 6 g
Fu Ling *Sclerotium Poriae cocos* 6 g
Chuan Bei Mu *Bulbus Fritillariae cirrhosae* 6 g
Sang Bai Pi *Cortex Mori albae radicis* 6 g
Xing Ren *Semen Pruni armeniacae* 9 g
Zhi Mu *Radix Anemarrhenae asphodeloidis* 6 g

REN SHEN HU TAO TANG
Ginseng-Juglans Decoction
Ren Shen *Radix Ginseng* 4.5 g
Hu Tao Ren *Semen Juglandis regiae* 5 pieces
Sheng Jiang *Rhizoma Zingiberis officinalis recens* 5 slices

REN SHEN YANG RONG TANG
Ginseng Nourishing and Flourishing Decoction
Ren Shen *Radix Ginseng* 9 g
Bai Zhu *Rhizoma Atractylodis macrocephalae* 9 g
Huang Qi *Radix Astragali membranacei* 9 g
Dang Gui *Radix Angelicae sinensis* 9 g
Bai Shao *Radix Paeoniae albae* 18 g
Shu Di Huang *Radix Rehmanniae glutinosae praeparata* 9 g
Rou Gui *Cortex Cinnamomi cassiae* 9 g
Wu Wei Zi *Fructus Schisandrae chinensis* 6 g
Yuan Zhi *Radix Polygalae tenuifoliae* 4.5 g
Fu Ling *Sclerotium Poriae cocos* 6 g
Chen Pi *Pericarpium Citri reticulatae* 9 g
Zhi Gan Cao *Radix Glycyrrhizae uralensis praeparata* 6 g

RUN CHANG WAN Variation
Moistening the Intestines Pill
Dang Gui *Radix Angelicae sinensis* 9 g
Sheng Di Huang *Radix Rehmanniae glutinosae* 12 g
Huo Ma Ren *Semen Cannabis sativa* 6 g
Tao Ren *Semen Persicae* 4.5 g
Zhi Ke *Fructus Citri aurantii* 6 g

SAN AO TANG
Three Break Decoction
Ma Huang *Herba Ephedrae* 6 g
Xing Ren *Semen Pruni armeniacae* 9 g
Zhi Gan Cao *Radix Glycyrrhizae uralensis praeparata* 3 g

SAN FENG CHU SHI TANG
Scattering Wind and Eliminating Dampness Decoction
Huang Bo *Cortex Phellodendri* 6 g
Cang Zhu *Rhizoma Atractylodis lanceae* 6 g
Fang Feng *Radix Ledebouriellae sesloidis* 6 g
Xi Xian Cao *Herba Siegesbeckiae orientalis* 4 g
Cang Er Zi *Fructus Xanthii* 4 g
Fu Ping *Herba Lemnae seu Spirodelae* 4 g
Bai Xian Pi *Cortex Radicis Dictami dasycarpi* 6 g
She Chuang Zi *Semen Cnidii monnieri* 4 g

SAN JIN TANG
Three-Gold Decoction
Jin Qian Cao *Herba Desmodii styracifolii* 15 g
Hai Jin Sha *Spora Lygodii japonici* 9 g

Ji Nei Jin *Endothelium Corneum Gigeraiae Galli* 6 g
Dong Kui Zi *Semen Abutiloni seu Malvae* 6 g
Shi Wei *Folium Pyrrosiae* 6 g
Qu Mai *Herba Dianthi* 6 g

SAN MIAO SAN
Three Wonderful Powder
Cang Zhu *Rhizoma Atractylodis lanceae* 15 g
Huang Bo *Cortex Phellodendri* 12 g
Niu Xi *Radix Cyathulae* 6 g

SAN ZI YANG QIN TANG
Three-Seed Nourishing the Parents Decoction
Su Zi *Fructus Perillae frutescentis* 9 g
Bai Jie Zi *Semen Sinapis albae* 6 g
Lai Fu Zi *Semen Raphani sativi* 9 g

SANG BAI PI TANG
Cortex Mori Decoction
Sang Bai Pi *Cortex Mori albae radicis* 9 g
Huang Qin *Radix Scutellariae baicalensis* 6 g
Huang Lian *Rhizoma Coptidis* 3 g
Zhi Zi *Fructus Gardeniae jasminoidis* 4 g
Chuan Bei Mu *Bulbus Fritillariae cirrhosae* 4 g
Xing Ren *Semen Pruni armeniacae* 6 g
Su Zi *Fructus Perillae frutescentis* 6 g
Ban Xia *Rhizoma Pinelliae ternatae* 6 g

SANG JU YIN
Morus-Chrysanthemum Decoction
Sang Ye *Folium Mori albae* 6 g
Ju Hua *Flos Chrysanthemi morifolii* 3 g
Bo He *Herba Menthae* 3 g
Xing Ren *Semen Pruni armeniacae* 6 g
Jie Geng *Radix Platycodi grandiflori* 6 g
Lian Qiao *Fructus Forsythiae suspensae* 6 g
Lu Gen *Rhizoma Phragmitis communis* 6 g
Gan Cao *Radix Glycyrrhizae uralensis* 3 g

SANG PIAO XIAO SAN
Ootheca Mantidis Pill
Sang Piao Xiao *Ootheca Mantidis* 9 g
Long Gu *Os Draconis* 15 g
Gui Ban *Plastrum Testudinis* 15 g
Dang Gui *Radix Angelicae sinensis* 9 g
Ren Shen *Radix Ginseng* 9 g
Fu Shen *Sclerotium Poriae cocos pararadicis* 6 g
Yuan Zhi *Radix Polygalae tenuifoliae* 6 g
Shi Chang Pu *Rhizoma Acori graminei* 6 g

SANG XING TANG
Morus-Prunus Decoction
Sang Ye *Folium Mori albae* 9 g
Xing Ren *Semen Pruni armeniacae* 9 g
Dan Dou Chi *Semen Sojae preaparatum* 9 g
Zhi Zi *Fructus Gardeniae jasminoidis* 6 g
Zhe Bei Mu *Bulbus Fritillariae thunbergii* 6 g
Nan Sha Shen *Radix Adenophorae* 6 g
Li Pi *Pericarpium Fructi Pyri* 6 g

SHA SHEN MAI DONG TANG
Glehnia-Ophiopogon Decoction
Bei Sha Shen *Radix Glehniae littoralis* 9 g
Mai Men Dong *Tuber Ophiopogonis japonici* 9 g
Yu Zhu *Rhizoma Polygonati odorati* 6 g
Tian Hua Fen *Radix Trichosanthis* 4.5 g
Sang Ye *Folium Mori albae* 4.5 g
Bian Dou *Semen Dolichoris lablab* 4.5 g
Gan Cao *Radix Glycyrrhizae uralensis* 3 g

SHAO FU ZHU YU TANG
Lower Abdomen Eliminating Stasis Decoction
Xiao Hui Xiang *Fructus Foeniculi vulgaris* 6 g
Gan Jiang *Rhizoma Zingiberis officinalis* 2 g
Rou Gui *Cortex Cinnamomi cassiae* 1.5 g
Yan Hu Suo *Rhizoma Corydalis yanhusuo* 6 g
Mo Yao *Myrrha* 6 g
Pu Huang *Pollen Typhae* 6 g
Wu Ling Zhi *Excrementum Trogopteri* 4.5 g
Dang Gui *Radix Angelicae sinensis* 9 g
Chuan Xiong *Radix Ligustici wallichii* 4.5 g
Chi Shao Yao *Radix Paeoniae rubrae* 6 g

SHAO YAO TANG
Paeonia Decoction
Bai Shao *Radix Paeoniae albae* 20 g
Dang Gui *Radix Angelicae sinensis* 9 g
Zhi Gan Cao *Radix Glycyrrhizae uralensis praeparata* 5 g
Huang Lian *Rhizoma Coptidis* 5 g
Huang Qin *Radix Scutellariae baicalensis* 9 g
Da Huang *Rhizoma Rhei* 9 g
Mu Xiang *Radix Saussureae* 5 g
Bing Lang *Semen Arecae catechu catechu* 5 g
Rou Gui *Cortex Cinnamomi cassiae* 2 g

SHE GAN MA HUANG TANG
Belamcanda-Ephedra Decoction
She Gan *Rhizoma Belamcandae chinensis* 6 g

Ma Huang *Herba Ephedrae* 9 g
Gan Jiang *Rhizoma Zingiberis officinalis* 3 g
Xi Xin *Herba Asari cum radice* 3 g
Ban Xia *Rhizoma Pinelliae ternatae* 9 g
Zi Wan *Radix Asteris tatarici* 6 g
Kuan Dong Hua *Flos Tussilaginis farfarae* 6 g
Gan Cao *Radix Glycyrrhizae uralensis* 3 g
Wu Wei Zi *Fructus Schisandrae chinensis* 3 g
Da Zao *Fructus Ziziphi jujubae* 3 dates

SHEN FU TANG
Ginseng-Aconitum Decoction
Ren Shen *Radix Ginseng* 9 g
Fu Zi *Radix Aconiti carmichaeli praeparata* 6 g

SHEN GE SAN
Ginseng-Gecko Powder
Ren Shen *Radix Ginseng* 12 g
Ge Jie *Gecko* 12 g

SHEN LING BAI ZHU SAN
Ginseng-Poria-Atractylodes Powder
Ren Shen *Radix Ginseng* 6 g (or **Dang Shen** *Radix Codonopsis pilosulae* 12 g)
Bai Zhu *Rhizoma Atractylodis macrocephalae* 9 g
Fu Ling *Sclerotium Poriae cocos* 12 g
Zhi Gan Cao *Radix Glycyrrhizae uralensis praeparata* 6 g
Bian Dou *Semen Dolichoris lablab* 12 g
Shan Yao *Radix Dioscoreae oppositae* 12 g
Lian Zi *Semen Nelumbinis nuciferae* 12 g
Sha Ren *Fructus seu Semen Amomi* 4.5 g
Yi Yi Ren *Semen Coicis lachryma jobi* 10 g
Jie Geng *Radix Platycodi grandiflori* 6 g

SHEN SU YIN
Ginseng-Perilla Decoction
Ren Shen *Radix Ginseng* 9 g
Zi Su Ye *Folium Perillae frutescentis* 3 g
Ge Gen *Radix Puerariae* 9 g
Qian Hu *Radix Peucedani* 3 g
Ban Xia *Rhizoma Pinelliae ternatae* 6 g
Fu Ling *Sclerotium Poriae cocos* 9 g
Chen Pi *Pericarpium Citri reticulatae* 3 g
Zhi Ke *Fructus Citri aurantii* 6 g
Jie Geng *Radix Platycodi grandiflori* 6 g
Zhi Gan Cao *Radix Glycyrrhizae uralensis praeparata* 3 g
Sheng Jiang *Rhizoma Zingiberis officinalis recens* 3 g

Da Zao *Fructus Ziziphi jujubae* 4 dates

SHEN TONG ZHU YU TANG
Body-Pain Eliminating Stagnation Decoction
Dang Gui *Radix Angelicae sinensis* 9 g
Chuan Xiong *Radix Ligustici wallichii* 6 g
Tao Ren *Semen Persicae* 9 g
Hong Hua *Flos Carthami tinctorii* 9 g
Mo Yao *Myrrha* 6 g
Wu Ling Zhi *Excrementum Trogopteri* 6 g
Xiang Fu *Rhizoma Cyperi rotundi* 3 g
Niu Xi *Radix Achyranthis bidentatae seu Cyathulae* 9 g
Di Long *Pheretima aspergillum* 6 g
Qin Jiao *Radix Gentianae macrophyllae* 3 g
Qiang Huo *Radix et Rhizoma Notopterygii* 3 g
Gan Cao *Radix Glycyrrhizae uralensis* 3 g

SHENG MAI SAN
Generating the Pulse Powder
Ren Shen *Radix Ginseng* 9 g
Mai Men Dong *Tuber Ophiopogonis japonici* 9 g
Wu Wei Zi *Fructus Schisandrae chinensis* 3 g

SHENG TIE LUO YIN
Frusta Ferri Decoction
Sheng Tie Luo *Frusta Ferri* 60 g
Dan Nan Xing *Rhizoma Arisaematis praeparata* 9 g
Zhe Bei Mu *Bulbus Fritillariae thunbergii* 9 g
Xuan Shen *Radix Scrophulariae ningpoensis* 9 g
Tian Men Dong *Tuber Asparagi cochinchinensis* 9 g
Mai Men Dong *Tuber Ophiopogonis japonici* 9 g
Lian Qiao *Fructus Forsythiae suspensae* 9 g
Dan Shen *Radix Salviae miltiorrhizae* 12 g
Fu Ling *Sclerotium Poriae cocos* 12 g
Chen Pi *Pericarpium Citri reticulatae* 6 g
Shi Chang Pu *Rhizoma Acori graminei* 6 g
Yuan Zhi *Radix Polygalae tenuifoliae* 6 g
Zhu Sha *Cinnabaris* 1.8 g

SHENG YU TANG
Sage-like Healing Decoction
Ren Shen *Radix Ginseng* 12 g
Huang Qi *Radix Astragali membranacei* 18 g
Dang Gui *Radix Angelicae sinensis* 15 g
Chuan Xiong *Radix Ligustici wallichii* 8 g
Shu Di Huang *Radix Rehmanniae glutinosae praeparata* 18 g
Bai Shao *Radix Paeoniae albae* 12 g

SHI PI YIN
Strengthening the Spleen Decoction
Fu Zi *Radix Aconiti carmichaeli praeparata* 6 g
Gan Jiang *Rhizoma Zingiberis officinalis* 6 g
Fu Ling *Sclerotium Poriae cocos* 6 g
Mu Gua *Fructus Chaenomelis lagenariae* 6 g
Bai Zhu *Rhizoma Atractylodis macrocephalae* 6 g
Hou Po *Cortex Magnoliae officinalis* 6 g
Mu Xiang *Radix Saussureae* 6 g
Da Fu Pi *Pericarpium Arecae catechu* 6 g
Cao Guo *Fructus Amomi Tsaoko* 6 g
Zhi Gan Cao *Radix Glycyrrhizae uralensis praeparata* 3 g

SHI QUAN DA BU TANG
Ten Complete Great Tonification Decoction
Ba Zhen Tang *Eight Precious Decoction* plus:
Huang Qi *Radix Astragali membranacei* 8 g
Rou Gui *Cortex Cinnamomi cassiae* 4 g

SHI WEI SAN
Pyrrosia Powder
Shi Wei *Folium Pyrrosiae* 9 g
Dong Kui Zi *Semen Abutiloni seu Malvae* 6 g
Qu Mai *Herba Dianthi* 6 g
Che Qian Zi *Semen Plantaginis* 6 g
Hua Shi *Talcum* 6 g

SHI WEI WEN DAN TANG
Ten-Ingredient Warming the Gall-Bladder Decoction
Ban Xia *Rhizoma Pinelliae ternatae* 6 g
Chen Pi *Pericarpium Citri reticulatae* 6 g
Fu Ling *Sclerotium Poriae cocos* 4.5 g
Zhi Shi *Fructus Citri aurantii immaturus* 6 g
Ren Shen *Radix Ginseng* 3 g (**Dang Shen** *Radix Codonopsis pilosulae* 9 g)
Shu Di Huang *Radix Rehmanniae glutinosae praeparata* 9 g
Suan Zao Ren *Semen Ziziphi spinosae* 3 g
Yuan Zhi *Radix Polygalae tenuifoliae* 3 g
Zhi Gan Cao *Radix Glycyrrhizae uralensis praeparata* 1.5 g
Sheng Jiang *Rhizoma Zingiberis officinalis recens* 5 slices
Hong Zao *Fructus Ziziphi jujubae* one date

SHI XIAO SAN
Breaking into a Smile Powder
Pu Huang *Pollen Typhae* 9 g
Wu Ling Zhi *Excrementum Trogopteri* 9 g

SHU ZAO YIN ZI
Dredging and Digging Decoction
Qiang Huo *Radix et Rhizoma Notopterygii* 6 g
Qin Jiao *Radix Gentianae macrophyllae* 6 g
Da Fu Pi *Pericarpium Arecae catechu* 6 g
Fu Ling Pi *Cortex Poriae cocos* 6 g
Sheng Jiang Pi *Cortex Rhizomae Zingiberis officinalis recens* 6 g
Ze Xie *Rhizoma Alismatis orientalis* 6 g
Mu Tong *Caulis Akebiae* 3 g
Jiao Mu *Fructus Zanthoxyli schinifolii* 1.5 g
Chi Xiao Dou *Semen Phaseoli calcarati* 6 g
Bing Lang *Semen Arecae catechu* 6 g

SI JUN ZI TANG
Four Gentleman Decoction
Ren Shen *Radix Ginseng* 9 g
Bai Zhu *Rhizoma Atractylodis macrocephalae* 6 g
Fu Ling *Sclerotium Poriae cocos* 6 g
Zhi Gan Cao *Radix Glycyrrhizae uralensis praeparata* 3 g

SI MIAO SAN
Four Wonderful Powder
Cang Zhu *Rhizoma Atractylodis lanceae* 6 g
Huang Bo *Cortex Phellodendri* 9 g
Niu Xi *Radix Achyranthis bidentatae seu Cyathulae* 6 g
Yi Yi Ren *Semen Coicis lachryma jobi* 9 g

SI NI SAN
Four Rebellious Powder
Chai Hu *Radix Bupleuri* 6 g
Bai Shao *Radix Paeoniae albae* 9 g
Zhi Shi *Fructus Citri aurantii immaturus* 6 g
Zhi Gan Cao *Radix Glycyrrhizae uralensis praeparata* 6 g

SI SHEN WAN
Four Spirits Pill
Bai Dou Kou *Fructus Cardamomi rotundi* 6 g
Bu Gu Zhi *Fructus Psoraleae corylifoliae* 12 g
Wu Wei Zi *Fructus Schisandrae chinensis* 6 g
Wu Zhu Yu *Fructus Evodiae rutaecarpae* 3 g
Sheng Jiang *Rhizoma Zingiberis officinalis recens* 3 slices
Hong Zao *Fructus Ziziphi jujubae* 3 dates

SI WU TANG
Four Substances Decoction

Shu Di Huang *Radix Rehmanniae glutinosae prae-parata* 12 g
Dang Gui *Radix Angelicae sinensis* 10 g
Bai Shao *Radix Paeoniae albae* 12 g
Chuan Xiong *Radix Ligustici wallichii* 8 g

SU HE XIANG WAN
Styrax Pill
Su He Xiang *Styrax liquidis* 30 g
She Xiang *Secretio Moschus moschiferi* 60 g
Bing Pian *Borneol* 30 g
An Xi Xiang *Benzoinum* 60 g
Mu Xiang *Radix Saussureae* 60 g
Tan Xiang *Lignum Santali albi* 60 g
Chen Xiang *Lignum Aquilariae* 60 g
Ru Xiang *Gummi Olibanum* 30 g
Ding Xiang *Flos Caryophylli* 60 g
Xiang Fu *Rhizoma Cyperi rotundi* 60 g
Bi Ba *Fructus Piperis longi* 60 g
Shui Niu Jiao *Cornu Bufali* 60 g
Zhu Sha *Cinnabaris* 60 g
Bai Zhu *Rhizoma Atractylodis macrocephalae* 60 g
He Zi *Fructus Terminaliae chebulae* 60 g

SU ZI JIANG QI TANG
Perilla Seed Lowering Qi Decoction
Su Zi *Fructus Perillae frutescentis* 9 g
Ban Xia *Rhizoma Pinelliae ternataee* 9 g
Hou Po *Cortex Magnoliae officinalis* 6 g
Qian Hu *Radix Peucedani* 6 g
Rou Gui *Cortex Cinnamomi cassiae* 3 g
Dang Gui *Radix Angelicae sinensis* 6 g
Sheng Jiang *Rhizoma Zingiberis officinalis recens* 2 slices
Su Ye *Folium Perillae frutescentis* 5 leaves
Zhi Gan Cao *Radix Glycyrrhizae uralensis prae-parata* 6 g
Da Zao *Fructus Ziziphi jujubae* one date

SUAN ZAO REN TANG
Ziziphus Decoction
Suan Zao Ren *Semen Ziziphi spinosae* 18 g
Chuan Xiong *Radix Ligustici wallichii* 6 g
Fu Ling *Sclerotium Poriae cocos* 12 g
Zhi Mu *Radix Anemarrhenae asphodeloidis* 9 g
Gan Cao *Radix Glycyrrhizae uralensis* 3 g

SUO QUAN WAN
Contracting the Spring Pill
Yi Zhi Ren *Fructus Alpiniae oxyphyllae* 9 g

Wu Yao *Radix Linderae strychnifoliae* 6 g
Shan Yao *Radix Dioscoreae oppositae* 9 g

TAO HE CHENG QI TANG
Persica Conducting Qi Decoction
Tao Ren *Semen Persicae* 12 g
Da Huang *Rhizoma Rhei* 12 g
Gui Zhi *Ramulus Cinnamomi cassiae* 6 g
Mang Xiao *Mirabilitum* 6 g
Zhi Gan Cao *Radix Glycyrrhizae uralensis prae-parata* 6 g

TAO HONG SI WU TANG
Persica-Carthamus Four Substances Decoction
Dang Gui *Radix Angelicae sinensis* 9 g
Chuan Xiong *Radix Ligustici wallichii* 6 g
Shu Di Huang *Radix Rehmanniae glutinosae prae-parata* 12 g
Bai Shao *Radix Paeoniae albae* 9 g
Tao Ren *Semen Persicae* 6 g
Hong Hua *Flos Carthami tinctorii* 6 g

TAO HONG YIN
Prunus-Carthamus Decoction
Tao Ren *Semen Persicae* 6 g
Hong Hua *Flos Carthami tinctorii* 6 g
Chuan Xiong *Radix Ligustici wallichii* 6 g
Dang Gui (Wei) *Radix Angelicae sinensis* ("tail" only) 6 g
Wei Ling Xian *Radix Clematidis chinensis* 6 g

TIAN MA GOU TENG YIN
Gastrodia-Uncaria Decoction
Tian Ma *Rhizoma Gastrodiae elatae* 9 g
Gou Teng *Ramulus Uncariae* 9 g
Shi Jue Ming *Concha Haliotidis* 6 g
Sang Ji Sheng *Ramulus Loranthi* 9 g
Du Zhong *Radix Eucommiae ulmoidis* 9 g
Chuan Niu Xi *Radix Cyathulae* 9 g
Zhi Zi *Fructus Gardeniae jasminoidis* 6 g
Huang Qin *Radix Scutellariae baicalensis* 9 g
Yi Mu Cao *Herba Leonori heterophylli* 9 g
Ye Jiao Teng *Caulis Polygoni multiflori* 9 g
Fu Shen *Sclerotium Poriae cocos pararadicis* 6 g

TIAN WANG BU XIN DAN
Heavenly Emperor Tonifying the Heart Pill
Sheng Di Huang *Radix Rehmanniae glutinosae* 12 g
Xuan Shen *Radix Scrophulariae ningpoensis* 6 g

Mai Men Dong *Tuber Ophiopogonis japonici* 6 g
Tian Men Dong *Tuber Asparagi cochinchinensis* 6 g
Ren Shen *Radix Ginseng* 6 g
Fu Ling *Sclerotium Poriae cocos* 6 g
Wu Wei Zi *Fructus Schisandrae chinensis* 6 g
Dang Gui *Radix Angelicae sinensis* 6 g
Dan Shen *Radix Salviae miltiorrhizae* 6 g
Bai Zi Ren *Semen Biotae orientalis* 6 g
Suan Zao Ren *Semen Ziziphi spinosae* 6 g
Yuan Zhi *Radix Polygalae tenuifoliae* 6 g
Jie Geng *Radix Platycodi grandiflori* 3 g

TIAO GAN TANG
Regulating the Liver Decoction
Dang Gui *Radix Angelicae sinensis* 9 g
Bai Shao *Radix Paeoniae albae* 9 g
Shan Yao *Radix Dioscoreae oppositae* 12 g
E Jiao *Gelatinum Corii Asini* 9 g
Shan Zhu Yu *Fructus Corni officinalis* 6 g
Ba Ji Tian *Radix Morindae officinalis* 9 g
Zhi Gan Cao *Radix Glycyrrhizae uralensis praeparata* 3 g

TIAO WEI CHENG QI TANG
Regulating the Stomach Conducting Qi Decoction
Da Huang *Rhizoma Rhei* 12 g
Mang Xiao *Mirabilitum* 9 g
Zhi Gan Cao *Radix Glycyrrhizae uralensis praeparata* 6 g

TIAO YING LIAN GAN YIN
Regulating Nutritive Qi and Restraining the Liver Decoction
Dang Gui *Radix Angelicae sinensis* 6 g
Chuan Xiong *Radix Ligustici wallichii* 6 g
E Jiao *Gelatinum Corii Asini* 6 g
Bai Shao *Radix Paeoniae albae* 9 g
Gou Qi Zi *Fructus Lycii chinensis* 6 g
Wu Wei Zi *Fructus Schisandrae chinensis* 3 g
Suan Zao Ren *Semen Ziziphi spinosae* 3 g
Fu Ling *Sclerotium Poriae cocos* 6 g
Chen Pi *Pericarpium Citri reticulatae* 4 g
Mu Xiang *Radix Saussureae* 3 g
Sheng Jiang *Rhizoma Zingiberis officinalis recens* 3 slices
Da Zao *Fructus Ziziphi jujubae* 3 dates

TONG GUAN WAN
Opening the Gate Pill
Huang Bo *Cortex Phellodendri* 30 g

Zhi Mu *Radix Anemarrhenae asphodeloidis* 30 g
Rou Gui *Cortex Cinnamomi cassiae* 1.5 g

TONG MAI SI NI TANG
Penetrating the Blood Vessels Four Rebellious Decoction
Fu Zi *Radix Aconiti carmichaeli praeparata* 15 g
Gan Jiang *Rhizoma Zingiberis officinalis* 9 g
Zhi Gan Cao *Radix Glycyrrhizae uralensis praeparata* 6 g

TONG QIAO HUA XUE TANG
Opening the Orifices and Moving Blood Decoction
Chi Shao Yao *Radix Paeoniae rubrae* 3 g
Chuan Xiong *Radix Ligustici wallichii* 3 g
Tao Ren *Semen Persicae* 9 g
Hong Hua *Flos Carthami tinctorii* 9 g
She Xiang *Secretio Moschus moschiferi* .15 g
Cong Bai *Herba Allii* 3 g
Hong Zao *Fructus Ziziphi jujubae* 7 red dates
Sheng Jiang *Rhizoma Zingiberis officinalis recens* 3 slices
Rice wine

TONG XIE YAO FANG
Painful Diarrhoea Formula
Bai Zhu *Rhizoma Atractylodis macrocephalae* 9 g
Bai Shao *Radix Paeoniae albae* 6 g
Chen Pi *Pericarpium Citri reticulatae* 4.5 g
Fang Feng *Radix Ledebouriellae sesloidis* 6 g

TONG XUAN LI FEI TANG
Penetrating Dispersing and Regulating Lung-Qi Decoction
Zi Su Ye *Folium Perillae frutescentis* 6 g
Ma Huang *Herba Ephedrae* 6 g
Xing Ren *Semen Pruni armeniacae* 6 g
Zhi Ke *Fructus Citri aurantii* 6 g
Jie Geng *Radix Platycodi grandiflori* 4 g
Qian Hu *Radix Peucedani* 4 g
Chen Pi *Pericarpium Citri reticulatae* 3 g
Fu Ling *Sclerotium Poriae cocos* 6 g
Ban Xia *Rhizoma Pinelliae ternatae* 6 g
Huang Qin *Radix Scutellariae baicalensis* 3 g
Gan Cao *Radix Glycyrrhizae uralensis* 3 g

TONG YOU TANG
Penetrating the Deep Decoction
Sheng Di Huang *Radix Rehmanniae glutinosae* 12 g

Shu Di Huang *Radix Rehmanniae glutinosae praeparata* 12 g
Dang Gui *Radix Angelicae sinensis* 12 g
Tao Ren *Semen Persicae* 4.5 g
Hong Hua *Flos Carthami tinctorii* 4.5 g
Sheng Ma *Rhizoma Cimicifugae* 3 g
Zhi Gan Cao *Radix Glycyrrhizae uralensis praeparata* 3 g

WEI LING TANG
Stomach Poria Decoction
Cang Zhu *Rhizoma Atyractylodis lanceae* 6 g
Hou Po *Cortex Magnoliae officinalis* 6 g
Chen Pi *Pericarpium Citri reticulatae* 4 g
Gan Cao *Radix Glycyrrhizae uralensis* 3 g
Bai Zhu *Rhizoma Atractylodis macrocephalae* 6 g
Fu Ling *Sclerotium Poriae cocos* 6 g
Zhu Ling *Sclerotium Polyperi umbellati* 6 g
Ze Xie *Rhizoma Alismatis orientalis* 6 g
Gui Zhi *Ramulus Cinnamomi cassiae* 3 g

WEN DAN TANG
Warming the Gall-Bladder Decoction
Ban Xia *Rhizoma Pinelliae ternatae* 6 g
Fu Ling *Sclerotium Poriae cocos* 5 g
Chen Pi *Pericarpium Citri reticulatae* 9 g
Zhu Ru *Caulis Bambusae in Taenis* 6 g
Zhi Shi *Fructus Citri aurantii immaturus* 6 g
Zhi Gan Cao *Radix Glycyrrhizae uralensis praeparata* 3 g
Sheng Jiang *Rhizoma Zingiberis officinalis recens* 5 slices
Da Zao *Fructus Ziziphi jujubae* one date

WEN JING TANG
Warm the Menses Decoction
Wu Zhu Yu *Fructus Evodiae rutaecarpae* 9 g
Gui Zhi *Ramulus Cinnamomi cassiae* 9 g
Sheng Jiang *Rhizoma Zingiberis officinalis recens* 6 g
Dang Gui *Radix Angelicae sinensis* 9 g
Chuan Xiong *Radix Ligustici wallichii* 4.5 g
Bai Shao *Radix Paeoniae albae* 9 g
Dang Shen *Radix Codonopsis pilosulae* 12 g
Mai Men Dong *Tuber Ophiopogonis japonici* 6 g
E Jiao *Gelatinum Corii Asini* 9 g
Mu Dan Pi *Cortex Moutan radicis* 4.5 g
Ban Xia *Rhizoma Pinelliae ternatae* 6 g
Zhi Gan Cao *Radix Glycyrrhizae uralensis praeparata* 3 g

WEN PI TANG
Warming the Spleen Decoction
Da Huang *Rhizoma Rhei* 9 g
Fu Zi *Radix Aconiti carmichaeli praeparata* 6 g
Gan Jiang *Rhizoma Zingiberis officinalis* 4.5 g
Ren Shen *Radix Ginseng* 9 g
Zhi Gan Cao *Radix Glycyrrhizae uralensis praeparata* 3 g

WU BI SHAN YAO WAN
Incomparable Dioscorea Pill
Shan Yao *Radix Dioscoreae oppositae* 15 g
Rou Cong Rong *Herba Cistanchis* 9 g
Tu Si Zi *Semen Cuscutae* 9 g
Ba Ji Tian *Radix Morindae officinalis* 6 g
Du Zhong *Cortex Eucommiae ulmoidis* 6 g
Shu Di Huang *Radix Rehmanniae glutinosae praeparata* 9 g
Shan Zhu Yu *Fructus Corni officinalis* 6 g
Niu Xi *Radix Achyranthis bidentatae seu Cyathulae* 6 g
Wu Wei Zi *Fructus Schisandrae chinensis* 4.5 g
Chi Shi Zhi *Halloysitum rubrum* 6 g
Ze Xie *Rhizoma Alismatis orientalis* 6 g
Fu Shen *Sclerotium Poriae cocos pararadicis* 6 g

WU FU MA XIN GUI JIANG TANG
Aconitum-Ephedra-Asarum-Cinnamomum-Zingiber Decoction
Wu Tou *Radix Aconiti carmichaeli* 3 g
Fu Zi *Radix Aconiti carmichaeli praeparata* 1.5 g
Ma Huang *Herba Ephedrae* 3 g
Xi Xin *Herba Asari cum radice* 1.5 g
Gui Zhi *Ramulus Cinnamomi cassiae* 3 g
Gan Jiang *Rhizoma Zingiberis officinalis* 1.5 g
Gan Cao *Radix Glycyrrhizae uralensis* 2 g

WU GE KUAN ZHONG SAN
Five-Diaphragm Relaxing the Middle Powder
Bai Dou Kou *Fructus Cardamomi rotundi* 1.5 g
Hou Po *Cortex Magnoliae officinalis* 9 g
Sha Ren *Fructus seu Semen Amomi* 4.5 g
Mu Xiang *Radix Saussureae* 3 g
Xiang Fu *Rhizoma Cyperi rotundi* 9 g
Qing Pi *Pericarpium Citri reticulatae viridae* 4.5 g
Chen Pi *Pericarpium Citri reticulatae* 4.5 g
Ding Xiang *Flos Caryophylli* 3 g
Zhi Gan Cao *Radix Glycyrrhizae uralensis praeparata* 6 g

Sheng Jiang *Rhizoma Zingiberis officinalis recens* 3 slices

WU JI SAN
Five Accumulations Powder
Ma Huang *Herba Ephedrae* 4 g
Bai Zhi *Radix Angelicae dahuricae* 3 g
Cong Bai *Herba Allii fistulosi* 4 g
Sheng Jiang *Rhizoma Zingiberis officinalis recens* 3 slices
Cang Zhu *Rhizoma Atractylodis lanceae* 12 g
Hou Po *Cortex Magnoliae officinalis* 3 g
Chen Pi *Pericarpium Citri reticulatae* 4 g
Gan Cao *Radix Glycyrrhizae uralensis* 3 g
Ban Xia *Rhizoma Pinelliae ternatae* 3 g
Fu Ling *Sclerotium Poriae cocos* 3 g
Jie Geng *Radix Platycodi grandiflori* 6 g
Zhi Ke *Fructus Citri aurantii* 4 g
Gan Jiang *Rhizoma Zingiberis officinalis* 2 g
Rou Gui *Cortex Cinnamomi cassiae* 2 g
Dang Gui *Radix Angelicae sinensis* 3 g
Bai Shao *Radix Paeoniae albae* 3 g
Chuan Xiong *Radix Ligustici wallichii* 3 g

WU LING SAN
Five "Ling" Powder
Fu Ling *Sclerotium Poriae cocos* 6 g
Zhu Ling *Sclerotium Polypori umbellati* 6 g
Bai Zhu *Rhizoma Atractylodis macrocephalae* 6 g
Ze Xie *Rhizoma Alismatis orientalis* 6 g
Gui Zhi *Ramulus Cinnamomi cassiae* 6 g

WU MO YIN ZI
Five Powders Decoction
Chen Xiang *Lignum Aquilariae* 6 g
Mu Xiang *Radix Saussureae* 3 g
Bing Lang *Semen Arecae catechu* 6 g
Wu Yao *Radix Linderae strychnifoliae* 6 g
Zhi Shi *Fructus Citri aurantii immaturus* 6 g
White Wine
Bai He *Bulbus Lilii* 6 g
He Huan Pi *Cortex Albizziae julibrissin* 6 g
Suan Zao Ren *Semen Ziziphi spinosae* 6 g
Yuan Zhi *Radix Polygalae tenuifoliae* 6 g

WU PI SAN
Five Peels Powder
Sheng Jiang Pi *Pericarpium Zingiberis officinalis recens* 9 g

Sang Bai Pi *Cortex Mori albae radicis* 9 g
Chen Pi *Pericarpium Citri reticulatae* 9 g
Da Fu Pi *Pericarpium Arecae catechu* 9 g
Fu Ling Pi *Cortex Poriae cocos* 9 g

WU REN WAN
Five Seeds Pill
Tao Ren *Semen Persicae*
Xing Ren *Semen Pruni armeniacae*
Bai Zi Ren *Semen Biotae orientalis*
Song Zi Ren *Semen Pini tabulaeformis*
Yu Li Ren *Semen Pruni*
Chen Pi *Pericarpium Citri reticulatae*

WU TOU TANG
Aconitum Decoction
Wu Tou *Radix Aconiti carmichaeli praeparata* 3 g
Ma Huang *Herba Ephedrae* 3 g
Bai Shao *Radix Paeoniae albae* 3 g
Gan Cao *Radix Glycyrrhizae uralensis* 3 g
Huang Qi *Radix Astragali membranacei* 3 g

WU WEI XIAO DU YIN
Five-Ingredient Resolving Poison Decoction
Jin Yin Hua *Flos Lonicerae japonicae* 9 g
Pu Gong Ying *Herba Taraxaci mongolici cum Radice* 3.5 g
Zi Hua Di Ding *Herba Violae cum radice* 3.5 g
Ju Hua *Flos Chrysanthemi morifolii* 3.5 g
Zi Bei Tian Kui *Herba Begoniae fimbristipulatae* 3.5 g

WU ZHU YU TANG
Evodia Decoction
Wu Zhu Yu *Fructus Evodiae rutaecarpae* 3 g
Ren Shen *Radix Ginseng* 6 g (or **Dang Shen** *Radix Codonopsis pilosulae* 12 g)
Sheng Jiang *Rhizoma Zingiberis recens* 18 g
Da Zao *Fructus Ziziphi jujubae* 4 pieces

WU ZI YAN ZONG WAN
Five-Seed Developing Ancestors Pill
Tu Si Zi *Semen Cuscutae* 12 g
Wu Wei Zi *Fructus Schisandrae chinensis* 3 g
Gou Qi Zi *Fructus Lycii chinensis* 6 g
Fu Pen Zi *Fructus Rubi* 6 g
Che Qian Zi *Semen Plantaginis* 3 g

XI JIAO DI HUANG TANG
Cornu Bufali-Rehmannia Decoction

Shui Niu Jiao *Cornu Bufali* 30 g
Sheng Di Huang *Radix Rehmanniae glutinosae* 30 g
Chi Shao *Radix Paeoniae rubrae* 12 g
Mu Dan Pi *Cortex Moutan radicis* 9 g

XI JIAO SAN
Cornu Bisontis Decoction
Sheng Di Huang *Radix Rehmanniae glutinosae* 9 g
Xi Jiao *Cornu bisontis* 12 g
Xuan Shen *Radix Scrophulariae ningpoensis* 6 g
Mai Men Dong *Tuber Ophiopogonis japonici* 6 g
Fang Ji *Radix Stephaniae tetrandae* 6 g
Jiang Huang *Rhizoma Curcumae longae* 6 g
Qin Jiao *Radix Gentianae macrophyllae* 6 g
Hai Tong Pi *Cortex Erythrinae variegatae* 3 g

XIANG LIAN WAN
Saussurea-Coptis Pill
Huang Lian *Rhizoma Coptidis* 6 g
Mu Xiang *Radix Saussureae* 13 g

XIANG SHA LIU JUN ZI TANG
Saussurea-Amomum Six Gentlemen Decoction
Ren Shen *Radix Ginseng* (or **Dang Shen** *Radix Codonopsis pilosulae*) 10 g
Bai Zhu *Rhizoma Atractylodis macrocephalae* 9 g
Fu Ling *Sclerotium Poriae cocos* 9 g
Zhi Gan Cao *Radix Glycyrrhizae uralensis praeparata* 3 g
Chen Pi *Pericarpium Citri reticulatae* 4.5 g
Ban Xia *Rhizoma Pinelliae ternatae* 12 g
Mu Xiang *Radix Saussureae* 6 g
Sha Ren *Fructus seu Semen Amomi* 6 g

XIANG SHA ZHI ZHU WAN
Saussurea-Amomum-Citrus-Atractylodes Pill
Mu Xiang *Radix Saussureae* 4.5 g
Sha Ren *Fructus seu Semen Amomi* 4.5 g
Zhi Shi *Fructus Citri aurantii immaturus* 4.5 g
Chen Pi *Pericarpium Citri reticulatae* 3 g
Ban Xia *Rhizoma Pinelliae ternatae* 6 g
Bai Zhu *Rhizoma Atractylodis macrocephalae* 6 g
Bo He *Herba Menthae* 3 g

XIAO CHAI HU TANG
Small Bupleurum Decoction
Chai Hu *Radix Bupleuri* 12 g
Huang Qin *Radix Scutellariae baicalensis* 9 g
Ban Xia *Rhizoma Pinelliae ternatae* 9 g

Ren Shen *Radix Ginseng* 6 g
Zhi Gan Cao *Radix Glycyrrhizae uralensis praeparata* 5 g
Sheng Jiang *Rhizoma Zingiberis officinalis recens* 9 g
Da Zao *Fructus Ziziphi jujubae* 4 dates

XIAO FENG CHONG JI
Clearing Wind Decoction
Jing Jie *Herba seu Flos Schizonepetae tenuifoliae* 6 g
Chan Tui *Periostracum Cicadae* 6 g
Niu Bang Zi *Fructus Arctii lappae* 4 g
Dang Gui *Radix Angelicae sinensis* 9 g
Hei Zhi Ma *Semen Sesami indici* 6 g
Sheng Di huang *Radix Rehmanniae glutinosae* 9 g
Ku Shen *Radix Sophorae flavescentis* 6 g
Cang Zhu *Rhizoma Atractylodis lanceae* 4 g
Mu Tong *Caulis Akebiae* 2 g
Zhi Mu *Radix Anemarrhenae asphodeloidis* 4 g
Shi Gao *Gypsum fibrosum* 12 g
Gan Cao *Radix Glycyrrhizae uralensis* 3 g

XIAO FENG SAN
Clearing Wind Powder
Jing Jie *Herba seu Flos Schizonepetae tenuifoliae* 3 g
Fang Feng *Radix Ledebouriellae sesloidis* 3 g
Chan Tui *Periostracum Cicadae* 3 g
Niu Bang Zi *Fructus Arctii lappae* 3 g
Ku Shen *Radix Sophorae flavescentis* 3 g
Mu Tong *Caulis Akebiae* 1.5 g
Cang Zhu *Rhizoma Atractylodis lanceae* 3 g
Sheng Di Huang *Radix Rehmanniae glutinosae* 5 g
Shi Gao *Gypsum fibrosum* 10 g
Zhi Mu *Radix Anemarrhenae asphodeloidis* 3 g
Dang Gui *Radix Angelicae sinensis* 3 g
Hei Zhi Ma *Semen Sesami indici* 3 g
Gan Cao *Radix Glycyrrhizae uralensis* 3 g

XIAO JI YIN ZI
Cephalanoplos Decoction
Xiao Ji *Herba Cephalanoplos segeti* 30 g
Ou Jie *Nodus Nelumbinis nuciferae rhizomatis* 6 g
Pu Huang *Pollen Typhae* 9 g
Hua Shi *Talcum* 15 g
Mu Tong *Caulis Akebiae* 9 g
Zhu Ye *Herba Lophatheri gracilis* 9 g
Zhi Zi *Fructus Gardeniae jasminoidis* 9 g
Sheng Di Huang *Radix Rehmanniae glutinosae* 30 g

Dang Gui *Radix Angelicae sinensis* 6 g
Gan Cao *Radix Glycyrrhizae uralensis* 6 g

XIAO JIAN ZHONG TANG
Minor Strengthening the Centre Decoction
Yi Tang *Saccharum granorum* 30 g
Bai Shao *Radix Paeoniae albae* 18 g
Gui Zhi *Ramulus Cinnamomi cassiae* 9 g
Sheng Jiang *Rhizoma Zingiberis officinalis recens* 10 g
Zhi Gan Cao *Radix Glycyrrhizae uralensis praeparata* 6 g
Da Zao *Fructus Ziziphi jujubae* 12 dates

XIAO QING LONG TANG
Small Green Dragon Decoction
Ma Huang *Herba Ephedrae* 9 g
Gui Zhi *Ramulus Cinnamomi cassiae* 6 g
Xi Xin *Herba Asari cum radice* 3 g
Gan Jiang *Rhizoma Zingiberis officinalis* 3 g
Ban Xia *Rhizoma Pinelliae ternatae* 9 g
Bai Shao *Radix Paeoniae albae* 9 g
Wu Wei Zi *Fructus Schisandrae chinensis* 3 g
Zhi Gan Cao *Radix Glycyrrhizae uralensis praeparata* 6 g

XIAO XIAN XIONG TANG
Small Sinking [Qi of the] Chest Decoction
Huang Lian *Rhizoma Coptidis* 6 g
Ban Xia *Rhizoma Pinelliae ternatae* 12 g
Gua Lou *Fructus Trichosanthis* 30 g

XIAO YAO SAN
Free and Easy Wanderer Powder
Bo He *Herba Menthae* 3 g
Chai Hu *Radix Bupleuri* 9 g
Dang Gui *Radix Angelicae sinensis* 9 g
Bai Shao *Radix Paeoniae albae* 12 g
Bai Zhu *Rhizoma Atractylodis macrocephalae* 9 g
Fu Ling *Sclerotium Poriae cocos* 15 g
Gan Cao *Radix Glycyrrhizae uralensis* 6 g
Sheng Jiang *Rhizoma Zingiberis officinalis recens* 3 slices

XIE BAI SAN
Draining Whiteness Powder
Di Gu Pi *Cortex Lycii chinensis radicis* 9 g
Sang Bai Pi *Cortex Mori albae radicis* 9 g
Zhi Gan Cao *Radix Glycyrrhizae uralensis praeparata* 3 g

Geng Mi *Semen Oryzae sativae* 6 g

XIE GAN AN SHEN WAN
Draining the Liver-Calming the Mind Pill
Long Dan Cao *Radix Gentianae scabrae* 9 g
Shan Zhi Zi *Fructus Gardeniae jasminoidis* 6 g
Huang Qin *Radix Scutellariae baicalensis* 6 g
Bai Ji Li *Fructus Tribuli terrestris* 4 g
Shi Jue Ming *Concha Haliotidis* 12 g
Ze Xie *Rhizoma Alismatis orientalis* 6 g
Che Qian Zi *Semen Plantaginis* 6 g
Dang Gui *Radix Angelicae sinensis* 6 g
Sheng Di Huang *Radix Rehmanniae glutinosae* 9 g
Mai Men Dong *Tuber Ophiopogonis japonici* 6 g
Zhen Zhu Mu *Concha margaritiferae* 12 g
Long Gu *Os Draconis* 12 g
Mu Li *Concha Ostreae* 12 g
Fu Shen *Sclerotium Poriae cocos pararadicis* 6 g
Yuan Zhi *Radix Polygalae tenuifoliae* 6 g
Bai Zi Ren *Semen Biotae orientalis* 6 g
Suan Zao Ren *Semen Ziziphi spinosae* 6 g
Gan Cao *Radix Glycyrrhizae uralensis* 3 g

XIE HUANG SAN
Draining Yellowness Powder
Shi Gao *Gypsum fibrosum* 15 g
Zhi Zi *Fructus Gardeniae jasminoidis* 6 g
Fang Feng *Radix Ledebouriellae sesloidis* 12 g
Huo Xiang *Herba Agastachis* 21 g
Gan Cao *Radix Glycyrrhizae uralensis* 9 g

XIE XIN TANG
Draining the Heart Decoction
Da Huang *Rhizoma Rhei* 9 g
Huang Lian *Rhizoma Coptidis* 6 g
Huang Qin *Radix Scutellariae baicalensis* 9 g

XIN YI QING FEI YIN
Magnolia Clearing the Lungs Decoction
Xin Yi Hua *Flos Magnoliae liliflorae* 9 g
Huang Qin *Radix Scutellariae baicalensis* 9 g
Shan Zhi Zi *Fructus Gardeniae jasminoidis* 6 g
Shi Gao *Gypsum fibrosum* 12 g
Zhi Mu *Radix Anemarrhenae asphodeloidis* 6 g
Jin Yin Hua *Flos Lonicerae japonicae* 6 g
Yu Xing Cao *Herba Houttuyniae cordatae* 6 g
Mai Men Dong *Tuber Ophiopogonis japonici* 6 g

XING SU SAN
Prunus-Perilla Leaf Powder
Xing Ren *Semen Pruni armeniacae* 9 g
Zi Su Ye *Folium Perillae frutescentis* 6 g
Jie Geng *Radix Platycodi grandiflori* 4.5 g
Chen Pi *Pericarpium Citri reticulatae* 3 g
Ban Xia *Rhizoma Pinelliae ternatae* 6 g
Fu Ling *Sclerotium Poriae cocos* 6 g
Zhi Ke *Fructus Citri aurantii* 6 g
Qian Hu *Radix Peucedani* 6 g
Sheng Jiang *Rhizoma Zingiberis officinalis recens*
3 slices
Gan Cao *Radix Glycyrrhizae uralensis* 3 g
Da Zao *Fructus Ziziphi jujubae* 3 dates

XUAN BI TANG
Clearing Painful Obstruction Syndrome Decoction
Fang Ji *Radix Stephaniae tetrandae* 6 g
Can Sha *Excrementum Bombycis mori* 6 g
Xing Ren *Semen Pruni armeniacae* 3 g
Hua Shi *Gypsum fibrosum* 12 g
Lian Qiao *Fructus Forsythiae suspensae* 6 g
Shan Zhi Zi *Fructus Gardeniae jasminoidis* 6 g
Yi Ren *Semen Coicis lachryma jobi* 6 g
Chi Xiao Dou *Semen Phaseoli calcarati* 6 g
Ban Xia *Rhizoma Pinelliae ternatae* 6 g

XUAN FU HUA TANG
Inula Decoction
Xuan Fu Hua *Flos Inulae* 9 g
Xiang Fu *Rhizoma Cyperi rotundi* 6 g
Su Geng *Radix Perillae frutescentis* 6 g
Yu Jin *Tuber Curcumae* 6 g
Zhi Ke *Fructus Citri aurantii* 6 g
Si Gua Luo *Fasciculus Luffae vascularis* 6 g

XUE FU ZHU YU TANG
Blood Mansion Eliminating Stasis Decoction
Dang Gui *Radix Angelicae sinensis* 9 g
Sheng Di Huang *Radix Rehmanniae glutinosae* 9 g
Chi Shao *Radix Paeoniae rubrae* 6 g
Chuan Xiong *Radix Ligustici wallichii* 5 g
Tao Ren *Semen Persicae* 12 g
Hong Hua *Flos Carthami tinctorii* 9 g
Chai Hu *Radix Bupleuri* 3 g
Zhi Ke *Fructus Citri aurantii* 6 g
Niu Xi *Radix Cyathulae* 9 g
Jie Geng *Radix Platycodi grandiflori* 5 g
Gan Cao *Radix Glycyrrhizae uralensis* 3 g

YANG WEI TANG
Nourishing the Stomach Decoction
Bei Sha Shen *Radix Glehniae littoralis* 9 g
Mai Men Dong *Tuber Ophiopogonis japonici* 6 g
Yu Zhu *Rhizoma Polygonati odorati* 6 g
Bian Dou *Semen Dolichoris lablab* 6 g
Sang Ye *Folium Mori albae* 4 g
Shi Hu *Herba Dendrobii* 6 g
Zhi Gan Cao *Radix Glycyrrhizae uralensis prae-parata* 3 g

YANG XIN TANG (I)
Nourishing the Heart Decoction
Ren Shen *Radix Ginseng* 6 g (or **Dang Shen** *Radix Codonopsis pilosulae* 12 g)
Huang Qi *Radix Astragali membranacei* 9 g
Fu Ling *Sclerotium Poriae cocos* 6 g
Zhi Gan Cao *Radix Glycyrrhizae uralensis prae-parata* 4.5 g
Dang Gui *Radix Angelicae sinensis* 6 g
Chuan Xiong *Radix Ligustici wallichii* 4.5 g
Wu Wei Zi *Fructus Schisandrae chinensis* 4.5 g
Bai Zi Ren *Semen Biotae orientalis* 6 g
Suan Zao Ren *Semen Ziziphi spinosae* 4.5 g
Yuan Zhi *Radix Polygalae tenuifoliae* 6 g
Rou Gui *Cortex Cinnamomi cassiae* 1.5 g
Ban Xia *Rhizoma Pinelliae ternatae* 4.5 g

YANG XIN TANG (II)
Nourishing the Heart Decoction
Huang Qi *Radix Astragali membranacei* 6 g
Ren Shen *Radix Ginseng* 6 g
Bai Zi Ren *Semen Biotae orientalis* 9 g
Fu Shen *Sclerotium Poriae cocos pararadicis* 6 g
Chuan Xiong *Radix Ligustici wallichii* 3 g
Yuan Zhi *Radix Polygalae tenuifoliae* 6 g
Mai Men Dong *Tuber Ophiopogonis japonici* 6 g
Wu Wei Zi *Fructus Schisandrae chinensis* 6 g
Zhi Gan Cao *Radix Glycyrrhizae uralensis prae-parata* 3 g
Sheng Jiang *Rhizoma Zingiberis officinalis recens*
one slice

YANG XUE DING FENG TANG
Nourishing Blood and Clearing Wind Decoction
Sheng Di Huang *Radix Rehmanniae glutinosae*
12 g
Dang Gui *Radix Angelicae sinensis* 9 g
Chi Shao *Radix Paeoniae rubrae* 6 g

Chuan Xiong *Radix Ligustici wallichii* 4 g
Tian Men Dong *Tuber Asparagi cochinchinensis* 6 g
Mai Men Dong *Tuber Ophiopogonis japonici* 6 g
Jiang Can *Bombyx batryticatus* 3 g
Shou Wu *Radix Polygoni multiflori* 9 g
Shan Zhi Zi *Fructus Gardeniae jasminoidis* 4 g
Mu Dan Pi *Cortex Moutan radicis* 4 g

YI DU YANG YUAN TANG
Benefiting the Governing Vessels and Nourishing the Original Qi Decoction
Gui Ban *Plastrum Testudinis* 15 g
Shu Di Huang *Radix Rehmanniae glutinosae praeparata* 9 g
Rou Cong Rong *Herba Cistanchis* 9 g
Bu Gu Zhi *Fructus Psoraleae corylifoliae* 6 g
Lu Jiao Jiao *Colla Cornu Cervi* 3 g
Wu Wei Zi *Fructus Schisandrae chinensis* 3 g
Zhi Mu *Radix Anemarrhenae asphodeloidis* 3 g
Huang Bo *Cortex Phellodendri* 3 g

YI GUAN JIAN
One Linking Decoction
Bei Sha Shen *Radix Glehniae littoralis* 10 g
Mai Men Dong *Tuber Ophiopogonis japonici* 10 g
Dang Gui *Radix Angelicae sinensis* 10 g
Sheng Di Huang *Radix Rehmanniae glutinosae* 30 g
Gou Qi Zi *Fructus Lycii chinensis* 12 g
Chuan Lian Zi *Fructus Meliae toosendan* 5 g

YI SHEN TONG MAI TANG
Benefit the Kidneys-Penetrate the Blood Vessels Decoction
Hong Shen *Radix Ginseng (Red Ginseng)* 6 g
Gou Qi Zi *Fructus Lycii chinensis* 10 g
Shan Zhu Yu *Fructus Corni officinalis* 6 g
Fu Ling *Sclerotium Poriae cocos* 15 g
Dang Gui *Radix Angelicae sinensis* 12 g
Chi Shao *Radix Paeoniae rubrae* 6 g
Hong Hua *Flos Carthami tinctorii* 6 g
Ze Lan *Herba Lycopi lucidi* 6 g
Wang Bu Liu Xing *Semen Vaccariae* 15 g
Chuan Xiong *Radix Ligustici wallichii* 12 g
Dan Shen *Radix Salviae miltiorrhizae* 12 g
Gui Zhi *Ramulus Cinnamomi cassiae* 6 g

YI WEI TANG
Benefiting the Stomach Decoction
Bei Sha Shen *Radix Glehniae littoralis* 9 g

Mai Men Dong *Tuber Ophiopogonis japonici* 9 g
Sheng Di Huang *Radix Rehmanniae glutinosae* 12 g
Yu Zhu *Rhizoma Polygonati odorati* 6 g
Bing Tang *Brown sugar* 3 g

YI YI REN TANG
Coix Decoction
Yi Yi Ren *Semen Coicis lachryma jobi* 6 g
Cang Zhu *Rhizoma Atractylodis lanceae* 6 g
Qiang Huo *Radix et Rhizoma Notopterygii* 3 g
Du Huo *Radix Angelicae pubescentis* 6 g
Fang Feng *Radix Ledebouriellae sesloidis* 6 g
Wu Tou *Radix Aconiti carmichaeli praeparata* 1.5 g
Ma Huang *Herba Ephedrae* 3 g
Gui Zhi *Ramulus Cinnamomi cassiae* 3 g
Dang Gui *Radix Angelicae sinensis* 6 g
Chuan Xiong *Radix Ligustici wallichii* 3 g
Sheng Jiang *Rhizoma Zingiberis officinalis recens* 3 slices
Gan Cao *Radix Glycyrrhizae uralensis* 3 g

YIN CHEN HAO TANG
Artemisia capillaris Decoction
Yin Chen Hao *Herba Artemisiae capillaris* 30 g
Zhi Zi *Fructus Gardeniae jasminoidis* 15 g
Da Huang *Rhizoma Rhei* 9 g

YIN CHEN WU LING SAN
Artemisia capillaris Five Ling Powder
Yin Chen Hao *Herba Artemisiae capillaris* 10 g
Wu Ling San *Five Ling Powder* 5 g

YIN MEI TANG
Attracting Sleep Decoction
Bai Shao *Radix Paeoniae albae* 30 g
Dang Gui *Radix Angelicae sinensis* 15 g
Long Chi *Dens Draconis* 6 g
Tu Si Zi *Semen Cuscutae* 9 g
Mai Men Dong *Tuber Ophiopogonis japonici* 15 g
Bai Zi Ren *Semen Biotae orientalis* 6 g
Suan Zao Ren *Semen Ziziphi spinosae* 9 g
Fu Shen *Sclerotium Poriae cocos pararadicis* 9 g

YIN QIAO SAN
Lonicera-Forsythia Powder
Jin Yin Hua *Flos Lonicerae japonicae* 9 g
Lian Qiao *Fructus Forsythiae suspensae* 9 g
Jie Geng *Radix Platycodi grandiflori* 6 g

Niu Bang Zi *Fructus Arctii lappae* 9 g
Bo He *Herba Menthae* 6 g
Jing Jie *Herba seu Flos Schizonepetae tenuifoliae* 5 g
Zhu Ye *Herba Lophatheri gracilis* 4 g
Dan Dou Chi *Semen Sojae praeparatum* 5 g
Gan Cao *Radix Glycyrrhizae uralensis* 5 g

YOU GUI WAN
Restoring the Right [Kidney] Pill
Fu Zi *Radix Aconiti carmichaeli praeparata* 3 g
Rou Gui *Cortex Cinnamomi cassiae* 3 g
Du Zhong *Cortex Eucommiae ulmoidis* 6 g
Shan Zhu Yu *Fructus Corni officinalis* 4.5 g
Tu Si Zi *Semen Cuscutae* 6 g
Lu Jiao Jiao *Colla Corni Cervi* 6 g
Shu Di Huang *Radix Rehmanniae glutinosae praeparata* 12 g
Shan Yao *Radix Dioscoreae oppositae* 6 g
Gou Qi Zi *Fructus Lycii chinensis* 6 g
Dang Gui *Radix Angelicae sinensis* 4.5 g

YOU GUI YIN
Restoring the Right [Kidney] Decoction
Shu Di Huang *Radix Rehmanniae glutinosae praeparata* 15 g
Shan Zhu Yu *Fructus Corni officinalis* 3 g
Shan Yao *Radix Dioscoreae oppositae* 6 g
Du Zhong *Cortex Eucommiae ulmoidis* 6 g
Rou Gui *Cortex Cinnamomi cassiae* 3 g
Fu Zi *Radix Aconiti carmichaeli praeparata* 3 g
Gou Qi Zi *Fructus Lycii chinensis* 6 g
Zhi Gan Cao *Radix Glycyrrhizae uralensis praeparata* 3 g

YU NU JIAN
Jade Woman Decoction
Shi Gao *Gypsum fibrosum* 30 g
Zhi Mu *Radix Anemarrhenae asphodeloidis* 4.5 g
Shu Di Huang *Radix Rehmanniae glutinosae praeparata* 9 g
Mai Men Dong *Tuber Ophiopogonis japonici* 6 g
Niu Xi *Radix Achyranthis bidentatae seu Cyathulae* 4.5 g

YU PING FENG SAN
Jade Wind Screen Powder
Huang Qi *Radix Astragali membranacei* 30 g
Bai Zhu *Rhizoma Atractylodis macrocephalae* 60 g
Fang Feng *Radix Ledebouriellae sesloidis* 30 g

YUE BI JIA ZHU TANG
Overstepping Maidservant Decoction plus Atractylodes
Ma Huang *Herba Ephedrae* 9 g
Shi Gao *Gypsum fibrosum* 18 g
Sheng Jiang *Rhizoma Zingiberis officinalis recens* 9 g
Gan Cao *Radix Glycyrrhizae uralensis* 5 g
Da Zao *Fructus Ziziphi jujubae* 5 dates
Bai Zhu *Rhizoma Atractylodis macrocephalae* 9 g

YUE JU WAN
Gardenia-Ligusticum Pill
Cang Zhu *Rhizoma Atractylodis lanceae* 6 g
Chuan Xiong *Radix Ligustici wallichii* 6 g
Xiang Fu *Rhizoma Cyperi rotundi* 6 g
Zhi Zi *Fructus Gardeniae jasminoidis* 6 g
Shen Qu *Massa Fermentata Medicinalis* 6 g

ZAI ZAO SAN
Renewal Powder
Dang Shen *Radix Codonopsis pilosulae* 12 g
Huang Qi *Radix Astragali membranacei* 15 g
Fu Zi *Radix Aconiti carmichaeli praeparata* 6 g
Qiang Huo *Radix et Rhizoma Notopterygii* 6 g
Fang Feng *Radix Ledebouriellae sesloidis* 6 g
Chuan Xiong *Radix Ligustici wallichii* 6 g
Xi Xin *Herba Asari cum radice* 3 g
Gui Zhi *Ramulus Cinnamomi cassiae* 6 g
Bai Shao *Radix Paeoniae albae* 6 g
Gan Cao *Radix Glycyrrhizae uralensis* 3 g
Sheng Jiang *Rhizoma Zingiberis officinalis recens* 6 g
Da Zao *Fructus Ziziphi jujubae* 3 dates

ZENG YE TANG
Increasing Fluids Decoction
Xuan Shen *Radix Scrophulariae ningpoensis* 18 g
Mai Men Dong *Tuber Ophiopogonis japonici* 12 g
Sheng Di Huang *Radix Rehmanniae glutinosae* 12 g

ZHEN GAN XI FENG TANG
Pacifying the Liver and Subduing Wind Decoction
Huai Niu Xi *Radix Achyrantis bidentatae* 15 g
Dai Zhe Shi *Haematitum* 15 g
Long Gu *Os Draconis* 12 g
Mu Li *Concha Ostreae* 12 g
Gui Ban *Plastrum Testudinis* 12 g
Xuan Shen *Radix Scrophulariae ningpoensis* 12 g
Tian Men Dong *Tuber Asparagi cochinchinensis* 12 g

Bai Shao *Radix Paeoniae albae* 12 g
Yin Chen Hao *Herba Artemisiae capillaris* 6 g
Chuan Lian Zi *Fructus Meliae toosendan* 6 g
Mai Ya *Fructus Hordei vulgaris germinatus* 6 g
Gan Cao *Radix Glycyrrhizae uralensis* 6 g

ZHEN WU TANG
True Warrior Decoction
Fu Zi *Radix Aconiti carmichaeli praeparata* 10 g
Bai Zhu *Rhizoma Atractylodis macrocephalae* 12 g
Fu Ling *Sclerotium Poriae cocos* 15 g
Bai Shao *Radix Paeoniae albae* 6 g
Sheng Jiang *Rhizoma Zingiberis officinalis recens*
3 slices

ZHEN ZHONG DAN
Bedside Pill
Gui Ban *Plastrum Testudinis* 10 g
Long Gu *Os Draconis* 10 g
Yuan Zhi *Radix Polygalae tenuifoliae* 10 g
Shi Chang Pu *Rhizoma Acori graminei* 10 g

ZHEN ZHU MU TANG
Concha margaritiferae Pill
Zhen Zhu Mu *Concha margaritiferae* 30 g
Long Chi *Dens Draconis* 18 g
Chen Xiang *Lignum Aquilariae* 3 g
Zhu Sha *Cinnabaris* 1.5 g
Shu Di Huang *Radix Rehmanniae glutinosae praeparata* 12 g
Dang Gui *Radix Angelicae sinensis* 6 g
Ren Shen *Radix Ginseng* 6 g
Suan Zao Ren *Semen Ziziphi spinosae* 6 g
Bai Zi Ren *Semen Biotae orientalis* 6 g
Fu Shen *Sclerotium Poriae cocos pararadicis* 6 g
Shui Niu Jiao *Cornu Bufali* 6 g

ZHENG QI TIAN XIANG SAN
Upright Qi Heavenly Fragrance Powder
Xiang Fu *Rhizoma Cyperi rotundi* 6 g
Wu Yao *Radix Linderae strychnifoliae* 6 g
Gan Jiang *Rhizoma Zingiberis officinalis* 3 g
Zi Su Ye *Folium Perillae frutescentis* 6 g
Chen Pi *Pericarpium Citri reticulatae* 4.5 g

ZHI BO DI HUANG WAN (or ZHI BO BA WEI WAN)
Anemarrhena-Phellodendron-Rehmannia Pill
(Anemarrhena-Phellodendron Eight-Ingredient Pill)

Shu Di Huang *Radix Rehmanniae glutinosae praeparata* 24 g
Shan Zhu Yu *Fructus Corni officinalis* 12 g
Shan Yao *Radix Dioscoreae oppositae* 12 g
Ze Xie *Rhizoma Alismatis orientalis* 9 g
Fu Ling *Sclerotium Poriae cocos* 9 g
Mu Dan Pi *Cortex Moutan radicis* 9 g
Zhi Mu *Radix Anemarrhenae asphodeloidis* 9 g
Huang Bo *Cortex Phellodendri* 9 g

ZHI GAN CAO TANG
Glycyrrhiza Decoction
Zhi Gan Cao *Radix Glycyrrhizae uralensis praeparata* 12 g
Ren Shen *Radix Ginseng* 6 g
Da Zao *Fructus Ziziphi jujubae* 10 dates
Sheng Di Huang *Radix Rehmanniae glutinosae* 30 g
Mai Men Dong *Tuber Ophiopogonis japonici* 10 g
E Jiao *Gelatinum Corii Asini* 6 g
Hu Ma Ren *Semen Sesami indici* 10 g
Sheng Jiang *Rhizoma Zingiberis officinalis recens* 9 g
Gui Zhi *Ramulus Cinnamomi cassiae* 9 g
Qing Jiu Rice wine 10 ml (added at the end)

ZHI SHI DAO ZHI WAN
Citrus aurantius Eliminating Stagnation Pill
Da Huang *Radix Rhei* 15 g
Zhi Shi *Fructus Citri aurantii immaturus* 12 g
Huang Lian *Rhizoma Coptidis* 6 g
Huang Qin *Radix Scutellariae baicalensis* 6 g
Fu Ling *Sclerotium Poriae cocos* 6 g
Ze Xie *Rhizoma Alismatis orientalis* 6 g
Bai Zhu *Rhizoma Atractylodis macrocephalae* 6 g
Shen Qu *Massa Fermentata Medicinalis* 12 g

ZHI SHI XIE BAI GUI ZHI TANG
Citrus-Allium-Cinnamomum Decoction
Zhi Shi *Fructus Citri aurantii immaturus* 12 g
Xie Bai *Bulbus Allii* 9 g
Gui Zhi *Ramulus Cinnamomi cassiae* 6 g
Gua Lou *Fructus Trichosanthis* 12 g
Hou Po *Cortex Magnoliae officinalis* 12 g

ZHI SHI ZHI ZI TANG
Citrus aurantium-Gardenia Decoction
Zhi Shi *Fructus Citri aurantii immaturus* 6 g
Zhi Zi *Fructus Gardeniae jasminoidis* 9 g
Dan Dou Chi *Semen Sojae praeparatum* 9 g

ZHI SOU SAN
Stopping Cough Powder
Jing Jie *Herba seu Flos Schizonepetae tenuifoliae* 6 g
Jie Geng *Radix Platycodi grandiflori* 4.5 g
Bai Qian *Radix et Rhizoma Cynanchii stautoni* 6 g
Chen Pi *Pericarpium Citri reticulatae* 3 g
Bai Bu *Radix Stemonae* 6 g
Zi Wan *Radix Asteris tatarici* 6 g
Gan Cao *Radix Glycyrrhizae uralensis* 3 g

ZHI ZI CHI TANG
Gardenia-Soja Decoction
Zhi Zi *Fructus Gardeniae jasminoidis* 9 g
Dan Dou Chi *Semen Sojae praeparatum* 9 g

ZHU SHA AN SHEN WAN
Cinnabar Calming the Mind Pill
Huang Lian *Rhizoma Coptidis* 3 g
Sheng Di Huang *Radix Rehmanniae glutinosae* 12 g
Dang Gui *Radix Angelicae sinensis* 6 g
Fu Ling *Sclerotium Poriae cocos* 6 g
Suan Zao Ren *Semen Ziziphi spinosae* 6 g
Zhu Sha *Cinnabaris* 3 g
Yuan Zhi *Radix Polygalae tenuifoliae* 6 g
Gan Cao *Radix Glycyrrhizae uralensis* 3 g

ZHU YE SHI GAO TANG
Zhu Ye *Herba Lophateri gracilis* 15 g
Shi Gao *Gypsum fibrosum* 30 g
Ban Xia *Rhizoma Pinelliae ternatae* 9 g
Mai Men Dong *Tuber Ophiopogonis japonici* 15 g

Ren Shen *Radix Ginseng* 5 g
Gan Cao *Radix Glycyrrhizae uralensis* 3 g
Geng Mi *Semen Oryzae sativae* 15 g

ZUO GUI WAN
Restoring the Left [Kidney] Pill
Shu Di Huang *Radix Rehmanniae glutinosae praeparata* 15 g
Shan Yao *Radix Dioscoreae oppositae* 9 g
Shan Zhu Yu *Fructus Corni officinalis* 9 g
Gou Qi Zi *Fructus Lycii chinensis* 9 g
Chuan Niu Xi *Radix Cyathulae* 6 g
Tu Si Zi *Semen Cuscutae* 9 g
Lu Jiao *Cornu Cervi* 9 g
Gui Ban Jiao *Colla Plastri Testudinis* 9 g

ZUO GUI YIN
Restore the Left [Kidney] Decoction
Shu Di Huang *Radix Rehmanniae glutinosae praeparata* 12 g
Shan Zhu Yu *Fructus Corni officinalis* 6 g
Gou Qi Zi *Fructus Lycii chinensis* 6 g
Shan Yao *Radix Dioscoreae oppositae* 6 g
Fu Ling *Sclerotium Poriae cocos* 6 g
Zhi Gan Cao *Radix Glycyrrhizae uralensis praeparata* 3 g

ZUO JIN WAN
Left Metal Pill
Huang Lian *Rhizoma Coptidis* 15 g
Wu Zhu Yu *Fructus Evodiae rutaecarpae* 2 g

Appendix V
Patent remedies

AN MIAN PIAN
Peaceful Sleep Tablet
Suan Zao Ren *Semen Ziziphi spinosae*
Yuan Zhi *Radix Polygalae tenuifoliae*
Fu Ling *Sclerotium Poriae cocos*
Shan Zhi Zi *Fructus Gardeniae jasminoidis*
Shen Qu *Massa Fermentata Medicinalis*
Quan Xie *Buthus Martensi*
Gan Cao *Radix Glycyrrhizae uralensis*

AN SHEN BU NAO PIAN
Calming the Mind and Tonifying the Brain Tablet
Huang Jing *Rhizoma Polygonati*
Nu Zhen Zi *Fructus Ligustri lucidi*
Dang Gui *Radix Angelicae sinensis*
He Huan Pi *Cortex Albizziae julibrissin*
Han Lian Cao *Herba Ecliptae prostratae*
Suan Zao Ren *Semen Ziziphi spinosae*
Fu Ling *Sclerotium Poriae cocos*
Shou Wu *Radix Polygoni multiflori*
Yuan Zhi *Radix Polygalae tenuifoliae*
Zhu Sha *Cinnabaris*

AN SHEN BU XIN PIAN
Calming the Mind and Tonifying the Heart Tablet
Zhen Zhu Mu *Concha margaritiferae*
Ye Jiao Teng *Caulis Polygoni multiflori*
Nu Zhen Zi *Fructus Ligustri lucidi*
Han Lian Cao *Herba Ecliptae prostratae*
He Huan Pi *Cortex Albizziae julibrissin*
Dan Shen *Radix Salviae miltiorrhizae*
Sheng Di Huang *Radix Rehmanniae glutinosae*

Shu Di Huang *Radix Rehmanniae glutinosae praeparata*
Wu Wei Zi *Fructus Schisandrae chinensis*
Shi Chang Pu *Rhizoma Acori graminei*

AN SHEN BU XIN WAN
Calming the Mind and Tonifying the Heart Pill
Zhen Zhu Mu *Concha margaritiferae*
Shou Wu *Radix Polygoni multiflori*
Nu Zhen Zi *Fructus Ligustri lucidi*
Han Lian Cao *Herba Ecliptae prostratae*
Dan Shen *Radix Salviae miltiorrhizae*
He Huan Pi *Cortex Albizziae julibrissin*
Tu Si Zi *Semen Cuscutae*
Wu Wei Zi *Fructus Schisandrae chinensis*
Shi Chang Pu *Rhizoma Acori graminei*

AN TAI WAN
Calming the Foetus Pill
Dang Gui *Radix Angelicae sinensis*
Bai Shao *Radix Paeoniae albae*
Huang Qin *Radix Scutellariae baicalensis*
Bai Zhu *Rhizoma Atractylodis macrocephalae*
Chuan Xiong *Radix Ligustici wallichii*

BA XIAN CHANG SHOU WAN
Eight Immortals Longevity Pill
Mai Men Dong *Tuber Ophiopogonis japonici*
Wu Wei Zi *Fructus Schisandrae chinensis*
Shu Di Huang *Radix Rehmanniae glutinosae praeparata*
Shan Yao *Radix Dioscoreae oppositae*
Shan Zhu Yu *Fructus Corni officinalis*
Ze Xie *Rhizoma Alismatis orientalis*
Fu Ling *Sclerotium Poriae cocos*
Mu Dan Pi *Cortex Moutan radicis*

BA ZHEN WAN
Eight Precious Pill
Dang Gui *Radix Angelicae sinensis*
Chuan Xiong *Radix Ligustici wallichii*
Bai Shao *Radix Paeoniae albae*
Shu Di Huang *Radix Rehmanniae glutinosae praeparata*
Ren Shen *Radix Ginseng*
Bai Zhu *Rhizoma Atractylodis macrocephalae*
Fu Ling *Sclerotium Poriae cocos*
Zhi Gan Cao *Radix Glycyrrhizae uralensis praeparata*

BAI HE GU JIN WAN
Lilium Consolidating Metal Pill
Bai He *Bulbus Lilii*
Mai Men Dong *Tuber Ophiopogonis japonicis*
Xuan Shen *Radix Scrophulariae ningpoensis*
Sheng Di Huang *Radix Rehmanniae glutinosae*
Shu Di Huang *Radix Rehmanniae glutinosae praeparata*
Dang Gui *Radix Angelicae sinensis*
Bai Shao *Radix Paeoniae albae*
Jie Geng *Radix Platycodi grandiflori*
Gan Cao *Radix Glycyrrhizae uralensis*

BAI ZI YANG XIN WAN
Biota Nourishing the Heart Pill
Ren Shen *Radix Ginseng* (or Dang Shen *Radix Codonopsis pilosulae*)
Huang Qi *Radix Astragali membranacei*
Dang Gui *Radix Angelicae sinensis*
Chuan Xiong *Radix Ligustici wallichii*
Fu Ling *Sclerotium Poriae cocos*
Bai Zi Ren *Semen Biotae orientalis*
Suan Zao Ren *Semen Ziziphi spinosae*
Yuan Zhi *Radix Polygalae tenuifoliae*
Wu Wei Zi *Fructus Schisandrae chinensis*
Ban Xia *Rhizoma Pinelliae ternatae*
Rou Gui *Cortex Cinnamomi cassiae*
Zhi Gan Cao *Radix Glycyrrhizae uralensis praeparata*

BAO HE WAN
Preserving and Harmonizing Pill
Shan Zha *Fructus Crataegi*
Shen Qu *Massa Fermentata Medicinalis*
Lai Fu Zi *Semen Raphani sativi*
Ban Xia *Rhizoma Pinelliae ternatae*
Chen Pi *Pericarpum Citri reticulatae*
Fu Ling *Sclerotium Poriae cocos*
Lian Qiao *Fructus Forsythiae suspensae*

BAO JI WAN
Protecting and Benefiting Pill
Chi Shi Zhi *Halloysitum rubrum*
Bai Zhi *Radix Angelicae dahuricae*
Ju Hua *Flos Chrysanthemi morifolii*
Bo He *Herba Menthae*
Ge Gen *Radix Puerariae*
Tian Hua Fen *Radix Trichosanthis*
Cang Zhu *Rhizoma Atractylodis lanceae*
Yi Yi Ren *Semen Coicis lachryma jobi*

Fu Ling *Sclerotium Poriae cocos*
Mu Xiang *Radix Saussureae*
Hou Po *Cortex Magnoliae officinalis*
Chen Pi *Pericarpium Citri reticulatae*
Shen Qu *Massa Fermentata Medicinalis*
Huo Xiang *Herba Agastachis*
Gu Ya *Fructus Oryzae sativae germinatus*

BAO JIAN MEI JIAN FEI CHA
Maintaining Vigour and Beauty and Reducing Fat Tea
Qing Cha *Green tea*
Shan Zha *Fructus Crataegi*
Chi Xiao Dou *Semen Phaseoli calcarati*
Mai Ya *Fructus Hordei vulgaris germinatus*
Chen Pi *Pericarpium Citri reticulatae*
Shen Qu *Massa Fermentata Medicinalis*
Jue Ming Zi *Semen Cassiae torae*
Qian Niu Zi *Semen Pharbitidis*
Ze Xie *Rhizoma Alismatis orientalis*
Lai Fu Zi *Semen Raphani sativi*

BI YAN PIAN
Rhinitis Tablet
Cang Er Zi *Fructus Xanthii*
Xin Yi Hua *Flos Magnoliae liliflorae*
Gan Cao *Radix Glycyrrhizae uralensis*
Huang Bo *Cortex Phellodendri*
Jie Geng *Radix Platycodi grandiflori*
Wu Wei Zi *Fructus Schisandrae chinensis*
Lian Qiao *Fructus Forsythiae suspensae*
Bai Zhi *Radix Angelicae dahuricae*
Zhi Mu *Rhizoma Anemarrhenae asphodeloidis*
Ju Hua *Flos Chrysanthemi morifolii*
Fang Feng *Radix Ledebouriellae sesloidis*
Jing Jie *Herba seu Flos Schizonepetae tenuifoliae*

BU NAO WAN
Tonifying the Brain Pill
Dang Gui *Radix Angelicae sinensis*
Suan Zao Ren *Semen Ziziphi spinosae*
Rou Cong Rong *Herba Cistanchis*
Bai Zi Ren *Semen Biotae orientalis*
Yuan Zhi *Radix Polygalae tenuifoliae*
Tao Ren *Semen Persicae*
Tian Nan Xing *Rhizoma Arisaematis praeparata*
Shi Chang Pu *Rhizoma Acori graminei*
Gou Qi Zi *Fructus Lycii chinensis*
Hu Po *Succinum*

Long Chi *Dens Draconis*
Wu Wei Zi *Fructus Schisandrae chinensis*

BU XUE TIAO JING PIAN
Tonifying Blood and Regulating Menses Tablet
Xiang Fu *Rhizoma Cyperi rotundi*
Jin Ying Zi *Semen Rosae laevigatae*
Ji Xue Teng *Caulis Millettiae seu Caulis Spatholobi*
Sang Ji Sheng *Ramus Loranthi*
Shang Cang Zi *Fructus Litseae*
Gang Nian *Herba Rhodomyrti*
Qian Jin Ba *Radix Moghaniae*
Yi Mu Cao *Herba Leonori heterophylli*
Gao Liang Jiang *Rhizoma Alpiniae officinari*
Wu Hua Guo Gen *Radix Fici*
Ai Ye *Folium Artemisiae*
Ji Cai *Herba Capsellae*
Dang Shen *Radix Codonopsis pilosulae*
Bai Zhu *Rhizoma Atractylodis macrocephalae*
Zhi Gan Cao *Radix Glycyrrhizae uralensis praeparata*
E Jiao *Gelatinum Corii Asini*
Rou Gui *Cortex Cinnamomi cassiae*
Bai Bei Ye *Herba Baipo*

BU ZHONG YI QI WAN
Tonifying the Centre and Benefiting Qi Pill
Huang Qi *Radix Astragali membranacei*
Dang Shen *Radix Codonopsis pilosulae*
Zhi Gan Cao *Radix Glycyrrhizae uralensis praeparata*
Bai Zhu *Rhizoma Atractylodis macrocephalae*
Dang Gui *Radix Angelicae sinensis*
Chen Pi *Pericarpium Citri reticulatae*
Sheng Ma *Rhizoma Cimicifugae*
Chai Hu *Radix Bupleuri*
Sheng Jiang *Rhizoma Zingiberis officinalis recens*
Da Zao *Fructus Ziziphi jujubae*

CAI FENG ZHEN ZHU AN CHUANG WAN
Colourful Phoenix Pearl Hiding Boils Pill
Zhen Zhu *Margarita*
Sheng Di Huang *Radix Rehmanniae glutinosae*
Nan Sha Shen *Radix Adenophorae*
Xuan Shen *Radix Scrophulariae ningpoensis*
Jin Yin Hua *Flos Lonicerae japonicae*
Huang Bo *Cortex Phellodendri*
Da Huang *Rhizoma Rhei*
Ling Yang Jiao *Cornu Antelopis*

CHUAN BEI PI PA GAO
Fritillaria-Eriobotrya Syrup

Pi Pa Ye *Folium Eriobotryae japonicae*
Chuan Bei Mu *Bulbus Fritillariae cirrhosae*
Nan Sha Shen *Radix Adenophorae*
Wu Wei Zi *Fructus Schisandrae chinensis*
Chen Pi *Pericarpium Citri reticulatae*
Jie Geng *Radix Platycodi grandiflori*
Ban Xia *Rhizoma Pinelliae ternatae*
Bo He *Herba Menthae*
Kuan Dong Hua *Flos Tussilaginis farfarae*
Xing Ren *Semen Pruni armeniacae*
Feng Mi *Mel*

CHUAN XIONG CHA TIAO WAN
Ligusticum-Green Tea Regulating Pill
Chuan Xiong *Radix Ligustici wallichii*
Qiang Huo *Radix et Rhizoma Notopterygii*
Bai Zhi *Radix Angelicae dahuricae*
Jing Jie *Herba seu Flos Schizonepetae tenuifoliae*
Xi Xin *Herba Asari cum radice*
Fang Feng *Radix Ledebouriellae sesloidis*
Bo He *Herba Menthae*
Gan Cao *Radix Glycyrrhizae uralensis*
Qing Cha (Green Tea) *Folia Cameliae*

DA BU YIN WAN
Big Tonifying the Yin Pill
Shu Di Huang *Radix Rehmanniae glutinosae praeparata*
Gui Ban *Plastrum Testudinis*
Zhi Mu *Rhizoma Anemarrhenae asphodeloidis*
Huang Bo *Cortex Phellodendri*

DA HUO LUO DAN
Great Invigorating the Connecting Channels Pill
An Xi Xiang *Benzonium*
Bing Pian *Borneol*
Cao Wu Tou *Radix Aconiti carmichaeli*
Chen Xiang *Lignum Aquilariae*
Chi Shao *Radix Paeoniae rubrae*
Chuan Niu Xi *Radix Cyathulae*
Chuan Xiong *Radix Ligustici wallichii*
Da Huang *Rhizoma Rhei*
Dang Gui *Radix Angelicae sinensis*
Di Long *Pheretima aspergillum*
Ding Xiang *Flos Caryophylli*
Cao Dou Kou *Semen Alpiniae katsumadae*
Fang Feng *Radix Ledebouriellae sesloidis*
Fu Ling *Sclerotium Poriae cocos*
Gan Cao *Radix Glycyrrhizae uralensis*

Ge Gen *Radix Puerariae*
Gu Sui Bu *Rhizoma Gusuibu*
Guan Zhong *Radix seu Herba Potentillae*
Gui Ban *Plastrum Testudinis*
Shou Wu *Radix Polygoni multiflori*
Hu Gu *Os Tigris*
Huang Lian *Rhizoma Coptidis*
Huang Qin *Radix Scutellariae baicalensis*
Huo Xiang *Herba Agastachis*
Jiang Can *Bombyx batryticatus*
Ma Huang *Herba Ephedrae*
Mo Yao *Myrrha*
Mu Xiang *Radix Saussureae*
Niu Huang *Calculus Bovis*
Qi She *Agkistrodon acutus*
Qiang Huo *Radix et Rhizoma Notopterygii*
Qing Pi *Pericarpium Citri reticulatae viridae*
Ren Shen *Radix Ginseng*
Rou Gui *Cortex Cinnamomi cassiae*
Ru Xiang *Gummi Olibanum*
She Xiang *Secretio Moschus moschiferi*
Shu Di Huang *Radix Rehmanniae glutinosae praeparata*
Song Xiang *Resina praeparata Pini*
Tian Ma *Rhizoma Gastrodiae elatae*
Dan Nan Xing *Rhizoma Arisaematis praeparata*
Wei Ling Xian *Radix Clematidis chinensis*
Wu Shao She *Zaocys dhumnades*
Wu Yao *Radix Lynderae strychnifoliae*
Shui Niu Jiao *Cornu Bufali*
Xi Xin *Herba Asari cum radice*
Xiang Fu *Rhizoma Cyperi rotundi*
Xuan Shen *Radix Scrophulariae ningpoensis*
Xue Jie *Sanguis draconis*

DAN SHEN PIAN
Salvia Tablet
Dan Shen *Radix Salviae miltiorrhizae*

DANG GUI PIAN
Angelica Tablet
Dang Gui *Radix Angelicae sinensis*

DING XIN WAN
Settling the Heart Pill
Dang Shen *Radix Codonopsis pilosulae*
Dang Gui *Radix Angelicae sinensis*
Fu Shen *Sclerotium Poriae cocos pararadicis*
Yuan Zhi *Radix Polygalae tenuifoliae*

Suan Zao Ren *Semen Ziziphi spinosae*
Bai Zi Ren *Semen Biotae orientalis*
Mai Men Dong *Tuber Ophiopogonis japonicis*
Hu Po *Succinum*

DU HUO JI SHENG WAN
Angelica pubescens-Loranthus Pill
Du Huo *Radix Angelicae pubescentis*
Xi Xin *Herba Asari cum radice*
Fang Feng *Radix Ledebouriellae sesloidis*
Qin Jiao *Radix Gentianae macrophyllae*
Sang Ji Sheng *Ramus Loranthi*
Du Zhong *Radix Eucommiae ulmoidis*
Niu Xi *Radix Achyranthis bidentatae seu Cyathulae*
Dang Gui *Radix Angelicae sinensis*
Chuan Xiong *Radix Ligustici wallichii*
Sheng Di Huang *Radix Rehmanniae glutinosae*
Bai Shao *Radix Paeoniae albae*
Ren Shen *Radix Ginseng*
Fu Ling *Sclerotium Poriae cocos*
Rou Gui *Cortex Cinnamomi cassiae*
Gan Cao *Radix Glycyrrhizae uralensis*

DU ZHONG BU TIAN SU
Eucommia Benefiting Heaven Pill
Du Zhong *Cortex Eucommiae ulmoidis*
Gou Qi Zi *Fructus Lycii chinensis*
Huang Qi *Radix Astragali membranacei*
Dang Shen *Radix Codonopsis pilosulae*
Dang Gui *Radix Angelicae sinensis*
Sheng Di Huang *Radix Rehmanniae glutinosae*
Ba Ji Tian *Radix Morindae officinalis*
Shan Zhu Yu *Fructus Corni officinalis*
Rou Cong Rong *Herba Cistanchis*
Lian Zi *Semen Nelumbinis nuciferae*
Bai Zi Ren *Semen Biotae orientalis*

DU ZHONG HU GU WAN
Eucommia-Tiger Bone Pill
Ren Shen *Radix Ginseng*
Bai Zhu *Rhizoma Atractylodis macrocephalae*
Dang Gui *Radix Angelicae sinensis*
Chuan Xiong *Radix Ligustici wallichii*
Ji Xue Teng *Caulis Millettiae seu Caulis Spatholobi*
San Qi *Radix Notoginseng*
Du Zhong *Cortex Eucommiae ulmoidis*
Hu Gu *Os Tigris*
Mu Gua *Fructus Chaenomelis lagenariae*
Yin Yang Huo *Herba Epimedii*

Wu Shao She *Zaocys dhumnades*
Lu Lu Tong *Fructus Liquidambaris taiwanianae*
Cang Zhu *Rhizoma Atractylodis lanceae*
Xun Gu Feng *Rhizoma seu Herba Aristolochiae*
Wei Ling Xian *Radix Clematidis chinensis*
Shi Nan Teng *Ramus Photiniae*
Sang Zhi *Ramulus Mori albae*

ER CHEN WAN
Two Old Pill
Ban Xia *Rhizoma Pinelliae ternatae*
Chen Pi *Pericarpium Citri reticulatae*
Fu Ling *Sclerotium Poriae cocos*
Zhi Gan Cao *Radix Glycyrrhizae uralensis praeparata*
Sheng Jiang *Rhizoma Zingiberis officinalis recens*
Wu Mei *Fructus Pruni mume*

ER MING ZUO CI WAN
Tinnitus Pill that is Kind to the Left [Kidney]
Shu Di Huang *Radix Rehmanniae glutinosae praeparata*
Shan Yao *Rhizoma Dioscoreae oppositae*
Shan Zhu Yu *Fructus Corni officinalis*
Ze Xie *Rhizoma Alismatis orientalis*
Fu Ling *Sclerotium Poriae cocos*
Mu Dan Pi *Cortex Moutan radicis*
Ci Shi *Magnetitum*
Chai Hu *Radix Bupleuri*

FENG SHI LING PIAN
Wind-Dampness Efficacious Tablet
Chuan Wu *Radix Aconiti carmichaeli*
San Qi *Radix Notoginseng*
Ren Shen *Radix Ginseng*
Duan Jie Shen *Radix Cynanchi wallichii*

FENG SHI PIAN
Wind-Dampness Tablet
Ma Huang *Herba Ephedrae*
Gui Zhi *Ramulus Cinnamomi cassiae*
Fang Feng *Radix Ledebouriellae sesloidis*
Du Huo *Radix Angelicae pubescentis*
Quan Xie *Buthus Martensi*
Ma Qian Zi *Semen Strychnotis*
Du Zhong *Cortex Eucommiae ulmoidis*
Niu Xi *Radix Achyranthis bidentatae seu Cyathulae*
Gan Cao *Radix Glycyrrhizae uralensis*

FU FANG DAN SHEN PIAN
Compound-Formula Salvia Tablet

Dan Shen *Radix Salviae miltiorrhizae*
Bing Pian *Borneol*

FU ZI LI ZHONG WAN
Aconitum Regulating the Centre Pill
Gan Jiang *Rhizoma Zingiberis officinalis*
Bai Zhu *Rhizoma Atractylodis macrocephalae*
Dang Shen *Radix Codonopsis pilosulae*
Gan Cao *Radix Glycyrrhizae uralensis*
Fu Zi *Radix Aconiti carmichaeli praeparata*

GAN MAO DAN
Common Cold Pill
Jin Yin Hua *Flos Lonicerae japonicae*
Lian Qiao *Fructus Forsythiae suspensae*
Shan Zhi Zi *Fructus Gardeniae jasminoidis*
Lu Gen *Rhizoma Phragmitis communis*
Chi Shao *Radix Paeoniae rubrae*
Bai Mao Gen *Rhizoma Imperatae cylindricae*
Dan Dou Chi *Semen Sojae praeparatum*
Bo He *Herba Menthae*
Sang Ye *Folium Mori albae*
Jing Jie *Herba seu Flos Schizonepetae tenuifoliae*
Zi Wan *Radix Asteris tatarici*
Jie Geng *Radix Platycodi grandiflori*
Chen Pi *Pericarpium Citri reticulatae*

GE JIE BU SHEN WAN
Gecko Tonifying the Kidneys Pill
Ge Jie *Gecko*
Lu Rong *Cornu Cervi parvum*
Ren Shen *Radix Ginseng*
Huang Qi *Radix Astragali membranacei*
Du Zhong *Cortex Eucommiae ulmoidis*
Gou Shen *Testis et Penis Canis*
Dong Chong Xia Cao *Sclerotium Cordicipitis chinensis*
Gou Qi Zi *Fructus Lycii chinensis*
Fu Ling *Sclerotium Poriae cocos*
Bai Zhu *Rhizoma Atractylodis macrocephalae*

GE JIE DA BU WAN
Gecko Big Tonifying Pill
Ge Jie *Gecko*
Dang Shen *Radix Codonopsis pilosulae*
Huang Qi *Radix Astragali membranacei*
Gou Qi Zi *Fructus Lycii chinensis*
Dang Gui *Radix Angelicae sinensis*
Fu Ling *Sclerotium Poriae cocos*

Shu Di Huang *Radix Rehmanniae glutinosae praeparata*
Nu Zhen Zi *Fructus Ligustri lucidi*
Gan Cao *Radix Glycyrrhizae uralensis*
Shan Yao *Radix Dioscoreae oppositae*
Mu Gua *Fructus Chaenomelis lagenariae*
Gou Qi Zi *Fructus Lycii chinensis*
Ba Ji Tian *Radix Morindae officinalis*
Bai Zhi *Radix Angelicae dahuricae*
Xu Duan *Radix Dipsaci*
Du Zhong *Cortex Eucommiae ulmoidis*
Huang Jing *Rhizoma Polygonati*
Gu Sui Bu *Rhizoma Gusuibu*

GU ZHE CUO SHANG SAN
Fracture and Contusion Powder
Ye Zhu Gu *Cranium Suis Scrofae*
Huang Gua Zi *Semen Cucumeris sativae*
Dang Gui *Radix Angelicae sinensis*
Hong Hua *Flos Carthami tinctorii*
Xue Jie *Sangui Draconis*
Da Huang *Rhizoma Rhei*
Ru Xiang *Gummi Olibanum*
Mo Yao *Myrrha*
Di Bie Chong *Eupolyphaga sue opishoplatia*

GUA LOU PIAN
Trichosanthes Tablet
Gua Lou *Semen Trichosanthis*

GUAN JIE YAN WAN
Arthritis Pill
Xi Xian Cao *Herba Siegesbeckiae orientalis*
Cang Zhu *Rhizoma Atractylodis lanceae*
Yi Yi Ren *Semen Coicis lachryma jobi*
Fang Ji *Radix Stephaniae tetrandae*
Huai Niu Xi *Radix Achyranthis bidentatae*
Qin Jiao *Radix Gentianae macrophyllae*
Rou Gui *Cortex Cinnamomi cassiae*
Sheng Jiang *Rhizoma Zingiberis officinalis recens*
Ma Huang *Herba Ephedrae*
Du Huo *Radix Angelicae pubescentis*

GUAN XIN SU HE WAN
Styrax Coronary Pill
Su He Xiang *Styrax liquidis*
Bing Pian *Borneol*
Tan Xiang *Lignum Santali albi*
Ru Xiang *Gummi Olibanum*
Mu Hu Die *Semen Oroxyli indici*

GUI PI WAN
Tonifying the Spleen Pill
Dang Shen *Radix Codonopsis pilosulae*
Huang Qi *Radix Astragali membranacei*
Bai Zhu *Rhizoma Atractylodis macrocephalae*
Fu Shen *Sclerotium Poriae cocos pararadicis*
Suan Zao Ren *Semen Ziziphi spinosae*
Yuan Zhi *Radix Polygalae tenuifoliae*
Dang Gui *Radix Angelicae sinensis*
Mu Xiang *Radix Saussureae*
Gan Cao *Radix Glycyrrhizae uralensis*
Long Yan Rou *Arillus Euphoriae longanae*

HE CHE DA ZAO WAN
Placenta Great Fortifying Pill
Gui Ban *Plastrum Testudinis*
Shu Di Huang *Radix Rehmanniae glutinosae praeparata*
Dang Shen *Radix Codonopsis pilosulae*
Huang Bo *Cortex Phellodendri*
Du Zhong *Cortex Eucommiae ulmoidis*
Zi He Che *Placenta hominis*
Niu Xi *Radix Achyranthis bidentatae seu Cyathulae*
Tian Men Dong *Tuber Asparagi cochinchinensis*
Mai Men Dong *Tuber Ophiopogonis japonici*
Fu Ling *Sclerotium Poriae cocos*
Sha Ren *Fructus seu Semen Amomi*

HU PO DUO MEI WAN
Succinum Good Sleep Pill
Hu Po *Succinum*
Yuan Zhi *Radix Polygalae tenuifoliae*
Fu Ling *Sclerotium Poriae cocos*
Dang Shen *Radix Codonopsis pilosulae*
Gan Cao *Radix Glycyrrhizae uralensis*
Ling Yang Jiao *Cornu Antelopis*

HUANG LIAN SHANG QING WAN (PIAN)
Coptis Upward-Clearing Pill (Tablet)
Huang Lian *Rhizoma Coptidis*
Chuan Xiong *Radix Ligustici wallichii*
Jing Jie *Herba seu Flos Schizonepetae tenuifoliae*
Fang Feng *Radix Ledebouriellae sesloidis*
Huang Qin *Radix Scutellariae baicalensis*
Jie Geng *Radix Platycodi grandiflori*
Shi Gao *Gypsum fibrosum*
Ju Hua *Flos Chrysanthemi morifolii*
Bai Zhi *Radix Angelicae dahuricae*
Gan Cao *Radix Glycyrrhizae uralensis*

Da Huang *Rhizoma Rhei*
Man Jing Zi *Fructus Viticis*
Lian Qiao *Fructus Forsythiae suspensae*
Xuan Fu Hua *Flos Inulae*
Huang Bo *Cortex Phellodendri*
Bo He *Herba Menthae*
Zhi Zi *Fructus Gardeniae jasminoidis*

HUANG LIAN YANG GAN WAN
Coptis-Goat's Liver Pill
Huang Lian *Rhizoma Coptidis*
Mi Meng Hua *Flos Buddleiae officinalis*
Jue Ming Zi *Semen Cassiae torae*
Shi Jue Ming *Concha Haliotidis*
Chong Wei Zi *Semen Leonori heterophylli*
Ye Ming Sha *Excrementum Vespertilionis*
Long Dan Cao *Radix Gentianae scabrae*
Huang Bo *Cortex Phellodendri*
Huang Qin *Radix Scutellariae baicalensis*
Hu Huang Lian *Radix Picrorhizae*
Chai Hu *Radix Bupleuri*
Qing Pi *Pericarpium Citri reticulatae viridae*
Mu Zei *Herba Equiseti hieinalis*
Yang Gan *Iecur Caprae seu Ovis*

HUO DAN WAN
Agastache-Bile Pill
Huo Xiang *Herba Agastachis*
Zhu Dan *Pig's bile*

HUO XIANG ZHENG QI WAN
Agastache Upright Qi Pill
Huo Xiang *Herba Agastachis*
Zi Su Ye *Folium Perillae frutescentis*
Bai Zhi *Radix Angelicae dahuricae*
Ban Xia *Rhizoma Pinelliae ternatae*
Chen Pi *Pericarpium Citri reticulatae*
Bai Zhu *Rhizoma Atractylodis macrocephalae*
Fu Ling *Sclerotium Poriae cocos*
Hou Po *Cortex Magnoliae officinalis*
Da Fu Pi *Pericarpium Arecae catechu*
Jie Geng *Radix Platycodi grandiflori*
Sheng Jiang *Rhizoma Zingiberis officinalis recens*
Da Zao *Fructus Ziziphi jujubae*
Zhi Gan Cao *Radix Glycyrrhizae uralensis praeparata*

HUANG LIAN SU PIAN
Coptis Extract Tablet
Huang Lian *Rhizoma Coptidis*

JI GU CAO WAN
Abrum Pill
Ji Gu Cao *Fructus Abri*
She Dan *Snake's bile*
Zhen Zhu *Margarita*
Niu Huang *Calculus Bovis*
Dang Gui *Radix Angelicae sinensis*
Gou Qi Zi *Fructus Lycii chinensis*
Dan Shen *Radix Salviae miltiorrhizae*

JI XUE TENG QIN GAO PIAN
Millettia Liquid Extract Tablet
Ji Xue Teng *Caulis Millettiae seu Caulis Spatholobi*

JIA WEI XIANG LIAN PIAN
Supplemented Saussurea and Coptis Tablet
Mu Xiang *Radix Saussureae*
Bing Lang *Semen Arecae catechu*
Zhi Ke *Fructus Citri aurantii*
Hou Po *Cortex Magnoliae officinalis*
Wu Zhu Yu *Fructus Evodiae rutaecarpae*
Huang Lian *Rhizoma Coptidis*
Huang Bo *Cortex Phellodendri*
Huang Qin *Radix Scutellariae baicalensis*
Yan Hu Suo *Rhizoma Corydalis yanhusuo*
Bai Shao *Radix Paeoniae albae*
Dang Gui *Radix Angelicae sinensis*
Gan Cao *Radix Glycyrrhizae uralensis*

JIAN BU HU QIAN WAN
Vigorous Walk [like] Stealthy Tiger Pill
Mu Gua *Fructus Chaenomelis lagenariae*
Huai Niu Xi *Radix Achyranthis bidentatae*
Hu Gu *Os Tigris*
Qin Jiao *Radix Gentianae macrophyllae*
Dang Gui *Radix Angelicae sinensis*
Ren Shen *Radix Ginseng*
Feng Mi *Mel*

JIAN NAO WAN
Strengthening the Brain Pill
Suan Zao Ren *Semen Ziziphi spinosae*
Shan Yao *Rhizoma Dioscoreae oppositae*
Rou Cong Rong *Herba Cistanchis*
Wu Wei Zi *Fructus Schisandrae chinensis*
Hu Po *Succinum*
Long Chi *Dens Draconis*
Tian Ma *Rhizoma Gastrodiae elatae*
Ren Shen *Radix Ginseng*

Dang Gui *Radix Angelicae sinensis*
Gou Qi Zi *Fructus Lycii chinensis*
Yi Zhi Ren *Fructus Alpiniae oxyphyllae*
Tian Zhu Huang *Concretio Siliceae Bambusae*
Jiu Jie Chang Pu *Rhizoma Anemonis altaicae*
Zhu Sha *Cinnabaris*
Bai Zi Ren *Semen Biotae orientalis*

JIAN PI WAN
Strengthening the Spleen Pill
Dang Shen *Radix Codonopsis pilosulae*
Shan Zha *Fructus Crataegi*
Bai Zhu *Rhizoma Atractylodis macrocephalae*
Zhi Shi *Fructus Citri aurantii immaturus*
Chen Pi *Pericarpium Citri reticulatae*
Mai Ya *Fructus Hordei vulgaris germinatus*

JIANG YA WAN
Lowering [Blood] Pressure Pill
Yi Mu Cao *Herba Leonori heterophylli*
Huai Niu Xi *Radix Achyranthis bidentatae*
Sheng Di Huang *Radix Rehmanniae glutinosae*
E Jiao *Gelatinum Corii Asini*
Dang Gui *Radix Angelicae sinensis*
Gou Teng *Ramulus Uncariae*
Chen Xiang *Lignum Aquilariae*
Chuan Xiong *Radix Ligustici wallichii*
Xia Ku Cao *Spica Prunellae vulgaris*
Mu Dan Pi *Cortex Moutan radicis*
Tian Ma *Rhizoma Gastrodiae elatae*
Da Huang *Rhizoma Rhei*
Hu Po *Succinum*
Huang Lian *Rhizoma Coptidis*
Ling Yang Jiao *Cornu Antelopis*

JIE JIE WAN
Dispel Swelling Pill
Sheng Di Huang *Radix Rehmanniae glutinosae*
Huang Qi *Radix Astragali membranacei*
Dang Shen *Radix Codonopsis pilosulae*
Nu Zhen Zi *Fructus Ligustri lucidi*
Che Qian Zi *Semen Plantaginis*
Huai Niu Xi *Radix Achyranthis bidentatae*
Dan Shen *Radix Salviae miltiorrhizae*
Ze Xie *Rhizoma Alismatis orientalis*
Tu Si Zi *Semen Cuscutae*
Sang Piao Xiao *Ootheca Mantidis*

JIN GU DIE SHANG WAN
Muscle and Bone Traumatic Injury Pill

San Qi *Radix Notoginseng*
Xue Jie *Sanguis Draconis*
Dang Gui *Radix Angelicae sinensis*
Ru Xiang *Gummi Olibanum*
Mo Yao *Myrrha*
Hong Hua *Flos Carthami tinctorii*

JIN GUI SHEN QI WAN
Golden Chest Kidney-Qi Pill
Gui Zhi *Ramulus Cinnamomi cassiae* (or Rou Gui *Cortex Cinnamomi cassiae*)
Fu Zi *Radix Aconiti carmichaeli praeparata*
Shu Di Huang *Radix Rehmanniae glutinosae praeparata*
Shan Yao *Radix Dioscoreae oppositae*
Shan Zhu Yu *Fructus Corni officinalis*
Ze Xie *Rhizoma Alismatis orientalis*
Fu Ling *Sclerotium Poriae cocos*
Mu Dan Pi *Cortex Moutan radicis*

JIN SUO GU JING WAN
Golden Lock Consolidating the Essence Pill
Qian Shi *Semen Euryales ferocis*
Lian Xu *Stamen Nelumbinis nuciferae*
Long Gu *Os Draconis* (calcined)
Mu Li *Concha Ostreae* (calcined)
Lian Zi *Semen Nelumbinis nuciferae*
Sha Yuan Ji Li *Semen Astragali membranacei*

KANG NING WAN
Health and Quiet Pill
Tian Ma *Rhizoma Gastrodiae elatae*
Bai Zhi *Radix Angelicae dahuricae*
Ju Hua *Flos Chrysanthemi morifolii*
Bo He *Herba Menthae*
Ge Gen *Radix Puerariae*
Tian Hua Fen *Radix Trichosanthis*
Cang Zhu *Rhizoma Atractylodis lanceae*
Yi Yi Ren *Semen Coicis lachryma jobi*
Fu Ling *Sclerotium Poriae cocos*
Mu Xiang *Radix Saussureae*
Hou Po *Cortex Magnoliae officinalis*
Chen Pi *Pericarpium Citri reticulatae*
Shen Qu *Massa Fermentata Medicinalis*
Huo Xiang *Herba Agastachis*
Gu Ya *Fructus Oryzae sativae germinatus*

LI DAN PIAN
Benefiting the Gall-Bladder Tablet

Huang Qin *Radix Scutellariae baicalensis*
Mu Xiang *Radix Saussureae*
Jin Qian Cao *Herba Desmodii styracifolii*
Jin Yin Hua *Flos Lonicerae japonicae*
Yin Chen Hao *Herba Artemisiae capillaris*
Chai Hu *Radix Bupleuri*
Da Qing Ye *Folium Isatidis seu Baphicacanthi*
Da Huang *Rhizoma Rhei*

LI FEI WAN
Benefiting the Lungs Pill
Dong Chong Xia Cao *Sclerotium Cordicipitis chinensis*
Ge Jie *Gecko*
Bai He *Bulbus Lilii*
Wu Wei Zi *Fructus Schisandrae chinensis*
Bai Ji *Rhizoma Bletillae striatae*
Bai Bu *Radix Stemonae*
Mu Li *Concha Ostreae*
Pi Pa Ye *Folium Eriobotryae japonicae*
Gan Cao *Radix Glycyrrhizae uralensis*

LI GAN PIAN
Benefiting the Liver Tablet
Jia Qian Cao *Herba Desmodii styracifolii*
Niu Dan *Fellis Bovis*

LI ZHONG WAN
Regulating the Centre Pill
Gan Jiang *Rhizoma Zingiberis officinalis*
Bai Zhu *Rhizoma Atractylodis macrocephalae*
Dang Shen *Radix Codonopsis pilosulae*
Gan Cao *Radix Glycyrrhizae uralensis*

LIAN QIAO BAI DU PIAN
Forsythia Expelling Poison Tablet
Lian Qiao *Fructus Forsythiae suspensae*
Jin Yin Hua *Flos Lonicerae japonicae*
Fang Feng *Radix Ledebouriellae sesloidis*
Bai Xian Pi *Cortex Radicis Dictami dasycarpi*
Chan Tui *Periostracum Cicadae*
Chi Shao *Radix Paeoniae rubrae*
Da Huang *Rhizoma Rhei*
Huang Qin *Radix Scutellariae baicalensis*
Zhi Zi *Fructus Gardeniae jasminoidis*

LING YANG SHANG FENG LING
Cornu Antelopis Influenza Formula
Ling Yang Jiao *Cornu Antelopis*

Tian Hua Fen *Radix Trichosanthis*
Lian Qiao *Fructus Forsythiae suspensae*
Zhu Yu *Herba Lophatheri gracilis*
Jing Jie *Herba seu Flos Schizonepetae tenuifoliae*
Ge Gen *Radix Puerariae*
Gan Cao *Radix Glycyrrhizae uralensis*
Jin Yin Hua *Flos Lonicerae japonicae*
Niu Bang Zi *Fructus Arctii lappae*
Bo He *Herba Menthae*

LING ZHI PIAN
Ganoderma Tablet
Ling Zhi *Fructus Ganodermae lucidi*

LIU JUN ZI WAN
Six Gentlemen Pill
Dang Shen *Radix Codonopsis pilosulae*
Bai Zhu *Rhizoma Atractylodis macrocephalae*
Fu Ling *Sclerotium Poriae cocos*
Zhi Gan Cao *Radix Glycyrrhizae uralensis praeparata*
Chen Pi *Pericarpium Citri reticulatae*
Ban Xia *Rhizoma Pinelliae ternatae*

LIU WEI DI HUANG WAN
Six-Ingredient Rehmannia Pill
Shu Di Huang *Radix Rehmanniae glutinosae praeparata*
Shan Yao *Radix Dioscoreae oppositae*
Shan Zhu Yu *Fructus Corni officinalis*
Ze Xie *Rhizoma Alismatis orientalis*
Fu Ling *Sclerotium Poriae cocos*
Mu Dan Pi *Cortex Moutan radicis*

LONG DAN XIE GAN WAN
Gentiana Draining the Liver Pill
Long Dan Cao *Radix Gentianae scabrae*
Huang Qin *Radix Scutellariae baicalensis*
Shan Zhi Zi *Fructus Gardeniae jasminoidis*
Ze Xie *Rhizoma Alismatis orientalis*
Mu Tong *Caulis Akebiae*
Che Qian Zi *Semen Plantaginis*
Sheng Di Huang *Radix Rehmanniae glutinosae*
Dang Gui *Radix Angelicae sinensis*
Chai Hu *Radix Bupleuri*
Gan Cao *Radix Glycyrrhizae uralensis*

MA XING ZHI KE PIAN
Ephedra-Prunus Cough Tablet
Ma Huang *Herba Ephedrae*

Xing Ren *Semen Pruni armeniacae*
Shi Gao *Gypsum fibrosum*
Gan Cao *Radix Glycyrrhizae uralensis*
Jie Geng *Radix Platycodi grandiflori*
Chen Pi *Pericarpium Citri reticulatae*
Hua Shi *Talcum*
Feng Mi *Honey*

MING MU SHANG QING PIAN
Brightening the Eyes Clearing Upward Tablet
Shan Zhi Zi *Fructus Gardeniae jasminoidis*
Dang Gui *Radix Angelicae sinensis*
Huang Lian *Rhizoma Coptidis*
Ju Hua *Flos Chrysanthemi morifolii*
Da Huang *Rhizoma Rhei*
Huang Qin *Radix Scutellariae baicalensis*
Lian Qiao *Fructus Forsythiae suspensae*
Bai Ji Li *Fructus Tribuli terrestris*
Chan Tui *Periostracum Cicadae*
Mai Dong *Tuber Ophiopogonis japonici*
Shi Gao *Gypsum fibrosum*

MU XIANG SHUN QI WAN
Saussurea Subduing Qi Pill
Mu Xiang *Radix Saussureae*
Bai Dou Kou *Fructus Amomi cardamomi*
Cang Zhu *Rhizoma Atractylodis lanceae*
Sheng Jiang *Rhizoma Zingiberis officinalis recens*
Qing Pi *Pericarpium Citri reticulatae viridae*
Chen Pi *Pericarpium Citri reticulatae*
Fu Ling *Sclerotium Poriae cocos*
Chai Hu *Radix Bupleuri*
Hou Po *Cortex Magnoliae officinalis*
Bing Lang *Semen Arecae catechu*
Zhi Ke *Fructus Citri aurantii*
Wu Yao *Radix Lynderae strychnifoliae*
Lai Fu Zi *Semen Raphani sativi*
Shan Zha *Fructus Crataegi*
Shen Qu *Massa Fermentata Medicinalis*
Mai Ya *Fructus Hordei vulgaris germinatus*
Gan Cao *Radix Glycyrrhizae uralensis*

NAN XING BU SHEN WAN
Male Gender Tonifying the Kidneys Pill
Shu Di Huang *Radix Rehmanniae glutinosae praeparata*
Shan Yao *Radix Dioscoreae oppositae*
Shan Zhu Yu *Fructus Corni officinalis*
Ze Xie *Rhizoma Alismatis orientalis*

Fu Ling *Sclerotium Poriae cocos*
Mu Dan Pi *Cortex Moutan radicis*
Rou Gui *Cortex Cinnamomi cassiae*
Fu Zi *Radix Aconiti carmichaeli praeparata*
Wu Wei Zi *Fructus Schisandrae chinensis*
Che Qian Zi *Semen Plantaginis*

NAO LI QING
Brain Erecting and Clearing
Ci Shi *Magnetitum*
Dai Zhe Shi *Haematitum*
Ban Xia *Rhizoma Pinelliae ternatae*
Bing Pian *Borneol*
Zhen Zhu Mu *Concha margaritiferae*
Niu Xi *Radix Achyranthis bidentatae seu Cyathulae*
Bo He *Herba Menthae*

NIU HUANG JIANG YA WAN
Calculus Bovis Lowering [Blood] Pressure Pill
Ling Yang Jiao *Cornu Antelopis*
Niu Huang *Calculus Bovis*
Zhen Zhu *Margarita*
Bing Pian *Borneol*
Yu Jin *Tuber Curcumae*
Huang Qi *Radix Astragali membranacei*

NIU HUANG JIE DU PIAN
Calculus Bovis Resolving Poison Tablet
Da Huang *Rhizoma Rhei*
Shi Gao *Gypsum fibrosum*
Huang Qin *Radix Scutellariae baicalensis*
Jie Geng *Radix Platycodi grandiflori*
Gan Cao *Radix Glycyrrhizae uralensis*
Bing Pian *Borneol*
Niu Huang *Calculus Bovis*

PING CHUAN WAN
Calming Breathlessness Pill
Dang Shen *Radix Codonopsis pilosulae*
Dong Chong Xia Cao *Sclerotium Cordicipitis chinensis*
Ge Jie *Gecko*
Xing Ren *Semen Pruni armeniacae*
Chen Pi *Pericarpium Citri reticulatae*
Gan Cao *Radix Glycyrrhizae uralensis*
Sang Bai Pi *Cortex Radicis Mori albae*
Bai Qian *Radix et Rhizoma Cynanchii stautoni*
Meng Shi *Lapis Chloritis*
Wu Zhi Mao Tao *Radix Fici simplicissimae*
Man Hu Tui Zi *Semen Elaeagni glabrae thunbergii*

PING WEI PIAN
Balancing the Stomach Tablet
Cang Zhu *Rhizoma Atractylodis lanceae*
Chen Pi *Pericarpium Citri reticulatae*
Hou Po *Cortex Magnoliae officinalis*
Zhi Gan Cao *Radix Glycyrrhizae uralensis praeparata*
Sheng Jiang *Rhizoma Zingiberis officinalis recens*
Da Zao *Fructus Ziziphi jujubae*

QI GUAN YAN KE SOU TAN CHUAN WAN
Bronchial Cough, Phlegm and Dyspnoea Pill
Qian Hu *Radix Peucedani*
Xing Ren *Semen Pruni armeniacae*
Yuan Zhi *Radix Polygalae tenuifoliae*
Sang Ye *Folium Mori albae*
Chuan Bei Mu *Bulbus Fritillariae cirrhosae*
Chen Pi *Pericarpium Citri reticulatae*
Pi Pa Ye *Folium Eriobotryae japonicae*
Kuan Dong Hua *Flos Tussilaginis farfarae*
Dang Shen *Radix Codonopsis pilosulae*
Ma Dou Ling *Fructus Aristolochiae*
Wu Wei Zi *Fructus Schisandrae chinensis*
Sheng Jiang *Rhizoma Zingiberis officinalis recens*
Da Zao *Fructus Ziziphi jujubae*

QI JU DI HUANG WAN
Lycium-Chrysanthemum-Rehmannia Pill
Gou Qi Zi *Fructus Lycii chinensis*
Ju Hua *Flos Chrysanthemi morifolii*
Shu Di Huang *Radix Rehmanniae glutinosae praeparata*
Shan Yao *Radix Dioscoreae oppositae*
Shan Zhu Yu *Fructus Corni officinalis*
Ze Xie *Rhizoma Alismatis orientalis*
Fu Ling *Sclerotium Poriae cocos*
Mu Dan Pi *Cortex Moutan radicis*

QI XING CHA
Seven Stars Tea
Zhu Ye *Herba Lophatheri gracilis*
Gou Teng *Ramulus Uncariae*
Chan Tui *Periostracum Cicadae*
Shan Zha *Fructus Crataegi*
Gu Ya *Fructus Oryzae sativae germinatus*
Yi Yi Ren *Semen Coicis lachryma jobi*
Gan Cao *Radix Glycyrrhizae uralensis*

QIAN JIN ZHI DAI WAN
Thousand Gold Pieces Stopping Leukorrhoea Pill

Da Qing Ye *Folium Isatidis seu Baphicacanthi*
Dang Shen *Radix Codonopsis pilosulae*
Mu Li *Concha Ostreae*
Mu Xiang *Radix Saussureae*
Dang Gui *Radix Angelicae sinensis*
Yan Hu Suo *Rhizoma Corydalis yanhusuo*
Xu Duan *Radix Dipsaci*
Bai Zhu *Rhizoma Atractylodis macrocephalae*
Xiao Hui Xiang *Fructus Foeniculi vulgaris*

QIAN LIE XIAN WAN
Prostate Gland Pill
Wang Bu Liu Xing *Semen Vaccariae segetalis*
Mu Dan Pi *Cortex Moutan radicis*
Chi Shao *Radix Paeoniae rubrae*
Huang Qi *Radix Astragali membranacei*
Bai Jiang *Herba Patriniae seu Thlaspi*
Qian Hu *Radix Peucedani*
Gan Cao *Radix Glycyrrhizae uralensis*
Mu Xiang *Radix Saussureae*
Mu Tong *Caulis Akebiae*

QING FEI YI HUO PIAN
Clearing the Lungs and Eliminating Fire Tablet
Huang Qin *Radix Scutellariae baicalensis*
Shan Zhi Zi *Fructus Gardeniae jasminoidis*
Da Huang *Rhizoma Rhei*
Qian Hu *Radix Peucedani*
Ku Shen *Radix Sophorae flavescentis*
Tian Hua Fen *Radix Trichosanthis*
Jie Geng *Radix Platycodi grandiflori*
Zhi Mu *Radix Anemarrhenae asphodeloidis*

QING QI HUA TAN WAN
Clearing Qi and Resolving Phlegm Pill
Dan Nan Xing *Rhizoma Arisaematis praeparata*
Gua Lou *Semen Trichosanthis*
Huang Qin *Radix Scutellariae baicalensis*
Zhi Shi *Fructus Citri aurantii immaturus*
Chen Pi *Pericarpium Citri reticulatae*
Fu Ling *Sclerotium Poriae cocos*
Xing Ren *Semen Pruni armeniacae*
Ban Xia *Rhizoma Pinelliae ternatae*

QIU LI GAO
Autumn Pear Syrup
Qiu Li *Fructus Pyri*
Mai Men Dong *Tuber Ophiopogonis japonici*
Zhe Bei Mu *Bulbus Fritillariae thunbergii*

Ou Jie *Nodus Nelumbinis neciferae rhizomatis*
Qing Luo Bo *Green turnip*

QUAN LU WAN
Whole-Deer Pill
Lu Rou *Caro Cervi*
Lu Rong *Cornu Cervi parvum*
Lu Wei *Penis et testis Cervi*
Lu Shen *Renes Cervi*
Lu Jiao Jiao *Colla Cornu Cervi*
Ren Shen *Radix Ginseng*
Bai Zhu *Rhizoma Atractylodis macrocephalae*
Fu Ling *Sclerotium Poriae cocos*
Gan Cao *Radix Glycyrrhizae uralensis*
Dang Gui *Radix Angelicae sinensis*
Chuan Xiong *Radix Ligustici wallichii*
Shu Di Huang *Radix Rehmanniae glutinosae praeparata*
Huang Qi *Radix Astragali membranacei*
Gou Qi Zi *Fructus Lycii chinensis*
Du Zhong *Cortex Eucommiae ulmoidis*
Niu Xi *Radix Achyranthis bidentatae seu Cyathulae*
Xu Duan *Radix Dipsaci*
Rou Cong Rong *Herba Cistanchis*
Suo Yang *Herba Cynomorii songarici*
Bai Ji Tian *Radix Morindae officinalis*
Tian Men Dong *Tuber Asparagi cochinchinensis*
Mai Men Dong *Tuber Ophiopogonis japonici*
Wu Wei Zi *Fructus Schisandrae chinensis*
Chen Xiang *Lignum Aquilariae*
Chen Pi *Pericarpium Citri reticulatae*

REN SHEN JIAN PI WAN
Ginseng Strengthening the Spleen Pill
Ren Shen *Radix Ginseng*
Bai Zhu *Rhizoma Atractylodis macrocephalae*
Zhi Shi *Fructus Citri aurantii immaturus*
Shan Zha *Fructus Crataegi*
Chen Pi *Pericarpium Citri reticulatae*
Mai Ya *Fructus Hordei vulgaris germinatus*

REN SHEN LU RONG WAN
Ginseng-Cornu Cervi Pill
Ren Shen *Radix Ginseng*
Du Zhong *Cortex Eucommiae ulmoidis*
Ba Ji Tian *Radix Morindae officinalis*
Huang Qi *Radix Astragali membranacei*
Lu Rong *Cornu Cervi parvum*
Dang Gui *Radix Angelicae sinensis*

Niu Xi *Radix Achyranthis bidentatae seu Cyathulae*
Long Yan Rou *Arillus Euphoriae longanae*

REN SHEN ZAI ZAO WAN
Ginseng Renewal Pill
Ren Shen *Radix Ginseng*
Huang Qi *Radix Astragali membranacei*
Shu Di Huang *Radix Rehmanniae glutinosae praeparata*
Shou Wu *Radix Polygoni multiflori*
Gui Ban *Plastrum Testudinis*
Hu Gu *Os Tigris*
Gu Sui Bu *Rhizoma Gusuibu*
Quan Xie *Buthus Martensi*
Di Long *Pheretima aspergillum*
Tian Ma *Rhizoma Gastrodiae elatae*
Jiang Can *Bombyx batryticatus*
Qi She Rou *Agkistrodon*
Sang Ji Sheng *Ramus Loranthi*
Bi Xie *Rhizoma Dioscoreae hypoglaucae*
Song Jie *Lignum Pini nodi*
Wei Ling Xian *Radix Clematidis chinensis*
Ma Huang *Herba Ephedrae*
Xi Xin *Herba Asari cum radice*
Fang Feng *Radix Ledebouriellae sesloidis*
Qiang Huo *Radix et Rhizoma Notopterygii*
Bai Zhi *Radix Angelicae dahuricae*
Ge Gen *Radix Puerariae*
Qing Pi *Pericarpium Citri reticulatae viridae*
Ding Xiang *Flos Caryophylli*
Xuan Shen *Radix Scrophulariae ningpoensis*
Da Huang *Rhizoma Rhei*
Hong Qu *Semen Oryzae cum Monasco*
Huang Lian *Rhizoma Coptidis*
Zhu Sha *Cinnabaris*
Tan Xiang *Lignum Santali albi*
Jiang Huang *Rhizoma Curcumae longae*
Huo Xiang *Herba Agastachis*
Chi Shao *Radix Paeoniae rubrae*
Fu Zi *Radix Aconiti carmichaeli praeparata*
Rou Gui *Cortex Cinnamomi cassiae*
Chuan Xiong *Radix Ligustici wallichii*
Chen Xiang *Lignum Aquilariae*
Wu Yao *Radix Linderae strychnifoliae*
Xiang Fu *Rhizoma Cyperi rotundi*
Xue Jie *Sanguis draconis*
Ru Xiang *Gummi Olibanum*
Mo Yao *Myrrha*
San Qi *Radix Notoginseng*

Dang Gui *Radix Angelicae sinensis*
Chen Pi *Pericarpium Citri reticulatae*
Bai Zhu *Rhizoma Atractylodis macrocephalae*
Fu Ling *Sclerotium Poriae cocos*
Gan Cao *Radix Glycyrrhizae uralensis*
Dou Kou *Semen Alpiniae katsumadai*
Shen Qu *Massa Fermentata Medicinalis*
Niu Huang *Calculus Bovis*
Shui Niu Jiao *Cornu Bufali*
Tian Zhu Huang *Secretio Siliceae Bambusae*
Bing Pian *Borneol*
She Xiang *Secretio Moschus moschiferi*

REN SHEN ZAI ZAO WAN (2)
Ginseng Renewal Pill
Chuan Shan Jia *Squama Manitis pentadactylae*
Wu Xiao She *Zaocys Dhumnades*
Quan Xie *Buthus Martensi*
Ren Shen *Radix Ginseng*
Hu Po *Succinum*
Hu Gu *Os Tigris*
Tian Ma *Rhizoma Gastrodiae elatae*
Shui Niu Jiao *Cornu Bufali*
Niu Huang *Calculus Bovis*

RUN CHANG WAN
Moistening the Intestines Pill
Huo Ma Ren *Semen Cannabis sativae*
Tao Ren *Semen Persicae*
Qiang Huo *Radix et Rhizoma Notopterygii*
Dang Gui *Radix Angelicae sinensis*
Da Huang *Rhizoma Rhei*

SAI MEI AN
Race [between] Rot and Peaceful [Health]
Ge Ke *Concha Cyclinae*
Han Shui Shi *Calcitum*
Wa Leng Zi *Concha Arcae*
Fu Long Gan *Terra Flava usta*
Bing Pian *Borneol*
Zhong Ju *Stalactitum*
Zhen Zhu *Margarita*

SANG JU GAN MAO PIAN
Morus-Chrysanthemum Common Cold Tablet
Sang Ye *Folium Mori albae*
Ju Hua *Flos Chrysanthemi morifolii*
Bo He *Herba Menthae*
Xing Ren *Semen Pruni armeniacae*

Jie Geng *Radix Platycodi grandiflori*
Lian Qiao *Fructus Forsythiae suspensae*
Lu Gen *Rhizoma Phragmitis communis*
Gan Cao *Radix Glycyrrhizae uralensis*

SHEN LING BAI ZHU WAN (PIAN)
Ginseng-Poria-Atractylodes Pill (Tablet)
Ren Shen *Radix Ginseng* (or Dang Shen *Radix Codonopsis pilosulae*)
Fu Ling *Sclerotium Poriae cocos*
Bai Zhu *Rhizoma Atractylodis macrocephalae*
Jie Geng *Radix Platycodi grandiflori*
Shan Yao *Radix Dioscoreae oppositae*
Chen Pi *Pericarpium Citri reticulatae*
Sha Ren *Fructus seu Semen Amomi*
Lian Zi *Semen Nelumbinis nuciferae*
Bian Dou *Semen Dolichoris lablab*
Yi Yi Ren *Semen Coicis lachryma jobi*
Zhi Gan Cao *Radix Glycyrrhizae uralensis praeparata*

SHEN QU CHA
Massa Fermentata Tea
Qing Hao *Herba Artemisiae apiaceae*
Huang Qin *Radix Scutellariae baicalensis*
Xiang Ru *Herba Elsholtziae splendentis*
Qiang Huo *Radix et Rhizoma Notopterygii*
Du Huo *Radix Angelicae pubescentis*
Qing Pi *Pericarpium Citri reticulatae viridae*
Hu Po *Succinum*
Cao Guo *Fructus Amomi Tsaoko*
Mu Gua *Fructus Chaenomelis lagenariae*
Jie Geng *Radix Platycodi grandiflori*
Shan Yao *Radix Dioscoreae oppositae*
Fu Ling *Sclerotium Poriae cocos*
Gan Cao *Radix Glycyrrhizae uralensis*
Shen Qu *Massa Fermentata Medicinalis*

SHEN RONG HU GU WAN
Ginseng-Cornu Cervi-Os Tigris Pill
Ren Shen *Radix Ginseng*
Lu Rong *Cornu Cervi parvum*
Dang Gui *Radix Angelicae sinensis*
Hu Gu *Os Tigris*
Fang Ji *Radix Stephaniae tetrandae*
Fang Feng *Radix Ledebouriellae sesloidis*

SHI QUAN DA BU WAN
Ten Complete Great Tonification Pill
Ba Zhen Wan *Eight Precious Pill*

Huang Qi *Radix Astragali membranacei*
Rou Gui *Cortex Cinnamomi cassiae*

SHU GAN WAN
Pacifying the Liver Pill
Chuan Lian Zi *Fructus Meliae toosendan*
Jiang Huang *Rhizoma Curcumae longae*
Chen Xiang *Lignum Aquilariae*
Yan Hu Suo *Rhizoma Corydalis yanhusuo*
Mu Xiang *Radix Saussureae*
Bai Dou Kou *Fructus Amomi cardamomi*
Bai Shao *Radix Paeoniae albae*
Fu Ling *Sclerotium Poriae cocos*
Zhi Ke *Fructus Citri aurantii*
Chen Pi *Pericarpium Citri reticulatae*
Sha Ren *Fructus seu Semen Amomi*
Hou Po *Cortex Magnoliae officinalis*

SHUANG LIAO HOU FENG SAN
Double-Ingredient Throat-Wind Powder
Niu Huang *Calculus Bovis*
Bing Pian *Borneol*
Gan Cao *Radix Glycyrrhizae uralensis*
Qing Dai *Indigo naturalis*
Zhen Zhu *Margarita*
Huang Lian *Rhizoma Coptidis*
Shan Dou Gen *Radix Sophorae subprostratae*

SU BING DI WAN
Styrax-Borneol Pill
Su He Xiang *Styrax liquidis*
Bing Pian *Borneol*

SU HE XIANG WAN
Styrax Pill
Su He Xiang *Styrax liquidis*

SU ZI JIANG QI WAN
Perilla-seed Descending Qi Pill
Su Zi *Fructus Perillae frutescentis*
Ban Xia *Rhizoma Pinelliae ternatae*
Hou Po *Cortex Magnoliae officinalis*
Qian Hu *Radix Peucedani*
Chen Pi *Pericarpium Citri reticulatae*
Chen Xiang *Lignum Aquilariae*
Dang Gui *Radix Angelicae sinensis*
Sheng Jiang *Rhizoma Zingiberis officinalis recens*
Da Zao *Fructus Ziziphi jujubae*
Gan Cao *Radix Glycyrrhizae uralensis*

SUAN ZAO REN TANG PIAN
Tablet of the Ziziphus Decoction
Suan Zao Ren *Semen Ziziphi spinosae*
Chuan Xiong *Radix Ligustici wallichii*
Fu Ling *Sclerotium Poriae cocos*
Zhi Mu *Rhizoma Anemarrhenae asphodeloidis*
Gan Cao *Radix Glycyrrhizae uralensis*

TE XIAO PAI SHI WAN
Especially-Effective Discharging Stones Pill
Jin Qian Cao *Herba Desmodii styracifolii*
Hai Jin Sha *Spora Lygodii japonici*
Bai Zhi *Radix Angelicae dahuricae*
Chuan Xin Lian *Herba Andrographis paniculatae*
Chuan Niu Xi *Radix Cyathulae*
Wu Hua Guo Gen *Radix Fici*
Huang Lian *Rhizoma Coptidis*
Da Huang *Rhizoma Rhei*
Niu Da Li *Radix Millettiae speciosae*
San Qi *Radix Notoginseng*
Hu Po *Succinum*

TE XIAO YAO TONG LING
Especially-Effective Back-ache Pill
Du Zhong *Cortex Eucommiae ulmoidis*
Ba Ji Tian *Radix Morindae officinalis*
Chuan Xiong *Radix Ligustici wallichii*
Hong Hua *Flos Carthami tinctorii*
Huai Niu Xi *Radix Achyranthis bidentatae*
Qin Jiao *Radix Gentianae macrophyllae*
Shou Wu *Radix Polygoni multiflori*
Du Huo *Radix Angelicae pubescentis*
Sang Ji Sheng *Ramulus Loranthi*
Dang Gui *Radix Angelicae sinensis*
Wei Ling Xian *Radix Clematidis chinensis*

TIAN MA HU GU WAN
Gastrodia-Tiger Bone Pill
Tian Ma *Rhizoma Gastrodiae elatae*
Gao Ben *Rhizoma et Radix Ligustici sinensis*
Hu Gu *Os Tigris*
Chuan Xiong *Radix Ligustici wallichii*
Du Zhong *Cortex Eucommiae ulmoidis*
Dang Gui *Radix Angelicae sinensis*
Ren Shen *Radix Ginseng*

TIAN MA QU FENG BU PIAN
Gastrodia Expelling Wind and Tonifying Tablet
Tian Ma *Rhizoma Gastrodiae elatae*

Dang Gui *Radix Angelicae sinensis*
Sheng Di Huang *Radix Rehmanniae glutinosae*
Rou Gui *Cortex Cinnamomi cassiae*
Huai Niu Xi *Radix Achyranthis bidentatae*
Du Zhong *Cortex Eucommiae ulmoidis*
Qiang Huo *Radix et Rhizoma Notopterygii*
Bai Fu Zi *Rhizoma Thyphonii gigantei*

TIAN MA SHOU WU PIAN
Gastrodia-Polygonum Pill
Tian Ma *Rhizoma Gastrodiae elatae*
Shou Wu *Radix Polygoni multiflori*
Yin Yang Huo *Herba Epimedii*
Ren Shen *Radix Ginseng*

TIAN WANG BU XIN DAN
Heavenly Emperor Tonifying the Heart Pill
Sheng Di Huang *Radix Rehmanniae glutinosae*
Xuan Shen *Radix Scrophulariae ningpoensis*
Mai Men Dong *Tuber Ophiopogonis japonicis*
Tian Men Dong *Tuber Asparagi cochinchinensis*
Ren Shen *Radix Ginseng*
Fu Ling *Sclerotium Poriae cocos*
Wu Wei Zi *Fructus Schisandrae chinensis*
Dang Gui *Radix Angelicae sinensis*
Dan Shen *Radix Salviae miltiorrhizae*
Bai Zi Ren *Semen Biotae orientalis*
Suan Zao Ren *Semen Ziziphi spinosae*
Yuan Zhi *Radix Polygalae tenuifoliae*
Jie Geng *Radix Platycodi grandiflori*

TONG JING WAN
Dysmenorrhoea Pill
Shu Di Huang *Radix Rehmanniae glutinosae praeparata*
Dang Gui *Radix Angelicae sinensis*
Dan Shen *Radix Salviae miltiorrhizae*
Xiang Fu *Rhizoma Cyperi rotundi*
Shan Zha *Fructus Crataegi*
Bai Shao *Radix Paeoniae albae*
Yan Hu Suo *Rhizoma Corydalis yanhusuo*
Wu Ling Zhi *Excrementum Trogopteri*
Chuan Xiong *Radix Ligustici wallichii*
Hong Hua *Flos Carthami tinctorii*
Mu Xiang *Radix Saussureae*
Qing Pi *Pericarpium Citri reticulatae viridae*
Rou Gui *Cortex Cinnamomi cassiae*
Gan Jiang *Rhizoma Zingiberis officinalis*
Yi Mu Cao *Herba Leonori heterophylli*

TONG JING WAN
Penetrating Menses Pill
E Zhu *Rhizoma Curcumae zedoariae*
San Leng *Rhizoma Sparganii*
Chi Shao *Radix Paeoniae rubrae*
Hong Hua *Flos Carthami tinctorii*
Chuan Xiong *Radix Ligustici wallichii*
Dang Gui *Radix Angelicae sinensis*
Dan Shen *Radix Salviae miltiorrhizae*

TONG XUAN LI FEI WAN
Penetrating, Dispersing and Regulating the Lungs Pill
Ma Huang *Herba Ephedrae*
Zhi Ke *Fructus Citri aurantii*
Jie Geng *Radix Platycodi grandiflori*
Fu Ling *Sclerotium Poriae cocos*
Qian Hu *Radix Peucedani*
Huang Qin *Radix Scutellariae baicalensis*
Chen Pi *Pericarpium Citri reticulatae*
Gan Cao *Radix Glycyrrhizae uralensis*
Ban Xia *Rhizoma Pinelliae ternatae*
Xing Ren *Semen Pruni armeniacae*
Zi Su Ye *Folium Perillae frutescentis*

WAN SHI NIU HUANG QING XIN WAN
Wan's Calculus Bovis Clearing the Heart Pill
Niu Huang *Calculus Bovis*
Zhi Zi *Fructus Gardeniae jasminoidis*
Huang Lian *Rhizoma Coptidis*
Huang Qin *Radix Scutellariae baicalensis*
Yu Jin *Tuber Curcumae*
Zhu Sha *Cinnabaris*

WU JIN WAN
Black Gold Pill
Yi Mu Cao *Herba Leonori heterophylli*
San Leng *Rhizoma Sparganii*
E Zhu *Rhizoma Curcumae zedoariae*
Xiang Fu *Rhizoma Cyperi rotundi*
Yan Hu Suo *Rhizoma Corydalis yanhusuo*
Wu Zhu Yu *Fructus Evodiae rutaecarpae*
Xiao Hui Xiang *Fructus Foeniculi vulgaris*
Mu Xiang *Radix Saussureae*
Bai Shao *Radix Paeoniae albae*
Chuan Xiong *Radix Ligustici wallichii*
Dang Gui *Radix Angelicae sinensis*
Shu Di Huang *Radix Rehmanniae glutinosae praeparata*

Bu Gu Zhi *Fructus Psoraleae corylifoliae*
Pu Huang *Pollen Typhae*
Ai Ye Tan *Folium Artemisiae carbonisatum*

WU LING SAN
Five "Ling" Powder
Bai Zhu *Rhizoma Atractylodis macrocephalae*
Fu Ling *Sclerotium Poriae cocos*
Zhu Ling *Sclerotium Polypori umbellati*
Ze Xie *Rhizoma Alismatis orientalis*
Gui Zhi *Ramulus Cinnamomi cassiae*

WU SHI CHA
Midday Tea
Huo Xiang *Herba Agastachis*
Bai Zhi *Radix Angelicae dahuricae*
Zi Su Ye *Folium Perillae frutescentis*
Fang Feng *Radix Ledebouriellae sesloidis*
Qiang Huo *Radix et Rhizoma Notopterygii*
Chai Hu *Radix Bupleuri*
Zhi Shi *Fructus Citri aurantii immaturus*
Chen Pi *Pericarpium Citri reticulatae*
Shan Zha *Fructus Crataegi*
Mai Ya *Fructus Hordei vulgaris germinatus*
Shen Qu *Massa Fermentata Medicinalis*
Hou Po *Cortex Magnoliae officinalis*
Cang Zhu *Rhizoma Atractylodis lanceae*
Qian Hu *Radix Peucedani*
Jie Geng *Radix Platycodi grandiflori*
Gan Cao *Radix Glycyrrhizae uralensis*
Hong Cha *Black tea*

XI HUANG WAN
Rhinoceros-Calculus Bovis Pill
Niu Huang *Calculus Bovis*
She Xiang *Secretio Moschus moschiferi*
Ru Xiang *Gummi Olibanum*
Mo Yao *Myrrha*

XIANG SHA LIU JUN ZI WAN
Saussurea-Amomum Six Gentlemen Pill
Dang Shen *Radix Codonopsis pilosulae*
Bai Zhu *Rhizoma Atractylodis macrocephalae*
Fu Ling *Sclerotium Poriae cocos*
Zhi Gan Cao *Radix Glycyrrhizae uralensis praeparata*
Chen Pi *Pericarpium Citri reticulatae*
Ban Xia *Rhizoma Pinelliae ternatae*
Mu Xiang *Radix Saussureae*
Sha Ren *Fructus seu Semen Amomi*

XIANG SHA YANG WEI PIAN (I)
Saussurea-Amomum Nourishing the Stomach Tablet
Dang Shen *Radix Codonopsis pilosulae*
Bai Zhu *Rhizoma Atractylodis macrocephalae*
Zhi Gan Cao *Radix Glycyrrhizae uralensis praeparata*
Chen Pi *Pericarpium Citri reticulatae*
Mu Xiang *Radix Saussureae*
Sha Ren *Fructus seu Semen Amomi*
Mai Ya *Fructus Hordei vulgaris germinatus*
Shen Qu *Massa Fermentata Medicinalis*
Bai Dou Kou *Fructus Amomi cardamomi*

XIANG SHA YANG WEI PIAN (II)
Saussurea-Amomum Nourishing the Stomach Tablet
Bai Zhu *Rhizoma Atractylodis macrocephalae*
Zhi Gan Cao *Radix Glycyrrhizae uralensis praeparata*
Chen Pi *Pericarpium Citri reticulatae*
Mu Xiang *Radix Saussureae*
Sha Ren *Fructus seu Semen Amomi*
Bai Dou Kou *Fructus Amomi cardamomi*
Fu Ling *Sclerotium Poriae cocos*
Ban Xia *Rhizoma Pinelliae ternatae*
Huo Xiang *Herba Agastachis*
Xiang Fu *Rhizoma Cyperi rotundi*
Hou Po *Cortex Magnoliae officinalis*
Zhi Ke *Fructus Citri aurantii*

XIAO CHAI HU TANG WAN
Small Bupleurum Pill
Chai Hu *Radix Bupleuri*
Huang Qin *Radix Scutellariae baicalensis*
Ban Xia *Rhizoma Pinelliae ternatae*
Ren Shen *Radix Ginseng*
Zhi Gan Cao *Radix Glycyrrhizae uralensis praeparata*
Sheng Jiang *Rhizoma Zingiberis officinalis recens*
Da Zao *Fructus Ziziphi jujubae*

XIAO CHAN WAN
Calming Tremor Pill
Tian Ma *Rhizoma Gastrodiae elatae*
Gou Teng *Ramulus Uncariae*
Zhen Zhu Mu *Concha margaritiferae*
Jiang Can *Bombyx batryticatus*

XIAO CHUAN CHONG JI
Asthma Granules
Da Qing Ye *Folium Isatidis seu Baphicacanthi*
Ping Di Mu (also called Zi Jin Niu) *Folium*

Ardisiae japonicae
Qian Hu *Radix Peucedani*
Sang Bai Pi *Cortex Mori albae radicis*
Ban Xia *Rhizoma Pinelliae ternatae*
Xuan Fu Hua *Flos Inulae*
Zhi Gan Cao *Radix Glycyrrhizae uralensis praeparata*
Ma Huang *Herba Ephedrae*
Bai Guo *Semen Ginkgo bilobae*

XIAO HUO LUO DAN
Small Invigorating the Connecting Vessels Pill
Chuan Wu *Radix Aconiti carmichaeli*
Cao Wu *Radix Aconiti kusnezoffii*
Dan Nan Xing *Rhizoma Arisaemae praeparata*
Ru Xiang *Gummi Olibanum*
Mo Yao *Myrrha*
Di Long *Pheretima aspergillum*

XIAO YAO WAN
Free and Easy Wanderer Pill
Chai Hu *Radix Bupleuri*
Bo He *Herba Menthae*
Dang Gui *Radix Angelicae sinensis*
Bai Shao *Radix Paeoniae albae*
Bai Zhu *Rhizoma Atractylodis macrocephalae*
Fu Ling *Sclerotium Poriae cocos*
Zhi Gan Cao *Radix Glycyrrhizae uralensis praeparata*
Sheng Jiang *Rhizoma Zingiberis officinalis recens*

YAN HU SUO ZHI TONG PIAN
Corydalis Stopping Pain Tablet
Yan Hu Suo *Rhizoma Corydalis yanhusuo*

YANG YIN QING FEI TANG JIANG
Nourishing Yin and Clearing the Lungs Syrup
Mu Dan Pi *Cortex Moutan radicis*
Zhe Bei Mu *Bulbus Fritillariae thunbergii*
Bai Shao *Radix Paeoniae albae*
Xuan Shen *Radix Scrophulariae ningpoensis*
Sheng Di Huang *Radix Rehmanniae glutinosae*
Mai Men Dong *Tuber Ophiopogonis japonici*
Gan Cao *Radix Glycyrrhizae uralensis*
Bo He *Herba Menthae*

YAO TONG PIAN
Back-ache Tablet
Dang Gui *Radix Angelicae sinensis*
Xu Duan *Radix Dipsaci*
Du Zhong *Cortex Eucommiae ulmoidis*

Gou Qi Zi *Fructus Lycii chinensis*
Bai Zhu *Rhizoma Atractylodis macrocephalae*
Bu Gu Zhi *Fructus Psoraleae corylifoliae*
Niu Xi *Radix Achyranthis bidentatae seu Cyathulae*

YIN QIAO JIE DU WAN (or PIAN)
Lonicera-Forsythia Expelling Poison Pill (or Tablet)
Jin Yin Hua *Flos Lonicerae japonicae*
Lian Qiao *Fructus Forsythiae suspensae*
Jie Geng *Radix Platycodi grandiflori*
Niu Bang Zi *Fructus Arctii lappae*
Bo He *Herba Menthae*
Jing Jie *Herba seu Flos Schizonepetae tenuifoliae*
Zhu Ye *Herba Lophatheri gracilis*
Dan Dou Chi *Semen Sojae praeparatum*
Gan Cao *Radix Glycyrrhizae uralensis*

YONG SHENG HE E JIAO
Eternally Vigorous Combination Donkey Skin Glue
E Jiao *Gelatinum Corii Asini*
Dang Gui *Radix Angelicae sinensis*
Huang Qi *Radix Astragali membranacei*
Mai Men Dong *Tuber Ophiopogonis japonici*
Fu Ling *Sclerotium Poriae cocos*
Shu Di Huang *Radix Rehmanniae glutinosae praeparata*
Rice wine
Sugar
Sesame oil

YOU GUI WAN
Restoring the Right [Kidney] Pill
Fu Zi *Radix Aconiti carmichaeli praeparata*
Rou Gui *Cortex Cinnamomi cassiae*
Du Zhong *Cortex Eucommiae ulmoidis*
Shan Zhu Yu *Fructus Corni officinalis*
Tu Si Zi *Semen Cuscutae*
Lu Jiao Jiao *Colla Cornu Cervi*
Shu Di Huang *Radix Rehmanniae glutinosae praeparata*
Shan Yao *Radix Dioscoreae oppositae*
Gou Qi Zi *Fructus Lycii chinensis*
Dang Gui *Radix Angelicae sinensis*

YUE JU WAN
Gardenia-Ligusticum Pill
Xiang Fu *Rhizoma Cyperi rotundi*
Cang Zhu *Rhizoma Atractylodis lanceae*

Shan Zhi Zi *Fructus Gardeniae jasminoidis*
Chuan Xiong *Radix Ligustici wallichii*
Shen Qu *Massa Fermentata Medicinalis*

YUNNAN BAI YAO
Yunnan White Medicine
San Qi *Radix Notoginseng*
Other ingredients not disclosed

YUNNAN TE CHAN TIAN QI PIAN
Yunnan Specially-Prepared Notoginseng Tablet
San Qi *Radix Notoginseng*

ZAI ZAO WAN
Renewal Pill
Chen Xiang *Lignum Aquilariae*
Hu Gu *Os Tigris*
Ren Shen *Radix Ginseng*
Mo Yao *Myrrha*
She Xiang *Secretio Moschus moschiferi*
Dang Gui *Radix Angelicae sinensis*
Niu Huang *Calculus Bovis*
Shui Niu Jiao *Cornu Bufali*
Huang Qi *Radix Astragali membranacei*
Rou Gui *Cortex Cinnamomi cassiae*
Xue Jie *Sangui Draconis*
Tian Ma *Rhizoma Gastrodiae elatae*
Hong Hua *Flos Carthami tinctorii*
Wu Xiao She *Zaocys Dhumnades*
Sheng Di Huang *Radix Rehmanniae glutinosae*
Bai Dou Kou *Fructus Amomi cardamomi*
Fang Feng *Radix Ledebouriellae sesloidis*
Chuan Xiong *Radix Ligustici wallichii*

ZHEN ZHU SAN
Zhen Zhu *Margarita*

ZHI BO BA WEI WAN
Anemarrhena-Phellodendron Eight-Ingredient Pill
Shu Di Huang *Radix Rehmanniae glutinosae praeparata*
Shan Zhu Yu *Fructus Corni officinalis*
Shan Yao *Radix Dioscoreae oppositae*
Ze Xie *Rhizoma Alismatis orientalis*
Fu Ling *Sclerotium Poriae cocos*
Mu Dan Pi *Cortex Moutan radicis*
Zhi Mu *Rhizoma Anemarrhenae asphodeloidis*
Huang Bo *Cortex Phellodendri*

ZHI SOU DING CHUAN WAN
Stopping Cough and Calming Breathlessness Pill
Ma Huang *Herba Ephedrae*
Xing Ren *Semen Pruni armeniacae*
Shi Gao *Gypsum fibrosum*
Zhi Gan Cao *Radix Glycyrrhizae uralensis praeparata*

ZHU SHA AN SHEN WAN
Cinnabar Calming the Mind Pill
Dang Gui *Radix Angelicae sinensis*
Sheng Di Huang *Radix Rehmanniae glutinosae*
Zhu Sha *Cinnabaris*
Huang Lian *Rhizoma Coptidis*
Gan Cao *Radix Glycyrrhizae uralensis*

ZHUANG YAO JIAN SHEN PIAN
Invigorating the Back and Strengthening the Kidneys Tablet
Gou Ji *Rhizoma Cibotii barometz*
Huai Niu Xi *Radix Achyranthis bidentatae*
Du Zhong *Cortex Eucommiae ulmoidis*
Jin Ying Zi *Fructus Rosae levigatae*
Sang Ji Sheng *Ramus Loranthi*
Dong Chong Xia Cao *Sclerotium Cordicipitis chinensis*
Fu Ling *Sclerotium Poriae cocos*
Fu Pen Zi *Fructus Rubi*

ZHUI FENG HUO XUE PIAN
Expelling Wind and Moving Blood Tablet
Gui Zhi *Ramulus Cinnamomi cassiae*
Du Huo *Radix Angelicae pubescentis*
Ma Huang *Herba Ephedrae*
Fang Feng *Radix Ledebouriellae sesloidis*
Di Feng *Cortex Illici*
Qiang Huo *Radix et Rhizoma Notopterygii*
Ru Xiang *Gummi Olibanum*
Zi Ran Tong *Pyritum*
Mo Yao *Myrrha*
Du Zhong *Cortex Eucommiae ulmoidis*
Qian Nian Jian *Rhizoma Homalomenae occultae*
Mu Gua *Fructus Chaenomelis lagenariae*
Niu Xi *Radix Achyranthis bidentatae seu Cyathulae*
Gan Cao *Radix Glycyrrhizae uralensis*
Feng Mi *Mel*

ZI SHENG WAN
Life-Providing Pill
Dang Shen *Radix Codonopsis pilosulae*
Bai Zhu *Rhizoma Atractylodis macrocephalae*
Yi Yi Ren *Semen Coicis lachryma jobi*
Shen Qu *Massa Fermentata Medicinalis*
Chen Pi *Pericarpium Citri reticulatae*
Shan Zha *Fructus Crataegi*
Qian Shi *Semen Euryales ferocis*
Shan Yao *Radix Dioscoreae oppositae*
Bian Dou *Semen Dolichoris lablab*
Mai Ya *Fructus Hordei vulgaris germinatus*
Fu Ling *Sclerotium Poriae cocos*
Lian Zi *Semen Nelumbinis nuciferae*
Jie Geng *Radix Platycodi grandiflori*
Huo Xiang *Herba Agastachis*
Gan Cao *Radix Glycyrrhizae uralensis*
Bai Dou Kou *Fructus Amomi cardamomi*
Huang Lian *Rhizoma Coptidis*

Glossary of Chinese terms

SYMPTOMS

喘	*Chuan*	Breathlessness
哮	*Xiao*	Wheezing
鼻渊	*Bi Yuan*	"Nose pool" (sinusitis)
胀	*Zhang*	Feeling of distension
满	*Man*	Feeling of fullness
闷	*Men*	Feeling of oppression
痞	*Pi*	Feeling of stuffiness
积	*Ji*	Blood masses
聚	*Ju*	Qi masses
实	*Shi*	Full, Fullness, Excess
虚	*Xu*	Empty, Emptiness, Deficiency
本	*Ben*	Root
杓	*Biao*	Manifestation
痹证	*Bi Zheng*	Painful Obstruction Syndrome
痿证	*Wei Zheng*	Atrophy Syndrome
中风	*Zhong Feng*	Wind-stroke
淋证	*Lin Zheng*	Painful Urination Syndrome
热毒	*Re Du*	Fire-Poison
心烦	*Xin Fan*	Mental restlessness
温病	*Wen Bing*	Warm disease

VITAL SUBSTANCES

神	*Shen*	Mind or Spirit
魂	*Hun*	Ethereal Soul
魄	*Po*	Corporeal Soul
意	*Yi*	Intellect
志	*Zhi*	Will-Power
精	*Jing*	Essence

原气	*Yuan Qi*	Original Qi
卫气	*Wei Qi*	Defensive Qi
营气	*Ying Qi*	Nutritive Qi
宗气	*Zong Qi*	Gathering Qi (of the chest)
真气	*Zhen Qi*	True Qi
正气	*Zheng Qi*	Upright Qi
中气	*Zhong Qi*	Central Qi
命门	*Ming Men*	Gate of Vitality

EMOTIONS

怒	*Nu*	Anger
思	*Si*	Pensiveness
悲	*Bei*	Sadness
忧	*You*	Worry
喜	*Xi*	Joy
恐	*Kong*	Fear
惊	*Jing*	Shock

CHANNELS AND POINTS

络脉	*Luo Mai (Xue)*	Connecting (point or channel)
别脉	*Bie Mai*	Divergent channels
原穴	*Yuan Xue*	Source point
希穴	*Xi Xue*	Accumulation point
会穴	*Hui Xue*	Gathering point

俞穴	*(Bei) Shu Xue*	Back-Transporting points
募穴	*Mu Xue*	Front-Collecting points
五输穴	*Wu Shu Xue*	Five Transporting points
任脉	*Ren Mai*	Directing Vessel
督脉	*Du Mai*	Governing Vessel
冲脉	*Chong Mai*	Penetrating Vessel
阳蹻脉	*Yang Qiao Mai*	Yang Heel Vessel
阳蹻脉	*Yin Qiao Mai*	Yin Heel Vessel
阳维脉	*Yang Wei Mai*	Yang Linking Vessel
阴维脉	*Yin Wei Mai*	Yin Linking Vessel
带脉	*Dai Mai*	Girdle Vessel
太阳	*Tai Yang*	Greater Yang
阳明	*Yang Ming*	Bright Yang
少阳	*Shao Yang*	Lesser Yang
太阴	*Tai Yin*	Greater Yin
少阴	*Shao Yin*	Lesser Yin
厥阴	*Jue Yin*	Terminal Yin
膝理	*Cou Li*	Space between skin and muscles

PULSE

寸	*Cun*	Front (pulse position)
关	*Guan*	Middle (pulse position)
迟	*Chi*	Rear (pulse position)

Bibliography

Ancient classics

1. 1979 The Yellow Emperor's Classic of Internal Medicine — Simple Questions (*Huang Ti Nei Jing Su Wen* 黄帝内经素问), People's Health Publishing House, Beijing. First published *c*. 100 BC.
2. 1981 Spiritual Axis (*Ling Shu Jing* 灵枢经), People's Health Publishing House, Beijing. First published *c*. 100 BC.
3. Nanjing College of Traditional Chinese Medicine 1960 An Explanation of the Classic of Difficulties (*Nan Jing Yi Shi* 难经译释), Shanghai Science Publishing House, Shanghai. First published *c*. AD 100.
4. Hua Tuo 1985 The Classic of the Secret Transmission (*Zhong Cang Jing* 中藏经), Jiangsu Science Publishing House, Nanjing. First published *c*. AD 198.
5. Nanjing College of Traditional Chinese Medicine — Shang Han Lun Research Group 1980 Discussion of Cold-induced Diseases (*Shang Han Lun* 伤寒论), Shanghai Science Publishing House, Shanghai. First published by Zhang Zhong Jing *c*. AD 220.
6. 1981 Discussion of the Essential Prescriptions of the Golden Chest (*Jin Gui Yao Lue Fang Lun* 金匮要略方论), Zhejiang Science Publishing House, Zhejiang. The "Essential Prescriptions of the Golden Chest" itself was written by Zhang Zhong Jing and first published *c*. AD 220.
7. He Ren 1979 A Popular Guide to the Essential Prescriptions of the Golden Chest (*Jin Gui Yao Lue Tong Su Jiang Hua* 金匮要略通俗讲话), Shanghai Science Publishing House, Shanghai.
8. He Ren 1981 A New Explanation of the Essential Prescriptions of the Golden Chest (*Jin Gui Yao Lue Xin Jie* 金匮要略新解), Zhejiang Scientific Publishing House.
9. Duan Guang Zhou et al 1986 A Manual of the Essential Prescriptions of the Golden Chest (*Jin Gui Yao Lue Shou Ce* 金匮要略手册), Science Publishing House.
10. Traditional Chinese Medicine Research Institute 1959 An Explanation of the Essential Prescriptions of the Golden Chest (*Jin Gui Yao Lue Yu Yi* 金匮要略语译), People's Health Publishing House, Beijing.

11. Shandong College of Traditional Chinese Medicine 1984 An Explanation of the Pulse Classic (*Mai Jing Jiao Shi* 脉经校释), People's Health Publishing House, Beijing. The "Pulse Classic" itself was written by Wang Shu He and first published *c.* AD 280.

12. Shandong College of Traditional Chinese Medicine 1979 An Explanation of the ABC of Acupuncture (*Zhen Jiu Jia Yi Jing Jiao Shi* 针灸甲乙经校释), People's Health Publishing House, Beijing. The ABC of Acupuncture was written by Huang Fu Mi and published in AD 282.

13. Li Jing Wei 1987 An Illustrated Manual of Acupuncture Points as shown on the Bronze Man (*Tong Ren Shu Xue Zhen Jiu Tu Jing* 铜人腧穴针灸图经), Chinese Bookshop Publishing House, Beijing. Written by Wang Wei Yi and first published in 1026.

14. Li Dong Yuan 1976 Discussion on Stomach and Spleen (*Pi Wei Lun* 脾胃论), People's Health Publishing House, Beijing. First published in 1249.

15. Wang Luo Zhen 1985 A Compilation of the "Study of the Eight Extraordinary Vessels" (*Qi Jing Ba Mai Kao Jiao Zhu* 奇经八脉考校注), Shanghai Science Publishing House, Shanghai. The "Study of the Eight Extraordinary Vessels" itself by Li Shi Zhen was first published in 1578.

16. Yang Ji Zhou 1980 Compendium of Acupuncture (*Zhen Jiu Da Cheng* 针灸大成), People's Health Publishing House, Beijing. First published in 1601.

17. Wu Zhan Ren, Yu Zhi Gao 1987 Correct Seal of Medical Circles (*Yi Lin Zheng Yin* 医林正印), Jiangsu Science Publishing House, Nanjing. Written by Ma Zhao Sheng and first published in 1605.

18. Zhang Jie Bin (also called Zhang Jing Yue) 1982 Classic of Categories (*Lei Jing* 类经), People's Health Publishing House, Beijing. First published in 1624.

19. Zhang Jing Yue 1986 Complete Book of Jing Yue (*Jing Yue Quan Shu* 景岳全书), Shanghai Science Publishing House, Shanghai. First published in 1624.

20. Traditional Chinese Medicine Research Group of Zhejiang Province 1977 An Explanation of the Discussion of Warm Epidemics (*Wen Yi Lun Ping Zhu* 温疫论评注), People's Health Publishing House, Beijing. The Discussion of Warm Epidemics was written by Wu You Xing and first published in 1642.

21. Yue Han Zhen 1990 An Explanation of Acupuncture Points (*Jing Xue Jie* 经穴解), People's Health Publishing House, Beijing. First published in 1654.

22. Lin Zhi Han 1987 The Essential Four Diagnostic Examinations (*Si Zhen Jue Wei* 四诊抉微), Chinese Bookshop Publishing House, Beijing. First published in 1723.

23. Wu Qian 1973 Golden Mirror of Medicine (*Yi Zong Jin Jian* 医宗金鉴), People's Health Publishing House, Beijing. First published in 1742.

24. Nanjing College of Traditional Chinese Medicine 1978 A Study of Warm Diseases (*Wen Bing Xue* 温病学), Shanghai Science Publishing House, Shanghai. Written by Ye Tian Shi and first published in 1746.

25. Wu Ju Tong 1978 Differentiation of Warm Diseases (*Wen Bing Tiao Bian* 温病条辨), People's Health Publishing House, Beijing. First published in 1798.

26. Tang Zong Hai 1979 Discussion of Blood Syndromes (*Xue Zheng Lun* 血证论), People's Health Publishing House, Beijing. First published in 1884.

Modern texts

1. Zhang Bo Yu 1986 Internal Medicine (*Zhong Yi Nei Ke Xue* 中医内科学), Shanghai Science Publishing House.

2. Yang Jia San 1989 Acupuncture (*Zhen Jiu Xue* 针灸学), People's Health Publishing House, Beijing.

3. Wang Ke Qin 1988 Theory of the Mind in Chinese Medicine (*Zhong Yi Shen Zhu Xue Shuo* 中医神主学说), Ancient Chinese Medical Texts Publishing House, Beijing.

4. Shi Zi Guang 1988 Essential Clinical Experience of Famous Modern Doctors — Asthma (*Dang Dai Ming Yi Ling Zhen Jing Hua* 当代名医临证精华), Ancient Chinese Medical Texts Publishing House, Beijing.

5. Shi Zi Guang 1988 Essential Clinical Experience of Famous Modern Doctors — Painful Obstruction Syndrome (*Dang Dai Ming Yi Ling Zhen Jing Hua* 当代名医临证精华), Ancient Chinese Medical Texts Publishing House, Beijing.

6. Shi Zi Guang 1988 Essential Clinical Experience of Famous Modern Doctors — Epigastric Pain (*Dang Dai Ming Yi Ling Zhen Jing Hua* 当代名医临证精华), Ancient Chinese Medical Texts Publishing House, Beijing.

7. Fei Bo Xiong et al 1985 Medical Collection from Four Families from Meng He (*Meng He Si Jia Yi Ji* 孟河四家医集), Jiangsu Science Publishing House, Nanjing.

8. Gu He Dao 1979 History of Chinese Medicine (*Zhong Guo Yi Xue Shi Lue* 中国医学史略), Shanxi People's Publishing House, Taiyuan.

9. 1981 Syndromes and Treatment of the Internal Organs (*Zang Fu Zheng Zhi* 脏腑证治), Tianjin Science Publishing House, Tianjin.

10. 1980 Concise Dictionary of Chinese Medicine (*Jian Ming Zhong Yi Ci Dian* 简明中医辞典), People's Health Publishing House, Beijing.

11. 1979 Patterns and Treatment of Kidney Diseases (*Shen Yu Shen Bing de Zheng Zhi* 肾与肾病的证治), Hebei People's Publishing House, Hebei.

12. Li Wen Chuan, He Bao Yi 1987 Practical Acupuncture (*Shi Yong Zhen Jiu Xue* 实用针灸学), People's Health Publishing House, Beijing.

13. Li Shi Zhen 1985 Clinical Application of Frequently-Used Acupuncture Points (*Chang Yong Shu Xue Lin Chuang Fa Hui* 常用输穴临床发挥), People's Health Publishing House, Beijing.

14. Shan Yu Dang 1984 Selection of Acupuncture Point Combinations from the Discussion of Cold-induced Diseases (*Shang Han Lun Zhen Jiu Pei Xue Xuan Zhu* 伤寒论针灸配穴选注), People's Health Publishing House, Beijing.

15. Ji Jie Yin 1984 Clinical Records of Tai Yi Shen Acupuncture (*Tai Yi Shen Zhen Jiu Lin Zheng Lu* 太乙神针灸临证录), Shanxi Science Publishing House, Shanxi.

16. Nanjing College of Traditional Chinese Medicine — Warm Diseases Research Group 1959 Teaching Reference Material on the School of Warm Diseases (*Wen Bing Xue Jiao Xue Can Kao Zi Liao* 温病学教学参考资料), Jiangsu People's Publishing House, Nanjing.

17. Shanghai College of Traditional Chinese Medicine 1979

Chinese Pediatrics (*Zhong Yi Er Ke Xue* 中医儿科学),
Shanghai Science Publishing House, Shanghai.

18. Cong Chun Yu 1988 Chinese Gynaecology (*Zhong Yi Fu Ke Xue* 中医妇科学), Ancient Medical Texts Publishing House, Beijing.

19. Chen You Bang 1990 Chinese Acupuncture Therapy (*Zhong Guo Zhen Jiu Zhi Liao Xue* 中国针灸治疗学), China Science Publishing House, Beijing.

20. Wang Xue Tai 1987 Great Treatise of Chinese Acupuncture (*Zhong Guo Zhen Jiu Da Quan* 中国针大全), Henan Science and Technology Publishing House, Henan.

21. He Shu Huai 1985 Acupuncture (*Zhen Jiu Xue* 针灸学), Ancient Chinese Medical Texts Publishing House.

22. Zhang Wen Jin 1988 Acupuncture Empirical Formulae (*Zhen Jiu Yan Fang* 针灸验方), Shanxi Science Publishing House, Shanxi.

23. Beijing College of Traditional Chinese Medicine 1975 Practical Chinese Medicine (*Shi Yong Zhong Yi Xue* 实用中医学), People's Health Publishing House, Beijing.

24. Hu Jiao Ming 1989 Great Treatise of Secret Chinese Medicine Prescriptions (*Zhong Guo Zhong Yi Mi Fang Da Quan* 中国中医秘方大全), Literary Publishing House, Shanghai.

25. Zhou Feng Yu 1989 Practical Study of Prescriptions (*Shi Yong Fang Ji Xue* 实用方剂学), Shandong Science Publishing House, Shandong.

26. Guangdong Institute of Traditional Chinese Medicine 1976 Chinese Internal Medicine (*Zhong Yi Nei Ke* 中医内科), People's Health Publishing House, Beijing.

27. Nanjing College of Traditional Chinese Medicine 1959 Concise Chinese Internal Medicine (*Jian Ming Zhong Yi Nei Ke* 简明中医内科), Shanghai Science Publishing House, Shanghai.

28. Ye Xian Chun 1976 Frequently-Used Chinese Patent Medicines (*Chang Yong Zhong Cheng Yao* 常用中成药), Shanghai People's Publishing House.

English language texts

1. Jake Fratkin 1986 Chinese Herbal Patent Formulas, Institute for Traditional Medicine, Portland, Oregon.
2. Zhu Chun Han 1989 Clinical Handbook of Chinese Prepared Medicines, Paradigm Publications, Brookline, Massachusetts.
3. D Bensky-A Gamble 1986 Chinese Herbal Medicine Materia Medica, Eastland Press, Seattle.

Western medicine textbooks

1. J Macleod 1974 Davidson's Principles and Practice of Medicine, Churchill Livingstone, Edinburgh.
2. H Jones-G Seegar 1982 Gynaecology, Williams and Wilkins, Baltimore.
3. P Kumar-M Clark 1987 Clinical Medicine, Bailliere Tindall, London.
4. P Hickling-J Golding 1984 An Outline of Rheumathology, Wright, Bristol.
5. J Crawford Adams-D Hamblen 1990 Outline of Orthopaedics, Churchill Livingstone, Edinburgh.
6. P Turner-A Richens 1973 Clinical Pharmacology, Churchill Livingstone, Edinburgh.
7. C Seward 1960 Bedside Diagnosis, Churchill Livingstone, Edinburgh.
8. DeGowin 1969 Diagnostic Examination, Macmillan, London.
9. B Bates 1983 A Guide to Physical Examination, J B Lippincott Company, Philadelphia.
10. N Bogduk-L Twomey 1987 Clinical Anatomy of the Lumbar Spine, Churchill Livingstone, Edinburgh.
11. J M Naish-A Read 1971 The Clinical Apprentice, John Wright & Sons Ltd, Bristol.

Index